TOTAL BURN CARE

TOTAL BURN CARE

Edited By

D N HERNDON

Chief of Staff, Shriners Burns Institute,
and
Jesse H Jones Distinguished Chair
in Burn Surgery at the
University of Texas Medical Branch,
Galveston, Texas

W B SAUNDERS COMPANY LTD

London Philadelphia Toronto Sydney Tokyo

W. B. Saunders Company Ltd 24–28 Oval Road
London NW1 7DX

The Curtis Center
Independence Square West
Philadelphia, PA 19106-3399, USA

Harcourt Brace & Company
55 Horner Avenue
Toronto, Ontario M8Z 4X6, Canada

Harcourt Brace & Company, Australia
30–52 Smidmore Street
Marrickville, NSW 2204, Australia

Harcourt Brace & Company, Japan
Ichibancho Central Building, 22–1 Ichibancho
Chiyoda-ku, Tokyo 102, Japan

This book is printed on acid-free paper

A catalogue record for this book is available from the British Library

ISBN 7–7020–1827–9

Typeset by Phoenix Photosetting, Chatham, Kent
Printed in Great Britain by The Bath Press, Bath, Avon

Contents

The colour plate section appears between pp 264 and 265

Contributors

N Aikawa MD DMSc FACS, Professor and Chairman, Department of Emergency and Critical Care Medicine, Keio University Hospital, Tokyo, Japan.

M I Alvarado MA OTR, Director of Rehabilitation Services, Shriners Burns Institute, Galveston, Texas, USA.

D Benjamin RN MSN, Research Nurse, Department of Clinical Research, Shriners Burns Institute, Galveston, Texas, USA.

P Q Bessey MA MD, Professor, Director of Trauma, Burns and Critical Care, Department of Surgery, University of Rochester Medical Center, Rochester, New York, USA.

P E Blakeney PhD, Director, Family Services, Shriners Burns Institute, Galveston Unit; and Clinical Associate Professor of Surgery, University of Texas Medical Branch, Galveston, Texas, USA.

J F Burke MD, Chief Trauma Services Emeritus, Massachusetts General Hospital; and Helen Andrus Benedict Professor of Surgery, Emeritus, Department of Surgery, Harvard Medical School, Boston, MA, USA.

J C Calhoun MD MEng, Chairman, Department of Orthopedics, University of Texas Medical Branch, Galveston, Texas, USA.

A Chavarria RN BSN, Case Manager, Nursing Department, Shriners Burns Institute, Galveston, Texas, USA.

W G Cioffi, Jr MD FACS, Chief of the Division of Trauma and Burns, Department of Surgery, Rhode Island Hospital, Providence, Rhode Island, USA.

M H Desai MD FRCS FACS FCCM, Professor of Surgery, University of Texas Medical Branch; and Director, Blocker Burn Unit and Assistant Chief of Staff, Department of Surgery, Shriners Burns Institute, Galveston, Texas, USA.

A R Dimick MD, Professor of Surgery, and Director, Burn Center, Department of Surgery, The University of Alabama at Birmingham, Birmingham, Alabama, USA.

P Edgar RN, Director of Infection Control/Emp. Health, Department of Infection Control, Shriners Burns Institute, Galveston, Texas, USA.

L H Engrav MD, Professor, and Chief, Department of Plastic Surgery, University of Washington, Seattle, Washington, USA.

E B Evans MD, Professor, Department of Orthopedics, University of Texas Medical Branch, Galveston, Texas, USA.

J C Fitzpatrick MD, Staff Surgeon, US Army Institute of Surgical Research, San Antonio, Texas, USA.

V Gilinsky RN BSN, Case Manager, Nursing Department, Shriners Burns Institute, Galveston, Texas, USA.

D Gilpin MB Bch FRCS, Department of Surgery, Institute of Clinical Science, The Queen's University of Belfast, Belfast, Northern Ireland, UK.

M Gottschlich PhD RD, Director, Nutrition Services, Shriners Hospitals for Crippled Children, Burns Institute - Cincinnati Unit, Cincinnati, Ohio, USA.

L Hannon CO, Morgan Prosthetics Orthotics, 625 University Boulevard, Galveston, Texas, USA.

R H C Harries MD, Professor of Surgery, Director of Burn Unit, Shriners Burns Institute, Wound Healing Department, Galveston, Texas, USA.

C E Hartford MD, Department of Surgery, University of Colorado Health Sciences Center, Denver, Colorado, USA.

J P Heggers BA MSc PhD ASPRS FAAM, Director, Clinical Microbiology, Shriners Burns Institute; and Professor of Surgery, Microbiology and Immunology, Department of Surgery, University of Texas Medical Branch, Galveston, Texas, USA.

D M Heimbach MD, Professor of Surgery, and Director, University of Washington Burn Center, Department of Surgery, Harborview Medical Center, Seattle, Washington, USA.

D N Herndon MD, Chief of Staff, Shriners Burns Institute, Galveston, Texas; and the Jesse H Jones Distinguished Chair in Burn Surgery, Professor of Surgery and Pediatrics at the University of Texas Medical Branch, Galveston, Texas, USA.

M A Hildreth BS RD, Director of Support Services, Shriners Hospitals for Crippled Children, Burns Institute - Galveston Unit, Galveston, Texas, USA.

F Hinder MD, Anesthesiology Resident, Klinik und Poliklinik für Anasthesiologie und Operative Intensivmedizin, Westfalische Wilhelms Universität, Münster, Germany.

M A Hollyoak MBBS MMedSc, General Surgical Registrar, Department of Surgery, Royal Brisbane Hospital, Brisbane, Queensland, Australia.

G L Klein MD MPH, Professor, Department of Pediatrics, University of Texas Medical Branch and Shriners Burns Institute, Galveston, Texas, USA.

G C Kramer PhD, Professor, Departments of Anesthesiology and Physiology, UTMB, Galveston, Texas, USA.

H A Linares MD DMSc, Chief of Research Pathology, Shriners Burns Institute, Galveston, Texas, USA; and Clinical Assistant Professor of Pathology, University of Texas Medical Branch, Galveston, Texas, USA.

W W Lingnau MD ESICM SCCM, Assistant Professor, Department of Anaesthesia and Intensive Care Medicine, The Leopold-Franzens-University of Innsbruck, Anichstrasse 35, A-6020 Innsbruck, Austria.

W G Lyle MD, Resident, University of Texas Medical Branch, Division of General Surgery, Galveston, Texas, USA.

K Macgill MBBS FRACS, Consultant Plastic Surgeon, Royal Children's and Royal Melbourne Hospitals, Melbourne, Victoria, Australia.

R Mann MD, Assistant Professor of Surgery and Assistant Director, Department of Surgery, University of Washington, Harborview Medical Center, Seattle, USA.

A J Manning MS RD, Clinical Dietitian, Shriners Burns Institute, Galveston, Texas, USA.

J A Marvin RN MN, Director of Nursing, Nursing Department, Shriners Burns Institute, Galveston, Texas, USA.

A D Mason, Jr MD, Chief, Laboratory Division, US Army Institute of Surgical Research, San Antonio, Texas, USA.

R L McCauley MD FACS, Associate Professor of Surgery and Pediatrics, and Chief, Plastic and Reconstructive Surgery, Department of Plastic Surgery/Medical Staff Admin., The University of Texas Medical Branch/Shriners Burns Institute, Galveston, Texas, USA.

B J McCoy RN MSN, Clinical Nurse Specialist, Nursing Department, Shriners Burns Institute, Galveston, Texas, USA.

K McElroy PT, Clinical Supervisor, Occupational Therapy/Physical Therapy Department, Shriners Burns Institute, Galveston, Texas, USA.

N Meyer MD, Resident, Department of Surgery, Medical College of Wisconsin, Milwaukee, Wisconsin, USA.

W J Meyer III MD, Gladys and R. Lee Kempner Professor of Child Psychiatry, Department of Psychiatry and Behavioral Sciences, University of Texas Medical Branch, Galveston, Texas, USA.

S M Milner MB BDS FRCS, Division of Plastic Surgery, The University of Texas Medical Branch, Galveston, Texas, USA; formerly Lieutenant Colonel, Trauma Section, Chemical and Biological Defence Establishment, Porton Down, Salisbury, Wiltshire, UK.

G Mlcak RN, Assistant Clinical Director, Nursing Service, Shriners Burns Institute, Galveston, Texas, USA.

R P Mlcak BA RRT RCP, Director Respiratory Care, Department of Respiratory Care, Shriners Burns Institute, Galveston, Texas, USA.

W W Monafo MD, Professor of Surgery, Department of Surgery, Washington University School of Medicine, St Louis, Missouri, USA.

D. Morgan CPO, Morgan Prosthetics Orthotics, 625 University Boulevard, Galveston, Texas, USA.

D W Mozingo MD, Clinical Assistant Professor of Surgery, The University of Texas Health Science Center at San Antonio; and Chief, Clinical Division, US Army Institute of Surgical Research, San Antonio, Texas, USA.

M J Muller MBBS FRACS, Deputy Director, Burns Unit, Royal Brisbane Hospital, Brisbane, Queensland, Australia.

A M Munster MD FACS (Eng & Ed) FRCS, Professor of Surgery and Plastic Surgery, and Director, Baltimore Burn Center, Department of Surgery, Johns Hopkins Bayview Medical Center, Baltimore, Maryland, USA.

T T Nguyen MD, Plastic Surgery Fellow, Department of Plastic Surgery, University of South Carolina, Charleston, South Carolina, USA.

R J Nichols, Jr MD, Professor of Anesthesiology, The University of Texas Medical Branch; and Chief of Anesthesiology, Shriners Burns Institute, Galveston, Texas, USA.

M W Nicolai RN CNOR, Clinical Research Nurse, Shriners Burns Institute, Galveston, Texas, USA.

S E Ott OTR BSc, Occupational Therapist III, Department of Occupational Therapy, University of Texas Medical Branch at Galveston, Galveston, Texas, USA.

S P Pegg FRCS(Eng) FRACS FRACMA, Associate Professor of Surgery, Royal Brisbane Hospital, Brisbane, Queensland, Australia.

L G Phillips MD FACS ASPRS, Truman G. Blocker, Jr, M.D., Distinguished Chair and Chief, Division of Plastic Surgery, Department of Surgery, University of Texas Medical Branch, Galveston, Texas, USA.

T Pickett RN, Case Manager, Nursing Department, Shriners Burns Institute, Galveston, Texas, USA.

E J Pierre MD, Research Burn Fellow, Department of Surgery, Shriners Burns Institute, Galveston, Texas, USA.

V Pollard FFARCSI, Assistant Professor, Department of Anesthesiology, The University of Texas Medical Branch, Galveston, Texas, USA.

D S Prough MD, Professor and Chairman, Department of Anesthesiology, The University of Texas Medical Branch, Galveston, Texas, USA.

B A Pruitt MD, US Army Institute of Surgical Reseach, Fort Sam Houston, San Antonio, Texas, USA.

R J Redelmeier BASc MBA AIChE, Shell Oil Products Company, Houston, Texas, USA.

D K Robie BASc MD, Chief of Pediatric Surgery, Walter Reed Army Medical Center, Washington, DC; and Assistant Professor of Surgery and Pediatrics, Departments of Surgery and Pediatrics, Uniformed Services University of the Health Sciences, Bethesda, Maryland, USA.

M C Robson MD FACS ASPRS, Chief, Surgical Services, Department of Surgery, Bay Pines VA Medical Center, Tampa, Florida, USA.

R L Rutan RN BSN, Research Coordinator, Department of Surgery, New Jersey Medical School, 185 South Orange Avenue, University Heights, Newark, New Jersey, USA.

L T A Rylah FRCA, Formerly Director, Clinical Care, The Regional Burn Unit, St Andrews Hospital, Billericay, Essex, UK.

J M Shaw MD, Resident, Division of Plastic Surgery, University of Texas Medical Branch, Galveston, Texas, USA.

R L Sheridan MD, Assistant Chief of Staff, Department of Surgery, Shriners Burns Institute and Massachusetts General Hospital Burn Center, Boston, Massachusetts, USA; and Assistant Professor of Surgery, Harvard Medical School.

Y Shinozawa MD DMSc, Associate Professor, Department of Emergency and Critical Care Medicine, Keio University Hospital, Tokyo, Japan.

D J Smith Jr MD, Professor of Surgery, Chief, Division of Plastic Surgery, University of Michigan, Ann Arbor, Michigan, USA.

L L Strock MD, Resident, Division of Plastic Surgery, University of Texas Medical Branch, Galveston, Texas, USA.

D M Tompkins RN BSN MBA, Nursing Consultant, Burn Care, Shriners Burns Institute, Massachussetts General Hospital, Boston, MA, USA.

R G Tompkins MD ScD, Chief of Staff, Shriners Burns Institute; and Chief, Burn and Trauma Services, Massachusetts General Hospital, Department of Surgery, Harvard Medical School, Boston, MA, USA.

D L Traber PhD, Professor, Department of Anesthesiology, Physiology and Biophysics, The University of Texas Medical Branch, Galveston, Texas, USA.

C G Villarreal BSc, Director of Pharmacy, Department of Pharmacy, Shriners Burns Institute, Galveston, Texas, USA.

T L Wachtel MD FACS FCCM, Clinical Associate Professor of Surgery, University of California, San Diego and Uniformed Services University for Health Sciences; and Medical Director, Department of Trauma Services, Sharp Memorial Hospital, San Diego, California, USA.

G D Warden MD, Chief of Staff, Shriners Burns Institute, Cincinnati, Ohio; and Professor of Surgery and Director of Burn Division, University of Cincinnati College of Medicine, Cincinnati, Ohio, USA.

W G Williams MD, Division of Plastic Surgery, University of Texas Medical Branch, Galveston, Texas, USA.

R Wiggins, Staff Nurse, Shriners Burns Institute, Galveston, Texas, USA.

R R Wolfe PhD, Professor of Surgery and Anesthesiology, Chief of Metabolism Unit, Shriners Burns Institute, Galveston, Texas, USA.

L C Woodson MD PhD, Assistant Professor of Anesthesiology, Department of Anesthesiology, The University of Texas Medical Branch at Galveston, Galveston, Texas, USA.

B E Zawacki MD, Director, Burn Service/Associate Professor of Surgery, Professor of Medicine and Religion, University of Southern California, 1200 North State Street, Room 12-650, Los Angeles, California, USA.

Foreword

Society's recognition of the frequency and complexity of burn injury has led to the development of the hierarchial regionalized network of burn centers in which multidisciplinary professional teams provide the care needed by severely burned patients. Dr Herndon, Chief of Staff of the Galveston Shriners Burns Institute, has recognized the need for a text that can be used to expand the physiologic understanding and enhance the clinical practice of the professionals who care for those patients. He has carefully selected authors distinguished by their expertise and clarity of exposition to insure concise yet complete coverage of each topic. The roster of authors which includes twelve past presidents of the American Burn Association has been given an international flavor by inclusion of European, Australian and Japanese authors.

The multisystem response to burn injury, thoroughly described in Chapters 19 through 37, which has influenced the organization of burn centers, and the composition of burn care teams, dictates the multidisciplinary care required by the extensively burned patient. Chapters 3 through 18 progress in measured logical fashion from the scene of injury through the pre-hospital emergency room phase, to the critical care unit, the operating room and finally, the rehabilitation services and the psychosocial support program.

A particular strength of the book is the emphasis that is placed on the total care of the burned patient, and the amplification of treatment effectiveness and efficiency by fully utilizing the special skills of each member of the burn team. The expertise of the editor's staff members, evident throughout the work is particularly well displayed in the section on Psychological and Social Issues which highlights the importance of establishing realistic goals and achieving full reintegration of the burned patient into the mainstream of society. Chapters 38 through 42, describing the treatment of patients with other forms of cutaneous damage, illustrate the universality of the multisystem response to extensive cutaneous injury and the applicability of the principles of burn wound care to patients with other forms of cutaneous damage.

This work fills a specific void in the surgical literature and is destined to become an international reference. It should be on the shelf of every medical school and burn center library, and in the personal library of all personnel involved in burn care.

Basil A. Pruitt, Jr, MD
Colonel, MC
US Army Institute of Surgical Research
Fort Sam Houston, Texas

PREFACE

In the last decade, burn care has improved to the extent that persons with burns covering 80% of their total body surface can frequently survive. In this book, advances in the treatment of burn shock, inhalation injury, sepsis, hypermetabolism, the operative excision of burn wounds, scar reconstruction and rehabilitation are reviewed. Burn care demands attention to every organ system as well as to the patient's psychological and social status. The scope of burn treatment extends beyond the preservation of life and function and the ultimate goal is the return of burn survivors, as full participants, back into their communities.

This book was prepared to consider the complex management of burned patients from injury through rehabilitation; it incorporates treatments of injuries from diverse sources and addresses the concerns of a variety of burn care professionals who act in concert. A major theme throughout is that advances defined in basic science laboratories need to progress through prospective randomized studies to their clinical application. *Total Burn Care* is designed as a text on the management of burned patients, not only for surgeons, anesthesiologists, and residents, but also nurses and allied health professionals. This book will hopefully serve as a sophisticated instruction manual to guide those with less experience through difficult experiences in burn care. It is anticipated that it will additionally stimulate knowledgeable scientists and experienced clinicians to pose new questions and to join together in pursuing randomized and prospective studies.

Contributors have been selected from a small number of institutions in order to provide a unified approach with a sharp focus and minimal duplication. Themes covered elsewhere in the literature have been condensed and the bibliographies selected to assure the reader ready access to the expanded literature on current burn care. The final organization of the book reflects neither the importance of the subject matter nor the order of application following injury.

The support of the staff of W.B. Saunders Company Limited is gratefully acknowledged, as is the Shriners Burns Institute, contributors' universities, and the teaching hospitals which have provided clinical opportunities and the laboratories for research.

DAVID N HERNDON
30 August 1995

Acknowledgment

Grateful acknowledgment is given to the many authors whose time and expertise made this book possible. Also, special thanks are offered to Dr Patricia Blakeney and Dr Michael Muller who reviewed many of the chapter manuscripts with me and to Dr Karina Stokes who applied her editorial expertise to every chapter in this book. I would also like to acknowledge those secretaries who were particularly diligent about typing manuscripts and taking care of details: Thomala Roberson and Laura Powledge. Finally, I wish to thank my wife, Rose, for her invaluable personal support.

CHAPTER ONE

Teamwork for Total Burn Care: Achievements, Directions and Hopes

David N. Herndon, Michael J. Muller and Patricia E. Blakeney

Major burn injury evokes strong emotional responses in most lay persons and health professionals who are confronted by the spectre of pain, deformity, and potential death associated with significant burns. Severe pain and repeated episodes of sepsis followed by predictable outcomes of either death or a survival encumbered by pronounced disfigurement and disability has been the expected pattern of sequelae to serious burn injury for most of mankind's history.[1] However, these dire consequences have, over time, been ameliorated so that, while burn injury is still intensely painful and sad, the probability of resultant death has been significantly diminished. As illustrated in **Table 1.1**, during the decade prior to 1952, a 50% mortality rate occurred in young adults (15–44 years of age) with total body surface area (TBSA) burns of 46% or greater.[2] Forty years later, statistics from the pediatric and adult burn units in Galveston, Texas indicated that the 50% mortality rate accompanied a 70% or greater TBSA for the same age group. Improved survival has been the primary focus of burn treatment advancement in the past few decades.

Such improvement in forestalling death is a direct result of the maturation of the science of burn care. Scientifically sound analyses of patient data have led to the development of formulas for fluid resuscitation[3–6] and nutritional support.[7,8] Clinical research has demonstrated the utility of topical antimicrobials in delaying onset of sepsis, thereby contributing to decreased mortality of burn patients.[8] Prospective randomized clinical trials have determined the efficacy of early surgical therapy in improving survival for many burned patients by decreasing blood loss and by diminishing the occurrence of sepsis.[10–15] Basic science and clinical research have contributed to decreased mortality by describing pathophysiology related to inhalation injury and suggesting treatment methods which have decreased the incidence of pulmonary edema and pneumonia.[16–19] Scientific investigations of the hypermetabolic response to major burn injury have led to improved management of this life-threatening phenomenon.[20–22]

Table 1.1 Percent of total body surface area (TBSA) burn for an expected 50% mortality in 1952 and 1993

Age (years)	1952 (% TBSA)	1993† (% TBSA)
0–14	49	98
15–44	46	72
45–64	27	51
>65	10	25

† Galveston Burn Unit.

Melding scientific research with clinical care has been promoted throughout the recent history of burn care, in large part because of the aggregation of burned patients into single purpose units staffed by dedicated health care personnel. Dedicated burn units were first established in Great Britain in order to facilitate nursing care.[23] The first US burn center was established at the Medical College of Virginia in 1947 followed that same year by the US Army Surgical Research Unit, later renamed the US Army Institute of Surgical Research.[23] Directors of both of these centers and later the founders of the Burn Institutes of Shriners Hospitals for Crippled Children emphasized the importance of collaboration between clinical care and basic scientific disciplines.[1] The organizational design of these centers stimulated the formation of a self-perpetuating feedback loop of clinical and basic scientific inquiry.[23] Scientists in such a system receive first-hand information about clinical problems while clinicians receive provocative ideas about patient responses to injury from experts of other disciplines.[1] Advances in burn care over the last 50 years attest to the value of a dedicated burn unit organized around the concept of a collegial group of basic scientists, clinical researchers, and clinical care givers, all asking questions of each other, sharing observations and information, and together seeking solutions to improve the welfare of their patients.

Findings of the group at the Army Surgical Research Institute pointed out the necessity of involving many disciplines in the treatment of patients with major burn injuries and stressed the utility of a team concept.[1] The International Society of Burn Injuries and its journal, *Burns*, and the American Burn Association with its publication, *Journal of Burn Care and Rehabilitation*, have publicized to widespread audiences the notion of successful multidisciplinary work by burn teams.

Members of a Burn Team

As illustrated by a perusal of the contents of either of the aforementioned journals and by the contents of this volume, the burn team can include epidemiologists, molecular biologists, microbiologists, physiologists, biochemists, pharmacists, pathologists, endocrinologists, nutritionists, and numerous other scientific and medical specialists. Burn injury is a complex systemic injury, and the search for improved methods of treatment leads to inquiry from many approaches. Each scientific finding stimulates new questions and potential involvement of additional specialists.

At times, the burn team can be thought of as including the environmental service workers responsible for cleaning the unit, the volunteers who may assist in a variety of ways to provide comfort for patients and families, the hospital administrator, and many others who support the day-to-day operations of a burn center and impact significantly on the well-being of patients and staff. The traditional concept of the burn team, however, connotes the multidisciplinary group of direct-care providers. Burn surgeons, nurses, dietitians, and physical and occupational therapists are the skeletal core; most burn units include anesthesiologists, respiratory therapists, pharmacists and social workers. In recent years, as mortality rates have decreased, interest has intensified in the quality of life for burn survivors, both acutely in the hospital and for the long term. Consequently, more burn units have added psychologists and psychiatrists to their burn team membership. In pediatric units, child life specialists and school teachers are significant members of the team of care takers as well.

Infrequently mentioned as members of the team, but obviously important in influencing the outcome of treatment, are the patient and the family of the patient. Persons with major burn injuries contribute actively to their own recovery, and each brings individual needs and agendas into the hospital setting which influence the ways in which treatment is provided by the professional care team.[24] The patient's family members often become active participants; obviously so in the case of children, but also in the case of adult patients. Family members often become conduits of information from the professional staff to the patient; they act, at times, as spokespersons for the patient, and at other times, they become advocates for the staff in encouraging the patient to cooperate with dreaded procedures.

With so many diverse personalities and specialists potentially involved, it may appear absurd to purport to know what or who constitutes a burn team. Yet references to the 'burn team' are plentiful, and there is common agreement on some specialists whose expertise is required for excellent care of significant burn injury.

Surgeons

A burn surgeon is the key figure of the burn team. Either a general surgeon or a plastic surgeon or, perhaps, both with expertise in providing emergency and critical care, as well as the techniques of skin grafting and amputations, provides leadership and guidance for the rest of the team which may include several surgeons. The surgeon's leadership is particularly important during the early phase of patient care when moment-to-moment decisions must be made based on the surgeon's knowledge of the physiological responses to the injury, the current scientific evidence, and the appropriate medical/surgical treatment. The surgeon must not only possess knowledge and skill in medicine, but also must be able to communicate clearly, both receiving and giving information, with a diverse staff of experts in other disciplines. The surgeon cannot alone provide comprehensive care but must be wise enough to know when and how to seek counsel as well as how to give directions clearly and firmly to direct activities surrounding patient care. The senior surgeon of the team is accorded the most authority and control of any member of the team and, thus, bears the responsibility and receives the accolades for the success of the team as a whole.[24]

Nurses

The nurses of the burn team represent the largest single disciplinary segment of the burn team, providing continuous coordinated care to a patient.[23] The nursing staff is responsible for technical management of the 24-hour physical treatment of the patient. As well, they provide emotional support to the patient and patient's family and control the therapeutic milieu that allows the patient to recover. The nursing staff is often the first to identify changes in the patient's condition and initiate therapeutic interventions.[23] Because recovery from a major burn is a rather slow process, the burn nurses combine the qualities of sophisticated intensive care nursing with the challenging aspects of psychiatric nursing. Nursing case management can play an important role in burn treatment, extending the coordination of care beyond the hospitalization through the lengthy period of out-patient rehabilitation.

Anesthesiologists

An anesthesiologist who is an expert in the altered physiological parameters of the burned patient is critical to the survival of the patient, who usually undergoes multiple surgical procedures acutely. Anesthesiologists on the burn team must be familiar with the phases of burn recovery and the physiological changes to be anticipated as the burn wounds heal.[1] Anesthesiologists play significant roles in facilitating comfort for burned patients, not only in the operating room but also in the painful ordeals of dressing changes, removal of staples, and physical exercise.

Respiratory Therapists

Inhalation injury, prolonged bed rest, fluid shifts, and the threat of pneumonia concomitant with burn injury render respiratory therapists essential to the patient's welfare.[23] They evaluate pulmonary mechanics, perform therapy to facilitate breathing, and closely monitor the status of the patient's respiratory functioning.

Rehabilitation Therapists

Occupational and physical therapists begin at the patient's admission to plan therapeutic interventions to maximize functional recovery. Burned patients require special positioning and splinting, early mobilization, strengthening exercises, endurance activities, and pressure garments to promote healing while controlling scar formation. These therapists must be very creative in designing and applying the appropriate appliances. Knowledge of the timing of application is necessary. In addition, rehabilitation therapists must become expert behavioral managers for their necessary treatments are usually painful to the recovering patient who will resist in a variety of ways. While the patient is angry, protesting loudly, or pleading for mercy, the rehabilitation therapist must persist with aggressive treatment in order to combat quickly forming and very strong scar contractures. The same therapist, however, typically is rewarded with adoration and gratitude from an enabled burn survivor.

Nutritionists

A nutritionist or dietitian monitors daily caloric intake and weight maintenance and recommends dietary interventions to provide optimal nutritional support to combat the hypermetabolic response of burn injury. Caloric intake as well as intake of appropriate vitamins, minerals, and trace elements must be managed to promote wound healing and facilitate recovery.

Psychosocial Experts

Psychiatrists, psychologists, and social workers with expertise in human behavior and psychotherapeutic interventions provide continuous sensitivity in caring for the emotional and mental well-being of patients and their families. These professionals must be knowledgeable about the process of burn recovery as well as human behavior in order to make optimal interventions. They serve as confidants and supports for the patients, families of patients, and on occasion, for other burn team members.[25] They often assist colleagues from other disciplines in developing behavioral interventions with problematic patients which allow the colleague and the patient to achieve therapeutic success. During initial hospitalization, these experts attend to managing the patient's mental status, pain tolerance, and anxiety level to provide comfort to the patient and also to facilitate physical recovery. As the patient progresses toward rehabilitation, the role of the mental health team becomes more prominent in supporting optimal psychological, social, and physical rehabilitation.

Functioning of a Burn Team

Gathering together a group of experts from diverse disciplines will not constitute a team. The group becomes a team when they have common goals and tasks to be accomplished and when they share, as individual members, overlapping values that will be served by accomplishing their goals.[26,27] The team becomes an efficient work group through a process of establishing mechanisms of collaboration and cooperation which facilitate focusing on explicit tasks rather than on covert distractions of personal need and interpersonal conflict.[27,28] Work groups seem to develop best in conditions which allow each individual to feel acknowledged as valuable to the team.[29,30]

A burn team has defined and shared goals with clear tasks. For the group of burn experts to become an efficient team, skillful leadership that facilitates the development of shared values among team members and ensures the validation of the members of the team as they accomplish tasks is necessary. The acknowledged formal leader of the team is the senior surgeon who may find the arduous job of medical and social leadership difficult and perplexing. Empirical studies, with remarkable consistency, indicate that the required functions for successful leadership can be grouped into two somewhat incompatible clusters:

- to direct the group toward tasks and goal attainment; and
- to facilitate the interaction of the group members, enhancing their feelings of worth.[27,30–33]

Task-oriented behavior by the leader may at times clash with the needs of the group for emotional support. During those times, the team may inadvertently impede the successful performance of both the leader and the team as the group seeks alternate means of establishing feelings of self-worth. When the social/emotional needs of the group are not met, the group begins to spend more time attempting to satisfy individual needs and less time pursuing task-related activity.

Studies of group behaviour demonstrate that high performance teams are characterized by synergy between task accomplishment and individual need fulfillment.[27,31] Since one formal leader cannot always attend to task and interpersonal nuances, groups allocate, informally or formally, leadership activities to multiple persons.[27,28,30,32] Current literature in organizational behavior indicates that the most effective leader is one who engages the talents of others and empowers them to utilize their abilities to further the work of the group.[27,28,32] Failure to empower the informal leaders limits their abilities to contribute fully.

For the identified leader of the burn team, i.e. the senior surgeon, to achieve a successful, efficient burn team, it is important that the leader be prepared to share leadership with one or more 'informal' leaders in such a way that all leadership functions are fulfilled.[27,28,30,32,34] The prominence and the identity of any one of these informal leaders will change according to situational alterations. The successful formal leader will encourage and support the leadership roles of other members of the team, developing a climate in which the team members are more likely to cooperate and collaborate toward achievement beyond individual capacity.

For many physicians, the concept of sharing leadership and power appears at first to be threatening, for it is the physician, after all, who must ultimately write the orders and be responsible for the patient's medical needs.[35] However, sharing power does not mean giving up control.[32] The physician shares leadership by seeking information and advice from other team members and empowers them by validating the importance of their expertise in the decision making process. The physician, however, maintains control of the patient's care and medical treatment.

Summary and Hopes for the Future

Centralized care provided in designated burn units has promoted a team approach to both scientific investigation and clinical care which has demonstrably improved the welfare of burn patients. Multidisciplinary efforts are imperative for the continued increase in understanding of and therapeutic responses to the emotional, psychological, and physiological recovery and rehabilitation of the burned person. Tremendous scientific and technological advances have led to dramatically increased survivability for burn victims.

Our hopes for the future are that by following the same model of collaboration, scientists and clinicians will pursue solutions to the perplexing problems which the burn survivor must encounter. Physical discomforts such as itching still interfere with rehabilitation of the patient. New techniques for controlling hypertrophic scar and for reconstructive surgeries could do much to diminish the resultant disfigurement.[36] Further development of psychological expertise within burn care and increased public awareness of the competence of burn survivors may ease the survivor's transition from incapacitated patient to functional member of society. We hope that burn care in the future will continue to devote the same energy and resources which have resulted in such tremendous advances in saving lives to improving the capacity for preserving optimal quality of life for survivors.

References

1. Artz C P, Moncrief J A. The burn problem. In: Artz C P, Moncrief J A, eds. *The Treatment of Burns* 2nd edition. Philadelphia, PA: W B Saunders Co, 1969: 1–21.

2. Bull J P, Fisher A J. A study of mortality in a burns unit: a revised estimate. *Ann Surg* 1954; **139:** 269–74.

3. Evans E I, Purnell O J, Robinett P W, Batchelor A, Martin M. Fluid and electrolyte requirements in severe burns. *Ann Surg* 1952; **135:** 804–17.

4. Baxter C R, Marvin J A, Curreri P W. Fluid and electrolyte therapy of burn shock. *Heart Lung* 1973; **2:** 707–13.

5. Artz C P. Burns updated. *J Trauma* 1976; **16:** 2–15.

6. Carvajal H F. Fluid therapy for acutely burned child. *Compr Ther* 1977; **3:** 17–24.

7. Curreri P W, Richmond D, Marvin J A, Baxter C R. Dietary requirements of patients with major burns. *J Am Diet Assoc* 1974; **65:** 415–17.

8. Hildreth M A, Herndon D N, Desai M H, Duke M A. Reassessing caloric requirements in pediatric burn patients. *J Burn Care Rehabil* 1988; **9:** 616–18.

9. Lindbergh R B, Pruitt B A Jr, Mason A D Jr. Topical chemotherapy and prophylaxis in thermal injury. *Chemotherapy* 1976; **3:** 351–9.

10. Janzekovic Z. A new concept in the early excision and immediate grafting of burns. *J Trauma* 1975; **15:** 42–62.

11. Burke J F, Bandoc C C, Quinby W C. Primary burn excision and immediate grafting: a method for shortening illness. *J Trauma* 1974; **14:** 389–95.

12. Engrav L H, Heimbach D M, Reus J L, Harnar T J, Marvin J A. Early excision and grafting vs. nonoperative treatment of burns of indeterminant depth: a randomized prospective study. *J Trauma* 1983; **23:** 1001–4.

13. Herndon D N, Barrow R E, Rutan R L, Rutan T C, Desai M H, Abston S. A comparison of conservative versus early excision therapies in severely burned patients. *Ann Surg* 1989; **209:** 547–53.

14. Desai M H, Herndon D N, Broemeling L, Barrow R E, Nichols R J Jr, Rutan R L. Early burn wound excision significantly reduces blood loss. *Ann Surg* 1990; **211:** 753–62.

15. Desai M H, Rutan R L, Herndon D N. Conservative treatment of scald burns is superior to early excision. *J Burn Care Rehabil* 1991; **12:** 482–4.

16. Shirani K Z, Pruitt B A Jr, Mason A D Jr. The influence of inhalation injury and pneumonia on burn mortality. *Ann Surg* 1987; **205:** 82–7.

17. Herndon D N, Barrow R E, Traber D L, Rutan T C, Rutan R L, Abston S. Extravascular lung water changes following smoke inhalation and massive burn injury. *Surgery* 1987; **102:** 341–9.

18. Herndon D N, Barrow R E, Linares H A, *et al.* Inhalation injury in burned patients: effects and treatment. *Burns* 1988; **14:** 349–56.

19. Cioffi W G Jr, Rue L W III, Graves T A, McManus W F, Mason A D Jr, Pruitt B A Jr. Prophylactic use of high-frequency percussive ventilation in patients with inhalation injury. *Ann Surg* 1991; **213:** 575–82.

20. Wilmore D W, Long J M, Mason A D Jr, Skreen R W, Pruitt BA Jr. Catecholamines: mediator of the hypermetabolic response to thermal injury. *Ann Surg* 1974; **180:** 653–69.

21. Herndon D N, Stein M D, Rutan T C, Abston S, Linares H. Failure of TPN supplementation to improve liver function, immunity, and mortality in thermally injured patients. *J Trauma* 1987; **27:** 195–204.

22. Herndon D N, Barrow R E, Stein M, *et al.*, Increased mortality with intravenous supplemental feeding in severely burned patients. *J Burn Care Rehabil* 1989; **10:** 309–13.

23. Rutan R L, On the shoulders of giants. Galveston, TX: Shriners Burns Institute, 1994, unpublished manuscript.

24. Shakespeare P G. Who should lead the burn care team? *Burns* 1994; **19**(6): 490–4.

25. Morris J, McFadd A. The mental health team on a burn unit: a multidisciplinary approach. *J Trauma* 1978; **18**(9): 658–63.

26. Miller E J, Rice A K. Selections from: Systems of organization. In: Colman A D, Bexton W H, eds. *Group Relations Reader* Sausalito, CA: Grex, 1975: 43–68.

27. Harris P R, Harris D L. High performance team management. *Leadership and Organization – Development Journal* 1989; **10**(4): 28–32.

28. Yank G R, Barber J W, Hargrove D S, Whitt P D. The mental health treatment team as a work group: team dynamics and the role of the leader. *Psychiatry* 1992; **55:** 250–64.

29. Pawlicki R E, Bertera J F, Nicholson M. Practice management: what constitutes an excellent team member. *Am J Pain M* 1994; **4**(4): 175–7.

30. Litterer J A, *The Analysis of Organizations, 2nd ed.* New York: John Wiley & Sons, 1973.

31. Fleishman E A, Mumford M D, Zaccaro S J, Levin K Y, Korotkin A L, Hein M B. Taxonomic efforts in the description of leader behavior: a synthesis and functional interpretation. *Special Issue: Individual Differences and Leadership: Leadership Quarterly* 1991; **2**(4): 245–87.

32. Hollander E P, Offermann L R, Power and leadership in organizations: relationships in transition. *Am Psychol* 1990; **45**(2): 179–89.

33. Krantz J. Lessons from the field: an essay on the crisis of leadership in contemporary organizations. *J Appl Behav Sci* 1990; **26**(1): 49–64.

34. Glaser E M, Van Eynde D F. Human resource development, team building, and a little bit of 'Kiem Tau': Part 1. *Organization Development Journal* 1989: 20–4.

35. Fiorelli J S. Power in work groups: team members' perspectives. *Hum Relat* 1988; **41**(1): 1–12.

36. Constable J D. The state of burn care: past, present, and future. *Burns* 1994; **20**(4): 316–24.

CHAPTER TWO

Epidemiological, Demographic and Outcome Characteristics of Burn Injury

Basil A. Pruitt, Jr and Arthur D. Mason, Jr

Introduction

The magnitude of the public health problem represented by burns is reflected in the fire and burn deaths which are reported by each state to the National Center for Injury Prevention and Control. In 1991, such deaths totaled 5053 in the United States and ranged from four in Hawaii and eight in Vermont to 337 in California and 359 in Texas. In 1991, the age-adjusted rate of fire and burn deaths, which excludes patients of unknown age, ranged from 0.164 per 100 000 population in Colorado to 3.75 per 100 000 population in Mississippi.[1]

Fire and burn deaths occur with greatest frequency in residential fires, especially in multi-family dwellings and in low income census tracts.[2] Four out of five unintentional deaths and almost three out of four (73%) of all deaths due to burns in fires result from house fires.[3] It has been reported that approximately 12 individuals die in a residential fire each day with young children and the elderly being the most likely victims,[4,5] the former have difficulty escaping because of dependency and the latter because of preexisting diseases and decreased agility.

Epidemiology and Demography

Geographic location, presumably because of regional differences in construction and heating devices, influences death rates from house fires. House fire death rates are higher in the east, particularly the southeast, as compared to the west.[3] Seasonal differences in house fire death rates are also evident, with the majority of such deaths occurring during the cold winter months when greatest use is made of heating and lighting devices. In recent years the house fire death rate has decreased; this trend has been attributed to the combined effects of improved building design, increased use of smoke and fire detectors, and use of safer appliances and heating devices. House fires cause only approximately 4% of burn admissions but the 12% fatality rate of patients hospitalized for burns sustained in house fires is higher than the 3% fatality rate for patients with burns from other causes. This difference is presumably the effect of associated inhalation injury.[6,7]

Playing with matches, cigarette lighters, or other ignition devices has been incriminated as the cause of one in ten residential fire deaths.[3] House fire death rates show little gender predominance except for an increased incidence in males age 2 to 5, a group which has the highest rate of nonfatal burns due to unsupervised play with matches.[8] Careless smoking, which accounts for one in four residential fire deaths, is the most common cause of such fatalities. Alcohol and drug intoxication, which contribute to careless smoking behavior by impairing mentation, have been reported to be a factor in 40% of residential fire deaths and appear to contribute to the high weekend frequency of house fires.[9] Arson is the second most common cause of residential fire deaths; and defective or inappropriately used heating devices, which are the third most common cause, account for one in six residential fire deaths overall and an even greater proportion in low income areas.[10] The effect of low income on fire and burn deaths also appears to be related to residence in older buildings, crowded living conditions, and absence of smoke detectors. As a reflection of the effect of economic status, minority children age 0–19 are more than three times as likely to die in a residential fire than white children.[5] As income increases, racial differences in house fire death rates decrease.[11]

The economic consequences of residential fires are also great. Property loss in 1991 due to such fires amounted to over 5.5 billion dollars, of which 1.5 billion dollars were lost in the Oakland, California fire alone, which occurred in a high income residential area.[4] Health care costs are also prodigious. Each year in the United States 60 000–80 000 people require in-hospital care for burns; and the average cost for hospital care of a patient injured by flame and/or smoke inhalation ranges from $36 452.00 to $117 506.00 with much higher costs incurred by patients with extensive burns.[12] The estimated cost of a fire-related death, which includes the loss of future productivity, ranges from $250 000.00 to $1.5 million.[12–14]

Unlike fire deaths, the precise number of burn injuries which occur in the United States is unknown. Twenty-one states require that burn injuries be reported; only two require reporting burns associated with assaults or arson, and seven require only that larger burns (usually those involving more than 15% of the total body surface) be reported.[15] Consequently, the total number of burns must be estimated by extrapolation to the entire population via data collected in less than one-half of the states. Such estimates range from 1.4 million to 2 million injuries due to burns in fires each year.[3,16] The majority of those burns are of limited extent (more than 80% of burns involve less than 20% of the total body surface area); but in the United States, 270–300 patients per million population (67 500–75 000) per year sustain burns which, because of extent, associated injury, or co-morbid conditions, require admission to a hospital.[2]

A smaller subset of approximately 20 000 burn patients with even more severe injuries, as defined by the American Burn Association (**Table 2.1**), are best cared for in a burn center.[17] Those patients consist of 42 per million population with major burns and

Table 2.1 American Burn Association major burn injury criteria

Second and third degree burns greater than 10% of the total body surface area in patients under 10 or over 50 years of age
Second and third degree burns greater than 20% of the total body surface area in other age groups
Significant burns of face, hands, feet, genitalia, or perineum and those that involve skin overlying major joints
Third degree burns greater than 5% of the total body surface area in any age group
Inhalation injury
Significant electric injury including lightning injury
Significant chemical injury
Burns with significant preexisting medical disorders that could complicate management, prolong recovery, or affect mortality (e.g. diabetes mellitus or cardiopulmonary disease)
Burns with significant concomitant trauma (may require initial treatment in a trauma center)
Burn injury in patients who will require special social and emotional or long-term rehabilitative support, including cases of suspected child abuse and neglect

40 per million population having lesser burns but a complicating co-factor.[2] There are 138 burn care facilities in the United States and 21 in Canada which are distributed in proportion to population density and contain a total of 1951 beds (**Figure 2.1**).[18] As described below, the geographic distribution of burn centers necessitates the use of aeromedical transfer by both rotary and fixed wing aircraft to transport patients requiring burn center care to those facilities from distant and remote areas.

In addition to economic status[19] and geographic location[19,20] the risk of being burned and the predominant cause of burn injury are related to age,[21] occupation, and participation in recreational activities.[22] Scald burns are the most frequent form of burn injury overall and cause over 100 000 patients to seek treatment in hospital emergency rooms each year.[23] Spill scalds are the most common cause of burn injury in children.[24] A survey of burn units in New York State found that 45% of hospital admissions for scalds occurred in children less than 5 years of age.[25] Hot beverages, particularly coffee, which may be dispensed at temperatures of up to 180°F (82.2°C), are the predominant cause of scald burns in children.

Based on data collected by the National Electronic Injury Surveillance System, it is estimated that approximately 3500 patients required emergency treatment in 1988 for scald burns sustained from hot tap water in showers and bath tubs. More than 66% of those 3500 patients were children below the age of 5; and one-fourth of the 3500 required admission to a hospital.[3] The occurrence of tap water scalds can be prevented by adjusting the temperature settings on hot water heaters or by installing special faucet valves so that water does not leave the tap at temperatures above 120°F (48.8°C). Thermostatic valves, which shut the hot water off if the cold water fails, are the most dependable.[26] The results of a survey in Denmark indicate that the kitchen, not the bathroom, is the most common site of burn injury (39% of burns).[27] Those burns were most commonly due to contact with hot liquids.

The disabled are a group of patients considered to be 'burn-prone'. The majority of burns in the disabled occur at home and are most often scalds. The effects of disability and the preexisting disease in those patients are evident in the duration of hospital stay (27.6 days on average) and in the death rate (22.2%) which is associated with the modest average extent of burn (10% of the total body surface area).[28]

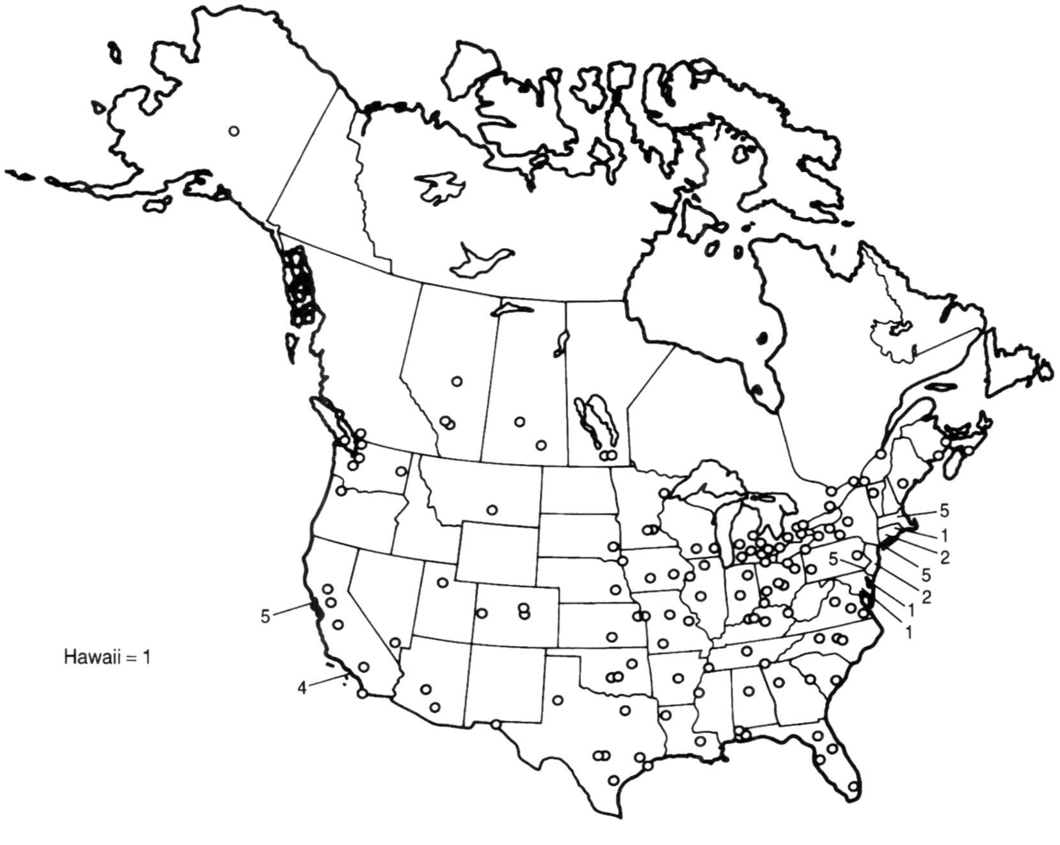

Fig. 2.1 Burn care facilities in North America 1993–1994. The numbers indicate facilities in areas where these are concentrated.

Burns from scalds and contacts with hot materials cause approximately 100 deaths per year.[3] The case fatality rate of scald injury is low (presumably due to the limited burn depth and amount of body surface involved), but scalds are major causes of morbidity and associated health care costs particularly in children less than 5 years of age and in the elderly. Although deaths from scalds are relatively rare in patients between the ages of 5 and 64, both rates of hospitalization for burn injury and death rates are three times greater for blacks than for caucasians.[29]

Even though the burns of 30% of all patients requiring admission to hospital are caused by scalding due to hot liquid,[30,31] flame is the predominant cause of burns in patients admitted to burn centers, particularly in the adult age group (**Table 2.2**). In one epidemiological study in New York state, the largest number of admissions in the teenage/early adult age group (15–24 years) were related to automobiles. Ignition of fuel following a crash, steam from radiators, and contact with hot engine and exhaust parts were the most frequent causes.[31] In a review of 178 patients who had been burned in an automobile crash it was noted that slightly more than one-third had other injuries, most commonly involving the musculoskeletal system, and that approximately one in six had inhalation injury (one in three of those who died).[32] A recent review from SBI–Galveston's burn center revealed that burns sustained while operating a vehicle involved an average of more than 30% of the total body surface and were associated with mechanical injuries (predominantly fractures) much more frequently than those burns incurred in the course of vehicle maintenance activities which involved an average of less than 30% of the total body surface.[33]

Automotive-related flame burns can also be caused by fires and explosions resulting from 'carburetor-priming' with liquid gasoline; and such burns have been reported to account for 2–5% of burn unit admissions.[34] The burns sustained in boating accidents are also most often flash burns due to an explosion of gasoline or butane and typically affect the face and hands.[22] Bonfire and barbecue burns caused by flash ignition of flammable liquid which is used to start or accelerate a fire affect those same areas as well as the anterior trunk.[35]

Table 2.2 Admissions to US Army Institute of Surgical Research Burn Center, 1989–1993

Cause of burn	Age groups (years) 0–15	16–40	Over 40
Hot liquids	150	80	40
Gasoline, diesel, and kerosene	30	115	58
Open flame	43	160	63
Electrical	4	49	11
Structural fires	25	46	33
Bomb, shell, simulator grenade, and gunpowder explosions	2	50	4
Contact	29	10	11
Motor vehicle crashes		21	3
Butane, propane, or natural/sewer gas explosions	6	29	7
Chemical	2	17	14
Self-inflicted		23	6
Welding		4	2
Smoking, clothes ignition			8
Other:			
Sunburn		1	
Totals	291	605	260

The ignition of clothing is the second leading cause of burn admissions for most ages.[31] The burn injury rate due to the ignition of clothing is influenced by poverty and is inversely related to income. The fatality rate of patients with burns due to the ignition of clothing is second only to that of patients with burns incurred in house fires.[31] Burns caused by the ignition of synthetic fabrics which melt and adhere to skin are commonly deeper than burns caused by other fabrics and typically exhibit a gravity dependent 'runoff' pattern. More than three-quarters of deaths due to the ignition of clothing occur in patients more than 64 years old.[3] Clothing ignition deaths, which were a frequent cause of death in young girls, have decreased as clothing styles have changed and are now rare among children with little overall gender difference at the present time. Since 1975, when it was mandated that sleepwear sizes 0 to 6x successfully pass a standard flame test, the percentage of clothing burns caused by sleepwear in children age 0–12 decreased from 55 to 27.[31,36]

Work-related burns account for 20–25% of all serious burns; and the Bureau of Labor Statistics survey in 1985 indicated that 6% of all work-related thermal burns occurred in adolescent workers (16–19 years).[37] In a 1986 study in Ohio, it was noted that the majority of hospital-treated burns in the teenage/young adult group occurred on the job.[38] A study in that same year revealed that 6 out of 10 hospitalized burn injuries in employed men in Massachusetts were work-related.[39] Restaurant-related burns, particularly those due to deep fryers, represent a major and preventable source of occupational burn morbidity and in restaurants account for 12% of work-related injuries.[40] Almost 700 deaths annually are caused by occupation-related burns.[40,41]

As would be anticipated, the risk of burn injury due to hot tar is greatest for roofers and paving workers. Of all accidents involving roofers and sheet metal workers, 16% are burns caused by hot bitumen, and 17% of those injuries are of sufficient severity to prevent work for a variable period of time. In the state of California, in 1979, 366 roofers and slaters sustained burn injuries.[42] The majority of hot tar burns involve the hand and upper limb.[43] Another occupation associated with an increased risk of burn injury is welding in which flash burns and explosions are the most common injury-producing events.

In the United States in 1988, there were 236 200 patients with chemical injuries of all types treated in emergency rooms. Of those patients, 35 000 or 15% were patients of all ages with chemical burns, and 6500 or 5% were children younger than 5 years with chemical burns. The limited extent of burns due to chemical contact is indexed by the fact that only 800, or 2%, of the chemical burns required admission to a hospital. The effect of age (in the very young, removal of the offending agent may be delayed) on the severity of chemical injury is evident in the fact that 400 of the patients requiring admission to hospital for the care of chemical burn injuries were children younger than 5 years.[44] The greatest risk of injury due to strong acids occurs in persons who are involved in plating processes and fertilizer manufacture. The greatest risk of strong alkali injury in the workplace is associated with soap manufacturing, and in the home with the use of oven cleaners. The greatest risk of phenol injury is associated with the manufacture of dyes, fertilizers, plastics, and explosives. The greatest risk of hydrofluoric acid injury is associated with etching processes, petroleum refining, and air conditioner cleaning. Anhydrous ammonia injury is most common in agricultural workers, and cement injury is most common in construction workers. Injury due to petroleum distillates, which cause dilapidation, is greatest in refinery and tank farm workers; while white phosphorus and mustard gas injuries are most frequent in military personnel.[45]

Nearly a thousand deaths are caused annually by electric current. One-third of electric injuries occur in the home and one-quarter occur on farms or industrial sites.[31] The greatest incidence of electric injury caused by household current exists in young children who insert uninsulated objects into electrical receptacles or bite or suck on electric cords and sockets.[2] Low-voltage direct current injury can be caused by contact with automobile battery terminals or by defective or inappropriately used medical equipment such as electrosurgical devices,[46] external pacing devices,[47] or defibrillators.[48] Although such injuries may involve the full-thickness of the skin, they are characteristically of limited extent. Caucasians, apparently because of employment patterns, are almost twice as likely to be injured by high-voltage electric current as are blacks.[41] Employees of utility companies, electricians, construction workers (particularly those working with cranes), farm workers moving irrigation pipe, oil field workers, truck drivers, and individuals installing antennae are at greatest risk of high-voltage electric injury.[2] The greatest incidence of electric injury occurs during the summer as a reflection of farm irrigation activity, construction work, and work on outdoor electrical systems and equipment.[8]

In the United States, approximately 80 people are killed by lightning each year.[3] The death rate from lightning is greatest between the 10th and 19th years of life and is seven times greater in males than females. Deaths rates are highest in mountainous and southern states; and deaths occur with greatest frequency during the summer months, apparently because more people are outdoors during thunder storms.[3] Most deaths occur in people who are in open fields or on the water and/or are touching metal equipment such as antennae. Out-of-doors workers, such as those on farms, construction sites, or other outdoor workplaces, are involved in up to one-third of fatal lightning strikes.[49] One of every six lightning deaths is related to recreation such as golfing, fishing, and camping.[50] The recent decrease in lightning-related deaths appears to be related to decreases in the farm population, better understanding of the pathophysiology of lightning injury, and improved resuscitation regimens.

Fireworks are another seasonal cause of burn injury. Approximately 10% of patients with fireworks injuries require in-hospital care and approximately 60% of those injuries are burns.[51] These data can be used to estimate that 1.86–5.82 fireworks-related burns per 100 000 persons occur in the United States during the Fourth of July holiday.[52] NEISS (National Electronic Injury Surveillance System) extrapolated data indicate that 13 263 patients sustained burns in 1992 from fireworks and flares.[53] Sparklers, firecrackers, and bottle rockets caused the greatest number of burn injuries requiring hospital care.[54] At the US Army Institute of Surgical Research, only four, or 0.1%, of 3628 burn patients admitted during a recent 15-year period had been burned by fireworks.

Burn injury can also be self-inflicted or caused by third party assault. A retrospective review of 5758 burn patients treated at a regional burn center during a 12-year period identified 51 patients (26 males and 25 females) with a diagnosis of self-inflicted burns.[55] In 42 patients, in whom the injury was an attempt at suicide, the burn involved from 1 to 84% of the total body surface with an average extent of 22%. Twelve, or 28% of those patients expired. There were nine patients in whom the injury was considered a form of self-mutilation. Those injuries involved from 1 to 5% of the total body surface with an average extent of 1.4%. Forty-three percent of all of the injuries occurred at home, and 14 occurred while the patient was in a psychiatric institution. Seventy-three percent of the patients had a history of psychiatric disease; and these were predominantly affective disorders or schizophrenia in the suicides, and personality disorders in the self-mutilators. Fifty-five percent of the suicides had previously attempted suicide; 66% of the self-mutilators had made at least one previous attempt at self-mutilation. The authors concluded that the very fact of self-burning warranted psychiatric assessment. Buddhist ritual burning caused by contact with smoldering incense is a traditional religious form of self-mutilation.[56] Squyres *et al.* reported their experience in treating 17 people over a 3-year period for self-inflicted burns.[57] The average extent of burn in those patients was 29.5% of the total body surface; and 59% of them had concomitant inhalation injury. All of those patients had a psychiatric disorder which, in 47% of the group, was related to substance abuse. The most frequently employed means of injury was ignition of a flammable liquid.

Assault by burning is most often caused by throwing liquid chemicals at the face of the intended victim or by the ignition of a flammable liquid with which the victim has been doused. Relatively uncommon is the infliction of burn injury by dousing the victim with hot water. Duminy and Hudson have reported their experience with 127 patients who had been intentionally injured with hot water.[58] The burns in those patients involved from 1 to 45% of the total body surface area with an average extent of 13.7%. The trunk and arms were burned in 116 of the patients, the head and neck in 84, and the legs in 27. The vast majority, 84, had only partial thickness injuries. Fifty-one of the male patients and 12 of the 33 females had been assaulted by their spouses. In cases of spouse abuse, the face or genitalia are characteristically splashed with chemicals or hot liquids while cases due to abuse or neglect in elderly, disabled, and handicapped adults resemble those in child abuse cases.[59,60] In India, a common form of spouse abuse is burning by intentional ignition of clothing. When such burns are fatal they have been called 'dowry deaths' since they have been used to establish the widower's eligibility for a new bride and dowry.

Child abuse represents a special form of burn injury most commonly inflicted by parents but also perpetrated by siblings and child care personnel. Child abuse has been associated with teenage parents, mental deficits in either the child or the abuser, illegitimacy, a single parent household, and low socioeconomic status (although child abuse can occur in all economic groups). Abuse is usually inflicted upon children younger than 2 years of age who, in addition to burns, may exhibit signs of poor hygiene, psychological deprivation, and nutritional impairment.[61] The most common form (approximately one-third of cases) of child abuse thermal injury is caused by cigarettes; such injuries, because of their limited extent, frequently do not require admission to a hospital.[62] Child abuse by burning has also been inflicted by placing a small child in a microwave oven. The burn injuries produced in that manner are typically present on the body parts nearest the microwave generating element, full-thickness in depth and sharply demarcated.[63] Child neglect, if not child abuse, is considered to be a factor in burns of the hand, particularly those on the dorsum of the hand, due to contact with a hot clothing iron.[64] Most often scalding causes the burns in abused children who require in-hospital care.[65] Such injuries are often associated with soft tissue trauma, fractures, and head injury. A distribution typical of child abuse immersion scald burns, i.e. feet, posterior legs, buttocks, and the hands, should heighten one's suspicion of child abuse; such observations mandate a complete evaluation of the circumstances surrounding the injury and the home situation. The importance of identifying child abuse in the cause of a burn injury resides in the fact that if such abuse goes undetected and the child is returned to the abusive environment, there is a high risk of fatality due to repeated abuse.

Patients may also sustain burns while in the hospital for diagnosis and treatment of other disease.[66] In addition to the electric injuries noted above, chemical burns have been produced by inadvertent application of glacial acetic acid, concentrated silver nitrate, iodine, or phenol solutions, and potassium permanganate crystals. Application of excessively hot soaks or towels or inappropriate use of heat lamps or a heating blanket are other causes of burn injury to patients.[67] Much more serious are the burns and inhalation injuries caused by electrocautery or laser devices, explosions of gases (including oxygen), or ignition of the instruments used for endotracheal and endobronchial procedures or anesthetic management.[68] A common cause of burn injury, particularly in disoriented hospital or nursing home patients, is the ignition of bed clothes and clothing by a smoking cigarette. Smoking should be banned in heath care facilities, or at least restricted to adequately monitored situations.

Outcome Characteristics

As noted above, the concordance of burn treatment facility and population densities necessitates that many patients requiring burn center care be transferred from other locations to such institutions. For transfer across short distances and in congested urban areas, ground transportation is frequently more expeditious than aeromedical transfer. Aeromedical transfer is indicated when the patient requires movement from a remote area or when such transfer will shorten the time during which the patient is in transit as compared to ground transportation. Helicopters are frequently employed for the aeromedical transfer of patients over distances of less than 200 miles. Vibration, poor lighting, restricted space, and noise make in-flight therapeutic interventions difficult, a fact which emphasizes the importance of carefully evaluating the patient and modifying treatment as needed to establish hemodynamic and pulmonary stability prior to undertaking the transfer. When transfer requires movement over greater distances, fixed wing aircraft are utilized, ideally those in which an oxygen supply is available to support mechanical ventilation. The patient compartment of such aircraft should be well lighted, permit movement of attending personnel, and have some measure of temperature control.

In general, burned patients travel best in the immediate postburn period as soon as hemodynamic and pulmonary stability have been attained by resuscitation. This avoids the instability caused by infection, secondary hemorrhage, sepsis, or cardiac insufficiency which occur later in the severely burned patient's hospital course.[69] The importance of an experienced burn physician accompanying a patient during aeromedical transfer is indicated by the findings of a study in which the management problems encountered during 124 flights to transfer 148 burn patients were reviewed.[70] More than half the patients required therapeutic interventions prior to undertaking aeromedical transfer. Such interventions most commonly involved placement or adjustment of a cannula or catheter, modification of fluid therapy, or endotracheal intubation and modification of ventilatory management. In slightly more than one-third of the patients, such interventions were considered necessary to correct physiologic instabilities which would have compromised patient safety during the transfer procedure. Six of the 124 patients required an escharotomy to relieve compression of the chest or a limb caused by a constricting eschar. The therapeutic alterations most commonly needed during the aeromedical transfer procedure itself were changes in fluid therapy, adjustment of a ventilator, and administration of parenteral medications exclusive of analgesics.

Physician-to-physician case review to assess the need for and safety of aeromedical transfer, prompt initiation of the aeromedical transfer mission, examination of the patient in the hospital of origin by a burn surgeon from the receiving hospital prior to undertaking aeromedical transfer, and in-flight monitoring by burn experienced personnel ensure both continuity and quality of care during the transport procedure. During the 16-year period 1977–1992, US Army Institute of Surgical Research personnel using such a regimen completed 1158 helicopter and fixed wing aeromedical transfers to transport 1386 burned patients within the continental United States without any in-flight deaths. During the same period, the Institute carried out 30 intercontinental aeromedical transfer missions in which 94 burned patients were transported with only one in-flight death.

Outcome Analysis in Burn Injury

The importance of extent of injury in determining burn outcome was recognized by Holmes in 1860, and discussions expressing that extent as either a measured surface area or as a fraction of body surface appeared early in this century.[71,72,73] Formal expression of burn size as a percentage of total body surface area, however, awaited the work of Berkow in 1924.[74] Though accorded little recognition as such, this single advance in the understanding of thermal injury, along with the corollary understanding that burn size is a crucial determinant of pathophysiological response, made burns the first form of trauma whose impact could be measured and easily communicated. Techniques based on this understanding produced what were in effect the first trauma indices. This made assessment of the relationship between burn size and mortality, direct comparison of populations of burned patients, and rational assessment of therapy possible long before rigorous outcome analysis became feasible for any other form of injury.

The earliest comprehensive statistical technique used for such assessment was univariate probit analysis.[75,76] This approach, laborious in the days of paper files and rotary calculators, required that the population studied be arbitrarily partitioned into groups which were relatively similar in burn size and age. Such analyses yield equations describing the effect of burn size on mortality which are valid for only the particular age group studied. An early attempt to develop a multivariate evaluation was made by Schwartz, who used probit plane analysis to estimate the relative contributions of partial and full thickness burns to mortality. This approach also required arbitrary partitioning of the population.[77]

The advent of computers of suitable power, and further development of statistical techniques, have reduced the difficulty of analysing burn mortality, removed the necessity for arbitrary partitioning, and made these techniques much more accessible.[78] Their use to assess outcome requires an understanding of the techniques themselves and of the population being analysed. The analysis of a population of 8448 patients admitted for burn care to the United States Army Institute of Surgical Research or to its predecessor, the US Army Surgical Research Unit, between January 1, 1950 and December 31, 1991 will be used to illustrate the concepts underlying modern outcome analysis and to depict the trends in mortality that have been characteristic of most major burn centers in this country.

For validity, an important first step in such studies is to achieve as much uniformity as possible in the population to be analysed. These patients reached the Institute between the day of injury and postburn day 531 (mean 5.86 d, median 1 d), with burns averaging 31% (range 1–100%, median 26%) of the total body surface. Their age distribution was biphasic, with one peak at one year of age and another at age 20; the mean age of the entire population was 26.5 years (range 0–97 years, median 23 years). From these patients, we first selected the 7893 (93.4%) who had flame or scald injuries, excluding other forms of thermal injury.

Included in this group were patients who sustained thermal injuries in Vietnam and were first transferred to Japan and then selectively transferred to the Institute. Arriving at the Institute relatively late in their courses, these survivors of a temporal cohort in which some deaths had already occurred exhibited inordinately low mortality. Outcome is inevitably biased toward survival as the postburn time of admission lengthens. To avoid this bias, the analysis focused on the 4870 patients with flame or scald injuries who reached the Institute on or before the second postburn day, excluding later arrivals. Burn size in these patients average 34% (range 1–100%, median 29%), and age was again biphasic, with peaks at 1 and 21 yrs and a mean of 27.1 yrs (range 0–93 yrs, median 24 yrs).

One object of the analysis was to evaluate changes in burn mortality during the four decades of experience included in the study. For reliable results, the techniques which were used required more subjects than were available in some single years; a moving 5-year interval, advancing one year at a time, was used to group the data. The number of patients in each of the overlapping 5-year intervals is shown in **Figure 2.2.** In this and subsequent plots, the data for a 5-year interval are plotted at the first year of the interval, reflecting that year and the succeeding four. The number of admissions meeting the selection criteria was small in the early years of the Institute's experience and rose in somewhat linear fashion during the second and third decades to a sustained plateau of approximately 800 (160/yr).

Mean patient age is shown in **Figure 2.3**. Between 1950 and 1965, most of the admissions were young soldiers; mean age approximated 22.5 years and was relatively stable. During the succeeding decade, this value rose to an irregular plateau centering on 30 years of age, a change reflecting a greater number of civilian emergency admissions and increasing age in the military population.

Figure 2.4 shows the variation in mean burn size during the study interval, and **Figure 2.5** shows the roughly parallel mortality. Mean burn size peaked in the two intervals spanning 1969 to 1974 and decreased steadily after that time. Mortality, principally due to burn wound sepsis, peaked at 46% during those years. The two data sets are shown together in **Figure 2.6** and suggest a crude index of the results of burn care in this population. There were two intervals in which percent mortality exceeded mean percent burn. The first occurred in the late 1950s and early 1960s, a time when burn wound sepsis due to *Pseudomonas aeruginosa* was uncontrolled. This was succeeded by a 6-year interval of good control of wound infection following the introduction of topical wound treatment with mafenide. In turn, this was followed by a second interval of poor control in the late 1960s and early 1970s, during which both *Pseudomonas* and a mafenide-resistant *Providencia stuartii* were major causes of sepsis; this endemic was controlled by the mid-1970s following changes in topical treatment and wound management.

Raw percent mortality, even in conjunction with burn size, is never an adequate index of the effectiveness of treatment, since the frequency of death after burn injury is also determined by prior patient condition, age, inhalation injury, and the occurrence of pneumonia and burn wound sepsis. Each of these elements, except for prior condition, can be addressed in analysis, but only burn size, age and the presence or absence of inhalation injury are known at the time of admission. In the present group, burn size and age are available for every patient, but data on inhalation injury are missing for patients admitted in the earlier years; we elected to use burn size

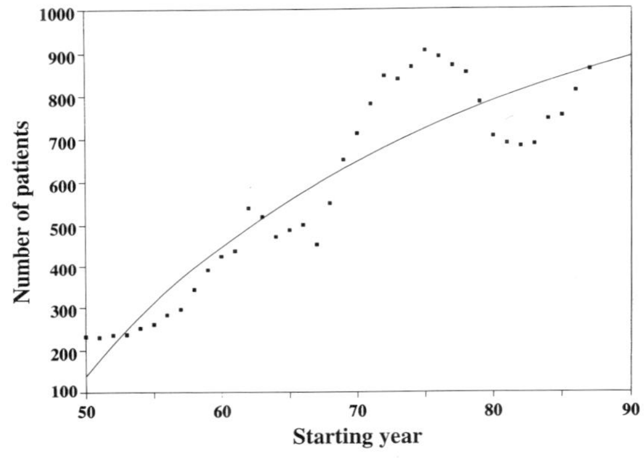

Fig 2.2 Number of patients meeting study criteria. Values are plotted at the first year of each moving 5-year interval.

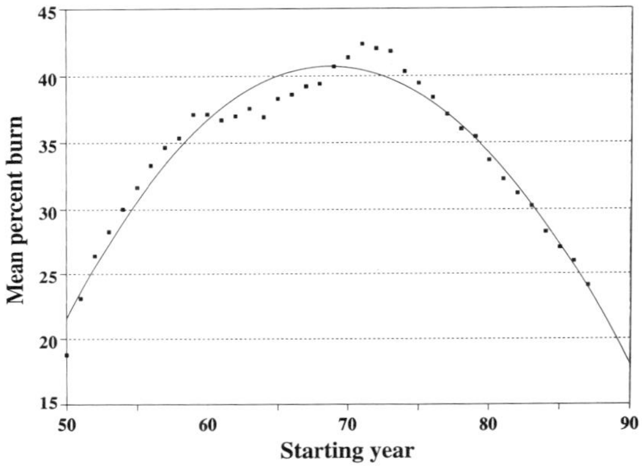

Fig 2.4 Mean burn size in study patients.

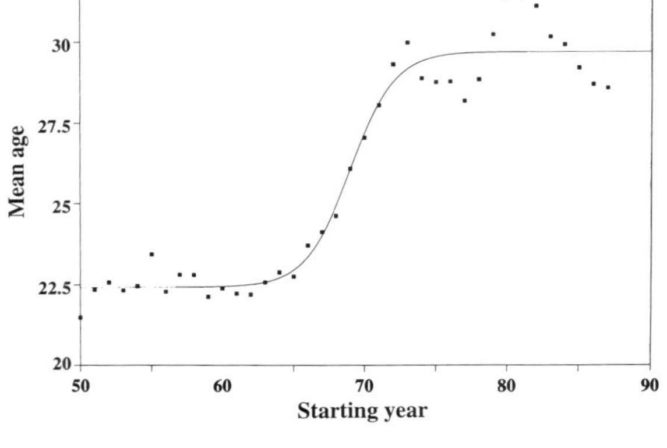

Fig 2.3 Mean age of study patients.

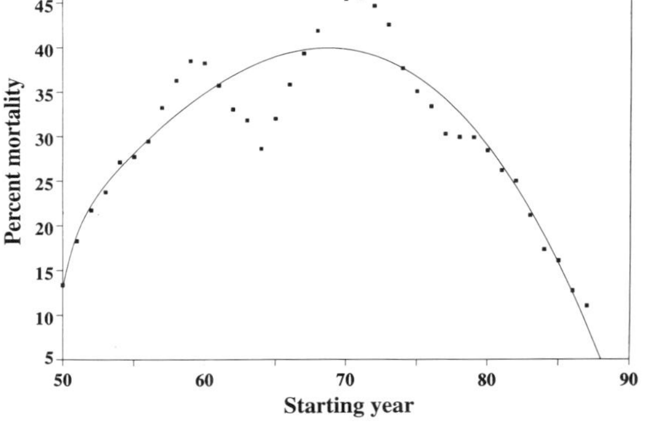

Fig 2.5 Percent mortality in study patients in each moving 5-year interval.

and age for analysis. This choice does not exclude the impact of the complications but does confound that impact with those of burn size and age.

For a uniform population of specific age, a plot of the relationship between burn size and percent mortality is S-shaped, or sigmoid – small burns produce relatively few deaths, but as burn size increases mortality rises steeply and then plateaus as it approaches its maximum of 100%. **Figure 2.7** illustrates this dose response relationship for 50-year-old patients admitted to the Institute between 1987 and 1991. Such curves are mathematically intractable and are usually transformed to more easily managed straight lines for analysis. Several mathematical transformations have been used to accomplish this. As previously noted, the one used in early analyses was probit transformation; in the present study, a logistic transformation was used as is illustrated in **Figure 2.8**. The choice between these is one of convenience as either yields essentially the same information.[79,80]

The locations of a sequence of such curves for groups of patients of increasing age move first to the right (toward larger burn size) as age increases from infancy to young adulthood, and then to the left, passing through the infant location at around age 45 and continuing inexorably leftward with increasing age. These differing locations reflect the greater risk of burn mortality at the extremes of age. The cubic curve in **Figure 2.9** describes this curvilinear effect of age on mortality; the effect is least at age 21. For this population, the age function was relatively stable over the entire interval of study.

As we have noted, earlier analyses began by dividing the studied population into arbitrary age and burn size groups; probit analysis of the relationship between burn size and percent mortality in each age group then permitted estimation of the LD50, the burn size lethal to half the selected age group. To accommodate both age and burn size simultaneously, without arbitrary partitioning of the population, multiple logistic regression was used for this study, with each member of the population entering the analysis as an individual data point.

The result of this 3-dimensional form of analysis is most readily visualized as a plane lying within a cube. **Figure 2.10** shows the sigmoid response of mortality to burn size for three discrete ages, and **Figure 2.11** shows the curvilinear variation of mortality with age in patients entering this study between 1987 and 1991. A best fitting plane which covers the tips of spikes representing all of the burn sizes and ages of interest is generated by the multiple logistic technique, and it is illustrated for these particular patients in **Figure 2.12**. The equation representing this plane is of the form shown below, in which L is the logistic of percent mortality and P the expected fractional mortality rate.

$$L = a_1 + a_2\,(\%burn) - a_3\,(age) + a_4\left(\frac{age^2}{100}\right) - a_5\left(\frac{age^3}{100^2}\right)$$

$$P = \frac{e^L}{1 + e^L}$$

The advantage of this approach, as opposed to previously used age and burn size partitioned analyses, is that it permits analysis of an entire population without artificial segmentation, and allows and explicit estimation of expected mortality for each member of the

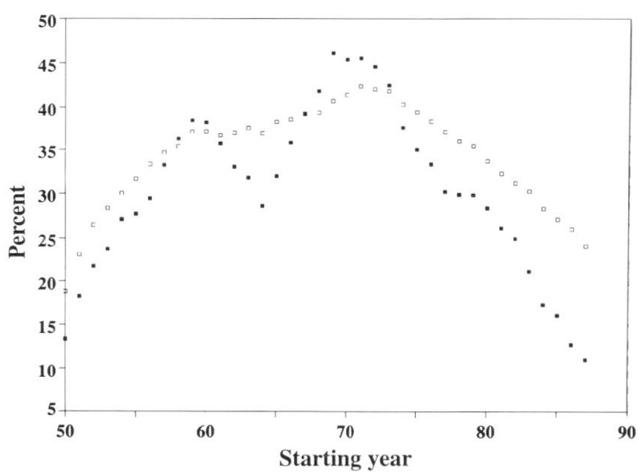

Fig 2.6 Comparison of mean burn size (open circles) and percent mortality (solid dots).

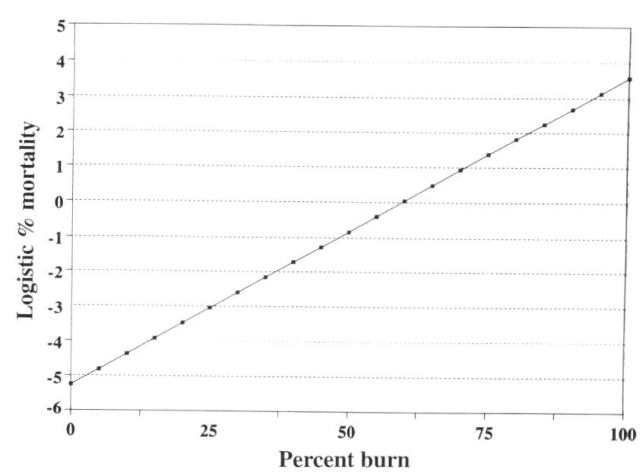

Fig 2.8 Logistic transformation of ordinate of Figure 2.6.

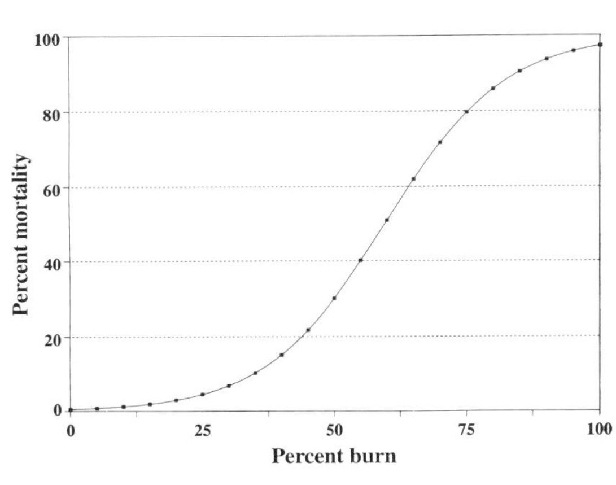

Fig 2.7 Effect of burn size on percent mortality.

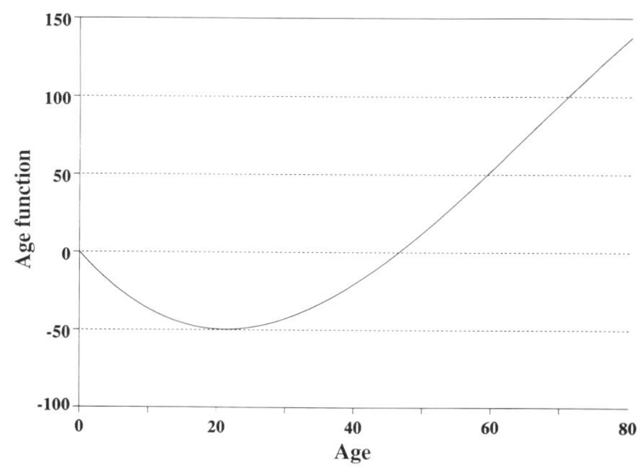

Fig 2.9 Effect of age on mortality. Effect is minimal at age 21. Note that horizontal intersects share a common effect.

population. Serial applications of the technique were used to assess mortality in each of the moving five year intervals of the study.

Figure 2.13 reflects the changes in LD50 which were experienced by young adult patients during the four decades of the study. This value, indexing the mean likelihood of survival after burn injury, has increased steadily in all age groups since the mid-1970s. Many aspects of care have changed and improved during these two decades:

- early resuscitation is more widely understood and better practiced;
- better infection control techniques have limited cross contamination of wounds;
- the clinical facility had been remodeled to permit single bed isolation;
- topical chemotherapy with alternating applications of mafenide acetate and silver sulfadiazine, coupled with the use of a chlorhexidine-based wash solution (Hibiclens), has permitted better control of wound infection;
- new antibiotics, more effective against gram-negative organisms, have become available;
- early wound excision is more generally practiced;
- inhalation injury and other pulmonary problems are better understood and are managed with better equipment;
- improved grafting techniques and the use of biological dressings facilitate earlier coverage of large wounds.

In essence, we have learned, through integrated clinical and laboratory research, how to apply ordinary principles of trauma and wound care to this extraordinary injury. No single innovation has produced a 'step' improvement in mortality, but the aggregate effect has been steadily improving survival.

This improvement in survival is reflected in **Figures 2.14** and **2.15**, which depict early (1950–1963) and recent (1987–1991) mortality planes, respectively. The improvement is not uniform for all burn sizes or ages, nor would one expect this to be so. Small burns have never been lethal, except at the extremes of age; little improvement in survival could occur with such injuries. At the other extreme, very large burns in older patients have always been lethal and remain so. To define the age and burn size coordinates of the improvement in survival, one must subtract one mortality plane from another; the result is itself a plane depicting the difference in

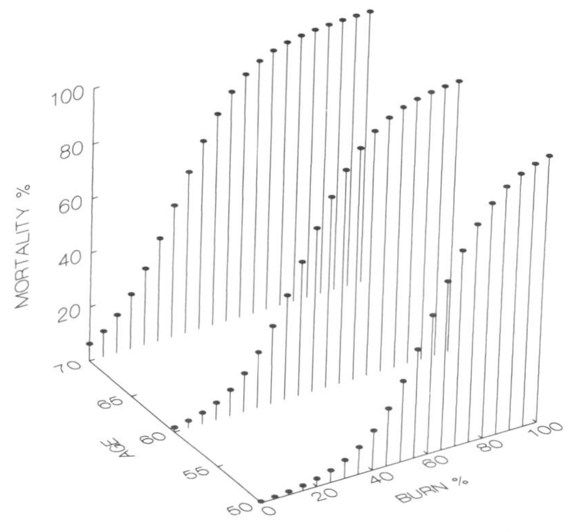

Fig 2.10 Effect of burn size on percent mortality at three discrete ages (1987–1991).

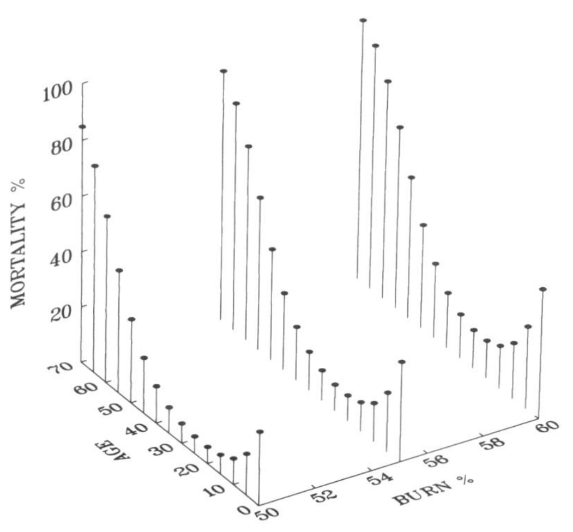

Fig 2.11 Effect of age on percent mortality at three discrete burn sizes (1987–1991).

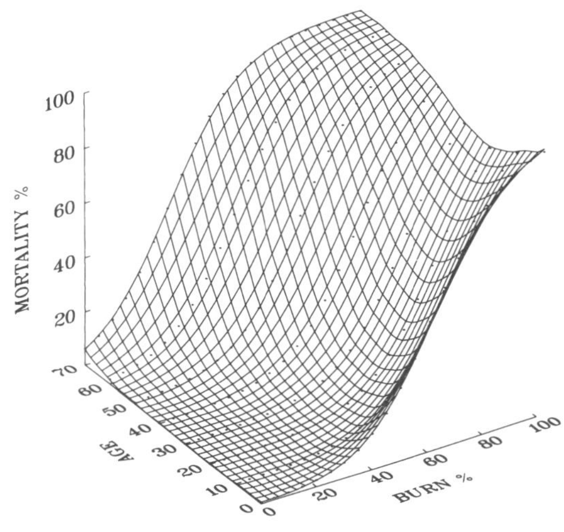

Fig 2.12 Plane of percent mortality with age and burn size coordinates (1987–1991).

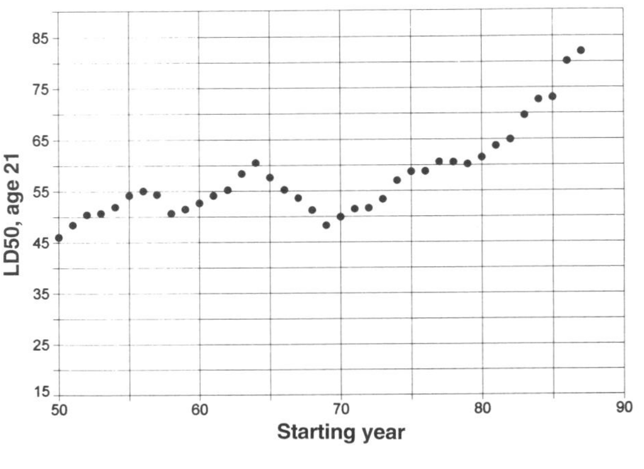

Fig 2.13 LD50 in moving 5-year intervals in patients 21 years of age. Increasing values indicates improving prognosis.

mortality in age and burn size coordinates (**Figure 2.16**). The greatest differences occurred in the area of the LD80 of the 1950–1963 mortality plane.

Though this improvement is consistent with the experience of most burn centers in the United States, it should be noted that there are still many areas of the world where the survival of patients with burns of more than 40% of the total body surface is rare. During the 42-year interval of this study, 1416 (29%) of the studied patients died. Had the mortality experienced between 1987 and 1991 prevailed through the whole interval, only half this number of deaths would have occurred.

As previously noted, estimates of the annual total number of burns in the United States, for which there is little reliable information, range as high as 2 000 000. A more reliable but still imperfect estimate is that approximately 70 000 acutely burned patients are admitted to US hospitals each year. **Figure 2.17** is based on composite data from several sources and depicts an estimate of the age and burn size distribution of these patients. Using the Institute's mortality experience between 1987 and 1991 as a basis for projecting expected mortality in these patients yields the data shown in **Figure 2.18**, which is an estimation of the age and burn size distribution of the 4856 (7%) expected deaths.

According to this model, patients over 50 years of age with burns of 50% or less of the total body surface account for 19% of admissions and 50% of deaths; at the other age extreme, children under five account for 19% of admissions and only 12.5% of deaths.

Much has been accomplished in acute burn care during the last half century, and further improvement in outcome will probably

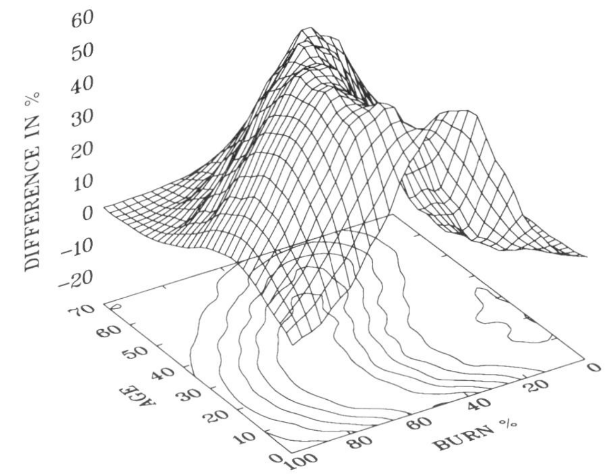

Fig 2.16 Plane of differences in percent mortality between 1950–1963 and 1987–1991. Note location of peak.

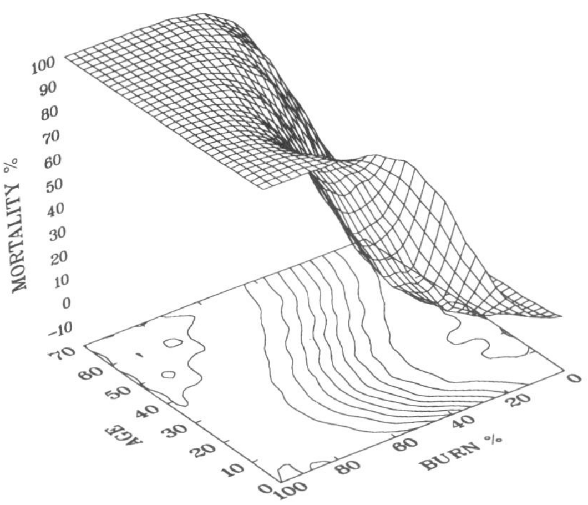

Fig 2.14 Mortality plane for patients admitted between 1950 and 1963. Note location of contour lines in base of cube.

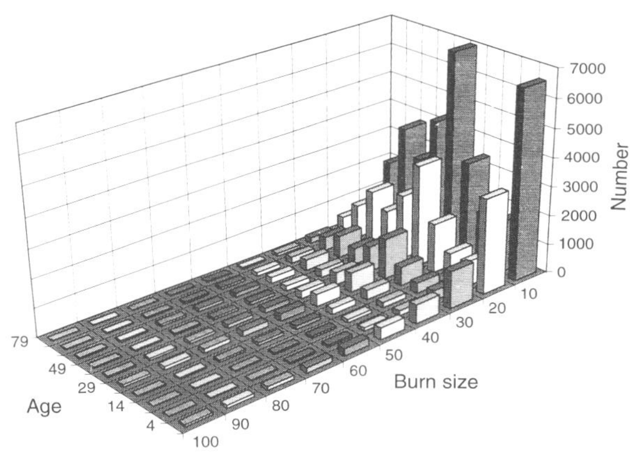

Fig 2.17 Estimated age/burn size distribution of 70 000 annual hospital admissions.

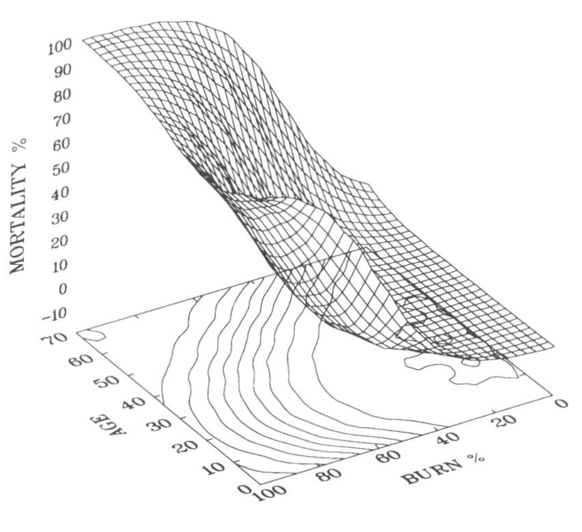

Fig 2.15 Mortality plane for patients admitted between 1987 and 1991. Note contour locations.

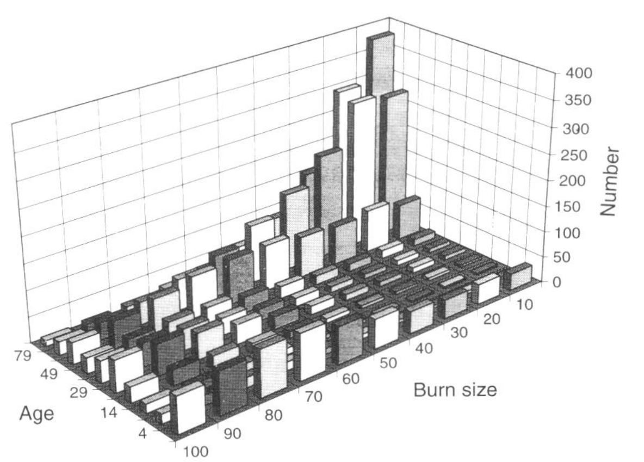

Fig 2.18 Estimated age and burn size distribution of expected deaths among patients depicted in Figure 2.16.

occur as inhalation injury and pneumonia come under control and new wound coverage techniques are developed, but such improvement will be harder won and smaller in magnitude. Preservation of function, reconstruction and rehabilitation, areas which have received less attention in the past, appear the more likely primary targets of future burn research and may be expected to materially enhance the quality of life for burn survivors.

REFERENCES

1. *Fire/Burn Deaths and Rates per 100 000.* E890–899, E923–E925. National Center for Health Statistics Mortality Data Tapes for number of deaths. Division of Unintentional Injury Prevention, National Center for Injury Prevention and Control, Centers for Disease Control and Prevention, Atlanta, GA, 1991.

2. Pruitt B A Jr, Mason A D Jr, Goodwin C W. Epidemiology of burn injury and demography of burn care facilities. In: Gann D S, ed. *Problems in General Surgery.* Vol. 7, No. 2. Philadelphia: J B Lippincott, 1990: 235–51.

3. Baker S P, O'Neill B, Ginsberg N J, Li G. Fire, burns and lightning. Chapter 12. *The Injury Fact Book.* 2nd ed. New York: Oxford University Press, 1992: 161–73.

4. Karter M J. 1991 U.S. fire loss. *NFPA Journal* 1992; **Sep–Oct:** 30–43.

5. US DoH. *Injury Mortality: National Summary of Injury Mortality Data, 1984–1990.* U.S. Department of Health and Human Services, Washington, DC, June 1993.

6. Feck G A, Baptiste M S, Tate C L Jr. Burn injuries: epidemiology and prevention. *Accid Anal Prev* 1979; **11:** 129–36.

7. Feck G A, Baptiste M S, Tate C L Jr. *An Epidemiologic Study of Burn Injuries and Strategies for Prevention.* Atlanta, GA: Department of Health and Human Services, Public Health Services, Centers for Disease Control, 1978.

8. Baker S P, O'Neill B, Ginsberg N J, Li G. Unintentional injury. Chapter 4. *The Injury Fact Book.* 2nd ed. New York: Oxford University Press, 1992: 39–64.

9. Runyan C W, Bangdiwala S I, Linzer M A, *et al.* Risk factors for fatal residential fires. *N Engl J Med* 1992; **327:** 859–63.

10. *Fire in the United States, 1983 to 1990.* 8th ed. National Fire Data Center, Emmitsburg, MD, October 1993.

11. Mierley M C, Baker S P. Fatal house fires in an urban population. *JAMA* 1983; **249:** 1466–8.

12. *Burns Causes and Costs: A Burn Foundation Report.* Burn Foundation, Philadelphia, PA, 1989.

13. Rice D P, MacKenzie E J, *et al. Costs of Injury in the United States: a Report to Congress.* Institute for Health and Aging, University of California, San Francisco, CA, An Injury Prevention Center, The Johns Hopkins University, 1989.

14. Hall J R. *The Total Cost of Fire in the United States through 1991.* Quincy, M A: National Fire Protection Association. 1993: 1–20.

15. Hammond J. The status of statewide burn prevention legislation. *J Burn Case Rehabil* 1993; **14:** 473–5.

16. Pruitt B A Jr, Goodwin C W. Thermal injuries. Chapter 71. In: Davis J H, Drucker W R, Foster RS Jr, *et al.*, eds. *Clinical Surgery.* St Louis: C V Mosby Company, 1987, 2823–2903.

17. Resources for optimal care of patients with burn injury. Chapter 14. In: *Resources for Optimal Care of the Injured Patient.* Chicago, IL: The American College of Surgeons, 1990: 58.

18. *Burn Care Resources in North America 1993–1994.* New York: American Burn Association, Office of the Secretary, 525 East 68th Street, New York, NY 10021.

19. Hedson D A, Rode H, Bloch C E. Primus stove burns in Cape Town: a costly but preventable injury. *Burns* 1988; **20:** 251–2.

20. Rioja L F, Alonso P E, Soria M D, *et al.* Incidence of ember burns in Andalusia (Spain). *Burns* 1993; **19:** 220–2.

21. Iregbulem L M, Nnabuko B E. Epidemiology of childhood thermal burns in Enugu, Nigeria. *Burns* 1993; **19:** 223–6.

22. Shergill G, Scerri G V, Regan P J Roberts AHN. Burn injuries in boating accidents. *Burns* 1993; **19:** 229–31.

23. Graitcer P L, Sniezek J E. Hospitalizations due to tap water scalds 1978–1985. MMWR 1988; **37:** 35–8.

24. Milo Y, Robinpour M, Glicksman A, Tamir G, Burvin R, Hauben D J Epidemiology of burns in the Tel Aviv area. *Burns* 1993; **19:** 352–7.

25. Baptiste M S, Feck G. Preventing tap water burns. *Am J Public Health* 1980; **70:** 727–9.

26. Stephen F R, Murray J P. Prevention of hot tap water burns – a comparative study of three types of automatic mixing valve. *Burns* 1993; **19:** 56–62.

27. Lindblad B E, Mikkelsen S S, Larsen T K, Steinke M S. A comparative analysis of burn injuries at two burns centers in Denmark. *Burns* 1994; **20:** 173–5.

28. Backstein R, Peters W, Neligan P. Burns in the disabled. *Burns* 1993; **19:** 192–7.

29. Rossignol A M, Boyle C M, Locke J A, Burke J F. Hospitalized burn injuries in Massachusetts: An assessment of incidence and product involvement. *Am J Public Health* 1986; **76:** 1341–3.

30. Clark W R, Fromm B S. Burn mortality experienced at a regional unit. Literature review, *Acta Chir Scand* 1987; **Suppl 357**.

31. Baker S P, O'Neill B, Karpf R S. *The injury Fact Book*, Lexington, MA: Lexington Books, 1984: 139–54.

32. Purdue G F, Hunt J L, Layton T R, *et al.* Burns in motor vehicle accidents. *J Trauma* **25:** 216–219, 1985.

33. Barillo D J, Cioffi W G, McManus W F, *et al.* Vehicle-related burn injuries. *Proceedings of Association for the Advancement of Automotive Medicine*, 2340 Des Plaines Avenue, Suite 106, Des Plaines, 11, 1993, pp 209–18.

34. Renz B M, Sherman R. Automobile carburetors – and radiator – related burns. *J Burn Care Rehabil*, 1992; **1:** 414–421.

35. Regan P J, Budny P G, Lavelle J R, *et al.* Bonfire and barbecue burns. *Burns*, 1991; **17:** 306–308.

36. *8th Annual Flammable Fabrics Report*, Consumer Product Safety Commission, Washington, DC, 1980.

37. Occupational Burns among restaurant workers – Colorado and Minnesota. *MMWR*, 1993; **42:** 713–16.

38. Chatterjee B F, Barancik J I, Fratianne R B, Waltz R C, Fife D. Northeastern Ohio Trauma Study: V. Burn Injury. *J Trauma*, 1986; **26:** 844–7.

39. Rossignol A M, Locke J A, Boyle C M, Burke J F: Epidemiology of work-related burn injuries in Massachusetts requiring hospitalization. *J Trauma*, 1986; **26:** 1097–101.

40. Personck M E. Profiles in safety and health: Eating and drinking places. *Monthly Labor Review*, 1991; **114:** 19–26.

41. Baker S P, O'Neill B, Ginsberg N J, *et al.* Occupational injury. Chapter 9. *The Injury Fact Book*, 2nd ed. Oxford University Press: New York, 1992; 114–33.

42. Pruitt B A Jr, Edlich R F. Treatment of bitumen burns (Letter) *JAMA*, 1982; **247:** 1565.

43. Renz B M, Sherman R: Hot tar burns: 27 hospitalized cases. *J Burn Care Rehabil*, 1994; **15:** 341–345.

44. Acute chemical hazards to children and adults. *NEISS Data Highlights.* Vol 12, January–December 1988. Washington, DC. Directorate for Epidemiology, US Consumer Product Safety Commission.

45. Mozingo D W, Smith A A, McManus W F, *et al.* Chemical burns. *J Trauma*, 1988; **28:** 642–7.

46. Leeming M N, Ray C Jr, Howland W S. Low-voltage direct current burns. *JAMA*, 1970; **214:** 1681–4.

47. Pride H B, McKinley D F. Third-degree burns from the use of an external cardiac pacing device. *Crit Care Med*, 1990; **18:** 572–3.

48. Reisin L, Baruchin A M: latrogenic defibrillator burns. *Burns*, 1990; **16:** 128.

49. Duclos P J, Sanderson L M. An epidemiological description of lightning-related deaths in the United States. *Int J Epidemiol*, 1990; **19:** 673–8.

50. Weigel E P. Lightning: the underrated killer. *National Oceanographic and Atmospheric Administration Magazine* 1976; 6.

51. Kale D, Harwood B. Fireworks injuries, 1981. *NEISS Data Highlights.* January–December, 1981. Washington, DC: Directorate for Epidemiology, US Consumer Products Safety Commission.

52. McFarland L V, Harris J R, Kobayashi J M, *et al.* Risk factors for fireworks-related injury in Washington state. *JAMA*, 1984; **251:** 3251–4.

53. Injuries associated with selected consumer products treated in hospital emergency departments calendar 1992. *NEISS Data Highlights*. Vol. 16, 1992. Washington, DC: Directorate for Epidemiology, US consumer Products Safety Commission.

54. Berger L R, Kalishman S, Rivara F P. Injuries from fireworks. *Pediatrics*, 1985; **75:** 877–82.

55. Sonneborn C K, Vanstraelen T M. A retrospective study of self-inflicted burns. *Gen Hosp Psychiatry*, 1992; **14:** 404–7.

56. Budny P G, Regan P J, Riley P, *et al.* Ritual burns – the Buddhist tradition. *Burns*, 1991; **17:** 335–7.

57. Squyres V, Law E J, Still J M Jr. Self-inflicted burns. *J Burn Care Rehabil*, 1993; **14:** 476–9.

58. Duminy F J, Hudson D A. Assault inflicted by water. *Burns*, 1993; **19:** 426–8.

59. Krob M J, Johnson A, Jordan M H. Burned-and-battered adults. *J Burn Care Rehabil*, 1986; **7:** 529–31.

60. Bowden M L, Grant S T, Vogel B, *et al.* The elderly, disabled and handicapped adult burned through abuse and neglect. *Burns*, 1988; **14:** 447–50.

61. O'Neill J A Jr, Meacham W F, Griffin P P, *et al.* Patterns of injury in the battered child syndrome. *J Trauma*, 1973; **13:** 332–9.

62. Showers J, Garrison K M. Burn abuse: A four year study. *J Trauma*, 1988; **28:** 1581–3.

63. Surrell J A, Alexander R C, Kohle S D, *et al.* Effects of microwave radiation on living tissues. *J Trauma*, 1987; **27:** 935–9.

64. Batchelor J S, Vanjari S, Budny P, Roberts A H N. Domestic iron burns in children: a cause for concern? *Burns*, 1994; **20:** 74–5.

65. Purdue G F, Hunt J L, Prescott P R. Child abuse by burning – an index of suspicion. *J Trauma*, 1988; **28:** 221–4.

66. Pegg S P. Can burns injuries occur in hospital? Presented at *9th Congress of the International Society for Burn Injuries, 30 June 1994, Paris, France.* Abstract 87 in 9th Congress of International Society for Burns Injuries, Abstracts Volume.

67. Sadove R C, Furgasen T G. Major thermal burn as a result of intraoperative heating blanket use. *J Burn Care Rehabil*, 1992; **13:** 443–5.

68. Chang B W, Petty P, Manson P N. Patient fire safety in the operating room. *Plast Reconstr Surg*, 1994; **93:** 519–21.

69. Pruitt B A Jr, FitzGerald B E. A military perspective. In: Bowers J Z, Purcell E F, eds. *Emergency Medical Services*: Measures to improve care. Port Washington, NY: Independent Publishers Group, 1980: 223–44.

70. Treat R C, Sirinek K R, Levine B E, Pruitt B A Jr. Air evacuation of thermally injured patients: principles of treatment and results. *J Trauma*, 1980; **20:** 275–9.

71. Holmes T, ed. *A System of Surgery, Theoretical and Practical.* vol. I. London: J W Parker & Son, 1860, p. 723.

72. Suzuki S. The injuries in modern naval warfare. *Boston Med Surg J* CXXXVII(24): 610, December 9, 1897.

73. Weidenfeld L B. *Medizinisches Vademecus.* 1912: pp. 206–24.

74. Berkow S G. Method of estimating extensiveness of lesions (burns and scalds) based on surface area proportions. *Arch Surg*, January 1924; **8**(pt. 1): 138–48.

75. Bull J P, Squire J R. A study of mortality in a burns unit: standards for the evaluation of alternative methods of treatment. *Ann Surg*, August 1949; **130**(2): 160–73.

76. Bull J P, Fisher A J. A study of mortality in a burns unit: a revised estimate. *Ann Surg*, 1954; **139**(3): 269–74.

77. Schwartz M S, Soroff H S, Reiss E, Artz C P. An evaluation of the mortality and the relative severity of second and third-degree injuries in burns. Research Report Nr. 12–56. In: *Research Reports*. US Army Surgical Research Unit, Form Sam Houston, TX, December 1956.

78. *BMDP Statistical Software*, version 7. Los Angeles: BMDP Statistical Software, Inc., 1992.

79. FInney D J. *Probit analysis*. 3rd ed. Cambridge: Cambridge University Press, 1971.

80. Hosmer D W, Lemeshow S. *Applied Logistic Regression*. New York: John Wiley & Sons, 1989.

Immediate Care

CHAPTER THREE

BURN DISASTER MANAGEMENT

THOMAS L. WACHTEL AND ALAN R. DIMICK

INTRODUCTION

Burns are among the worst trauma problems which can befall man. The larger a burn injury, the more severe the consequences and the higher the chance of an adverse outcome or even death. The utilization of resources for burned patients is extraordinarily high as well, when compared to other trauma victims.[1] Advances in science and technology have increased the risk of accidents which result in a transfer of thermal energy to people located nearby. As more powerful sources of energy are harnessed, the numbers of casualties from such accidents increase.[2] As a result of expansion in the fields of transportation and technology, we are now confronted with a rapid growth in the absolute number of burns and their mass incidence as well as an increase in the potential dangers surrounding the use of thermic energy of unprecedented power such that the magnitude and consequences can be appalling.[3,4] The potential for modern day fire catastrophes involving high rise buildings, worldwide terrorism, and large crowds collected at community events poses a serious challenge to fire technology and to society.[5] Such disasters normally exceed the resources of local health care providers and facilities.[2]

A disaster is a situation where there are unforeseen serious and immediate threats to public health.[6] Masellis has divided the management of rescue operations into two separate entities – thermal agent (fire) disaster and burn disaster. They are linked by the common denominator of fire as well as causal force. The former includes losses of material goods and losses of human life as a result of massive heat production (**Figure 3.1**) and can be quantified by the extent of damage to material goods and the number of people who are dead and injured.[7] Burn disaster can be defined as the overall effect on living people which is caused by massive action from a known thermal agent. It is characterized by a high number of fatalities and by seriously burned patients with a high rate of potential mortality and disability[7] (**Figure 3.1**). A fire causing 25 or more deaths is termed a fire catastrophe.

Fire disasters with large numbers of burned victims will escalate problems severalfold and require application of the principles of disaster management. Disaster medicine is the study of collaborative applications of various health disciplines to the prevention, immediate response to, and rehabilitation of health problems which arise from a disaster.[8] The consequences of a major fire disaster can be broadly predicted, even though specific measures for dealing with injured victims will vary from region to region.[9] In terms of numbers of wounded, the worst disasters have occurred outdoors. None of the indoor incidents resulted in more than 50 hospital

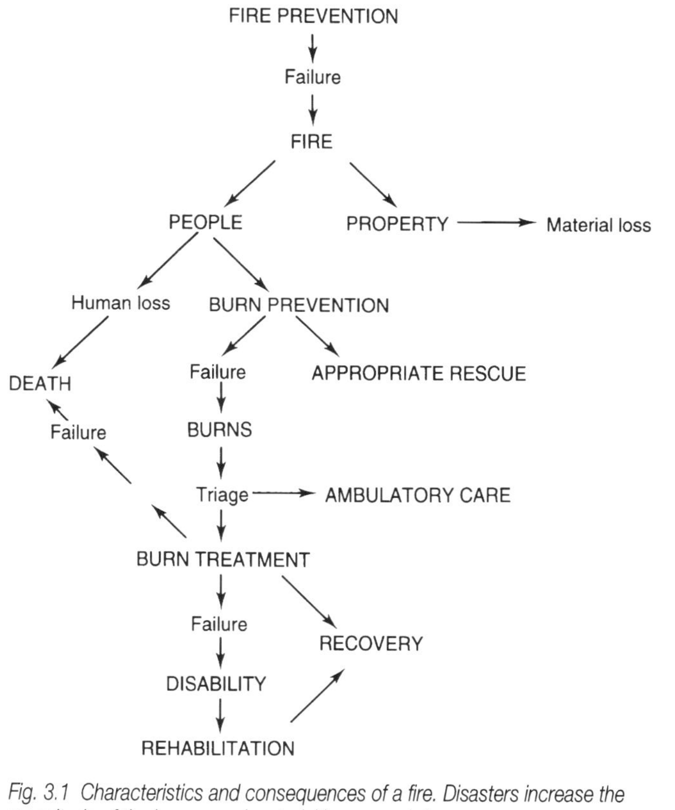

Fig. 3.1 Characteristics and consequences of a fire. Disasters increase the magnitude of the human and material losses and damages.

admissions, while the smallest number admitted to a hospital following an outdoor incident was 71.[9] A fire disaster is a serious and sudden vast ecological breakdown in the relation between man and his environment on such a scale that the stricken community needs extraordinary efforts to cope with it, and often requires outside help or international aid.[8] There have been 25 such fires in the United States in the twentieth century which have caused tremendous destruction of life and property and have led to changes in public opinion and important advances in fire prevention.[5]

Burn disasters are most frequently man-made as opposed to natural disasters (e.g. an earthquake) and, in general, are comparatively confined to a limited geographical area (**Figure 3.2**). The initial information needed in order to respond to a disaster revolves around a definition of the geography in question. This includes information about the location as well as means of access to the location, such as points of egress from a building or room.[10] A major disaster plan is intended to provide optimal treatment of victims of a major accident when there are too many patients to be treated by routine emergency services.[11] Burn disaster management is necessary when the number of burn casualties exceeds local resources. The number of people injured in a burn disaster is defined as the sum of the number admitted to hospitals with burns and the number killed outright.[6,9] For rural or wilderness areas, that number may be as few as one or two. For an urban burn center, in a large tertiary hospital, the number of burn victims may be much larger; but eventually even the resources of a sophisticated burn center in a multi-specialty hospital with a mature trauma system will become exhausted, and the planning, preparedness, training, response, relief, rehabilitation, and reconstruction of a major emergency or disaster situation will be overcome.[12] The solution will require either secondary triage of burn victims to other more distant burn facilities or transportation of staff, supplies, and equipment to the site of the disaster.[1] Very large disasters remain uncommon.[9] When fire comes in contact with objects and materials which burn, they are destroyed in a relatively short time; but the action of fire on living organisms is lethal within a few seconds. If a fire is not immediately lethal, it determines a pathologic condition called a burn which is considered to be the most complex trauma which can strike a human organism.[7] One specific aspect of a fire disaster is that the number of people involved is always high. The aspects of a burn disaster are shown in **Table 3.1**.

Despite the potential for mass disasters, conflagrations have become less frequent in the USA since the 1940s.[5] The incidence of major fires in Europe has increased in recent years.[9] The severity of injuries among those admitted to hospitals suggests that either victims were able to escape rapidly and, thus, sustained relatively small burns (<30% total body surface area) typically to exposed areas of skin, or that timely escape was impossible and victims were engulfed and sustained lethal injuries (70% TBSA).[9] The management of mass burns still remains a highly complex problem of organization.[3] In the worst burn disasters, which occur outdoors, a considerable number of lethally injured patients reached hospitals alive; but the subsequent death rate was high. Following indoor burn disasters, a smaller number of patients were admitted, and most of them had sustained relatively small burns of less than 30% TBSA.[6] A great number of victims are trapped in indoor fires and fail to escape. They suffer from the combination of hypoxia and inhalation of poisonous compounds.[6,13] The effect of hydrogen cyanide and carbon monoxide has been postulated as a cause of incapacity and inability to react, and accounts for high indoor death rates.[6] The high immediate death rate in indoor disasters was mainly due to inhalation injuries and intoxication. No rescue people reached the severely injured in time.[6]

The diversity of the incidence of fire disasters serves to illustrate the scale and nature of problems faced by medical services in dealing with mass burn casualties.[9,14–16] For truly effective disaster management, the key is prevention and preparedness rather than a post hoc firefighting type of emergency response.[8,17] For this kind of scientific approach and technical underpinning, special studies, surveys and applied research, social and natural science investigations, and managerial applications are necessary[8] (**Table 3.2**).

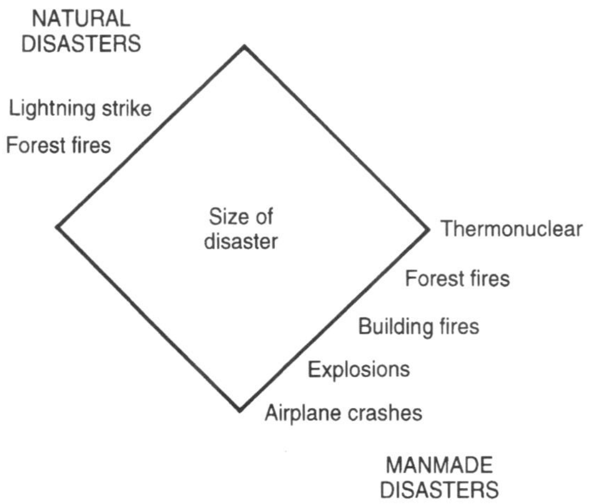

Fig. 3.2 Burn disaster sources and magnitude of destruction.

Table 3.1 Characteristics and principles of a burn disaster[7]

The burns are mainly very extensive and the general condition of the victims is precarious
The place the disaster occurs is not always assessable and care and assistance may not be adequate
The time interval between the accident and initiation of care must be less than 2 hours
Triage of victims must be effected only by specialists, as only specialists are able to evaluate the immediate gravity of the burn
Inhalation of combustion gases, fumes and hot air causes damage to the airways: and this alone can jeopardize survival
Hypovolemic shock induces a state of tissue hypoxia with irreversible damage to various organs and systems
The burn is often associated with other serious problems such as vast wounds, fractures, electrocution, or blast injury lesions
The overall assessment of the damage to persons must be made not only on the basis of the number of dead, but also the number of people burned and suffering risk of disability

Table 3.2 The ten principles for the scientific basis of disaster management[8]

Prevention
Preparedness
Disaster profiles
Disease patterns
Planning and preparation for effective multidisciplinary response
Mobilization of multisectorial manpower resources
Risk assessment
Post-emergency phase
Reconstructive phase
Community and local/national institution involvement

Epidemiology has proved most promising in disaster management.[8] Disaster epidemiology links data collection, analysis of disaster, analysis of risk factors for adverse social and health effects, clinical investigation of the impact of diagnostic and therapeutic methods, the effectiveness of various types of assistance, and the long-term influence of relief operations on restoration of predisaster conditions.[8] Training people for disaster management requires courses on disaster health, in addition to innate humanitarian compassion.[8] Of all disasters with more than 20 dead at the scene, 70% are classified as fires and explosions due to train crashes, air accidents, and underground disasters.[6] The most severe of such fires are liquefied petroleum gas disasters.[6]

The Disaster Plan

Few people will have a chance to exercise their disaster plan in a real burn disaster, but everyone must plan for such a contingency. The burn component must be integrated into overall local, regional, national and international disaster plans. Despite evidence available from past disasters, adequate provision for the management of burn casualties is still lacking in most disaster plans.[9] Effective disaster planning will not only lessen property loss and social disruption caused by disaster impacts, but will also reduce suffering and the distress of casualties.[18] Disaster planning should emphasize that most burns are either minor or very extensive.[18] New developments in the organization of emergency medical service systems dictate that new approaches to disaster planning and preparedness are essential in order to implement current concepts of emergency medical care delivery.[10] The important aspects of modern disaster management from the medical perspective include:

- the utilization of medical triage and treatment protocols in order to effect control and transportation of patients;
- early notification of all hospitals which could potentially receive patients; and
- transportation of patients to appropriate hospitals utilizing an existing point-of-entry plan.

This enables burn victims to be transported to facilities with burn treatment capability and available beds.[10] Three distinct phases of relief operations are necessary: immediate assistance, first aid, and organized relief. Immediate assistance is provided in the first 2–3 hours by people on the spot (trained volunteers, physicians, and nurses) and is fundamental to the prognosis of fire disaster victims. A timely, rational, safe and effective intervention is the main guarantee *quo ad vitam* for the victims of a fire disaster.[8] A more complex body of organized relief will not be able to reach a disaster scene for at least 6 or 7 hours. Entire systems must be tested in training programs which are made intelligible to the public, supported by management resources, implemented properly, and promulgated to all potential first rescue workers.[19] A major disaster should be declared so that facilities can prepare for upcoming casualties.[1]

A survey of modern disasters has shown that fire incidents occurring outdoors result in larger numbers of hospital admissions, with more severe injuries, than incidents occurring indoors.[9] The majority of burn casualties sustained burns covering less than 30% of the total body surface area, but outdoor disasters resulted in admissions of burns covering more than 70% TBSA.[9] Not all fire disasters result in mass burn casualties.[9] When a burn disaster involves many hundreds of patients, it will usually be necessary to have burn teams from many countries participate in order to achieve optimal care for victims.[2] Collaboration is possible, especially when such teams have made advance plans for transporting their teams and equipment to a site many thousands of kilometers from their home bases.[2] The joint work of the Soviet and US physicians during the Ufa train explosion demonstrates the efficacy of international cooperation. In planning for the care of victims of future disasters, such international cooperation should be noted.

Planning aimed at mitigating the effects on people (in terms of suffering, disability, and risk to life) must be related to a more complete evaluation of involved damage.[7] The operational rescue plan must be developed along three lines: immediate care, medical rescue within 3 hours, and use of specific equipment and means for the rescue of burned patients. Factors which influence the evolution of a disaster include:[7]

- the unpredictability of when disasters occur;
- the moment of a disaster (day/night, festivity, etc.);
- the characteristics of a disaster (explosion, collapse of building, production of toxic gases and fumes, forest fire, etc.);
- the area where a disaster occurs (city, nonurban area, accessibility, presence of material suitable for relief operations, etc.);
- the type of building involved (civil dwelling, hotel, office, hospital, etc.);
- the number of people injured and the type of trauma;
- the population's degree of preparedness to manage a disaster situation.

Communication

On-line voice communication with a trauma center, trauma surgeon, burn coordinator, and burn surgeon is important. Disaster plans should utilize existing communication venues and have the ability to expand (i.e. bring in additional equipment and staff). It must be fast, practiced, and limited in scope. A point-of-entry plan must communicate the type of disaster: burns, burns and other trauma, trauma, spinal cord injuries, acute medical complication, poisoning, behavioral crisis, neonatal, or pediatric. A consideration which impacts on incident management is the existence and utilization of a centralized reporting and notification mechanism,[10] such as the 911 centralized communication system for fire, police, and emergency medical services in the United States. The system should have the capability to contact metropolitan area ambulance services and hospitals individually or collectively through the centralized communication system. This feature allows for central collection of hospital bed availability data, relay of relevant information on the status of disaster to hospitals, centralized coordination of disaster response, and direction of ambulances carrying triaged patients to appropriate facilities.[10] The benefits of a comprehensive system with a centralized communications component are shown in **Table 3.3**.

A central bank which stores up-to-date information on the capacity of each burn center to accept patients is imperative for disaster management. Valuable information is also provided concerning hospital capability, intensive care/burn intensive care availability, equipment availability (fluidized beds, etc.) and technical procedures. The information must be utilized on a daily basis for the distribution of burns within the geographical area and can then be extremely useful in the event of a disaster when the distribution of patients is acute. The French telematic data bank for burns also includes an epidemiologic file which forms the basis for prevention campaigns. It is compatible with the International Society for Burn Injuries and the European organization.[20] A German system which

Table 3.3 Benefits of a comprehensive system with a centralized communications component[10]

Improved notification of the incident
Consistent initial and follow-up information
Timeliness of response
Better management of the incident
Accuracy in the collection of pertinent information concerning the incident
Analysis of the information to determine the correct level of response, triage to hospitals and specialty centers
Utilization of transport vehicles
Ultimate outcome of burned victims

is used on a daily basis responds extremely well. It was not used primarily in the Ramstein air disaster, and that was a reason for criticism of their disaster management. It was used for secondary triage and for consultation on burned patients. The United States' system, National Disaster Management System (NDMS), was activated during Operation Desert Storm and is used regionally for the distribution of burn patients. The Italian ARGO satellite system combines a coordination center, data collection center, data transportation center, and burn center into a mesh sub-network. It is expandable and allows the organization to care for severely burned patients. The telecommunication system has high standards of reliability and survival to guarantee continuity of communications from and to a disaster area. It is expandable and allows the organization to care for severely burned patients. The telecommunication system has high standards of reliability and survival to guarantee continuity of communications from and to a disaster area. It is divided into telephone, fax, and video telecommunications networks, and a territorial data collection network. The information is continually updated and links with a national organization capable of rapid mobilization of carriers for the transport of patients. It allows immediate contact between specialized burn centers and the physicians treating patients in the disaster area so that support is available for staff in the field. It functions as a radio telephone in an ambulance and as an ordinary portable telephone carried by a physician.[21]

The Plan for a Disaster Scene

There is a practical need for a disaster plan.[22] Of the 14 disasters studied by Arturson, only in the San Juanico tragedy was a disaster plan in place.[6] Preventive measures were usually lacking in all disasters investigated, and mistakes were observed frequently.[6] Advance planning includes availability of well trained leadership for disaster situations.[6] Sorting or triage is performed most effectively by a clinician experienced in the care of burns, as doctors without such experience frequently overestimate the proportion of the body surface burned.[1] Expert triage may minimize the requirement for specialized burn beds since moderate to severe burns, which are best cared for in specialized burn centers, seem to be fewer in numbers following severe fire disasters.[6] The French burn system, for example, incorporates this philosophy into a uniform triage system.[20]

The initial task for a disaster plan is to identify all burned victims. Search and rescue in disaster primarily involves the finding, extricating, and/or transportation of victims, including the dead and injured as well as the non-injured.[18] Fire services are well placed and structured to undertake this search and rescue role. There should be significant predisaster planning and training for organized search and rescue, involving the fire service and a variety of local groups. Seldom does one specific community group assume responsibility. Timeliness is essential and stress is inherent. Widespread damage to structures will result in large numbers of casualties and trapped people within an immediate disaster zone. It can be anticipated that people who are trapped will attempt to free themselves, and untrapped survivors will go to their aid. A concentrated effort to rescue trapped persons during the first few hours after a disaster will yield greater dividends in lives saved than any effort made later.[18] A large burn disaster may require that trained rescuers operate solely in a supervisory role while large numbers of untrained workers are added to a trained nucleus in order to rapidly expand rescue capability.

Most disaster plans emphasize a restriction of treatment, at the site or in the emergency department/accident ward, to lifesaving measures and initial prioritization with early transfer to more sophisticated resources where reassessment can take place.[23] Prior disasters and international responses to them underscore the need for a coordinated response to major burn disasters and the positive results of international cooperation.[2] Delays in the dispersal of casualties may be avoided by prior planning, especially if international transfer of patients is envisioned.[9] Recent incidents involving mass burn casualties have demonstrated that the specific needs of severely burned victims demand a comprehensive plan which provides initial care which follows the guidelines of advanced burn life support courses for resuscitation, assessment of burn size and depth, evaluation for other injuries, care of the burn wound, etc.[24]

The positive effect of a previous disaster on preparedness of people involved is substantial. A disaster plan must incorporate details of disasters occurring in several scenarios. These may be unique to an individual area, but all should include explosions.[6,15,22,23,25–29] Particular procedures regarding both medical assistance and general behavior, and those which rescue workers have to perform, must include campaigns, educational campaigns, refresher courses, and training sessions aimed at citizens of every social extraction starting at school age.[7] As an example, burn disaster from a forest fire would depend on the fire typology; and the variability depends on meteorological conditions. The essential figure is usually a firefighter, but other victims may be involved.[30] The number of victims may range from only a dozen (France, 1986) to very many (71 dead, 2000 injured – Australia, 1983; 50 000 homeless – China, 1987).

A disaster response system can be activated for industrial accidents, such as petrochemical industries, foundries, and the like.[31] The preparation phase is characterized by mapping the industries at risk of potential flammable or toxic substances most frequently used in an area and which transit avenues are used. This requires a collaboration of other experts such as engineers, chemists, physicists, toxicologists, etc., in order to coordinate all necessary data for potential fire disasters. A training phase should be carried out in close collaboration with agencies and people likely to be involved in self-protection, extinguishing of a fire, and rescue of burn victims. A didactic phase through organized meetings of volunteer personnel is required.[31] Burn centers whose catchment area includes oil rigs or hazardous materials should plan for appropriate contingencies.[32]

A disaster plan may have to be tailored to meet specific needs of an area or a site. In a fire disaster, the number of people involved may be so high that it is impossible to consider their immediate transfer to existing specialized burn centers. Because of the limited number of beds available and because a disaster may occur some distance away,[2,33–35] the organization and establishment of a field hospital may be required. To be effective, a field hospital must have easy transport, rapid assembly, and the possibility of administering complete and effective treatment to patients. Multi-unit nomadic tents may offer the best facilities.[34,35] The reduced weights of these tents, their ease of packing, and their limited bulk represent considerable advantages, especially with regard to transportation and rapidity and simplicity of assembly. The modular composition means that their sizes can be adapted according to the effective needs of a disaster situation.[35] The organization and establishment of a field hospital must be based on a very precise predetermined plan which defines all the logistic and sanitary activities of a field hospital which are required to manage a disaster immediately and long term.[35]

It is important to exercise a disaster plan through coordination of simulated disasters involving all of the relevant public safety agencies, prehospital ambulance providers, hospital-based personnel, and proceed-out teams.[10,17] As one team reported: 'The whole operation went very smoothly. This was partly because the staff had been through several "dummy runs" of a detailed civil accident procedure and partly because they had several hours to prepare for the first casualties to arrive.'[36]

Effective disaster management can only be accomplished when a thorough disaster planning process has been conducted.[37] Such a process must include all elements and all recognized emergency response and relief agencies which could play a role in responding to a disaster.[10,38,39] The most important outcome of a planning exercise is that each of the agencies be educated as to the roles and responsibilities of the others so that essential links between agencies can be established.[10]

Transportation: How Will They Arrive?

Transportation considerations depend on the number of victims and their conditions, identification of toxic substances, and other factors. Emergency transport of burn victims may be sporadic and *de novo* in a fire disaster, but more often it will involve medical rescue services such as fully equipped ambulances, helicopters, fixed wing aircraft, and water rescue craft. Most victims are transported by ground vehicles (ambulances, private vehicles, commandeered buses, trucks, etc.) For fire disasters up to 100 miles from medical facilities, the use of helicopter services which are fully equipped flying ambulances, often permanently based at hospitals and used exclusively for emergency purposes, are an invaluable mechanism for transport. Numerous factors have led to the creation and development world wide of medical air rescue services and, in particular, to the widespread use of helicopter services.[40] Over 300 hospitals in the world have their own helicopter ambulances and fixed wing aircraft used exclusively for emergency transport.[40] The Italian model of helicopter rescue service is acquiring growing recognition.[40] The Italian medical evacuation is made through a single nationwide telephone number in Italy which connects qualified multilingual personnel, including physicians and other specialists, to local rescue services, hospitals, civil and military authorities, and other organizations involved in disaster relief. A sophisticated software program provides, in real time, all necessary information for rescue operations within a specific region, and if the need arises, for inter-regional coordination and transport.[40,41]

The main aim of a helicopter rescue service is to guarantee a prompt arrival (maximum time 20 minutes) of a medical team specialized in resuscitation and provided with all the equipment normally available in a hospital intensive care unit. The necessary emergency therapy can be carried out on the spot or continued during transport of a patient. The transport is not necessarily to the nearest hospital, but to the hospital best equipped to receive a patient.[40] The communication coordination system, activated by the regional operative headquarters, coordinates transportation by ground, helicopter, or a fixed wing aircraft for long distance transport.

In some circumstances, transportation must be carried out in coordination with other rescue organizations. The transport of a victim to the nearest hospital for more thorough assessment and treatment may occur pending possible placement in a specialized burn center. This phase is often difficult because of lack of beds for burn patients in a region, especially in the case of those requiring extensive care, and must be planned in the transportation phase of a disaster plan.

Timing and coordination of transport of burned patients is critical;[42] and delays may occur, especially if national or international transportation by air is envisioned, unless communication and cooperation are assured.[9] The personnel and material conditions, as well as the mode of transport, should be an integral part of an emergency disaster plan. A burn team must consider the consequences of aeromedical transport in order to determine whether it is safe for a burned patient and what measures should be used in order to effect a safe transfer.[43] Burn casualties can best tolerate transfer on the day of the accident, so long as it does not take more than 60 minutes; and later transfers should take place by the end of the third or fourth post-accident day before sepsis can fully develop.[3] The result of an extensive traffic jam must be anticipated in a disaster plan since it may hinder the arrival of patients as well as physicians and staff who are not on duty.[22] Long delays in transportation of patients have been obvious in most disasters.[6]

Facilities

It is vital to plan for supporting hospitals in a primary inner circle and further designated hospitals in an outer circle[6,44] (**Figure 3.3**). The scarcity of burn facilities is such that involvement of distant centers may be anticipated following large disasters.[9] The relative scarcity of specialized facilities and expertise for treatment of extensive burns is of particular concern.[9] Even a moderate disaster might fill all available burn beds and saturate the total burn capacity of a wide area. Following very large disasters, optimal care of severely burned victims will be achieved only if distant burn centers are also involved.[45] The successful dispersal of casualties will, therefore, be enhanced by prior awareness of the location and capacity of specialized facilities.[46] Accurate triage by clinicians experienced in burns will minimize the requirements for scarce burn facilities.[9]

The role played by specialized burn treatment units is significant.[3] Burn centers seldom plan to have low levels of occupancy which would enable them to accommodate mass burn casualties, so the emergency plan for a burn center must include emergency evacuation of existing surgical, trauma, and other patients in order to have available beds for mass burn casualties. The hospital must establish a control center, discharge or move patients to alternate care, organize beds for the incoming mass casualties, and pull in extra staff, often without the knowledge of how many casualties to expect. Multiple injuries, including burns and inhalation injuries, may occur in mass casualties from explosions. A burn center should receive logistical support from the sponsor hospital in order to provide the best treatment for a large number of burn casualties. Logistical support requires work of the hospital staff who are concerned with sterilization, pharmacy, medical and nursing care, radiological diagnosis, and intensive care.[22] Little things, such as availability of urine dosimeters, are important!

Traditionally, hospitals have seen their role, during a burn disaster, as related to the medical management of patients admitted to them as a result of an incident. An expanded role has included sending teams of physicians and nurses to disaster scenes in order to aid

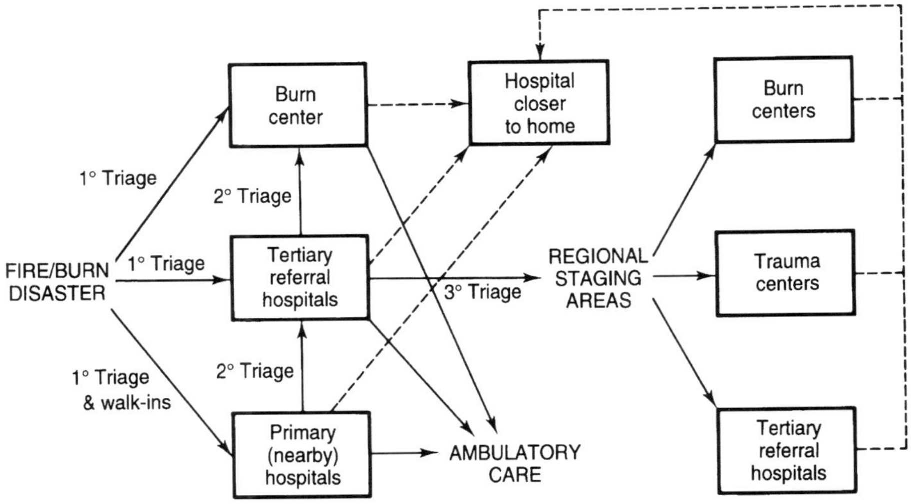

Fig. 3.3 Triage scheme for a fire/burn disaster: 1°, primary; 2°, secondary; 3°, tertiary.

in triage and medical management.[47,48] The role of a hospital in disaster management can be expanded further to include a strong focus on leadership within the medical component of a disaster. On-site medical management can be organized in one of two ways:

- via proceed-out 'teams of physicians who go directly to the scene'; or
- through voice medical direction given by radio to trained prehospital life support teams at the scene.[10]

Another responsibility which may be given to a hospital is the coordination with and medical guidance of the fire, rescue, police, and public safety components of a disaster response.[10] Few major hospitals have full comprehensive specialty services, including burn units; and major disaster plans should recognize such limitations and obtain prior consent for referral.[11] Within a hospital the disaster plan must bring additional operating rooms on-line as needed for semi-urgent care of burn victims, while reserving one or two for lifesaving procedures which may be required. The goal is to match hospital resources with the needs of burned victims. In some cases, this will be driven by priorities; in others, a first-come-first-served basis will be installed.

Trauma systems

Burn centers should be integrated in large hospitals which are able to provide assistance from several units.[22] Trauma centers must begin to fill the gap which exists between resources for emergency medical systems and a disaster response.[10] With leadership from trauma systems, meaningful planning can be accomplished among hospitals, prehospital emergency medical systems, and the public safety community.[10] This shift in disaster management responsibility from the public safety sector to the medical community incorporates advances made in the organization of emergency medical services.[10]

Personnel

As part of an overall disaster plan, it must be ensured that sufficient numbers of people have adequate training for initial resuscitation of burned victims. Often the medical and hospital staff who are willing to help have little experience in burn care. It has been found that training of personnel is rare, especially concerning communication links.[6] Training in preventive measures typically is absent, and disasters display the lack of training of personnel to cope with a tragedy.[6,26] Education concerning simple management of minor and moderate burns should be given on a broad basis to doctors and nurses outside of burn care facilities.[6] The Advanced Burn Life Support Course is an excellent tool for training such individuals.[24] Burn center staff must be available for advisory and consultation services by telephone or telex.[3] Expert triage is important, but health care professionals must be able to work effectively in primitive conditions together with other emergency helpers.[6] When admitting patients and rendering qualified specialized medical aid at a hospital, the participation of mixed physician teams (surgeon, burn specialist, resuscitation, therapist, etc.) is advisable.

A plan which places a single caregiver, usually a nurse, with each patient is optimal. That nurse, then, stays with a burned patient through all of the initial steps of care and insures intravenous fluid administration, pain control, tetanus toxoid administration, airway maintenance, ventilation, and documentation.

Often the first thing that is asked by a burn patient is to contact relatives.[36] That task should be delegated to someone other than hands-on caregivers for a burn casualty. The handling of families, as well as mass media,[49,50] must be an integral part of a disaster plan. Major mass burn casualties, such as the Piper Alpha and Ramstein tragedies, involve casualties and relatives from many countries.[32,36,51-53] Multilingual support personnel are essential under these circumstances.

Research on human behavior in critical situations has identified three different kinds of reaction: panic, rational action, and resignation. When positive action will lead to safety, resignation is a pathologic form of behavior. The two normal reactions when a way of escape can be seen are panic and rational action.[54] It is difficult to plan for the psychological reactions to a fire/burn disaster. The two main elements of this drama which have to be understood are the mass of people and the actual fire.[54] Nevertheless, experts with psychological training should be utilized for the development of psychological support for burn victims, their families and friends, rescue workers, and health care workers. Immediate sessions for debriefing of the rescue workers should be put in place. Psychological support for health care workers will be necessary because of their high levels of stress and extended hours of work. The psychological support teams in fire and burn disaster simulations can help a team rehearse the decisions which must be made in the care of large numbers of burn casualties so that the team is less likely to suffer emotional stress at the precise moment when technical skill and emotional equilibrium are most needed.[54]

As an alternative to designated burn centers, patients with burns may be managed in a general hospital without any particular facility for the management of burns.[55] In this case, a hospital disaster plan must be activated. The reception area and initial treatment area must be available for the majority of burned victims. Additional personnel must be summoned. A hospital must set into action the clearing of hospital beds, particularly on surgical wards and intensive care units, by transfer or discharge.

The effect of a previous disaster can have a profound effect on responsible staff. The recent disasters in Armenia and Chernobyl emphasized to the Soviet Health Ministry officials the importance of having contingency plans made in advance of any accident. That experience led to the rapid triage and transport of victims from the accident site to medical centers in surrounding towns following the Ufa train disaster. The Soviet experience during the Ufa response demonstrated that such an organization of public health services permitted the rendering of aid to the majority of victims in a rapid and appropriate time frame.[2] The Italian military have become interested in their role in disaster relief.[38,39] Physicians and other staff members who are not familiar with burn care must have some means to assess the extent of burns and initiate therapy. Vitale *et al.* have prepared a clinical file and protocol for general doctors and for nonspecialized hospital physicians to assist burn patients.[56] Such a file would be incorporated into a disaster plan.

Supplies/Equipment

A disaster plan must be tailored to the supplies and equipment which are available. For example, fiberoptic bronchoscopy may be useful in the early diagnosis of inhalation injury, but may not be available for use during a disaster[22] so that an alternate plan for an individual hospital or the need for transport of burn victims to facilities which have the capability of proper care due to the availability of appropriate equipment is required. Problems in rendering aid in such extreme situations exemplify the necessity of having an organization with separate departments of catastrophe medicine.[2] A plan must assure that the management of individual patients will be optimal under a variety of organizational structures. Compromises may be necessary in extreme circumstances, but the ideal is to develop a plan to avoid them whenever possible (i.e. patients with eyelid/facial burns are seen within 4 hours by an ophthalmic surgeon or physiotherapy is started within 48 hours).[55] Even when personnel are available, there is generally a lack of specific materials. A practical kit for various procedures in the first few hours after severe burns is helpful.[57] It must incorporate the following basic features:[58]

- easy to transport to the scene of a disaster;
- easy to keep in good condition at a medical/surgical post;
- long lasting;
- simple to use;
- robust and lightweight enough for air transport.

The contents of an emergency kit should be an integral part of a disaster preparation and be approved by burn experts on a planning committee. The logistics of preparing a kit, which includes all the necessary supplies for initial care, is a significant investment in time and money to initiate and maintain. Prepositioned supplies were of significant benefit at Landstuhl Army Hospital during the Ramstein air disaster.

Education

Health education and training programs assume particular importance in burn disaster planning. They must encompass the technical aspect, the clinical aspect, and the operational aspect of a disaster. Implementation of these plans must follow well defined programs of teaching at schools, starting with primary school level through education at civil defense courses, periodic refresher courses for physicians, nurses, volunteers, Red Cross personnel, fire brigades, police, etc., in addition to periodic exercises with simulated fire disasters which involve the general population and local rescue forces.[19,41] Training methods may use brochures, stickers, coloring albums, posters, notices, and a variety of audiovisual means, particularly videotapes. Videotapes can recreate and simulate situations and propose actions for assistance to victims.[19] An interactive video using ordinary documentary film with educational elements can train a student in prevention as well as every element of burn care. Multimedia presentations improve a user's attention and achieve greater educational effectiveness than a usual monomedium message; and they should be used in initial as well as refresher courses.[19]

The level of prevention achieved depends on the number and effectiveness of public education and information programs which have been pursued.[59] The role of health education is to facilitate the learning of behavior patterns which will reduce risk factors and increase protection factors by means of identification of motivational elements related to behavior.[59] An educational program must be based on a precise method which starts with analysis of a problem of health and safety and then encompasses epidemiological, behavioral, and educational diagnosis.[59]

Prevention

The most notable immediate reward for good burn disaster planning is the template which is established for burn prevention programs. Inspection of public buildings at the time of their initial construction and after any remodeling is necessary in order to ensure proper fire prevention methods. Failure to observe this axiom was crucial in the Stardust disaster.[60] Attention should be paid to methods of egress, as well as fire-fighting capability such as water hose reels and fire-resistant materials.[60] Posting fire escape plans within rooms of public buildings, providing adequate fire egress instructions and facilities, having fire drills in public facilities (schools, office buildings, hospitals,[15] operating rooms,[17] ships, airplanes,[14] etc.) are important aspects of training as well as prevention. There must be proper liaison between disaster planning departments and fire services. A fire department must ensure that they have proper equipment to fight fires and rescue victims from all facilities in their catchment area, including high rise buildings, hospitals, and schools. They should be aware of buildings with hazardous materials, fuel, and explosives in their area. Inspections must include adherence to statutory building regulations and the laws which make these regulations effective. Fire services and local authorities must be adequately staffed, properly equipped, and appropriately trained.

The Disaster

A disaster plan is especially important for burned patients; and thus, it may be helpful to illustrate the operation of such plans through actual major burn disasters. Most burn disasters and burn casualties occur in more urban and populated areas.[6,22,26,34,51,53,61] The Ural train/gas pipeline catastrophe was an exception.[2,27,28,62–64] Thus, the arrival of the first casualty will usually occur shortly after an incident; and the flow thereafter will be proportional to the number of casualties, the distance from the receiving facilities, the ease of triage, and the transportation available. The aim of all health workers concerned with mass burns is to give each burned patient the same care he/she would receive if he/she were the only patient burned and to save and cure as many of those affected as possible.[3] There may be overriding conditions which may not make this possible. It is imperative when this situation occurs that a reassessment about secondary triage to other burn care facilities be entertained. The operation of a rescue plan must take into account the types, kinds, and numbers of burn victims and the type of intervention required.[7]

Putting the Disaster Plan into Action

Immediate care is usually delivered by people on the scene of a disaster – relatives, friends and passersby – all people who have witnessed the disaster and who have arrived immediately at the scene. Generally speaking, their help is an automatic reaction derived from affection, friendship, or a spirit of human solidarity.[7] In the case of burn disasters, the first responders must know how to approach a fire, how to enter a burning building which may be full of smoke or toxic fumes, how to rescue a person whose clothes are on fire, how to treat burn wounds and the associated lesions immediately, and how to provide medical relief.[7] One of the most troublesome confounding problems is establishing the number of casualties and the size of their burns.

Often the major management problem is a lack of information from the site of the accident.[23] The focus of patient assessment and care responsibilities has shifted from hospitals to the scene of a disaster where triage, evaluation, and medical management of multiple casualties occur.[10,65] Burn disaster activities should all be centrally coordinated through one resource center utilizing a centralized communication hub with central medical emergency direction capabilities (see Table 3.3). On-scene patient management is generally organized in two distinct phases: patient triage; and ambulance staging.[10] On-scene management, when organized and conducted properly, allows for controlled treatment of patients, optimal allocation of resources, and maximization of the utility of these resources for patients.[66] Guidelines for immediate care of burn victims include:

- self-control;
- self protection;
- qualitative assessment of burns;
- quantitative assessment of a patient's burns;
- intravenous fluid therapy;
- analgesic therapy;
- bladder catheterization;
- pressure relieving incisions;
- re-examination of a patient;
- hospital transfer.[19]

All assistance to patients who have been exposed to fire and have extensive burns must be specific, precise, considerate, and timely.[19]

Triage – The Inflow

Triage, treatment, and transport are the three basic problems which confront health care workers caring for mass burns. Triage ought to be conducted in a simple, straightforward and experienced manner. Triage should be prognostic with a view to singling out those among the burned who are likely to survive.[3] The two most important aspects of triage have to do with who will perform triage and where. The initial triage will most likely be at the site of a burn disaster by bystanders followed shortly by other first responders. The triage area is an important consideration. A safe triage area must be secured so that additional burn victims are not created because of lack of scene safety. The lobby of a hotel might serve as a good triage area, since it has good access and egress, appropriate space to work, and serves as a known location to all rescue workers and medical personnel. With lack of sophistication at the scene, burn victims may be taken to the nearest hospital emergency department or accident ward for triage[10] before they are transported to tertiary burn centers.[10,23,27,52,53,64] Sorting should ideally be performed at the site by an expert in burns.[1,53,67] Expert triage may minimize the requirement for specialized burn beds.[9] Few casualties with burn wounds of 30–70% TBSA (14% of those admitted) were encountered following fire disaster.[9] Since bed availability in specialized centers is limited, it is clear that accurate triage is essential.[9] The rapid evacuation of casualties to nearby hospitals is a realistic aim for all but the most isolated locations, aided by the fact that most burn victims are themselves initially mobile and cooperative.[38]

The organization of salvage work is affected by the number of casualties, the seriousness of their injuries, and the general conditions of a disaster.[3] The actual triage of patients will be influenced not only by the total number of casualties and bed availability, but also by such factors as depth and location of wounds, complications such as inhalation injury, and extremes of age.[9,20] With effective triage, the demand for specialized burn care can be minimized. In the cast of the Ramstein disaster, the triage sites formed *de novo* where large numbers of patients were encountered and medical personnel congregated naturally and supplies could be obtained for initial resuscitation. The patients were then carried a short distance to staging areas for helicopter pick up or for ambulance or bus loading. In the Ramstein disaster, complete triage on the scene was not possible. Most of the victims were transported by a 'load and go' system to nearby hospitals. The response of emergency services at the air base was criticized.[6,52,53] Because of the nature of some burn disasters, it is important to establish triage stations somewhat removed from an immediate scene.[10] This would be in response to hazards to the rescue and triage personnel such as bomb threats and potential explosions, interference by a crowd, or simply the fact that better facilities for triage are nearby and available.

Patients must be triaged into categories for systematic referral to appropriate facilities. The triage category is based on the severity of injury and the potential for salvage. The overall goal is to do the most good for the most people. In general, when resources are unlimited and a disaster plan incorporated additional resources, even the most severely injured burn victim will receive optimal care if the triage is accomplished in an optimal pattern. Where resources are limited, triage may require a method for selecting casualties on a true priority basis. It may mean developing an expectant category for those so severely injured that they are unlikely to survive. The problem of triage can be simplified and facilitated by a flexible adaptation of certain formulas. The gravity of burns can be expressed in terms of extent and age. In Czechoslovakia, the sum of age and extent of burn which is greater than 90 has established an empirical 50% chance of survival. By flexibility bringing this number up or down, depending on the overall situation, one can extend or narrow the number of burn casualties who ought to be transported first.[3] Immediate triage is essential in the presence of large numbers of burned patients. It has been observed that if a long period of time elapses before rescue teams could start triage and resuscitation, most of the severely injured die and many of the initially moderately injured develop serious complications.[6]

For victims of burn disasters, triage may identify five important groups:[1]

- Minor burns/non-critical sites (<10% TBSA for children; <20% TBSA for adults). Dress wounds; tetanus prophylaxis; out-patient care.
- Minor burns/critical sites (hands, face, perineum). Admit, early operations, special wound care, short hospital stay.
- 20–60% TBSA (requires intravenous fluids/careful monitoring). Burns units, trained personnel.
- Extensive burns (>60% TBSA); mortality high.
- Minor burns/inhalation injury/associated injuries. Administer oxygen, measure carboxyhemoglobin, + or – intubate, ventilate, care of injuries.

Initial Care, the ABCs

The first order of treatment is to ensure an adequate airway and respiration for each burn victim. This is most often a problem in patients with inhalation injury or mechanical trauma to the face, neck or chest. Patients with respiratory problems must be identified immediately; those with inhalation injuries must be noted very early in order to reduce mortality and morbidity.[55] Intubation and ventilation may be required at the scene and at any time thereafter for inadequate airway or breathing. Firemen are usually the best trained rescue personnel and are capable of initiating care of burned victims. The kind of assistance provided by the first rescuers is of primary importance for the prognosis of casualties. They must carry out the first triage of urgent cases, taking into consideration a high number of poly-traumatized patients. They must also initiate all medical and surgical procedures necessary for a preliminary resuscitative therapy and an initial local treatment of burns.[7]

Patients with all but minor burns should receive prompt fluid replacement in order to counteract the loss of protein-rich fluid from veins into interstitial tissues.[1] In the Ufa train disaster, first aid was rendered to victims at the site of the accident by local inhabitants and the medical staff of hospitals located in nearby settlements. Within 12 hours, 25 teams of emergency first aid personnel from the city of Ufa and Civil Defense Medical Brigades provided additional care. Effective early management extends the time available for dispersal of casualties.[9] The two fundamental conditions for prognosis are the time interval between the accident and commencement of infusion therapy and the quality of therapy administered.[56] Effective fluid therapy during the first 24 hours provides an interval in which a transfer of patients may be organized.[9] Fluid therapy should be based on the simplest, most expedient effective way of treating a problem. The Baxter-Shires formula of 4 ml Ringer's lactate/kg body weight/1% TBSA second and third degree burn with maintenance of diuresis at 0.5–0.7 ml/kg/h is effective and should be started within half an hour for adults with burns greater than 20% TBSA, for children with burns greater than 10% TBSA, and patients up to the age of 4 years with burns greater than 5% TBSA.[3] The substitution of intravenous resuscitation by enteral therapy is possible for smaller burns.[3] No colloids should be administered for the first 24 hours.

Junior staff can set up intravenous infusion, administer analgesics, obtain baseline blood samples and radiographs, arrange photographic documentation, begin monitoring fluid balance and prepare chronological documentation.[1] Adequate resuscitation was the key to a better survival rate among similar groups of patients whose medical treatment was otherwise the same in two burn units in Spain.[6,25] The Ufa train disaster provided an example of the consequences of a long delay in fluid resuscitation.[6]

The extent of a burn should be assessed in terms of the percentage of the total body surface area (TBSA) using a patient's hand (fingers together) as representing 1%.[1] It is unnecessary to separate partial-thickness from full-thickness burns when calculating fluid requirements. Initially, burned areas should be simply covered with a sterile sheet. If a patient must remain for a period of time, the initial facility may wish to cover a wound with gauze and impregnate it with silver sulfadiazine or some other effective topical agent. The efficient work of a nursing staff in treating patients with silver sulfadiazine cream before an exact diagnosis and depth and extent of burns is known wastes time, because the wounds need to be uncovered in order to allow medical staff to confirm a diagnosis.[22] One must exercise judgment as to how long to leave a burn wound unprotected from topical antimicrobials so that a physician can evaluate the burn wound. Physicians may well be consumed in lifesaving measures for other burned victims for some extended period of time. The same could be said for the need for escharotomies. Detailed assessment of casualties will obviously take some time; such assessment is, therefore, only practical in a clinical environment where facilities and personnel are available for management of fluid therapy and for treatment of urgent complications.[9] Early debridement of burn tissue is not necessary initially, but can be carried out within the first 5 days postburn once a patient has reached an appropriate facility. The management of burns should involve debridement and wound coverage as soon as possible,[22] but this is a function of the tertiary referral hospital/burn center and should only be considered as part of the eventual care of the patient, not the initial resuscitation.

Methods of treatment must be modified, and medications must be standardized and reduced to basics.[6] Initially, no prophylactic antibiotics are administered, but prophylaxis against stress ulcers should be given. Although antibiotics are not used in many burn centers for prophylaxis because of the development of resistant organisms,[68] in a situation where a large number of patients with burns arrive at a general hospital, which would be unlikely to have an endogenous supply of resistant organisms (or the capability of early detection of burn wound sepsis), it would seem advisable to use prophylaxis.[55]

Staffing

Initial staffing

Medical staff on duty must be able to undertake emergency care of initial victims prior to arrival of additional staff, as was the case with the Hipercor victims when traffic conditions delayed the arrival of off-duty burns and surgical staff as well as additional hospital staff to care for burned patients.[22] This can create an overwhelming task for health care providers. In the Ufa train disaster the average number of patients per health care team was 12–15.[2] Within a very short period of time, initial medical people (physicians, nurses, and members of voluntary organizations) must respond to victims of a burn disaster site. These medical personnel are supported by public and private organizations in the area, hospitals, casualty departments, clinics, fire brigades, and police; and they are coordinated by local authorities.[7]

When admitting patients and rendering qualified, specialized medical aid at a hospital, the participation of mixed physician teams is advisable.[2] A senior surgeon should calculate the number of hours of operating room time required for the proper care of all patients. A priority must be established for initial care and for any dressing changes and reoperations which are required. From that calculation, staffing requirements for the operating rooms, as well as for postoperative anesthetic care, intensive care and ward care, can be established. A senior surgeon should act as coordinator and get surgeons working as soon as patients arrive, keeping two operating theaters reserved for life-saving operations.[11] Such calculations will drive the requirements for equipment and supplies and, with some foresight, drive the resupply rate.

In the San Juanico tragedy, in which about 7000 people were injured, 2000 were hospitalized, 625 had severe burns, 300 died immediately, 250 died in hospitals later, and 60 000 were evacuated; 7000 people were involved in the rescue work during the first 48 hours. Of these, 200 were firefighters, 1000 were physicians, 1300 were paramedics, 1800 were nurses, 2000 were military personnel, and 750 were drivers and helicopter pilots.[6,26]

Volunteers will come! Assistance from volunteers may occur spontaneously from a crowd or community as it did at Ramstein and Piper Alpha or respond to a formal request as in the Ufa train disaster. 'You'll see the basic goodness in people when this sort of thing happens. Everyone rallies around. They don't think of payment. We had no problem with staffing, people just appeared'.[36] Although only a skeleton staff was on duty, the switchboard was flooded with nurses offering their services.[36]

At Ramstein, the townspeople in Landstuhl heard the jet airplanes stop flying and many helicopters start flying and sensed a disaster. They responded to the Landstuhl Army Hospital and served as clean-up crews, traffic control, stretcher bearers and many other functions without being asked and often without any supervision. They just did the right things to help the effort. After needs were assessed, two pediatric burn teams were sent to assist in the care of burned children. These teams integrated with the host nation's medical personnel to care for the burn victims.[27,64] The US team arrived 2 weeks after the disaster.[64] The cooperative effort allowed an increased frequency of dressings and more aggressive, rapid, and complete debridement of wounds. New techniques were introduced such as the use of a free hand skin graft knife, an air-driven dermatome, a skin graft mesher, and the use of dilute epinephrine solution for topical control of bleeding. Additional splints were made. One aspect of the burn care at Children's Hospital Nine was the role of parents in providing much of the care of their children. They were present virtually all of the time on the wards. For those children whose parents were missing or children orphaned as a result of a disaster, others acted as surrogates. They fed the children, changed the beds and clothing, transported them around the hospital and received them directly from the dressing and operating rooms still partially anesthetized.[64] Soviet medical and paramedical staff slowly realized the large number of patients involved, the extent of their injuries, and the logistics of their care. The result was acceptance of medical help offered by burn care teams from the US, United Kingdom, France, Israel, and Cuba, which illustrated the importance of having access to international medical support following disasters of such magnitude that local (regional and national) medical resources were exhausted.[6] Full and immediate use should be made of colleagues called out under a major disaster plan or they will disappear.

Relief

After initial staff become exhausted, formal relief personnel must replace or be assigned to the effort. With so many serious cases, often the usual number of staff must be doubled. Usually there is no difficulty in finding them. Nurses often volunteer their services and the response is great.[36] A plastic surgeon who had been attending a burn conference heard news of the Piper Alpha disaster and was accompanied by six burn specialists from all over the country to help treat burns. At Ramstein, off-duty hospital personnel augmented initial staff and provided the relief staff needed to care for burned and mechanically traumatized victims.

Organized relief refers to the mobilization of all military and civil defense forces which are ready to intervene in the event of a burn disaster.[38,39] These forces arrive at the scene of an accident as rapidly as possible, but usually not within the first 3 hours. They are equipped with the necessary means and structures to enable them to perform their rescue action during the first 48–72 hours after a disaster until all the people have been evacuated.[7] These forces are generally trained to manage the general details of fire disasters. These special units are composed of personnel trained in the emergency care of severely burned patients and equipped with specific means and materials. These units should be in charge of preliminary triage, preparing a preliminary evacuation plan, contacting dispatching stations, selecting means of transport, organizing first aid posts, and clearing the area of the dead.[7]

Supply

Replenishing supplies used up in the care of many burn patients initially comes from warehousing facilities at or near a hospital or burn unit. Transport of additional supplies becomes crucial since the care of burned patients has high resource requirements for intravenous fluids, topical antibiotics, pain medications, and the like. If resupply cannot be effected, then there will be a decline in the care of burn victims or a need for secondary triage to a facility equipped and supplied to provide optimal care.

As the US team joined burn surgeons at Children's Hospital Nine in caring for children from the Ufa train disaster, certain ideas and materials also necessarily came along. Project Hope provided over 7000 kg of badly needed medical supplies, drugs, and equipment, all of which arrived during the 2 weeks while the US team was in the then Soviet Union. Such material aid permitted the Soviet surgeons to carry out usual therapy more effectively and the US team to introduce some new ideas and techniques.[64] The Brooke Army team brought tons of much needed supplies with them as well. Authorities need to act on the basis of guidelines which provide for the stockpiling of specific mobilization materials in the most convenient location, the management of ambulance services, traffic control, the use of local and regional mass media, and the general means of transportation.[7] At Ramstein, contingency supplies specifically for a mass disaster were brought in and used for the care of burned patients.

Secondary Triage

The Ural mountain train/gas pipeline explosion (Ufa train disaster) was a classic example of the need for secondary triage. During the initial stages follow the Ufa train accident, victims were evacuated to nearby settlements where first aid was rendered, aseptic bandages placed, and fluid resuscitation started. During the second stage, victims were evacuated by medical vehicles and helicopters to Ufa and Techelyabinsk. Total evacuation took 16 hours and 45 minutes, and 806 people were admitted to hospitals and burn centers.[2] Helicopters from a nearby military training base airlifted survivors to hospitals in the regional cities of Ufa, Asha, Gorky and Chelyabinsk. Aeroflot organized a series of special flights, evacuating 160 of the most badly burned, including 37 children, to hospitals in Moscow.[64] In the Ramstein disaster, rapid initial transport to supporting hospitals was instituted, but further transport to designated hospitals was not thought to have been carried out properly. The result was that some hospitals and burn centers were overloaded with patients while nearby hospitals did not get any patients at all[6,52,53]. Secondary or tertiary transfers could have relieved the problem.

A region-wide disaster network could be developed, linking the communications of multiple hospitals so that each could receive all communications relevant to a disaster from the central communications center and air and group transportation units would be included in the link. This requires rigid communications discipline in order to ensure that only pertinent voice communication is transmitted. Through this system, secondary patient triage, hospital notification, and medical control of patients coming from a disaster, as well as mobilization of ground and aeromedical transportation, can be effected. Priority triage of victims can be accomplished by radio contact between central communication physicians and referring physicians in local hospitals. Through such a system, burned patients can be secondarily transferred to burn centers with available beds, equipment, and personnel so that optimal care can be delivered to each patient. The end result of good secondary triage is that none of the institutions will be overly taxed in providing disaster response; this will allow uninterrupted care of all patients, including the patients who are already in a facility.

Once patients are re-triaged to a specialty center, a surgeon directing a major disaster plan may not be able to personally see and assign priorities to a large number of patients because the true priority cannot be assigned until the last patient has arrived. Therefore, a first-come-first-served policy may be effective, reserving some resources for severe emergency problems. To reexamine each of the patients thoroughly by removing all dressings is distressing for the patients and time-consuming for surgeons. Surgeons, therefore, may make hurried and incomplete examinations from which some minor mistakes may result. Further, the senior surgeon directing the surgical management of a major accident should stay out of the operating theater, freeing himself of all routine commitments for the day until the last patient has left the operating theater.[11] He must, however, keep control of the surgical needs of the patients, interface with relatives, and arrange for transfers of patients to other hospitals if an overload occurs in a receiving hospital and also to eventually transfer patients closer to their homes when their care can be directed safely and appropriately from a hospital closer to home (see **Figure 3.3**).

Forty-seven patients from the Ramstein disaster were re-triaged at the trauma center of Homburg-Saar using Plan A (natural disasters, fires and explosions/departments of surgery, anesthesia, and radiology), Level II (20–50 victims, activates additional staff and an executive team of department chairs) of their hospital disaster plan. The secondary triage took place in the triage zone of the trauma center by six emergency room shock teams. Patients were dismissed to nearby hospitals; but this proved to be unnecessary. Four intensive care units were reinforced with additional staff. Forty-two patients arrived together on a bus less than 1 hour after the crash and activated the main secondary triage. Twenty-four victims had deep thermal or full-thickness burns up to 90%. Eleven had additional trauma. Twenty-two were classified second priority and eight with minor injuries went home after first aid treatment in the out-patient department. Six burn victims were transferred by helicopter to German and American burn centers during the following 48 hours. After discussion with burn center physicians, five patients with severe injuries (burns in combination with other injuries) were not transferred and expired of multiple organ failure.[53] Secondary triage or tertiary triage may occur when burn victims can be transferred to their domestic hospitals. Eleven of the 22 hospitalized patients at the Homburg trauma center following the Ramstein disaster were transferred to their domestic hospitals.

Psychological Considerations

Patients admitted to a hospital should have supportive psychological counseling given early, throughout their hospital stay, and for follow-up after discharge in order to minimize late emotional disturbances.[55] Professionally trained teams of experienced rescue workers help to control emotional problems such as panic caused by a fire disaster.[55] Most of these patients will have major emotional problems.[32,36] 'They are agitated, anxious, very dependent, and out of action. Their faces are not looking good. They have seen their friends go up in flames. Some survivors had heard hundreds of men screaming that they were going to die. Psychologists and social workers were drafted to offer emotional and practical help to survivors and brief families, as well as support the nurses looking after them.'[36] It is only later, as the drama of the first days dies down, that nurses start to feel the strain. Talking among the health caregivers about an incident helps.[36] Advisors from Bradford and Kent, who had developed special services to help the bereaved in response to the Bradford fire and the Zeebrugge ferry disasters were available to help.[36] Apart from the casualties themselves, the greatest concern was for the bereaved relatives, most of them with no body to grieve over and no ritual funeral rites to help them mourn. Many bereaved families were desperate to speak to persons in the hospital in order to find out all they could about missing relatives now presumed dead.[36] Professionals must be available to help these people during and after a disaster.

Psychological training must be given by expert psychoanalysts using group work techniques.[54] An effort should be made to reduce psychological interference which might hinder the organization of rescue work and burn care. Initially, people must trust their rescue workers and be guided by them. This assists in the escape from disaster and lessens the psychological impact. The best psychological first aid is to assist and organize escape from a disaster. During and immediately after a fire/burn disaster, civic education in schools by mass media and through other means of communication may help lessen the psychological impact of a disaster on a community. Psychological support must be tailored to the situation of a fire/burn disaster. As in the case of the Ramstein disaster, the audience at the air show was family oriented with many schoolchildren witnessing the holocaust and experiencing the panic of the event. Therefore, great energy was spent in psychological debriefs in the schools where the children attended and in other public forums.

Control/Communications Center

Accounting for patients is the main function of the control/communication center after initial communications between a disaster scene and facilities have diminished. Transmittal of pertinent information regarding the condition of those patients being transferred from one facility to another tertiary care facility is important. Equally important is to accurately account for the dead. This information is crucial for handling families and friends. Appropriate communication to the press media is an issue of public trust but must follow approved public relations protocols.[49]

Transportation

Coordination and mobilization of necessary transportation mechanisms (i.e. ground ambulance and/or aeromedical helicopter) and avoidance of calling in unneeded ambulances to a scene, which tends to confuse scene management, are essential.[10] The same control may be necessary for leapfrogging facilities so as to not overload one hospital at any given time.[69] Most patients will be transported by ground vehicles, particularly if a disaster is in an urban area. Remoteness of areas, traffic congestion, and the need for secondary triage may provide good reasons for aeromedical transfer. For a helicopter service in Italy, 2.5% of approximately 2500 flights concerned the secondary transport of burn victims while 0.5% provided direct medical assistance to burned patients at the scene of accidents.[70] Careful preparation by a hospital requesting transfers can be performed prior to air medical evacuation (**Table 3.4**). The size of a helicopter (or airplane) effects the optimal therapeutic access to various anatomical parts, monitoring of a patient, ventilatory assistance, and the number of patients that can be transported at one time. Larger helicopters with advanced instrumentation and excellent air speed effect the transportation during adverse meteorological conditions.[70]

Table 3.4 Specific protocol for preparing burned patients for medical evaluation[70]

Cannulation of several venous routes of which one should be central if possible (followed by chest radiograph)
Monitoring of diuresis
Insertion of nasogastric probe
Sedation and/or analgesia
Cleansing of wounds
Tracheal intubation (if necessary)
Application of sanitary devices to prevent excessive heat loss

After-action Requirements

Disaster management cannot leave out consideration of overall assessment of the consequences of a disaster. This assessment must be as accurate as possible whether it refers to a presumed or actual event.[7] Awareness of the scale and nature of past disasters may aid in the formulation of plans for dealing with mass burn casualties in the future.[9] The use of a uniform language and framework to report and analyse disaster incidents is important and will contribute to a more accurate evaluation of results.[10] Continuing to make modifications and revisions to a disaster plan and disaster management can be effectively accomplished by initiating a mechanism of post-incident evaluation of actual disaster responses. The central coordination of the response can be the focal point for this evaluation which must include all of the emergency medical services and the resources involved in a disaster response.[47]

All of the agencies and individuals involved in a burn disaster should be assembled routinely immediately following incidents in order to critique the events while the facts are clear in the minds of the providers.[10] Information included in these sessions, although sometimes subjective, is usually quite candid and complete; and when combined with taped and written recordings of the incidents, it provides important lessons about the strengths and weaknesses of the management of the response.[10] Relevant lessons learned include the knowledge that all public service agencies are integrally involved in a successful management of a burn disaster and must be kept informed of the current burn disaster plans. Such a critique depends on reliable information for successful management of the next disaster. From such a critique, individual facilities are able to affect changes such as directing on-line communications to an admitting office, preparing intensive care units and operating rooms, as well as establishing a person with the authority to make decisions for the hospitals' ability to accept patients without questioning their fiscal resources. Major internal changes can be effected, based on data and corrections made to allow a hospital to accept burn disaster victims at any hour that a disaster may occur. The practical benefit of these evaluation sessions is the fact that changes in disaster plans and operational management are made based on information learned during a disaster response critique.[10] Critiques often identify problems on notification of hospitals and burn centers concerning the nature and extent of injuries, as well as the number of patients they should expect. Organized relay of pertinent patient information to hospital staff or mobilization of appropriate physicians, specialists and staff is key. Matching of patients with specific injuries, such as burns, to facilities capable of treating these specific problems, such as burn centers, is the mark of a well designed disaster plan which is effectively managed.

Some important, but previously unknown, statistics have been generated from after-action reports. The total number of injured patients was more than six times higher and the number of casualties admitted to hospitals was nearly 20 times greater following outdoor disasters than indoor disasters.[6] The immediate death rate at the site was very high (74%) in indoor fires compared to outdoor disasters (35%), but the hospital death rate was lower following indoor disasters.[6,9] Sixty percent of burn victims sustained burns covering less than 30% of their total body surface area.[6] A significant number of patients with very extensive burns (greater than 70% TBSA) occurred after outdoor burns, while very few were admitted with extensive burns after indoor fires.[1] Those who failed to escape from indoor fires died rapidly from a combination of hypoxia and inhalation of poisonous compounds.[71,72] The poor prognosis of burn victims with large burns sustained in mass disasters has been emphasized and is reflected in the high mortality following outdoor disasters.[9,25,73] The number of burn victims admitted with burns in the 30–70% TBSA range was consistently low, which is more important since patients with this burn size potentially obtain the greatest benefit from referral to a burn center.[9] In an indoor disaster of another kind, the MGM Grand Hotel fire in Las Vegas resulted in 300 hospital admissions for smoke inhalation, but no injuries.[74] After-action reports will allow analysis of the environmental impact of the disaster, the vulnerability of the territory, and the information, education, and participation of the population.[59] In emergencies, human behavior is a decisive factor in the creation of dangerous or harmful situations and it plays a basic role in the evolution of the effects of a disaster.[59]

A bonus lesson learned from after-action reporting was that burn teams working together can exchange new ideas and techniques with colleagues from other parts of the world who are not familiar with such techniques.[2] The history of the combined efforts of the Soviet and US Army medical teams who worked together at the largest hospital in the city of Ufa, in which neither the hospital nor the Soviet physicians working at the hospital had had significant burn care experience prior to the disaster, was that the team was able to effectively care for a large number of patients.[2] All of these data are important in planning for the next burn disaster.

Acknowledgment

The authors would like to thank Rhonda Glazebrook for her assistance in preparing this chapter.

References

1. Griffiths R W. Management of multiple casualties with burns. *BMJ* 1985; **291:** 917–18.

2. Kulyapin A V, Sakhautdinov V G, Temerbulatov V, Becker W, Waymack J. Bashkiria train-gas pipeline disaster: a history of the joint USSR/USA collaboration. *Burns* 1990; **16**(5): 339–42.

3. Simko S. Reflections on the organization of mass burns treatment. *Acta Chir Plast* 1981; **23**(3): 197–200.

4. Sorensen B. Management of burns occurring as mass casualties after nuclear explosion. *Burns* 1979; **6:** 33–6.

5. Layton T R, Elhauge E R. U.S. fire catastrophes of the 20th century. *J Burn Care Rehabil* 1982; **3:** 21–8.

6. Arturson G. Analysis of severe fire disasters. Chapter 4. In: Masellis M, Gunn S W A, eds. *The Management of Mass Burn Casualties and Fire Disasters: Proceedings of the First International Conference on Burns and Fire Disasters.* Dordrecht/Boston/London: Kluwer Academic Publishers, 1992: 24–33.

7. Masellis M. Thermal agent disaster and fire disaster: definition, damage, assessment and relief operations. Chapter 1. In: Masellis M, Gunn S W A, eds. *The Management of Mass Burn Casualties and Fire Disasters: Proceedings of The First International Conference on Burns and Fire Disasters.* Dordrecht/Boston/London: Kluwer Academic Publishers, 1992: 7–12.

8. Gunn S W A. The scientific basis of disaster medicine. Chapter 2. In: Masellis M, Gunn S W A, eds. *The Management of Mass Burn Casualties and Fire Disasters: Proceedings of The First International Conference on Burns and Fire Disasters.* Dordrecht/Boston/London: Kluwer Academic Publishers, 1992: 13–18.

9. Mackie D P, Koning H M. Fate of mass burn casualties: implications for disaster planning. *Burns* 1990; **16**(3): 203–6.

10. Jacobs L M, Goody M M, Sinclair A. The role of a trauma center in disaster management. *J Trauma* 1983; **23:** 697–701.

11. Bliss A R Major disaster planning. *Br Med J* 1984; **288:** 1433–4.

12. Gunn S W A. *Multilingual Dictionary of Disaster Medicine and International Relief.* Dordrecht: Kluwer Academic Publishers, 1990.

13. Woolley W D, Smith P C, Fardell P J, Murrell J M, Rogers S P. The Stardust Disco Fire. Dublin 1981: Studies of combustion products during simulation experiments. *Fire Safety Journal* 1984; **7:** 267.

14. Hill I R. An analysis of factors impeding passenger escape from aircraft fires. *Avia Space Environ Med* 1990; **61**(3): 261–5.

15. Servais J. Fire emergency in a hospital. Chapter 17. In: Masellis M, Gunn S W A, eds. *The Management of Mass Burn Casualties and Fire Disasters: Proceedings of the First International Conference on Burns and Fire Disasters.* Dordrecht/Boston/London: Kluwer Academic Publishers, 1992: pp 113–15.

16. Trovato B. Fire services at a motor racing track. Chapter 16. In: Masellis M, Gunn S W A, eds. *The Management of Mass Burn Casualties and Fire Disasters: Proceedings of the First International Conference on Burns and Fire Disasters.* Dordrecht/Boston/London: Kluwer Academic Publishers, 1992: pp 110–12.

17. Halstead M A. Fire drill in the operating room. Role playing as a learning tool. *AORN J* 1993; **58**(4): 697–706.

18. Alley E E. Problems of search and rescue in disasters. Chapter 26. In: Masellis M, Gunn S W A, eds. *The Management of Mass Burn Casualties and Fire Disasters: Proceedings of the First International Conference on Burns and Fire Disasters.* Dordrecht/Boston/London: Kluwer Academic Publishers, 1992: pp 175–6.

19. Masellis M L. Management of mass burn casualties in disasters. *Ann Medit Burns Club* 1988; **1:** 155–9.

20. Costagliola M, Laguerre J, Rouge D. Infobrul – the value of a telematic databank for burns and burns centres in the event of a disaster. Chapter 32. In: Masellis M, Gunn S W A, eds. *The Management of Mass Burn Casualties and Fire Disasters: Proceedings of the First International Conference on Burns and Fire Disasters.* Dordrecht/Boston/London: Kluwer Academic Publishers, 1992: pp 190–4.

21. Martinelli G. The ARGO satellite system: a network for severe burns and disasters. Chapter 44. In: Masellis M, Gunn S W A, eds. *The Management of Mass Burn Casualties and Fire Disasters: Proceedings of the First International Conference on Burns and Fire Disasters.* Dordrecht/Boston/London: Kluwer Academic Publishers, 1992: pp 7–12.

22. Morrell P A G, Nasif F E, Domenech R P, Carol E S, Roda J A B. Burns caused by the terrorist bombing of the department store hipercor in Barcelona: Part I. *Burns* 1990; **16**(6): 423–5.

23. Allister L, Hamilton G M. Cardowan coal mine explosion: experience of a mass burns event. *BMJ* 1983; **287:** 403–5.

24. Demuthi M W, Dimich A R, Gillespie R W, *et al. Advanced Burn Life Support Course.* Lincoln, NE: National Burn Institute, 1990.

25. Arturson G. The Los Alfaques disaster: a boiling-liquid, expanding-vapour explosion. *Burns* 1981; **7:** 233–51.

26. Arturson G. The tragedy of San Juanico – the most severe LPG disaster in history. *Burns* 1987; **13:** 87–102.

27. Herndon D N. A survey of the primary aid response to the Bashkir train-gas pipeline disaster. *Burns* 1990; **16:** 323–4.

28. Benmeir P, Levine I, Shostak A, Oz V, Shemer J, Sokolova T. The ural train-gas pipeline catastrophe: the report of the IDF medical corps assistance. *Burns* 1991; **17**(4): 320–2.

29. Brusco M. Fire in port. Chapter 13. In: Masellis M, Gunn S W A, eds. *The Management of Mass Burn Casualties and Fire Disasters: Proceedings of the First International Conference on Burns and Fire Disasters.* Dordrecht/Boston/London: Kluwer Academic Publishers, 1992: pp 89–92.

30. Bovio G. Forest fires and the danger to firefighters. Chapter 7. In: Masellis M, Gunn S W A, eds. *The Management of Mass Burn Casualties and Fire Disasters: Proceedings of the First International Conference on Burns and Fire Disasters.* Dordrecht/Boston/London: Kluwer Academic Publishers, 1992: pp 51–9.

31. Colombo D, Foti F, Volonte M, Micucci G. Rescue of the burn patients and on-site medical assistance by a helicopter rescue service. Chapter 42. In: Masellis M, Gunn S W A, eds. *The Management of Mass Burn Casualties and Fire Disasters: Proceedings of the First International Conference on Burns and Fire Disasters.* Dordrecht/Boston/London: Kluwer Academic Publishers, 1992: pp 249–50.

32. Rayner C. Offshore disaster on a fixed installation – the Piper Alpha disaster of 6 July 1988. In: Zellner P R, ed. *Die Versorgung des brandverletzten in Katastrophenfall,* Darmstadt: Steinkopff Verlag, 1990, 33–7.

33. Dioguardi D, Brienza E, Altacera M. The role of information sciences in the management of disasters. *Ann Medit Burns Club* 1988; **1:** 165–167.

34. Dioguardi D, Brienza E, Portincasa A, Di Lonardo A, Matarrese V. A proposal for the strategic planning of medical services in the case of major fire disasters in the city of Bari. *Ann Medit Burns Club* 1989; **2**(3): 147–50.

35. Brienza E, Madami L M, Catalano F, Del Zotti M. Organizational criteria for setting up a field hospital after a fire disaster. Chapter 33. In: Masellis M, Gunn S W A, eds. *The Management of Mass Burn Casualties and Fire Disasters: Proceedings of the First International Conference on Burns and Fire Disasters.* Dordrecht/Boston/London: Kluwer Academic Publishers, 1992: pp 195–7.

36. Hicks C. No stranger to disaster. *Nurs Times* 1988; **84**(29): 16–17.

37. Jenkins A L. Disaster planning. Chapter 15. In: *Emergency Department Organization and Management.* St Louis: Mosby, 1978; 243–61.

38. Cucciniello G. The commitment of the Italian Army Medical Corps to relief of the civilian population in the event of public disasters. Chapter 29. In: Masellis M, Gunn S W A, eds. *The Management of Mass Burn Casualties and Fire Disasters: Proceedings of the First International Conference on Burns and Fire Disasters.* Dordrecht/Boston/London: Kluwer Academic Publishers, 1992: pp 133–9.

39. Di Martino M. The organization of the Italian Army Medical Corps in relation to contributions to civil defense in the event of disasters. Chapter 30. In: Masellis M, Gunn S W A, eds. *The Management of Mass Burn Casualties and Fire Disasters: Proceedings of the First International Conference on Burns and Fire Disasters.* Dordrecht/Boston/London: Kluwer Academic Publishers, 1992: pp 185–6.

40. Bianchi M, Minniti U. The use of helicopters in integrated rescue work and medical transport. Chapter 41. In: Masellis M, Gunn S W A, eds. *The Management of Mass Burn Casualties and Fire Disasters: Proceedings of the First International Conference on Burns and Fire Disasters.* Dordrecht/Boston/London: Kluwer Academic Publishers, 1992: pp 246–8.

41. Meurant J. Communications in the prevention of natural and man-made disasters: the role of the national and international Red Cross and Red Crescent organizations. Chapter 60. In: Masellis M, Gunn S W A, eds. *The Management of Mass Burn Casualties and Fire Disasters: Proceedings of the First International Conference on Burns and Fire Disasters.* Dordrecht/Boston/London: Kluwer Academic Publishers, 1992: pp 317–27.

42. Judkins K C. Aeromedical transfer of burned patients: a review with special reference to European civilian practice. *Burns* **14:** 1988; 171–9.

43. Heredero F X S. Physiopathology of burn disease during air evacuation. Chapter 40. In: Masellis M, Gunn S W A, eds. *The Management of Mass Burn Casualties and Fire Disasters: Proceedings of the First International Conference on Burns and Fire Disasters.* Dordrecht/Boston/London: Kluwer Academic Publishers, 1992: pp 243–5.

44. Wachtel T L, Cowan M L, Reardon J D. Developing a regional and national burn disaster response. *J Burn Care Rehabil* 1989; **10**(6): 561–675.

45. Bayer M. Rampenbestrijiding verliep uitzonderlijk snel. *Alert* 1988; **10:** 2.

46. Editorial. Burn care facilities in the UK. *Burns* 1989; **15:** 183.

47. Baker F. The management of mass casualty disasters. *Top Emerg Med* 1979; **1:** 149–157.

48. Orr S, Robinson W. The Hyatt disaster: two physicians' perspectives. *J Emerg Nursing* 1982; **8:** 6–11.

49. Melorio E. Mass media and serious emergencies. Chapter 56. In: Masellis M, Gunn S W A, eds. *The Management of Mass Burn Casualties and Fire Disasters: Proceedings of the First International Conference on Burns and Fire Disasters.* Dordrecht/Boston/London: Kluwer Academic Publishers, 1992: pp 301–4.

50. Mosca A, Amico M, Geraci V, Masellis M. The role of the mass media in burn prevention campaigns – psychological considerations. Chapter 58. In: Masellis M, Gunn S W A, eds. *The Management of Mass Burn Casualties and Fire Disasters: Proceedings of the First International Conference on Burns and Fire Disasters.* Dordrecht/Boston/London: Kluwer Academic Publishers, 1992: pp 311–13.

51. Ellinger K, Quintel M. Das Ramstein Ungluck. *Notarzt* 1989; **5:** 68.

52. Kossmann T, Trentz O. Das Flugschau–Ungluck in Ramstein: Erfahrungsbericht uber die Akutversorgung des Verletztenkontingents des Universitatsklinikums Homburn/Saar. In: Zellner P R, ed. *Die Versorgung des Brandvenietzten in Katastrophenfall.* Darmstadt: Steinkopff Verlag, 1990, 79–83.

53. Kossmann T, Wittling I, Buhren V, Sutter G, Trantz O. Transferred triage to a level 1 trauma center in a mass catastrophe of patients; many of them burns. *Acta Chir Plast.* 1991; **33**(3): 145–150.

54. Amico M, Geraci V, Mosca A, Masellis M. Psychological reactions in fire disaster emergencies: hypotheses and operative guidelines. Chapter 50. In: Masellis M, Gunn S W A, eds. *The Management of Mass Burn Casualties and Fire Disasters: Proceedings of the First International Conference on Burns and Fire Disasters.* Dordrecht/Boston/London: Kluwer Academic Publishers, 1992: pp 278–81.

55. Duignan J P, McEntee G P, Scully B, Corrigan T P. Report of a fire disaster – management of burns and complications. *Irish Med J* 1984; **77:** 8–10.

56. Vitale R, D'Arpa N, Conte F, Cucchiara P, Guzzetta C, Masellis M. Clinical file and protocol for general doctors and for non-specialized hospital doctors to assist burn patients. Chapter 34. In: Masellis M, Gunn S W A, eds. *The Management of Mass Burn Casualties and Fire Disasters: Proceedings of the First International Conference on Burns and Fire Disasters.* Dordrecht/Boston/London: Kluwer Academic Publishers, 1992: pp 198–221.

57. Di Salvo L, Vitale R, Masellis M. Therapeutic kit and procedures for fluid resuscitation in disasters. Chapter 38. In: Masellis M, Gunn S W A, eds. *The Management of Mass Burn Casualties and Fire Disasters: Proceedings of the First International Conference on Burns and Fire Disasters.* Dordrecht/Boston/London: Kluwer Academic Publishers, 1992: pp 231–8.

58. Caruso E, Crabai P, Donati L, Klinger M, Garbin S, Zaza R. Ready-to-use emergency kit for treatment of severe burns: definition and specifications. Chapter 39. In: Masellis M, Gunn S W A, eds. *The Management of Mass Burn Casualties and Fire Disasters: Proceedings of the First International Conference on Burns and Fire Disasters.* Dordrecht/Boston/London: Kluwer Academic Publishers, 1992: pp 239–42.

59. Costanzo S. Health education in disaster medicine. Chapter 20. In: Masellis M, Gunn S W A, eds. *The Management of Mass Burn Casualties and Fire Disasters: Proceedings of the First International Conference on Burns and Fire Disasters.* Dordrecht/Boston/London: Kluwer Academic Publishers, 1992: pp 133–9.

60. McCollum S T. Lessons from the Dublin 1981 fire catastrophe. Chapter 6. In: Masellis M, Gunn S W A, eds. *The Management of Mass Burn Casualties and Fire Disasters: Proceedings of the First International Conference on Burns and Fire Disasters.* Dordrecht/Boston/London: Kluwer Academic Publishers, 1992: pp 45–50.

61. Pietersen C M, Huerta S C. *Analysis of the LPG Incident at San Juan Ixhuatepec, Mexico City.* The Hague: TNO, 1984.

62. Pietersen C M. De ramp met de pepleiding in de Sovjet Unie. *Alert,* 1989; **9:** 3.

63. Fedorov V D, Alekseev A A. Medical care of mass burn victims: the Vishnevsky principles and organization in the Ufa disaster. Chapter 35. In: Masellis M, Gunn S W A, eds. *The Management of Mass Burn Casualties and Fire Disasters: Proceedings of the First International Conference on Burns and Fire Disasters.* Dordrecht/Boston/London: Kluwer Academic Publishers, 1992: pp 222–3.

64. Remensnyder J P, Ackroyd F P, Astrozjnikova S. *et al.* Burned children from the Bashkir train-gas pipeline disaster II. Follow-up experience at Children's Hospital 9, Moscow, USSR. *Burns* 1990; **16**(5): 333–6.

65. Mazzarella B, Scanni E, Carideo P, Maresca A, Vivona G, Sorrentino A. On-site treatment of severely burned patients. Chapter 36. In: Masellis M, Gunn S W A, eds. *The Management of Mass Burn Casualties and Fire Disasters: Proceedings of the First International Conference on Burns and Fire Disasters.* Dordrecht/Boston/London: Kluwer Academic Publishers, 1992: pp 224–6.

66. Cohen E. Triage 1982. *J Emerg Med Serv* 1982; **7:** 24–8.

67. Barclay T L. Planning for mass burn casualties. In: Wood, C, *Accident and Emergency Burns: Lessons from the Bradford Disaster.* London: Royal Society of Medicine Services Roundtable III, 1986.

68. Alexander J W. Control of infection following burn injury. *Arch Surg* 1971; **103:** 435–43.

69. Jacobs L M, Ramp J, Breay J. An emergency medical system approach to disaster planning. *J Trauma,* 1979; **19:** 157–62.

70. Landiscina M, Bile L, Bollini C, Magatti M F. The burn patient and medically assisted helicopter transport. Chapter 43. In: Masellis M, Gunn S W A, eds. *The Management of Mass Burn Casualties and Fire Disasters: Proceedings of the First International Conference on Burns and Fire Disasters.* Dordrecht/Boston/London: Kluwer Academic Publishers, 1992: pp 251–2.

71. Davies J W L. Toxic chemicals versus lung tissue – an aspect of inhalation injury revisited. *J Burn Rehabil* 1986; **7:** 213.

72. Clark W R, Nieman G F. Smoke inhalation. *Burns* 1988; **14:** 472.

73. Sharpe D T, Roberts A H, Barclay T L, *et al.* Treatment of burns casualties after fire at Bradford City football ground. *BMJ* 1985; **291:** 945–8.

74. Buerk C A, Batdorf J W, Cammack K V, *et al.* The MGM Grand Hotel fire. *Arch Surg* 1982; **117:** 641–5.

CHAPTER FOUR

Pre-hospital Management, Transportation and Emergency Care

Ronald P. Mlcak, Alan R. Dimick and Glenda Mlcak

Advances in trauma and burn management over the past three decades have resulted in improved survival and reduced morbidity from major burns. The cost of such care, however, is high; it requires conservation of resources such that only a limited number of burn intensive care units with the capabilities of caring for such labor-intensive patients can be found – hence regional burn care has evolved. This regionalization has led to the need for effective pre-hospital management, transportation and emergency care. Progress in the development of rapid, effective transport systems has resulted in marked improvement in the clinical course and survival for victims of thermal trauma.

For burn victims, there are usually two phases of transport. The first is the entry of the burn patient into the emergency medical system with treatment at the scene and transport to the initial care facility. The second phase is the assessment and stabilization of the patient at the initial care facility and transportation to a burn intensive care unit.[1] With this perspective in mind, this chapter reviews current principles of optimal pre-hospital management, transportation, and emergency care.

Pre-hospital Care

Prior to any specific treatment, a patient must be removed from the source of injury and the burning process stopped. As the patient is removed from the injuring source, care must be taken so that a rescuer does not become another victim.[2] All caregivers should be aware of the possibility that they may be injured by contact with the patient or the patient's clothing. Universal precautions, including wearing gloves, gowns, masks, and protective eye wear, should be used whenever there is likely contact with blood or body fluids. Burning clothing should be removed as soon as possible to prevent further injury.[3] All rings, watches, jewelry and belts should be removed as they can retain heat and produce a tourniquet-like effect with digital vascular ischemia.[4] If water is readily available, it should be poured directly on the burned area. Early cooling can reduce the depth of the burn and reduce pain, but cooling measures must be used with caution, since a significant drop in body temperature may result in hypothermia with ventricular fibrillation or asystole. Ice or ice packs should never be used, since they may cause further injury to the skin or produce hypothermia.

Initial management of chemical burns involves removing saturated clothing, brushing the skin if the agent is a powder, and irrigation with copious amounts of water. Irrigation with water should continue from the scene of the accident through emergency evaluation in the hospital. Efforts to neutralize chemicals are contraindicated due to the additional generation of heat, which would further contribute to tissue damage. A rescuer must be careful not to come in contact with the chemical, i.e. gloves, eye protectors, etc. should be worn.

Removal of a victim from an electrical current is best accomplished by turning off the current and by using a non conductor to separate the victim from the source.[5]

On-site Assessment of a Burned Patient

Assessment of a burned patient is divided into primary and secondary surveys. In the primary survey, immediate life-threatening conditions are quickly identified and treated. The primary survey is a rapid, systematic approach to identify life-threatening conditions. The secondary survey is a more thorough head-to-toe evaluation of the patient. Initial management of a burned patient should be the same as for any other trauma patient, with attention directed at airway, breathing, circulation, and cervical spine immobilization.

Primary Assessment

Exposure to heated gases and smoke resulting from the combustion of a variety of materials results in damage to the respiratory tract.

Direct heat to the upper airways results in edema formation which may obstruct the airway. Initially, 100% humidified oxygen should be given to all patients even when no obvious signs of respiratory distress are present. Upper airway obstruction may develop rapidly following injury, and the respiratory status must be continually monitored in order to assess the need for airway control and ventilator support. Progressive hoarseness is a sign of impending airway obstruction. Endotracheal intubation should be done early before edema obliterates the anatomy of the area.[3]

The patient's chest should be exposed in order to adequately assess ventilatory exchange. Circumferential burns may restrict breathing and chest movement. Airway patency alone does not assure adequate ventilation. After an airway is established, breathing must be assessed in order to insure adequate chest expansion. Impaired ventilation and poor oxygenation may be due to smoke inhalation or carbon monoxide intoxication. Endotracheal intubation is necessary for unconscious patients, for those in acute respiratory distress, or for patients with burns of the face or neck which may result in edema which causes obstruction of the airway.[3] The nasal route is the recommended site of intubation. Assisted ventilation with 100% humidified oxygen is required for all intubated patients.

Blood pressure is not the most accurate method of monitoring a patient with a large burn because of the pathophysiologic changes which accompany such an injury. Blood pressure may be difficult to ascertain because of edema in the extremities. A pulse rate may be somewhat more helpful in monitoring the appropriateness of fluid resuscitation.[6]

If a burn victim was in an explosion or deceleration accident, there is the possibility of a spinal cord injury. Appropriate cervical spine stabilization must be accomplished by whatever means necessary, including a cervical collar to keep the head immobilized until the condition can be evaluated.

Secondary Assessment

After completing a primary assessment, a thorough head-to-toe evaluation of a patient is imperative.[7] A careful determination of trauma other than obvious burn wounds should be made. As long as no immediate life-threatening injury or hazard is present, a secondary examination can be performed before moving a patient; precautions such as cervical collars, backboards, and splints should be used.[8] Secondary assessment should examine a patient's past medical history, medications, allergies, and the mechanism of injury.

There should never be a delay in transporting burn victims to an emergency facility due to an inability to establish intravenous (IV) access. If the local/regional emergency medical system (EMS) protocol prescribes that an IV line be started, then that protocol should be followed. The pre-hospital burn life support course recommends that if a patient is less than 60 minutes from a hospital, an IV is not essential and can be deferred until a patient is at a hospital. If an IV line is established, Ringer's lactate solution should be infused at 500 ml/h in an adult and 250 ml/h in a child 5 years of age or over. In children younger than 5 years of age no IV lines are recommended.[4]

Pre-hospital care of burn wounds is basic and simple, because it requires only protection from the environment with an application of a clean dressing or sheet to cover the involved part. Covering wounds is the first step in diminishing pain. If it is approved for use by the local/regional EMS, narcotics may be given for pain, but only intravenously in small doses and only enough to control pain. Intramuscular or subcutaneous routes should never be used, since fluid resuscitation could result in unpredictable patterns of uptake.[4] No topical antimicrobial agents should be applied in the field.[4, 9] The patient should then be wrapped in a blanket to minimize heat loss and to control temperature during transport.

Transport to Hospital Emergency Department

Rapid, uncontrolled transport of a burn victim is not the highest priority, except in cases where other life-threatening conditions coexist. In the majority of accidents involving major burns, ground transportation of victims to a hospital is available and appropriate. Helicopter transport is of greatest use when the distance between an accident and a hospital is 30–150 miles or when a patient's condition warrants.[10] Whatever the mode of transport, it should be of appropriate size, and have emergency equipment available as well as trained personnel, such as a nurse, physician, paramedic, or respiratory therapist.

Assessment and Emergency Treatment at Initial Care Facility

The assessment of a patient with burn injuries in a hospital emergency department is essentially the same as outlined for a pre-hospital phase of care. The only real difference is the availability of more resouces for diagnosis and treatment in an emergency department. As with other forms of trauma, the primary survey begins with the ABCs, and the establishment of an adequate airway is vital. Endotracheal intubation should be accomplished early if impending respiratory obstruction or ventilatory failure is anticipated, because it may be impossible after the onset of edema following the initiation of fluid therapy. Securing an endotracheal tube may be difficult because traditional methods often do not adhere to burned skin, and tubes are easily dislodged. One method of choice includes securing an endotracheal tube with woven tape under the ears as well as over the ears.[11] While doing assessments and making interventions for life-threatening problems in the primary survey, precautions should be taken to maintain cervical spine immobilization until injuries to the spine can be ruled out.

Following a primary survey, a thorough head-to-toe evaluation of a patient should be done. This includes obtaining a history as thorough as circumstances permit. The history should include the mechanism and time of the injury and a description of the surrounding environment, such as whether injuries were incurred in an enclosed space, the presence of noxious chemicals, the possibility of smoke inhalation, and any related trauma. A complete physical examination should include a careful neurological examination as evidence of cerebral anoxic injury can be subtle. Patients with facial burns should have their corneas examined with fluorescent staining. Routine admission laboratories should include a complete blood count, serum electrolytes, glucose, blood urea nitrogen (BUN), and creatine. Pulmonary assessment should include arterial blood gases, chest x-rays, and carboxyhemoglobin.[12]

All extremities should be examined for pulses, especially with circumferential burns. Evaluation of pulses can be assisted by use of a Doppler ultrasound flowmeter. If pulses are absent, the involved limb may need urgent escharotomy for release of the constrictive, unyielding eschar (**Figure 4.1**). In circumferential chest burns, escharotomy may also be necessary to relieve chest wall restriction and improve ventilation. Escharotomies may be performed at the bedside under intravenous sedation using electrocautery. Mid-axial incisions are made through the eschar but not into subcutaneous tissue of the eschar in order to assure adequate release. Limbs should be elevated above the heart level. Pulses should be monitored for 48 hours.[12]

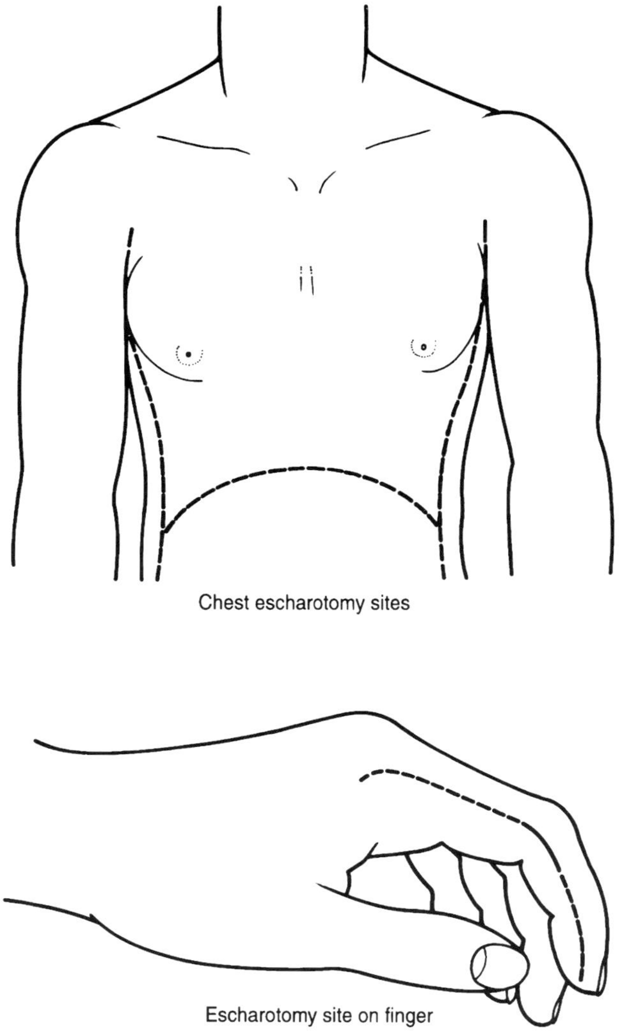

Fig. 4.1 Possible escharotomy sites.

If pulses are still present, but appear endangered, chemical escharotomy with sutilains ointment (Travase) can be effective. Enzymatic escharotomy in hand burns may be preferred since surgical incisions risk exposure of superficial nerves, vessels, and tendons. Enzymatic escharotomy is indicated only during the first 24–48 hours postburn, and it should be used only in combination with a topical antimicrobial agent or sepsis can occur. With enzymatic escharotomy, there is usually a spike in temperature which subsides after the enzyme is removed.

Evaluation of Wounds

After the primary and secondary surveys are completed and resuscitation is underway, a more careful evaluation of burn wounds is performed. The wounds are gently cleaned, and loose skin and blisters are debrided. Blister fluid contains high levels of inflammatory mediators which increase burn wound ischemia. The blister fluid is also a rich media for subsequent bacterial growth. Deep blisters on the palms and soles are generally aspirated instead of debrided in order to improve patient comfort. After burn wound assessment is complete, the wounds are covered with a topical antimicrobial agent and an appropriate burn dressing or a biological dressing is applied.

An estimate of burn size and depth assists in making a determination of severity, prognosis, and disposition of a patient. Burn size directly affects fluid resuscitation, nutritional support and surgical interventions. The size of a burn wound is most frequently estimated by using the rule-of-nines method (**Figure 4.2**). A more accurate assessment can be made of a burn injury, especially in children, by using the Lund and Browder chart, which takes into account changes brought about by growth (**Figure 4.3**).[4,9] The American Burn Association identifies certain injuries as usually requiring a referral to a burn center. Patients with these burns should be treated in a specialized burn facility after initial assessment and treatment at an emergency department. Questions about specific patients should be resolved by consultation with a burn center physician (**Table 4.1**).[4,13]

Fluid Resuscitation

Establishment of intravenous lines for fluid resuscitation is necessary for all patients with major burns including those with inhalation injury or other associated injuries. These lines are best started in the upper extremity peripherally. A minimum of two large caliber IV catheters should be established through nonburned tissue if possible, or through burns if no unburned areas are available. Ringer's lactate solution should be infused at 2–4 ml/kg/% total body

Adult body	% of total
Part	BSA
Arm	9%
Head	9%
Neck	1%
Leg	18%
Anterior trunk	18%
Posterior trunk	18%

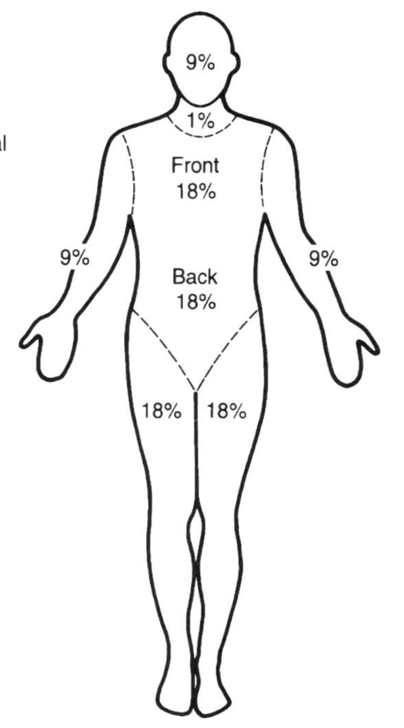

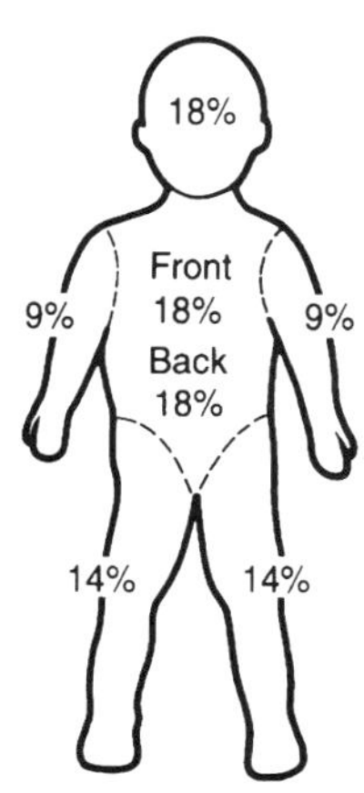

Child body	% of total
Part	BSA
Arm	9%
Head and neck	18%
Leg	14%
Anterior trunk	18%
Posterior trunk	18%

Fig. 4.2 Estimation of burn size using the Rule of Nines.

Age	0–1	1–4	5–9	10–14	15
A – 1/2 of head	9 1/2%	8 1/2%	6 1/2%	5 1/2%	4 1/2%
B – 1/2 of one thigh	2 3/4%	3 1/4%	4%	4 1/4%	4 1/2%
C – 1/2 of one leg	2 1/2%	2 1/2%	2 3/4%	3%	3 1/4%

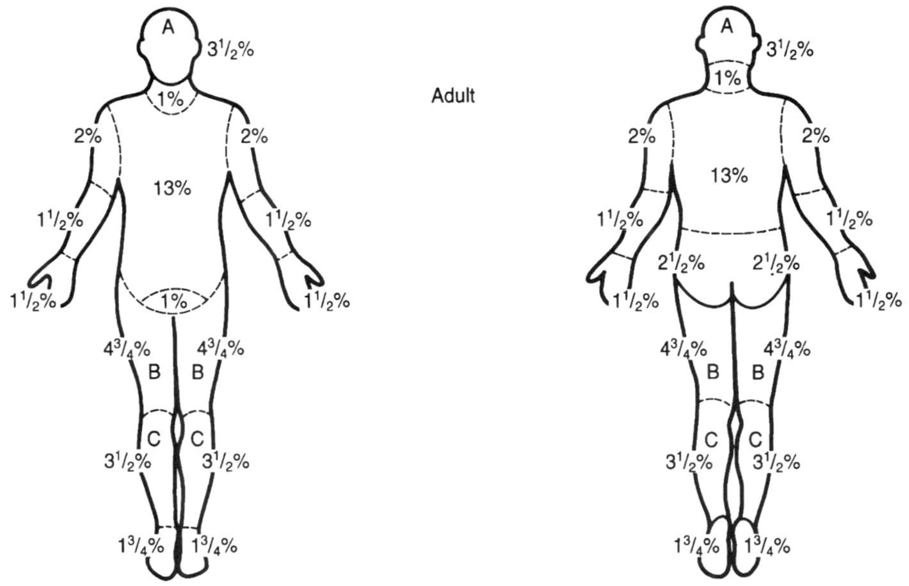

Fig. 4.3 Estimation of burn size using the Lund and Browder method.

Table 4.1 Criteria for transfer of a burn patient to a burn center

Second and third degree burns of 10% TBSA in children <10 years of age or adults >50 years of age
Second and third degree burns of 20% TBSA at any age
Third degree burns ≥10% in any age group
Second and third degree burns that involve and threaten functional or cosmetic impairment of the face, hands, feet, genitalia, perineum and major joints
Chemical burns that involve or threaten functional or cosmetic impairment in the face, hands, feet, genitalia, perineum and major joints
Electrical burns including lightning injuries
Any second or third degree burn with concomitant trauma in which the burn injuries pose the greatest risk to the patient
Burns with inhalation injury
Patients with preexisting medical disorders that could adversely effect patient care and outcome
Hospitals without qualified personnel or equipment for the care of critically burned children

surface area (TBSA) which is burned.[1,4,9] Children must have additional fluid for maintenance.[14]

Taking into account the increased evaporative water loss in the formula for fluid resuscitation for pediatric patients, the initial resuscitation should begin with 5000 ml/m²/% TBSA burned/day + 2000 ml/m²/BSA total/day 5% dextrose in Ringer's lactate. This formula calls for one-half of the total amount to be given in the first 8 hours post-injury with the remainder given over the following 16 hours (**Table 4.2**).[14]

All resuscitation formulas are designed to serve as a guide only. The response to fluid administration and physiologic tolerance of a

Table 4.2 Burn fluid resuscitation formula

Fluid administration – Ringer's lactate
First 24 hours: 5000 ml/m² burn + 2000 ml/body area m²; administer half in 8 hours and the remaining half in 16 hours
Second 24 hours: 3750 ml/m² + 1500 ml/body area m² administer half in 8 hours and the remaining half in 16 hours
Adjust the above rates to maintain a urine output of 1 ml/kg/h

patient is the most important determinant. Additional fluids are commonly needed with inhalation injury, electrical burns, associated trauma, and delayed resuscitation. The appropriate resuscitation regimen administers the minimal amount of fluid necessary for maintenance of vital organ perfusion; the subsequent response of the patient over time will dictate if more or less fluids are needed so that the rate of fluid administration can be adjusted accordingly. Inadequate resuscitation can cause diminished perfusion of renal and mesenteric vascular beds. Fluid overload can produce undesired pulmonary or cerebral edema.

Urine Output Requirements

The single best monitor of fluid replacement is urine output. Acceptable hydration is indicated by a urine output of more than 30 ml/h in an adult (0.5 ml/kg/h) and 1 ml/kg/h in a child. Diuretics are generally not indicated during an acute resuscitation period. Patients with high voltage electrical burns and crush injuries with myoglobin and/or hemoglobin in the urine have an increased risk of renal tubular obstruction. Sodium bicarbonate should be added to IV fluids in order to alkalinize the urine, and urine output should be maintained at 1–2 ml/kg/h as long as these pigments are in the urine.[1,4] The addition of an osmotic diuretic such as mannitol may also be needed to assist in clearing the urine of these pigments.

Additional Assessments and Treatments

Decompression of stomach

To combat the problem of gastric ileus, a nasogastric tube should be inserted in all patients with major burns in order to decompress the stomach. This is especially important for patients being transported at high altitudes.[13] Additionally, all patients should be restricted from taking anything by mouth until after the transfer has been completed. Decompression of the stomach is usually necessary because an anxious, apprehensive patient will swallow considerable amounts of air and distend the stomach. Narcotics also diminish peristalsis of the gastrointestinal tract and result in distension.

A patient must be kept warm and dry. Hypothermia is detrimental to traumatized patients and can be avoided or at least minimized by the use of blankets. Wet dressings should be avoided.

The degree of pain experienced initially by the burn victim is inversely proportional to the severity of the injury.[8] No medication for pain relief should be given intramuscularly or subcutaneously. For mild pain, aspirin 650 mg orally every 4–6 hours may be given. For severe pain, morphine, 1–4 mg intravenously every 2–4 hours, is the drug of choice, although meperidine (Demerol) 10–40 mg by intravenous push every 2–4 hours may be used.[10] Recommendations for tetanus prophylaxis are based on the condition of the wound and the patient's immunization history. All patients with burns >10% TBSA should receive 0.5 ml of tetanus toxoid. If prior immunization is absent or unclear, or if the last booster was more than 10 years ago, 250 units of tetanus immunoglobulin is also given.[4]

Transportation Guidelines

The primary purpose of any transport team is not to bring a patient to an intensive care unit but to bring that level of care to the patient as soon as possible. Therefore, the critical time involved in a transport scenario is the time it takes to get the team to the patient. The time involved in transporting a patient back to a burn center becomes secondary. Communication and teamwork are the keynotes to an effective transport system.

When transportation is required from a referring facility to a specialized burn center, a patient can be fairly well stabilized before being moved. Initially, the referring facility should be informed that all patient referrals require physician-to-physician discussion. Pertinent information needed will include patient demographic data; time, date, cause and extent of burn injury; weight and height; baseline vital signs; neurological status; laboratory data; respiratory status; previous medical and surgical history; and allergies.

A referring hospital is informed of specific treatment protocols regarding patient management prior to transfer. To ensure patient stability the following guidelines are offered:

- Establish two IV sites, preferably in an unburned upper extremity, and secure IV tubes with sutures.
- Insert a foley catheter and monitor for acceptable urine output (30 ml/h adult, 1 ml/kg/h child).
- Insert a nasogastric tube and ensure that the patient remains NPO.
- Maintain body temperature between 38 and 39.0°C rectally.
- Stop all narcotics.
- For burns less than 24 hours old, only use lactated Ringer's solution. The staff physician will advise on the infusion rate which is calculated based on the percentage of total body surface area which is burned.

Following physician-to-physician contact and collection of all pertinent information, the physicians will make recommendations regarding an appropriate mode of transportation. The options are based on distance to a referring unit, patient complexity, and comprehensiveness of medical care required. Options include:

- Full medical intensive care unit transport with a complete team, consisting of a physician, a nurse, and a respiratory therapist from the burn facility.
- Medical intensive care transport via fixed wing or helicopter with a team from a referring facility.
- Private plane with medical personnel to attend patient.
- Commercial airline.
- Private ground ambulance.
- Transport van with appropriate personnel.

Transport Team Composition

Because stabilization and care for a burn patient is so specialized, team selection is of the utmost importance. Traditionally, these patients were placed in an ambulance with an emergency medical technician and transported with few efforts made to stabilize the patient prior to transfer. As levels of care and technology have evolved, the need for specialized transport personnel has been increasingly observed. Today most transport teams are made up of one or more of the following health care members: a registered nurse, a respiratory therapist, and/or a staff physician or house resident. Because a large number of burned patients require some type of respiratory support due to inhalation injury or carbon monoxide intoxication, the respiratory therapist and nurse team has proven to be an effective combination. The background and training of nurses and therapists differ in many ways, so such a team provides a larger scope of knowledge and experience when both are utilized. Team members ideally should be cross-trained so that each member can function at the other's level of expertise.

Training and Selection

Since the transport team will work in a high stress environment, often with life or death consequences, these individuals must be carefully selected. The selection process should involve interviews with a nursing administrator, a director of respiratory therapy, and a medical director of a transport program.

Minimum requirements for transport team members should include:

1. Transport nurse qualifications:
    - a registered nurse;
    - minimum of 6 months burn care experience;
    - current cardiopulmonary resuscitation (CPR) certification;
    - advanced cardiac life support (ACLS) or pediatric advanced life support (PALS) certification;
    - able to demonstrate clinical competency;

- observe two transports;
- a valid passport for international response.

2. Transport respiratory therapist qualifications:
   - Registered/certified respiratory therapist with 6 months burn care experience;
   - licensed by appropriate regulatory agency as a respiratory care practitioner;
   - have current CPR certification;
   - have ACLS or PALS certification;
   - able to demonstrate clinical competency;
   - observe two transports;
   - demonstrate a working knowledge of transport equipment;
   - a valid passport for international response.

Because all of the care rendered by a transport team outside a hospital is given as an extension of care from a transporting/receiving facility, specific steps must be taken to protect staff and physicians from medical liability and to provide consistent care for all patients. Strict protocols are used to guide all patient care; team members should be in constant communication with an attending physician regarding a patient's condition and the interventions to be considered. Team members must be proficient at a number of procedures which may be needed during transport or while stabilizing a patient prior to transport. To keep up with current technology and changes, team members should be included in discussions of recent transports and current management techniques, so that they can discuss patient care issues, receive ongoing in-service education, and participate in a review of the quality of transports.

Modes of Transportation

Once the need for transport of a burned patient is established, the decision must be rendered concerning what type of transportation vehicle is to be used (**Table 4.3**). There are two modes of transport commonly used: ground (ambulance/transport vehicle), air (helicopter, fixed wing), or a combination of both. Factors to be considered when selecting a mode of transportation are the condition of the patient and the distance involved. The level of the severity of the burn mandates the speed with which the team must arrive in order to stabilize and transport a patient.[15]

Ground transport

Ground transport should be considered to cover distances of 70 miles or less; however, sometimes a patient's condition may require air transport, particularly helicopter transport, even though the distance is within the 70 mile range. The ground transport vehicle should be modified with special equipment needed for intensive care transport, and there must be enough room to comfortably seat team members and equipment.

Air transport

Air transport is used primarily when long distances or the critical nature of an injury separate a team from a patient. Air transport, however, does present its own unique set of problems. Aviation physiology is a specialty unto itself, and the gas laws play an important role in air transport and must be taken into consideration.

Table 4.3 Transport criteria: Mode and team composition, burns ≤ 6 days postburn

Weight	% Burn	Distance (miles)	Team*	Transport mode
≤3	Any	75	C	Van, helicopter
		76–250	C	Turboprop airplane
		≥251	C	Learjet
3.1–20	≤10	75	N-RT	Van, helicopter
		76–500	N-RT	Commercial flight or turboprop airplane
		≥501	N-RT	Commercial airplane or Learjet
	≥10	75	C	Van, helicopter
		76–250	C	Turboprop airplane
		≥251	C	Learjet
20≥20	≤20	75	N	Commercial flight or turboprop airplane
		76–500	N-RT	
		≥501	N-RT	Commercial airplane or Learjet
	≥20	75	N	Van, helicopter
		76–500	C	Turboprop plane
		≥501	C	Jet

*C, Complete team (doctor, nurse, respiratory therapist); N, nurse; RT, respiratory therapist.
If any of the following criteria exist, the transport shall be changed to the fastest mode with a complete team:
- depressed mental status,
- drug depression,
- respiratory support,
- unstable cardiovascular system,
- presence of associated diseases,
- decreased urine output unresponsive to appropriate fluid administration,
- absent or marginal venous access,
- hypothermia unresponsive to corrective measures.

Dalton's law states that in a mixture of gases, the total pressure exerted by the mixture is equal to the sum of the pressures each would exert alone.[16] This is important when changing a patient's altitude because as altitude increases, barometric pressure decreases. The percentages of nitrogen, oxygen and carbon dioxide remain the same, but the partial pressures they exert change (**Table 4.4**).[17]

Altitude is an important factor in the oxygenation of a transported patient and constant monitoring by a team is required under such circumstances. Boyle's law states that the volume of gas is inversely proportional to the pressure to which it is subject at a constant temperature. This gas law significantly affects patients with air leaks and free air in the abdomen because as altitude increases, the volume of air in closed cavities also increases.[18] For this reason, all air which can be reached should be evacuated prior to an increase in altitude. Intrathoracic air and gastric air must be

Table 4.4 Altitude's effects on blood gas values

Altitude	Pressure	Tracheal Po_2	Alveolar Po_2	Alveolar Pco_2
Sea level	760	149	103	40
5000 feet	632	122	79	38
10 000 feet	523	100	61	36
15 000 feet	429	80	46	33
20 000 feet	349	63	33	30

removed via functional chest tubes or nasogastric tubes and periodically checked during transport. Other factors which should be considered during air transport are reduced cabin pressure, turbulence, noise and vibration, changes in barometric pressure, and acceleration/deceleration forces. Physiologic changes which affect a patient and team members include middle ear dysfunction, pressure-related problems with sinuses, air expansion in a gastrointestinal tract and motion sickness. Utilizing transport vehicles which have pressurized cabins can reduce or eliminate most of these problems.[19]

Helicopters and fixed wing aircraft

Helicopters and fixed wing aircraft both have advantages and disadvantages related to patient care. Helicopters are widely used for short distance medical air transport. Medical helicopters, because they are usually based on hospital premises, have no need to use airport facilities or ambulance services and, thereby, reduce team response time. Helicopters are able to land close to a referring hospital. Additionally, helicopters provide ease in loading and unloading patients and equipment.[15] The disadvantages of helicopter transport include its limited range, usually less than 150 miles[20] and its nonpressurized cabin which limits the altitude at which patients can be safely carried. The low altitude capabilities also subject the aircraft to variability in weather (i.e fog, rain, reduced visibility); therefore, helicopter flights experience much more interference due to weather. Other disadvantages include noise, vibrations, reduced air speed, small working space, lower weight accommodation, and high maintenance requirements.[15]

When long distances must be traveled (greater than 150 miles) or when increased altitude is necessary, fixed wing aircraft are considered as a viable mode of transport for patients. The advantages of using fixed wing aircraft include: long range capabilities, increased speed, ability to fly in most weather conditions, control of cabin pressure and temperature, larger cabin space, and more liberal weight restrictions. Disadvantages of fixed wing aircraft include the need for an airport with adequate runway length, difficulty in loading and unloading patients and equipment, and the pressure of air turbulence and noise.

EQUIPMENT

Because medical equipment used in intensive care units has evolved tremendously in the last 10 years, there is no reason that these advances should not be extended to the equipment which is used in a transport program. **Tables 4.5** and **4.6** outline the drugs and equipment which are used in our successful transport system. The transport team must be able to provide ICU level care whenever needed. Most hospitals are well stocked and able to provide necessary supplies for initial patient stabilization and resuscitation; however, specialty items relating to the care of burn patients may not be present or adequate to meet the needs of burn victims. It is imperative that adequate equipment be available to handle any situation which may arise during a transport process (**Figure 4.4**). Extra battery packs and electrical converters on fixed wing aircraft are recommended due to long transport times and delays caused by unforseeable circumstances of weather or logistics.

Portable Monitor

A portable ECG monitor capable of monitoring two pressure channels should accompany all patients in transport. This allows for continuous monitoring of heart rate, rhythm, and arterial blood

Table 4.5 Medical equipment used in a transport system

Monitor bag	Quantity
Pressure bag	1
EKG cable	1
Pressure cable	2
Oxygen saturation cables	2
Oxygen saturation probes	2
Stapler	1
Staple remover	1
Stethoscope	1
EKG pads (adult/pedi)	9 each
Blood pressure tubing (NIBP)	1
Safe-cuff (NIBP – various sizes)	1 each
Automatic blood pressure cuffs	1 each
Temperature cable – Foley	1
Temperature probe – rectal	1
Thermometer	1
Thermometer covers	1 Box
Defibrillator jell tube	1
Sphygmomanometer	1
GI/GU bag	
Salem sumps (10,12,14,16fr)	1 each
Feeding tube 8fr	1
Surgilube	5
Clean gloves	20
Umbilical tape	1 jar
60ml catheter tip syringe	2
Guaiac cards	10
Guaiac reagent	1 bottle
Diastix	1 bottle
Benzoin swabs	5
Cal stat	1 bottle
Tongue blades	10
Cotton swabs	10
Foley's temp. (8,10,12,16fr)	1 each
Sterile gloves	10
pH paper	1
Respiratory equipment	
Resuscitation bag adult/pedi	1 each
Oxygen mask adult/pedi	1 eacg
Venturi mask adult/pedi	1 each
T-Tube adapters	2
CPR microshield	1
Cricothyrotomy catheter sets	1
Tracheostomy tubes (00–8.0)	1 each
Endotracheal tubes (3.0–8.0)	2 each
Laryngoscope handles (1g.sm.)	2 each
Laryngoscope blades (Miller – sizes 0–4)	1 each
Laryngoscope blades (MacIntosh – sizes 0–4)	2
Magill forceps adult/pedi	1
Stylets adult/pedi	1
Airways (sm, med, lg)	1
PEEP valves	2
Wright respirometer	1
Pleural drainage set	1
Heimlick valves	2
Siemens Minimed III	1
Defibrillator	1
Batteries (C & D)	4 each
Prepodyne swabs	4
Skin degreaser	1 bottle
Nebulizer kit	2
1″ tape roll	1
Nipple adapters	2
E cylinder regulator	2
E cylinder wrench	2
Suction catheters (8–14fr)	5 each
Suction pump	1
Hard tip suction device	1
Adapters (15 & 22MM)	2 each
Normal saline vials	10
Vaponephrine solution	1 bottle
Goggles	1
Clean gloves	10
Humid vent adapters	2
Oxygen tanks aluminum	6
Oxygen tubing	2
Transport ventilator	1
Protocol Propag 106	1
Defibrillator battery support system	1

Table 4.6 Burn transport supply list

Medications	Quantity	Medications	Quantity
Epinephrine	2	Compazine	2
Atropine sulfate	2	Hep-Lock flush	5
Sodium bicarbonate	2	Heparin	1
Calcium chloride	2	Lidocaine	
D50	2	(injectable/cardiac strip)	1
Lidocaine	2	Narcan	4
Bretylol	2	Albumin	2
Isoproterenol	2	Regular insulin	1
Dopamine	4	Benadryl	4
Dobutrex	2	Chloral hydrate suppository	2
Calcium gluconate	2	Chloral hydrate 500 mg/10 ml	2
Lasix	10	Tylenol 650 mg/25 ml	2
Potassium chloride	4	Tylenol suppository	2
Ranitidine	2	Lacri-Lube tube	2
Benadryl (injectable)	4	Maalox	1
Polysporin ointment	2	Phenergan	2
Travase ointment	2	Thorazine	2
Medical equipment	**Quantity**	**Medical equipment**	**Quantity**
IV bag 1			
D5.3NS 1000 ml	2	Needle holder	1
D10W 500 ml	1	Hemostat	1
Lactated Ringer's solution	2	0-silk suture	3
48″ Pressure tubing	2	Staples (10, 11, 15)	1
IV start pack	2	Solution sets (10 gtts/ml)	2
T-piece	4	Solution sets (60 gtts/ml)	2
Stopcocks	4	Minimed full set	2
Y-ports	2	Minimed half set	2
Scissors	1	Betadine (bottle)	1
IV bag 2			
D5W 250 ml	2	Syringes (1, 3, 5, 10, 35 ml)	10 each
Normal saline 250 ml	2	Needles (22g, 20g, 19g, 16g)	10 each
Pressure transducers	2	IV catheters (16g, 18g, 20g, 22g)	6 each
60 ml Luer-lock syringe	2	Medicuts (18g, 20g, 22g)	1 each
Side pouch			
Kerlix 6″	10	Burn dressing (lg)	2
Ace wraps (6″, 4″, 3″)	6 each	1″ tape roll	1
Space blanket	1	2″ tape roll	1
Urometer	1	4 × 4's (box)	2

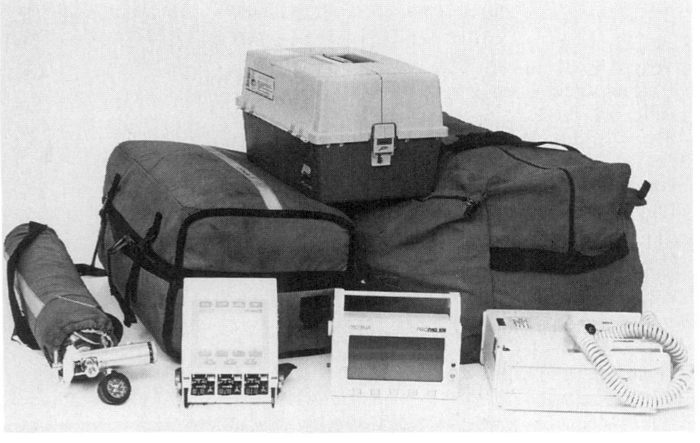

Fig. 4.4 Typical equipment used in transport of a patient.

pressure. The second pressure channel may be used for patients with a pulmonary artery catheter or those who need intracranial pressure monitoring. This monitor should be small and lightweight but able to provide a display bright enough to be seen from several feet away. The monitor should have its own rechargeable power supply which continuously charges while connected to an alternating current (AC) power supply. One suitable unit is the Protocol Systems Propaq 106 portable monitor (**Figure 4.5**). This monitor has two pressure channels; it provides a continuous display of ECG, heart rate, systolic, diastolic, and mean blood pressure; it can display temperature and oxygen saturation; and it is also capable of operating a noninvasive blood pressure cuff. High and low alarms for each monitored parameter can be set, silenced, or disabled by a trained operator.

Infusion Pump

Continuous delivery of fluids and pharmacological agents must not be interrupted during transport. Infusion pumps can be easily attached to stretchers and are usually capable of operating for several hours on internal batteries. These devices should have alarms to warn of infusion problems and should be as small and lightweight as possible (**Figure 4.6**).

Ventilator

Size, weight, and oxygen consumption are the primary concerns in selecting transport ventilators. A weight under 5 pounds (2.2 kg) is desirable, and a ventilator's dimensions should make it easy to

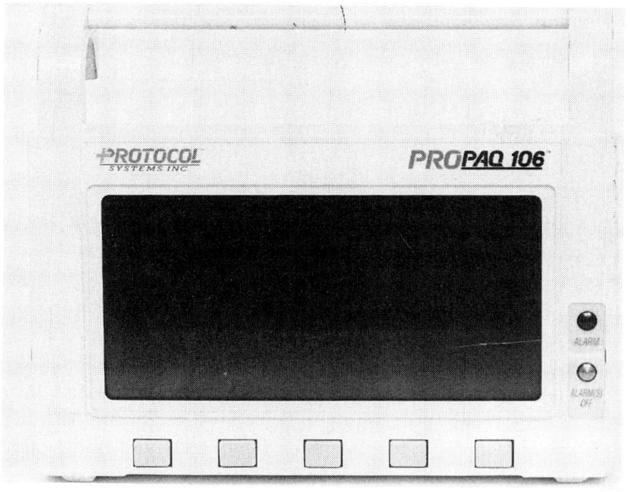

Fig. 4.5 Portable ECG monitor used in transport.

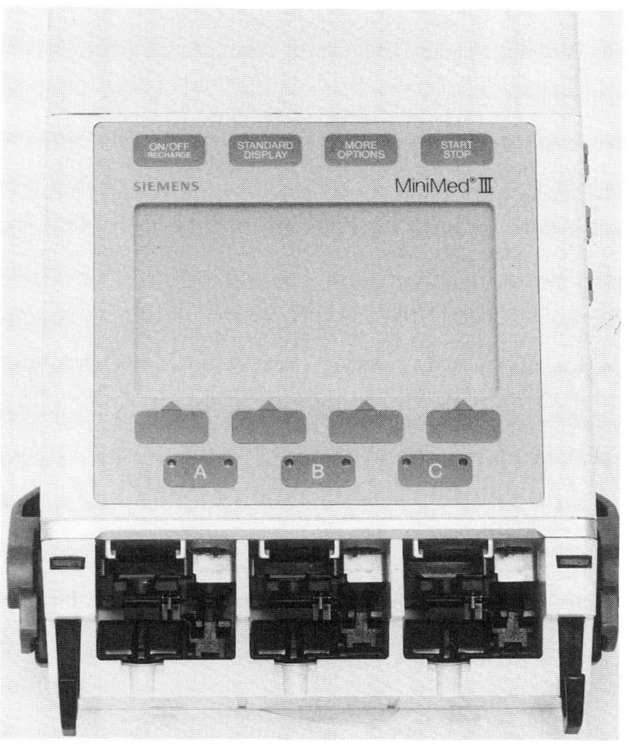

Fig. 4.6 Portable IV pump used in transport.

mount or to place on a bed. Orientation of controls should be along a single plane, and inadvertent movement of dials should be difficult.[21] The ventilator breathing circuit and exhalation valve should be kept simple, and incorrect assembly should be impossible. The Hamilton MAX (**Figure 4.7**) ventilator is acceptable for transport purposes and easy to use. This ventilator is a pressure or flow controller which can be time-, pressure-, or manually triggered, pressure or flow-limited, and time- or pressure-cycled. It is pneumatically and electronically powered and allows both electronic and pneumatic controls. The ventilator allows an operator to set tidal volume (V_T) and frequency; and it also allows a manual breath to be delivered. The MAX operates in the intermittent mandatory ventilation (IMV) mode. Respiratory rate is adjusted from 2 to 30 breaths/min, and the inspiratory time is fixed at 1 second. Tidal volume is adjustable from 50 to 1500 ml with an inspiratory flow from 30 to 90 liters/minute.[22]

STABILIZATION

One of the primary reasons for a specialized transport team is to be able to transport a patient in as stable condition as possible. Current practice has evolved to embrace the concept that events during the first few hours following burn injury may affect the eventual outcome of the patient; this is especially true with regard to fluid management and inhalation injury. Stabilization techniques performed by the transport team have been expanded to include procedures which are usually not performed by nursing or respiratory personnel. Such techniques include interpreting radiographs and laboratory results and then conferring with fellow team members, referring physicians, and the team's own medical staff in order to arrive at a diagnosis and plan for stabilization. The transport team may perform such procedures as venous cannulation, endotracheal intubation, arterial blood gas interpretation, and management of mechanical ventilators. Team members may request new radiographs, in order to assess catheter or endotracheal tube placement or to assess the pulmonary system's condition. Team members may aid in the diagnosis of air leaks (pneumothorax) and evacuate the pleural space of the lung by needle aspiration as indicated. All of these procedures may be immediately necessary and lifesaving. Cross-training of all team members to be able to perform the others' jobs is recommended in order to safeguard patients in the event that any team member becomes incapacitated during transport. All these skills can be learned via experience in a burn intensive care unit, through formal training seminars, and via a thorough orientation program. Mature judgment, excellent clinical skills, and the ability to function under stress are characteristics needed when selecting candidates for a transport program.

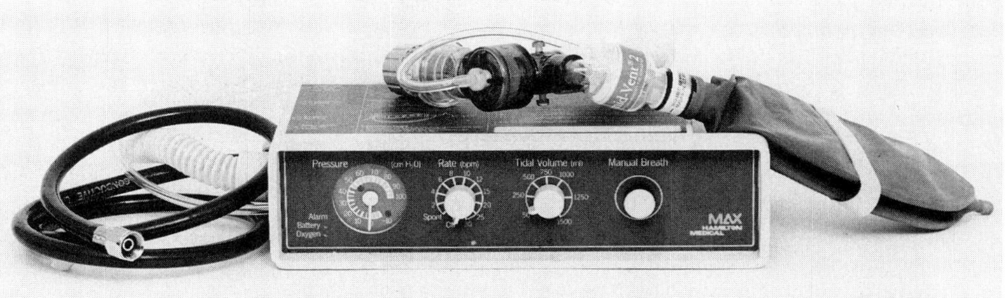

Fig. 4.7 Transport ventilator.

Patient Assessment Prior to Transport to a Specialized Burn Care Unit from a Referring Hospital

Initial assessment upon arrival of a flight team should include a list of standard procedures for determining a burned patient's current condition. First, a thorough review of the patient's history concerning the accident and past medical history must be done. This process provides the transport team with an excellent base from which to begin to formulate a plan of action. The patient will certainly have been diagnosed by a referring physician; however, a transport team often finds problems overlooked in initial evaluations. Since burn care is a specialized field, modes of treatment may vary greatly outside the burn treatment community. Frequently, a referring hospital is not well versed in the treatment of burn victims and should not be expected to display the expertise found among clinicians who work with such patients every day. Thus, the next step in stabilizing a burn patient is a physical assessment done by a transport team. These procedures should always be performed in the same order and in a structured fashion. Assessment of a burn patient begins with the ABCs of a primary survey, including airway, breathing, circulation, cervical spine immobilization, and a brief baseline neurological examination. All patients should be placed on supplemental oxygen prior to transport in order to minimize the effects of altitude changes on oxygenation. Two intravenous lines should be started peripherally with a 16 gauge catheter or larger. Ideally, IV lines should be placed in non-burn areas but may be placed through a burn if they are the only sites available for cannulation. Intravenous lines should be sutured in place because venous access may not be available after the onset of generalized edema. The fluid of choice for initial resuscitation is lactated Ringer's solution.

In addition to initial stabilization procedures, blood should be obtained for initial laboratory studies if not already done. Initial diagnostic studies should include hematocrit, electrolytes, urinalysis, chest x-ray, arterial blood gas and carboxyhemoglobin levels. Any correction of laboratory values must be done prior to transfer and verified with repeat studies. Electrocardiographic monitoring should be instituted on any patient prior to transfer. Electrode patches may be a problem to place because the adhesive will not stick to burned skin. If alternate sites for placement cannot be found, an option for monitoring is to insert skin staples and attach the monitor leads to them with alligator clips. This provides a stable monitoring system, particularly for the agitated or restless patient who may displace needle electrodes. A Foley catheter with a urimeter should be placed to accurately monitor urine output. Acceptable hydration is indicated by a urine output of more than 30 ml/h in an adult (5 ml/kg/h) and at least 1 ml/kg/h in a child.

With the exception of escharotomies, open chest wounds, and actively bleeding wounds, management during transport consists of simply covering wounds with a topical antimicrobial agent or a biological dressing. Wet dressings are contraindicated because of the decreased thermoregulatory capacity of patients sustaining large burns and the possibility of hypothermia. To combat the problem of a gastric ileus, a nasogastric tube should be inserted in all burn patients in order to decompress the stomach. This is especially important for patients being transported at high altitudes. Hypothermia can be avoided or minimized by the use of heated blankets and/or aluminized mylar space blankets. The patient's rectal temperature must be kept between 37.5 and 39.0 °C.

A clear, concise, chronological record of the mechanism of injury and assessment of airway, breathing, and circulation should be kept in the field and en route to the hospital. This information is vital for a referring facility to better understand and anticipate the condition of the patient. Additionally, all treatment, including invasive procedures, must be recorded, along with a patient's response to these interventions.

Summary

Burn injuries present a major challenge to a health care team, but an orderly, systematic approach can simplify stabilization and management. A clear understanding of the pathophysiology of burn injuries is essential for providing quality burn care in the pre-hospital setting, at the receiving health care facility, and at the referring hospital prior to transport. After a patient has been rescued from an injury-causing agent, assessment of the burn victim begins with a primary survey. Life-threatening injuries must be treated first, followed by a secondary survey which documents and treats other injuries or problems. Intravenous access may be established in concert with local/regional medical control and appropriate fluid resuscitation begun. Burn wounds should be covered with clean, dry sheets; and the patient should be kept warm with blankets to prevent hypothermia. The patient should be transported to an emergency room in the most appropriate mode available.

At the local hospital, it should be determined if a burn patient needs burn center care according to the American Burn Association Guidelines. In preparing for and organizing a transfer of a burn victim, consideration must be given to the continued monitoring and management of the patient during transport. In transferring burn patients, the same priorities developed for pre-hospital management remain valid. During initial assessment and treatment and throughout transport, the transport team must ensure that the patient has an adequate airway, breathing, circulation, fluid resuscitation, urine output, and pain control. Ideally, transport of burn victims will occur through an organized, protocol-driven plan which includes specialized transport mechanisms and personnel. Successful transport of burn victims, whether in the pre-hospital phase or during interhospital transfer, requires careful attention to treatment priorities, protocols, and details.

References

1. Boswick J A, ed. *The Art and Science of Burn Care*. Rockville, MD: Aspen Publishers, 1987.

2. Dimick A R. Triage of burn patients. In: Wachtel T L, Kahn V, Franks H A, eds. *Currents Topics in Burn Care*. Rockville, MD: Aspen Systems, 1983: 15–18.

3. Wachtel T L. Initial care of major burns. Postgrad Med 1989; **85**(1): 178–96.

4. Nebraska Burn Institute. *Advanced Burn Life Support Providers Manual*, Lincoln, NE: Nebraska Burn Institute, 1987.

5. Nebraska Burn Institute. Radiation injury. *Advanced Burn Life Support Manual*. Appendix 1 Lincoln, NE: Nebraska Burn Institute, 1987.

6. Bartholome C W, Jacoby W D. Cutaneous manifestations of lightning injury. *Arch Dermatol* 1975; **26:** 1466–8.

7. Committee on Trauma, American College of Surgeons. Burns. In: *Advanced Trauma Life Support Course Book*. Chicago: American College of Surgeons, 1984: 155–63.

8. Rauscher L A, Ochs G M. Pre-hospital care of the seriously burned patient. In: Wachtel T L, Kahn V, Franks H A, eds *Current Topics in Burn Care*. Rockville, MD: Aspen Systems, 1983: 1–9.

9. Goldfarb J W. The burn patient, Air Medical Crew National Standards Curriculum, Phoenix, 1988, ASHBEAMS.

10. Marvin J A, Heinback D M. Pain control during the intensive care phase of burn care. *Crit Care Clin* 1985; **1:** 147–57.

11. Mlcak R P, Helvick B. Protocol for securing endotracheal tubes in a pediatric burn unit. *J. Burn Care* 1987; **8:** 233–7.

12. Herndon D, *et al*: Desai, M H, Abston, S. *Residents Manual.* Galveston: Shriners Burns Institute, and the University of Texas Medical Branch, 1992: 1–17.

13. Collini F J, Kealy G P. Burns: a review and update. *Contemp Surg* 1989; **34:** 75–7.

14. Herndon D, Rutan: R, Rutan T. The management of burned children. *J. Burn Care Rehabil* 1993; **14:** 3–8.

15. Roy L R, Cunningham W. Transport. *Neonatal and Pediatric Respiratory Care.* St Louis: CV Mosby Company, 1988: 321.

16. McPhearson S P. *Respiratory Therapy Equipment.* 3rd ed. St Louis: CV Mosby Company, 1986.

17. *US Navy Flight Surgeons' Manual.* Government publication, 1968.

18. Jacobs B. *Emergency Patient Care, Pre-hospital Ground and Air Procedures.* New York: Macmillan, 1983.

19. McNeil E L. *Airborne Care of the Ill and Injured.* New York: Springer–Verlag, 1983.

20. *Federal Regulations for Pilots.* Government publication, 1987.

21. Branson R D. Intrahospital transport of critically ill; mechanical ventilation of patients. *Resp Care* 1992; **37:** 775–93.

22. Johanningman J A, Branson R D, Cambell R S, Hurst J M. Laboratory and clinical evaluation of the Max transport ventilator. *Resp Care* 1990; **35:** 952–9.

CHAPTER FIVE

Pathophysiology of Burn Shock and Burn Edema

George C. Kramer and Thuan T. Nguyen

Introduction and Historical Notes

Cutaneous thermal injury greater than 35–40% of total body surface area (TBSA) invariably results in the severe and unique derangements of cardiovascular function called burn shock. Shock is defined as an abnormal physiologic state in which the flow of blood is insufficient to maintain adequate nutritive perfusion at the capillary level. Before the nineteenth century, ineffective procedures such as bleeding and purging were advocated for severe burns.[1] During the nineteenth century, the development of bacteriology suggested the importance of combating and avoiding infection.[1] It was also demonstrated that after a burn, fluid was lost from blood so that the blood became thicker; and in 1897, saline infusions were first advocated for severe burns.[2] However, a real understanding of burn pathophysiology was not reached until the work of Frank Underhill.[3] He demonstrated that unresuscitated burn shock correlated with the greatly increased hematocrits of burned patients, which are secondary to fluid and electrolyte loss after burn injury. Increased hematocrit values soon after severe burns were thereafter interpreted as a plasma volume deficit. Cope and Moore[4] showed that the hypovolemia of burn injury resulted from fluid and protein translocation into burned and nonburned tissues.

Through the twentieth century, the importance of fluid resuscitation for burn shock has been established by both animal and clinical studies. Investigations have focused on the rapid and massive fluid sequestration in the burn wound and the resultant hypovolemia. We now have an extensive experimental database on the circulatory and microcirculatory alterations associated with burn shock and edema in both the burn wound and nonburned tissues. Most recently, research has focused on identifying and defining the release mechanisms and the effects of the many inflammatory mediators produced and released after burn injury.

It is now recognized that burn shock is a complex process of circulatory and microcirculatory dysfunction, not easily or fully repaired by fluid resuscitation. Severe burn injury results in significant hypovolemic shock and tissue trauma, both of which cause the formation and release of many local and systemic mediators.[5–7] Burn shock results from the interplay of hypovolemia and mediator action and continues as a significant pathophysiologic state, even if hypovolemia is corrected. Increases in pulmonary and systemic vascular resistance, together with myocardial depression, occur despite adequate preload and volume support.[7–11] These physiologic changes can further exacerbate the whole body inflammatory response into a vicious cycle of accelerating organ dysfunction.[6,7,12]

This chapter examines our present understanding of the pathophysiology of the early events in burn shock, focusing on the many facets of organ and systemic effects directly resulting from the hypovolemia and circulating mediators. Inflammatory shock mediators, both local and systemic, that are implicated in the pathogenesis of burn shock include histamine, serotonin, kinins, oxygen free radicals, products of the eicosanoid acid cascade, prostaglandins, thromboxanes and interleukins. Additionally, certain hormones and mediators of cardiovascular function are elevated severalfold after burn injury; these include epinephrine, norepinephrine, vasopressin, angiotensin II, and neuropeptide Y. Understanding the complex mechanism of the pathophysiologic actions of these mediators is necessary before optimally effective therapies can be designed. The hope is that better early treatment of burn shock, perhaps through mediator blockade, can be developed to ameliorate or eliminate the incidence of developing organ dysfunction. Effective burn resuscitation and treatment of burn shock remain major challenges in modern medicine.

Hypovolemia and Rapid Edema Formation

Burn shock is, first, hypovolemic shock and is characterized by hemodynamic changes similar to those that occur after hemorrhage, including decreased plasma volume, cardiac output, urine output, and an increased systemic vascular resistance with resultant reduced peripheral blood flow[5,7,13–15] As in the treatment of other forms of hypovolemic shock, the primary initial therapeutic goal is to promptly restore vascular volume and preserve tissue perfusion in order to minimize tissue ischemia. However, burn resuscitation is complicated not only by severe burn wound edema but also by severe and sustained edema in nonburned soft tissues that is unique to thermal trauma. Large volumes of resuscitation solutions are required to maintain vascular volume during the first few hours after a large burn. The rapid edema formation and weight gain slows during the first few hours, but can continue for the first 24 hours.[15,16]

By definition, edema develops when the rate by which fluid is filtered out of the microvessels exceeds the flow in the lymph vessels draining the same tissue mass. The edema formation appears to follow a biphasic pattern. An immediate and rapid increase in the water of burn tissue is seen in the first hour after injury.[14,16] A second and more gradual increase in fluid flux of both burned skin and nonburned soft tissue follows the first 12–24 hours after burn.[6,16] The amount of edema formation in burned skin depends on the type and extent of injury[14,17] and whether fluid resuscitation is given.[18] Without sustained fluid infusion, the edema fluid is somewhat self-limited as plasma volume and capillary pressure decrease. During resuscitation, however, maintenance of blood volume, blood flow, and capillary pressure can continue to cause fluid extravasation. The edema development in thermally injured skin is characterized by an extremely rapid onset and can double the tissue water content within the first hour after burn.[14,19] Leape[15,20,21] found a 70–80% increase in water content of a full-thickness burn wound in 30 minutes with 90% of this change occurring in the first 5 minutes. There was little increase in burn wound water after the first hour in these nonresuscitated animals. In resuscitated animals or animals with small wounds, adequate tissue perfusion continues to 'feed' the edema for several hours. Demling *et al.*[16] used dichromatic absorptionmetry to measure edema development during the first week after an experimental partial-thickness burn injury on one hind limb in sheep. Although edema was rapid, with over half occurring in the first hour, maximum water content did not occur until 12–24 hours after burn.

Normal Microcirculatory Fluid Exchange

An understanding of the mechanism of the rapid formation of burn edema requires a review of normal microvascular physiology. Under normal physiologic conditions, the pressure in arterioles and capillaries causes a filtration of fluid into the interstitial space of all tissues. This fluid is then partially reabsorbed into the circulation at the venous end of the capillaries and venules, while the remaining net filtration is removed by lymphatic drainage.[22] Fluid transport across the microcirculatory wall in normal and pathological states is quantitatively described by the Landis–Starling equation:

$$J_v = K_f\,[P_c - P_{if}) - \sigma\,(\Pi_p - \Pi_{if})]$$

This equation describes the physical forces and physiologic mechanisms which govern fluid transfer between vascular and extravascular compartments. J_v is the volume of fluid that crosses the microvasculature barrier; K_f is the capillary filtration coefficient, which is the product of the capillary surface area and the hydraulic conductivity; P_c is the capillary hydrostatic pressure; P_{if} is the interstitial fluid hydrostatic pressure; Π_p is the colloid osmotic pressure of plasma; Π_{if} is the colloid osmotic pressure of interstitial fluid; σ is the osmotic reflection coefficient. Edema occurs when the lymphatic drainage (J_L) does not keep pace with the increased J_v.

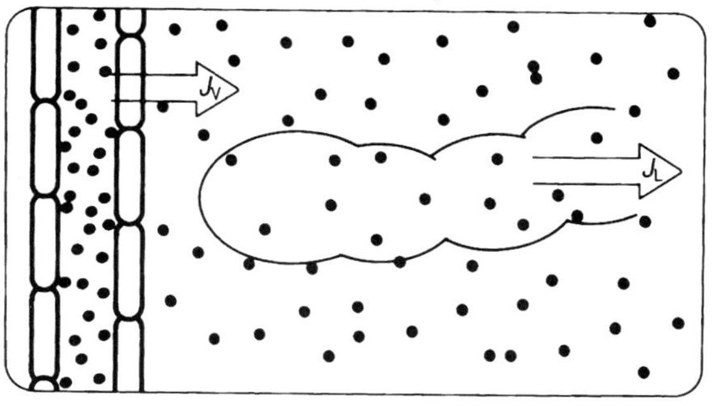

Fig. 5.1 The normal pressures of the Starling equation for skin result in a slight imbalance favoring filtration with lymph flow (J_L) exactly equal to fluid filtration (J_v). In burn skin all Starling factors are increased creating a large net filtration which exceeds lymph flow and causes rapid edema. Data shown represent filtration forces in skin before and after burn injury.

Mechanisms of Burn Edema

By analysing the factors in this equation that govern fluid flux, edema may theoretically be formed by:

- decreased σ;
- increased K_f;
- increased P_c;
- decreased P_{if};
- decreased Π_p; and
- increased Π_{if}.

Burn edema may be unique among other types of edema, since only in burn edema do all of the above variables change significantly in the direction required to increase fluid filtration. Each of the variables is discussed individually.

Capillary Filtration Coefficient (K_f)

Burn injury causes direct and indirect mediator-modulated changes in the barrier properties of the capillary wall, which are reflected as large increases in the transendothelial permeability of both protein and water permeability. Arturson[23] showed that K_f in the scalded hind limb immediately increases two to three times, suggesting that water permeability or hydraulic conductivity of the capillary wall is increased; however, K_f is a function of both hydraulic conductivity and capillary surface area. Thus, local vasodilation and microvascular recruitment will also likely contribute to the increased K_f in addition to an increased hydraulic conductivity. Measuring K_f and the rate of edema formation (J_v) allowed Arturson to calculate the changes in transcapillary pressures required to account for the capillary filtration. Arturson assumed that $\Delta J_L = 0$ in the first 10 minutes after injury. His calculation indicated that transcapillary pressure gradients of 100–250 mmHg occurred in the first 10 minutes after scald. He concluded that only a small fraction of the early formation of burn edema could be attributed to K_f and the changes in permeability. He suggested that osmotically active molecules were released from burn-damaged cells which generated sufficiently large osmotic reabsorption pressures. On the other hand, recent studies described below show that very large increases in filtration force can be directly attributed to changes in P_c and P_{if} in burn-injured skin.

Capillary Pressure (P_c)

In most forms of shock, capillary pressure decreases as a result of arteriolar vasoconstriction. However, studies in which P_c was estimated by vascular occlusion methods, in the scalded hind limb of dogs, showed that P_c doubled to 45–50 mmHg during the first 30 minutes after burn and slowly returned to baseline over 3 hours.[24] We are unaware of studies that have measured P_c in nonburned skin, but it is likely that P_c decreases in nonburned tissues as a result of the documented increase in peripheral resistance.

Interstitial Hydrostatic Pressure (P_{if})

A surprising but well verified recent finding has established that P_{if} in dermis becomes very negative after thermal injury. Using micropipettes and tissue oncometers, Lund[17,25] has demonstrated that dermal P_{if} is reduced from its normal value of −1 mmHg to less than −100 mmHg in isolated skin preparations. *In vivo* measurements show temporary reductions to −20 to −30 mmHg; presumably, this number is less negative because fluid extravasation relieves the imbibition pressure. After resuscitation, P_{if} increases to the slightly positive value of 1–2 mmHg which is usually associated with edema.[25,26] The mechanism of this negative-pressure generation may be related to the denaturation of collagen.[28] These data suggest that the highly negative P_{if}, coupled with increased P_c, are the predominant mechanisms responsible for the rapid development of burn edema.

Osmotic Reflection Coefficient (σ)

The osmotic reflection coefficient is an index of the proportion of the full osmotic pressure generated by plasma proteins that is effectively exerted across the capillary wall. A σ of 1.0 represents a membrane impermeable to protein; a σ of 0 represents a membrane that is completely permeable to protein. In skin, the normal σ of albumin is reported to be between 0.85 and 0.95.[26,27] Reduction of σ is associated with increased protein permeability and would cause an effective reduction in the reabsorptive oncotic gradient across the capillary wall and would increase net fluid filtration. Studies of lymph sampled from burned skin are consistent with large and sustained reductions in capillary permeability,[14,27,28] while a transient increase in capillary permeability over 8–12 hours is indicated in other soft tissues not directly burned.[27] Pitt[24] estimated σ for skin from dog hind paw using the lymph washdown technique and reported a normal σ of 0.87 for albumin and a reduction to 0.45 after scald injury.

Plasma Colloid Osmotic Pressure (Π_p)

The normal plasma protein concentration of 6–8 g/dl and its associated Π of 25–30 mmHg produces a significant transcapillary reabsorptive force limiting fluid filtration out of the microvasculature.[32] Plasma colloid osmotic pressure decreases in non-resuscitated burned animals as a protein-rich fluid extravasates into burn wounds, while a protein-poor transcapillary reabsorption takes place in nonburned tissues.[30–33] Plasma is further diluted and Π_p is further reduced after crystalloid resuscitation. Zetterström and Arturson[30] found that plasma oncotic pressure was reduced to half of the normal values (25–30 mmHg) in burn patients. Π_p can decrease so rapidly with resuscitation that the Π_p–Π_{if} colloid osmotic pressure gradient reverses to actually favor filtration and edema.[33] Although it is likely that some hypoproteinemia after major burn injury is inevitable, it is well established in both animal and clinical studies that early use of colloid can maintain Π_p at higher levels than crystalloid resuscitation alone.[6,31,34] Also, it is clear that the degree of hypoproteinemia and reduced Π_p correlate with the magnitude of edema.[31] Colloid therapy is begun immediately by some clinicians,[6] while others wait 8–24 hours after injury, believing that normalization of soft tissue permeability must occur before colloid is cost effective.[7]

Interstitial Colloid Osmotic Pressure (Π_{if})

The Π_{if} in skin is normally about 10–15 mmHg, or about one-half that of plasma in humans.[29,32] Experimental studies in animals using lymph to sample interstitial fluid show that Π_{if} in burned skin initially increases 4–8 mmHg because of increased permeability.[27] However, more direct measurements of Π_{if} using wick sampling[18,32] or tissue sampling[35] show only modest initial increases in Π_{if} of 1–4 mmHg in the early nonresuscitated phase of burn injury. With resuscitation, Π_p falls and then Π_{if} decreases as the protein concentration of capillary filtrate remains less than plasma despite an increased permeability and a reduced σ. Compared to nonburned skin, Π_{if} remains significantly higher in the burn wound, supporting the view that sustained increases in protein permeability contribute to the persistence of the burn edema.[18,32,35] However, compared with the large changes in P_c and P_{if}, increased capillary protein permeability is not likely to be the predominant mechanism for the early rapid rate of edema formation in burn-injured skin.

Nonburned Tissue

Generalized edema in soft tissue not directly injured is characteristic after a major burn. Brouhard *et al.*[36] reported an increased water content in nonburned skin even after a 10% burn, with the maximum increase occurring at 12 hours. Arturson[14,19,28] reported an increased transcapillary fluid flux (lymph flow) from nonburned tissue, and a transient increase in permeability, as measured in acute animal experiments. Harms[27] extended these findings by measuring changes in lymph flow and protein transport of noninjured soft tissue for 3 days after injury. He found that skin and muscle permeability were elevated for up to 12 hours postburn for molecules the size of albumin and immunoglobulin G, while capillary permeability of the lung's microvascular showed no increase. Maximum increased lymph flow and tissue water content were observed to correlate with the severe hypoproteinemia occurring during the early resuscitation period.[7,34] The sustained increase in water content and the elevated lymph flow of these tissues is probably caused by the sustained hypoproteinemia.[27,31]

Demling and colleagues[37] also postulated that the edema can be partially attributed to an alteration in the interstitium. They suggested that interstitial protein washout increases the compliance of the interstitial space and that water transport and hydraulic conductivity across the entire blood–tissue–lymph barrier are increased with hypoproteinemia. Several clinical and animal studies have established that the overall edema formation can be ameliorated by maintaining more normal protein levels.[6,38] Nonburn edema can also be prevented by using nonprotein colloids such as dextran, if the colloid osmotic gradients are increased above normal.[7,34] After the dextran infusions are discontinued and dextran is cleared from the circulation by the kidneys, over 12–36 hours, the edema again develops, due to the unmasking of the hypoproteinemic state.[7]

ALTERED CELLULAR MEMBRANES AND CELLULAR EDEMA

In addition to a loss of capillary endothelial integrity, thermal injury also causes changes at the membrane level of other cells. Baxter[9] demonstrated that in burns of >30% TBSA, there is a systemic decrease in cellular transmembrane potentials as measured in skeletal muscle away from the site of injury. It would be expected that the directly injured cell would have a damaged cell membrane, increasing sodium and potassium fluxes, resulting in cell swelling. However, this process also appears in cells that are not directly heat-injured. Micropuncture techniques have demonstrated a decrease in the normal cell membrane potential of −90 mV to levels of −70 to −80 mV; cell death occurs at −60 mV. The decrease in membrane potentials is associated with an increase in intracellular water and sodium.[39,40] Similar alterations in membrane functions and cellular edema have been reported in hemorrhagic shock,[39,41] also in liver and endothelial cells.[42,43] Recent data suggest that a circulating shock factor is responsible for the membrane depolarization.[44] Early investigators of this phenomenen postulated that a decrease in ATP levels or ATPase activity was responsible for membrane depolarization. Recent research suggests that it may result from an increased sodium conductance in membranes or an increase in sodium–hydrogen antiport activity.[40,45] Resuscitation of hemorrhage rapidly restores depolarized membrane potentials to normal, but resuscitation of burn injury only partially restores the membrane potential and intracellular sodium concentrations to normal levels, demonstrating that hypovolemia with its attendant ischemia is not totally responsible for the cellular swelling seen in burn shock.[46] Very little is known about the time course of the changes in membrane potential in clinical burns. More importantly, we do not know the extent to which altered membrane potentials affect organ function in burn injury or shock in general.

MEDIATORS OF BURN INJURY

Several local and circulating mediators are produced or released after thermal injury. These mediators play important roles in the pathogenesis of edema and the cardiovascular abnormalities of burn injury. Many mediators alter vascular permeability directly or indirectly by increasing microvascular hydrostatic pressure and surface area, via arteriolar vasodilation superimposed on an already altered membrane. The exact mechanisms of mediator-induced injury are of considerable clinical importance, as this understanding would allow for development of pharmacologic modulation of burn edema and shock by mediator inhibition.

Histamine

Histamine is the likely mediator responsible for an early phase of increased capillary permeability immediately after burn. Histamine causes large endothelial gaps to transiently form as a result of contraction of venular endothelial cells.[47] Histamine is released from heat-injured skin mast cells; however, the increase in histamine levels and its actions are only transient. Histamine can also cause arteriolar dilation and venular contraction.[47] Statistically significant reductions in burn edema have been achieved with histamine blockers and mast cell stabilizers when tested in acute animal models.[48,49] Recently Friedl *et al.*[50] demonstrated that the pathogenesis of burn edema in the skin of rats appears to be related to the interaction of histamine with xanthine oxidase and oxygen radicals. Histamine and its metabolic derivatives increased the catalytic activity of xanthine oxidase (but not xanthine dehydrogenase) in rat plasma and in rat pulmonary artery endothelial cells. In thermally injured rats, levels of plasma histamine and xanthine oxidase rose in parallel, in association with increases in uric acid. Burn edema was greatly attenuated by treating rats with:

- the mast cell stabilizer, cromolyn;
- complement depletion; and
- the H_2 receptor antagonist, cimetidine;

but was unaffected by neutrophil depletion.[48,51] Despite these encouraging results in animals, the long-term benefit of antihistamine treatment of burn injury has not been clinically demonstrated.

Prostaglandins

Prostaglandins are potent vasoactive autocoids synthesized from arachidonic acid released from burned tissue and inflammatory cells. They are at least in part responsible for the inflammatory response of burn injury.[52,53] Macrophages and neutrophils infiltrate the wound and release prostaglandin as well as thromboxanes, leukotrienes, and interleukin-1. These wound mediators have both local and systemic effects. Prostaglandin E_2 (PGE_2) and leukotrienes LB_4–LD_4 directly and indirectly increase microvascular permeability.[54] Prostacyclin (PGI_2) is produced in burn injury and is also a vasodilator, but may cause direct increases in capillary permeability as well. PGE_2 appears to be one of the most important inflammatory prostaglandins, causing the postburn vasodilation in wounds, which, when coupled with increased microvascular permeability, contributes to edema.[55,56]

Thromboxane

Thromboxane A_2 (TXA_2) and its metabolite, thromboxane B_2 (TXB_2), are produced locally at the burn wound by platelets.[47] Vasoconstrictor thromboxanes may be less important in edema formation, but by decreasing blood flow they can contribute to a growing zone of ischemia under the burn wound and can cause conversion of a partial-thickness wound to a deeper full-thickness wound. The serum level of TXA_2 and TXA_2/PGI_2 ratios are increased significantly in burn patients.[57] Heggers[58,59] showed the release of TXB_2 at the burn wound was associated with local tissue ischemia, and thromboxane inhibitors prevented the progressive dermal ischemia associated with thermal injury and thromboxane release. The TXA_2 synthesis inhibitor anisodamine also showed beneficial effects by restoring the hemodynamic and rheological disturbances towards normal. Demling[60] showed that topically applied ibuprofen (which inhibits the synthesis of prostaglandins and thromboxanes) decreases both local edema and prostanoid production in burned tissue without altering systemic production. On the other hand, systemic administration of ibuprofen did not modify early edema, but did attenuate the postburn vasoconstriction that impaired adequate oxygen delivery to tissues in burned sheep.[61]

Kinins

Kinins, specifically the bradykinins, are known to increase venular permeability. It is likely that bradykinin production is increased after burn injury, but detection in blood or lymph can be very difficult owing to the simultaneous increase in kininase activity and the rapid inactivation of free kinins. The generalized inflammatory response after burn injury certainly favors the release of bradykinin.[62] Pretreatment of burn-injured animals with aprotinin (Trasylol), a general protease inhibitor, should have decreased the release of free kinin, but no effect on edema was noted.[63]

Serotonin

Serotonin is also released early after burn injury.[64] This agent is a smooth-muscle constrictor and may increase capillary permeability. Antiserotonin agents, such as ketanserin, have been found to decrease peripheral vascular resistance after burn injury, but have not been reported to decrease edema.[64]

Catecholamines

Catecholamines are also released in massive amounts after burn injury.[6,65,66] These agents act primarily on the arteriolar side of the microvessels, causing vasoconstriction that would tend to reduce capillary pressure.[47] It is likely that catecholamine effects and reduced capillary pressure occur primarily in nonburned skin, skeletal muscle, and visceral organs, where they may limit edema and actually reasorb interstitial fluid in nonresuscitated burn shock. Catecholamines, via β-agonist activity, may also partially inhibit the increased capillary permeability induced by histamine and bradykinin.[47] These potentially beneficial effects may not be operative in the directly injured tissue and may also be offset in nonburned tissues by the deleterious vasoconstrictor effects of catecholamines. The hemodynamic effects of catecholamines will be discussed later in the chapter.

Oxygen Radicals

Oxygen radicals probably play an important inflammatory role in all types of shock, including burn. These short-lived elements are highly unstable reactive metabolites of oxygen; each one has an unpaired electron, making them strong oxidizing agents.[67] Superoxide anion (O_2^-, hydrogen peroxide (H_2O_2), and hydroxyl ion (OH^-) are produced and released after any inflammatory reaction or reperfusion of ischemic tissue. The hydroxyl ion is likely the most potent and damaging of the three. The formation of the hydroxyl radical requires free ferrous iron (Fe^{2+}) and H_2O_2. Evidence that these agents are released after burn injury is the increased lipid peroxidation found in circulating red cells and biopsied tissues.[51,67,68]

Antioxidants, namely agents that either directly bind to the oxygen radicals (scavengers) or cause their further metabolism, have been evaluated in several experimental studies.[69,70] Catalase, which removes H_2O_2, and superoxide dismutase (SOD), which does the same for O_2, have been reported to decrease the vascular loss of plasma after burn injury in dogs.[51,69] Demling[71] showed that large doses of deferoxamine (DFO), an iron chelator, when used for burn resuscitation of 40% TBSA burn in sheep, prevented systemic lipid peroxidation and decreased the vascular leak in nonburned tissues while also increasing oxygen utilization. However, DFO may have accentuated burned tissue edema, possibly by increasing perfusion of burned tissue.

The plasma of thermally injured rats showed dramatic increases in levels of xanthine oxidase activity, with peak values appearing as early as 15 minutes after thermal trauma. Excision of the burned skin immediately after thermal injury significantly diminished the increase in plasma xanthine oxidase activity.[50,51] The skin permeability changes were attenuated by treating the animals with antioxidants (catalase, SOD, dimethyl sulfoxide, dimethylthiourea) or an iron chelator (DFO), thus supporting the role of oxygen radicals in the development of vascular injury, as defined by greatly increased vascular permeability.[51] Allopurinol, a xanthine oxidase inhibitor, markedly reduced both burn lymph flow and levels of circulating lipid peroxides, and further prevented all pulmonary lipid peroxidation and inflammation. This suggests that the release of oxidants from burn tissue was in part responsible for local burn edema, as well as distant inflammation and oxidant release.[68] The failure of neutrophil depletion to protect against the vascular permeability changes and the protective effects of the xanthine oxidase inhibitors (allopurinol and lodoxamide tromethamine) suggests that xanthine oxidase is the more likely source of the oxygen radicals involved in edema formation. Lodoxamide was found to have some hydroxyl-scavenging ability but no iron-chelating activity. Some of the protective effects of lodoxamide and allopurinol may be linked to their hydroxyl-scavenging abilities. These data suggest that the vascular injury, defined by an increased vascular permeability of burn injury, is in part related to the activation of xanthine oxidase and the generation of toxic oxygen metabolites that damage microvascular endothelial cells.[50,51]

Platelet Aggregation Factor

Platelet aggregation (or activating) factor (PAF) can increase capillary permeability and is also released after burn injury.[63,72]. Ono *et al.*[72] showed in scald-injured rabbits that TCV-309 (Takeda Pharmaceutical Co Ltd, Japan), a PAF antagonist, infused soon after the burn, blocked edema formation in the wound and significantly inhibited PAF increase in the damaged tissue in a dose-dependent manner. In contrast, the superoxide dismutase content in the group treated with TCV-309 was significantly higher than that of the control group. These findings suggest that the administration of large doses of a PAF antagonist immediately after injury may reduce burn wound edema and the subsequent degree of burn shock by suppressing PAF and superoxide radical formation.

Angiotension II and Vasopressin

Angiotensin II and vasopressin or antidiuretic hormone (ADH) are two hormones that participate in the normal regulation of extracellular fluid volume by controlling sodium balance and osmolality through renal function and thirst.[47] In the shock state, however, where, sympathetic tone is high and volume receptors are stimulated, both hormones can be found in supranormal levels in the blood. Both are potent vasoconstrictors of the terminal arterioles and yet have little effect on the venules. Angiotensin II may be responsible for the selective gut ischemia; and gut mucosal ischemia may play a pivotal role in bacterial translocation and the development of sepsis and even multiorgan failure.[73] In severely burn-injured patients angiotensin II levels were elevated two to eight times normal in the first 1–5 days after burn injury with peak levels occurring on day 3.[74] Vasopressin had peak levels of 50 times normal upon admission and declined towards normal over the first 5 days after burn injury. Vasopressin, along with catecholamines, may be largely responsible for increased system vascular resistance and left heart afterload which can occur in resuscitated burn shock.

Sun *et al.*[75] used vasopressin-receptor antagonist in rats with burn shock to improve hemodynamics and survival time, while vasopressin infusion exacerbated burn shock.

Corticotrophin-releasing Factor

Corticotrophin-releasing factor (CRF) has proven to be efficacious in reducing protein extravasation and edema in burned rat paw. CRF may be a powerful natural inhibitory mediator of the acute inflammatory response of the skin to thermal injury.[76]

Hemodynamic Consequences of Acute Burns

The cause of the reduction of cardiac output during the resuscitative phase of burn injury has been the subject of considerable debate. There is an immediate depression of cardiac output before any detectable reduction in plasma volume. The rapidity of this response suggests a neurogenic response to receptors in the thermally injured skin. After thermal injury, there is a near immediate release of vasopressin, angiotensin II, neuropeptide Y, catecholamines, and perhaps other circulating vasoconstrictor mediators.[74,75] Soon after injury a developing hypovolemia and reduced venous return play major roles in depressed cardiac output. But the subsequent persistence of reduced cardiac output (CO) after apparently adequate fluid therapy, as evidenced by a reduction in heart rate and restoration of both arterial blood pressure and urinary output, has been attributed to circulating myocardial depressant factor(s), which possibly originate from the burn wound.[10,11] Demling *et al.*[16] showed a 15% reduction in CO even with an aggressive volume replacement protocol after a 40% scald burn in sheep. However, there are also sustained increases in catecholamine secretion and elevated systemic vascular resistance for up to 5 days after burn injury.[65,74] Michie *et al.*[77] measured CO and SVR in anesthetized dogs resuscitated after burn injury. They found that CO fell shortly after injury, then returned toward normal, while further decreases of blood volume occurred, i.e. blood volume deficit was not paralleled by reduced CO. They concluded that the depression of CO results not only from blood volume decreases, but also from an increased SVR and from the presence of a circulating myocardial depressant substance. Thus, there are at least two factors other than reduced volume and venous return that significantly affect cardiac output after burn injury: SVR and depressed myocardial contractility.

Increased Systemic Vascular Resistance

Cardiac output remains depressed after adequate volume replacement in burned patients and experimental animals. Sympathetic stimulation and hypovolemia result in the release of catecholamines, vasopressin, angiotensin II, and neuropeptide Y after burn injury. These agents act primarily on arteriolar smooth muscle, causing vasoconstriction which is systemically manifested by increased SVR. Hilton and others[11,66,78] performed a series of experiments in anesthetized dogs in which infusion of various peripheral vasodilators improved CO after burn injury. Using a strain gauge placed on the left ventricle, they demonstrated reduction in peripheral vascular resistance using a verapamil augmented CO, but myocardial force of contraction remained depressed. Pruitt *et al.*[79] examined the hypothesis that increased sympathetic activity is responsible partly for reduced CO in a group of burned patients. They showed an improvement of CO with the vasodilator hydralazine and fluid resuscitation; namely CO increased from 77% of expected after-burn levels to 110% with treatment, and SVR decreased to 51% of expected after-burn levels. Hydralazine was also shown to improve CO in experimental animals subjected to burn injury.[77] The increase in SVR, after burn injury, results from a summation of peripheral vasoconstriction and increased blood viscosity secondary to hemoconcentration.

Pulmonary Edema

In large burns, there is also a pronounced increase in pulmonary vascular resistance (PVR) that corresponds with the increase in SVR.[7,34] Pulmonary edema is not an uncommon occurrence after the fluid-resuscitation phase of burn injury. It results from increased capillary pressure secondary to the increased PVR, which has components of both pre- and postcapillary vasoconstriction. Pulmonary wedge pressure is increased more than left atrial pressure after experimental burn injury due to postcapillary venular constriction.[34,80] It is clear that initially some left heart failure also contributes to the increased capillary pressure. However, the developing hypoproteinemia may be the greatest contributing factor to postburn pulmonary edema.[81] There is no evidence of increased capillary permeability from analysis of lung lymph sampled, in large animal models, after severe burn injury, although studies in rats suggest that albumin sequestration increases in the lungs after a 30% cutaneous scald.[51] Clinical studies suggest that in the absence of inhalation injury, the lungs do not necessarily develop edema, a finding that is consistent with little or no change in the microvascular permeability of the lung.[82,83]

Myocardial Dysfunction

Myocardial function can be compromised after burn injury due to right heart overload and direct depression of contractility.[84,85] Increases in the afterload of the left and right heart result from the increases in SVR and PVR. The left ventricle compensates by increasing both contractility and myocardial oxygen extraction. The right ventricle has minimal capacity to compensate for increased afterload. In severe cases, desynchronization of the right and left ventricles is deleteriously superimposed on a depressed myocardium.[84] Burns greater than 45% BSA can produce intrinsic contractile defects. Horton[85-87] *et al.*[87] showed that aggressive crystalloid fluid resuscitation, initiated immediately after burn and continued for 24 hours, failed to correct left ventricular contractile and compliance defects. These data suggest that hypovolemia is not the sole mechanism underlying the myocardial defects observed with burn shock. Sera from patients failing to sustain a normal CO, after thermal injury, have exhibited a marked negative inotrophic effect on *in vitro* heart preparations[88] In patients with larger burn injuries and normal cardiac indices, little or no depressant activity was detected.

The mechanism by which burn shock alters myocardial cell membrane integrity and impairs mechanical function remains unclear. Oxygen-derived free radicals may play a key causative role in the cell membrane dysfunction that is characteristic of several low-flow states. Baxter *et al.*[89] showed that combination therapy of free radical scavengers SOD and catalase significantly improved burn-mediated defects in left ventricular contractility and relaxation when administered along with adequate fluid resuscitation (4 ml/kg/% burn). Antioxidant therapy did not alter the volume of fluid resuscitation required after burn injury.

Sugi *et al.*[90,91] studied intact, chronically instrumented sheep after a 40% TBSA flame burn injury and smoke inhalation injury and then with smoke inhalation injury alone. They found that maximal elastance (E_{max}) was reduced after either burn injury or inhalation injury showing decreased contractility in an intact animal. Horton *et al.*[92] demonstrated decreased left ventricular contractility in isolated, coronary perfused, guinea-pig hearts harvested 24 hours after burn injury. This dysfunction was more pronounced in hearts from aged animals and was not totally reversed by resuscitation with isotonic fluid. It was largely reversed by treatment with 4 ml/kg of hypertonic saline dextran (HSD) if administered during the first 4–6 hours of resuscitation. Persistent myocardial depression after burn was not identified by Cioffi and colleagues[93] in a similar model when the animals received resuscitation synchronous with the burn injury. In these studies, timely resuscitation totally reversed abnormalities of contraction and relaxation after burn injury. Such studies emphasize the importance of early intervention and suggest that myocardial depression after burn may not occur in all patients.

SUMMARY AND CONCLUSION

Thermal injury results not only in massive fluid shifts that cause hypovolemia but also in the release of inflammatory mediators from burn wounds; these mediators deleteriously affect cardiovascular function and lead to burn shock. The end result of a complex chain of events is decreased intravascular volume, increased systemic vascular resistance, decreased cardiac output, end-organ ischemia, and metabolic acidosis. Without early and full resuscitation therapy, these derangements result in acute renal failure, cardiovascular collapse, and death.

Resuscitation itself is not without complications. Burn edema is worsened by resuscitation, particularly with crystalloid solutions. This edema itself is a serious complication. Burn edema most likely contributes to decreased tissue oxygen diffusion and further ischemic insult to already damaged cells. The increased tissue pressure caused by the edema may further compromise blood flow, again potentiating the tissue damage and increasing the risk of infection. Research should continue to be focused on methods to ameliorate the severe edema and vasoconstriction that exacerbate tissue ischemia. The success of this research will require identification of all the circulatory factors that alter capillary permeability, cause vasoconstriction, depolarize cellular membranes, and depress myocardial function. Then methods to prevent the release and to block the activity of specific mediators can be developed and thus offer hope for reducing the great morbidity and mortality rates of burn shock.

REFERENCES

1. Cockshott W P. The history of the treatment of burns. *Surg Gynecol Obstet* 1956; **102:** 116–24.

2. Haynes B W. The history of burn care. In: Boswick J A Jr, ed. *The Art and Science of Burn Care* Rockville, MA: Aspen, 1987: 3–9.

3. Underhill F P, Carrington G L, Kapsinov R, Pack G T. Blood concentration changes in extensive superficial burns, and their significance for systemic treatment. *Arch Intern Med* 1923; **32:** 31–49.

4. Cope O, Moore F D. The redistribution of body water and fluid therapy of the burned patient. *Ann Surg* 1947; **126:** 1010–45.

5. Aulick L H, Wilmore D W, Mason A D Jr, Pruitt B A. Influence of the burn wound on peripheral circulation in thermally injured patients. *Am J Physiol* 1977; **233:** H520–6.

6. Settle J A D. Fluid therapy in burns. *J R Soc Med* 1982; **75** (Suppl 1): 7–11.

7. Demling R H, Fluid replacement in burned patients. *Surg Clin North Am* 1987; **67:** 15–30.

8. Demling R H, Will J A, Belzer F O. Effect of major thermal injury on the pulmonary microcirculation. *Surgery* 1978; **83:** 746–51.

9. Baxter C R. Fluid volume and electrolyte changes in the early post-burn period. *Clin Plast Surg* 1974; **1**(4): 693–709.

10. Baxter C R, Cook W A, Shires G T. Serum myocardial depressant factor of burn shock. *Surg Forum* 1966; **17:** 1–3.

11. Hilton J G, Marulllo D S. Effects of thermal trauma on cardiac force of contraction. *Burns Incl Therm Inj* 1986; **12:** 167–71.

12. Clark W R. Death due to thermal trauma In: Dolecek R, Brizio-Molteni L, Molteni A, Traber D, (eds). *Endocrinology of Thermal Trauma.* Philadelphia, PA: Lea & Febiger, 1990: 6–27.

13. Lund T, Reed R K. Acute hemodynamic effects of thermal skin injury in the rat. *Circ Shock* 1986; **20:** 105–14.

14. Arturson G. Pathophysiological aspects of the burn syndrome. *Acta Chir Scand* 1961; **274** (Supp 1): 1–135.

15. Leape L L. Kinetics of burn edema formation in primates. *Ann Surg* 1972; **176:** 223–6.

16. Demling R H, Mazess R B, Witt R M, Wolberg W H. The study of burn wound edema using dichromatic absorptiometry. *J Trauma* 1978; **18:** 124–8.

17. Lund T, Wiig H, Reed R K. Acute after burn edema: role of strongly negative interstitial fluid pressure. *Am J Physiol* 1988; **255** (*Heart, Circ Physiol* **24**): H1069–74.

18. Onarheim H, Lund T, Reed R K. Thermal skin injury: II. Effects on edema formation and albumin extravasation of fluid resuscitation with lactated Ringer's, plasma and hypertonic (2400 mosm/l) saline in the rat. *Circ Shock* 1989; **27:** 25–37.

19. Arturson G, Jakobsson O P. Oedema measurements in a standard burn model. *Burns* 1985; **1:** 1–7.

20. Leape L L. Early burn wound changes. *J Pediatr Surg* 1968; **3:** 292–9.

21. Leape L L. Initial changes in burns: tissue changes in burned and unburned skin of rhesus monkeys. *J Trauma* 1970; **10:** 488–92.

22. Landis E M, Pappenheimer J R. Exchange of substances through the capillary walls. In: Hamilton W F, Dow P, eds. *Handbook of Physiology.* Baltimore: Williams and Wilkins, 1963; sect 2, vol 2: 961–1034.

23. Arturson G, Mellander S. Acute changes in capillary filtration and diffusion in experimental burn injury. *Acta Physiol Scand* 1964; **62:** 457–63.

24. Pitt R M, Parker J C, Jurkovich G J, Taylor A E, Curreri P W. Analysis of altered capillary pressure and permeability after thermal injury. *J Surg Res* 1987; **42:** 603–702.

25. Lund T, Onarheim H, Reed R K. Pathogenesis of edema formation in burn injuries. *World J Surg* 1992; **16:** 2–9.

26. Taylor A E, Granger D N. Exchange of macromolecules across the microcirculation. In: Renkin E M, Michel C C eds. *Handbook of Physiology. The Cardiovascular System. Vol. IV. Microcirculation. Part 1.* Bethesda, MD: The American Physiological Society, 1984: 467–520.

27. Harms B A, Bodia B I, Kramer G C, Demling R H. Microvascular fluid and protein flux in pulmonary and systemic circulations after thermal injury. *Microvasc Res* 1982; **23:** 77–86.

28. Arturson G. Microvascular permeability to macromolecules in thermal injury. *Acta Physiol Scand* 1979; **463** (Suppl): 111–222.

29. Noddeland H. Colloid osmotic pressure of human subcutaneous interstitial fluid sampled by nylon wicks: evaluation of the method. *Scand. J Clin Lab Invest* 1982; **42:** 123–30.

30. Zetterström H, Arturson G. Plasma oncotic pressure and plasma protein concentration in patients following thermal injury. *Acta Anaesth Scand* 1980; **24:** 288–94.

31. Demling R H, Kramer G C, Harms B. Role of thermal injury induced hypoproteinemia on fluid flux and protein permeability in burned and nonburned tissue. *Surgery* 1984; **95:** 136–43.

32. Lund T, Reed R K. Microvascular fluid exchange following thermal skin injury in the rat: changes in extravascular colloid osmotic pressure, albumin mass and water content. *Circ Shock* 1986; **20:** 91–104.

33. Pitkänen J, Lund T, Ananderud L, Reed R K. Transcapillary colloid osmotic pressures in injured and non-injured skin of seriously burned patients. *Burns* 1987; **13:** 198–203.

34. Kramer G C, Gunther R A, Nerlich M L, Zweifach S S, Demling R H. Effect of dextran-70 on increased microvascular fluid and protein flux after thermal injury. *Circ Shock* 1989; **9:** 29–41.

35. Kinsky M P, Guha S C, Button B, *et al.* Initial resuscitation of burn injury with hypertonic saline dextran (HSD) prevents the reversal of the plasma-interstitial oncotic gradient in non-burned skin. *Shock* 1993; **1** (Suppl): 9.

36. Brouhard B H, Carvajal H F, Linares H A. Burn edema and protein leakage in the rat. I. Relationship to time of injury. *Microvasc Res* 1978; **15:** 221–8.

37. Neumann M R, Demling H. Colloid vs crystalloid: a current perspective. *Intens Crit Care Dig* 1990; **9:** 36.

38. Kramer G C, Harms B A, Bodai B I, Demling R H, Renkin E M. Mechanisms for redistribution of plasma protein following acute protein depletion. *Am J Physiol* 1982; **243:** H803–H809.

39. Shires G T, Cunningham J N, Baker C R F, *et al.* Alterations in cellular membrane function during hemorrhagic shock in primates. *Ann Surg* 1972; **176:** 288–295.

40. Nakayama S, Kramer G C, Carlsen R C, Holcroft J W, Cala P M. Amiloride blocks membrane potential depolarization in rat skeletal muscle during hemorrhagic shock. *Circ Shock* 1984; **13:** 106–7.

41. Arango A, Illner H, Shires G T. Roles of ischemia in the induction of changes in cell membrane during hemorrhagic shock. *J Surg Res* 1976; **20:** 473–6.

42. Holliday R L, Illner H P, Shires G T. Liver cell membrane alterations during hemorrhagic shock in the rat. *J Surg Res* 1981; **31:** 506–15.

43. Mazzoni M C, Borgstrom P, Intaglietta M, Arfors K E. Lumenal narrowing and endothelial cell swelling in skeletal muscle capillaries during hemorrhagic shock. *Circ Shock* 1989; **29:** 27–39.

44. Evans J A, Darlington D N, Gann D S. A circulating factor(s) mediates cell depolarization in hemorrhagic shock. *Ann Surg* 1991; **213:** 549–57.

45. Mazzoni M C, Intaglietta M, Cragoe E J J, Arfors K E. Amiloride-sensitive Na^+ pathways in capillary endothelial cell swelling during hemorrhagic shock. *J Appl Physiol* 1992; **73:** 1467–3.

46. Button B, Brodwick M, Baker R, Kramer G C. Evidence of circulating membrane depolarization factor(s) in hemorrhagic shock. *Shock* 1994; **1** (Suppl): 15.

47. Goodman Gilman A, Rall T W, Nies A S, Taylor P. *The Pharmacological Basis of Therapeutics*. New York: Pergamon Press, 1990.

48. Boykin J V Jr, Manson N H. Mechanisms of cimetidine protection following thermal injury. *Am J Med* 1987; **83**(6A): 76–81.

49. Bramblecombe R. Histamine H_2 receptor antagonists in thermal injury in rats. *Burns* 1976; **3:** 8–13.

50. Friedl H P, Till G O, Trentz O, Ward P A. Roles of histamine, complement and xanthine oxidase in thermal injury of skin. *Am J Pathol* 1989; **1:** 203–17.

51. Till G O, Guilds L S, Mahrougui M, *et al.* Role of xanthine oxidase in thermal injury of skin. *Am J Pathol* 1989; **1:** 195–202.

52. Harms B, Bodai B, Demling R. Prostaglandin release and altered microvascular integrity after burn injury. *J Surg Res* 1981; **31:** 274–280.

53. Anggard E, Jonsson C E. Efflux of prostaglandins in lymph from scalded tissue. *Acta Physiol Scand* 1971; **81:** 440–3.

54. Arturson G. Anti-inflammatory drugs and burn edema formation. In: May R, Dogo G, eds. *Care of the Burn Wound*. Basel: Karger, 1981: 210–24.

55. Arturson G, Hamberg M, Jonsson C E. Prostaglandins in human burn blister fluid. *Acta Physiol Scand* 1973; **87:** 270–6.

56. LaLonde C, Knox J, Daryani R, *et al.* Topical flurbiprofen decreases burn wound-induced hypermetabolism and systemic lipid peroxidation. *Surgery* 1991; **109:** 645–51.

57. Huang Y S, Li A, Yang Z C. Roles of thromboxane and its inhibitor anisodamine in burn shock. *Burns* 1990; **4:** 249–53.

58. Heggers J P, Loy G L, Robson M C, Del Beccaro E J. Histological demonstration of prostaglandins and thromboxanes in burned tissue. *J Surg Res* 1980; **28:** 110–15.

59. Heggers J P, Robson M C, Zachary L S. Thromboxane inhibitors for the prevention of progressive dermal ischemia due to thermal injury. *J Burn Care Rehabil* 1985; **6:** 466–8.

60. Demling R H, LaLonde C. Topical ibuprofen decreases early postburn edema. *Surgery* 1987; **5:** 857–61.

61. LaLonde C, Demling R H. Inhibition of thromboxane synthetase accentuates hemodynamic instability and burn edema in the anesthetized sheep model. *Surgery* 1989; **5:** 638–44.

62. Jacobsen S, Waaler B G. The effect of scalding on the content of kininogen and kininase in limb lymph. *Br J Pharmacol* 1966; **27:** 222–9.

63. Hafner J A, Fritz H. Balance antiinflammation: the combined application of a PAF inhibitor and a cyclooxygenase inhibitor blocks the inflammatory take-off after burns. *Int J Tissue React* 1990; **12:** 203.

64. Carvajal H, Linares H, Brouhard B. Effect of antihistamine, antiserotonin, and ganglionic blocking agents upon increased capillary permeability following burn edema. *J Trauma* 1975; **15:** 969–75.

65. Wilmore D W, Long J M, Mason A D, Skreen R W, Pruitt B A. Catecholamines: mediator of the hypermetabolic response to thermal injury. *Ann Surg* 1974; **80:** 653–9.

66. Hilton J G. Effects of sodium nitroprusside on thermal trauma depressed cardiac output in the anesthesized dog. *Burns Incl Therm Inj* 1984; **10:** 318–22.

67. McCord J, Fridovich I. The biology and pathology of oxygen radicals. *Ann Intern Med* 1978; **89:** 122–7.

68. Demling R H, LaLonde C. Early postburn lipid peroxidation: effect of ibuprofen and allopurinol. *Surgery* 1990; **107:** 85–93.

69. Slater T F, Benedetto C. Free radical reactions in relation to lipid peroxidation, inflammation and prostaglandin metabolism. In: Berti F, Veto G, eds. *The Prostaglandin System*. New York: Plenum Press, 1979: 109–26.

70. McCord J M. Oxygen-derived free radicals in post ischemic tissue injury. *N Engl J Med* 1979; **312:** 159–63.

71. Demling R, LaLonde C, Knox J *et al.* Fluid resuscitation with deferoxamine prevents systemic burn-induced oxidant injury. *J Trauma* 1991; **4:** 538–43.

72. Ono I, Gunji H, Hasegawa T, Harada H, Kaneko F, Matsuzaki M. Effects of a platelet activating factor antagonist on edema formation following burns. *Burns* 1993; **3:** 202–7.

73. Fink M P. Gastrointestinal mucosal injury in experimental models of shock, trauma and sepsis. *Crit Care Med* 1991; **19:** 627–41.

74. Crum R L, Dominic W, Hansbrough J F, *et al.* Cardiovascular and neurohumoral responses following burn injury. *Arch Surg* 1990; **125:** 1065–70.

75. Sun K, Gong A, Wang C H, Lin B C, Zhu H N. Effect of peripheral injection of arginine vasopressin and its receptor antagonist on burn shock in the rat. *Neuropeptides* 1990; **1:** 1720.

76. Kiang J G, Wei E T. Corticotropin-releasing factor inhibits thermal injury. *J Pharmacol Exp Ther* 1987; **2:** 517–20.

77. Michie D D, Goldsmith R S, Mason A D Jr. Effects of hydralazine and high molecular weight dextran upon the circulatory responses to severe thermal burns. *Circ Res* 1963; **13:** 468.

78. Hilton J G. Effects of verapamil on thermal trauma depressed cardiac output in the anesthetized dog. *Burns Incl Therm Inj* 1984; **10:** 313–17.

79. Pruitt B A, Mason A D Jr, Moncrief J A. Hemodynamic changes in the early postburn patient: the influence of fluid administration and of a vasodilator. *J Trauma* 1971; **11:** 36–46.

80. Demling R H, Wong C, Jin L, *et al.* Early lung dysfunction after major burns: role of edema and vasoactive mediators. *J Trauma* 1985; **25:** 959–66.

81. Demling R H, Niehaus G, Perea A, Will J A. Effect of burn-induced hypoproteinemia on pulmonary transvascular fluid filtration rate. *Surgery* 1979; **85:** 339–43.

82. Tranbaugh R F, Elings V B, Christensen J M, Lewis F R. Effect of inhalation injury on lung water accumulation. *J Trauma* 1983; **23:** 597.

83. Tranbaugh R F, Lewis F R, Christensen J M, Elings V B. Lung water changes after thermal injury: the effects of crystalloid resuscitation and sepsis. *Ann Surg* 1980; **192:** 479.

84. Martyn J A J, Wilson R S, Burke J F. Right ventricular function and pulmonary hemodynamics during dopamine infusion in burned patients. *Chest* 1986; **89:** 357–60.

85. Adams H R, Baxter C R, Izenberg S D. Decreased contractility and compliance of the left ventricle as complications of thermal trauma. *Am Heart J* 1984; **108**(6): 1477–87.

86. Merriman T W Jr, Jackson R. Myocardial function following thermal injury. *Circ Res* 1962; **11:** 669.

87. Horton J W, White J, Baxter C R. Aging alters myocardial response during resuscitation in burn shock. *Surg Forum* 1987; **38:** 249–51.

88. Baxter C R, Shires G T. Physiological response to crystalloid resuscitation of severe burns. *Ann NY Acad Sci* 1968; **150(3):** 874–94.

89. Horton J W, White J, Baxter C R. The role of oxygen-derived free radicals in burn-induced myocardial contractile depression. *J Burn Care Rehabil* 1988; **9**(6):589–98.

90. Sugi K, Newald J, Traber L D, *et al.* Smoke inhalation injury causes myocardial depression in sheep. *Anesthesiology* 1988; **69:** A111.

91. Sugi K, Theissen J L, Traber L D, Herndon D N, Traber D L. Impact of carbon monoxide on cardiopulmonary dysfunction after smoke inhalation injury. *Circ Res* 1990; **66:** 69–75.

92. Horton J W, Baxter C R, White D J. Differences in cardiac responses to resuscitation from burn shock. *Surg Gynecol Obstet* 1989; **168:** 201–6.

93. Cioffi W G, DeMeules J E, Gamelli R L. The effects of burn injury and fluid resuscitation on cardiac function in vitro. *J Trauma* 1986; **26:** 638–43.

CHAPTER SIX

Fluid Resuscitation and Early Management

Glenn D. Warden

Proper fluid management is critical to the survival of a victim of a major thermal injury. In the 1940s, hypovolemic shock or shock-induced renal failure was the leading cause of death after burn injury. Today, with our current knowledge of the massive fluid shifts and vascular changes which occur during burn shock, mortality related to burn-induced volume loss has decreased considerably. Although a vigorous approach to fluid therapy has ensued in the last 20 years and fewer deaths are occurring in the first 24–48 hours postburn, the fact remains that approximately 50% of the deaths occur within the first 10 days following burn injury from a multitude of causes, one of the most significant being inadequate fluid resuscitation therapy.[1] Knowledge of fluid management following burn shock resuscitation is also important and is often overlooked in burn education.

Burn Shock Resuscitation

The history of burn resuscitation began over a century ago; however, complete appreciation of the severity of fluid loss in burns was not apparent until the enlightening studies of Frank P. Underhill,[2] who studied the victims of the Rialto Theater fire in 1921. His concept that burn shock was due to intravascular fluid loss was further elucidated by Moore[3] who conducted studies on patients from the Coconut Grove disaster in 1942. They developed the concept of burn edema and introduced the body-weight burn budget formula for fluid resuscitation of burn patients. In 1952, Artz and Moncrief[1] developed a burn surface area–weight formula for computing fluid replacement in burns which became the first simplified formula for fluid resuscitation for burn patients. Surgeons at the Brooke Army Medical Center modified the original Evans formula and this became the standard for the next 15 years.

A number of methods for accomplishing adequate volume replacement therapy have been advocated in the more than 40 years since the introduction of the Evans' formula in 1952. This chapter reviews the various methods advocated and presents the rationale of each. Importantly, when properly utilized, each resuscitation formula can be effective in the resuscitation of a burn patient in the immediate postburn period, provided that close attention is paid to the individual's clinical response to therapy and that fluid replacement therapy is modified according to this response. The fact that patients respond to a wide variety of resuscitative efforts is testimony to the fact that burned patients are very resilient and can be overwhelmed only under the most unfavorable circumstances.[4]

Pathophysiology of Burn Injury

Modern fluid resuscitation formulas originate from experimental studies in the pathophysiology of burn shock. Burn shock is both hypovolemic shock and cellular shock, and is characterized by specific hemodynamic changes including decreased cardiac output, extracellular fluid, plasma volume, and oliguria. As in the treatment of other forms of shock, the primary goal is to restore and preserve tissue perfusion in order to avoid ischemia. However, in burn shock, resuscitation is complicated by obligatory burn edema, and the voluminous transvascular fluid shifts which result from a major burn are unique to thermal trauma.

Although the exact pathophysiology of the postburn vascular changes and fluid shifts is unknown, one major component of burn shock is the increase in total body capillary permeability. Direct thermal injury results in marked changes in the microcirculation. Most of the changes occur locally at the burn site, when maximal edema formation occurs at about 8–12 hours post-injury in smaller burns and 12–24 hours post-injury in major thermal injuries. The rate of progression of tissue edema is dependent upon the adequacy of resuscitation.

Multiple mediators have been proposed to explain the changes in vascular permeability seen postburn. The mediators can produce either an increase in vascular permeability or an increase in microvascular hydrostatic pressure.[5,6] Most mediators act to increase permeability by altering membrane integrity in the venules. The early phase of burn edema formation, lasting for minutes to an hour, has been thought by some investigators to be the result of mediators, particularly histamine and bradykinin. Other mediators implicated in the changes in vascular permeability seen postburn include vasoactive amines, products of platelet activation and the complement cascade, hormones, prostaglandins, and leukotrienes. Vasoactive substances are also released which may act primarily by increasing microvascular blood flow or vascular pressures, further accentuating the burn edema.[7,8] Histamine is released in large quantities from mast cells in burned skin immediately after injury.[9] Histamine has been clearly demonstrated to increase the leakage of fluid and protein from systemic microvessels, its major effect being on venules in which an increase in the intracellular junction space is characteristically seen.[10] However, the increase in serum histamine levels after burn is transient, peaking in the first several hours post-injury, indicating that histamine is only involved in the very early increase in permeability. The use of H_1 receptor inhibitors, e.g. diphenhydramine, has only limited success in decreasing edema.

Recently, the use of an H_2 receptor antagonist has been reported to decrease burn edema in an animal model.[11]

Serotonin is released immediately postburn as a result of platelet aggregation and acts directly to increase the pulmonary vascular resistance and indirectly to amplify the vasoconstrictive effect of norepinephrine, histamine, angiotensin-II, and prostaglandin.[12] The use of ketanserin, a specific serotonin antagonist in a porcine burn shock model, improved cardiac index, decreased pulmonary pressure, and reduced arteriovenous oxygen content differences compared to a control group in the early postburn period. Serotonin antagonists should be investigated further as possible adjuvant therapeutic agents during burn shock resuscitation.[13] Prostaglandins, vasoactive products of arachidonic acid metabolism, have been reported to be released in burn tissue and to be at least in part responsible for burn edema. Although these substances do not directly alter vasopermeability, increased levels of vasodilator prostaglandins such as PGE2 and prostacyclin PGI2 result in arterial dilatation in burned tissue, increased blood flow and intravascular hydrostatic pressure in the injured microcirculation, and thus accentuate the edema process. Concentrations of PGI2 and the vasoconstrictor thromboxane A2 have been demonstrably found in burned tissue, burn blister fluid, lymph, and wound secretion.[14,15] The use of prostaglandin inhibitors has produced variable results in animal studies. Arturson[16] reported a decrease in burn lymph and protein flow with the use of a prostaglandin inhibitor, indomethacin. Those results have not been corroborated by other investigators and the role of thromboxane and the prostaglandins still needs to be elucidated.

The activation of the proteolytic cascades, including those of coagulation, fibrinolysis, the kinins, and the complement system, has been demonstrated to occur immediately following thermal injury. Kinins, specifically bradykinins, are known to increase vascular permeability, primarily in the venule. Roeha and coworkers[17] report increased kinin levels in burn edema fluid in rats. The release of other mediators and the generalized inflammatory response after burns favors the activation of the kallikrein–kinin system, with the release of bradykinin into the circulation.[18] Elevation of proteolytic activity has been demonstrated in both animals and in burn patients.[19] Pretreatment with protease inhibitors significantly decreases free kinin levels but appears to have little effect on the edema process.

The end result of the changes in the microvasculature due to thermal injury is disruption of normal capillary barriers separating intravascular and interstitial compartments, and rapid equilibrium of these compartments. This results in severe depletion of plasma volume with a marked increase in extracellular fluid, clinically manifested as hypovolemia.

In addition to a loss of capillary integrity, thermal injury also causes changes at the cellular level. Baxter[20] has demonstrated that in burns of >30% total body surface area (TBSA), there is a systemic decrease in cell transmembrane potential, also involving nonthermally injured cells. This decrease in cell transmitting potential, as defined by the Nernst equation, results from an increase in intracellular sodium concentration. The cause of this is thought to be a decrease in sodium ATPase activity responsible for maintaining the intracellular–extracellular ionic gradient. Baxter further demonstrated that resuscitation only partially restores the membrane potential and intracellular sodium concentrations to normal levels, demonstrating that hypovolemia with its attendant ischemia is not totally responsible for the cellular swelling seen in burn shock. In fact, the membrane potential may not return to normal for many days postburn despite adequate resuscitation. If resuscitation is inadequate, cell membrane potential progressively decreases, resulting ultimately in cellular death. This may be the final common denominator in burn shock during the resuscitation period.

Although the etiology of burn shock is not totally understood, many authors have studied the fluid volume shifts and hemodynamic changes which accompany burn shock. Early work by Moyer, and Baxter and Shires, established the definitive role of crystalloid solutions in burn resuscitation and delineated the fluid volume changes in the early postburn period. Moyer's original studies[21] in 1965, demonstrated that burn edema sequestered enormous amounts of fluid, resulting in the hypovolemia of burn shock. In addition, he described the first crystalloid-only resuscitation formula used to treat burn shock. He noted that burn shock recovery occurred in the majority of patients studied, although hemoconcentration remained unchanged and the hematocrit was unresponsive to fluid administration despite adequate resuscitation. This became the first objective evidence that burn shock is not simply due to hypovolemia but is also influenced by extracellular sodium depletion. Baxter and Shires[22] in 1968, using radioisotope dilution techniques, defined the fluid volume changes of the postburn period in relation to cardiac output. They first demonstrated that edema fluid in the burn wound is isotonic with respect to plasma fluid and contains protein in the same proportions as that found in blood. This confirmed Arturson's earlier findings that in major burns there is complete disruption of the normal capillary barrier, with free exchange between plasma and extravascular extracellular compartments. They measured changes in fluid compartment volumes in burned primates and dogs and demonstrated that in untreated (unresuscitated) animals, a 30–50% extracellular fluid (ECF) defect persisted at 18 hours postburn. Plasma volume decreased 23–27% below controls, although red cell mass changed only about 10% over the same 18 hour period. Thus, the greatest volume loss was functional intravascular extracellular fluid. Cardiac output was initially depressed very soon after injury to a level of about 25% of controls at 4 hours after a 30% TBSA burn. By 18 hours, however, the cardiac output had stabilized at around 40% of control, despite persistent defects in plasma and ECF volumes. On the basis of studies using different volumes of resuscitation fluids, they arrived at an optimal response in terms of cardiac output and restoration of ECF at the end of 24 hours in a canine model. Clinical studies using similar sodium and fluid loads immediately followed, confirming efficacy in restoring ECF to within 10% of controls within 24 hours. This became the basis for the Baxter or Parkland formula.[20] Mortality was comparable to that obtained with a colloid-containing resuscitation formula.

Baxter went on to demonstrate that during the first 24 hours postburn, plasma volume changes were independent of the type of infused fluid, whether crystalloid or colloid, but at approximately 24 hours post-injury, an infused amount of colloid would increase the plasma volume by the same amount. His findings prove that colloid-containing solutions are an unnecessary component of fluid resuscitation in the first 24 hours. He recommended their use only after capillary integrity was restored, to correct the persistent plasma volume deficit of about 20% as measured externally. While the fluid shifts were being defined by Baxter in terms of crystalloid resuscitation, Moncrief and Pruitt[4] worked to characterize the hemodynamic alterations that occur in burn shock with and without fluid resuscitation. Their efforts culminated in the Brooke formula modification which utilized 2 ml/kg/% burn during the first 24 hours. Fluid needs were initially estimated according to the modified Brooke formula, but the actual volume for resuscitation was based on clinical response. In their study, resuscitation permitted an average decrease of about 20% in both extracellular fluid and plasma volume, but no further loss accrued in the first 24 hours. In the second 24 hours postburn, plasma volume restoration occurred with the administration of colloid. Blood volume, however, was only partially restored and an ongoing loss of 9% of the red cell mass per day was found. Cardiac output, initially quite low, rose over the first 18 hours postburn, despite plasma volume and blood volume defects. These results were quite consistent with those demonstrated by Baxter in his animal studies. Peripheral vascular resistance during the initial 24 hours was initially very high but decreased as cardiac output improved, and in fact the changes were reciprocal. Once plasma volume and blood volume loss ceased, cardiac output rose to supranormal levels where it remained until healing or grafting occurred.

In 1973, Moylan and associates,[23] using a canine model, defined the relationships between fluid volumes, sodium concentration, and colloid in restoring cardiac output during the first 12 hours post-injury. No significant colloid effect on cardiac output was noted in the first 12 hours post-injury. In addition, 1 mEq of sodium was found to exert an effect on cardiac output equal to 13 times that of 1 ml of salt-free volume. This experiment established the fact that any combination of sodium and volume within the broad limits of the study would effectively resuscitate a thermally injured patient.

Arturson's landmark studies in 1979[16] on vascular permeability characterized the nature of the 'leaky capillary' in the postburn period. He demonstrated in a canine model that increased capillary permeability is found both locally and in nonburned tissue at distant sites when the TBSA burn exceeded 25%. He proposed that the burn wound is characterized by rapid edema formation due to dilatation of the resistance vessels (precapillary arterioles); increased extravascular osmotic activity, due to the products of thermal injury; and increased microvascular permeability to macromolecules. The increased permeability permits molecules of molecular weight up to 350 000 daltons to escape from the microvasculature, a size which allows essentially all elements of the vascular space except red blood cells to escape from it. Further studies by Demling and coworkers[24] have demonstrated that in 50% TBSA burns, one-half of the initial fluid resuscitation requirement may end up in nonthermally injured tissues.

Resuscitation from Burn Shock

Fluid resuscitation is aimed at supporting the patient throughout the initial 24–48 hour period of hypovolemia. The primary goal of therapy is to replace the fluid sequestered as a result of thermal injury. The critical concept in burn shock is that massive fluid shifts can occur even though total body water remains unchanged. What actually changes is the volume of each fluid compartment, intracellular and interstitial volumes increasing at the expense of plasma volume and blood volume. In light of all the studies on different fluid regimens, the question still remains: 'What is the best formula for resuscitation of the burn patient?'

It is quite clear that the edema process is accentuated by the resuscitation fluid. The magnitude of edema will be affected by the amount and type of fluid administered.[25] The National Institutes of Health consensus summary on fluid resuscitation in 1978 was not in agreement with regard to a specific formula; however, there was consensus with regard to two major issues: the guidelines used during the resuscitation process and the type of fluid used. With regard to the guidelines, the consensus was to give the least amount of fluid necessary to maintain adequate organ perfusion. The volume infused should be continually titrated so as to avoid both under-resuscitation and over-resuscitation.[26,27] As for the optimum type of fluid, there is no question that replacement of the extracellular salt lost into the burned tissue and into the cell is essential for successful resuscitation.[19,21]

Crystalloid resuscitation

Crystalloid, in particular lactated Ringer's solution with a sodium concentration of 130 mEq/l, is the most popular resuscitation fluid currently utilized. Proponents of the use of crystalloid solution alone for resuscitation report that other solutions, specifically colloids, are no better and certainly more expensive than crystalloid for maintaining intravascular volume following thermal injury.[4] The most common reason given for not using colloids is that even large proteins leak from the capillary following thermal injury. However, capillaries in nonburned tissues do continue to sieve proteins, maintaining relatively normal protein permeability characteristics.

The quantity of crystalloid needed is in part dependent upon the parameters used to monitor resuscitation. If a urinary output of 0.5 ml/kg body weight/hour is considered to indicate adequate perfusion, approximately 3 ml/kg/% burn will be needed in the first 24 hours. If 1 ml/kg body weight/hour of urine is deemed necessary, then of course considerably more fluid will be needed and in turn more edema will result. The Parkland formula recommends 4 ml/kg/% burn in the first 24 hours, with one-half of that amount administered in the first 8 hours[9] (**Table 6.1**). The modified Brooke

Table 6.1 Formulas for estimating adult burn patient resuscitation fluid needs[48]

Colloid formulas	Electrolyte	Colloid	D5W
Evans	Normal saline 1.0 ml/kg/% burn	1.0 ml/kg/% burn	2000 ml
Brooke	Lactated Ringer's 1.5 ml/kg/% burn	0.5 ml/kg	2000 ml
Slater	Lactated Ringer's 2 l/24 h	Fresh frozen plasma 75 ml/kg/24 h	
Crystalloid formulas			
Parkland	Lactated Ringer's	4 ml/kg/% burn	
Modified Brooke	Lactated Ringer's	2 ml/kg/% burn	
Hypertonic saline formulas			
Hypertonic saline solution (Monafo)	Volume to maintain urine output at 30 ml/h		
	Fluid contains 250 mEq Na/l		
Modified hypertonic (Warden)	Lactated Ringer's + 50 mEq $NaHCO_3$ (180 mEq Na/l) for 8 hours to maintain urine output at 30–50 ml/h		
	Lactated Ringer's to maintain urine output at 30–50 ml/h beginning 8 hours postburn		
Dextran formula (Demling)	Dextran 40 in saline – 2 ml/kg/h for 8 hours		
	Lactated Ringer's – volume to maintain urine output at 30 ml/h		
	Fresh frozen plasma – 0.5 ml/kg/h for 18 hours beginning 8 hours postburn		

formula recommends beginning burn shock resuscitation at 2 ml/kg/% burn in the first 24 hours (Table 6.1). In major burns, severe hypoproteinemia usually develops with these resuscitation regimens. The hypoproteinemia and interstitial protein depletion may result in more edema formation.

Hypertonic saline

Hypertonic salt solutions have been known for many years to be effective in treating burn shock.[28,29] Monafo[28] reported that the resuscitation of burn patients with salt solution of 240–300 mEq/l resulted in less edema because of the smaller total fluid requirements than with lactated Ringer's solution. Urine output was the indicator used during resuscitation. Demling and colleagues[30] in an animal model demonstrated that the net fluid intake was less if burned animals were resuscitated with hypertonic saline to the same cardiac output compared with lactated Ringer's. Urine output was much higher with hypertonic solution. Interestingly, soft tissue interstitial edema in burned and nonburned tissue, as reflected by lymph flow, was increased with hypertonic saline similar to that of lactated Ringer's. This can be explained by a shift of intracellular water into extracellular space as the result of the hyperosmolar solution. Extracellular edema can therefore occur at the same time as intracellular fluid defect. This may give the external appearance of less edema. Although several studies to date have reported that this intracellular water depletion does not appear to be deleterious, the issue remains controversial. Current recommendations are that the serum sodium levels should not be allowed to exceed 160 mEq/dl during its use. Of interest, Gunn and associates,[31] in a prospective randomized study of patients with 20% TBSA burns evaluating hypertonic sodium lactate versus lactated Ringer's solution, were not able to demonstrate decreased fluid requirements, improved nutritional tolerance, or decreased percent weight gain.

One burns institute in Cincinnati has utilized a modified hypertonic solution in major thermal injuries >40% TBSA burn. The resuscitation fluid contains 180 mEq Na^+ (lactated Ringer's + 50 mEq $NaHCO_3$). The solution is utilized until the reversal of metabolic acidosis has occurred, usually by 8 hours postburn. The volume administered is begun at a rate calculated by the Parkland formula (4 ml/kg/% burn); however, volume is titrated to maintain urine output at 30–50 ml/hr. After 8 hours the resuscitation is completed utilizing lactated Ringer's to maintain urine output at 30–50 ml/h. This hypertonic formula can be used in infants and in the elderly without the accompanying risk of hypernatremia.[32,33]

Colloid resuscitation

Plasma proteins are extremely important in the circulation since they generate the inward oncotic force that counteracts the outward capillary hydrostatic force. Without protein, plasma volume could not be maintained and massive edema would result. Protein replacement was an important component of early formulas for burn management. The Evans formula, advocated in 1952, used 1 ml/kg body weight/% burn each for colloid and lactated Ringer's over the first 24 hours. The Brooke formula clearly was based on estimate rather than determined scientifically, but the formula used 0.5 ml/kg/% burn as colloid and 1.5 ml/kg/% burn as lactated Ringer's. The burn budget of Moore similarly used a substantial amount of colloids[3]. Considerable confusion exists concerning the role of protein in a resuscitation formula. There are three schools of thought:

- Protein solutions should not be given in the first 24 hours because during this period they are no more effective than salt water in maintaining intravascular volume and they promote accumulation of lung water when edema fluid is being absorbed from the burn wound;[34]
- Proteins, specifically albumin, should be given from the beginning of resuscitation along with crystalloid; they should usually be added to salt water; and
- Protein should be given between 8 and 12 hours postburn using strictly crystalloid in the first 8–12 hours because of the massive fluid shifts during this period.

Demling demonstrated experimentally that restoration and maintenance of plasma protein contents were not effective until 8 hours postburn, after which adequate levels can be maintained with infusion.[35] Because nonburned tissues appear to regain normal permeability very shortly after injury and because hypoproteinemia may accentuate the edema, the action advocated by the first school appears to be least appropriate.

The choice of the type of protein solution can be confusing. Heat-fixed protein solutions, e.g. Plasmanate, are known to contain some denatured and aggregated protein, which decreases the oncotic effect. Albumin solutions would clearly be the most oncotically active solutions. Fresh frozen plasma, however, contains all the protein fractions that exert both the oncotic and the nononcotic actions. The optimal amount of protein to infuse remains undefined. Demling[35] uses between 0.5 and 1 ml/kg/% burn of fresh frozen plasma during the first 24 hours, beginning at 8–10 hours postburn.[36,37] He emphasizes that all major burns require large amounts of fluid, but notes that older patients with burns, patients with burns and concomitant inhalation injury, and patients with burns in excess of 50% TBSA not only develop less edema but also better maintain hemodynamic stability with the addition of protein.

Slater and coworkers[32] have recently utilized fresh frozen plasma during burn shock. They use lactated Ringer's, 2 liters for 24 hours, and fresh frozen plasma, 75 ml/kg/24 h (**Table 6.1**). Although the volume of fresh frozen plasma is calculated, the volume infused is titrated to maintain an adequate urine output. Although the authors are utilizing colloid early in the burn shock period, they emphasize that most burned patients have received lactated Ringer's in significant volumes during field management.

In the young pediatric burned patient with major burn injury, colloid replacement is frequently required as serum protein concentration rapidly decreases during burn shock.

Dextran resuscitation solutions

Dextran is a colloid consisting of glucose molecules which have been polymerized into chains to form high molecular weight polysaccharides.[37] This compound is commercially available in a number of molecular sizes. Dextran, which has an average molecular weight of 40 000 daltons, is referred to as low molecular weight dextran. British dextran has a mean molecular weight of 150 000 daltons whereas the dextran used predominantly in Sweden has a molecular weight of 70 000 daltons. Dextran is excreted at the kidneys, with 40% removed within 24 hours. The remainder is slowly metabolized. Demling and associates have utilized dextran 70 in a 6% solution to prevent edema in nonburned tissues. Dextran 70 carries some risk of allergic reaction and can interfere with blood typing. Dextran 40 actually improves the microcirculatory flow by decreasing red cell aggregation.[38] Demling and colleagues[37] demonstrated that the net requirements to maintain vascular pressure at the baseline levels with dextran 40 were about half those seen with lactated Ringer's alone during the first 24 hours postburn. These authors have used an infusion rate of dextran 40 and saline of

2 ml/kg/h along with sufficient lactated Ringer's to maintain adequate perfusion. At 8 hours an infusion of fresh frozen plasma at 0.5–1.0 ml/kg/% TBSA burn over 18 hours is instituted along with necessary additional crystalloid (**Table 6.1**).

Special Considerations in Burn Shock Resuscitation

Fluid resuscitation in the thermally injured pediatric patient

The burned child continues to represent a special challenge, since resuscitation therapy must be more precise than that for an adult with a similar burn. In addition, children have a limited physiologic reserve. One burns institute has demonstrated that children require more fluid for burn shock resuscitation than adults with similar thermal injury; fluid requirements for children averaged 5.8 ml/kg/% burn.[39] In addition, children commonly require intravenous resuscitation for relatively small burns of 10–20% TBSA. Baxter[33] found similar resuscitation requirements in the pediatric age group. Graves and associates[40] substantiated that children received 6.3 ± 2 ml/kg/% TBSA burn. At the Shriners Burns Institute, Cincinnati Unit, we have utilized the Parkland formula with the addition of maintenance fluid, to the resuscitation fluid volume, 4 ml/kg/x% TBSA burn per 24 hours + 1500 ml/m^2 BSA per 24 hours. This is the formula used to begin burn shock resuscitation and to compare the amount of fluid needed by a particular pediatric burned patient with that needed by an unburned pediatric patient (**Table 6.2**). This is similar to the results reported by Graves and coworkers[40] who found that if maintenance fluids were subtracted from the resuscitation fluid requirements, the resulting resuscitation volumes would approach 4 ml/kg/% burn. At the Shriners Burns Institute in Galveston, fluid requirements are estimated according to a formula based on total BSA and BSA burned in square meters.[41] Total fluid requirements for the first day are estimated as follows: 5000 ml/m^2 BSA burned per 24 hours + 2000 ml/m^2 BSA per 24 hours.

Inhalation injury

The presence of inhalation injury increases the fluid requirements for resuscitation from burn shock after thermal injury.[42] We have demonstrated that patients with documented inhalation injury require 5.7 ml/kg/% burn, as compared to 3.98 ml/kg/% burn in patients without inhalation injury. These data confirm and quantitate that inhalation injury accompanying thermal trauma increases the magnitude of total body injury and requires increased volumes of fluid and sodium to achieve resuscitation from early burn shock.

Choice of Fluids and Rate of Administration

It is clear that all the solutions reviewed are effective in restoring tissue perfusion. However, it makes no more sense to use one particular fluid for all patients than it does to use one antibiotic for all infections. Most patients with burns of <40% TBSA and patients with no pulmonary injury can be resuscitated with isotonic crystalloid fluid. In patients with burns of >40% TBSA and in patients with pulmonary injury, hypertonic saline can be utilized in the first 8 hours postburn, following which lactated Ringer's is infused to complete burn shock resuscitation. In the pediatric and elderly burn patient population, utilizing a lower but still hypertonic concentration of sodium, i.e. 180 mEq/l, still gives the benefits of hypertonic resuscitation without the potential complications of excessive sodium retention and hypernatremia.

In patients with massive burns, young pediatric patients, and burns complicated by severe inhalation injury, a combination of fluids may be utilized to achieve the desired goal of tissue perfusion while minimizing edema. In treating such patients, we have utilized the regimen of modified hypertonic (lactated Ringer's + 50 mEq $NaHCO_3$) saline fluid containing 180 mEq Na/l for the first 8 hours. After correction of the metabolic acidosis, which generally requires 8 hours, the patients are given lactated Ringer's only for the second 8 hours. In the last 8 hours, a 5% albumin in lactated Ringer's is utilized to complete resuscitation. The resuscitation solution used in Galveston for pediatric patients is an isotonic glucose-containing solution to which a moderate amount of colloid (human serum albumin) is added. The solution is prepared by mixing 50 ml of 25% human serum albumin (12.5 g) with 950 ml of 5% dextrose in a lactated Ringer's solution.

The volume of resuscitation fluid infused should be adequate for tissue perfusion. The volume of infused fluid should maintain a urine output of 30–50 ml/h hour in adults and 1 ml/h in children. It is important to remember that in children weighing >50 kg, the urine volume should not exceed 30–50 ml/h. Heart rate and blood pressure are not necessarily indicative of fluid volume status in the burn patient. Fluid volume status and cardiac output may be measured directly via thermodilution pulmonary artery catheterization. However, a low measured filling pressure with evidence of adequate perfusion is common. Placement of a Swan–Ganz catheter to monitor burn shock resuscitation should be reserved for burn patients with limited cardiac reserve, such as the elderly or patients with significant co-morbid diseases. In addition, burned patients who require volumes that are extremely excessive may require monitoring by thermodilutional pulmonary artery catheterization.

It is important to emphasize that all of the resuscitation formulas are only guidelines for burn shock resuscitation. The Parkland formula, for instance, decreases the volume administered by 50% at 8 hours postburn. The relationship between the fluid volume required

Table 6.2 Formulas for estimating pediatric resuscitation needs

Cincinnati Unit,	4 ml × kg × % TBSA burn	1st 8 hours	Lactated Ringer's + 50 mg $NaHCO_3$
Shriners Burns Institute	+		
	1500 ml × m^2 BSA	2nd 8 hours	Lactated Ringer's
		3rd 8 hours	Lactated Ringer's + 12.5 g albumin
Galveston Unit,	5000 ml/m^2 BSA burn	DS Ringer's lactate	
Shriners Burns Institute	+	+	
	2000 ml/m^2 BSA	12.5 g albumin	

and time postburn depicted by the smooth curve in **Figure 6.1** represents the influence of temporal changes in microvascular permeability and edema volume on fluid needs. That curve is contrasted with the abrupt changes in fluid infusion rate as prescribed by the formula. The formulas are utilized as starting points for volume replacement and to compare the individual patient with the 'average' burned patient.

An interesting question is: 'When has burn shock resuscitation been completed successfully?' It is obvious that resuscitation is completed when there is no further accumulation of edema fluid, which generally occurs between 18 and 30 hours postburn. The resuscitation fluids are utilized until the volume of infused fluid needed to maintain adequate urine volume of 30–50 ml/h in adults and 1 ml/kg/h in children equals the maintenance fluid volume. The maintenance fluid requirements following burn shock resuscitation include the patient's normal maintenance volume plus evaporative water loss.

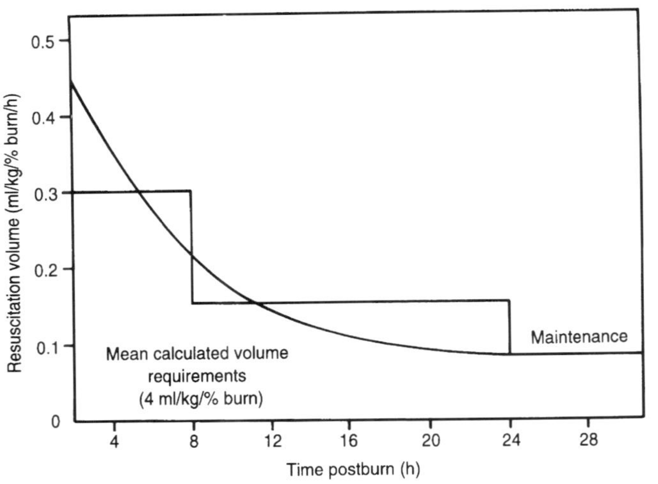

Fig. 6.1 Physiologic curve of fluid requirements compared to Parkland formula, emphasizing that formulas are only guidelines for fluid therapy during burn shock. Adapted from Warden,[48] with permission.

Failure of Burn Shock Resuscitation

In certain patients, failure of burn shock resuscitation still occurs despite administration of massive volumes of fluid. Such patients are characterized by either extreme age and exceptionally extensive tissue trauma or by major electrical injury, major inhalation injury, delay in initiating adequate fluid resuscitation or underlying disease that limits metabolic and cardiovascular reserve.[43] In these patients, refractory burn shock and resuscitation failure remain major causes of early mortality despite advances in emergency care and transport, resuscitation regimens, and physiologic stabilization.

A burns institute in Cincinnati has used plasma exchange in patients with major thermal injuries who failed to respond to conventional fluid volumes during resuscitation from burn shock.[44] The indications for plasma exchange are ongoing fluid requirements exceeding twice those predicted by the Parkland formula despite conversion to hypertonic lactated saline resuscitation fluid. During a 3-year period, 22 patients underwent plasma exchange during burn shock resuscitation. A therapeutic response was documented in 21 of the 22 patients, characterized by a sharp decrease in fluid requirements from a mean of 260% above the predicted hourly volume by the resuscitation formula to within calculated requirements at a mean time of 2.3 hours following plasma exchange. Only one patient, who had a 100% TBSA burn (88% full thickness), failed to respond to plasma exchange and expired at 18 hours postburn. Slater and Goldfarb[45] have substantiated the beneficial effect of plasma exchange in sustaining patients during the immediate postburn period when patients fail to respond appropriately to conventional fluid resuscitation. This modality offers an alternative management technique for the treatment of refractory burn shock.

Fluid Replacement Following Burn Shock Resuscitation

Although the heat-injured microvessels may continue to manifest increased vascular permeability for several days, the rate of loss is considerably less than that seen in the first 24 hours. Burn edema by this time is near maximal and the interstitial space may well be saturated with sodium. Additional fluid requirements will depend on the type of fluid used during the initial resuscitation. If hypertonic salt resuscitation has been utilized during the entire burn shock period, a hyperosmolar state is produced and the addition of free water will be required to restore the extracellular space to an iso-osmolar state.

If colloid has not been utilized during burn shock and the serum oncotic pressure is low due to intravascular protein depletion, protein repletion is frequently needed. The amount of protein varies with the resuscitation utilized. Requirements of 0.3–6.5 ml/kg/TBSA burn of 5% albumin during the second 24 hours are utilized with the modified Brooke formula. The Parkland formula replaces the plasma volume deficit with colloid. This deficit varies from 20% to 60% of the circulating plasma volume. We have utilized colloid replacement based on a 20% plasma volume deficit during the second 24 hours (circulating plasma volume × 20%).

In addition to colloid, the patients should receive maintenance fluids. In burned patients the maintenance fluids include an additional amount for evaporative water loss. The total daily maintenance fluid requirements in the adult patient following burn shock can be calculated by the following formula: Basal (1500 ml/m^2) + evaporative water loss [(25 + % burn) × m^2 × 24] = total maintenance fluid (m^2 = total body surface area in square meters). This fluid may be given via the intravenous route or with enteral feeding. The solution infused intravenously should be 50% normal saline with potassium supplements. With the loss of intracellular potassium during burn shock, the potassium requirements in adults are about 120 mEq/day. In the pediatric patient, increased fluids are required due to the differences in TBSA to weight ratios compared to adults. In addition, children also require relatively larger volumes of urine for excretion of waste products. At the Cincinnati Shriners' Unit, the maintenance fluid requirements are calculated by the following formula: (35 + % burn × TBSA × 24 (evaporative water loss) + 1500 ml × TBSA per day (maintenance fluids). In Galveston, the recommended fluid needs are estimated as follows: 3750 ml/m^2 TBSA per day (burn-related losses) + 1500 ml/m^2 BSA per day (maintenance fluids).

Following the initial 24–48 hours postburn period of resuscitation, urinary output is an unreliable guide to adequacy of hydration.[46] Respiratory water losses, osmotic diuresis secondary to accentuated glucose intolerance, osmotic diuresis secondary to high protein, high caloric feedings and derangements in the ADH mechanisms all contribute to increased fluid losses despite an adequate urine output. In general, patients with major thermal injuries will require a urine output of 1500–2000 ml/24 hours in adults, and 3–4 ml/kg/h in children.

The measurement of serum sodium concentration is not only a means of diagnosing dehydration, but the best guide for planning and following successful fluid replacement. Other useful laboratory indices of the state of hydration and guides of therapy include body weight change, serum and urine nitrogen concentrations, serum and urine glucose concentrations, the intake and output record, and clinical examination. Continuous colloid replacement may be required to maintain colloid oncotic pressure in very large burns and in the pediatric burn patient. Maintaining serum albumin levels above 2.0 g/dl is desirable. The electrolytes calcium, magnesium and phosphate must also be monitored. Although the replacement of these electrolytes has been studied in detail in burn patients, maintaining the values within normal limits is desirable and vary in each patient.

Summary

The volume necessary to resuscitate burn patients depends upon injury severity, age, physiologic status, and associated injury. Consequently, the volume predicted by a resuscitation formula must commonly be modified according to the individual's response to therapy. In optimizing fluid resuscitation in severely burned patients, the amount of fluid should be just enough to maintain vital organ function without producing iatrogenic pathological changes. The composition of the resuscitation fluid, within limitations, in the first 24 hours postburn probably makes very little difference; however, it should be individualized to the particular patient. The utilization of the beneficial properties of hypertonic, crystalloid, and colloid solutions at various times postburn will minimize the amount of edema formation. The rate of administration of resuscitation fluids should maintain urine outputs of 30–50 ml in adults and 1–2 ml/kg in children. When a child weighs 30–50 kg, the urine output should be maintained at the adult level. Fluid resuscitation based on our current knowledge of the massive fluid shifts and vascular changes which occur following burn injury has markedly decreased mortality related to burn-induced volume loss. The failure rate for adequate resuscitation is <5% even for patients with burns >85% TBSA. These improved statistics, however, are derived from experience in burn centers where there is substantial knowledge of the pathophysiology of burn injury. Inadequate volume replacement in major burns is, unfortunately, common when clinicians lack sufficient knowledge and experience in this area.

Areas of burn shock research which need further attention include:

- the definition of the postburn course of capillary permeability changes and identification of humoral or cellular factors influencing these changes;
- the identification and evaluation of pharmacologic agents which can significantly alter capillary leakage;
- elucidation of the relationships between resuscitation fluid composition and pulmonary function changes; and
- the effect of resuscitation on late organ dysfunction, such as post-resuscitation wound, renal, and pulmonary complications.[47]

References

1. Artz C P, Moncrief J A. The burn problem. In: Artz C P, Moncrief J A, eds. *The Treatment of Burns*. Philadelphia: W B Saunders, 1969: 1–22.

2. Underhill F P. The significance of anhydremia in extensive surface burn. *JAMA* 1930; **95:** 852–7.

3. Moore F D. The body-weight budget: basic fluid therapy for the early burn. *Surg Clin North Am* 1970; **50:** 1249–65.

4. Pruitt B A Jr, Mason A D Jr, Moncrief J A. Hemodynamic changes in the early post burn patients: the influence of fluid administration and of a vasodilator (hydralazine). *J Trauma* 1971; **11:** 36–46.

5. Majno G, Palide G E. Studies on inflammation. I. The effect of histamine and serotonin on vascular permeability. *J Cell Biol* 1961; **11:** 571–8.

6. Majno G, Shea S M, Leventhal M. Endothelial contractures induced by histamine type mediators. *J Cell Biol* 1969; **42:** 647–72.

7. Anggard E, Jonsson C E. Eflux of prostaglandins in lymph from scalded tissue. *Acta Physiol Scand* 1971; **81:** 440–7.

8. Sevitt S. Local blood flow in experimental burns. *J Pathol Bact* 1949; **61:** 427–34.

9. Leape L. Initial changes in burns: tissue changes in burned and unburned skins of Rhesus monkeys. *J Trauma* 1970; **10:** 488–92.

10. Carvajal H F, Brouhard B H, Linares H A. Effect of antihistamine-antiserotonin and ganglionic blocking agents upon increased capillary permeability following burn trauma. *J Trauma* 1975; **15:** 969–75.

11. Boykin J V Jr, Crute S L, Haynes B W Jr. Cimetidine therapy for burn shock: a quantitative assessment. *J Trauma* 1985; **25:** 864–70.

12. VanNeuten J M, Janssen P A J, VanBeck J. Vascular effects of ketanserin (R 41 468), a novel antagonist of 5-HT_2 serotonergic receptors. *J Pharmacol Exp Ther* 1981; **218:** 217–80.

13. Holliman C J, Meuleman T R, Larsen K R, *et al.* The effect of ketanserin, a specific serotonin antagonist, on burn shock hemodynamic parameters in a porcine burn model. *J Trauma* 1983; **23:** 867–74.

14. Heggers J P, Loy G L, Robson M C, DelBaccaro E J. Histological demonstration of prostaglandins and thromboxanes in burned tissue. *J Surg Res* 1980; **28:** 110–17.

15. Herndon D N, Abston S, Stein M D. Increased thromboxane B_2 levels in the plasma of burned and septic burned patients. *Surg Gynecol Obstet* 1984; **159:** 210–13.

16. Arturson G. Microvascular permeability to macromolecules in thermal injury. *Acta Physiol Scand Suppl* 1979; **463:** 111–22.

17. Roeha E, Silva M, Antonio A. Release of bradykinin and the mechanisms of production of thermic edema (45°C) in the rat's paw. *Med Exp* 1960; **3:** 371–8.

18. Holder I A, Neely A N. Hageman factor-dependent kinin activation in burns and its theoretical relationship to postburn immunosuppression syndrome and infection. *J Burn Care Rehabil* 1990; **11**(6): 496–503.

19. Neely A N, Nathan P, Highsmith R F. Plasma proteolytic activity following burns. *J Trauma* 1988; **28:** 362–7.

20. Baxter C R. Fluid volume and electrolyte changes in the early postburn period. *Clin Plast Surg* 1974; **1:** 693–703.

21. Moyer C A, Margraf H W, Monafo W W. Burn shock and extravascular sodium deficiency: treatment with Ringer's solution with lactate. *Arch Surg* 1965; **90:** 799–811.

22. Baxter C R, Shires G T. Physiological response to crystalloid resuscitation of severe burns. *Ann NY Acad Sci* 1968; **150:** 874–94.

23. Moylan J A, Mason A B, Rogers P W, Walker H L. Postburn shock: a critical evaluation of resuscitation. *J Trauma* 1973; **13:** 354–8.

24. Demling R H, Mazess R B, Witt R M, Wolbert W H. The study of burn wound edema using dichosmatic absorptionmetry. *J Trauma* 1978; **18:** 124–8.

25. Hilton J G. Effects of fluid resuscitation on total fluid loss following thermal injury. *Surg Gynecol Obstet* 1981; **152:** 441–7.

26. Schwartz S L. Consensus summary on fluid resuscitation. *J Trauma* 1979; **19**(11 Suppl): 876–7.

27. Shires G T. Proceedings of the second NIH Workshop on Burn Management. *J Trauma* 1979; **19**(11 Suppl): 862–3.

28. Monafo W W. The treatment of burn shock by the intravenous and oral administration of hypertonic lactated saline solution. *J Trauma* 1970; **10:** 575–86.

29. Monafo W W, Halverson J D, Schechtman K. The role of concentrated sodium solutions in the resuscitation of patients with severe burns. *Surgery* 1984; **95:** 129–35.

30. Demling R H, Gunther R A, Haines B, Kramer G. Burn edema. Part II: Complications, prevention, and treatment. *J Burn Care Rehabil* 1982; **3:** 199–206.

31. Gunn M L, Hansbrough J F, Davis J W, Furst S R, Field T O. Prospective randomized trial of hypertonic sodium lactate vs. lactated Ringer's solution for burn shock resuscitation. *J Trauma* 1989; **29:** 1261–7.

32. Du G, Slater H, Goldfarb I W. Influence of different resuscitation regimens on acute weight gain in extensively burned patients. *Burns* 1991; **17:** 147–50.

33. Baxter C R. Problems and complications of burn shock resuscitation. *Surg Clin North Am* 1978; **58:** 1313–22.

34. Goodwin C W, Dorethy J, Lam V, Pruitt B A Jr. Randomized trial of efficacy of crystalloid and colloid resuscitation on hemodynamic response and lung water following thermal injury. *Ann Surg* 1983; **197:** 520–31.

35. Demling R H. Fluid resuscitation. In: Boswick J A Jr, ed. *The Art and Science of Burn Care*. Rockville: Aspen, 1987: 189–202.

36. Demling R H, Kramer G D, Harms B. Role of thermal injury-induced hypoproteinemia on edema formation in burned and non-burned tissue. *Surgery* 1984; **95:** 136–44.

37. Demling R H, Kramer G C, Gunther R, Nerlich M. Effect of non-protein colloid on post-burn edema formation in soft tissues and lung. *Surgery* 1985; **95:** 593–602.

38. Gelin L E, Solvell L, Zederfeldt B. The plasma volume expanding effect of low viscous dextran and Macrodex. *Acta Chir Scand* 1961; **122:** 309–23.

39. Merrell S W, Saffle J R, Sullivan J J, Navar P D, Kravitz M, Warden G D, Fluid resuscitation in thermally injured children. *Am J Surg* 1986; **152:** 664–9.

40. Graves T A, Cioffi W G, McManus W F, Mason A D Jr, Pruitt B A Jr. Fluid resuscitation of infants and children with massive thermal injury. *J Trauma* 1988; **28:** 1656–9.

41. Carvajal H F. Fluid therapy for the acutely burned child. *Compr Ther* 1977; **3**(3): 17–24.

42. Navar P D, Saffle J R, Warden G D. Effect of inhalation injury on fluid resuscitation requirements after thermal injury. *Am J Surg* 1985; **150:** 716–20.

43. Pruitt B Jr. Fluid and electrolyte replacement in the burned patient. *Surg Clin North Am* 1978; **58:** 1291–312.

44. Warden G D, Stratta R, Saffle J R Jr, Kravitz M, Ninnemann J L. Plasma exchange therapy in patients failing to resuscitate from burn shock. *J Trauma* 1983; **23:** 945–51.

45. Schnarrs R, Cline C, Goldfarb I, *et al.* Plasma exchange for failure of early resuscitation in thermal injuries. *J Burn Care Rehabil* 1986; **7:** 230–3.

46. Warden G D, Wilmore D, Rogers P, Mason A D, Pruitt B. Hypernatremic state in hypermetabolic burn patients. *Arch Surg* 1973; **106:** 420–3.

47. Pruitt B A Jr. Fluid resuscitation of extensively burned patients. *J Trauma* 1981; **21** (Suppl): 690–2.

48. Warden G D. Burn shock resuscitation. *World J Surg* 1992; **16:** 16–23.

The Burn Wound

CHAPTER SEVEN

Pathophysiology of the Burn Wound

William G. Williams and Linda G. Phillips

The burn wound is the source of virtually all ill effects, local and systemic, seen in a burned patient. Removal of the burn wound (excision) results in a much improved patient and, when done early, results in improvements in survival as well as a decline in morbidity. It could be said that a burn wound and all of the subsequent events observed in the patient represent a continuum, without any clear points of separation. While recognizing this, the focus of this chapter concerns the events occurring in and surrounding the burned skin and subcutaneous tissues during the acute and subacute period. Only brief references are made to remote systemic effects and to healing and scarring, all of which are covered in other chapters.

Anatomy and Physiology of Normal Skin (Figure 7.1)

The surface area of the skin ranges from 0.2 to 0.3 m^2 in an average newborn to 1.5 to 2.0 m^2 in an adult. The skin consists of two layers: the epidermis, ranging from 0.05 mm thick (in areas such as the eyelids) to over 1 mm thick on the soles; and the dermis, usually at least 10 times thicker than the associated epidermis. An average total skin depth is 1–2 mm. Males generally have thicker skin than females. Skin is very thin in infants, increasing in thickness until age 30 or 40, and then progressively thinning with age. The

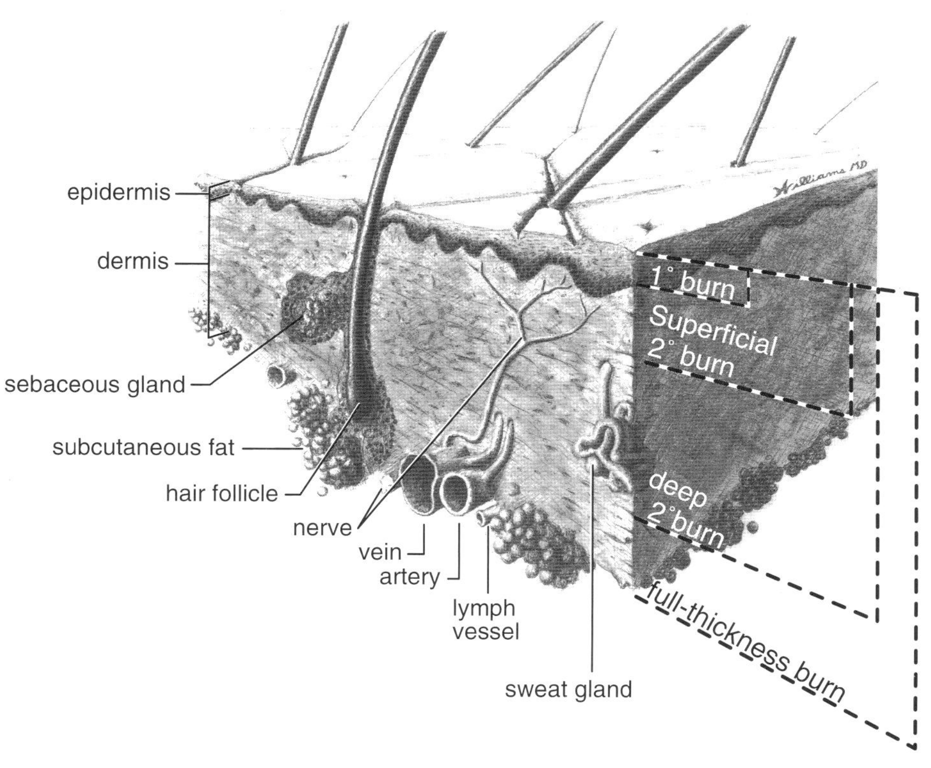

Fig. 7.1 Diagram of the skin including description of the various depths of burn injury. (Reproduced with permission from William G. Williams MD.)

epidermis, originating from ectoderm, is composed primarily of epithelial cells, specifically keratinocytes, as well as other cell types, including: melanocytes, which function to produce pigment for the purpose of ultraviolet radiation protection; Langerhans cells which serve an immune function; and Merkel cells which serve as mechanoreceptors.

The basal layer of keratinocytes is called the stratum germinativum and contains young cells which are mitotically active, providing generation of outwardly migrating epidermal cell layers. From this layer, cells migrate outward and mature along the way to become the stratum spinosum, a layer where mitosis no longer occurs but protein synthesis is prominent. The next outward layer of maturation is the stratum granulosum where specialization into keratin production predominates. The next stage of migration is the stratum lucidum, where cells lose their nuclei and flatten, evolving into a dead layer called the stratum corneum. This layer, composed of keratin, along with cellular debris, is a compact, relatively impervious layer which eventually desquamates. The entire process of epidermal maturation and turnover from the basal layer to desquamation takes approximately 2–4 weeks. Epidermal appendages (i.e. hair follicles, sebaceous glands, and sweat glands) are comprised of special cell types but are also lined with epidermal cells. These structures extend from the epidermis downward, residing mostly in the dermis.

The dermis, derived from mesoderm, is a relatively thick layer comprised of fibrous connective tissue. The primary cell type is the fibroblast, a spindle-shaped cell which does not frequently replicate but is very active in producing extracellular protein, primarily collagen and elastin. Collagen is secreted into the intercellular matrix, where it undergoes maturation (cross-linking and coiling) into strong fibers oriented so as to allow stretchability while providing tensile strength. Elastin is processed to form elastic fibers, imparting a degree of resting tension to the skin. Constant turnover (i.e. degradation, remodeling, and production of collagen) occurs at a low rate in unstressed skin and at higher rates when chronic mechanical stress is applied or when healing is occurring. This, along with plasticity in the arrangement of cells, grants the skin a great capacity to comply, over time, with two- and three-dimensional stresses. The ground substance of the skin is a non-fibrous bulk of glycosaminoglycans, proteoglycans and similar macromolecules. Hyaluronic acid is an example of a well known and important glycosaminoglycan. The ground substance provides a semifluid matrix which lubricates the cellular and fibrillar components; it is through this ground substance that inflammatory and other cells may migrate and nutrients diffuse.

The dermis is subdivided into a thin, superficial layer known as the papillary dermis and a thicker, deep portion called the reticular dermis. A large plexus of vessels beneath the dermis, known as the subdermal plexus, sends vessels upward to again form a plexus between the reticular and papillary dermis. More superficial yet, exists a network of smaller vessels, the papillary plexus. Other structures found in the dermis include lymphatics and also nerve fibers which are either bare-ended or receptor-associated. At the dermoepidermal junction exists a basement membrane, a layer composed of mucopolysaccharides but also rich in fibronectin. Cells of the basal epidermal layer are joined to the basement membrane by hemidesmosomes. The basement membrane, in turn, is anchored to the dermis with the aid of specialized fibrils.

Although the skin is often not thought of as an organ, its specific and vital functions clearly define it as such. These include:

- Protective – guards the body from harmful environmental entities, including radiation, weather, etc.
- Immunological – assists in the presentation of antigens to immune cells. Sebum possesses antibacterial properties owing to its high levels of long-chain fatty acids, particularly oleic acid.[1] Skin prevents entry of microorganisms and actually disposes of invasive bacteria through the desquamation process.
- Fluid, protein, and electrolyte homeostasis – prevents the excessive loss of these substances and participates in the control of fluid and electrolyte excretion.
- Thermoregulation – along with its appendages, prevents heat loss but also allows for rapid cooling during times of exercise through evaporation of sweat as well as vasodilation of dermal vessels.
- Neurosensory – possesses nerve endings and receptors which enable the nervous system to process and interpret information (pain, touch, hot and cold) from the environment.
- Social-interactive – when intact, aids in certain social, interpersonal reactions (sexual identity and attraction, body image, etc.).
- Metabolism – vitamin D production.

Thermal Energy and its Early Molecular, Cellular and Tissue Effects

Thermal energy or heat is a manifestation of random molecular kinetic energy. This energy is easily transferred from high energy molecules to those of lower energy during contact, via a process referred to as *conduction* of heat. An example of this process is a hot stove coil transferring heat to a pot. Conduction is greatly enhanced when the molecules which are giving up heat to a body or, alternatively, removing heat from a body are rapidly whisked away and replaced. This occurs when currents of air or liquid are involved; and the process is referred to as *convection*. An example would be the cooling of a hot object in a cool wind. *Radiation* describes a process whereby a molecule may give up kinetic energy through conversion to electromagnetic energy. The electromagnetic energy then travels through space to where it may be absorbed by another molecule, imparting kinetic energy (i.e. heat) again to a receiving molecule. An example would be the electric coil of a light bulb emitting infrared electromagnetic radiation which travels through space to heat an observer's hand several inches away.

All of these mechanisms affecting heat transfer may deliver heat to or away from living tissues. Radiation is a relatively inefficient method of heat transfer; and, for significant tissue injury to occur it must involve either a very hot temperature source such as an electric arc flash, or a long duration of exposure such as lying under a heat lamp. Conduction is more efficient, as is the case of burning a hand with a hot iron or by immersion in scalding water. In many burn injuries more than one of these mechanisms may be a factor as is the case when ignition of clothing is involved. Intense infrared radiation is emitted from a source of ignition (the clothing), heat is conducted from the hot fabric to the skin, and hot gases liberated from the flame heat the skin through convection.

When contemplating the effect of heat on a cell, one must consider the temperature to which the cell is heated as well as the time period for which the temperature is sustained. These two factors together determine the degree of damage incurred by a cell. Moritz and Henriquez[2] were among the first to work out the time–temperature relationship in thermal injury to skin (**Figure 7.2**). At sustained temperatures between 40 and 44°C,[2] various enzyme systems begin to malfunction, and early denaturation of protein

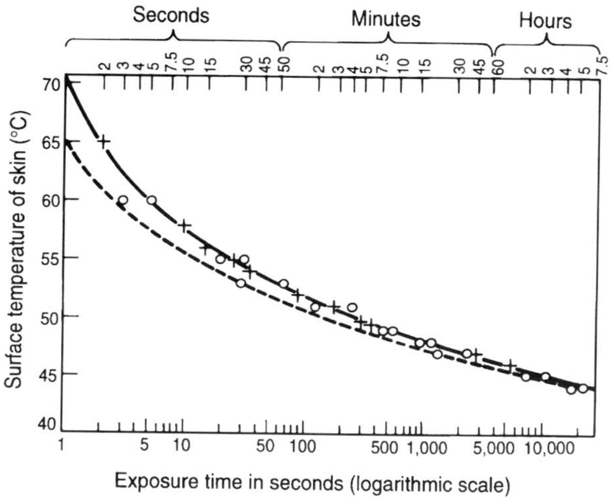

Fig. 7.2 Time–surface temperature thresholds at which cutaneous burning occurs. The broken line indicates the threshold at which irreversible epidermal injury of porcine skin is first sustained. The solid line indicates the threshold at which epidermal necrosis of porcine skin occurs. Critical exposures of porcine skin are represented by crosses. Each cross denotes the shortest exposure time at the temperature indicated which resulted in trans-epidermal necrosis. The results of critical experimental exposures of human skin are indicated by circles. The open circles represent the longest exposure at the temperature indicated that failed to destroy the epidermis, and the solid circles represent the shortest exposure at the temperature indicated that resulted in trans-epidermal necrosis. (Reproduced with permission from Moritz A R and Henriques F C. Studies of thermal injury II. The relative importance of time and surface temperature in the causation of cutaneous burns. Am J Pathol *1947;* ***23:*** *695–720.)*

occurs. Cellular functions are impaired, one of which is the membrane Na^+ pump; and the result is a high intracellular Na^+ concentration and concomitant swelling. As the temperature reaches 44°C and higher, damage accumulation outruns the cell's inherent repair mechanisms, assuming exposure time is long enough, and leads to eventual necrosis. Plasma membrane modifications which are significant enough to cause necrosis have been observed in cells exposed to 45°C for 1 hour.[3] Also occurring as part of the damage process is the production of oxygen free radicals, a class of oxygen species exhibiting an unpaired electron. These highly reactive molecules are capable of promoting further cell membrane abnormalities, leading to cell death. If the heat source is suddenly withdrawn, damage accumulation will continue until the cooling process brings cells back down to a tolerable temperature range. If, therefore, the cell is rapidly cooled, a significant amount of damage is obviated, which may determine whether a cell survives or dies.

As temperature increases, protein destruction increases in severity. The early denaturation described above gives way to severe alteration of protein, a process referred to as coagulation. This phenomenon involves destruction of all levels of protein architecture. New aberrant bonds are formed, creating macromolecules not resembling original structures. This condition may be reached immediately in cases where skin is exposed to high temperatures or, alternatively, where lower temperature is applied for longer duration. In either case cell necrosis is universal and complete, usually beginning at the skin surface where the heat energy was most directly received, and extending downward. This zone is called the *zone of coagulation* and is the first of three zones of burn injury (**Figure 7.3**) described by Jackson.[4] This zone comprises the initial burn eschar. Lying deep and peripheral to the zone of coagulation is a zone of lesser injury where most cells are initially viable. Here, however, circulation becomes progressively impaired; leading to cessation of blood flow and hence the term, *zone of stasis*. The development of ischemia within this zone is devastating to already compromised cells. Necrosis follows and in some cases may convert the entire zone of stasis to essentially dead eschar. Impairment of blood flow begins[5] with events occurring in the microvasculature, including platelet microthrombus formation, neutrophil adherence to vessel walls, fibrin deposition, endothelial swelling, and vasoconstriction.[6] Heat-injured erythrocytes lose the ability to deform,[7] impeding their passage through microvessels. Impairment of blood flow ensues within a couple of hours in more severe areas of a burn and is delayed for up to 16–24 hours[8] in less severe regions. Impairment of blood flow progressing to cessation in this region proceeds for up to 48 hours postburn.[6] This should not be confused with the coagulation of blood vessels seen immediately in severe injuries. Given optimal conditions, stasis may be reversed with cell recovery occurring within 1 week.[9] Even if recovery does occur, epithelial cell loss is high throughout this zone. During the recovery period, the tissues are very tenuous and susceptible to additional insult. Dehydration, pressure, hypovolemia, over-resuscitation and infection may lead to further necrosis. The burn physician, therefore, should take extra care to address these concerns. Zawacki[9] accordingly has demonstrated that, through rigorous but careful wound care, progressive burn wound ischemia may be reversed and necrosis prevented. Nondesiccating dressings, topical antimicrobial agents, and adequate but careful fluid resuscitation, along with frequent monitoring of a wound are all essential.

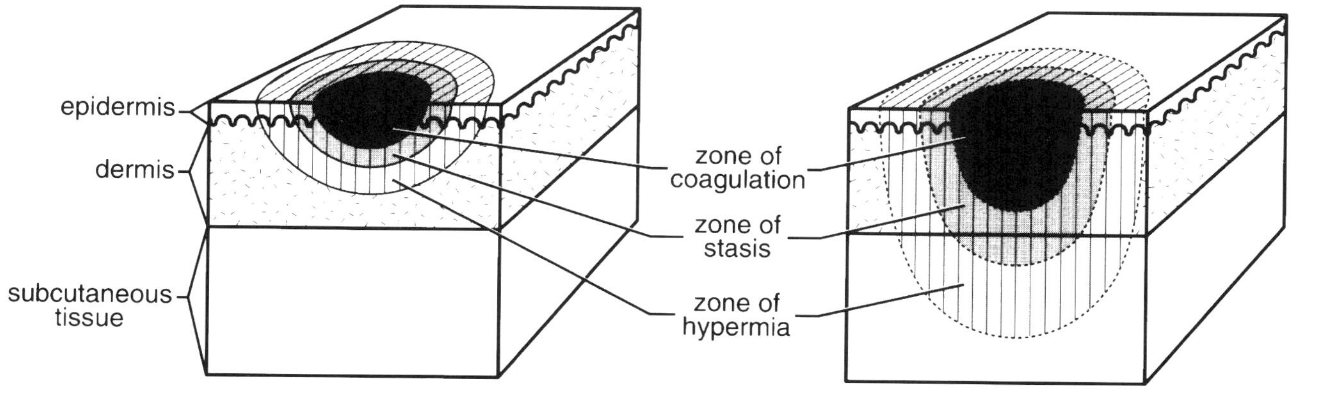

Fig. 7.3 Diagrammatic rendition of Jackson's three zones of burn injury. Superficial 2° injury on left, deeper 2° injury on right. (In deep 2° burn note potential for conversion to full-thickness tissue loss if zone of stasis progresses to necrosis.)

Robson *et al.*[4] have explored extensively the pathophysiology of progressive burn wound ischemia, looking for more specific treatments. This work was preceded by the knowledge that various vasoactive inflammatory mediators are formed in burned tissues, most notably thromboxane A_2 and prostaglandin F_2.[10] In using specific thromboxane inhibitors, Robson[4] and others[11] have been able to demonstrate significant improvement in dermal perfusion as well as reduced necrosis within the wound. Platelet adherence and vasoconstriction, known effects of thromboxane,[12] were all ameliorated. More generalized inhibitors of prostanoids including steroidal and nonsteroidal anti-inflammatory agents,[13] have been tried, with some success, but are problematic because of the blockage of some related beneficial events. Peripheral to the zone of stasis lies the *zone of hyperemia*, characterized by minimal cellular injury but also prominent vasodilation with increased blood flow due to vasoactive mediators produced as part of the inflammatory response. Complete cellular recovery usually prevails in this zone, barring complications such as infection or trauma. The concept of the three zones of the burn wound is important because it underscores the three-dimensional aspect of this injury as well as providing a framework for understanding its progressive nature.

Burn Wound Edema

Burn wound edema is a concept of paramount importance owing to its deleterious effect on oxygen and nutrient delivery as well as its role in systemic hypovolemia. Edema formation is a process which, in many nonburn injuries, may serve a useful purpose by delivering bacteria-fighting substances into the interstitium[14] and providing a mechanism (with the aid of lymphatics) for bacteria and debris removal. These beneficial effects are heavily outweighed by negative ones in a burn wound, where edema, most dramatic in the zone of ischemia, further compromises oxygen delivery to already ischemic tissues.[15]

Burn wound edema formation has been clearly documented[16,17] using a model wherein lymph flow from scalded dog and cat paws was measured and found to be elevated soon after burning. Furthermore, large amounts of protein in the draining lymph were noted, suggesting that the microvasculature in burned tissue had become much more permeable so as to allow leakage of plasma proteins into the interstitium. This was further documented by workers using radiolabeled albumin.[18] The causes of increased vessel permeability are poorly elucidated but are vital to understand if this process is to be modulated. One cause may be heat-mediated damage to capillary and venular endothelial cells. This results in cell swelling which disrupts intercellular connections and creates avenues for fluid loss (**Figure 7.4**).[19] Chemical mediators liberated within a burn wound have also received attention as causes of increased vessel permeability, primarily in postcapillary venules. These include histamine,[20] bradykinins,[21] as well as oxygen free radicals.[22]

Casting doubt on vessel permeability as the sole cause of burn edema formation is evidence that larger protein molecules are retained within the vasculature to a greater degree than are smaller ones,[23] despite the knowledge that capillary pore sizes are much larger[24,25] than the largest protein molecule (**Figure 7.4**). Specifically, analysis of burn edema fluid revealed a disproportionately low ratio of large molecules such as globulins and fibrinogens compared to small molecules such as albumin. These facts suggest that despite large vessel pore sizes, there remains an apparent degree of selective permeability against larger molecules and a tendency to retain them within the vessel. Possible explanations lie within the interstitium. For instance, the capillary basement membrane, which often appears to remain intact after heat injury, may

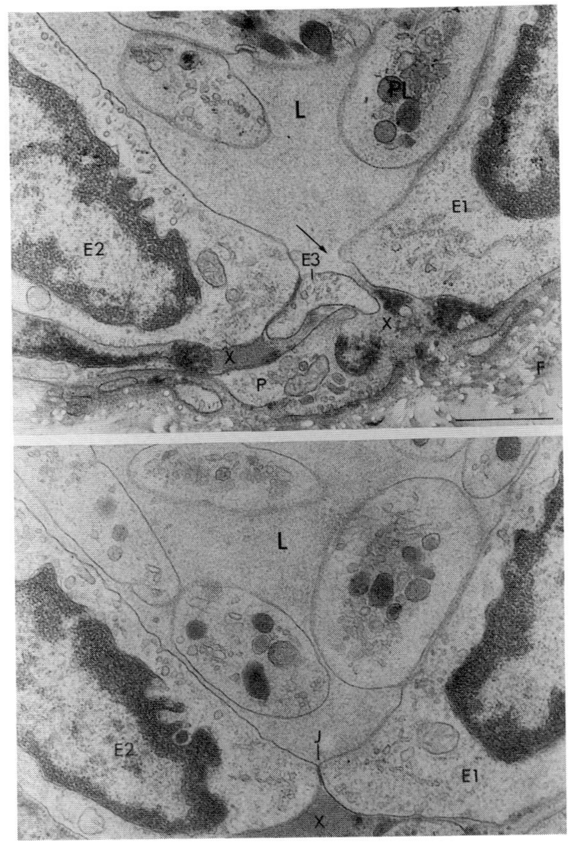

Fig. 7.4 Electron micrograph showing burn-induced endothelial cell gap. (Reproduced with permission from Cotran R S. The delayed and prolonged vascular leakage in inflammation. II. An electron microscope study of the vascular response after thermal injury. Am J Pathol *1965;* ***46:*** *589–620.)*

function as a back-up permeability barrier, retaining molecules which were allowed initial passage by damaged endothelium. Further evidence for an interstitial role is the observation that edema can arise in special settings where the endothelium remains intact but the interstitium is selectively injured as occurs in oxygen free radical damage of hyaluronic acid and collagen.[26] Creating a need for further explanations of edema formation were Arturson's calculations which suggest that in order to develop the massive amounts of edema seen in burn wounds, fluid-driving pressures in the ranges of 200–300 mmHg would be needed.[27] Attention was soon turned to elevated capillary hydrostatic pressure as a possible additional cause. Indeed, Pitt[28] found that capillary pressures are nearly doubled early after burn injury. One of the first proposed mechanisms for this process was the involvement of chemical mediators such as histamine, known for its ability to dilate arterioles[29] and also known to be released from mast cells upon injury.[30] Accordingly, histamine receptor antagonists have been studied in burn edema models. Several reports of success, especially with H_2 blockers, have come forth.[31,32] Adding more knowledge regarding histamine is the recent finding that its vasodilatory effect is mediated through nitric oxide release.[33] Yet another mechanism for histamine's role in the production of burn edema may occur through its stimulation of oxygen free radical formation[34–36] (to be discussed later in this chapter).

Various prostanoids (**Figure 7.5**) found in burn fluid[37–39] may also have roles in edema production. This line of thinking is supported by several studies using inhibitors of prostaglandin production, including indomethacin,[17] nicotinic acid,[40] and ibuprofen.[41] Results show that edema formation within a burn is reduced but without a significant change in lymph protein content. This suggests that the size of capillary pores is unchanged by the drug, pointing to increased capillary pressure through vasodilation, rather than increased permeability, as the prostaglandins' primary mechanism of action in causing edema.[38] Capillary filtration pressures may also be raised by impairment of venular outflow caused by erythrocyte sludging and agglutination[42] in postcapillary venules. This sludging could be a result of fluid loss from a more proximal capillary as well as heat-damaged erythrocytes having lost some of their ability to bend and deform for passage through small vessels.[6] Adherence of platelets and neutrophils to capillary and venular endothelial surfaces probably also contributes. Yet another cause of elevated capillary filtration pressure may be venular constriction, caused by mediators such as serotonin. Systemic conditions which may increase capillary filtration pressure include hypertension and fluid overload.

Remaining explanations for burn edema formation deal with events and conditions existing in the interstitium. Perhaps the most relevant recent discovery in this area is by Lund and coworkers[43] who found that interstitial hydrostatic pressures are dramatically reduced in the early postburn period, depending on the severity of the burn. The explanation given is that collagen fibers are damaged, resulting in an unraveling phenomena. The result is a mechanical expansion of the interstitial space which creates a vacuum effect. These negative pressures, measured by micropipette to be as much as 120 mmHg in severe burns, may explain the rapid achievement of significant edema levels seen in burn wounds by 2–3 hours. Additionally, these high negative pressures, when added to other forces present, are severe enough to account for Arturson's calculated pressure requirements for the formation of burn edema. In addition to hydrostatic pressure changes, interstitial osmotic pressure increases significantly through several mechanisms. The breakdown of collagen and other interstitial proteins into smaller more osmotically active particles,[44] the sequestration of sodium by damaged collagen,[45] and the flux of plasma proteins through enlarged vessel pores into the interstitium, may be involved.

The causes of burn wound edema may be summarized as follows:

- increased capillary and venular permeability resulting from direct effects of heat on endothelium as well as from the action of mediators produced in a burn wound;
- increased hydrostatic pressure within microvessels as a result of chemical mediators causing proximal vasodilation or distal vasoconstriction, as well as impedance of flow distally by endothelial damage and related events;
- dramatic decreases in interstitial hydrostatic pressure resulting from heat-related disturbances of collagen architecture; and
- relative increases in interstitial oncotic pressure due to creation of a greater osmotic load in the interstitium.

It is important to summarize the time course of burn edema since the ability of the tissues to receive oxygen[15] and nutrients is reduced during this period, while susceptibility to infection is increased.[46] Edema formation is rapid, achieving significance within 2–3 hours. This process is generally biphasic, with an immediate, transient phase lasting 10–15 minutes followed by a sustained phase. The rapidity and extent of edema formation is dependent upon the severity of burn injury. Lymphatic resorption begins immediately (although evidence suggests that it may be impeded early-on due to blockage from fibrinous debris)[47] and continues as long as the edema is present. The amount of edema in a wound is maximal by 12–24 hours after injury and persists at a high level for 48–72 hours. Subsequently, a slow resolution of edema occurs, depending on the physiological condition of the wound and the patient.

Burn Inflammation

Many of the above processes are either part of or a result of the inflammation process. For example, mediators responsible for the increased vessel permeability and hydrostatic pressure leading to burn edema arise from inflammation within the wound. Inflammation begins via several mechanisms, most notably when cell membrane phospholipids are destroyed or altered by thermal insult. Phospholipase A, stimulated by a number of burn injury byproducts,[48] then acts to convert the phospholipids to arachidonic acid which then feeds into the arachidonic acid cascade (**Figure 7.5**). The various prostanoids and leukotrienes which are produced go on to mediate vasodilation or in some cases vasoconstriction, increased capillary permeability, neutrophil chemotaxis, and diapedesis, as well as chemoattraction of other inflammatory cells. Several of these phenomena, in particular neutrophil activity, are stimulated by another set of key reactions, the complement cascade (**Figure 7.5**) which is activated in heat-damaged tissues.[49] Cellular infiltration,[50] initiated by inflammatory mediators from the burn wound, begins with the arrival of neutrophils at 4–5 days postburn,

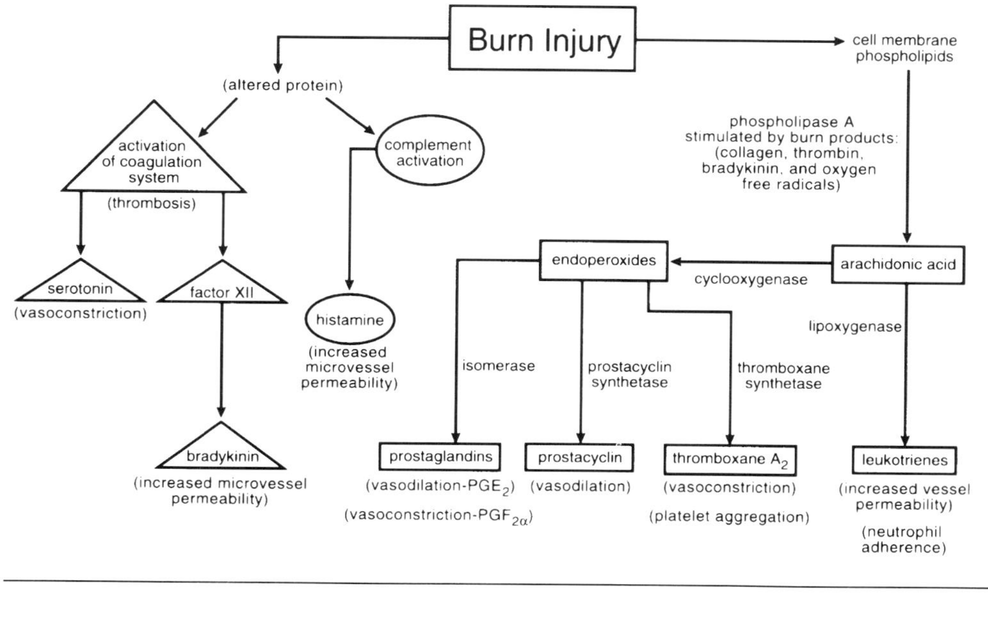

Fig. 7.5 Flow diagram showing several of the major molecular pathways activated and resultant mediators produced by thermal injury. (End responses listed in parentheses.)

followed by macrophages. The neutrophil, long known to be an important component of burn inflammation, has continued to be the center of much interest. Recent work has shown that postburn administration of antibodies which block neutrophil adherence to endothelial walls significantly reduces local edema and necrosis.[51] A means by which neutrophils mediate damage is through their release of oxygen free radicals[52] which in turn react with cell components, primarily membrane lipids, to create detectable lipid peroxidation products. Superoxide dismutase, an enzyme which inactivates the hydroxyl radical, has been found to reduce lipid peroxidation in burn settings,[53] suggesting a role for oxygen radical antagonists in ameliorating damage to cell membranes. Oxygen free radicals not only inflict damage directly on cell membranes, but also stimulate the activity of phospholipase A which triggers the arachidonic acid cascade and thus furthers inflammation. In addition to being produced by neutrophil-specific mechanisms, oxygen radicals are produced in microvascular endothelial cells as byproducts when hypoxanthine is converted to xanthine via the enzyme xanthine oxidase. This fact was linked to burn wound pathophysiology by Ward's group of investigators[32] who discovered that oxidative damage was reduced by the drug, allopurinol, a xanthine oxidase inhibitor. They further identified histamine as a promoter of xanthine oxidase activity and, thus, established a link between histamine and oxygen free radical production.[34] This was verified by observing a decreased production of lipid peroxidation products when H_2 receptor antagonists as well as cromolyn, a mast cell stabilizer, were administered.[30] Reestablishment of blood flow in the zone of stasis is yet another setting wherein oxygen free radicals are produced.[26] This phenomenon occurs as oxygen, a driving force in oxygen free radical production, is restored to the tissues. Part of this process involves ischemia-related alterations in purine metabolism which results in increased xanthine oxidase activity.[54] The renewed oxygen free radical production and subsequent damage in this and other post-ischemic settings is known as ischemia-reperfusion injury and may account for some of the late necrosis occurring in the burn wound.

After the arrival of inflammatory cells and the propagation of the above events within the burn wound, inflammation becomes prominent at 7–10 days. Consequently, blood flow is maximal at this stage, creating a troublesome and hazardous setting for surgical excision of the eschar. Accordingly, many surgeons plan surgery much earlier in order to avoid high operative blood loss.

Burn Wound Depth

First Degree Burns

First degree injury involves damage to only the epidermis and is rarely clinically significant other than being painful. The involved area is initially erythematous due to vasodilation. Eventually, desquamation ensues but is followed by complete scarless healing within 7 days.

Second Degree Burns

Second degree burns are partial thickness by definition but are further categorized into superficial and deep. In superficial injuries, all of the epidermis is destroyed as well as varying superficial portions of the dermis. These lesions are usually very painful due to survival of nerve endings in the mid and superficial dermis. Blistering is often present. Healing will generally occur rapidly and completely through migration to the surface of epithelial cells which survive in deeper portions of hair follicles as well as sweat and sebaceous glands.[55] Relatively little scarring occurs in a superficial injury, owing to the contracted inflammatory phase, which is cut short by wound closure (reepithelialization) occurring within 2 weeks. It is, however, this type of injury which may have a significant zone of stasis underlying the superficial necrosis and be, thus, predisposed to further necrosis and possible conversion to a much deeper wound. Unless complications occur, the treatment for superficial wounds consists of supportive dressing changes. Deep partial-thickness wounds are a very different story and, for all intents and purposes, are treated like full-thickness injuries. Most of the dermis is destroyed, and what few epithelial cells remain are located in the deepest recesses of the epidermal appendages. Heat kills the nerve endings, rendering a wound relatively insensate. Pressure sensation may remain owing to survival of deeply situated pressure receptors. Blistering is usually absent due to the thicker adherent overlying eschar which prevents the lifting effect of edema. Due to the depth from which migrating epithelial cells must travel, reepithelialization is greatly retarded in these wounds. When healing does occur, often weeks down the road, the epidermis is very thin, tenuous and sometimes nonfunctional. Due to the prolonged period before wound closure, the inflammatory phase is protracted, allowing extensive deposition of collagen which is manifested as copious scarring.

Third Degree Burns

Third degree or full-thickness burns involve necrosis of the entire thickness of skin, leaving no chance for healing except for very small wounds which may heal by contraction and epithelialization from the wound edges. Third degree wounds routinely are treated with excision and grafting.

Fourth Degree Burns

Fourth degree injury refers to situations where heat damage extends to deep structures, such as muscle, tendon, bone, etc. Treatment may require elaborate debridement or even amputation.

The Burn Eschar

There are several issues involving the burn eschar itself which must be addressed. Essentially the eschar represents an open wound. Nearly all of the properties of, and benefits provided by, normal skin are lost. The eschar no longer provides a barrier – mechanical, immunological, or otherwise – to infection. In fact, it provides a medium for bacterial growth.[56] This problem may be enhanced as the eschar takes up water from surrounding tissues or from topically applied drug vehicles. The ability of skin to prevent loss of fluids, electrolytes, and plasma components likewise is absent in the eschar due to its high degree of permeability.[57] It has been shown that ongoing protein loss occurs at a high rate through the eschar even after capillary permeability decreases.[58] The loss of complement components[59] and immunoglobulins[60] aggravates burn-induced immune suppression, while loss of protein in general impairs nitrogen balance and wound healing. The eschar may at times play a role in impairment of hemostasis as it promotes consumption of clotting and related factors, i.e. platelets, fibrinogen, etc.[61] This process may, in turn, give rise to some of the burn wound mediators discussed earlier, namely bradykinins and serotonin. The thermoregulatory function provided by normal skin is absent in eschar. Although the tissue within the eschar is metabolically dead, it contains heat-derived products and toxins which may diffuse into the circulation, causing distant organ dysfunction and other problems. Excision of the eschar and grafting of autogenous or nonautogenous skin greatly ameliorates many of these problems. The eschar may additionally contribute to regional morbidity (i.e. cause compression syndromes), requiring escharotomy. Even breathing may be mechanically impaired by a tight thoracic eschar.

The Blister

The blister arises usually in the setting of superficial partial-thickness injury. An exception is in infants and the elderly because of their thinner skin. Here, a relatively deep second degree burn may have a thin eschar which may allow for blister accumulation. A blister is formed by leakage of fluid from heat-injured vessels deep to the zone of coagulation. The fluid enters and collects, usually in the area of the damaged dermoepidermal junction, lifting the epidermis away from the underlying dermis. Release of plasma proteins and skin degradation products into the blister osmotically draws yet more fluid, causing enlargement of the blister over time. Many of the mediators located in the blister are harmful;[59] contributing to the concept that blisters should generally be debrided and the bed carefully dressed. Like the eschar, the blister does not generally provide the function of intact skin and therefore should not be considered a closed wound.

Systemic Effects

As alluded to previously, many of the systemic phenomena observed in burn patients are direct results of either toxins produced by heat damage, or of mediators produced by inflammation and related processes within the burn wound. These systemic effects, summarized in **Figure 7.6**, will be dealt with in detail in other chapters.

Conclusion

The burn wound is a serious injury, progressive in nature, causing a myriad of effects far beyond its bounds. Much knowledge has been gleaned regarding its pathophysiology, yet more remains to be uncovered. As more information is uncovered, much morbidity and mortality surrounding this dreadful injury can be controlled.

References

1. Ricketts C R, Squire J R, Topley E. Human skin lipids with particular reference to the self-sterilizing power of the skin. *Clin Sci Mol Med* 1951; **10:** 89–111.

2. Moritz A R, Henriquez F C. Studies of thermal injury II. The relative importance of time and surface temperature in the causation of cutaneous burns. *Am J Pathol* 1947; **23:** 695–720.

3. Bass H, Moore J L, Conkley W T. Lethality in mammalian cells due to hyperthermia under oxic and hypoxic conditions. *Int J Radiat Biol* 1978; **33:** 57–67.

4. Robson M C, Del Becarro E J, Heggers J P, *et al.* Increasing dermal perfusion after burning by decreasing thromboxane production. *J Trauma* 1980; **20:** 722–5.

5. Boykin J V, Eriksson E, Pittman R N. Microcirculation of scald burn: an *in vivo* experimental study of the hairless mouse ear. *Burns* 1980; **7:** 335–8.

6. Johnson G S, Lineberger T, Hothem A L, Adams K, Hinson T, Winkenwerder W. Erythrocyte flexibility in the burned patient. *Burns* 1979; **6:** 91–5.

7. Zawacki B E. The local effects of burn injury. In: Boswick J A, ed. *The Art and Science of Burn Care*. Rockville, MD: Aspen, 1987: 27.

8. Zawacki B E. The local effects of burn injury. In: Boswick J A, ed. *The Art and Science of Burn Care*. Rockville, MD: Aspen, 1987: 29.

9. Zawacki B E. Reversal of capillary stasis and prevention of necrosis in burns. *Ann Surg* 1974; **180:** 98–102.

10. Johnson C E, Granström E, Hamburg M. Prostaglandins and thromboxane in burn injury in man. *Scand J Plast Reconstr Surg* 1979; **13:** 45–7.

11. Del Becarro E J, Robson M C, Heggers J P, *et al.* The use of specific thromboxane inhibitors to preserve the dermal microcirculation after burning. *Surgery* 1980; **87:** 137–41.

12. Robson M C, Del Becarro E J, Heggers J P. The effect of prostaglandins on the dermal microcirculation after burning and the inhibition of the effect by specific pharmacological agents. *Plast Reconstr Surg* 1979; **63:** 781–7.

13. Jackson D M. The diagnosis of the depth of burning. *Br J Surg* 1953; **40:** 588–96.

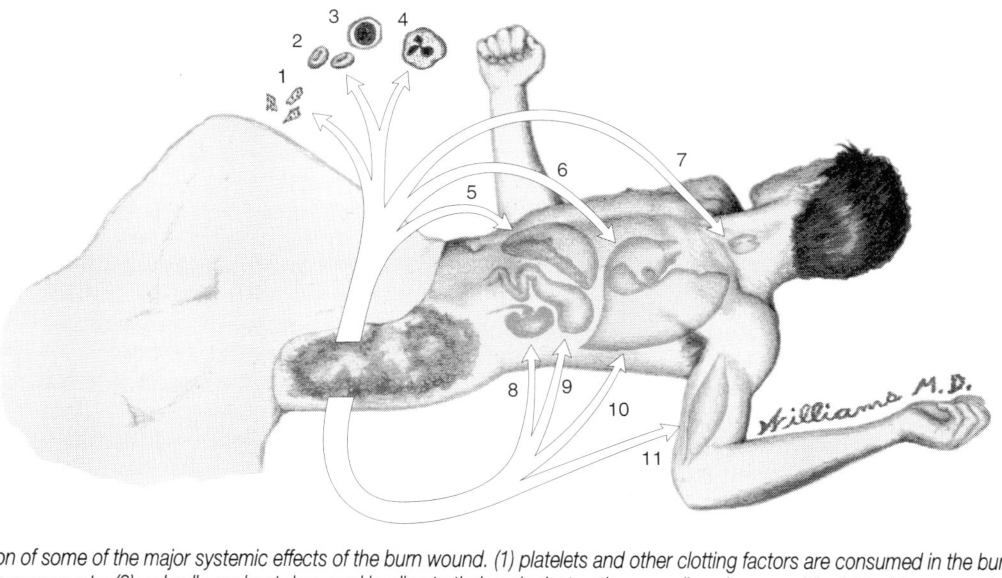

Fig. 7.6 Summarization of some of the major systemic effects of the burn wound. (1) platelets and other clotting factors are consumed in the burned tissue leading to systemic clotting derangements; (2) red cells are heat damaged leading to their early destruction as well as decreased flexibility; (3) suppression of cellular immunity by various burn-related by-products and mediators; (4) impairment of neutrophil function by burn mediators; (5) peroxidation of hepatocytes; (6) myocardial depression mediated by unknown factors produced in the burn wound; (7) multiple endocrine aberrations including hypermetabolism, produced in part by inflammatory mediators from the burn wound; (8) renal tubule damage from various burn wound products; (9) decreased blood flow to gut caused by burn mediators; (10) pulmonary hypertension and edema caused by burn inflammatory products; (11) fat and skeletal muscle catabolism caused by events initiated in the burn wound. (Reproduced with permission from William G. Williams MD.)

14. Warden G. Immunological response to burn injury. In: Boswick J A, ed. *The Art and Science of Burn Care*. Rockville, MD: Aspen, 1987: 113.

15. Remensnyder J P. Topography of tissue oxygen tension changes in acute burn edema. *Arch Surg* 1972; **105:** 477–82.

16. Arturson G. The changes in transcapillary leakage during healing of experimental burns. *Acta Chir Scand* 1967; **133:** 609–14.

17. Arturson G. Microvascular permeability to macromolecules in thermal injury. *Acta Physiol Scand Suppl* 1979; **463:** 111–22.

18. Brouhard B H, Carvajal H F, Linares H A. Burn edema and protein leakage in the rat. I. Relationship of time to injury. *Microvasc Res* 1978; **15:** 221–8.

19. Cotran R S. The delayed and prolonged vascular leakage in inflammation II. An electron microscope study of the vascular response after thermal injury. *Am J Pathol* 1965; **46:** 589–620.

20. Robson M C, Smith D J, Heggers J P. Innovations in burn wound management. In: Habal M B, ed. *Adv Plast Reconstr Surg*. Chicago, IL: Year Book, 1987; **4:** 149.

21. Demling R H. Pathophysiology of burn injury. In: Richardson J D, ed. *Trauma, Clinical Care and Pathophysiology*. Chicago, IL: Year Book, 1987: 128.

22. Hatherill J R, Till G O, Bruner L H, Ward P A. Thermal injury, intravascular hemolysis and toxic oxygen products. *J Clin Invest* 1986; **78:** 629–36.

23. Davies J W L. Capillary permeability, oedema and lymph PG1. In: *Physiological Responses to Burn Injury*. London: Academic Press, 1982: 61.

24. Demling R H, Kramer G C, Gunther R, *et al.* Effect of nonprotein colloid on postburn edema formation in soft tissues and lung. *Surgery* 1984; **95:** 593–602.

25. Honeycutt D, Traber L, Toole D, Herndon D N, Traber D L. Colloid resuscitation of ovine burn shock. *Circ Shock* 1990; **31:** 72.

26. Kaufman T, Neuman R A, Weinberg A. Is postburn dermal ischemia enhanced by oxygen free radicals? *Burns* 1989; **15:** 291–4.

27. Arturson G, Mellander S. Acute changes in capillary filtration and diffusion in experimental burn injury. *Acta Physiol Scand* 1964; **62:** 457–63.

28. Pitt R M, Parker J C, Jurkovich G J, Taylor A E, Curreri P W. Analysis of altered capillary pressure and permeability after thermal injury. *J Surg Res* 1987; **42:** 693–702.

29. Douglas W W. Histamine and 5-hydroxytryptamine (serotonin) and their antagonists. In: Gilman A G, Goodman L S, Rall T W, Murad F, eds. *The Pharmacological Basis of Therapeutics*. New York, NY: Macmillan, 1985: 605.

30. Friedl H P, Till G O, Trentz O, Ward P A. Roles of histamine, complement and xanthine oxidase in thermal injury of the skin. *Am J Pathol* 1989; **135:** 203–17.

31. Brimblecombe R W, Farrington H W. Histamine H_2 receptor antagonists and thermal injury in rats. *Burns* 1976; **3:** 8–13.

32. Till G O, Guilds L S, Mahrougui M, Friedl H P, Trentz O, Ward P A. Role of xanthine oxidase in thermal injury of skin. *Am J Pathol* 1989; **135:** 195–202.

33. Leurs R, Brozius M M, Jansen W, Bast A, Timmerman H. Histamine H-1 receptor-mediated cyclic GMP production in guinea pig lung tissue is an L-arginine-dependent process. *Biochem Pharmacol* 1991; **42:** 271–7.

34. Friedl H P, Till G O, Ryan V S, Ward P A. Mediator-induced activation of xanthine oxidase in endothelial cells. *FASEB J* 1989; **3:** 2512–18.

35. Granger D N, McCord J M, Parks D A, Hollwarth M E. Xanthine oxidase inhibitors attenuate ischemia-induced vascular permeability changes in the cat intestine. *Gastroenterology* 1986; **90:** 80–4.

36. Granger D, Rutili G, McCord J. Superoxide radicals in feline intestinal ischemia. *Gastroenterology* 1981; **81:** 22–9.

37. Änggard E, Arturson G, Jonsson C E. Efflux of prostaglandins in lymph from scalded tissues. *Acta Physiol Scand* 1970; **80:** 46A–47A.

38. Arturson G, Hamberg M, Jonsson C E. Prostaglandins in human burn blister fluid. *Acta Physiol Scand* 1973; **87:** 270–6.

39. Heggers J P, Loy G L, Robson M C, Del Beccaro E J. Histological demonstration of prostaglandins and thromboxanes in burned tissue. *J Surg Res* 1980; **28:** 110–17.

40. Hilton J G, Wells C H. Nicotinic acid reduction of plasma volume loss after thermal trauma. *Science* 1976; **191:** 861–2.

41. Demling R H, LaLonde C. Topical ibuprofen decreases early postburn edema. *Surgery* 1987; **102:** 857–61.

42. Robb H J. Dynamics of the microcirculation during a burn. *Arch Surg* 1967; **94:** 776–80.

43. Lund T, Wiig H, Reed R K. Acute postburn edema: role of strongly negative interstitial fluid pressure. *Am J Physiol* 1988; **255:** H1069–74.

44. Lund T, Onarheim H, Wiig H, Reed R H. Mechanisms behind increased dermal inbibition pressure in acute burn edema. *Am J Physiol* 1989; **256:** H940–8.

45. Leape L. Tissue changes in burned and unburned rhesus monkeys. *J Trauma* 1970; **10:** 488–92.

46. Knighton D, Halliday B, Hunt T K. Oxygen as an antibiotic. *Arch Surg* 1984; **119:** 199–204.

47. Glenn W W L, Gilbert H H, Drinker C K. The flow of lymph from burned tissue with particular reference to the effects of fibrin formation upon lymph drainage and composition. *Surgery* 1942; **12:** 685–95.

48. Arturson G. The pathophysiology of severe thermal injury. *J Burn Care Rehabil* 1985; **6:** 129–46.

49. Fjellstrom K E, Arturson G. Changes in the human complement system following burn trauma. *Acta Pathol Microbiol Scand* 1963; **59:** 257–70.

50. Shilling J A. Wound healing. *Physiol Rev* 1968; **48:** 374–423.

51. Bucky L P, Vedder N B, Hong C H Z, May J W, Ehrlich H P. A monoclonal antibody which blocks neutrophil adhesion prevents second degree burn becoming third degree burns. *Proc Am Burn Assn* 1991; **23:** 133.

52. Gasser H, Paul E, Redl H, Schlag G, Traber D, Herndon D N. Loss of plasma antioxidants after burn injury. *Circ Shock* 1991; **34:** 13.

53. Thomson P D, Till G O, Woolliscroft J O, Smith D J, Prasad J K. Superoxide dismutase prevents lipid peroxidation in burned patients. *Burns* 1990; **16:** 406–8.

54. Fantone J C, Ward P A. *Oxygen-derived Radicals and their Metabolites: Relationship to Tissue Injury*. Kalamazoo, MI: Upjohn, 1985: 32.

55. Zawacki B E. The natural history of reversible burn injury. *Surg Gynecol Obstet* 1974; **139:** 867–72.

56. Pruitt B A, Moncrief J A. Current trends in burn research. *J Surg Res* 1967; **7:** 280–93.

57. Jelenko C III, Ginsburg J M. Water holding lipid and water transmission through homeothermic and poikilothermic skins. *Proc Soc Exp Biol Med* 1971; **139:** 1059–62.

58. Waxman K. Protein loss across burn wounds. *J Trauma* 1987; **27:** 136–40.

59. Heggers J P, Ko F, Robson M C, Heggers R, Craft K E. Evaluation of burn blister fluid. *Plast Reconstr Surg* 1980; **65:** 798–804.

60. Heggers J P, Heggers R, Robson M C. The immunological deficit encountered in thermal injury. *J Am Med Technol* 1982; **44:** 99–102.

61. Simon T L, Curreri P W, Harker L A. Kinetic characterization of hemostasis in thermal injury. *J Lab Clin Med* 1977; **89:** 702–11.

CHAPTER EIGHT

CARE OF OUT-PATIENT BURNS

C. EDWARD HARTFORD

Each year in the United States, approximately 1.4 million individuals sustain burn injuries. Of this group, 54 000 patients need hospitalization and ultimately about 5000 die from burn-related injuries.[1] As these data show, thermal trauma typically results in an injury of low mortality in which the majority of care can safely be rendered in an ambulatory setting. The outcome of burns treated in an out-patient setting is usually good. If care is suboptimal, however, these patients can suffer protracted morbidity or compromised function. The goals of therapy are to minimize the risk of infection, achieve wound healing in a timely fashion, preserve physical function, minimize cosmetic deformity, and affect physical and psychosocial rehabilitation in the most expeditious manner.

WHO CAN BE MANAGED AS AN OUT-PATIENT?

In some instances, it is prudent to initiate care in a hospital so that potential, complicating medical problems can be sorted out. Information is immediately available when a patient is first evaluated from which an accurate prognosis can be derived. These prognostic factors – and a huge amount of common sense – are used to determine the initial treatment venue. The prognostic factors include: age of patient; extent of the burn; depth of the burn; premorbid diseases; and co-morbid disorders, including respiratory complications, associated trauma, distribution of the burn, and the injuring agent. Additionally, a patient's social situation needs to be assessed.

Age

Patients between 5 and 34 years of age have the most favorable outcome from burns.[2] Younger individuals, especially infants, have an increase in morbidity as well as mortality from burn injury. In this group, child abuse or neglect must also be included in the psychosocial analysis.[3,4] The peak incidence of nonaccidental burn injury is 13–24 months of age.[5] Burns which are particularly suspicious are those whose appearance suggests an injury from a cigarette, hot iron, or immersion in hot water. The latter injury is identified by sharp demarcation between burned and unburned skin. The absence of splash marks should also heighten one's suspicion. Additionally, scalding which has occurred in an institution is always cause for concern. Even with trivial injury, if a burn was sustained under suspicious circumstances or the history does not correspond with the nature or distribution of the burn, the patient should be hospitalized for protection. Cases of suspected abuse or neglect should be referred to the appropriate social services agency for investigation.

Patients of advanced age also have a substantial increase in burn mortality.[2] Any burned patient over the age of 60 years is in danger of dying regardless of the extent of a burn. Therefore, one should consider admitting older patients to a hospital in order to make certain that they can tolerate the injury before treatment is continued as an out-patient.

Extent of the Burn

The larger the percentage of body surface area involved by the burn, the worse the prognosis. The percentage of body surface area can be roughly estimated by the 'rule of nines',[6] or more accurately by the technique of Lund and Browder[7] (**Figures 8.1**). A helpful adjunct to estimating the area of a burn is the fact that the area of the palm approximates 1% of an individual's body surface area.

Patients with burns which require intravenous fluid resuscitation should be admitted to a hospital. This includes adults and older children with burns in excess of 15% of their total body surface area (TBSA) and younger children and infants with burns in excess of 10% of their total body surface area.[8] In some instances, due to premorbid dehydration caused by physical activity, an arid climate, alcohol, or diuretics, some patients with smaller burns may need supplemental intravenous fluids for optimal care.

Depth of the Burn

The deeper a burn, the worse is the prognosis. However, depth of small area burns is less important in determining the need to initiate care in a hospital than the extent of the burn. When a burn is first evaluated, it is often difficult to accurately determine its depth. The

BURN DIAGRAM Shriners Burns Institute – Galveston Unit

Age:__________ Sex: __________ Date of admission ____________________

Type of burn: Flame ☐ Electrical ☐ Scald ☐ Chemical ☐ Inhalation injury ☐

Date of burn: ________________

Date completed: ______________

Completed by: ________________

Date revised: ________________

Revised by: _________________

Approved by: ________________

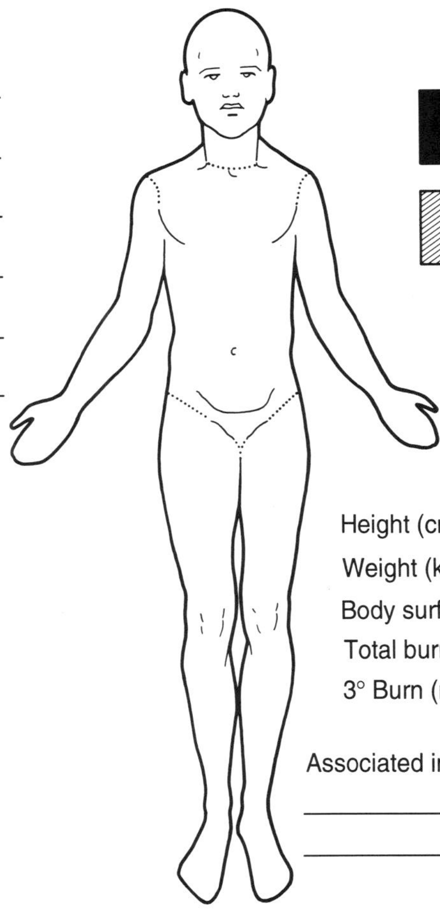

3rd°

2nd°

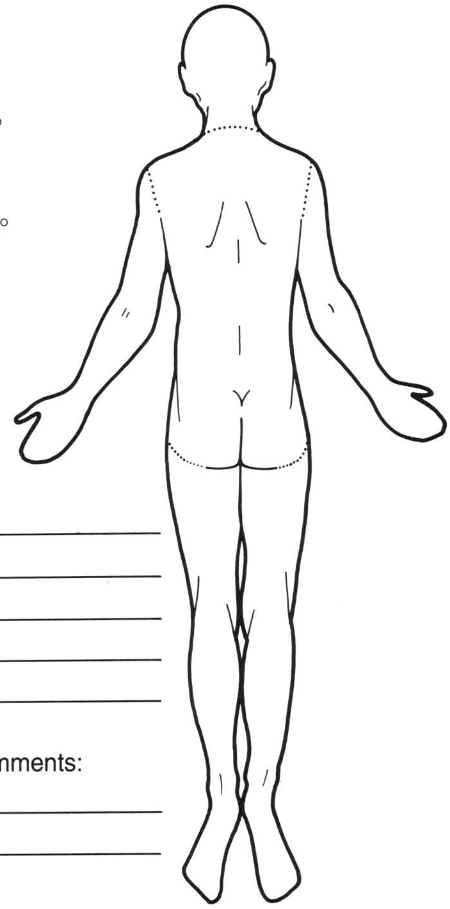

Height (cm) ________________

Weight (kg) ________________

Body surface (m^2) ____________

Total burn (m^2) ______________

3° Burn (m^2) ________________

Associated injuries/comments:

____

____

BURN ESTIMATE – AGE VS. AREA

Area	Birth–1 year	1–4 years	5–9 years	10–14 years	15 years	Adult	2°	3°	TBSA %
Head	19	17	13	11	9	7			
Neck	2	2	2	2	2	2			
Ant. trunk	13	13	13	13	13	13			
Post. trunk	13	13	13	13	13	13			
R. buttock	2.5	2.5	2.5	2.5	2.5	2.5			
L. buttock	2.5	2.5	2.5	2.5	2.5	2.5			
Genitalia	1	1	1	1	1	1			
R.U. arm	4	4	4	4	4	4			
L.U. arm	4	4	4	4	4	4			
R.L. arm	3	3	3	3	3	3			
L.L. arm	3	3	3	3	3	3			
R. hand	2.5	2.5	2.5	2.5	2.5	2.5			
L. hand	2.5	2.5	2.5	2.5	2.5	2.5			
R. thigh	5.5	6.5	8	8.5	9	9.5			
L. thigh	5.5	6.5	8	8.5	9	9.5			
R. leg	5	5	5.5	6	6.5	7			
L. leg	5	5	5.5	6	6.5	7			
R. foot	3.5	3.5	3.5	3.5	3.5	3.5			
L. foot	3.5	3.5	3.5	3.5	3.5	3.5			
						TOTAL			

Fig. 8.1 Modified from Lund and Browder.[7] Chart used to calculate the surface area involved by burn. It takes into account that, as one grows from infancy to adulthood, the relative surface area of the head decreases while the relative surface area of the lower extremities increases.

superficial injury of sunburn or its equivalent is easy to identify. Likewise, it is easy to discern a waxen, dry, inelastic, insensate, cadaveric-appearing wound as a full-thickness burn. However, it is extremely difficult to distinguish the subtle differences between a superficial partial-thickness burn, which will heal spontaneously in 3 or 4 weeks, and a deep partial-thickness burn which takes longer to heal. This is especially true for weeping wounds in which the blisters have ruptured. Initially, these wounds appear superficial and are perfused. However, with time, as injured small blood vessels in a wound thrombose, the wound takes on the ischemic, cadaveric appearance of a much deeper injury.[9,10] This change does not reflect invasive infection but merely the natural evolution of a wound.

Premorbid Diseases

Preexisting medical conditions often have a profound influence on the clinical course and outcome of a burn injury. While any medical disorder may have an adverse effect, there are a number of conditions which occur frequently among the burned and which may play a significant role in causation or outcome. For instance, any condition or habit which alters any individual's mental state may lead to a burn injury. These include the use of medication (especially sedatives), controlled substances, alcohol, seizure disorders, senility and psychiatric illnesses. These conditions usually obligate hospital admission. Medical conditions which are known to enhance morbidity of patients with burns include renal failure, congestive heart failure, cardiac dysrhythmias, hypertension, chronic obstructive pulmonary disease, diabetes mellitus, sequelae of alcoholism, conditions which require the use of steroids, and morbid obesity.[11] The clinical status of any of these disorders must be determined and their potential influence on the outcome must be assessed before determining whether a patient can be safely managed as an out-patient.

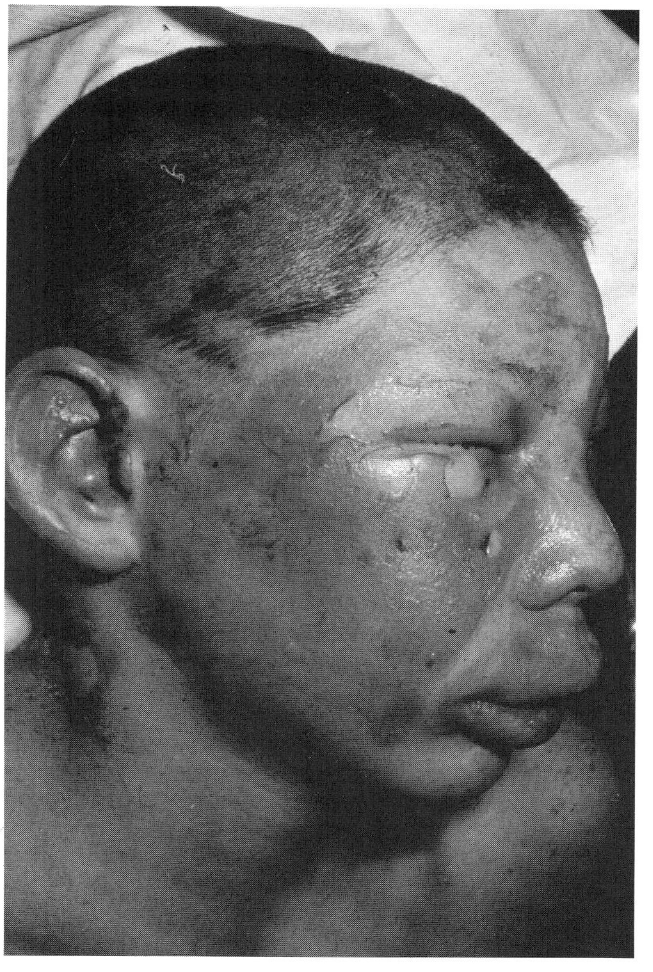

Fig. 8.2 Swelling caused by a burn that healed spontaneously without scar. For several days the edema of the eyelids prevented the patient from seeing.

Co-morbid Disorders

Respiratory complications

Synchronous lung injury substantially magnifies a burned patient's risk of morbidity and death.[12,13] Patients exposed to smoke are at risk of significant pulmonary dysfunction from inhalation injury, upper respiratory obstruction from edema, and carbon monoxide poisoning.[12] These potentially lethal complications may occur even with trivial burn injury. Since the adverse sequelae of these disorders may not be immediately apparent,[14] a period of monitored observation is warranted; an overnight admission is usually sufficient.

Associated trauma

Burns frequently occur with other forms of trauma. If a burn involves only a small area of the body, the associated trauma will dictate whether a patient needs to be hospitalized.

Distribution of a burn

The location of a burn may have a profound effect on a patient's activities of daily living, and dictate the setting in which the patient must receive care. For instance, the edema from a small area superficial burn of the face may result in swelling of the eyelids, hampering a patient's vision (**Figure 8.2**). Likewise, burns of the hands, feet, or those involving the perineum or adjacent areas may severely limit an individual's autonomy. While burns in these areas may not necessarily demand care in a hospital, consideration of the assistance available to a patient must be given when contemplating ambulatory care.

Because of fluid flux into tissues beneath a burn, patients with circumferential burns of an extremity are in danger of ischemia of underlying and distal tissues from increased tissue pressure.[15] Except for those with very superficial burns, all patients with circumferential burns of an extremity should be admitted to a hospital and monitored for evidence of elevated tissue pressure. Since the clinical signs of compartment syndrome and ischemia in a burned extremity are unreliable,[16] the author advocates measuring the tissue pressure by direct methods. Alternatively, the circulatory status of an extremity can be assessed by using a Doppler ultrasonic flowmeter.[16] Burns across joints do not, for that reason alone, require admission to a hospital.

Injuring agent

Special circumstances exist when an injury is caused by electricity or a chemical. Patients exposed to low-voltage electricity, arbitrarily defined as below 1000 volts (the most frequent source being household currents of 110 or 220 volts), are in great danger of dying at the accident scene from a cardiac dysrhythmia, usually ventricular fibrillation.[17] Following low-voltage electrical exposure, the most frequent residual electrocardiographic abnormality is a nonspecific change in the ST-T wave segment,[18] and the most troublesome dysrhythmias are among the atrial fibrillation–flutter group[19]. If the electrocardiogram is normal or becomes normal during observation, the chances of a subsequent dysrhythmia or cardiac arrest are virtually nil. The tissue damage from low levels of electrical energy is usually small and most patients do not need to be hospitalized. Conversely, patients who sustain tissue damage from contact with high-voltage electricity generally require admission.

Chemical injury can be minimized by removing the chemical within 15 seconds after contact. Brushing off dry chemicals or copious lavage with water of wet chemicals are the appropriate emergency treatments.[20,21] No one knows exactly how long lavage should be continued; up to 1 hour has been recommended.[22] One guide is the presence of pain, with the supposition being that, as long as there is pain, the chemical is still active and there is persistent need for lavage. In some instances, there are specific antidotes for pain. For example, with hydrofluoric acid, injured tissues should be injected with calcium gluconate.[23] Hydrofluoric acid also serves as a good example of the many chemicals which are absorbed into the body with the potential to cause organ injury. Exposure of concentrated hydrofluoric acid to as little as 3% of the body surface area can result in a fatal dysrhythmia from hypocalcemia due to calcium binding to absorbed fluoride ions.[24] Since it is impossible to remember the systemic sequelae of all the chemicals to which an individual might be exposed, the physician should identify the chemical and seek information from a local poison control center. After emergency local wound care, the treatment of the residual wound from a chemical is the same as the treatment for any burn wound.

Social Circumstances

Patients whose injuries appear to be nonaccidental need to be admitted to a hospital for their own protection. Before a patient is discharged from emergency care, the physician should ascertain that there are satisfactory resources available for supervision and care and that the patient can readily reaccess medical care. A visiting nurse can be invaluable in providing wound care and monitoring for wound complications as well as assessing the patient's physical progress and social situation after discharge.

TREATMENT

Cooling a Burn

The first objective in burn wound care is to dissipate heat and reduce the temperature in injured tissues below an injurious level, i.e. below 45°C.[25] After eliminating the source of heat, active cooling of a wound may help dissipate heat. The period of time active cooling is beneficial for reducing heat is brief.[26] Typically, by the time most patients present for care, the tissues have already cooled spontaneously.

However, active cooling also has several potential advantages beyond dissipation of heat. First, cooling stabilizes skin mast cells which decrease histamine release; and cooling, thereby, decreases edema of a wound. Second, in the first several hours after an injury, cooling is an effective way of controlling the pain of partial-thickness burns.[27,28]

In the cooling for pain control, cool, but not ice cold,[29,30] moist compresses are applied to a painful wound. This method is applicable in the management of virtually all patients whose wounds can be safely cared for in an ambulatory setting. Because of the limited surface area of burns among these patients, the detrimental systemic effects of active cooling, e.g. hypothermia from accelerated heat loss, usually do not occur. However, since water conducts heat 23 times faster than air, it makes good sense to monitor a patient's core temperature during active cooling of a wound.

Pain Control

Burn wounds are painful. The greatest pain is seen with partial thickness wounds devoid of the superficial layers of epithelium. The pain, initially intense and virtually unbearable, spontaneously moderates after several hours but intensifies when wounds are manipulated with dressing changes, wound care, and physical activity. While eschar-covered burns may be insensate, when the eschar is removed or cut, the exposed viable tissues are painful.[31]

Most patients will require analgesics. Narcotics are typically required as first-line treatment. In the emergency setting, small incremental doses of morphine can be given intravenously and titrated to effect. Clearance of analgesics is accelerated among those who regularly use alcohol or abuse controlled substances.[32,33] Subsequently, acetaminophen with codeine or similar analgesics, alone or in combination, are usually effective. Most patients will require supplemental analgesics for sleep, wound dressing changes, and physical therapy.

If a patient's pain cannot be controlled by oral medication, then the patient may need to be admitted to a hospital. In a hospital setting, effective pain control can be obtained by the patient-controlled analgesic method. Even with patient-controlled analgesia, supplemental analgesic will often be required when wound dressings are changed. Topically applied or injected local anesthetics are not recommended in the management of burns.

Local Burn Wound Care

After the initial patient assessment and institution of measures to control pain, attention is turned to local care of wounds. Loose, devitalized tissue is generally trimmed away, a practice known as epluchage. Pain and bleeding are kept to a minimum.

Blisters

There is no uniform agreement on the management of blisters. Recommendations range from leaving blisters intact and allowing underlying wounds to heal spontaneously,[34] to removing blistered skin immediately.[35] Other recommendations include needle aspiration of fluid and leaving collapsed blistered skin as a protective covering of a wound until healing occurs. Still others advocate removing blistered skin after several day[36] or if the blister ruptures.

Arguments for removal of blistered skin cite laboratory studies of the fluid in burn blisters which have shown it to exhibit several potentially detrimental effects.[35] Immune function is depressed by impaired function of polymorphonuclear leukocytes and lymphocytes. Neutrophil chemotaxis, opsonization and intracellular killing are all adversely affected by blister fluids. Inflammation is enhanced by the metabolites of arachidonic acid. A plasmin inhibitor in blister fluid decreases vascular patency. Finally, blister fluid may provide a medium for the growth of bacteria. Based on these considerations, the case can be made that blistered skin should be removed in order to facilitate healing.

Conversely, the author finds the rationale for leaving burn blisters intact to be more persuasive. Noting that blisters form in the stratum spinosum layer of the epidermis, an intact blister usually indicates a superficial partial-thickness wound which will heal spontaneously within 3 weeks. If, under these circumstances, the blister is removed, then a wound is converted from an absolutely painless one to a painful, open wound exposed to colonization by bacteria and potential infection.[34] An infection in a burn wound covered by an intact blister rarely occurs. Therefore, the author prefers to leave blisters intact, and recommends that they be dressed protectively and not covered with medication. Blistered skin violated by needle aspiration or by spontaneous rupture also has the potential for bacterial contamination and infection. Attempts to use the loose skin of a blister as a protective dressing are generally ineffective.

If the blister remains intact, and the wound is a superficial partial-thickness burn, spontaneous resorption of the fluid will begin in about 1 week. The blistered skin will wrinkle. Gradually, it will collapse onto the healing wound surface and become firm and inelastic. One should not be in a hurry to remove this protective layer. Persistence of a blister with no signs of spontaneous resorption of the fluid after several weeks, usually signifies that the underlying wound is either deep partial-thickness or full-thickness. There is often concern about large blisters in locations which limit range of motion, such as in the palm of the hand. Many advocate needle aspiration of the fluid. The author does not. Experience has shown that full range of motion of the hand is virtually always restored.

Cleansing a wound

For cleansing, and to remove residual dirt, a wound is gently washed with room temperature or tepid (100°C) water and a mild, bland soap. Chlorhexidine gluconate soap is desirable because of its antimicrobial activity against common skin flora.[37] In the treatment of burns from tar and asphalt, after cooling to dissipate heat, the solidified tar and asphalt should be removed by solvents which have a close structural affinity to these solutes. Therefore, substances related to petrolatum (an oleaginous colloid suspension of solid microcrystalline waxes in petroleum oil) are effective. Stratta and colleagues recommend De–Solv-it® (Orange–Sol, Inc. Chandler, AZ), a citrus and petroleum distillate (base oil) 25–27% limonene (orange oil), 2–3% lanolin and 1% surfactant (diocytl sodium sulfosuccinate), as the most satisfactory product available.[38] This nontoxic, nonirritating, odorless solvent is liberally applied and then removed by gentle wiping. Polysorbates alone or in combination with topical antibiotics[39] and topical antibiotics in petrolatum base[40] can be used; but they are less effective.

Topical agents

There is a long tradition of applying substances to burn wounds in an attempt to prevent infection.[41] A large variety of antiseptics, antibiotics, and topical antibacterial (antimicrobial) agents have been advocated. Most of these agents have adverse local or systemic effects or impede wound healing or both. Additionally, there is no published evidence that the use of any topical agent which is designed to prevent or control infection will favorably influence the outcome of small burns.[42–44] In spite of this, many physicians feel obligated to apply one of these agents to wounds. All published comparative studies show no advantage to these agents over petrolatum-impregnated gauze.[45] If a treating physician believes that the use of a topical antimicrobial agent is desirable, 1% silver sulfadiazine ointment is probably the current best recommendation. It has the fewest side effects of any available drug. If a patient is allergic to sulfa products, silver sulfadiazine should not be used. Because sulfonamide therapy is known to increase the possibility of kernicterus, silver sulfadiazine is not used on pregnant women, nursing mothers, and infants younger than 2 months of age. Because silver sulfadiazine impedes epithelialization, it should be discontinued when healing partial-thickness wounds are devoid of necrotic tissue and evidence of reepithelialization is seen (see **Figure 8.3**).

Dressing a wound

Dogmatic recommendations for dressing small burn wounds cannot be made because there are virtually no objective studies on the subject. Dressings serve three purposes: to absorb drainage; to provide protection and isolation of a wound from the environment; and to decrease wound pain. There are several situations in which wound dressings are impractical or not necessary. Otherwise, the author prefers to dress wounds and makes the following suggestions.

Superficial partial-thickness burns, the equivalent of sunburn, with intact epidermis, require neither topical medication nor a dressing. For relatively small superficial partial-thickness burns devoid of epithelium, it is generally conceded that topical antibacterial agents are not necessary.[42–44] Nonmedicinal white petrolatum-impregnated fine mesh or porous mesh gauze (Adaptic®), or fine mesh absorbent gauze impregnated with 3% bismuth tribro-

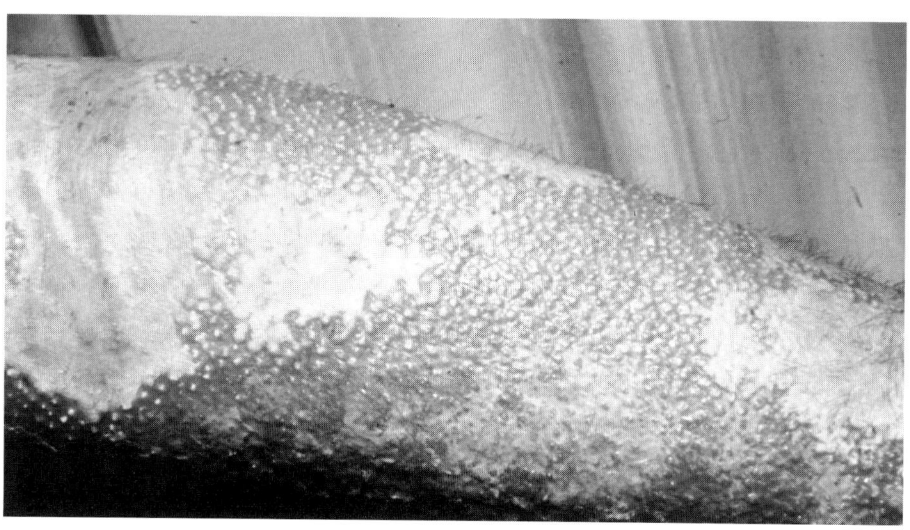

Fig. 8.3 Healing partial-thickness burn showing prominent islands of squamous epithelium that have emerged from epidermal appendages. Epithelium will expand to resurface the wound. When islands of squamous epithelium appear in a wound, spontaneous reepithelization is imminent.

mophenate in nonmedicinal petrolatum blend (Xeroform®) are satisfactory wound covers. If the burn is deeper and contains adherent necrotic tissue, a topical antimicrobial agent may be used.

For practical reasons, most burns of the face are treated without dressing. These wounds may also be treated without topical medication so as to allow the wounds to dry and form a crust. Because a dry wound is often uncomfortable, many physicians prefer to use a thin layer of bland ointment combined with a topical antibiotic, e.g. Baciquent® (bacitracin in anhydrous lanolin, mineral oil and white petrolatum) applied to the wound after gentle cleansing twice daily. Bacitracin has activity against gram-positive bacteria. Occasionally, it causes a contact dermatitis which impedes wound healing.

Since one purpose of dressings is to absorb drainage, the thickness of the dressing is determined by the amount of drainage generated between dressing changes. In weeping, superficial, partial-thickness wounds, the amount of drainage is greatest soon after the injury. As the character of a wound changes and healing begins, drainage decreases. Lint-free, coarse mesh gauze, usually starting with about 20 thicknesses, is preferred by the author. The dressing is held in place with an elastic gauze bandage (e.g. Kling® or Kerlix®) wrapped with sufficient tightness to hold the gauze in place but not so tightly as to impede circulation. Many use Flexinette®. In addition, the author often uses an outer layer of stockinette, which is relatively impervious to liquid, in order to prevent the drainage from soaking through a dressing. Joints are dressed to facilitate range of motion. Fingers are dressed individually (**Figure 8.4**).

The frequency with which dressings are changed is arbitrary. Recommendations range from twice daily to as infrequently as once a week. Those who advocate twice daily dressing changes do so based on the use of topical antimicrobials whose half-life is about 8 hours. Those who use petrolatum or bismuth-impregnated petrolatum gauze recommend less frequent dressing changes, some extending the period to as long as 5 or 7 days.[45,46] The author prefers once daily dressing changes in order to permit daily inspection and cleansing of the wound. Moreover, after about 24 hours, wound dressings are often saturated or disheveled. Daily dressing changes are recommended even if the patient or another lay person is responsible for the inspection, cleansing and redressing of a wound. Cleansing of a wound can often be incorporated into general body cleansing each day. The person responsible for wound care should also be instructed in the clinical manifestations of wound infections.

Synthetic wound dressings

Some advocate the covering of very superficial partial-thickness burn wounds, devoid of visible necrotic tissue, with one of several synthetic wound coverings, such as Biobrane®,[47] Opsite®,[48] or Tegaderm®. The purported advantages are decreased pain and cost and more rapid reepithelialization. Biobrane® is a bilayer fabric composed of an inner layer of knitted nylon threads coated with porcine collagen and an outer layer of rubberized silicone, pervious to gases but not to liquids and bacteria.[49] It is applied snugly to a cleansed wound, overlapping itself or unburned skin, and held in place with sterile strips of adhesive tape. The key to the successful use of Biobrane® is adherence to the wound. Therefore, a burned area must be dressed or splinted, especially across a joint, to prevent shearing of the Biobrane® from the wound surface. Satisfactory adherence usually occurs in about 3 or 4 days. If, in follow-up, the Biobrane® is found to be loose, the nonadherent area can be trimmed away and new Biobrane®, applied. If sterile fluid accumulates beneath the synthetic dressing, it can be aspirated; however, if the fluid is purulent, the Biobrane® must be opened to permit complete drainage. Biobrane® is left intact until a wound has reepithelialized, then it can be gently teased away. If the wound surface has residual necrotic tissue, Biobrane® will not adhere. Thin, transparent, elastic, adhesive-coated film derived from polyurethane, e.g. Opsite®[48] or Tegaderm®, may also be used much like Biobrane®. A wound must be covered completely with a wide purchase on uninjured skin, and perfect wound isolation must be maintained. Fluid which accumulates beneath the film is aspirated in order to prevent detachment from the surrounding uninjured skin. After aspiration, the puncture site should be patched with a small piece of film. It is important to note that, should the film become detached, the wound will be exposed to potential contamination. If the underlying fluid becomes turbid, the film should be removed; otherwise, it is left intact until the wound is reepithelialized and then removed.

Elevation of the Burned Area

One of the most effective ways to reduce the incidence of infection in burns is to eliminate edema from a burned part. Burn injury elicits edema in the tissues immediately subjacent to a wound. Additionally, there is a great tendency for a patient to hold an injured part immobile in a dependent position. To eliminate edema,

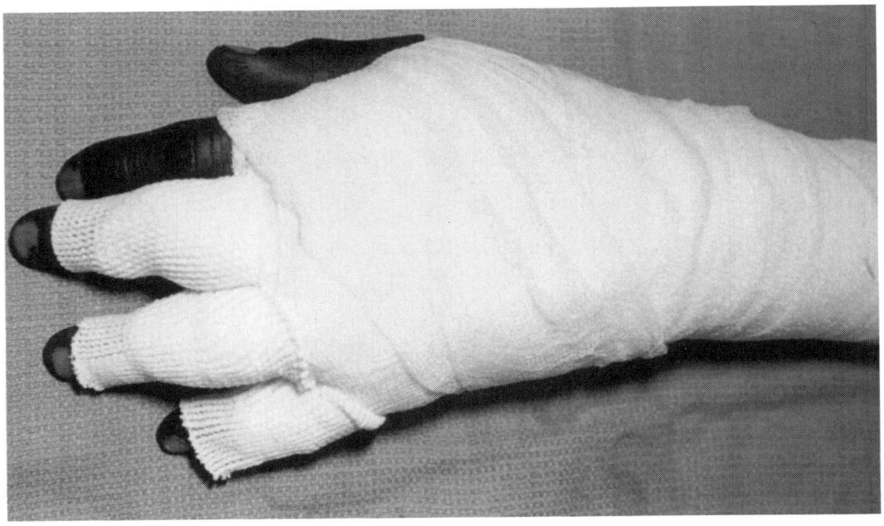

Fig. 8.4 Completed dressing of the hand. All joints should be dressed to allow as much functional range of motion as possible.

an injured part should be exercised regularly and, when not in use, maintained slightly above the level of the heart. Merely elevating a leg off the floor to the level of the hip when in a sitting position is not sufficient. Holding the burned forearm flexed and dependent in a sling will enhance edema. Specific instructions and a demonstration of the position should be explicit.

The most efficient position for an injured part is just slightly above the level of the heart. To elevate a burned part higher above the heart does not further enhance removal of excess tissue fluid. Furthermore, for every 1.3 cm of elevation above the heart, there is a decrease in arterial perfusion pressure of 1 mmHg.[50] Patients with small burns who experience persistent edema beyond 3 days are spending too much time with the part dependent. With burns of the lower extremity, holding a leg dependent and ambulation often elicit severe pain. To diminish this effect, rubberized, elastic bandages (Ace Bandage®) should be applied from the level of the toes to above the burn. This will also aid in reducing edema formation during walking.

Instructions and Follow-up Care

Before a patient is released from emergency care, he or she is instructed in wound care, positioning, physical therapy, clinical manifestations of infection, a convenient way to reaccess medical care (usually by telephone); and he or she is given pain medication. Most patients are examined the next day. This allows reinspection of a wound in order to assess a patient's compliance with instructions and to reinforce the principles of wound care. Often, because of pain during emergency care, a patient has been distracted from fully understanding instructions. If concern remains, daily return visits are scheduled until a physician is certain that care is being followed appropriately. After that, a patient can be seen at weekly intervals.

Definitive Wound Closure

An objective in burn care is to have *all wounds* healed within 1 month. Usually, this goal is easily achieved in an ambulatory setting. Burn wounds which heal spontaneously from the depth of the wound within 3 weeks have an excellent result. When this occurs, the skin functions normally with good elasticity, a nil incidence of hypertrophic scarring (scars which are red, raised and indurated), and little, if any, alteration in pigmentation. The longer that spontaneous healing takes, the worse the result usually is. With longer healing periods, there is an increasing likelihood of developing hypertrophic scarring[51] and unsightly alterations in pigmentation. In addition, wounds which take a very long time to heal may have unstable epithelium.

It is a surgeon's responsibility to make certain that burn wounds either heal spontaneously or are closed surgically in a timely fashion. If it is apparent that a wound will not heal spontaneously within 3 or 4 weeks, a better outcome[52,53] can be anticipated by surgically removing residual necrotic tissue and any granulation tissue by tangential excision[54] and applying a skin graft. In many instances it is obvious immediately or within several days as to whether spontaneous healing will occur within 3 or 4 weeks. Among wounds in which the subtle differences between superficial and deep partial-thickness burns are not initially discernible, it usually is apparent at 2 weeks after injury whether the wound will heal spontaneously within the next 7–10 days. At 2 weeks after injury, those wounds which are devoid of necrotic tissue and have evidence of squamous reepithelialization, can be expected to heal spontaneously within the desirable time frame. The beginning of reepithelialization can be detected by seeing tiny opalescent islands of epithelium throughout the wound (**Figure 8.3**).

Infection and Use of Systemic Antibiotics

There is no evidence that systemic antibiotic prophylaxis will decrease the incidence of infection in small burn wounds;[55] however, antibiotics should be used for the specific indication of infection. Burn elicits inflammation. The early manifestation of infection in a wound may be quite subtle as a result. Mild erythema, edema, pain, and tenderness, all classic signs of infection, may be present without infection. However, when these manifestations increase over a baseline, especially in the presence of lymphangitis and fever, treatment for infection should be instituted. Mainstays of treatment for infection include rest, elevation of the infected wound to control swelling, and systemic antibiotic therapy. If an infection progresses, the patient should be hospitalized and antibiotics given intravenously.

Infections in the out-patient setting are usually caused by common skin flora. Those most frequently implicated are staphylococci. A wound surface culture should be obtained to identify the offending organism and to narrow the spectrum of antibiotic therapy. While some burn care physicians advocate the use of burn wound biopsy quantitative culture rather than a wound surface culture,[56] the author has not found biopsy cultures to be necessary in the treatment of out-patient burns.

Among patients with burns treated in an ambulatory setting, it is quite unusual to develop systemic sepsis. In any case, patients should be instructed to take their temperature twice daily: once in the morning shortly after they get up from sleep and again late in the afternoon before they eat supper. Localized infection will be reflected in fever in the afternoon. Sustained fever is suggestive of systemic sepsis. Temperatures above 38°C and symptoms of malaise and anorexia should be reported to a physician, and the patient should be called in for an examination.

A change in the appearance of a wound during the first several days is more likely to indicate a decrease in perfusion of the wound than wound infection. This is frequently observed with scald burns. Any further burn wound discoloration, such as the appearance of gray or black spots, especially if there are other manifestations of infection, should raise concern for invasive infection. This rarely occurs among patients treated as out-patients; but, if it does occur, the patient should be hospitalized, the wound biopsied for histologic and microbiological studies,[57] and treatment for infection instituted. Burns, even minor ones, are tetanus-prone wounds.[58] Tetanus prophylaxis should be provided unless the patient has received tetanus immunization within 5 years.[59]

Pruritus

Itching is an annoying manifestation in healing and healed burn wounds. It interferes with everything. Scratching often results in repetitive superficial wounding of both skin grafted and spontaneously healed wounds. Triggered and enhanced by environmental extremes, especially heat, physical activity, and stress, pruritus is most intense in the period immediately after wounds are healed. In most instances, it gradually diminishes and eventually stops. There are a few patients in whom it persists beyond 12–18 months. Patients with prolonged and chronic itching may harbor a psychogenic component.

Whether the sensation of pruritus is a primary sensory modality[60] or, as widely held in the past, a 'forme fruste' of pain, is not clear. Histamine, whose synthesis is known to be increased in healing wounds,[61] as well as a series of endopeptides and bradykinin, have all been implicated in the genesis of itching.[62,63] Because the precise mechanism of pruritus is not known, the likelihood is that there are multiple causative factors. Since there are no controlled trials defining the best treatment, management is by trial and error. The antihistaminic diphenhydramine hydrochloride is the most frequently prescribed first treatment.[64] This drug has an added benefit of providing mild sedation. Other antihistamines, such as cyproheptadine hydrochloride, may also be tried. Analgesics of any kind may be helpful by altering perception of itching in the central nervous system. Combinations of antihistamines and analgesics may be tried. Many patients find comfort in an air-conditioned environment. Cool compresses also may temporarily interrupt the itching cycle. A variety of topical agents, including aloe vera[65] which has anti-inflammatory properties, and skin moisturizing creams, such as Vaseline Intensive Care®, Eucerin®, Nivea®, mineral oil, cocoa butter, and even lard have been effective. Hydroxyzine hydrochloride, a drug used to provide relief from anxiety and emotional tension, is used to help ameliorate itching. In addition, loose soft clothing made from cotton is preferred by many patients.

Traumatic Blisters in Reepithelialized Wounds

As wounds reepithelialize, the delicate thin layer of epithelium is fragile and easily damaged. Scratching and other mild forms of trauma may cause small blisters. Patients need to be cautioned about this potential, assured that the epithelium will gain strength and that this will not be a long-term problem. If these blisters rupture, leaving small superficial wounds, the wounds may be left exposed to form a crust. Alternatively, Adaptic® or Xeroform® and a light dressing may be used.

Rehabilitative Physical Care

Measures to preserve strength and restore function should be incorporated into a treatment plan when a patient is first seen.[66] Before leaving emergency care, a patient's physical activity should be discussed; and a program for range of motion exercises and muscle strengthening should be outlined – both verbally and in writing. At each subsequent follow-up visit, function and strength should be assessed. If there is lack of compliance or if a patient's function begins to deteriorate, then the patient should be referred for supervised physical therapy or occupational therapy, or both. If an injury extends across a joint, or involves a hand or distal portion of the lower extremity, it is advisable to have therapists involved from the beginning. When there are burns of the face which have the potential for facial dysfunction, it may be prudent to have the patient evaluated and treated by a speech pathologist. The potential for development of contractures and hypertrophic scars among the burned treated as out-patients is the same for those treated as in-patients.[66] The principles of prevention and treatment of these complications apply in both settings.

Out-Patient Treatment of Moderate and Major Burns

It is generally conceded that most individuals with minor burns, as defined by the American Burn Association,[67] can be safely treated as out-patients. Some patients, classified as having moderate or even major burn injuries (**Table 8.1**), are suitable for treatment in an ambulatory setting.[68] The purported advantages include less cost, less chance of exposure to antibiotic-resistant microorganisms which are common to burn care facilities, and a more normal environment for the patient. In spite of these benefits, caution should be exercised in selecting patients with moderate and major thermal injury for early discharge from a hospital. On the other hand, as convalescence progresses, many of these patients can have the terminal phase of their acute burn care completed safely as out-patients.

Table 8.1 Classification of burn severity

Minor burn
15% TBSA* or less 1st and 2nd degree burn in an adult
10% TBSA or less 1st and 2nd degree burn in a child
2% TBSA or less 3rd degree burn in child or adult not involving eyes, ears, face or genitalia
Moderate burn
15–25% TBSA 2nd degree burn in an adult
10–20% TBSA 2nd degree burn in a child
2–10% TBSA 3rd degree burn in child or adult not involving eyes, ears, face or genitalia
Major burn
Greater than 25% TBSA 2nd degree burn in adult
Greater than 20% TBSA 2nd degree burn in a child
Greater than 10% TBSA 3rd degree burn in child or adult
All burns involving eyes, ears, face, hands, feet or genitalia
All inhalation injuries
Electrical burns
Complicated burn injuries involving fractures, head injury, or other major trauma
All poor risk patients – preexisting conditions such as cerebrovascular accidents, psychiatric disability, emphysema and other lung diseases, cancer, diabetes, etc.

* Total body surface area.

The conditions which need to be met in order to consider ambulatory care for patients with either moderate or major burns include:

- intravenous fluid resuscitation must be completed;
- there must be no ongoing complications;
- there must be no wound or systemic manifestations of sepsis;
- adequate enteral nutrition must be established; and
- pain control must be satisfactory with medication taken by mouth.

Additionally, arrangements need to be made for wound care and physical and/or occupational therapy.

Acknowledgment

Martha George, BA and Alden H. Harken, MD provided valuable assistance in the preparation of this manuscript.

References

1. National Center for Health Statistics. *Health, United States, 1990.* Publication No. PHS 91–1232. Washington, DC, Public Health Service, 1991.

2. Feller I, Flora J D Jr, Bawol R. Baseline results of therapy for burned patients. *JAMA* 1976; **236:** 1943–7.

3. Rosenburg N M, Marino D. Frequency of suspected abuse/neglect in burn patients. *Pediatr Emerg Care* 1989; **5:** 219–21.

4. Guzzetta P C, Randolph J. Burns in children: 1982. *Pediatr Rev* 1983; **4:** 271–8.

5. Uchiyama N, German J. Pediatric considerations. In: Achauer B M, ed. *Management of the Burned Patient.* Norwalk, CT: Appleton & Lange, 1987: 203–9.

6. Evans E I, Purnell O J, Robinett P W, Batchelor A, Martin M. Fluid and electrolyte requirements in severe burns. *Ann Surg* 1952; **135:** 804–15.

7. Lund C C, Browder N C. The estimate of area of burns. *Surg Gynecol Obstet* 1944; **79:** 352–8.

8. Herdon D N, Rutan R L, Rutan T C. Management of the pediatric patient with burns. *J Burn Care Rehabil* 1993; **14:** 3–8.

9. deCamara D L, Raine T J, London M D, Robson M C, Heggers J P. Progression of thermal injury: a morphologic study. *Plast Reconstr Surg* 1982; **69:** 491–9.

10. Gatti J E, LaRossa D, Silverman D G, Hartford C E. Evaluation of the burn wound with perfusion fluorometry. *J Trauma* 1983; **23:** 202–6.

11. Krob M J, D'Amico F J, Ross D L. Do trauma scores accurately predict outcomes for patients with burns? *J Burn Care Rehabil* 1991; **12:** 560–3.

12. Heimbach D M, Waeckerle J F. Inhalation injuries. *Ann Emerg Med* 1988; **17:** 1316–20.

13. Thompson P B, Herndon D N, Traber D L, Abston S. Effect of mortality of inhalation injury. *J Trauma* 1986; **26:** 163–5.

14. McManus W F, Pruitt B A Jr. Thermal Injuries. In: Mattox K L, Moore E E, Feliciano D V, eds. *Trauma.* Norwalk, CT: Appleton & Lange, 1988: 675–89.

15. Waymack J P, Pruitt B A Jr. Burn wound care. *Adv Surg* 1990; **23:** 261–89.

16. Moylan J A Jr, Inge W W Jr, Pruitt B A Jr. Circulatory changes following circumferential extremity burns evaluated by the ultrasonic flowmeter: an analysis of 60 thermally injured limbs. *J Trauma* 1971; **11:** 763–70.

17. Hooker D R, Kouvenhoven W B, Langworthy O R. The effect of alternating electrical currents on the heart. *Am J Physiol* 1993; **103:** 444–54.

18. Solem L, Fischer R P, Strate R G. The natural history of electrical injury. *J Trauma* 1977; **17:** 487–92.

19. Baxter C R. Present concepts in the management of major electrical injury. *Surg Clin North Am* 1970; **50:** 1401–18.

20. Curreri P W, Asch M J, Pruitt B A Jr. The treatment of chemical burns: specialized diagnostic, therapeutic, and prognostic considerations. *J Trauma* 1970; **10:** 634–42.

21. van Rensburg L C. An experimental study of chemical burns. *S Afr Med J* 1962; **36:** 754–9.

22. Gruber R P, Laub D R, Vistnes L M. The effect of hydrotherapy on the clinical course and pH of experimental cutaneous chemical burns. *Plasr Reconstr Surg* 1975; **55:** 200–4.

23. Dibbell D G, Iverson R E, Jones W, Laub D R, Madison M S. Hydrofluoric acid burns of the hand. *J Bone Joint Surg* 1970; **52A:** 931–6.

24. Greco R J, Hartford C E, Haith L R Jr, Patton M L. Hydrofluoric acid-induced hypocalcemia. *J Trauma* 1988; **28:** 1593–6.

25. Moritz A R, Henriques F C Jr. Studies of thermal injury II. The relative importance of time and surface temperature in the causation of cutaneous burns. *Am J Pathol* 1947; **23:** 695–720.

26. Demling R H, Mazess R B, Wolberg W. The effect of immediate and delayed cool immersion on burn edema formation and resorption. *J Trauma* 1979; **19:** 56–60.

27. King T C, Zimmerman J M. First-aid cooling of the fresh burn. *Surg Gynecol Obstet* 1965; **120:** 1271–3.

28. Ofeigsson O J. Watercooling: first-aid treatment for scalds and burns. *Surgery* 1965; **57:** 391–400.

29. Pushkar N S, Sandorminsky B P. Cold treatment of burns. *Burns Incl Therml Inj* 1982; **9:** 101–10.

30. Purdue G F, Layton T R, Copeland C E. Cold injury complicating burn therapy. *J Trauma* 1985; **25:** 167–8.

31. Osgood P F, Szyfelbein S K. Management of burn pain in children. *Pediatr Clin North Am* 1989; 36: 1001–13.

32. Goldstein J A. Mechanism of induction of hepatic drug metabolizing enzymes: recent advances. *Trends Pharmacol Sci* 1984; **5:** 290.

33. Jaffe J H. Drug addition and drug abuse. In: Gilman A G, Rall T W, Nies A S, Taylor P, eds. *Goodman and Gilman's The Pharmacological Basis of Therapeutics.* 8th ed. New York: Pergamon Press, 1990: 522–73.

34. Swain A H, Azadian B S, Wakeley C J, Shakespeare P G. Management of blisters in minor burns. *Br Med J (Clin Res)* 1987; **295:** 181.

35. Rockwell W B, Ehrlich H P. Should burn blister fluid be evacuated? *J Burn Care Rehabil* 1990; **11:** 93–5.

36. Demling R H, LaLonde C. Burn trauma. In: Blaisdell F W, Trunkey D D, eds. *Trauma Management.* Vol IV. New York: Thieme Medical Publishers, Inc., 1989: 55–6.

37. Demling R H, Burns. *N Engl J Med* 1985; **313:** 1389–98.

38. Stratta R J, Saffle J R, Kravitz M, Warden G D. Management of tar and asphalt injuries. *Am J Surg* 1983; **146:** 766–9.

39. Demling R H, Buerstatte W R, Perea A. Management of hot tar burns. *J Trauma* 1980; **20:** 242.

40. Ashbell T S, Crawford H H, Adamson J E, Horton C E. Tar and grease removal from injured parts. *Plast Reconstr Surg* 1967; **40:** 330–1.

41. Hartford C E. The bequests of Moncrief and Moyer: an appraisal of topical therapy of burns – 1981 American Burn Association presidential address. *J Trauma* 1981; **21:** 827–34.

42. Hunter G R, Chang F C. Outpatient burns: prospective study. *J Trauma* 1976; **16:** 191–5.

43. Miller S F. Outpatient management of minor burns. *Am Fam Physician* 1977; **16:** 167–72.

44. Nance F C, Lewis V L Jr, Hines J L, Barnett D P, O'Neill J A. Aggressive outpatient care of burns. *J Trauma* 1972; **12:** 144–6.

45. Heinrich J J, Brand D A, Cuono C B. The role of topical treatment as a determinant of infection in outpatient burns. *J Burn Care Rehabil* 1988; **9:** 253–7.

46. Haynes B W Jr. Outpatient burns. *Clin Plast Surg* 1974; **1:** 645–51.

47. Gerding R L, Emerman C L, Effrom D, Lukens T, Imbembo A L, Fratianne R B. Outpatient management of partial-thickness burns: Biobrane® versus 1% silver sulfadiazine. *Ann Emerg Med* 1990; **19:** 121–4.

48. Poulsen T D, Freund K G, Arendrup K, Nyhuss P, Pedersen O D. Polyurethane film (Opsite*) vs. impregnated gauze (Jelonet*) in the treatment of outpatient burns: a prospective, randomized study. *Burns Incl Therm Inj* 1991; **17:** 59–61.

49. Tavis M J, Thornton J W, Bartlett R H, Roth J C, Woodroof E A. A new composite skin prosthesis. *Burns Incl Therm. Inj* 1980; **7:** 123.

50. Matsen F A III. *Compartmental Syndromes.* New York: Grune & Stratton, 1980: 57–8.

51. Deitch E A, Wheelahan T M, Rose M P, Clothier J, Cotter J. Hypertrophic burn scars: analysis of variables. *J Trauma* 1983; **23:** 895–98.

52. Engrav L H, Heimbach D M, Reus J L, Harnar T J, Marvin J A. Early excision and grafting vs. nonoperative treatment of burns of indeterminant depth: a randomized prospective study. *J Trauma* 1983; **23:** 1001–4.

53. Burke J F, Bondoc C C, Quinby W C Jr, Remensnyder J P. Primary surgical management of the deeply burned hand. *J Trauma* 1976; **16:** 593–8.

54. Janvekovic Z. A new concept in the early and immediate grafting of burns. *J Trauma* 1970; **10:** 1103–8.

55. Durtschi M B, Orgain C, Counts G W, Heimbach D M. A prospective study of prophylactic penicillin in acutely burned hospitalized patients. *J Trauma* 1982; **22:** 11–14.

56. Loebl E D, Marvin J A, Heck E L, Curreri P W, Baxter C R. The method of quantitative burn-wound biopsy cultures and its routine use in the care of the burned patient. *Am J Clin Pathol* 1974; **61:** 20–4.

57. Pruitt B A Jr. The diagnosis and treatment of infection in the burn patient. *Burns Incl Therml Inj* 1984; **11:** 79–91.

58. Larkin J M, Moylan J A. Tetanus following a minor burn. *J Trauma* 1975; **15:** 546–8.

59. Committee on Trauma, American College of Surgeons. *A Guide to Prophylaxis against Tetanus in Wound Management.* 1984 revision. Chicago, IL: The American College of Surgeons, 1984.

60. Herndon J H Jr. Itching: the pathophysiology of pruritus. *Int J Dermatol* 1975; **14:** 465–84.

61. Kahlsen G, Rosengren E. New approaches to the physiology of medicine. *Physio Rev* 1968; 48: 155–96.

62. Keele C A, Armstrong D. *Substances Producing Pain and Itch.* London: Edward Arnold Publishers, 1964: 297–8.

63. Robson M C, Jellema A, Heggers J P, Hagstrom W J. Care of the healed burn wound: a prospective randomized study. Abstract. San Antonio: American Burn Association, 1980: 94.

64. Gordon M D. Pruritus in burns. *J Burn Care Rehabil* 1988; **9:** 305–11.

65. Heimbach D M, Engrav L H, Marvin J. Minor burns: guidelines for successful outpatient management. *Postgrad Med* 1981; **69:** 22–32.

66. Helm P A, Kevorkian G, Lushbaugh M, Pullium G, Head M D, Cromes G F. Burn injury: rehabilitation management in 1982. *Arch Phys Med Rehabil* 1982; 63: 6–16.

67. *Specific Optimal Criteria for Hospital Resources for Care of Patients with Burn Injury*. New York: American Burn Association, 1976.

68. Warden G D, Kravtiz M, Schnebly A. The outpatient management of moderate and major thermal injury. *J. Burn Care Rehabil* 1981; **2:** 159–61.ss

CHAPTER NINE

Evaluation of the Burn Wound. Management Decisions

David Heimbach, Roberta Mann and Loren Engrav

In addition to the extent of burn and the age of the patient, the depth of burn is a primary determinant of mortality following thermal injury. Burn depth is also the primary determinant of the patient's long-term appearance and function. For many years burns were treated by daily washing, removal of loose dead tissue, and some sort of topical nostrum until they healed by themselves or, eventually, granulation tissue appeared in the base of the wound. Superficial dermal burns healed within 2 weeks and deep dermal burns healed over many weeks if infection was prevented. Full-thickness burns lost their eschar in 2–6 weeks by collagenase production from bacteria and mechanically by daily debridement. When the granulating bed became free of debris and relatively uninfected, split-thickness skin grafts were applied, usually some 3–8 weeks after injury, and a 50% graft take was considered to be acceptable. Repeated graftings eventually closed the wound. The prolonged and intense inflammatory response made hypertrophic scar and contractures part of normal burn treatment. Vigorous physical therapy, nutritional support, psychosocial support, and pain management were required on a daily basis for many weeks in order to yield a satisfactory result.

Modern treatment involves early surgical removal of the burn. Rather than waiting for spontaneous separation, the eschar is now surgically removed early in the burn course and the wound closed with grafting techniques and acute flaps individualized to each patient.

When non-operative treatment is the routine, the accurate assessment of burn depth is of little importance save for predicting mortality. On the other hand, with aggressive surgical treatment, an accurate estimation of burn depth becomes crucial. Burns which heal within 3 weeks generally do so without hypertrophic scarring or functional impairment, although long-term pigment changes are common. Burns which take longer than 3 weeks to heal often produce unsightly hypertrophic scars and frequently lead to functional impairment, as well as providing only a thin, fragile epithelial cover for many weeks or months. State of the art care now, at least in patients with small and moderate burns, involves early excision and grafting of all burns which will not heal within 3 weeks.[1–5] The challenge is to determine which burns will heal within 3 weeks.

An understanding of burn depth requires an understanding of skin thickness. The anatomy and pathophysiology of the skin is well covered in another chapter. The standard technique for determining burn depth has long been clinical observation of the wound. Unfortunately, the difference in burn depth between a burn which heals in 3 weeks and a deep dermal burn which will heal only after many weeks, or a full-thickness burn which won't heal at all may be only a matter of only a few tenths of a millimeter. Further, a burn is a dynamic process for the first few days, and a burn which appears shallow on day 1 may appear deep by day 3. Finally, the kind of topical wound care used can dramatically change the appearance of the burn. Because of these limitations, and because of its increased importance in planning definitive burn wound care, interest has been stirred and technology has brought numerous devices and techniques to determine burn depth more precisely than clinical observation.

Estimation of Burn Depth

Clinical Observation

Despite modern technology, clinical observation still remains the standard for diagnosis. Very shallow (heal in less than 2 weeks) and very deep (full-thickness charred burns) present little difficulty even to inexperienced observers. Superficial dermal burns involve only the papillary dermis and characteristically form blisters with fluid collection at the interface of the epidermis and dermis. Blistering may not occur for some hours following injury and burns thought to be first degree may subsequently be diagnosed as superficial dermal burns by day 2. Once blisters are removed, the wound is pink and wet and is quite painful as currents of air pass over it. The wound is hypersensitive to touch and the patient will rarely permit more than one diagnostic adventure with a pin to test sensation. These wounds blanch with pressure, and the blood flow to the dermis is increased over that of normal skin. Obvious charred full-thickness burns are leathery, firm, depressed when compared to adjoining normal skin, and are insensitive to light touch and pinprick. Unfortunately for the clinician, there are many burns whose depth is intermediate between these obvious ones.

Deep dermal burns extend into the reticular dermis and generally will take 3 or more weeks to heal. They also blister, but the wound surface is usually a mottled pink and white color immediately following the injury. The patient complains of discomfort rather than pain. When pressure is applied to the burn, capillaries refill slowly or not at all. The wound is often less sensitive to pinprick than the surrounding normal skin.[6,7] By the second day the wound may be white and is usually fairly dry.

Noncharred full-thickness burns can masquerade with many of the clinical findings of a deep dermal burn. Like deep dermal burns, they may be mottled in appearance. They rarely blanch on pressure, and may have a dry, white appearance. In some cases the burn may be translucent with clotted vessels visible in the depths. Some full-thickness burns, particularly immersion scalds, may have a red appearance, and can be confused by the uninitiated as a superficial dermal burn. They can be distinguished, however, because these red, full-thickness burns do not blanch with pressure.

Evaluation by an experienced surgeon as to whether an apparent deep dermal burn will heal in 3 weeks is about 50% accurate[8] – tossing a coin is about as useful a technique. In experienced hands, however, early excision and grafting provides better results than non-operative care for such 'indeterminate' burns.[2]

An intense search for a more precise diagnosis of burn depth has been mounted ever since it became important to determine whether the patient would benefit from early operation. A number of techniques have been used based on the physiology of the skin and alterations produced by burning. These techniques take advantage of:

- the ability to detect dead cells or denatured collagen (biopsy, ultrasound, vital dyes);
- altered blood flow (fluorescein, laser Doppler, and thermography);
- the color of the wound (light reflectance); and
- physical changes, such as edema (magnetic resonance imaging). A brief review of each follows.

Burn Wound Biopsy

Histologic wound biopsy would seem to be the most precise diagnostic tool.[9] However, biopsies leave permanent scars in partial-thickness wounds, they are expensive, and they require an experienced pathologist to tell live from denatured collagen and cells. Further, the burn wound is dynamic during the first several days, and even in the 1950s Douglas Jackson reported that 7 days were necessary to obtain reproducible results.[10] Another day or two is required to obtain permanent sections, and there is no guarantee that areas adjacent to the biopsy are the same depth. For these reasons, biopsies are rarely used in clinical practice; to the authors' knowledge, no studies have determined correlation with biopsy and time to healing.

Ultrasound

Moserová, using an industrial ultrasound device in 1982, was able to detect differences between normal pig skin and that scalded for 5 and 15 seconds.[11] His initial work was expanded as technology improved. Cantrell[12] was able to detect denatured from normal collagen in pigskin. One problem with this technique is that collagen denatures at 65°C while the epidermal cells, from which the burn must heal, are killed at about 47°C. As a result, apparent depth is likely to be underestimated by ultrasound. Further refinements in instrumentation have enabled Brink[13] to reach a significant correlation between ultrasound burn depth and histology in pigs (r=0.90). Unfortunately, in the clinical arena Wachtel,[14] in five burned patients, reported that ultrasound comparisons with clinical evaluation and histopathological studies of burn wound biopsies of the same burned areas failed to show any substantive improvement in predicting the depth of burn by ultrasonic scanning techniques. Perhaps more precise instruments will continue to improve resolution.

Vital Dyes

In experimental small mammal models, India ink can provide a one-time demonstration of blood flow to the skin.[15,17] India ink, however, kills the animal on injection; so, while a useful experimental technique, it has no role in patient wound assessment.

A vital dye directly applied to the burn wound would be useful in detecting dead tissue and also in determining the depth of excision. Davies[18] described important characteristics of such a dye. It should stain only dead tissue, not be removable with wound treatment, be nontoxic, provide a sharp demarcation between living and dead tissue, penetrate all dead tissue, and be compatible with topical treatments usually used in burn care. Zawacki[19] in 1970 studied patent blue V and tetracycline for the diagnosis of burn depth but the results were subjective. In a rat model, Davies and his coworkers evaluated methylene blue, toluidine blue, trypan blue, Evans blue and Disulphine Blue sulphan blue marker dyes. Methylene blue, which is metabolized to a colorless compound by living cells, was selected for preliminary testing in patients. When mixed with silver sulphadiazine and applied topically, a significant blue discoloration appeared within 48 hours which remained after vigorous washing. Excision was carried down to dermis which was unstained. They reported 'encouraging' results in this preliminary study, but the authors have no more recent reports listed in the Index Medicus. Immediately following this report with methylene blue, brief clinical use of this technique in our burn center did not produce a satisfactorily sharp demarcation to guide excision.

Fluorescein Fluorometry

Fluorescein, injected systemically, is delivered through a patent circulation and fluoresces under ultraviolet light. It has been widely used to determine viability of flaps,[20,21] intestine, and even whole extremities.[22] The use of fluorescein fluorescence to determine burn depth was first reported in 1943.[23] Because treatment plans were not altered based on burn depth, the technique lay fallow until more precise instruments could measure the magnitude of fluorescence – a fiberoptic perfusion fluorometer. Gatti[24] studied 63 burns with the fluorometer after intravenous administration of sodium fluorescein. The fluorescein kinetics were monitored for 1 hour within the first 48 hours and again between the third and sixth days postburn, and compared them to the kinetics in adjacent normal skin. Depth of burn was confirmed by biopsy and healing characteristics. Fluorometric analysis during both study periods consistently distinguished between partial-thickness and full-thickness burns. Partial-thickness burns uniformly exhibited fluorescence within 10 minutes; full-thickness burns showed nil. Enthusiasm for this technique must be tempered by the knowledge that when this technique was reported in 1982, most burn surgeons excised only full-thickness burns, leaving partial-thickness burns to heal on their own. Therefore, there was an advantage to distinguishing between partial and full-thickness burns. Gatti's report was confirmed with high speed Polaroid photography in 1984, but again the fluorescein technique was best at distinguishing full-thickness (no fluorescence) from nonfull-thickness burns.[25,26]

A report by Black[27] in 1986 could not confirm significant differences between partial and full-thickness burns using a similar technique. In both rat and human models, 59 burn sites (eight rats) and 37 burn sites (seven patients) were assessed. Readings were taken for 3 hours on the rats and 1 hour on the patients during the first 48 hours, and the procedure was repeated for 5 days postburn. Maximum values during these periods were determined for burn and nonburn sites, and background levels were subtracted from these values. The rate of fluorescein uptake and the peak times for burn and nonburn sites were then compared. Actual depth of burn was determined by whether or not healing had occurred. The results showed no significant difference between partial-thickness and full-thickness burns using fluorometry, as standard deviations in both models for both depths of burn were too large to distinguish between groups, let alone be predictive in any given burn.

The studies remain inconclusive. Our own experience with fluorescein indicates that it confirms the clinical diagnosis in very deep and very shallow burns, areas where there is little confusion, but that it cannot distinguish between intermediate and deep dermal burns, where the distinction is crucial in operative planning.

Laser Doppler Flowmetry

The laser Doppler has been used since 1975 for monitoring the cutaneous circulation. Light from a helium–neon laser is carried by fiberoptics to the skin where it interacts with both stationary structures and moving blood cells within a sample volume of approximately 1 mm^3. Back-scattered light from the moving cells is shifted in velocity using the Doppler principle, while back-scattered light from stationary objects remains at its original frequency. The mixing of these light waves is translated to an electrical signal, and mathematical estimation of blood flow can be made in normal versus study areas of skin. The laser Doppler has the advantage of being easy to use, non-invasive (although the probe must be held against the skin), and provides immediate results. In some studies, the skin was heated to >40°C (to ensure maximal vasodilatation).

Sorensen's group in Denmark first reported the use of a laser Doppler on a burn unit. In a first study, the investigators measured skin blood flow in burned patients at rest and after applying a topical heat load at 44°C and found a close relationship between burn depth and the combination of flow level and ability to vasodilate[28]. They also measured skin blood flow in 15 burned patients on the third day postburn and compared results to a punch biopsy taken from the same point. They found an excellent correlation between biopsy and laser, but only good correlation between laser and clinical assessment for full-thickness burns. Nonetheless the authors felt that their results were encouraging.

Initial studies in our burn center showed excellent correlation with full-thickness burns (no flow) and shallow burns (normal or increased flow) but considerable variation from patient to patient with comparable burns as well as at different times in the same area in the same patient with moderate and deep dermal burns. Readings varied particularly with temperature (immediately after bathing, in a warm room, etc.); the state of anxiety (catecholamine response); and elevation of an extremity (cutaneous blood flow essentially disappeared as the hands were elevated).

In further studies, we followed the cutaneous circulation over time in burned patients and rats[29]. We asked whether measuring changes in cutaneous blood flow might help predict the ultimate fate of burns which were not obviously shallow or deep. A laser Doppler flowmeter was used to study cutaneous perfusion for at least 72 hours in partial-thickness wounds on patients with burns of less than 15% TBSA and in experimental wounds of similar size on rats. Clinical wounds which healed without grafting consistently showed elevated perfusion levels which increased further within 72 hours. Wounds which eventually required grafting had lower perfusion levels with no obvious pattern of increase. Differences between average flow levels for healing and nonhealing burns were statistically significant throughout the study period. Perfusion levels in experimental wounds were stratified according to burn severity (scalds for 1, 3, 5, 10 seconds), with shallower wounds showing a pattern of increase similar to the clinical wounds. While the means were significantly different in these studies ($p < 0.05$), individual burns showed enough overlap that absolute levels of flow were not predictive for any given patient; however, the trend toward increased flow for healing burns and flat flow for nonhealing burns was quite constant, and if the patient can be followed for several days, the method has merit in deciding who would benefit from excision and grafting after day 3. Similar findings (significant group differences but considerable individual overlap) were reported recently by O'Reilly and colleagues[30]. Clinical studies using the laser Doppler to determine burn depth are ongoing, and refinements of the technology continue; however, its use has not become standard in everyday clinical decision-making (to graft or not to graft).

Thermography

Diminished blood flow to deep dermal and full thickness burns makes them cooler to touch,[31] a finding confirmed by thermography in 1974 by Hackett.[32] Initial studies of thermography as a tool for predicting the need for excision and grafting of deep dermal wounds in 30 patients were presented with guarded optimism by Mason in 1981, suggesting that thermography might be more accurate than clinical judgment.[33] Thermography, like the laser Doppler, is highly dependent on room and patient temperature, the patient's anxiety and stress level, and area of the body considered.[34] Despite these drawbacks, Cole[35,36] compared thermography to clinical assessment of 32 burned hands. Superficial and deep partial-thickness burns were treated conservatively, with excision and grafting of those which had not healed only after 2–3 weeks after injury. This delayed surgery group and the healed group were retrospectively analysed to determine the predictive value of the initial clinical and thermographic assessments of the depth of the burns. Full-thickness burns were excised and grafted within 5 days and were not included in the study. Initial thermographic assessment correctly predicted the outcome (whether healed or excised and grafted) in 33 of 36 burns. This relationship was highly significant. Initial clinical assessment of depth had no significant relationship with the time taken to heal.

Light Reflectance

The skin is relatively transparent to short wavelength infrared light, and reduced hemoglobin absorbs more of the light than oxygenated hemoglobin. Anselmo and Zawacki in 1973[37] reasoned that thrombosed vessels in full-thickness burns would become visible in infrared light and could be distinguished from the open vessels of partial-thickness burns. Computer analysis of infrared photographs was encouraging, and they extended their work, publishing results in 1977[38] of computer analyses of photographs taken with red, green, and infrared filtered light. A mainframe computer generated ratios of the green/infrared, red/infrared, and red/green images point by point over the entire surface. The authors felt that these images could accurately distinguish shallow, deep dermal, and full-thickness burns. Unfortunately, wound analysis was very expensive and time consuming, so it was too slow for clinical decision-making.

Based on their work, we devised a portable, non-invasive (the wound is not touched) electronic device which could instantaneously measure the spectral characteristics of red, green, and infrared light reflected from the burn.[39] The burn depth indicator (BDI) was essentially 100% accurate for shallow and full-thickness wounds. For intermediate wounds, using the endpoint of wound healing as less than or more than 3 weeks, clinical assessments by two experienced surgeons were compared to readings from the device. In about one-third of cases the surgeons were unwilling to commit themselves to a prediction. In the cases where the surgeons were willing to make a prediction, they were incorrect about 25% of the time. The BDI was significantly more accurate than the clinical assessment in those predicted not to heal by the surgeons and maintained an accuracy of 79% in the wounds where the surgeons would not make a prediction. Of importance, and not usually addressed in many other studies, are the dynamic qualities of the burn wound. The light reflectance device clearly showed changes each day for the first 3–4 days, and its accuracy, like that of the surgeons, was best on day 3.

We have extended our studies with light reflectance[40,41] and now can produce real-time false-colored television and Polaroid pictures of the wound, providing green colored wounds which will certainly heal, yellow colored wounds if unlikely to heal in 3 weeks, and red colored wounds which will definitely not heal in 3 weeks.

Magnetic Resonance Imaging (MRI)

Full-thickness burns result in slower resorption of wound edema than partial-thickness burns. Since proton MRI parameters correlate with tissue water content, Koruda[42] determined whether proton MRI could distinguish them. Early after burning the MRI could distinguish higher water content in partial and full-thickness rat burns than in adjacent normal skin. By 48 hours the partial-thickness burn had returned to control values, while the full-thickness burn remained edematous. Unfortunately the rat skin had to be excised in order to use the MRI, so useful clinical application is still some time away.

Based on this review of widely differing techniques, it becomes apparent that precise determination of burn depth awaits further refinement of instrumentation, and clinical assessment remains the not-so-golden standard. In addition to the appearance of the wound, other factors can help determine the need for operation. These factors are discussed below and include the type of burn, the age of the patient, and the circumstances surrounding the injury.

Scalds

In civilian practice, scalds, usually due to hot water, are the most common cause of burns. Despite educational programs, the epidemiology and incidence of scalds world wide changes very little.[43–50] Water at 140°F (60°C) will create a deep dermal or full-thickness burn in 3 seconds, and at 156°F (68.8°C) the same burn will occur in 1 second.[51] Freshly brewed coffee from an automatic percolator is generally about 180°F (82.2°C). Boiling water always causes deep burns; soups and sauces, which are thicker in consistency and remain in contact longer with the skin, invariably cause deep burns. In general, exposed areas tend to be burned less deeply than areas covered with clothing. Clothing retains the heat and keeps the liquid in contact with the skin for a longer period of time. As a result scalds are generally a mosaic of superficial and indeterminate dermal burns.[52] Therefore, unless the burns are obviously deep, we treat them nonoperatively for 10–14 days and then excise areas which will be unlikely to heal within the 3-week window. The wisdom of this plan was confirmed by Desai[53] who randomized children with scald burns to early (within 72 hours) versus late excision (waiting 2 weeks), showing that early operation required considerably more blood replacement without any clinical benefit.

Immersion scalds are deep and serious burns.[54–57] Although the water may not be as hot as with a spill scald, the duration of contact is usually longer and these burns frequently occur in small children or in elderly or infirm patients with thin skin. For this reason, many states have initiated legislation to set home and public hot water heaters to maximum temperatures below 130°F (54.4°C).[58]

Intentional scalds and head injuries are the most common forms of reported child abuse,[59–63] and in our burn center, deliberate scalds occur in about 2% of all the children admitted. Detailed descriptions of this tragic consequence are available elsewhere in this book, but the physician must be alert that the history provided matches the distribution and probable cause of the burn. Such burns are usually deep, and many will require excision and grafting. Although water temperature may not be as high as a spill scald, the duration of the burn is considerably longer. Deliberate scalds have also been reported as a form of female-to-male assault.[64,65]

Scald burns from grease or hot oil are generally deep dermal or full thickness. Cooking oil and grease, when hot enough to use for cooking, may be in the range of 350°F (176.7°C). Often the victim tries to carry a burning pot of grease out of doors and douses himself. In this circumstance, the grease is at about 400°F (204.4°C), and the burns are invariably suitable for early excision and grafting.[66,67]

Tar and asphalt burns are a special kind of scald. The 'mother pot' at the back of the roofing truck maintains tar at a temperature of 400–500°F (204–260°C). Burns caused by tar directly from the 'mother pot' are invariably full thickness. By the time the tar is spread on the roof, its temperature has diminished to the point where most of the burns are deep dermal in nature.[68–70] Unfortunately, initial evaluation is difficult because of the adherent tar.[71] Tar can be removed by application of a petroleum base ointment under a dressing. The dressing is changed and the ointment reapplied every 2–4 hours until the tar has dissolved. Only then can the extent of the injury and the depth of the burn be accurately estimated. Most tar burns are suitable for early excision and grafting.

Flame Burns

Flame burns are the next most common injuries seen. Although the incidence of injuries from house fires has decreased with the advent of smoke detectors, careless smoking, improper use of flammable liquids, automobile accidents, and clothing ignited from stoves or space heaters still exact their toll. In one study of several burn centers, 28% of flame burns occurred in patients with high blood ethanol levels, and 51% of victims in fires behaved inappropriately when trying to escape.[72] Patients whose bedding or clothes have been on fire rarely escape without some full-thickness burns.

Flash Burns

Flash burns are next in frequency. Explosions of natural gas, propane, gasoline and other flammable liquids cause intense heat for a very brief time. For the most part, clothing, unless it ignites, is protective in flash burns, and flash burns generally have a distribution involving all exposed skin, with the deepest areas facing the source of ignition. For the most part, flash burns are dermal in depth, being superficial or deep in proportion to the amount and kind of fuel that explodes. While such burns will generally heal without extensive skin grafting, they may be very large in extent and may be associated with significant thermal damage to the upper airway.

Contact Burns

Contact burns result from hot metals, plastic, glass, or hot coals. Such burns are usually limited in extent but are invariably very deep. Contact burns, especially in patients who were unconscious at the time of injury, or in patients dealing with molten materials, are frequently fourth degree. It is common for patients involved in industrial accidents to have both severe contact burns and crush injuries since these accidents commonly occur from presses or from hot, heavy objects. The increased use of wood-burning stoves with surface temperatures hot enough to ignite paper or wood brings an increasing number of toddlers with deep palm burns, as the toddler trips and falls with hands outstretched against the stove.[73] Left alone, such burns heal from the edges with contracture of the palm leading to permanent disability. An aggressive approach with excision and grafting using thick split-thickness grafts[73] or full thickness grafts[74] is warranted. Particularly vexing are contact burns following motor vehicle accidents where the patient is trapped against a muffler or engine block. Such burns are often fourth degree, and may well require acute flap coverage.[75]

Electrical Burns

Electrical burns are in reality thermal burns from very high intensity heat and from explosion of cell membranes.[76] Electricity as it meets the resistance of body tissues is converted to heat in direct proportion to the amperage of the current and the electrical resistance of the body parts through which it passes.[77] The smaller the size of the body parts through which the electricity passes, the more intense the heat and the less the heat is dissipated. Therefore, fingers, hands, forearms, feet, and lower legs are frequently totally destroyed whereas larger volume areas, like the trunk, usually dissipate enough current to prevent extensive damage to viscera unless the entrance or exit wound is on the abdomen or chest.[78–80] Arc electrical burns are common in addition to the usual entrance and exit wounds. These occur when current takes the most direct path, rather than a longer path of seeming less resistance. These deep and destructive wounds occur at joints which are in close apposition at the time of injury. Most common are burns of the volar aspect of the wrist, the antecubital fossa when the elbow is flexed, and the axilla if the shoulder is adducted as current passes from upper extremity to trunk. While cutaneous manifestations of electrical burns may appear limited, the skin injury is only the tip of the iceberg; massive underlying tissue destruction may take place.

There are two reasons for early operation in the patient with electrical burns. Massive deep tissue necrosis may lead to acidosis or myoglobinuria which will not clear with standard resuscitation techniques. In this unusual circumstance, major debridement and amputations may be needed urgently. Far more commonly, the deep tissues undergo swelling and the risk of compartment syndrome further compromising damaged tissue is real. Careful monitoring is mandatory and escharotomies and fasciotomies should be performed at the slightest suggestion of progression.[81] Any progression of median or ulnar nerve deficit in the electrically injured hand is an indication for immediate median and ulnar nerve release at the wrist. The use of a technetium scan to help identify damaged and necrotic muscle has been advocated,[82,83] but has not achieved widespread use. In our experience, they have been overly sensitive in detecting damage to deep, unexposed muscle groups which, left alone, will fibrose and not require excision.

If immediate decompression or debridement is not required, we feel that definitive operations can be done between days 3 and 5, before bacterial contamination occurs and after the tissue necrosis is delineated. Extraordinary measures, such as vascular grafts[84,85] to replace clotted arteries, and emergent free flaps[86,87] may sometimes be indicated, but the surgeon is cautioned that they may actually increase morbidity and prolong the patient's recovery when one of the newer prostheses might give better function than a hand or foot with poor sensation and motor function.

Chemical Burns

Chemical burns, usually caused by strong acids or alkali, are most often the result of industrial accidents, drain cleaners, assaults, and the improper use of harsh solvents. In contrast to thermal burns, chemical burns cause progressive damage until the chemicals are inactivated by reaction with the tissue or dilution by flushing with water. Although individual circumstances vary, acid burns may be more self-limiting than alkali burns. Acid tends to 'tan' the skin, creating an impermeable barrier which limits further penetration of the acid. Alkalis, on the other hand, combine with cutaneous lipids to create soap and thereby continue 'dissolving' the skin until they are neutralized. A full-thickness chemical burn may appear deceptively superficial, clinically causing only a mild brownish discoloration of the skin. The skin may appear to remain intact during the first few days postburn, and only then begin to slough spontaneously. Unless the observer can be absolutely sure, chemical burns should be considered deep dermal or full thickness until proven otherwise.

Burns caused by wet cement can be vexing.[88–90] Workers often kneel in wet cement or spill cement inside boots or gloves and do not become symptomatic for some hours. By the time they seek medical help, the wounds are often deep and, in our experience, most often need grafting.

Hydrofluoric acid (HF) burns are potentially very destructive. HF penetrates through the skin and causes deep tissue destruction by combining with cellular calcium.[91,92] HF is widely used in the computer chip industry, in cleaning solvents, and paint removers. As with cement, the worker may not become symptomatic for several hours after exposure, when severe pain develops, usually of involved fingers. Delayed or inadequate treatment can lead to amputation. Older recommendations of calcium-containing topical gels[93,94] and direct injection of calcium gluconate into the involved tissue, has now largely been replaced by intra-arterial perfusion of calcium ions into vessels serving the injured area.[95–98] Such treatment is almost magical with immediate cessation of pain and minimal tissue destruction.

Burns in the Elderly

As people age, their skin atrophies with thinning of the dermis and disappearance of skin appendages.[99] These are some of the many factors which make burn mortality in the geriatric patient disproportionate to the rest of the population with similar burns.[100–103] The thin skin also makes the diagnosis of burn depth difficult, although the best rule of thumb is to assume that there are no shallow burns in the elderly. Survivors with burns larger than 40% TBSA are rare, and modern surgical and intensive care techniques have only marginally influenced mortality in smaller burns.[102–105] The dilemma of nonoperative versus aggressive early operation is not resolved for the elderly population. An aggressive surgical approach[1,106–108] appears to cut down on hospital time, as it does in all patients, but does not appear to have any better survival nor function than a conservative approach[109] which emphasizes early discharge and home care for smaller burns.

In the elderly, grafts on fat often do not survive; all donors, even when taken at 0.008 inch are very slow to heal. Our current plan is to excise to fascia full-thickness burns which will not heal from the periphery or by contraction, and to graft them with 2:1 meshed grafts taken at 0.008 inch from the back. Indeterminate burns are generally left to heal or granulate, as out-patients if possible. Occasionally narrow burns can be excised and the skin surgically closed,[110] but closure with any tension invites dehiscence and infection.

Conclusion

Although there are many different types of burn wounds, the extent of tissue destruction is always a function of the temperature of the heat source, the duration of contact, and the thickness of the involved skin. Burns which are unlikely to heal in less than 3 weeks should be treated by early excision and grafting (within 7 days of injury). Benefits of this approach include reduction in length of hospital stay, earlier return to work or school, and optimal functional and cosmetic results. Research is ongoing to determine reliable methods of defining burn depth, so that those patients who need grafting may be treated expeditiously and so that the risks of operation can be avoided in those who do not.

References

1. Deitch E. A policy of early excision and grafting in elderly burn patients shortens the hospital stay and improves survival. *Burns Incl Therml Inj* 1985; **12:** 109–14.

2. Engrav L, Heimbach D, Reus J, Harner T, Marvin J A. Early excision and grafting vs. nonoperative treatment of burns of indeterminant depth: a randomized prospective study. *J Trauma* 1983; **23:** 1001.

3. Frist W, Ackroyd F, Burke J, Bondoc C. Long-term functional results of selective treatment of hand burns. *Am J Surg* 1985; **149:** 516–21.

4. Gray D, Pine R, Harner T. Early excision versus conventional therapy in patients with 20 to 40% burns. *Am J Surg* 1982; **149:** 76.

5. Thompson, P, Herndon D N, Abston S, Rutan T. Effect of early excision on patients with major thermal injury. *J Trauma* 1987; **27:** 205–7.

6. Jackson D. Second thoughts on the burn wound. *J Trauma* 1969; **9:** 839.

7. Bajaj S P, Nield D V, Rayment R, Khoo C T. A simple modification of the pin-prick test for the assessment of burn depth in children. *Burns Incl Therml Inj* 1988; **14:** 468–72.

8. Hlava P, Moserov A J, Konigov A R. Validity of clinical assessment of the depth of a thermal injury. *Acta Chir Plast* 1983; **25:** 202–8.

9. Sevitt S. *Burns Pathology and Therapeutic Applications.* London: Butterworth, 1910: 57.

10. Jackson D. The diagnosis of the depth of burning. *Br J Surg* 1953; **40:** 588–96.

11. Moserová J, Hlava P, Malinsky J. Scope for ultrasound diagnosis of the depth of thermal damage. Preliminary report. *Acta Chir Plast* 1982; **24:** 235–42.

12. Cantrell J H. Can ultrasound assist an experienced surgeon in estimating burn depth? *J Trauma* 1984; **24:** S64–70.

13. Brink J A, Sheets P W, Dines K A. Quantitative assessment of burn injury in porcine skin with high-frequency ultrasonic imaging. *Invest Radiol* 1986; **21:** 645–51.

14. Wachtel T L, Leopold G R, Frank H A, Frank D H. B-mode ultrasonic echo determination of depth of thermal injury. *Burns Incl Therml Inj* 1986; **12:** 432–7.

15. Zawacki B. Reversal of capillary stasis and prevention of necrosis in burns. *Ann Surg* 1974; **180:** 98.

16. Robson M C, Heggers J P. The effect of prostaglandins on the dermal microcirculation after burning, and the inhibition of the effect by specific pharmacological agents. *Plast Reconstr Surg* 1979; **63:** 781.

17. Kaufman T, Hurwitz D, Heggers J. The india ink injection technique to assess the depth of experimental burn wounds. *Burns* 1984; **10:** 405.

18. Davies M, Adendorff D, Rode H, van de Reit I S. Colouring the damaged tissues on the burn wound surface. *Burns* 1980; **6:** 156.

19. Zawacki B E, Walker H L. An evaluation of patent blue V, brophenol blue and tetracycline for the diagnosis of burn depth. *Plast Reconstr Surg* 1970; **54:** 459–65.

20. Silverman D, LaRossa D, Barlow C. Quantification of tissue fluorescein delivery and prediction of flap viability with the fiberoptic dermofluorometer. *Plast Reconstr Surg* 1980; **66:** 545.

21. Silverman D, Norton K, Brousseau D. Serial fluorometric documentation of fluorescein dye delivery. *Surgery* 1985; **97:** 185.

22. Hurford W E, Silverman D G. Evaluation of ischemic extremities by quantitative fluorescence assessment. *Surg Forum* 1982; **323:** 442–3.

23. Dingwall J A. A clinical test for differentiating second from third degree burns. *Ann Surg* 1943; **118:** 427–9.

24. Gatti J, LaRossa D, Silverman D, Hartford C. Evaluation of the burn wound with perfusion fluorometry. *J Trauma* 1983; **23:** 202–6.

25. Grossman A, Zuckerman A. Intravenous fluorescein photography in burns. *J Burn Care Rehabil* 1984; **5:** 65.

26. Zuckerman A. Fluorescein fluorescence photography for the evaluation of burns. *J Biol Photogr* 1983; **51:** 33–5.

27. Black K S, Hewitt C W, Miller D M. Burn depth evaluation with fluorometry: is it really definitive? *J Burn Care Rehabil* 1986; **7:** 313–17.

28. Alsbjoørn B, Micheels J, Soørensen B. Laser Doppler flowmetry measurements of superficial dermal, deep dermal and subdermal burns. *Scand J Plast Recon, Surg* 1984; **18:** 75–9.

29. Green M, Holloway G A, Heimbach D M. Laser Doppler monitoring of microcirculatory changes in acute burn wounds. *J Burn Care Rehabil* 1988; **9:** 57–62.

30. O'Reilly T J, Spence R J, Taylor R M, Scheulen J J. Laser Doppler flowmetry evaluation of burn wound depth. *J Burn Care Rehabil* 1989; **50:** 1–60.

31. Watson A C, Vasilescu C T. Thermography in plastic surgery. *J R Coll Surg Edinb* 1972; **17:** 247.

32. Hackett M E J. The use of thermography in the assessment of depth of burn and blood supply of flaps, with preliminary reports on its use in Dupuytren's contracture and treatment of varicose ulcer. *Br J Plas Surg* 1974; **27:** 311.

33. Mason B, Graff A, Pegg S. Colour thermography in the diagnosis of the depth of burn injury. *Burns* 1981; **7:** 197.

34. Henane R, Bittel J, Banssilon V. Partitional calorimetry measurements of energy exchanges in severely burned patients. *Burns* 1981; **7:** 180.

35. Cole R, Jones S, Shakespeare P. Thermographic assessment of hand burns. *Burns* 1990; **16:** 60–3.

36. Cole R, Shakespeare P, Chissell H, Jones S. Thermographic assessment of burns using a nonpermeable membrane as wound covering. *Burns* 1991; **17:** 117–22.

37. Anselmo V J, Zawacki B E. Infrared photography as a diagnostic tool for the burn ward. *Proc Soc Photo-optical Instr Engrs* 1973; **8:** 181.

38. Anselmo V J, Zawacki BE. Multispectral photographic analysis – a new quantitative tool to assist in the early diagnosis of thermal burn injury. *Ann Biomed Eng* 1977: 179–83.

39. Heimbach D, Afromowitz M, Engrav L. Burn depth estimation – man or machine. *J Trauma* 1984; **24:** 373.

40. Afromowitz M A, Van L G S, Heimbach D M. Clinical evaluation of burn injuries using an optical reflectance technique. *IEEE Trans Biomed Eng* 1987; **34:** 114–27.

41. Afromowitz M A, Callis J B, Heimbach D M, DeSoto L A, Norton M K. Multispectral imaging of burn wounds: a new clinical instrument for evaluating burn depth. *IEEE Trans Biomed Eng* 1988; **35:** 842–50.

42. Koruda M J, Zimbler A, Settle R G. Assessing burn wound depth using in vitro nuclear magnetic resonance (NMR). *J Surg Res* 1986; **40:** 475–81.

43. Cason C. A study of scalds in Birmingham. *J R Soc Med* 1990; **83:** 690–2.

44. Fallat M E, Rengers S J. The effect of education and safety devices on scald burn prevention. *J Trauma* 1993; **34:** 560–3.

45. Chen T, Yang J, Tsai Y, Noordhoff M. Pediatric burns – 2 year survey of cases admitted to the Chang Gung Memorial Hospital. *Chang Keng I Hsueh* 1989; **12:** 45–50.

46. Langley J, Dodge J, Silva P. Scalds to preschool children. *NZ Med J* 1981; **93:** 84–7.

47. Lindblad B, Terkelsen C. Scalding accidents among children – an epidemiologic study. *Ugeskr Laeger* 1990; **152:** 1590–1.

48. Langley J, Tobin P. Childhood burns. *NZ Med J* 1983 **96:** 681–4.

49. Raine P, Azmy A. A review of thermal injuries in young children. *J Pediatr Surg* 1983; **18:** 21–6.

50. Tejerina C, Reig A, Codina A. An epidemiological study of burn patients hospitalized in Valencia, Spain during 1989. *Burns* **18:** 15–18.

51. Moritz A, Henriques F. Studies of thermal injury II. The relative importance of time and surface temperature in the causation of cutaneous burns. *Am J Path* 1947; **23:** 695.

52. Irei M, Baston S, Bonds E. The optimal time for excision of scald burns in toddlers. *J Burn Care Rehab* 1986; **7:** 508–10.

53. Desai M H, Rutan R L, Herndon D N, Conservative treatment of scald burns is superior to early excision. *J Burn Care Rehabil* 1991; **12:** 482.

54. Ding Y I, Pu S S, Pan Z L. Extensive scalds following accidental immersion in hot water pools. *Burns Incl Therm Inj* 1987; **13:** 305–3.

55. Graitcer P L, Sniezek J E. Hospitalizations due to tap water scalds. *MMWR CDC Surveill Summ* 1987; **37:** 35–8.

56. Tennant W G, Davison P M. Bath scalds in children in the south-east of Scotland. *J R Coll Surg Edinb* 1991; **36:** 319–22.

57. Walker A. Fatal tapwater scald burn in the USA 1979–1986. *Burns* 1990; **16:** 49–52.

58. Erdmann T, Feldman K, Rivara F, Heimbach D, Wall H. Tap water burn prevention: the effect of legislation. *Pediatrics* 1991; **88:** 572–7.

59. Caniano D, Beaver B, Boles E. Child abuse: an update on surgical management in 256 cases. *Ann Surg* 1986; **203:** 219–24.

60. Kumar P. Child abuse by thermal injury – a retrospective study. *Burns* 1984; **10:** 344.

61. Ledbetter D, Tapper D. Injuries caused by child abuse. *Compr Ther* 1989; **15:** 9–13.

62. Renz B M, Sherman R. Child abuse by scalding. *J Med Assoc Ga* 1992; **81:** 574–8.

63. Renz B M, Sherman R. Abusive scald burns in infants and children: a prospective study. *Am Surg* 1993; **59:** 329–34.

64. Purdue G, Hunt J. Adult assault as a mechanism of burn injury. *Arch Surg* 1990; **125:** 268–9.

65. Krob M J, Johnson A, Jordan M H. Burned-and-battered adults. *J Burn Care Rehabil* 1986; **7:** 529–31.

66. Pegg S, Seawright A. Burns due to cooking oils – an increasing hazard. *Burns Incl Therm Inj* 1983; **9:** 362–9.

67. Hayes L C, Ward R S, Suffle J R, *et al.* Grease burns at fast-food restaurants. Adolescents at risk. *J Burn Care Rehabil* 1991; **12:** 203–8.

68. Wachtel T L, Frank H A, Shabbazz A. Scalds from molten tar: an industrial hazard. *J Burn Care Rehabil* 1988; **9:** 218–19.

69. Hill M, Achauer B, Martinez S. Tar and asphalt burns. *J Burn Care Rehabil* 1984; **5:** 271.

70. Demling R, Buerstatte W, Perea A. Management of hot tar burns. *J Trauma* 1980; **20:** 242.

71. James N, Moss A. Review of burns caused by bitumen and the problems of its removal. *Burns* 1990; **16:** 214–16.

72. Byrom R, Word E, Tewksbury C, Edlich R. Epidemiology of flame burn injuries. *Burns Incl Therm Inj* 1984; **11:** 1–10.

73. Yanofsky N. Upper extremity burns from wood stoves. *Pediatrics* 1984; **73:** 722–6.

74. Merrell S, Saffle J, Schnebly A. Full-thickness skin grafting for contact burns of the palm in children. *J Burn Care Rehabil* 1986; **7:** 501–7.

75. Gibran N S, Engrav L H, Heimbach D M, Swiontkowski M F, Foy H M. Engine block burns: Dupuytren's 4th, 5th and 6th burns. *J Trauma* 1994; **37**(2): 176–81.

76. Lee R C, Kolodney M S. Electrical injury mechanisms: electrical breakdown of cell membranes. *Plast Reconstr Surg* 1987; **80:** 672–9.

77. Sances A, Myklebust J, Larson S. Experimental electrical injury studies. *J Trauma* 1981; **21:** 589.

78. Xue-Wei W. Successful treatment of a case of electrical burn of the abdomen complicated with intestinal perforation. *Burns* 1981; **8:** 28.

79. Yang J, Tasi Y C, Noordhoff M S. Electrical burn with visceral injury. *Burns* 1985; **11:** 207.

80. Zhu Z X, Yu D C, Wang Y, Zhao L. Successful treatment of a severe electrical injury involving the stomach. *Burns* 1993; **19:** 80–2.

81. Edlich R, Rodeheaver G, Halfacre S. Technical consideration for fasciotomies in high voltage electrical injuries. *J Burn Care Rehabil* 1980; **1:** 22.

82. Holliman C, Saffle J, Kravitz M, Warden G. Early surgical decompression in the management of electrical injuries. *Am J Surg* 1982; **144:** 733.

83. Hunt J, Lewis S, Parkey R, Baxter C. The use of technetium-99m stannous pyrophosphate scintigraphy to identify muscle damage in acute electric burns. *J Trauma* 1979; **19:** 409.

84. Bartle E J, Wang X W, Miller G J. Early vascular grafting to prevent upper extremity necrosis after electrical burns: anastomotic false aneurysm, a severe complication. *Burns Incl Therm Inj* 1987; **13:** 313–17.

85. Wang X W, Bartle E J, Roberts B B. Early vascular grafting to prevent upper extremity necroses after electric burns: additional commentary on indications for surgery. *J Burn Care Rehabil* 1987; **8:** 391–4.

86. Wang X W, Barle E J, Roberts B B, *et al.* Free skin flap transfer in repairing deep electrical burns. *J Burn Care Rehabil*, 1987; **8:** 111–14.

87. Yang J Y, Noordhoff M S. Early adipofascial flap coverage of deep electrical burn wounds of upper extremities. *Plast Reconstr Surg* 1993; **91:** 819–25.

88. Early S, Simpson R. Caustic burns from contact with wet cement. *JAMA* 1985; **254:** 528–9.

89. Feldberg L, Regan P J, Roberts A H. Cement burns and their treatment. *Burns* 1992; **18:** 51–3.

90. Peters W. Alkali burns from wet cement. *Can Med Assoc J*, 1984; **130:** 902–4.

91. Bertolini J C. Hydrofluoric acid: a review of toxicity. *J Emerg Med* 1992; **10:** 163–68.

92. Anderson W J, Anderson J R. Hydrofluoric acid burns of the hand: mechanism of injury and treatment. *J Hand Surg* 1988; **13:** 52–7.

93. Bracken W, Cuppage F, McLaury R, Kirwin C, Klaassen C. Comparative effectiveness of topical treatments for hydrofluoric acid burns. *J Occup Med* 1985; **27:** 733–9.

94. Chick L, Borah G. Calcium carbonate gel therapy for hydrofluoric acid burns of the hand. *Plast Reconstr Surg* 1990; **86:** 935–40.

95. Siegel D C, Heard J M. Intra-arterial calcium infusion for hydrofluoric acid burns. *Aviat Space Environ Med* 1992; **63:** 206–22.

96. Vance M V, Curry S C, Kunkel D B, Ryan P J, Ruggeri S R. Digital hydrofluoric acid burns: treatment with intraarterial calcium infusion. *Ann Emerg Med* 1986; **15:** 890–6.

97. Velvart J. Arterial perfusion for hydrofluoric acid burns. *Hum Toxicol* 1983; **2:** 233–8.

98. Pegg S, Siu S, Gillett G. Intra-arterial infusions in the treatment of hydrofluoric acid burns. *Burns Incl Therm Inj* 1985; **11:** 440–3.

99. Gilchrest B A. Age-associated changes in the skin. *J Am Geriat Soc* 1982; **20:** 139–42.

100. Ostrow L B, Bongard F S, Sacks S T, McGuire A, Trunkey D D. Burns in the elderly. *Am Fam Physician* 1987; **35:** 149–54.

101. Saffle J, Larson C, Sullivan J, Shelby J. The continuing challenge of burn care in the elderly. *Surgery* 1990; **108:** 534–43.

102. Tejerina C, Reig A, Codina J, Safont J, Mirabet V. Burns in patients over 60 years old: epidemiology and mortality. *Burns* 1992; **18:** 149–52.

103. Zoch G, Meissl G, Bayer S, Kyral E. Reduction of the mortality rate in aged burn patients. *Burns* 1992; **18:** 153–6.

104. Anous M M, Heimbach D M. Causes of death and predictors in burned patients more than 60 years of age. *J Trauma* 1986; **26:** 135–9.

105. Li B, Hsu W, Shih T. Causes of death in aged burn patients: analysis of 36 cases. *Burns* 1990; **16:** 207–10.

106. Tompkins R, Burke J, Schoenfeld D. Prompt eschar excision: a treatment system contributing to reduced burn mortality. *Ann Surg* 1986; **204:** 272–81.

107. Deitch E, Clothier J. Burns in the elderly: an early surgical approach. *J Trauma* 1983; **23:** 891–4.

108. Kara M, Peters W J, Douglas L, Morris S. An early surgical approach to burns in the elderly. *J Trauma* 1990; **30:** 430–2.

109. Housinger T, Saffle J, Ward S, Warden G. Conservative approach to the elderly patient with burns. *Am J Surg* 1984; **148:** 817–20.

110. Ikeda J, Sugamata A, Jimbo, Yukioka T, Makino K. A new surgical procedure for aged burn victims: applications of dermolipectomy for burn wounds and donor sites. *J Burn Care Rehabil* 1990; **11:** 27–31.

CHAPTER TEN

WOUND CARE

WILLIAM W. MONAFO AND PALMER Q. BESSEY

After a burne the scarre which remaineth is commonly rough, unequall and ill-favoured. (Ambrose Paré, 1510–1590)

INTRODUCTION

Wound care comprises only one of the many burn care components, as the size of this volume attests; but it is arguably the most pivotal one. The management of extensive burn wounds is one of the last areas in surgical practice which still relies largely on uncontrolled clinical observations or on anecdotal personal experience. There are innumerable procedural details which, alone or in some combination or order, may be important or not, and which may either help or hinder, but which must – and sooner rather than later – result in a closed wound. It is, of course, impossible to communicate these details fully or in a precise chronological sequence even were space unlimited. What follows is necessarily incomplete; it is meant, however, to communicate the essentials of burn wound care, at least from one viewpoint. Major reasonable alternatives are commented upon at appropriate times as the treatment algorithm unfolds during the days or weeks (not months, any longer!) of acute phase convalescence, which ends when wounds are closed, or nearly so, and the focus of care shifts to rehabilitation and the recovery or maintenance of function.

When possible, the biological basis or the perceived rationale of a particular method, or procedure is stated. Hopefully, these explanations will satisfy more than those offered to surgical house officers by a prominent burn surgeon who, when asked why he was proceeding so, would respond: 'Because it's the best way we have.'

CUTANEOUS WOUND HEALING

It is axiomatic that intelligent wound management is not possible unless it is guided by the clinically relevant biology of wound healing, a subject which is presently in a phase of phenomenal growth on the biochemical and molecular level. A few brief comments about cutaneous wound healing are therefore in order.

Dermal or Partial-thickness Burns

Epidermis provides an important physical barrier to environmental microorganisms; its lipid components constitute another, if somewhat imperfect barrier – this to the loss of water vapor. Epidermal cells lining the skin appendages and at the perimeter provide the reservoir from which reepithelialization occurs. Notably, skin appendages are more sparse in the deep reticular dermis than in the superficial, papillary layer. So-called 'deep thermal' burns extending into the reticular dermis, therefore, require longer for reepithelialization – 3 weeks or more by clinical convention. Hypertrophic scar and contractures, which limit function, are common sequelae of these burns. (A useful clinical rule of thumb is that the longer the time required for epithelialization of dermal burns, the worse the functional or cosmetic result.) **Table 10.1** lists some of the principal distinguishing clinical characteristics of the two types of dermal burns.

Table 10.1 Clinical characteristics of superficial dermal and deep dermal burns

	Superficial	Deep
Blisters	Yes	Yes
Anatomical depth	Papillary dermis	Reticular dermis
Early analgesia	No	Yes
Color	Pink	Ivory, white, mottled
Capillary refill	Yes	No
Reepithelialization time	<21 days	>21 days
Hypertrophic scar	Rare	Frequent
Wound contraction	Minimal	Potentially significant

The colour plates for this chapter appear between pp 264 and 265.

Complex interactions, mediated by various cytokines and peptide growth factors, take place at the molecular level between epidermis and the subjacent extracellular dermal matrix and its population of fibroblasts, mesenchymal and endothelial cells.[1,2] As these interactions become more fully understood, pharmacological therapy which accelerates reepithelialization will likely become available. For example, a recent clinical trial has demonstrated a modest reduction in reepithelialization time of split thickness skin graft donor sites in burned patients; an approximately 10% reduction in 'healing' time was achieved with topically applied epidermal growth factor.[3] In another study, systemically administered recombinant human growth hormone also appeared to speed the reepithelialization of donor sites in severely burned children.[4] The use of growth factors, hormonal or other pharmacological therapy to promote epithelialization of burns is presently only in the developmental stage, but holds future promise.[1,5,6]

Full-thickness Burns (Subdermal, or Third Degree Burns)

Full-thickness burns require a surgical procedure for closure unless they are of limited area. The devitalized soft tissue ('eschar') which forms varies in thickness depending on the wound depth, but may extend well into the subcutaneous fat or even to the periosteum. Wound closure cannot occur while eschar remains *in situ*. Spontaneous eschar separation is due primarily to the action of bacterial proteases and, therefore, does not occur in full-thickness burns in the absence of wound bacterial colonization and is greatly delayed in proportion to the efficacy of the wound antiseptic measures employed.[7] For example, full-thickness burn eschars in gnotobiotic rodents do not slough spontaneously and remain in place for 8 months or more![8] (The less substantial and thinner eschar which forms over deep dermal burns will separate spontaneously as epithelialization proceeds, however, even in the absence of microorganisms.)

Wound Contraction

If eschar is left to fragment and separate spontaneously during several weeks, the wound area will be seen to progressively decrease – provided at least that infection is reasonably controlled and significant nutritional deficits are prevented. This decrease in the surface area is termed 'wound contraction'. The phenomenon may be due to contractile forces generated in granulation tissue by highly differentiated fibroblasts containing contractile protein – the so-called 'myofibroblasts'.[2] The contribution of epithelial ingrowth from the perimeter in reducing wound area is small, usually less than 10% during the first 6 weeks.

Contraction is, of course, desirable in one sense, because as it proceeds, both the risk of infection and the metabolic drain which results from the percutaneous loss of water vapor and body fluids decrease.[9] From a functional and/or cosmetic standpoint, however, wound contraction near important joints or cosmetically significant areas, such as the eyelid or lip, is evidently highly undesirable. Some of the factors which alter the rate of contraction are schematically indicated in **Figure 10.1**. Successful split-thickness skin grafts will impede subsequent contraction, while full-thickness grafts essentially abolish it. The clinical reality is, of course, that split-thickness grafts are mainly necessary in burn wound treatment because their donor sites will reepithelialize, can be recropped and do not require surgical closure. Small full-thickness grafts may be necessary during acute phase care on the eyelids and periorbital regions in order to correct severe ectropion or on deep palmar burns in infants.[10]

Hypertrophic Scar

Burns are the prototypical injury associated with hypertrophic scar, a phenomenon which is unique to man. The lack of an experimental animal model of hypertrophic scar explains the paucity of fundamental biological information about this distressing phenomenon, which occurs regularly in injuries of the reticular dermis, but with unpredictable and highly variable severity. The one widely used therapy for hypertrophic scar is the near-continuous wearing for many months of elastic compression garments, as discussed elsewhere in this volume, although a comparatively rapid therapeutic response with the use of topical silicone gel has also been noted.[11,12]

From the point of view of acute wound care, however, there is an important feature of which the clinician should be aware: hypertrophic scar rarely forms beneath split-thickness sheet grafts; and it will typically form in deep dermal burns which have been allowed to heal, in the interstices of expanded meshed grafts and at the perimeter of sheet grafts (**Plate 1a,b**). The mesh graft technique yields even less satisfactory cosmetic results than sheet grafts –

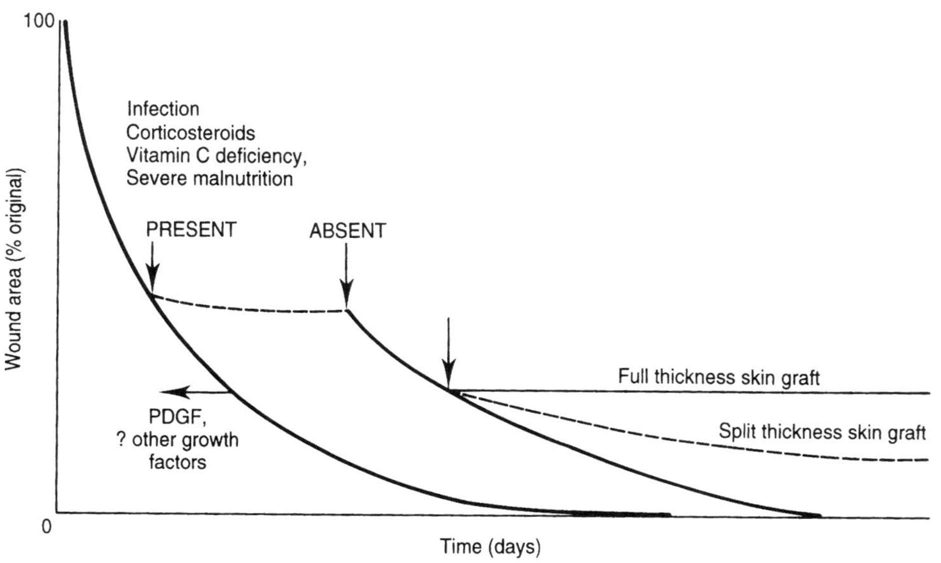

Fig. 10.1 A schematic representation of wound contraction showing the effects of infection, severe malnutrition[67] and other factors which impede spontaneous decrease in wound surface area. As shown, split-thickness skin grafts impede but do not prevent subsequent wound contraction, while full-thickness skin grafts essentially abolish it. The shift of the curve to the right by platelet derived growth factor (PDGF) is also shown.

which themselves frequently are unsatisfactory because of their poor color match and the unsightly halo of hypertrophic scar which may frame them.

WOUND CARE

Initial Assessment: an Individualized Care Plan is Essential

The clinical assessment of burn depth frequently changes during the first week post-injury. This has particular significance if early surgical wound closure is planned. Whether an apparent increase in depth is due to an inevitable, progressive occlusion of the circulation in the 'zone of stasis' at the wound periphery where endothelial vascular injury has occurred, or to compression of the dermal circulation by the edema attending intravenous fluid resuscitation, or whether it represents the ± 30% inaccuracy of most clinical observations cannot be determined in a given instance. Conversely, superficial dermal burns, especially those on the dorsum of the hand, may initially be diagnosed as deep dermal.

The clinician should formulate an appropriate individualized care plan within the first few days postburn which includes an achievable timetable for wound closure. The plan must include which burns are to be treated surgically, in what sequence, and using which donor sites. In the interim preceding wound closure, a protocol of daily wound care – based to the extent possible on physiologic principles – is also necessary, as is a team of nurses and other paramedical personnel to carry it out. A single set of standard procedures for bedside care is highly desirable, as multiple methods or variations typically lead to confusion and anxiety among nursing personnel and are important factors in staff turnover. Attending surgeons should agree upon the essentials of their protocol and ensure that the rationale of its components is clearly understood by all team members. When variance is necessary, as is often so, the team members need to be informed of the reasons for change.

The Bandage

A burn dressing has three principal functions:

- *Protective*. When skin is thermally injured, the physical barrier to microorganisms of the epidermis is lost, as well as its mild antiseptic property. The result is that the environmental flora will much more readily proliferate on the wound surface. In smaller burns, a dressing can effectively isolate the wound so that few, if any, organisms aside from those normally resident are ever recoverable. As the wound surface area increases, however, the efficacy of this barrier function of a dressing decreases concomitantly.

- *Metabolic*. An occlusive dressing will reduce evaporative heat loss and minimize cold stress and shivering. Because the principal cutaneous water vapor barrier resides in the epidermal lipids, even the most superficial burns result in increased water vapor loss (with its attendant caloric requirement of 0.58 kcal/g of water lost).[9] Intact eschar provides only a partial impediment, while excised or granulating wounds lose water vapor maximally.[13] Evaporative losses from exposed burns may be several-fold higher than the normal 'insensible' loss of about 150 ml/24 hours; and the air currents generated by air-fluidized beds may increase the evaporative loss by as much as 10-fold and, thus, impose an unnecessarily large caloric demand and fluid replacement requirement. An occlusive dressing (usually of cotton gauze) of reasonable thickness will impede water vapor loss appreciably, particularly if it is, in turn, covered with a dry blanket. Biological dressings, such as cadaver allograft and an increasing variety of commercially available (but generally expensive) synthetic dressing materials, can also be used; but their cost-effectiveness is often questionable and their overall efficacy not clearly documented, particularly for use on major burn wounds. Minimizing the nutritional demand is vital in the supportive care of patients with major burns, as discussed in detail elsewhere in this book.

- *Comfort*. Superficial dermal burns are initially extraordinarily sensitive to air currents; and deeper burns become progressively more tender with time. Open wounds drain. A bandage eliminates air currents from the wound surface, absorbs and contains wound secretions which would otherwise soil bed linens, etc. and, properly constructed, may also provide a splinting action to help maintain a desirable position of function.

Dressing Materials

A convenient, satisfactory dressing which can be rapidly applied consists of rolls of 36-layer, loose-weave cotton gauze, 9 inches in width pre-cut into 5 foot lengths (Hermitage Hospital Products, Niantac, CT). For smaller limbs, rolls of the same material, 4.5 inches in width are convenient. These dressings are in turn held in place with a spiral bandage of bias-cut stockinette, usually 6 inches in width, which is also pre-cut and rolled. The dressings and stockinette are sterilized in packages of 10. For dressing the face, an inner layer of 1 inch vaginal packing is useful for accurately covering the bridge of the nose, the chin, and for padding the ears to avoid pressure necrosis.

Over fresh skin grafts, a nonadherent synthetic plastic gauze (Exudry™, Frastec Corporation, New York, NY) can be used. This material is available either in rolls over which the aforementioned gauze dressing can be applied, or as a self-contained, prefabricated dressing which contains an absorbent pad bonded to the inner layer of the Exudry™. This material adheres minimally to the wound surface and, therefore, is convenient for use over freshly applied skin grafts. It is available in a wide variety of configurations.

Despite their cost, the physiologic (and psychological) benefits of occlusive burn dressings speak persuasively for their routine use. Alternative burn wound coverings, including the use of 'biological' dressings such as skin allograft or xenograft or the use of synthetic or biological materials for wound coverage are discussed in detail in Chapters 17 and 19.

Wound Hygiene

The French word *débridement* ('unbridling', i.e. as in escharotomy or fasciotomy, originally) has, in North America at least, come to signifty both the formal surgical excision of devitalized tissues (including, but not limited to burns) as well as the simple piecemeal removal of bits and fragments of separating eschar, ruptured bleb fragments, foreign material, etc. during the routine dressing change. The burn dressing is usually changed daily and, at times with apparent benefit, two or three times daily if the wound drainage is profuse. The thin eschar which forms over deep second degree burns also tends to separate in piecemeal fashion as epithelialization occurs beneath it. Systematic gentle wound cleansing with removal of bits of slough, exudate, etc. would seem to be eminently reasonable, although these maneuvers are not, to our knowledge, substantiated by valid scientific data. Hopefully, they are worth the not inconsiderable pain and discomfort with which they are associated.

Topical Agents

General Background

Burn injury not only damages the normal skin barrier, but also disrupts host immunological defenses. Because the avascular eschar is frequently several centimeters or more distant from patent microvasculature, systemically administered antimicrobial agents may not achieve reliable therapeutic levels. Topically applied antimicrobials will provide a high concentration of the agent on the wound surface where microbial numbers are usually highest. This is the rationale for their use. Topical agents will penetrate eschar to a variable extent, a property which should be considered in their selection.

Normal cutaneous bacterial flora are sparse, consisting mainly of diphtheroids and *Staphylococcus epidermidis*, although some normal individuals carry *Staphylococcus aureus*. Gram-negative bacteria are not usually present. The burn wound flora changes with time and with the topical and systemic antimicrobial therapy employed. After a variable initial period (days) when only normal flora are recovered or the cultures are apparently sterile, gram-positive organisms, mainly *S. aureus*, will typically predominate. Gram-negative opportunistic species subsequently appear. Most frequently, and in most centers, these include *Proteus, Klebsiella* and coliform species as well as *Pseudomonas*.[14–16] Anaerobes are infrequently isolated, although clostridial myositis may be encountered, particularly in high-voltage electrical injuries.

The goal of prophylactic topical antimicrobial therapy is initially to delay and later to minimize wound microbial colonization.[17] If successful, this will reduce, in turn, the frequency of invasive burn infection. Prophylactic usage should be distinguished from the treatment of established infection. Prophylactic agents do not need to penetrate the burn eschar deeply. They should have activity against common pathogens, should not retard wound healing (although all of them probably do so, to some extent[18]), and they should have acceptable toxicity, the latter implying that systemic absorption is low. Prophylactic topical antimicrobials have been a mainstay of burn therapy during the past 25 years.

None of the topical antimicrobials, either alone or in combination, will *eliminate* colonization of major burn wounds. Frequent clinical observation is essential in order to ensure that the basic wound hygienic measures (i.e. cleansing, 'debridement') are being satisfactorily and continually carried out and that the frequency of dressing changes is appropriate.

When an established invasive burn wound infection is present, the spectrum of activity of a proposed agent must, of course, include the responsible organism(s). Concerns about toxicity, cost, patient comfort, and other factors need to be weighed against the therapeutic goal. In most instances, eradication of an invasive infection will require the use of a topical agent (or combination of agents) which deeply penetrates eschar, as invasion of previously normal tissue at the eschar–body interface is present. Systemic and/or subeschar antibiotic infusions are also frequently employed, as is excision of the infected area when feasible. Invasive burn wound infections with Staphylococci or pseudomonads have frequently been treated in the recent past with topical mafenide acetate, which penetrates eschar freely.[19] Other topical agents may also be used to successfully treat invasive wound infections.

Specific Agents

In most instances, as noted above, the topical therapy is prophylactic. Frequent clinical observation is the best method of observing the therapeutic response. Wound surveillance culture results require clinical correlation because the distinction between colonization, which is frequent, and invasive wound infection, which is uncommon, is largely clinical. In general, quantitative wound biopsy cultures which exceed 10^5 organisms per gram of tissue are consistent with (but not necessarily diagnostic of) the presence of invasive infection. The microscopic visualization of organisms invading normal tissue on a wound biopsy specimen is diagnostic of an invasive burn infection but gives no information as to the extent to which this is occurring.

Silver sulfadiazine

Silver sulfadiazine is easily the most frequently used prophylactic topical antimicrobial in burn patients. Silver sulfadiazine is a white, highly insoluble compound which is synthesized from silver nitrate and sodium sulfadiazine.[17,20] It is available in 1% concentration in a water-soluble cream base. The cream is relatively painless to apply and does not stain bed linens or other objects which contact it. Silver sulfadiazine has *in vitro* activity against a wide range of organisms, including *S. aureus, E. coli, Klebsiella* species, *Pseudomonas aeruginosa*, the Enterobacteriaceae, *Proteus*, and *Candida albicans*. The drug penetrates eschar poorly. Its precise mechanism of action is unclear.

The toxic effects commonly associated with other sulfonamides, such as crystalluria or methemoglobinemia, are rare after silver sulfadiazine treatment. The most common toxic effect is a transient leukopenia, which occurs typically within 2–3 days after the initiation of therapy and is associated with a disproportionate decrease in the circulating neutrophil population. The incidence of this phenomenon is somewhere between 5 and 15%.[21,22] The leukopenia may reach alarmingly low levels (less than 1000 mm^2). Despite this, no increased incidence of infectious complications has been identified. The leukopenia tends to recover whether or not the agent is withdrawn. It has been suggested that leukocyte margination in the burn may, in itself, explain the leukopenia. However, recent data suggest that there is a direct toxic effect on bone marrow.[23] Cutaneous sensitivity reactions, typically a maculopapular rash, occur in less than 5% of patients and rarely require discontinuing the agent. Acute hemolytic anemia has been reported in a burned patient with the rare congenital absence of glucose-6-phosphate dehydrogenase whose wounds were treated with silver sulfadiazine.[24]

Although clinical trials suggest that silver sulfadiazine reduces wound bacterial numbers and delays colonization with gram-negative bacteria, treatment failures still occur with some frequency in large burns (<50% body surface area). The agent is usually applied on a daily or twice daily basis. When it is used on superficial second degree burns, a yellow-gray 'pseudo-eschar' may form after several days, which can be confusing to inexperienced personnel. This film, several millimeters thick, results from interaction between the cream and the wound exudate; it is easily lifted away, typically revealing a pink, superficial wound bed.

Mafenide (α-amino-*p*-toluene sulfonamide monoacetate)

Mafenide (α-amino-*p*-toluene sulfonamide monoacetate) was introduced as a topical burn treatment in the mid-1960s.[25] It is available in a water-soluble cream base at 11.1% concentration. It has excellent antibacterial activity against most gram-positive species, including clostridia, but has limited activity against some staphylococci, particularly methicillin-resistant strains. It has a broad spectrum of activity against most gram-negative burn pathogens, but minimal antifungal activity.[17] Early enthusiasm for its prophylactic use was tempered by its systemic toxicity and by the pain which results from its application. The drug is so rapidly absorbed that wound concentrations are markedly reduced within several hours, so that it is usually applied twice daily. A 5% solution has been used to wet the dressings over fresh skin grafts, but is not presently available commercially.

Mafenide is a potent carbonic anhydrase inhibitor; and hyperchloremic metabolic acidosis is frequent when it is used continuously on large burns.[19] Moderate to severe hyperventilation as respiratory compensation for the acidosis is characteristic, with a subnormal $Pa\text{CO}_2$. Minute ventilations as high as 50 liters may be observed. Pulmonary complications are frequent with the continuous use of mafenide in large burns. The risk of systemic toxicity increases in proportion to the wound area being treated and the duration of treatment. A maculopapular rash occurs in about 5% of patients, but this reaction is usually controlled with antihistamines and may not require discontinuing the drug.

Although the use of mafenide as a prophylactic topical agent has decreased in recent years, its excellent eschar penetration makes it useful for the short-term control of invasive infections. In some centers, toxicity is minimized or avoided in patients with large burns by alternating the topical therapy between mafenide and silver sulfadiazine.[15] Careful monitoring of pulmonary function and acid–base balance is essential in patients with large burns.

0.5% Silver nitrate solution

One-half percent silver nitrate solution was introduced as an effective topical burn therapy in the mid-1960s.[7] This signaled the beginning of the present era of topical therapy with silver compounds. The agent is effective against most strains of staphylococci and also has activity against *Pseudomonas aeruginosa* and other common gram-negative burn wound colonizers. Concentrations of silver nitrate much above the 0.5% are histotoxic. Most biologically important salts of silver, especially the chloride and proteinates, are highly insoluble. The agent, therefore, does not penetrate eschar to a significant extent and systemic absorption of silver is minimal. Although silver is detectable in blood and tissues, especially in patients with large burns who are treated for several weeks, no significant direct toxicity from it has been observed. But the hypotonic solution (29.4 mmol Ag/l) tends to leach electrolytes, especially sodium, from the wound surface. Up to 350 mmol of sodium per day may be lost per square meter of body surface area treated. Continuous oral or intravenous electrolyte supplementation is therefore essential. Hyponatremia may occur rapidly, especially in infants or children with major burns.

The other important, but fortunately infrequent, complication attending the use of silver nitrate is methemoglobinemia, which occurs as a result of the reduction of nitrate anions by wound bacteria (usually gram-negative), with subsequent absorption of the toxic nitrite. This diagnosis should be suspected if the skin or blood appear cyanotic or 'gray' but the $Pa\text{O}_2$ is normal. If the diagnosis is confirmed by measurement of the blood methemoglobin level, the silver nitrate should be discontinued promptly. Rarely, treatment with reducing agents may be required.

Silver nitrate is relatively painless to apply. It is typically used with the thick gauze dressings described elsewhere in this chapter. The dressings should be re-wet every several hours so as to prevent concentrations of silver reaching histotoxic levels. Silver nitrate stains everything which it touches brown or black, including the linens, floors, etc. Although the drug is a highly effective prophylactic agent, it is not presently widely used, principally because of its staining properties. Its therapeutic effect approximates that obtained with silver sulfadiazine, which is simpler to use.

Cerium nitrate–silver sulfadiazine

Since the mid-1970s, silver sulfadiazine modified by the addition of the lanthanide salt cerium nitrate has been used.[26] An increased efficacy of wound bacteriostasis in patients with large burns was noted then and has been observed by others subsequently.[27,28] The lanthanons, or 'rare earth' elements, one of which is the relatively non-toxic cerium, all have antimicrobial activity *in vitro*.[29] The antimicrobial spectrum of cerium nitrate–silver sulfadiazine *in vitro* is qualitatively similar to that of silver sulfadiazine or silver nitrate.

Some investigators have suggested that the efficacy of the cerium nitrate–silver sulfadiazine combination might be due in part to an effect on immune function. The cell-mediated immune response appears to be preserved in burned mice treated with cerium nitrate alone or in combination with silver sulfadiazine.[30] Others have immersed patients with major burns in a cerium nitrate bath shortly after their admittance to a burn center, also with favorable results, which they suggest may be due to a favorable effect on immune function.[31] The compound is not commercially available in the USA, but it is available in several western European countries as Flammacerium™ (Duphar Corporation, The Netherlands). It is easily prepared, however, by adding a concentrated aqueous solution of cerium nitrate to silver sulfadiazine cream.[32] Methemoglobinemia, due to the absorption of reduced nitrate from the combination cream, has been only rarely seen. Cerium nitrate–silver sulfadiazine cream is not associated with electrolyte disturbances. Absorption of cerium has been documented, but is minimal in patients with large burns treated continuously with it for several weeks. Recently, Wassermann has reported excellent results in patients with massive burns using cerium nitrate–silver sulfadiazine cream.[32] His report parallels earlier documented experience in patients with very large, ostensibly 'lethal' injuries.[33] Boeckx *et al.* also have reported favorable results clinically, although other investigators are less enthusiastic.[28,34]

Nitrofurazone

A water-soluble cream base containing 0.2% nitrofurazone is available. The agent has *in vitro* activity against a number of burn wound pathogens including staphylococci, but does not have significant activity against *Pseudomonas*. Severe allergic cutaneous reactions may occur with this drug. It may be useful in treating invasive staphylococcal wound infections.[35]

Chlorhexidine

Chlorhexidine gluconate combined with 0.5% silver nitrate appears to be comparable in terms of efficacy to silver sulfadiazine.[36] A newer, diphosphanilate chlorhexidine conjugate appears to have an even broader antimicrobial spectrum, but pain on application posed a problem in clinical trials.[37] Plasma-mediated resistance does not appear to occur with chlorhexidine in contrast to the sulfonamides.

Povidone–iodine

Povidone–iodine is an inappropriate compound for use on major burns both because of its relative inactivation by wound exudates and because of renal dysfunction associated with systemic absorption of iodine.[38] More rarely, iodine-induced thyroid dysfunction can also occur.[39]

Nystatin

The topical antifungal nystatin can be useful in controlling *candidal* growth on burn wounds.[40] Yeast and/or fungal colonization of burn wounds is not uncommon and may often be related to selection pressures exerted by systemic antibiotic use and/or the use of topical agents ineffective against these organisms. Fortunately, invasive yeast or fungal infections are relatively rare and colonization by *C. albicans* does not appear to increase mortality.

Other agents

Mupirocin, a recently introduced topical antibiotic, may be particularly useful against methicillin-resistant *staphylococci*; but, as it has not been widely used, its toxicity may not yet be fully apparent.[41,42] Polymyxin B and Bacitracin ointments may be used occasionally on small areas or on minor burns, but nephrotoxicity and/or ototoxicity preclude their prolonged use over wide areas.

Combination therapy

Using various topical agents in combination is not an unreasonable approach in selected patients, although there is evidence that antimicrobial efficacy, paradoxically, may be decreased with certain combinations (e.g. the simultaneous use of mafenide acetate and nystatin).[40] The use of *in vitro* sensitivity testing methods such as the agar well procedure to determine the optimal antimicrobial or combination of antimicrobials needs to be interpreted cautiously.[43] The results of this test depend importantly on the solubility in agar of the agent(s) being tested rather than reflecting the *in vitro* sensitivity of the organism. Silver or cerium compounds, for example, tend to fare poorly in this system.

Surgical Wound Closure

Perspective

During the last 25 years, the treatment of deep burns by experienced burn surgeons has changed dramatically.[44] Previously, nearly all large, deep burns were treated expectantly: eschar was permitted to slough spontaneously, and open wounds were left to granulate. Split-thickness skin grafts were then applied using a variety of free-hand techniques, including the placement of small patches or 'stamps' arranged a centimeter or more apart, or the even less efficient 'pinch' grafts. Weeks or, frequently, months passed before permanent wound closure could be achieved with these methods. Survival was essentially unprecedented when the burn surface area exceeded about two-thirds of the body surface area.

Perceptive surgeons were, of course, cognizant of the many disadvantages associated with passive, expectant therapy, which was recognized as being contrary to the fundamental principle in the treatment of other traumatic wounds which had been learned, forgotten, then relearned during two World Wars: the prompt excision of all devitalized tissue appeared to be ideal for deep burns, but the debate remained largely hypothetical because of numerous practical clinical constraints.

In the early years following World War II, surgical therapy was still being applied in practice only in burns which, by today's standard, would be considered trivial.[45] In extensive burns, because effective measures for the control of burn wound infection were lacking, dense colonization with microorganisms almost invariably occurred within a few days and often became the source of locally invasive or systemic sepsis. Physiologic monitoring was near nonexistent and ventilatory support consisted primarily of the administration of oxygen and the performance of tracheostomy. Finally, the importance of aggressive nutritional support and physical therapy was ill-appreciated. Those few who were fortunate enough to survive a major injury typically had severely impaired function.

The terrible odors which emanated from the hospitalized burn patients disappeared virtually overnight with the introduction of topical antimicrobial therapy in the mid-1960s.[7] This one advance, more than any other, stimulated widespread and general interest in the many, previously largely unaddressed problems of the burn patient: *pari passu*, there were many other advances, particularly in the area of critical care medicine, which itself was becoming a recognized subspecialty; an ever-growing menu of potent and relatively safe antibiotics was appearing; precision power dermatomes which made it easy to procure large skin grafts of precise thickness became widely available; mesh-expansion techniques which improved graft take and minimized the requisite donor site area were rediscovered;[46] sophisticated intra- and preoperative monitoring techniques became standard; and perhaps most importantly, the incalculable value of concentrating severely burned patients in dedicated burn treatment centers where experienced and interested personnel could interact was recognized and implemented. These and many other factors have contributed to the dramatic improvement in burn care which has occurred. It is, of course, not possible to calculate the individual contributions of those advances to the reduction in burn morbidity and mortality, but we suspect that they are perhaps generally underestimated, especially by enthusiastic surgeons.[47,49]

The Modern Era

A more aggressive, earlier and more frequent use of surgical therapy for deep burns is the norm today in the Western world.[47–53] The vastly better early physiologic status of the modern-day patient and the availability of in-depth logistic support now permits the complete excision of even near-total deep burns in one or more stages without incurring mortality in the perioperative period. What was a frustrating hypothetical debate 25 years ago has become surgical reality. When the deep burn injury is not life-threatening, early, aggressive surgical wound closure clearly has benefit. *The question remains open, however, as to when and to what extent it is best to utilize surgical wound closure in patients with burns so extensive that their survival is problematic.* Before discussing the various surgical options, it is useful to briefly outline the most commonly used operative techniques.

Methods of Surgical Wound Closure

General anesthesia is usually required for surgical wound closure, although regional anesthesia may occasionally be suitable, as for limb burns with adjacent available donor skin. We prefer to utilize the main hospital operating suite because of the rapid availability of personnel and expertise should problems develop intraoperatively. Depending on the magnitude of the wound area to be treated, an appropriate supply of cross-matched blood must be available. Estimates ranging from 172 to 616 ml of blood loss/1% total body surface area (TBSA) excised have been reported.[54,55] When appreciable blood loss is anticipated, we frequently utilize preoperative transfusion with packed RBCs in order to minimize the intraoperative transfusion requirement. The use of ketamine anesthesia rather than inhalation techniques is favored by some; and we have also found it useful. Succinylcholine administration is contraindicated in a burn patient because of the potentially lethal hyperkalemia which it can trigger. Anesthesia in burned patients is addressed in detail in another chapter of this book.

The operating room ambient temperature should be maintained in the low 90s (°F) in patients with large burns so as to avoid hypothermia, which is a particular hazard in children, with their relatively larger surface area, and in all patients with extensive burns. Recent data suggest that the rate at which body temperature returns to normal postoperatively may correlate with survival.[56] In order to reduce the severity of the intraoperative temperature drift, our practice is to change dressings preoperatively on those burns which are not to be treated surgically so that only the wound to be excised and the planned skin graft donor site remain exposed intraoperatively.

Primary closure of excised burns and/or donor sites

Small but deep burns on lax skin areas, such as the buttock, the female breast or the limbs or torso in the elderly can, on occasion, be excised and closed by suture or staple, particularly if cosmesis is not a major issue. In the elderly, it may also be possible to excise just-harvested donor sites from lax skin areas and close them primarily as well; delayed healing of donor sites or their eventual conversion to full thickness skin loss, two not uncommon complications in the elderly, can thus be avoided.

Amputation

When a major portion of a limb or digit has been destroyed, as in electrical injury or in some very deep thermal burns, amputation may be appropriate and necessary in order to eliminate the deep wound.

Tangential excision

The 'tangential' or so-called 'laminar' method of sequentially shaving the eschar from the burn surface until a viable tissue plane is reached was introduced in the USA about 20 years ago.[57,58] This procedure is suitable for the excision of many deep dermal and/or relatively shallow full-thickness burns. It is often performed using a hand-held blade mounted in a handle equipped with a calibrated depth guard. The small Goulian knife or the larger and somewhat more cumbersome Humby knife is ordinarily used (**Plate 2**). In experienced hands, tangential excision is rapid and effective, although hemorrhage from the dermis or deeper tissues may be considerable. Some believe that the use of a tourniquet may minimize blood loss, but the differentiation of viable from nonviable tissue is then more difficult.[59]

Dermatome excision

For broad, flat, deeply burned surfaces, a power dermatome such as the Brown, with its depth gauge set at the maximum, is conveniently used to perform what amounts to a laminar excision, usually at the level of the subcutaneous fat. The method is useful for the rapid excision of wounds from confluent areas above the wrist or ankle and on the torso, but is insufficiently precise for use on hands or digits.

Degloving (avulsion)

In deep full-thickness burns which extend well into the subcutaneous fat and are circumferential, a degloving technique is rapid and highly effective, if aesthetically disturbing. Linear escharotomies placed at about 180° apart on a limb facilitate this maneuver, which is usually best terminated using transverse circumferential incisions at or just above the level of the wrist or ankle. Very deep wounds on scalp or torso may also be rapidly removed in this manner.

Cold scalpel, electrocautery

Formal excision to any depth using the scalpel or the Bovie radiofrequency coagulation unit is also commonly used. Laser excision is not widely used presently because of the safety precautions necessary and the lack, to date, of a clear advantage in either operative time or in homeostasis.

Enzymatic wound debridement

The use of proteases (sutilains) elaborated by the *Bacillus subtilis* (Travase™ Boots Laboratories) as enzymatic debriding agents have not gained wide acceptance, and appropriately so, as bacteremia is associated with their use. Further, enzymatic proteolysis occurring in zones of otherwise reversible tissue injury could increase burn depth unnecessarily. It has also been proposed that enzymatic 'debridement' with sutilains can substitute for surgical escharotomy. We have no personal experience with this application of enzymatic debridement, which seems to be less certain, rapid, and definitive than simple surgical escharotomy; and the latter provides certain and immediate tissue decompression.

Hemostasis

As noted above, the blood loss associated with burn excision and skin grafting is brisk. The use of tourniquets for excising limb burns and topical dilute epinephrine on graft donor sites help to minimize hemorrhage.[59] Manual compression, elevation of limbs, electrocautery, and occasionally topical thrombin spray are also useful adjuncts. Large blood vessels are occasionally formally ligated with absorbable suture material. We limit total operative time, including graft harvest, to approximately 2 hours, as blood loss correlates strongly with the length of operation. The observation that intraoperative blood loss is lessened as the interval between injury and wound excision decreases has not been confirmed.[54]

Clearly, surgical wound closure increases the overall transfusion requirement and hence increases the risk of viral disease transmission. Although there is likely also to be an immunosuppressive effect of transfusion, the risk of lethal sepsis in healthy patients with relatively small burns should be low. The use of 'fibrin glue' as a topical hemostatic agent has not yet been approved by the Federal Food and Drug Agency, possibly in part because the commercial product is prepared from multiple donors.

Skin graft procurement

A variety of precision dermatomes, most of them gas-powered, are presently available. A detailed description of these instruments is beyond the scope of this chapter. It is worth mentioning, however, that the hand-held Goulian instrument, when equipped with a guard (shim) of appropriate width is extremely useful in procuring split-thickness grafts from the scalp and other relatively inaccessible anatomical areas (**Plate 3**). Since the introduction of the Tanner–Vandeput instrument for the meshing of skin grafts, other similar devices which provide a variety of expansion ratios and easily permit meshing of long sheets of graft have become available. For most purposes, a 2:1 expansion ratio provides a reasonable compromise between the necessary donor site area and the time required for final wound closure by epithelialization of the graft interstices. In patients with very extensive burns, larger expansion ratios can be useful. Cadaver allografts are also useful as a protective temporary dressing over widely expanded (4:1 or 6:1) autograft.[60,61] In most circumstances, an expansion ratio greater than 3:1 unduly prolongs final wound closure.

Surgical Wound Closure in Patients with Non-life-threatening Burns

Most burned patients do not have injuries which carry a significant mortality risk. The average burn size in a typical US burn center is about 20% TBSA, or somewhat less.[62] About two-thirds of burn center patients have burns of 30% TBSA or less.[63] In such patients who are under the age of 50, the survival rate exceeds 97%, as deaths from these relatively small burns occur almost exclusively either in the elderly or if severe inhalation injury coexists. Further, the total body surface area involved by deep burns will frequently be appreciably less than the total burn size. But even if all of the burns are full thickness, ample skin graft donor sites are present; and few patients will have a physiologic status contraindicating an operative procedure, even one characteristically associated with brisk hemorrhage.

In short, delaying the surgical therapy which will inevitably be necessary for wound closure in patients with small but deep burns is unnecessary and merely prolongs the hospitalization time, increases pain and discomfort, interferes with the necessary physical therapy, and increases cost. The two essential prerequisites for the surgical treatment of these injuries are a sufficiently skilled surgical team and an ample supply of compatible blood.

The excision and grafting of such injuries within a few days postburn is routine in many, if not most, centers including ours, where it has been practiced for more than 20 years. The take of skin grafts in such patients is (or should be) uniformly good or excellent so that prompt, permanent wound closure is regularly accomplished with one, or occasionally two, operative procedures.[48,49]

Is a Short Delay in Surgical Therapy Harmful in 'Small' Burns?

The question whether 'complete' surgical closure within a few days (or less) provides superior functional or cosmetic results compared to complete surgical closure which is delayed for 2 weeks or more when survival is not an issue remains. Enthusiastic advocates of early surgical therapy have tended to disregard the evidence that intensive, aggressive physical therapy continued well beyond the acute phase of convalescence may well be the one most important determinant of the end functional result.[64,65] Early functional recovery is clearly more rapid in patients with burns which have been successfully closed surgically because painless joint movement is facilitated; this difference narrows toward imperceptibility with time, provided that appropriate physical therapy is continued in those whose surgical closure is delayed or in whom deep dermal burns are permitted to heal.[66]

Disappointingly, the severity of residual hypertrophic scarring does not appear to be importantly influenced by the rapidity with which surgical closure of deep burns has been achieved; closure within a few days or within a few weeks seems to make little difference.

In sum, there is ample evidence that reasonably prompt (within 2 weeks) surgical therapy for deep burns of less than 20–25% TBSA in healthy patients is safe in experienced hands. Intraoperative hemorrhage is significant, and an experienced operative team is essential. With early surgical wound closure, hospital stay is appreciably shortened, of the order of 30–35% for those with the smallest burns (although the decrease in stay is progressively less as burn size increases); and there is earlier functional recovery. There is at best a marginal difference, however, either in the long-term functional outcome or in the appearance of the scars compared to expectant therapy in which surgical wound closure is either delayed for up to about 2 weeks or, for deep partial-thickness burns, is avoided altogether. Thus, initial enthusiasm (which we once shared) for the earliest tangential excision of deep partial-thickness burns has waned somewhat as controlled follow-up data have become available.

Burns Greater than 30% Body Surface Area: Staged Versus Early Total Surgical Wound Closure

Although only about one-third of the burn population have injuries exceeding 30% TBSA, one-half or more of all burn deaths occur in this cohort.[62] As burn size increases within the cohort, and/or if there is concomitant inhalation injury, the mortality probability, of course, also increases.

Early total excision

Would mortality be reduced if all the deep burns (i.e. full-thickness plus deep dermal) were surgically excised within a few days post-injury before wound bacterial growth becomes well established? This approach has a not inconsiderable number of credible advocates, including the Editor of this volume. But given the tendency to overdiagnose deep partial-thickness burns in the early post-injury phase, such very early surgical therapy would be expected to sacrifice some considerable burn areas which would otherwise heal, and thus treatment mode would further increase an already wide donor–recipient skin disparity. One or more lengthy operative procedures are necessary within the first 5–7 days post-injury; in those with the largest burns, unburned skin is not in sufficient supply to provide immediate closure, even with widely expanded autologous mesh grafts. Until sufficient donor skin becomes available, temporary coverage of much of the excised area must be accomplished with allograft or other nonviable temporary materials because there is consensus that extensive excised wounds should not be left open for long. This approach clearly requires an experienced team, and is logistically demanding of both personnel and resources.

Only two prospective, randomized trials of total early excision have been reported. In one, there was no survival advantage with excision which was performed within 24 hours following injury.[53] In the controls, the surgical treatment was delayed until the 10th to the 14th day postburn. Although there was a small reduction in hospital stay (3.3 days in those patients treated by the early excision), this was truly only in patients with relatively small injuries (<15% TBSA). The authors abandoned early total excision based on their results.

In another, more recent trial, 85 adults with burns ranging from 30 to 98% TBSA were treated either by excision of all deep burns within 72 hours or by a method described as 'conservative operative debridements with gradual wound closure', a method which would appear to be appreciably less aggressive than the staged excisional approach described below in this chapter, as the wounds in these control patients were not treated surgically until *at least 3 weeks* post-injury.[61] There were no intergroup differences in survival in the series as a whole, whether or not inhalation injury coexisted. (Advocates of early total excision had early expressed the hope that the excessive mortality from large burns and coexisting inhalation injury might be reduced by aggressive therapy.) In a subgroup of patients, aged 17–30 without inhalation injury, the death rate in 22 excised patients was 9% versus a significantly higher rate (45%) in 11 conservatively treated patients. Although these data might reappear to support early total excision, the passive and essentially outmoded surgical approach used in the control group, together with the wide range of burn size (30–98% TBSA) and the small number of patients, particularly in the controls, suggest that the benefits of early total surgical wound closure were not clearly established in this study.

The alternative: staged surgical wound closure

An alternative and only qualitatively less aggressive approach is used in many, and probably in most, burn centers, including our own, for patients with major burns in whom unburned skin is in scant supply. This is the staged excision of unequivocally deep burns at intervals of approximately 7 days, with immediate coverage of all exposed areas by autologous skin grafts. The timing of the first surgical procedure is dependent on physiologic status and on the clinical estimate of burn depth, but is preferably not delayed for more than 10 days. Progressive wound closure is thus achieved in a series of planned operative procedures in which areas of unequivocal full-thickness burn are treated first and in which some or all burns of indeterminate depth may be permitted to epithelialize. Careful planning of the sequence in which available donor sites will be utilized is essential, as is ingenuity in the harvesting of relatively inaccessible skin donor areas. An interval of 7–10 days between operative procedures is usual. We and others have found that topical therapy using 1% silver sulfadiazine cream modified by the addition of 2.2% cerium nitrate is useful because the adherent, thick eschar which typically forms with this topical agent is relatively resistant to bacterial colonization and can safely be left in place until it can be excised and the resultant wound closed with autologous skin grafts.[27,32]

It needs emphasis that, whatever their beliefs or bias, few, if any, contemporary burn surgeons delay for long the excision and grafting of large areas of unequivocally full-thickness burn, irrespective of the total burn extent. A recent review of a large series of 200 patients with burns of 30% TBSA or more is perhaps representative of the experience at large with staged excision.[50] Eighty-eight percent of those who survived had excision of full-thickness areas between the 4th and 31st day postburn (mean 13.5 days). Survivors in whom the excision was performed relatively late had a predominance of deep partial-thickness injury, which was permitted to heal, and smaller areas of full-thickness injury which were grafted later. The nonsurvivors had bigger burns and a higher incidence of inhalation injury, as might be expected or predicted. Excision could be performed in only 43% of the nonsurvivors, as the remainder were judged to be too unstable to tolerate surgery. Thus, outcome in these patients appeared to be determined principally by factors other than the surgical approach to wound therapy.

Envoi

The quotation heading this chapter is meant to emphasize that, notwithstanding the numerous advances in supportive care which have made surgical burn wound closure at a time of election a realistic option, the attendant scarring after a burn is unfortunately still frequently 'rough, unequall and ill-favoured', much as it was 400 years ago. The risk of death from burn injury is far less today than it was only 25 years ago, but the hope that more prompt surgical therapy would greatly reduce severity of the residual scarring has unfortunately not been realized.

Reasonably prompt surgical closure of deep burns which pose no major threat to life shortens the painful, arduous acute phase convalescence and speeds the recovery of function, although not as dramatically as some had hoped. In patients with massive or life-threatening burns, early total wound excision provides no clear-cut survival advantage and is logistically demanding of resources compared to staged surgical excision, in which some areas of deep dermal burn are permitted to heal spontaneously. The combination of massive burns and inhalation injury is still a highly lethal one.

References

1. Lynch S E, Colvin R B, Antoiniades N H. Growth factors in wound healing. *J Clin Invest* 1989; **84:** 640–64.

2. Pierce G F, VandeBerg J, Rudolph R, Tarpley J, Mustoe T A. PDGF-BB and TGF-β1 selectively modulate glycosaminoglycans, collagen, and myofibroblasts. *Am J Pathol* 1991; **138:** 629–46.

3. Brown G L, Nanney L B, Griffen J. *et al.* Enhancement of wound healing by topical treatment with epidermal growth factor. *N Engl J Med* 1989; **321:** 76–9.

4. Herndon D N, Barrow R E, Kunkel K R, Broemeling L, Rutan R L. Effects of recombinant human growth hormone on donor-site healing in severely burned children. *Ann Surg* 1990; **212:** 424–9.

5. Robson M C, Phillips L G, Thomason A, Robson L E, Pierce G F. Platelet-derived growth factor BB for the treatment of chronic pressure ulcers. *Lancet* 1992; **339:** 23–5.

6. Herndon D N, Nguyen T T, Gilpin D A. Growth factors: Local and systemic. *Arch Surg* 1993; **128:** 1227–33.

7. Moyer C A, Brentano L, Gravens D L, Margraf H W, Monafo W W. Treatment of large human burns with 0.5% silver nitrate solution. *Arch Surg* 1965; **90:** 812–67.

8. Dugan R C, Nance F C. Enzymatic burn wound debridement in conventional and germ-free rats. *Surg Forum* 1977; **28:** 33–4.

9. Cone J B, Wallace B H, Caldwell F T. The effect of staged burn wound closure on the rates of heat production and heat loss of burned children and young adults. *J Trauma* 1988; **28:** 968–72.

10. Schwanholt C, Greenhalgh D G, Warden G D. A comparison of full-thickness versus split-thickness autografts for the coverage of deep palm burns in the very young pediatric burn patient. *J Burn Care Rehabil* 1993; **14:** 29–33.

11. Ahn S T, Monafo W W, Mustoe T A. Topical silicone gel: a new treatment for hypertrophic scars. *Surgery* 1989; **106:** 781–7.

12. Ahn S T, Monafo W W, Mustoe T A. Topical silicone gel for the prevention and treatment of hypertrophic scar. *Arch Surg* 1991; **126:** 499–504.

13. Caldwell F T. Etiology and control of postburn hypermetabolism: the 1991 Presidential address to the American Burn Association. *J Burn Care Rehabil* 1991; **12:** 385–401.

14. Frame J D, Kangesu L, Malik W M. Changing flora in burn and trauma units: experience in the United Kingdom. *J Burn Care Rehabil* 1992; **13:** 281–6.

15. Heggers J P, McCauley R L, Herndon D N. Antimicrobial therapy in burn patients: Part II. *Surgical Rounds* 1992; **August:** 699–708.

16. Smith D J, Thomson P D. Changing flora in burn and trauma units: Historical perspective – experience in the United States. *J Burn Care Rehabil* 1992; **13:** 276–80.

17. Monafo W W, West M A. Current treatment recommendations for topical burn therapy. *Drugs* 1990; **40:** 364–73.

18. McCauley R L, Linares H A, Pelligrini V. *et al.* In vitro toxicity of topical antimicrobial agents to human fibroblasts. *J Surg Res* 1989; **46:** 267–74.

19. White M G, Asch M J. Acid base effects of topical mafenide acetate in the burned patient. *Arch Surg* 1984; **119:** 183–8.

20. Fox C L. Silver sulfadiazine: a new topical therapy for *Pseudomonas* in burns. *Arch Surg* 1968; **96:** 184–8.

21. Fuller F W, Engler P E. Leukopenia in non–specific burn patients receiving topical 1% silver sulfadiazine cream therapy: A survey. *J Burn Care Rehabil* 1988; **9:** 606–9.

22. Smith–Choban P, Marshall W J. Leukopenia secondary to silver sulfadiazine: frequency, characteristics and clinical consequences. *Am Surg* 1987; **53:** 515–17.

23. Gamelli R L, Paxton T P, O'Reilly M. Bone marrow toxicity by silver sulfadiazine. *Surg Gynecol Obstet* 1993; **177:** 115–20.

24. Eldad A, Neuman A, Weinberg A, Benmeir P, Rotem M, Wexler M R. Silver sulphadiazine-induced haemolytic anaemia in a glucose-6 phosphate dehydrogenase-deficient burn patient. *Burns* 1991; **17:** 430–2.

25. Lindbergh R B, Moncrief J A, Mason A D. Control of experimental and clinical burn wound sepsis by topical application of Sulfamylon compounds. *Ann N Y Acad Sci* 1968; **150:** 950–72.

26. Fox C L, Monafo W W, Ayvazian V H, *et al.* Topical chemotherapy for burns using cerium salts and silver sulfadiazine. *Surg Gynecol Obstet* 1977; **144:** 668–72.

27. Hermans R P. Topical treatment of serious infections with special reference to the use of a mixture of silver sulfadiazine and cerium nitrate: two clinical studies. *Burns* 1984; **11:** 59–62.

28. Boeckx W, Blondeel P N, Vandersteen K, Wolf-Peeters C D, Schmitz A. Effect of cerium nitrate–silver sulphadiazine on deep dermal burns: a histological hypothesis. *Burns* 1992; **18:** 456–62.

29. Burkes S, McCleskey C S. The bacteriostatic activity of cerium, lanthanum and thallium. *J Bacteriol* 1947; **54:** 417–24.

30. Peterson V M, Hansbrough J F, Wang X W, Zapata–Sirvent R, Boswick J A. Topical cerium nitrate cream prevents postburn immunosuppression. *J Trauma* 1985; **25:** 1039–44.

31. Scheidegger D, Sparkes B G, Luscher N, Schoenenberger G A, Allgöwer M. Survival in major burn injuries treated by one bathing in cerium nitrate. *Burns* 1992; **18:** 296–300.

32. Wassermann D, Schlotterer M, Lebreton F, Levy J, Guelfi M C. Use of topically applied silver sulphadiazine plus cerium nitrate in major burns. *Burns* 1989; **15:** 257–60.

33. Monafo W W, Robinson H N, Toshioka T, Ayvazian V H. Lethal burns: a progress report. *Arch Surg* 1978; **113:** 397–401.

34. Munster A M, Helvig E, Rowland S. Cerium nitrate–silver sulfadiazine cream in the treatment of burns: a prospective evaluation. *Surgery* 1980; **88:** 658–60.

35. Munster A M. Treatment of invasive *Enterobacter cloacae* burn wound sepsis with topical nitrofurazone. *J Trauma* 1984; **24:** 524–5.

36. Lawrence J C, Cason J S, Kidson A. Evaluation of phenoxetol-chlorhexidine cream as a prophylactic agent in burns. *Lancet* 1982; **1:** 1037–49.

37. McManus A T, Denton C L, Mason A D. Topical chlorhexidine diphosphanilate (WP-973) in burn wound sepsis. *Arch Surg* 1984; **119:** 206–11.

38. Hunt J L, Sato R, Heck E L, Baxter C L. A critical evaluation of povidine-iodine absorption in thermally injured patients. *J Trauma* 1980; **20:** 127–31.

39. Rath T, Meissi G. Induction of hyperthyroidism in burn patients treated topically with povidone-iodine. *Burns* 1988; **14:** 320–22.

40. Heggers J P, Robson M C, Herndon D N, Desai M H. The efficacy of nystatin combined with topical microbial agents in the treatment of burn wound sepsis. *J Burn Care Rehabil* 1989; **10:** 508–11.

41. Rode H, Ce Wet P M, Millar A J W, Cywes S. Bactericidal efficacy of muciprocin and multi-antibiotic *Staphylococcus aureus* burn wound infection. *J Antimicrob Chemother* 1988; **21:** 589–95.

42. Strock L L, Lee M M, Rutan R L, *et al.* Topical Bactroban (muciprocin): efficacy in treating burn wounds infected with methicillin-resistant staphylococci. *J Burn Care Rehabil* 1990; **11:** 454–60.

43. Nathan P, Law E J, Murphy D F, MacMillan B G. A laboratory method for selection of topical antimicrobial agents to treat infected burn wounds. *Burns* 1977; **4:** 177–87.

44. Monafo W W. Then and now: 50 years of burn treatment. *Burns* 1992; **18:** S7–S10.

45. Cope O, Langohr J L, Moore F D, Webster R C. Expeditious care of full-thickness burn wounds by surgical excision and grafting. *Ann Surg* 1947; **125:** 1–21.

46. Klasen H J. *History of free skin grafting.* Berlin/Heidelberg: Springer-Verlag, 1981, 190 pp.

47. Demling R H. Improved survival after massive burns. *J Trauma* 1983; **23:** 179–84.

48. Engrav L H, Heimbach D M, Reus J L, Narnar T J, Marvin J A. Early excision and grafting vs. nonoperative treatment of burns of indeterminate depth: a randomized prospective study. *J Trauma* 1983; **23:** 1001–4.

49. Gray D T, Pine R W, Harnar T J, Marvin J A, Engrav L H, Heimbach D M. Early surgical excision versus conventional therapy in patients with 20 to 40 percent burns. *Am J Surg* 1982; **144:** 76–80.

50. McManus W F, Mason A D, Pruitt B A. Excision of the burn wound in patients with large burns. *Arch Surg* 1989; **124:** 718–20.

51. Monafo W W, Bessey P Q. Benefits and limitations of burn wound excision. *World J Surg* 1992; **16:** 37–42.

52. Tompkins R G, Remensnyder J P, Burke J F, *et al.* Significant reductions in mortality for children with burn injuries through the use of prompt eschar excision. *Ann Surg* 1988; **208:** 577–85.

53. Sorensen B, Fisker N P, Steensen J P, Kalaja E. Acute excision or exposure treatment. Final results of a three-year-old randomized controlled clinical trial. *Scand J Plast Reconstr Surg* 1984; **18:** 87–93.

54. Desai M H, Herndon D N, Broemeling L, Barrow R E, Nichols R J, Rutan R L. Early burn wound excision significantly reduces blood loss. *Ann Surg* 1990; **211:** 753–62.

55. Housinger T A, Lang D, Warden G D. A prospective study of blood loss with excisional therapy in pediatric burn patients. *J Trauma* 1993; **34:** 262–3.

56. Shiozaki T, Kishikawa M, Hiraide A, *et al.* Recovery from postoperative hypothermia predicts survival in extensively burned patients. *Am J Surg* 1993; **165:** 326–31.

57. Monafo W W. Tangential excision. *Clin Plast Surg* 1974; **1:** 591–601.

58. Monafo W W, Aulenbacher C E, Pappalardo C. Early tangential excision of the eschars of major burns. *Arch Surg* 1972; **104:** 503–8.

59. Marano M A, O'Sullivan G, Madden M, Finkelstein J, Goodwin C W. Tourniquet technique for reduced blood loss and wound assessment during excisions of burn wounds of the extremity. *Surg Gynecol Obstet* 1990; **171:** 249–50.

60. Alexander J W, MacMillan B G, Law E, Kittur D S. Treatment of severe burns with widely meshed skin autograft and meshed skin allograft overlay. *J Trauma* 1981; **21:** 433–8.

61. Herndon D N, Barrow R E, Rutan R L, Rutan T C, Desai M H, Abston S. A comparison of conservative versus early excision: therapies in severely burned patients. *Ann Surg* 1989; **209:** 547–53.

62. Curreri P W, Luterman A, Braun D W, Shires G T. Burn Injury: analysis of survival and hospitalization time for 937 patients. *Ann Surg* 1980; **192:** 472–8.

63. Feller I, Tholen D, Cornell R G. Improvements in burn care, 1965 to 1979. *JAMA* 1980; **244:** 2074–8.

64. Salisbury R E, Wright P. Evaluation of early excision of dorsal burns of the hand. *Plast Reconstr Surg* 1982; **69:** 670–5.

65. Goodwin C W, Maguire M S, McManus W F, Pruitt B A. Prospective study of burn wound excision of the hands. *J Trauma* 1983; **23:** 510–17.

66. Edstrom L E, Robson M C, Macchiaverna J R, Scala A D. Prospective randomized treatments for burned hands: nonoperative vs. operative. Preliminary report. *Scand J Plast Reconstr Surg* 1979; **13:** 131–5.

67. Law N W, Ellis H. The effect of parenteral nutrition on the healing of abdominal wall wounds and colonic anastomoses in protein-malnourished rats. *Surgery* 1990; **107:** 449–54.

CHAPTER ELEVEN

Treatment of Infections in Burns

John Heggers, Hugo A. Linares, Patricia Edgar, Cynthia Villarreal and David N. Herndon

Microbial Identification of the Burn Wound Pathogen

Infection is a most undesirable partner in any operative procedure, and more particularly in the thermal injury. There are several major benchmarks which must be closely followed in order to achieve reliable clinical microbiology results in association with the thermal injury. The first and most important canon to remember concerns the selection of a proper specimen for culture. This entails obtaining a culture which is free from contamination by the normal flora which may be present on the surface of the injured skin after the injury. This should include any leukocyte laden exudate.[1] Secondly, the size or amount of the specimen plays a very significant role in the appropriate identification of the etiologic agent. The use of prophylactic antimicrobials, both topical and systemic, should be noted so that appropriate inhibitors or sufficient dilutions can be prepared or so that reagents can be added to negate drug interactions. The specimen should be collected and placed in a sterile container for appropriate transport media to the laboratory.[2] Most, if not all, burn wound specimens should be examined immediately. Tissue specimens should be homogenized or impression smears should be prepared; and other body fluids, transudates, and exudates should be examined immediately after collection.

Presumptive Examination of Burn Wound Specimens

One of the most important techniques available to the burn surgeon is the Gram stain. This procedure is the primary road sign which provides presumptive evidence as to the potential etiologic agent responsible for infection, as well as a possible opportunity for empirical use of both topical and systemic antibacteria therapy to control or eliminate the microbe, and, most importantly, what approach the laboratory should employ for successful isolation and identification of the etiologic agent of infection. The preparation of the specimen for staining is made by aseptically transferring the suspect material to an aseptically clean clear glass slide. If the specimen is dry, a drop of water is placed on the slide first in order to emulsify the specimen for proper staining. *Caution*: One must make sure that there is sufficient specimen for the Gram stain and the culture as well. If the quantity of the specimen is insufficient, one creates a culture first, then a Gram stain if possible. A thin film is made, fixed by drying air and then by heat fixation, by passing the slide a few times through a flame or placing the slide on a rack above the incinerator (Oxford Labware, St Louis, MO).

The Gram stain procedure is simple, consisting of four basic steps:

1. Flood the slide with crystal violet for 10 seconds to 1 minute. (Times vary depending on each stain employed, age of stain, authors' procedure, and outline.) Rinse with tap water.[2]
2. Flood then with Gram's iodine for 10 seconds to 1 minute. Rinse with tap water.
3. Carefully decolorize with 95% ethanol or acetone alcohol combination 10–20 seconds. (Acetone–alcohol may be used for a more rapid decolorization.)
4. Counterstain with safranin 10–30 seconds. Air dry or blot with bibulous paper.

Two basic reactions will be noted. Organisms which stain blue or purple are classified gram-positive (e.g. staphylococci) and those which stain red are classified gram-negative e.g. *Escherichia coli*).[2]

The colour plates for this chapter appear between pp 264 and 265.

For an explanation concerning the mechanisms of the Gram reaction, it is suggested that the reader review *Medical Microbiology* by Baron *et al.*, pages 28–34.[3] Specimens collected should be placed in an appropriate sterile container, transport, or holding medium. There are several options available for the more fastidious and anaerobic pathogens. Further discussion concerning the proper media will be addressed during the description of the frequently encountered pathogens.

All burn wound specimens taken at the time of surgical intervention should be inoculated to a variety of solid and liquid media. However, the only reliable method is a tissue biopsy which is the true indicator of the potential pathogen in surgical sepsis. Quantitative counts should be performed using the Robson–Heggers technique.[4] The liquid medium employed is generally an enriched thioglycolate medium (THIO) or brain heart infusion broth (BHIB), supplemented to facilitate the recovery of anaerobes as well as the aerobic pathogens.[2,3,5] Aliquots of the serial diluted specimens are subsequently inoculated to sheep blood agar plate (SBAP) with phenethyl alcohol (PEA), and MacConkey agar (MAC). SBAP is an enriched medium which contains nutrient supplements, allowing a wide variety of organisms to reproduce. The SBAP with PEA is a selective medium, in that it will permit the growth of *Bacteroides fragilis, B. melaninogenicus, Clostridium perfringens* (*welchii*), and *Peptostreptococcus anaerobius*; it should inhibit the growth of facultative enterics such as *Proteus mirabilis* and *Escherichia coli*. MAC, on the other hand, is a differential medium, which distinguishes between lactose and non-lactose fermenting enteric organisms. Each inoculated plate should be incubated in the suspected organism's appropriate atmospheric conditions. A review of the resident and transient microbial flora which live as parasites and/or symbionts in and on man will help to evaluate their significance as potential pathogens when encountered in surgical specimen (**Tables 11.1** and **11.2**).

MICROBIAL IDENTIFICATION

It is the design of the remaining portion of this chapter to reacquaint burn surgeons with some of the major distinguishing characteristics of those pathogens encountered in burn wound sepsis. The nomenclature and listing of the following microorganisms is a composite of *Bergey's Manual*[6] and NCDC's proposed changes:

A. Gram-positive cocci = facultative aerobic to anaerobic
   1. Spherical cells in pairs and clusters, no chains
      a. *Micrococcus* spp. – differentiation from *Staphylococcus aureus*
      b. *Staphylococcus* spp.
      c. *Peptococcus* spp. (anaerobe)
   2. Spherical cells in pairs, clumps and chains
      a. *Streptococcus* spp.
      b. *Enterococcus* spp.
      c. *Peptostreptococcus* spp. (anaerobe)

B. Gram-positive bacilli
   1. Aerobic (asporogenous) bacilli
      a. *Corynbacterium*
      b. *Listeria*
   2. Spore-forming bacilli
      a. *Bacillus* (aerobe)
      b. *Clostridium* (anaerobe)

C. Gram-negative aerobic rods
   1. Nonfermentors
      a. *Pseudomonas aeruginosa*
      b. *Pseudomonas* spp.
      c. Other miscellaneous aerobic gram-negative rods

D. Gram-negative facultatively anaerobic rods (glucose fermentors)
   1. Enterobacteriaceae
      a. *Escherichia coli*
      b. *Enterobacter cloacae*
      c. *Klebsiella pneumoniae*
      d. *Serrafia marcescens*
      e. Other enteric organisms
   2. Vibrionaceae
      a. *Aeromonas hydrophila*
   3. Other miscellaneous gram-negative rods

Gram-positive Cocci–pairs, Clusters

The *Micrococcus* spp. as a rule are considered amphibionts or nonpathogenic; however, with the increasing frequency of prosthetic valve transplants, these organisms are becoming more

Table 11.1 Frequently encountered gram-positive organisms according to organ association and probability of pathogenesis found in burn wounds*

Organism	Soft tissue skin	Upper respiratory tissue	Lower respiratory tissue	Endocardial	Gastro-intestinal tissue	Urogenital tract	Bone and joint
S. aureus	NF, P	P, NF	P	P	P	NF, P	P
S. epidermidis	NF, P	NF, P	P	P	P	NF, P	P
S. spp.	NF	NF, P	P	P	NF, P	NF, P	P
Str. pyogenes	P, NF	P, NF	P	P	P	P	P
Other strep	NF	NF	P	P	NF	NF, P	P
Enterococcus	P	P	P	P	NF, P	NF, P	P
Corynebacterium	NF	P	P	P	–	P	–
Diphtheroids	NF	NF	–	P	NF	NF	–
Micrococci	NF	NF	–	–	–	–	–
Candida albicans	NF	NF	P	P	NF	P, NF	P

NF, Normal flora; P, Pathogens; – normally not found; however, these organisms should not be ignored when encountered.
* Modified from Heggers J. Microbiology for surgeons. In: Kerstein M D, ed. *Management of Surgical Infections.* Mt Kisco, NY: Futura Publishing Co, 1980: 27–55.

Table 11.2 Frequently encountered gram-negative organisms according to tissue association and potential of pathogenesis found in burn wounds*

Organism	Soft tissue skin	Upper respiratory tissue	Lower respiratory tissue	Endocardial	Gastro-intestinal tissue	Urogenital tract	Bone and joint
Fermentors (enterics)							
Escherichia coli	NF, P	NF, P	P	P	NF, P	NF, P	P
Klebsiella pneumoniae; Enterobacter cloacae, aerogenes	NF, P	NF, P	P	P	NF, P	NF, P	P
Proteus spp.	NF, P	P	P	P	NF, P	NF, P	P
Morganella morganii	P	–	P	–	P	P	P
Serratia marcescens	NF, P	–	P	P	P	P	P
Providencia spp.	P	–	P	–	P	P	P
Other enterics	NF, P	NF, P	P	P	NF, P	P	P
Nonfermentors							
Aeromonas hydrophilia	P	P	P	P	NF, P	P	P
Pseudomonas aeruginosa	P	NF, P	P	P	NF, P	P	P
Acinetobacter spp.	NF	NF	P	–	NF	NF	P
Achromobacter xylosoxidans	P	P	P	P	NF, P	P	P

* NF, normal flora; P, pathogens; –, normally not found; however, these organisms should not be ignored when encountered. Modified from Heggers J. Microbiology for surgeons. In: Kerstein M D, ed. *Management of Surgical Infections*. Mt Kisco, NY: Futura Publishing Co, 1980: 27–55.

important. Another major reason for differentiating this genus is because of its similarity to the staphylococci. Micrococci are gram-positive cocci which generally form tetrads as opposed to the grape-like clusters often seen mixed with staphylococci. Nonhemolytic colonies are prevalent and produce a wide variety of color (i.e. *M. luteus*). Colonies vary from yellow and orange to red and even violet in color. There are three distinct species to be considered, and they are *M. luteus*, *M. roseus*, and *M. varians*. Cultural differences are presented in **Table 11.3**.[7] The micrococci are normal inhabitants of the skin and the frequency of isolation in a burn wound is between 5 and 10%. They are considered non-pathogenic in a burn wound and are more frequently considered wound contaminants. While all are catalase positive, their distinct growth requirements are essential components of delineating the specific organisms.

The genus *Staphylococcus* is composed of several important pathogens which include *S. aureus*, *S. epidermidis*, *S. saprophyticus*, *S. haemolyticus*, *S. hyicus hyicus*, *S. simulans*, and *S. cohnii*. All have variable hemolytic activity. Although *S. aureus* usually produces golden or cream-colored colonies and *S. epidermidis* produces white to dull gray colonies as do the other staphylococci, the color is not trustworthy for identification. The coagulase test is usually the differential test for separating these two species. It can be implemented best by either slide or tube method. However, should the slide method prove negative, then true coagulase negativity must be confirmed by the tube test. **Tables 11.4a** and **b** compare some of the major key reactions for proper identification among the staphylococci. The slide screening test using human plasma is a presumptive determination which examines for 'bound' coagulase. The confirmatory tube test employs rabbit

Table 11.3 Characteristics differentiating *Micrococcus* species from *Staphylococcus aureus**

Test	*M. varians*	*M. roseus*	*M. luteus*	*S. aureus*
Catalase	+	+	+	+
Coagulase	–	–	–	+
Acid from glucose aerobically	+	–	–	+
Acid from glucose anaerobically	–	–	–	+
15% NaC1	–	–	–	+
5% NaC1	+	+	+	+

+, positive; –, negative.
* Modified from Heggers J. Microbiology for surgeons. In: Kerstein M D, ed. *Management of Surgical Infections*. Mt Kisco, NY: Futura Publishing Co, 1980: 27–55.

plasma which tests for 'free' coagulase. One must be sure, however, that the microbe being tested is gram-positive cocci, since citrate-positive organisms such as *Pseudomonas*, *Serratia*, and *Enterococcus* species utilize citrate and release calcium, which can cause a clot to form.

Strains of *S. aureus*, as well as other *Staphylococcus* species, produce a wide variety of metabolites. Some are pathognomionic and also toxigenic, while those with minimal toxicity

Table 11.4 Differentiation of clinically important *Staphylococcus* species+

(a) Clinically important species

Character	*S. aureus*	*S. epidemidis*	*S. saprophyticus*
Coagulase*	+	–	–
Hemolysis	+	V	–
Novoabiocin resistance**	–	–	+
Phosphatase*	+	+	V
Acid, aerobically, from D-(+)-trehalose*	+	–	+
D-Mannitol	+	–	V
Maltose	+	+	+
Sucrose*	+	+	+
D-(+)-xylose* or L-(+)-arabinose	–	–	–
Xylitol	–	–	V
Anaerobic growth in thioglycollate	+	+	+>–
Nitrate/DNase	+/+	+w/–w	–/–
Identification accuracy based on the above characters	>95%	>95%	>90%

(b) Other clinically important *Staphylococcus* species+

Character	*S. simulans*	*S. haemolyticus*	*S. hyicus hyicus*	*S. hominis*
Coagulase*	–	–	V	–
Hemolysis	V	+>+	V	–>+
Novoabiocin resistance**	–	–	–	–
Phosphatase*	V	–>+	V	–>+
Acid, aerobically, from D-(+) trehalose*	+>–	+	+	+>–
D-Mannitol*	+>–	+,–	+	–
Maltose	–>+	+	+	+
Sucrose*	+	+	V	+
D-(+)-xylose* or L-(+)-arabinose	–	–	V	–
Xylitol	–	–	V	–
Anaerobic growth in *thioglycollate*	+	+>+,+	+	–>+
Nitrate/DNase	+/w	d/ds	+/+	d/–w
Identification accuracy based on the above characters	>90%	>85%	>85%	>80%

+ Modified from Holt J, Krieg N R, Sneath P H A, Staley J T, Williams S T, eds. *Bergey's Manual of Determinative Bacteriology*. 9th ed. Baltimore, MD: Williams & Wilkins, 1994.
* Characters recommended by the ICSB Subcommittee on the Taxonomy of Staphylococci and Micrococci.
** Minimal inhibitory concentration > 1.6 ug/ml.
V, Variable; w, weak reaction; +w, positive to weak reaction; –w, negative to weak reaction; d, delayed reaction; ds, tests differentiates subspecies; +, positive reaction; –, negative reaction.

or no toxic effects at all, are of some diagnostic significance. Most of the human pathogens produce α and β lysins. Some exotoxins which are produced by the pathogenic strains of staphylococci include a pyrogenic toxin, a dermonecrotizing toxin, a lethal toxin, and leukocidin which is presumably similar to the δ-lysin. Only *S. aureus* produces an enterotoxin which is the cause of staphylococcal food poisoning. Alpha hemolysin does not lyse human red cells, but will lyse sheep red blood cells and rabbit red cells; horse red cells are lysed only by δ-lysin. Other antigenic nontoxic metabolites produced by the staphylococci include: coagulase, protease, lipase, deoxyribonuclease, fibrinolysin, gelatinase, in addition to hyaluronidase, phosphate and staphylokinase.

S. aureus and the other members of the *Staphylococcus* species usually will develop resistance to antibiotics rather rapidly. The majority of the staphylococci strains which are isolated from hospital patients are resistant to penicillin, methicillin, cephalosporins and the aminoglycosides. The former resistance is mediated by a β-lactamase or penicillinase, whereas methicillin is considered resistant to β-lactamase.[8] *S. epidermidis* is a resident of human skin and mucous membranes and resembles *S. aureus* microscopically. *S. epidermidis* is tolerant of high concentrations of NaCl as is *S. aureus*. However, it differs from *S. aureus* in that it is mannitol, coagulase, and thermonuclease negative. It is equally as pathogenic as is *S. aureus*, and has been the principal etiologic agent in disease entities such as bacterial endocarditis, infected surgical prosthesis, infections following bone marrow transplantation, or other states of immunosuppression such as occur in the thermal injury. Typically *S. epidermidis* is resistant to penicillinase-resistant penicillins such as methicillin and cephalosporins as is the case with *S. aureus*. Methicillin resistance is genetically mediated through a transposon.[8,9] Methicillin-resistant *S. epidermidis* (MRSE) delivers its genetically resistant code to a previously labile *S. aureus* which subsequently becomes methicillin resistant (MRSA).[9] *S. saprophyticus* resembles the other staphylococci but it is distinguished from them because of its resistance to monobiocin. Further, *S. saprophyticus* is also resistant to nalidixic acid (**Table 11.4a**).

In burn wound infections, the predominate gram-positive agent responsible during 1988 and 1989 was *S. aureus* (53.8%) followed by *S. hyicus hyicus* (24.0%), while the other staphylococci accounted for the remaining 22.2% (**Table 11.5**). The staphylococci accounted for over 82% of the gram-positive isolates (SBAP). The staphylococci, more especially the MRSA and MRSE, are responsible for graft loss when the colony count of the graft bed is $>10^5$ CFUs per gram of tissue.

Staphylococcal diseases

All *Micrococcus* and *Staphylococcus* grow especially well on sheep blood agar. Suspect colonies should be tested for catalase from a nutrient agar culture because blood agar can give a positive catalase reaction leading to an incorrect presumptive identification. Mannitol salt sugar (7.5% NaCl), with a nutrient agar overlay, may be employed to confirm anaerobic fermentation of mannitol and NaCl tolerance, as previously discussed above and represented in Table 11.3.[6,7,10] Most common infections where the etiologic agent *Staphylococcus* spp. is encountered and considered pathognomonic are septicemia, cellulitis, impetigo, scalded skin syndrome, and postoperative wound infections. However, the most serious staphylococcal infections are puerperal sepsis, pneumonia, osteomyelitis, endocarditis and burn wound infections. Staphylococcal pseudomembranous enterocolitis will occur most frequently as a complication of antibiotic therapy.

Table 11.5 Gram-positive bacteria isolated from pediatric burn wounds

Organisms	Number 1993 Jan–Sept	%	1988–1989*	%	Overall % of group
S. aureus	810	29.2	4402	44.2	53.8
S. epidermidis	783	28.3	1305	13.1	
S. hyicus hyicus	19	0.7	1961	19.7	24.0
Other staphylococci	400†	14.5	517	5.2	
Total staphylococci	2012	72.7	8185	**82.2**	
Ec. faecalis	474	17.3	925	9.3 }	67.1
Ec. faecium	134	4.8	269	2.6 }	
Other streptococci	*145*	*5.2*	*584*	*5.9*	32.9
Total streptococci	753	27.3	1778	**17.8**	
Total Gram-positives	2765	100.0	9963	**100.0**	
Total isolates tested	5026	55.0	14 696	67.8	

* Heggers J P, McCauley R L, Herndon D N. Antimicrobial therapy in burn patients: part I. *Surgical Rounds* 1992; **July:** 613–17.
† Includes *S. hominis* and *S. haemolyticus*.

Toxic shock syndrome

The toxic shock syndrome (TSS) was first described as such in 1978.[11] The disease is adumbrated by sudden onset of fever, vomiting, diarrhea, shock, and a diffuse macular erythematous rash, followed by desquamation of the skin on the hands and feet as well as hyperemia of various mucous membranes. Unfortunately, the role of TSS has not been completely elucidated in burn patients. It has been our experience that while burned patients may be infected with a potential TSS-causing *S. aureus*, no other serious or untold complications have been observed. In fact, treatment of burn wounds was not any different for patients infected with a nontoxic *S. aureus*.

Streptococcaceae

The *Streptococcus* spp. appears as short and long chains of cocci and sometimes as diplococci, notably in the case of *Str. (Diplococcus) pneumoniae*, which often appear as teardrop or lancet diplococci. The streptococci are catalase negative and produce a variety of hemolytic activity in the presence of blood. The types of hemolysis produced on SBAP are frequently used as an initial means of identification for the streptococci; hemolytic streptococci manifest a green discoloration of blood agar surrounding a small grayish colony which is resistant to dissolution by bile (*Str. pneumoniae*). *Str. pneumoniae*, now classified as a member of the *Streptococcus* family, produces an α-hemolysis which is characteristic of the viridans group. It is bile soluble (autolysis by bile) and optochin sensitive (TAXO P disk, BBL). The optochin disk is impregnated with ethylhydrocupreine HCl and then placed on a SBAP inoculated with *Str. pneumoniae*. Inhibition of growth is observed after overnight incubation at 37°C in a 5–10% CO_2 atmosphere. Other α-hemolytic streptococci are not inhibited.[2,3,6] Both the enterococci and viridans streptococci fall into this particular group of multifarious streptococci.[11] The viridans group is obviously more susceptible to penicillin than is the enterococci group. Another dominant characteristic of this variety is that the hemolysis produced is considered a virulence factor; and quantitatively, this group of organisms does not lend itself to the standard rule that if there are more than 10^5 bacteria per gram of tissue in a wound, then a graft applicant will be likely to fail in any particular tissue closure.[12] The mere presence of a few β-hemolytic streptococci can cause a wound infection, failure of a primary closure, and loss of a skin graft.[12] The major species that can be diagnosed with this particular type of hemolysis are *Str. pyogenes*, β-hemolytic group A streptococci, *Str. agalactiae*, and β-hemolytic group C streptococci, just to mention a few.[13,14] There are those which subsist in the remaining Lancefield groups which demonstrate the same type of hemolytic action.[2,5] Presumptive identification of *Str. pyogenes* can be made by sensitivity to bacitracin, since 90% of all *Str. pyogenes* are sensitive to bacitracin. *Str. agalactiae*, however, is CAMP positive and hippurate positive (**Table 11.6**). The remaining streptococci are variable in their ability to tolerate salt and temperature requirements. They all proliferate well in a reduced O_2 environment, with a CO_2 tension of 3–5%, on SBAP. As recounted earlier, hemolysis is the passport for identifying these microbes. For proper discriminating characteristics and sensitivity to sulfamethoxazole – trimethoprim (SXT), see **Table 11.6**.[14]

While it is important to recognize the pathogenicity of the streptococci, it must be understood that the enterococci are the predominant etiologic agents of burn wound infections, accounting for 67.1% of such infections (**Table 11.5**). Among the other streptococci. *Str. mitis*, *Str. anguis*, and others are responsible for the remaining 32.9% of burn wound infections caused by the streptococci. The genus *Enterococcus (Ec.)* was established in 1984.[3,6] However, *Ec. faecalis* and *Ec. faecium* were the only two recognized species. Since that time 12 additional species have been classified within the enterococci group, but only *Ec. durans* and *Ec. avium* have been isolated from human infections.[2,6,11] The majority of the enterococci are non-hemolytic, termed γ-hemolysis. However, there are some strains that produce a β or α-hemolysis on blood agar. These microorganisms are distinguished by their capability to grow in high salt concentrations and hydrolyze esculin, resulting in black discoloration of the medium.[2,3,6] All members of the enterococci group, besides tolerating 6.5% NaCl and being bile esculin (BE) positive, are also pyrrolidonylarylamidase (PYR) and leucine aminopeptidase positive (LAP). The species are separated into three groups based on specific biochemical reactions. Group I does not hydrolyze arginine but forms acid in a mannitol, sorbitol and sorbose broth. The important species here is *Ec. avium*. Group II, on the other hand, hydrolyzes arginine and forms acid in mannitol and sorbitol broth. The significant species in this group are *Ec. faecalis* and *Ec. faecium*. Group III, which includes *Ec. durans*, is

Table 11.6 Biological characteristics of the *Streptococcus* spp.*

Lancefield group	Representative species	Hemolytic reaction	Bacitracin sensitivity	CAMP reaction	Na hippurate	Bile esculin	6.5% NaCl	SXT sensitivity	Optochin bile solubility
A	*Str. pyogenes*	b[a](rarely[b])	S	–	–	–	–	V	–
B	*Str. agalactiae*	b>a[c]>g[b]	R	+	+	–	V	R	–
C	*Str. equi*	b>a>g	R	–	–	–	–	S	–
D	Enterococci								
	Ec. faecalis	g>b>a	R	–	V	+	+	S	–
	Ec. faecium								
	Other								
	Ec. bovis	g>b>a	R	–	–	+	–	S	–
	Ec. equinus								
G	*Str. canis*	b>g>a	R	–				S	
H	*Str. sanguis*	a>b>g	R	–				S	
K	*Str. salivarius*	a>b>g	R	–				S	
Nongroupable	Viridans	a>b>g	V	–	–	–	–	S	–
E	*Str. uberis*	g>a	R	V	+	+	–	S	–
None	*Str. pneumoniae*	a	V	–	–	–	–	–	+

* Modified from Heggers J. Microbiology for surgeons. In: Kerstein M D, ed. *Management of Surgical Infections*. 1980, Mt Kisco, NY: Futura Publishing Co, 1980: 27–55.
[a] Beta hemolysis (b);
[b] gamma hemolysis (g);
[c] alpha hemolysis (a).
V, Variable; R, resistant; S, sensitive; –, negative; +, positive.

negative for all tests described above.[2,6] The clinical isolates of the enterococci will be *Ec. faecalis* about 80–90% of the time and *Ec. faecium* around 5–10%.[2,11] This is consistent with our burn wound isolates, 80% versus 20% respectively (**Table 11.5**).

While this portion of the chapter deals with the identification and isolation of gram-positive organisms, it has been our experience over the years that the major offenders of the burn wound infection predominantly include only the gram-positive cocci. In a recent 9-month evaluation of gram-positive clinical isolates, the staphylococci predominated, followed by the streptococci for a total number of gram-positive isolates of 2765. Among the staphylococci, *S. aureus* and *S. epidermidis* were predominant (1593), and the other staphylococci accounted for 419 isolates; among the streptococci, the enterococci predominated – particularly *Ec. faecalis* (474). This same trend was also observed in a 2-year study previously addressed (**Table 11.5**).

Peptococcaceae

The anaerobic gram-positive cocci are a part of the indigenous microflora of the skin, gastrointestinal, genitourinary, and oral cavity systems. They have been reported as pathogens in almost every type of human infection.[3,11] The anaerobic gram-positive cocci are divided into two respective genera which include the *Peptococcus* spp. (*Staphylococcus*-like) and the *Peptostreptococcus* spp. (*Streptococcus*-like). As the names indicate, their morphological features are similar to their aerobic counterparts of infection.[15] The *Peptococcus* genus contains six diverse species and the *Peptostreptococcus* genus contains five different species. The distinguishing reactions are presented in **Table 11.7**. On anaerobic blood agar plates, both genera appear as small gray to white colonies after 48–72 hours incubation. Occasional strains of both may be β-hemolytic or α-hemolytic. *Peptococcus*, unlike *Peptostreptococcus*, does not produce a sharp pungent odor which is believed to be an identifying characteristic. In thioglycolate (THIO) broth, colonies appear as small discrete compact bodies uniformly growing throughout the medium and sometimes producing gas[15] (**Table 11.7**). With early excision and grafting, however, these agents are rarely encountered in today's burn wound infections. Yet, in developing countries where early excision and grafting is not a reality, such organisms could be potentially dangerous.

Nonsporogenous Gram-positive Rods

The major asporogenous bacillus most frequently encountered is the *Corynebacterium* spp. which is felt to be a normal inhabitant of the skin, respiratory tract and/or vaginal tract (see **Table 11.1**). They are small, gram-positive rods which form Chinese-like characters or palisades. Methylene blue stains often are helpful in identifying the metachromatic granules of these microbes. The colonies on blood agar are usually very small, dry, and nonhemolytic; and they are often referred to as diphtheroids. The only *Corynebacterium* sp. which is considered to be of the pathogenic type is *C. diphtheriae*. When this organism is suspected as the etiologic agent, specimens should be inoculated in Loeffler's medium and blood tellurite agar. Colonies emerge as black or gray in color. Though fluorescent antibodies can identify the organism as *C. diphtheriae*, only the Elek plate will identify the toxigenic groups responsible for the infection.[3,6,7] (**Table 11.8**). A strip filter paper is impregnated with diphtheria antitoxin (100 U/ml) and is placed on a plate of enrichment medium with tellurite. Then the suspected microbe is inoculated in the plate perpendicular to the strip. The toxin from the organism diffuses through the medium as does the antitoxin. At the point of contact, a thin precipitate forms at a 45°

Table 11.7 Biological reactions of the anaerobic gram-positive cocci*

	Hemolysis	Catalase	Esculin hydrolysis	Gas	Indole	Nitrate	Tween 80 growth stimulant	Gelatin liquid
Peptococcus species								
P. ascaccharolyticus	–	–	–	+	+	–	+	–
P. constellatus	–	–	+	–	–	V	–	–
P. magnus	–	–	–	–	–	–	+	+
P. morbillorum	b[a]	–	–	–/+	–	–	+	–
P. prevotii	b	V	–/+	–/+	–	–	+	–
P. variables	–	–	–	–/+	–	–	+	+
Peptostreptococcus species								
P. anaerobius	b	–	–	+	–	–	+	–
P. intermedius	a[b]	–	+	+	–	–	+	–
P. micros	b	–	–	–/+	–	–	+	–
P. parvulus	–	–	–	+	–	–	+	+
P. productus	a or b	–	+	+	–	–	–	–

* Modified from Heggers J. Microbiology for surgeons. In: Kerstein M D, ed. *Management of Surgical Infections*. Mt Kisco, NY: Futura Publishing Co, 1980: 27–55.
[a] Beta hemolysis (b); [b] alpha hemolysis (a).
V, variable; –, negative; +, positive; –/+, reaction more negative than positive.

angle to the inoculation. Diphtheria antitoxin (DAT) is essential in the treatment of these infections.

An organism which provokes a monocytic response in rabbits, but usually not in humans, can cause a severe meningitis in humans. This organism, called *Listeria monocytogenes*, stains equally as a gram-positive rod or coccobacillus, and often forms palisades like those observed with the diphtheroids. *L. monocytogenes* is β-hemolytic on blood agar, and the specimen may require a few days at 4°C before primary isolation. *Listeria* is motile at room temperature, and this feature is not shared by the *Corynebacterium*[3,6,7] (**Table 11.8**). *Nocardia* is a gram-variable or gram-positive branching filamentous rod. This organism, like its anaerobic partner (*Actinomyces*) produces sulfur granules which appear as tiny, pale yellowish flecks composed of dainty branching hyphae. The media of choice for this microbe is Sabouraud's dextrose agar and SBAP. Species belonging to the *Nocardia* genus are acid fast or partially acid fast. (**Table 11.8** presents some of the predominant characteristics of *Nocardia*.)[3,6] *Erysipelothrix rhusiopathiae* (*insidiosa*), the etiologic agent of erysipeloid in man, is adumbrated as a slender gram-positive rod with a tendency to form filaments. On SBAP it produces an α-hemolysis and the colonies are translucent with a bluish sheen when seen by reflected light. It grows better on horse blood agar combined with a trypticase soy agar overlay. Indole is negative and its catalase is not produced[3,6] (**Table 11.8**). One of the anaerobic partners of the asporogenous gram-positive rods is the *Actinomyces* genus. This group of microbes resembles the *Corynebacterium* in that they produce diphtheroid-like characters. But, filamentous compositions are usually present after 18–48 hours of incubation. Like *Nocardia*, *Actinomyces* requires several days to a few weeks in order to make its demeanor obvious. Therefore, any specimen processed without an initial Gram stain will most decidedly disclose a negative

Table 11.8 Some characteristics of the gram-positive nonsporogenous bacilli*

Genus	Hemolysis	Aerobic 5–10% CO_2	Anaerobic	Facultative	Esculin	Catalase	Indole	Acid fast	Motility
Corynebacterim	V	+	+	+		+	V	–	–
Listeria	b[a]	+	–	+	+	+	–	–	+[b]
Nocardia	–	+	–	–	+			–	–
Erysipelothrix	a	+	–	–	–	–	–	+	–
Lactobacillus	–	–	+	+		–	–	–	–
Actinomyces	+[c]	–	+	+	+	–	–	–	–
Propionibacterium	–	–	+	–	+		V	–	
Bifidobacterium	–	–	–		+	–	–	–	–

* Modified from Heggers J. Microbiology for surgeons. In: Kerstein M D, ed. *Management of Surgical Infections*. Mt Kisco, NY: Futura Publishing Co, 1980: 27–55.
[a] *L. monocytogenes* only; [b] at 20–25°C; [c] Rabbit blood alpha>beta.
V, variable; –, negative; +, positive.

response after 48 hours of incubation.[3,6,15] *Propionibacterium* (*Corynebacterium*) *acnes* and species of *Bifidobacterium* (*Endobacterium* and *Arachnia*) are generally categorized as anaerobic diphtheroids. This class of microbes is often encountered with other facultative or anaerobic organisms, thus questioning their pathogenic potential. If, however, any of these microbes are isolated with relative frequency during an active disease process (acute or chronic), the clinician must consider them as the etiologic agent until further evidence to the contrary is obtained.[3,6,15]

The etiologic agents of infection described herein are notorious and have a world-wide distribution. Such infections may possibly be encountered in a burn injury. The frequency of occurrence has been negligible; but this might be explained by the fact that most of these agents are sensitive to penicillin G, except in the case of *Erysipelothrix* which is sensitive to erythromycin.

Spore-forming Bacilli

The endospore-forming rods exist in two separate genera: those which are aerobic and those which are anaerobic. The aerobic variety is the *Bacillus* sp. which has been given the *nom de plume* of contaminant because of its ubiquitousness which has but one exception: *B. anthracis*, the cause of anthrax. The *Bacillus* sp. grows readily on solid media. A ground glass look and 'Medusahead' colony formation is characteristic. It is extremely unlikely to be found in burn wound infections, unless contact with contaminated soil has occurred. A Gram stain often unveils a bacillus with square ends. Kingsley[16] employed a phenylethylalcohol (PEA) and chloral hydrate (CH) combination as a selective medium to identify *B. anthracis* from other *Bacillus* spp. (**Table 11.9**). *Bacillus* spp. other than *B. anthracis* have recently been implicated as etiologic agents which are found in burn wounds and are involved in bacteremia, septicemia, meningitis, and bronchopneumonia.[17,18] Turnball *et al.* provided evidence of a severe necrotic enterotoxin being produced by *B. cereus*.[19] As with the diphtheroids, the frequent isolation of a *Bacillus* sp. in any specimen must not be taken lightly. The anaerobic correlate is the genus *Clostridium*. Clostridia, like the aerobic gram-positive *Bacillus*, are also ubiquitous in nature. All species can produce *spores*; however, they are rarely seen in clinical specimens unless the tissue samples are necrotic. Those infections considered as exogenous are caused by this group: tetanus, gas gangrene (myonecrosis), botulism, food-borne gastrointestinal symptoms, and cellulitis. Predisposing constituents giving rise to endogenous infections include surgery, and any underlying disease entities such as leukemia, carcinoma, diabetes, as well as the use of immunosuppressive drugs. The necrotizing and hemolytic exotoxin of *Cl. perfringens* can be seen by an opalescence with the use of an egg yolk agar. *Cl. perfringens* is commonly associated with myonecrosis and can probably be differentiated from *Cl. bifermentans*, *Cl. novyi*, and *Cl. septicum*, because of its distinctive 'double zone' hemolysis.[15]

Table 11.9 Biological characteristics of the genus *Bacillus**

	SBAP hemolysis	Nitrate reduction	Motility	CH	PEA
B. anthracis	–	+	–	–	–
B. cereus	+	+	V	+	+
B. subtilis	+	+	+	V	+
B. megaterium	+	–	+	+	–

*Modified from Heggers J. Microbiology for surgeons. In: Kerstein M D, ed. *Management of Surgical Infections*. Mt Kisco, NY: Futura Publishing Co, 1980: 27–55.
SBAP, Sheep blood agar; CH, chloral hydrate; PEA, phenylethyl alcohol; V, variable; –, negative; +, positive.

Anaerobic infections in burned patients are usually associated with avascular muscle found in electrical injuries, frost bite, or cutaneous flame burns with concomitant crush type injuries.[20–24] The high risk of developing tetanus (*Cl. tetani*), even with small burns, has led to the accepted practice of tetanus prophylaxis (tetanus toxoid 0.5 ml) as a routine part of the admission protocol for most burn centers.[25,26] In addition, if prior immunization is absent or unclear, or the patient's last booster was more than 10 years ago, 250 units of tetanus is also given. This procedure is not unlike the administration of DAT.

Gram-negative Aerobic Rods

This family of gram-negative rods contains a distinctive group of etiologic agents of burn wound infections. Of this group aggregation, the *Pseudomonas* species are most repeatedly encountered and are chronic or acute. Earlier confrontations with this group of microbes were ignored as they were categorized as 'saprophytes'. This group of organisms are gram-negative and motile. They utilize carbohydrates oxidatively rather than via fermentation. Since 1960, *Pseudomonas aeruginosa* has been recognized as a major burn pathogen.[27,28] It has subsequently increased its presence not only in burns but in other forms of trauma.[29] *Ps. aeruginosa* is not the only documented pathogen among this group, however; other *Pseudomonas* species have been involved in nosocomial infections. After employing solutions of aqueous chlorhexidine, numerous infections caused by *Ps. cepacia* occurred in a London hospital.[30] The microorganism had somehow contaminated the chlorhexidine solution. The contamination of a water supply in a hospital by *Ps. multivorans* gave rise to a sequence of infections within that environment.[31] Twenty-two multiformities of surgical wounds and urinary tract conditions yielded *Ps. maltophila*, as reported by Gilardi,[32] with all species of *Pseudomonas* showing alterations in their susceptibility patterns and a prominent tendency toward resistance to newly developed antibiotics. This organism, however, is no longer called a pseudomonad but has been placed in the genus *Xanthomonas*.[2,3,6] While similar to *Ps. aeruginosa*, it is oxidase negative, whereas *Ps. aeruginosa* is positive in this respect. *X. maltophila* is the second most commonly isolated organism compared with *Ps. aeruginosa*. It is very adept at rapidly developing a broad spectrum antibiotic resistance. This resistance can emerge by changes to the expression of the chromosomal β-lactamase inducible populations and can be selected during therapy with broad spectrum cephalosporins, which sometimes cause clinical failure. Those organisms which fall into this select group include: *Ps. aeruginosa, Xanthomonas, Enterobacter, Serratia, Citrobacter*, and *Morganella* to mention only a few.[2,3,6]

Alcaligenes faecalis, another gram-negative motile rod, is often considered *persona non grata* among the pathogenic organisms; however, it must be taken seriously as an opportunistic pathogen[3,6] (**Table 11.10**). Its natural habitat is similar to that of *Ps. aeruginosa* in that it maintains a very close relationship with soil and water. Additionally, in hospital settings, it has been isolated from respirators, nebulizers, intravenous solutions, and hemodialysis systems.

Acinetobacter spp. are part of the indigenous flora of the skin as well as the respiratory, gastrointestinal, and genitourinary tracts of man and animals. They have been isolated from a diversity of clinical sources, including upper and lower respiratory tracts, urinary tract, surgical and burn wounds, and in bacteremias secondary to intravenous catheterization. Furthermore, occasional cases of

Table 11.10 Biological responses of *Pseudomonas* and other gram-negative rods*

Genus	Hemolysis	Motile	Oxidase	Citrate	Urea	Nitrate	Oxidase glucose	Arginine dehydrolase	Growth on SS
Pseudomonas	b	+	+	+	V	+	+	V	+
Alcaligenes	a	+	+	–/+	–	–	–	–	–
Acinetobacter		–	–	–	–	–	+	–	+
Achromobacter		+	+		+		+		+
Aeromonas		+	+		–	+	– (acid/gas) fermented	–	+

* Modified from Heggers J. Microbiology for surgeons. In: Kerstein M D, ed. *Management of Surgical Infections*. Mt Kisco, NY: Futura Publishing Co, 1980: 27–55.
SS, Shigella Salmonella Agar; a, alpha hemolysis; b, beta hemolysis; V, variable; +, positive; –, negative; –/+, more negative than positive.

septicemia or pneumonia have occurred in attenuated patients. Many of these patients who develop infections with this microorganism have had various manipulations including respiratory therapy equipment, tracheal intubation, or bladder or central venous line catheterization (**Table 11.10**). While it is an agent of low virulence, it has a predilection for infecting patients with deterred host defense mechanisms. It develops a high degree of antimicrobial resistance. This resistance may be a direct result of previous antimicrobial therapy. While current taxonomy for *Acinetobacter* accepts only one species, *A. calcoaceticus*, it should be recognized that two biochemically distinct varieties exist within the species. Those species which form acid from dextrose are called *A. calcoaceticus* var. *anitratus* while those that do not are called var. *Iwoffi*. It has been our experience at SBI–Galveston that the *anitratus* variety is the one most resistant to antibiotics; however, to date, we have not experienced any major problems with this agent. In fact, its incidence has been negligible.

Achromobacter spp. are frequently isolated from blood, ears, urine, respiratory tracts, surgical and burn wounds, as well as from feces. Some of the *Achromobacter* features necessary for identification can be found in **Table 11.10**. *Achromobacter* spp. are opportunistic pathogens which are frequently found in a hospital's water supply. As with all of the agents discussed above, it has a predilection for water.

Aeromonas (*Ae. hydrophila*) has been implicated as an etiologic agent of human gastroenteritis. It produces several types of enterotoxins. Based on the results of laboratory studies, *Ae. hydrophila* has been shown to produce additional factors such as hemolysins (cytotoxins), endotoxin,[33] leukocidin,[34] and phospholipases.[35] Each of these factors, as well as any combination, may contribute to the pathogenesis of disease mediated by *Ae. hydrophila*. Fatal and nonfatal water-borne *Aeromonas* infections are associated with various clinical manifestations including septicemia,[36–39] meningitis,[40] endocarditis,[41] corneal ulcers,[42] peritonitis,[43] and wound infections.[43,44] Most strains of *Ae. hydrophila* are hemolytic on blood agar and their culture filtrates lyse 1% suspensions of rabbit blood cells. These observations indicate that hemolysin produced by *Ae. hydrophila* may play an important role in the pathogenesis of disease. The significance of this microorganism as a human pathogen is better recognized now as more clinical laboratories are using proper diagnostic tests such as the indophenol oxidase test. In addition, *Ae. hydrophila* has been shown to be invasive in HEp-2 cell monolayers[45] and adherent to human blood cells.[46] These facts may also be important virulence properties of the organism. Three cases of *Ae. hydrophila* burn wound infection have been reported by Purdue and Hunt.[47] Because of the aquatic nature of these organisms, infections may be related to trauma and concomitant exposure to water and soil. All three of the cases included a history of extinguishing the fire with dirty water or by rolling in dirt. These actions should alert the physician to consider *Ae. hydrophila* as a possible etiologic agent of infection.

Gram-negative Facultatively Anaerobic Rods (Enteric Bacteria)

The largest and most repeatedly encountered group of microorganisms populating any burn wound environment along with the *Staphylococcus* spp. are the enterics; and they are found in the family of Enterobacteriaceae. This family contains 12 individual genera. Many of these organisms were previously categorized as non-pathogens, and among these were the *Klebsiella–Enterobacter* group, *Serratia marcescens, Providencia* species and *Erwinia* species.[3,6,48] *Escherichia coli*, probably the best known enteric, has been responsible for a wide diversity of infectious processes. Among these are:

- frequently severe and sometimes fatal infections such as appendicitis, cystitis, pyelitis, peritonitis, septicemia, and gallbladder infections;
- surgical and burn wound sepsis, and epidemic diarrhea of children and adults; and
- 'travelers' diarrhea'.

E. coli can be distinguished from other members of Enterobacteriaceae by its response to the classical IMVC (indole, methyl red, Voges–Proskauer and citrate) reaction (++––) (**Table 11.11**). The *Klebsiella–Enterobacter* group (K–E) are also gram-negative rods and can be either motile or nonmotile. Fifty-one percent of moderately ill hospitalized patients in one study had either *Kl. pneumoniae, Ent. aerogenes* or *Ent. cloacae* isolated from their oropharyngeal space.[49] *Kl. pneumoniae* and its family are fast becoming regular pathogens in nosocomial infections.[50] It is interesting that earlier isolation of the K–E group flora was thought to be part of the normal flora of the bronchial tree. The tribe Klebsiella is currently comprised of the genera *Klebsiella, Enterobacter*, and *Serratia*. Since the initial identification of *Ser. marcescens* in 1823, it has maintained a valueless position as a 'saprophyte'.[51] Initially, it was considered so harmless that it was used to examine bacterial drift and settling rates in 1964.[52] The idea seems quite logical since it produces a predominant chromogenic red pigment. However, 3 years later, Davis *et al.* reported that 94% of all the isolates from urinary tract infections were due to *Ser. marcescens*.[52] He also discovered that the mortality rate in these patients was 33%.

Table 11.11 Biological responses of some of the major Enterobacteriaceae*

Organism	Indole	MR	VP	Citrate	Urease	Motility	Arginine dihydrolase	KCN	H_2S
E. coli	+	+	–	–	–	V	V	–	–
Citrobacter	V	+	–	+	V	+	+	V	V
Klebsiella spp.	–	–	+	+	V	–	–	+	–
Enterobacter spp.	–	V	V	+	V	+	V	V	–
Ser. marcescens	–	V	+	+	–	+	–	+	–
Proteus spp.	+	+	–	V	+	+	?	V	V
Providencia	+	+	–	+	–	+	?	+	–
Morganella	+	+	–	–	+	+	–	+	–

* Modified from Heggers J. Microbiology for surgeons. In: Kerstein M D, ed. *Management of Surgical Infections.* Mt Kisco, NY: Futura Publishing Co, 1980: 27–55.
MR, Methyl red test; VP, Voges–Proskauer test; V, variable; –, negative; +, positive; ?, uncertain.

Thirty-five occurrences of *Ser. marcescens* bacteremia were reported in military personnel returning from Vietnam with accompanying burn wound infections.[53] The ubiquitousness of this microorganism has made it a serious pathogenic agent. It has been isolated on heart valves after cardiac surgery,[54,55] in surgical and burn wound infections, in sepsis after splenectomy, and repeatedly in nosocomial outbreaks in addition to being disseminated by poor hygienic practices.[56,57] **Table 11.11** examines some of its predominant biochemical responses. The remaining enterics consist of three additional genera, *Proteus, Providencia*, and *Morganella*.

The genus *Proteus* is composed of two species; *P. mirabilis* and *P. vulgaris*. Both species can be found in massive concentrations in the feces of individuals undergoing oral antibiotic therapy. This group of organisms is often accountable for surgical and burn wound infections, intra-abdominal infections, as well as bacteremias and urinary tract infections. Some key biological features can be found in **Table 11.11**. The genus *Providencia* is comprised of three species; *Prv. alcalifaciens, Prv. stuartii* and *Prv. rettgeri* which were formerly in the genus *Proteus*. The *Providencia* species, like *Ser. marcescens*, have a broad range of pathologic involvement from nosocomial infections[57,58] to septicemias, postoperative incisional wounds, burn wounds, pneumonias and urinary tract infections.[59] These gram-negative bacilli fall into the general category of the paracolon bacteria and are categorized as members of the genus *Proteus*, which is classified in Bergey's manual as *Proteus inconstans*.[6,48] The biological responses of this group of organisms is displayed in **Table 11.11**. *Prv. stuartii* has been incriminated in numerous infections of patients in a burn unit, and includes some urinary tract infections as well.

Morganella morganii is the only species in the genus *Morganella* and was considered earlier a member of the genus *Proteus*. *M. morganii* has been conjoined with wound infections as well as urinary tract infections.

The *Erwinia* genus consists of 13 distinct species, all of which have been identified as plant pathogens; however, *E. herbicola* has managed to become pathogenic for man. The principal controversy ruminating around this organism lies in its ability to mimic *Escherichia coli*. *Erwinia* are identical to all other gram-negative motile bacteria belonging to the Enterobacteriaceae.[6,48] Von Graevenitz and Strouse have found *Erwinia* in human wound infections.[60,61] The enterics are not fastidious and require minimal medium for growth. These organisms will grow on SBAP, MacConkey's agar (MACA), gram-negative enrichment broth (GN broth), eosin methylene blue agar (EMB), as well as nutrient agar. On MACA and EMB, lactose fermenters incorporate the dye contained in the media, while the nonlactose fermenters do not and appear colorless. Triple sugar iron agar (TSI) slants are used to further identify the enterics based on biochemical changes in the medium[6,48] (**Table 11.12**).

Table 11.12 TSI reaction for some Enterobacteriaceae

Organism	Slant	Butt	H_2S	Gas
Escherichia	A[b](K)[c]	A	–	+(–)
Citrobacter	A or K	A	V	+
K/E[a] group	A or K	A	–	+
Serratia spp.	K or A	A	–	–
Proteus vulgaris	A(K)	A	+	+
P. mirabilis	K(A)	A	+	+
M. morganii	K	A	–	–
Providencia	K	A	–	+/–
Prv. rettgeri	K	A	–	–

Butt, bottom of the test tube;
[a] *Klebsiella/Enterobacter* group; [b], acid reaction; [c], alkaline reaction; (), occasional; V, variable; –, negative; +, positive; +/–, more positive than negative.

Like the gram-positive clinical isolates, the gram-negative isolates from the burn wound are equally selective. While man's environment is overwhelmed with microbes, only a select smattering of gram-negative rods predominate which specifically include the pseudomonads and enterics. *Ps. aeruginosa* is the predominant isolate, followed by *E. coli* and the other enterics. A recent 9-month evaluation of these gram-negative pathogens, compared to a 1988–1989 study, shows essentially little or no difference in the predominating organisms. *Ps. aeruginosa* accounted for 30–40% of the gram-negative isolates (**Table 11.13**).

Miscellaneous Gram-negative Rods

Two species of gram-negative rods which are noteworthy in burn wound infections of man are *Flavobacterium meningosepticum* and *Chromobacterium violaceum*. Other members of this genera are natural inhabitants of soil, water, and vegetation; and are classified as contaminants.[6,48] *Fl. meningosepticum* is a gram-negative bacillus which is non-motile and aerobic with a strictly respiratory type of metabolism. It grows at 37°C and produces a yellow to orange

Table 11.13 Gram-negative bacteria isolated from pediatric burn wounds

Organisms	Number 1993 (9 mo.)	%	1998–1999*	%
Ps. aeruginosa	899	39.8	1591	33.6
E. coli	375	16.6	990	21.0
Kl. pneumoniae	216	9.6	714	15.1
Ent. cloacae	335	14.8	384	8.1
Ser. marcescens	53	2.3	304	6.4
Other enterics†	383	16.9	723	15.8
Total Gram-negatives	2261	100.0	4.733	100.0
Total isolates tested	5026	45.0	14 696	32.2

* Heggers JP, McCauley RL, Herndon DN. Antimicrobial therapy in burn patients: Part I. *Surgical Rounds* 1992; **July**: 613–17.
† Includes several different enterics and other pseudomonads.

pigment on solid media. It is catalase, oxidase and phosphatase positive. It produces acid from carbohydrates but no gas. It is widely distributed in soil and water, and also found in raw meats, milk, and other foods, as well as in the hospital environment and in human clinical material. Biochemical identification is displayed in **Table 11.14**. It is consistently resistant to many antibiotics. It has been isolated from burn wounds with relative inconsistency; but when isolated, it should be regarded as a pathogen. *Chr. violaceum* is also a gram-negative bacillus which is motile and produces a violet ring in nutrient broth. Its ideal growth occurs at 30–35°C and usually requires 7 days for its total growth at 37°C. On the other hand, *Fl. meningosepticum* also requires 7 days for full development; however, this can occur at room temperature. No pigment is produced at 37°C nor is there hemolysis, though the agar may exhibit a lavender/green discoloration as a result of proteolytic enzymatic activity. One major problem with this group of organisms is their natural habitat. Their close living arrangements with their human hosts give them a tactical advantage, not only for the development of tolerance, but for resistance. Misuse or abuse of parenteral or enteral antibiotics can provide an environment for the formation of resistance. Consumers of food products, generated through antibiotic feeding as well as unlicensed antibiotic usage, are prime targets for the development of resistant organisms.

Gram-negative Anaerobic Bacilli

The most repeatedly confronted organisms in the gram-negative anaerobic bacilli group which may play a fearful role in surgical and burn wound infections are *Bacteroides* spp. and *Fusobacterium* spp. They are considered normal flora of the human body, beginning at the oropharyngeal cavity and ending at the gastrointestinal and urogenital tracts. Numerically, they account for the major population in the oropharyngeal region in a 5:1 ratio over the aerobes and facultative anaerobes; while in the urogenital and gastrointestinal tract, the ratio is more dynamic at 1000:1.[2,6,15,48] Yet when one scrutinizes the current statistics of anaerobic infections related to locality, all but 2–5% of surgical wound infections occurring in the oropharyngeal area are caused by the anaerobic flora.[62] Those occurring in the gastrointestinal and urogenital tract are only responsible for about 10–15% of these wound infections.[62,63] Prior surgery, malignant neoplasms, arteriosclerosis, diabetes mellitus, prior antibiotic therapy, alcoholism, improper debridement, and steroid and immunosuppressive therapy are commonly major contributors associated with these types of wound infections.[63,64]

Specimens collected for anaerobic organisms should be placed in appropriate transport tubes void of atmospheric O_2 or should remain in syringes with attached needles containing suspect aspirates sealed off with a rubber stopper. **Table 11.15** examines some of the biochemical responses of this group of organisms. However, with the advent of the early excision and grafting the incidence of anaerobic infections in the thermal injury has been reduced to a nonentity; therefore, anaerobic cultures are uneconomical. Culturing for these anaerobes would be futile, since they require avascular tissue for survival. Their presence would only be observed if such tissue were to remain.

Fungi (Eumycetes)

Until the advent of topical antimicrobial agents, fungal infections were not common in burned patients. However, the incidence of mycotic invasion has doubled since the implementation of topical antimicrobial agents to control bacterial colonization.[65,66] The burn wound is the most commonly infected site, although local or disseminated fungal infections of the respiratory tract, urinary tract, gastrointestinal tract and vagina are increasingly common.[65,67,68] *Candida* spp. are the most common non-bacterial colonizers of the burn wound, although true fungi such as *Aspergillus*, *Penicillium*, *Rhizopus*, *Mucor*, *Rhizomucor*, *Fusarium* and *Curvularia* are not uncommon and have a much greater invasive potential than the yeast.[69–72] (**Table 11.16**).

Early diagnosis of fungal infection is difficult as clinical symptoms frequently mimic low grade bacterial infections. Routine culture techniques may require from 7 to 14 days to identify fungal contaminants; this fact delays the initiation of treatment as these pathogens are frequently not recovered in culture.[66] In contrast to bacterial sepsis, venous blood cultures may not reflect the causative organism.[72,73] Arterial blood cultures and retinal examination for characteristic candidal lesions can be useful. The isolation of candida from three organs is usually required for the diagnosis of candidal sepsis.[67] Serum antibody titers to *Candida* have recently been advocated to assist in the early diagnosis.[74] Premortem diagnosis, confirmed with sufficient time to implement appropriate treatment,

Table 11.14 Key biochemical responses for the pathogenic genera *Chromobacterium* and *Flavobacterium*

Species	Oxidase	Motility	Growth at 37°C	Indole	NO_2 to NO_3	Casein	Arginine dihydrolase	H_2S lead acetate strip	O-F media glucose maltose
Chr. violaceum	V	+	+	–	+	+	+	–/W[a]	–
Fl. meningosepticum	+	–	+	+	–	+	–	+	+

[a] = Weak reaction.
O-F, oxidation fermentation; V, Variable; +, positive; –, negative.

Table 11.15 Biochemical responses of the Bacteroidaceae

Organism	Hemolysis	Fermenter glucose	Indole	Catalase	20% Bile agar	Esculin hydrolysis	Black pigment	Kanamycin (1 MG Disc)	H_2S
Bacteroides									
distasonis	–	+	–	+	+	+	–	R	–
fragilis	–	+	–	+	+	+	–	R	–
vulgatus	–	+	–	V	+	V	–	R	–
melaninogenicus	+	+	+	–	–	–	+	R	–
Fusobacterium									
mortiferum	V	+	–	–	+	+	–	S	–
necrophorum	–	–	+	–	–	–	–	S	+
nucleaturm	Green	–	+	–	–	–	–	S	+

V, variable; R, resistant; S, sensitive; +, positive; –, negative.

Table 11.16 Colonization, infection, and invasive potential of the fungi

	Filamentous fungi	Candida
Incidence		
Colonization	2–4.4%	30–40%
Infection	1–2%	5–7%
Dissemination	1–2%	2–4%
Time of occurrence	Early	Late
Mortality		
With invasive infection	90–100%	80–100%

occurs in less than 40% of infected patients.[75] Because of their relatively large size, *Candida* are usually filtered out of blood at the capillary level. Organisms are typically seen in the urine when sepsis from a distant site occurs. Candidal sepsis is suspected when *C. albicans* can be isolated from three different tissue sites, i.e. blood, wound, urine, bronchial washings, or along retinal examination.

Candidal spores are omnipresent in the burned patient. They appear in stools, nasopharynx swabs, urine samples, and cultures of intact integument; however, fewer than 20% of patients with candidal wound colonization develop widespread candidiasis.[71,76] Only when the controlling bacterial populations are eradicated by systemic antibiotics or the host becomes immunosuppressed does candidal infection occur,[77] this frequently follows a bacterial sepsis. There is a 3–5% incidence of candidemia in the burned population[67,69,76,78] and a comparable rate of burn wound invasion.[69] Candidal infections occur most commonly in patients with large burn injuries who are hospitalized for long periods of time and receive multiple courses of antibiotics. Thus, prophylactic treatment with oropharyngeal and topical nystatin are recommended.[67] Fluconazole, however, may be a more effective treatment.

Unlike candidal infections, true fungal infections occur early in the hospital course of patients with specific predisposing characteristics. Most frequently, burned patients infected with fungi are exposed to spores in the environment by either rolling on the ground or jumping into surface water at the time of injury. Other environmental foci have been cited as sources of nosocomial fungal infection, including bandaging supplies left open to air, heating and air conditioning ducts, and floor drains.[79–81]

Once colonized, broad nonbranching hyphae extend into subcutaneous tissue and stimulate an inflammatory response. This phenomenon is diagnostic of fungal wound infection. Vascular invasion is common and often accompanied by thrombosis and avascular necrosis which are clinically observed as rapidly advancing dark discolorations of the wound margins or well described lesions.[66,70] Systemic dissemination of the infection occurs with invasion of the vasculature.

Viruses

Viral infections are being clinically recognized in burned patients with increasing frequency. Prospective and retrospective assays of sera have documented a large incidence of subclinical viral infection. Retrospectively, Linneman[82] assayed stored sera of burned children and found a fourfold increase in antibodies to cytomegalovirus (CMV) in 22% of patients, 8% had increased herpes simplex titers and 5% demonstrated a rise in varicella zoster titers. The study continued in a prospective manner, revealed that 33% of the burn injured children developed CMV infection, 25% developed herpetic infections and 17% developed adenovirus infection. These infections can be life-threatening in burn patients.

CMV infection typically occurs approximately 1 month postburn and clinically presents as a fever of unknown origin and lymphocytosis.[83] Rarely are patients with less than 50% total body surface area (TBSA) burn infected. CMV infection frequently occurs concurrently with bacterial and fungal infections, but it rarely alters the patient's clinical course. CMV inclusions may be identified in the cells of multiple organs, but they are not being found in burn wounds.[84] The burned patients who most commonly contract the infection are known to have received multiple blood transfusions which may represent a source of contamination.

Most commonly, herpetic lesions appear in healing partial-thickness burns or split-thickness donor sites, although other epithelial surfaces such as the oral or intestinal mucosa can be involved. In the latter case, herpetic lesions may lead to erosion and perforation. The clinical manifestations of lesions may be preceded by unexplained fever which is unresponsive to routine antibiotic coverage.[85] Partial-thickness burns and donor sites infected with herpes may 'convert' to full-thickness injuries requiring skin grafting for ultimate closure. Necrotizing hepatic and adrenal lesions may lead to multisystem organ failure. Mortality in patients with disseminated infection is about twice that which is expected for patients of similar age and burn size. Split-thickness grafts provide adequate coverage of previously infected herpetic wound.

Chickenpox (varicella zoster) infection is a frequent occurrence in school-aged children and is rapidly spread through inhalation of the virus. Varicella infections can be life-threatening in an immunocompromised host, and mini-epidemics have occurred within pediatric burn units.[86] The characteristic fluid-filled lesions appear in healed or healing partial-thickness burns, as well as uninjured epithelium and mucous membranes. Due to the fragility of the newly healed or healing skin, the vesicles are much more destructive in the injured than in the uninjured skin, and may present as hemorrhagic, oozing pockmarks which are prone to secondary infection and subsequent scarring. New, neovascularized skin grafts may be lost; further grafting procedures should be delayed until the lesions are quiescent. Herpes simplex and zoster are consistently treated with systemic acyclovir.

Histopathologic Approach Based on Clinical Findings

Obviously, an open wound is an easy and favorable target for bacterial colonization either from the environment or from the patient himself. This bacterial colonization indicates only the presence of microorganisms within the necrotic burn tissue. This colonization or 'contamination' of the burn wound, although potentially dangerous, does not imply an unavoidable and active, local or systemic infection. If the microorganisms actively reach viable tissue (invasion), they will produce either a local infection (septic burn wound) or a systemic hematological or lymphatic dissemination of the microorganisms themselves or its toxic products (burn wound sepsis).

Evidently, the progression from a simple eschar colonization to an invasive process is favored by a series of factors related to the patient (i.e. extension and depth of the burn, age, presence of previous disease, local conditions of the wound), the microorganism (i.e. density, motility, toxins, antimicrobial resistance), or to iatrogenic causes. Health care providers must also be aware that systemic signs of infection may be masked by metabolic dysfunctions encountered in a major burn. Therefore, it is essential to recognize the early signs of local burn wound infection. The burn wound should be examined at least once a day for signs of local wound infection[14,17,18] (**Table 11.17**).

Burn wound sepsis is suspected when a burn wound is the site of proliferating microorganisms exceeding 10^5/g tissue, and when there is invasion of subjacent unburned tissue.[28,87] The presence of microorganisms within the necrotic eschar cannot be considered evidence of burn wound sepsis; but, as a site of primary colonization, such eschar has a potential for bacterial overgrowth and invasion of viable tissue. Besides, although a bacterial count of 10^5/g of tissue or more is likely to indicate bacterial invasion, this is not invariably true. Only the histologic sections can indicate the level of infection. Both studies are usually complementary; the microbiological cultures define the type and quantity of microorganisms, and the histologic sections help define the level of infection. Therefore, burn wound cultures should always be accompanied by histologic sections from the same area.[88,89]

It is strongly advised that a continuous monitoring of the burn wound be conducted to determine the possibility of bacterial metastasis. The burned and unburned areas should be inspected daily for the presence of hemorrhagic, vesicular or necrotic areas, and for gray, dark brown, or black spots as well as other unusual changes (**Table 11.17**). The suspected areas should be biopsied and the sample subjected to microbiological cultures and histopathologic studies. The specimens for both laboratories should be taken from adjacent areas (one biopsy sample divided in half usually suffices). The only requisite is that the specimen for histology must include surrounding viable tissue (**Figure 11.1a,b**).

At least two methods are likely to ensure rapid histologic sections with minimum distortion. In the SBI–Galveston laboratory, we use either one:

- *56°C oven*. The fixation and embedding are performed with preheated solutions (total time, about 2.5 hours).
  1. 10% Formalin–buffer 20 min.
  2. 70% Alcohol 15 min.
  3. 95% Alcohol 15 min.
  4. Absolute alcohol 15 min.
  5. Xylene 15 min.
  6. Paraffin 20 min.
  7. Microtomization at 4–5 μm
  8. Stains: hematoxylin–eosin (general structure), McCallum–Goodpasture or similar for bacteria, and PAS or Groccott for fungal elements.[90]
- *Microwave* (specimens 1–2 mm in thickness; total time, about 1 hour).
  1. Normal saline, 135°F 2 min.
  2. Ethyl alcohol, 150°F 7–8 min.
  3. Isopropanol, 165°F 6 min.
  4. Paraffin, 150°F 3 min.
  5. Paraffin, 180°F 10 min.
  6. Microtomization and stains similar to oven method.

The evaluation of sepsis should include microbiological and histopathologic findings along with the clinical assessment of the patient. Blood cultures may be negative or the cultured organisms may be altered due to antibiotic therapy. The burn wound biopsy is a valuable procedure as it can also detect other local or systemic complications and uncover the presence of fungal or viral infections, usually seen or suspected without major difficulties in hematoxylin–eosin sections (**Figure 11.2a,b,c,d**). These infections have a low yield of culture isolation, require a specific technique for detection, and are frequent laboratory contaminants; thus, without the benefit of wound biopsy, these infections are difficult to recognize early.

The histologic diagnosis of burn wound sepsis requires precise differentiation between tissue necrosis due to thermal injury and that due to invading microorganisms. The presence of polymorphonuclear leukocytes is not always indicative of infection as they may accumulate and persist in the aseptic wound. If a viral infection is suspected, a Tzanck smear is very valuable and simple to perform.[91] The material from the suspected lesion is smeared on a microscopic slide and stained with methylene blue, Wright's, or Giemsa stain. The smear is examined under high power (400×) for the presence of multinucleated giant cells. This procedure can diagnose a herpes infection (**Figure 11.2d**). The likelihood of infection and invasion increases with burn depth. The morphologic sequence includes the presence of microorganisms over the surface and burn

Table 11.17 Burn wound infection: local signs*

Black or dark brown focal areas of discoloration
Enhanced sloughing of burned tissue or eschar
Partial-thickness injury converted to full-thickness necrosis
Purplish discoloration or edema of skin around the margins of the wound
Presence of ecthyma gangrenosa
Pyocyanotic appearance of subeschar tissue
Subcutaneous tissue with hemorrhagic discoloration
Variable-sized abscess formation and focal subeschar inconsistency

* Reproduced with permission from Heggers J P, Robson M C. Infection control in burn patients. *Clin Plas Surg* 1986; **13:** 39–47.

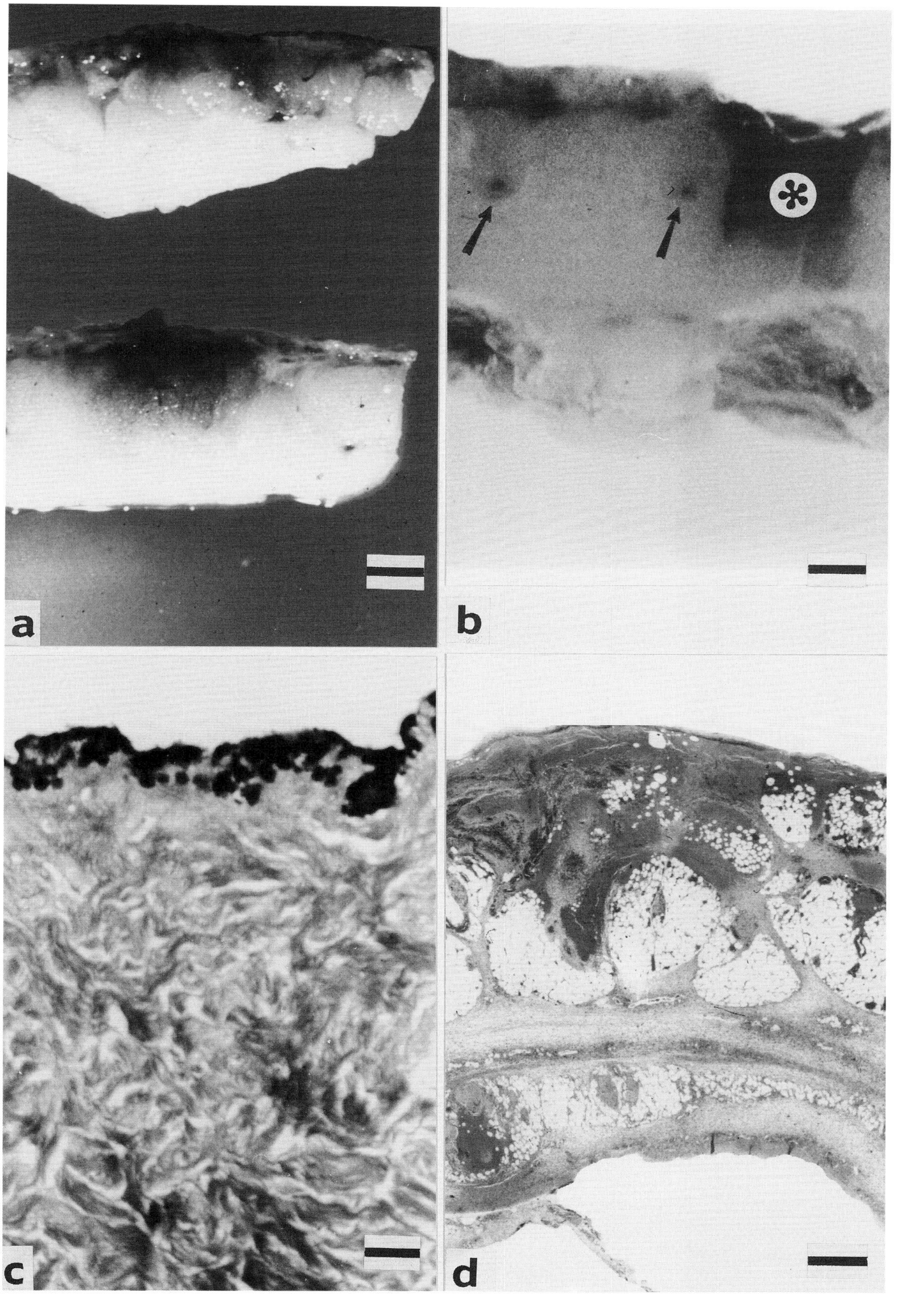

Fig. 11.1 Burn wound infection. (a) Discoloration of the subcutaneous tissue associated with Pseudomonas *sp. invasion of viable tissue in a full-thickness burn. Gross anatomy. Bar = 3 mm. (b) Burn wound infection with bacterial vasculitis (arrows). The asterisk indicates the site of the punch biopsy. Note that the lower level of the punch biopsy reaches the viable tissue beyond the vasculitis level. Gross anatomy. Bar = 2 mm. (c) Superficial bacterial colonization (black discoloration). Gram stain. Bar = 50 μm. (d) Sections of skin showing necrosis and bacterial invasion reaching subcutaneous adipose tissue. Gram stain. Bar = 500 μm.*

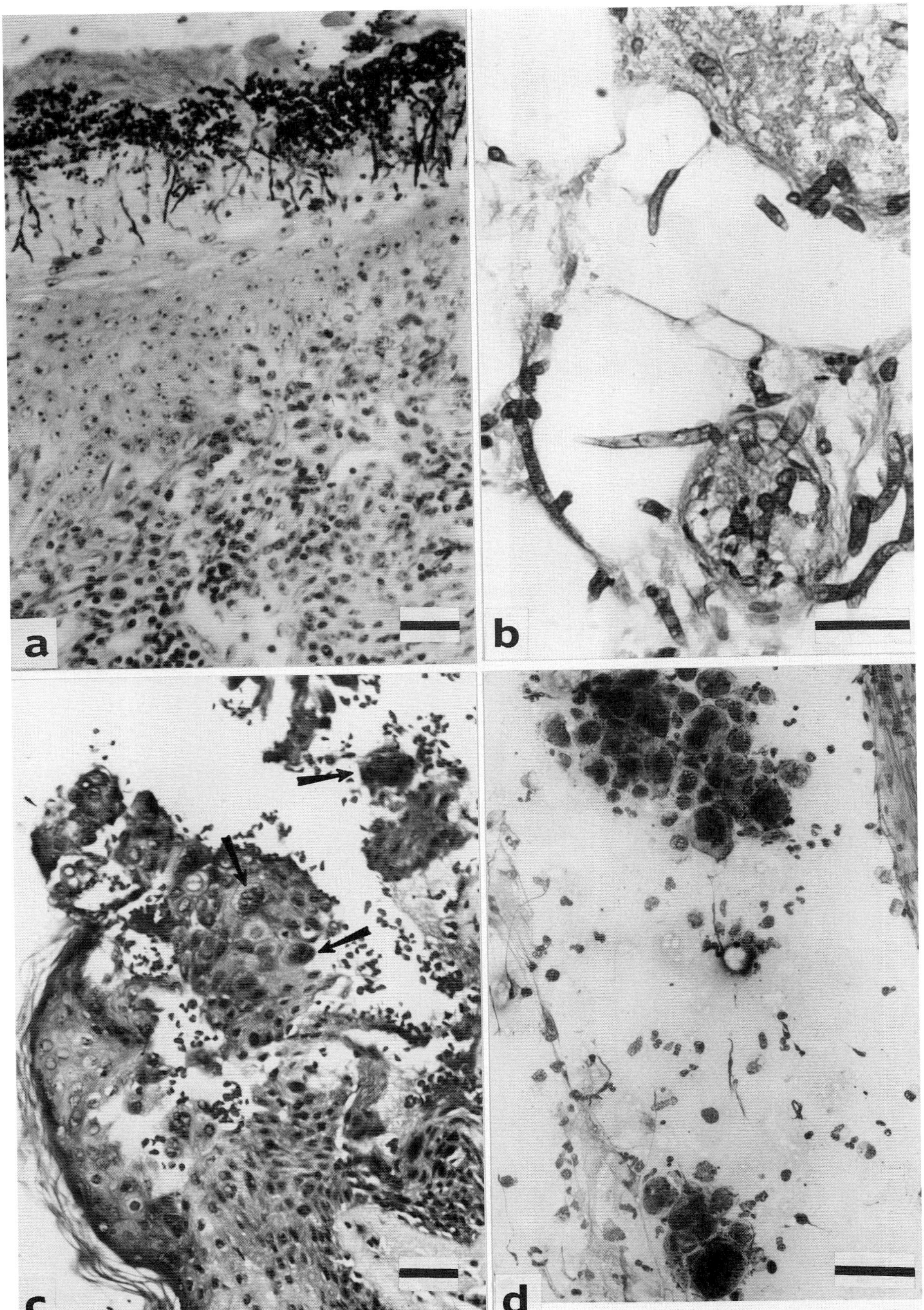

Fig. 11.2 Burn wound infection. (a) Superficial fungal colonization involving superficial areas of epidermis. PAS stain. Bar = 50 μm. (b) Fungal invasion of subcutaneous adipose tissue. PAS stain. Bar = 50 μm. (c) Herpes virus infection. The arrows indicate some inclusion bodies. HE stain. Bar = 50 μm. (d) Herpes virus infection. Tzanck smear. Bar = 50 μm.

eschar (colonization), within the surrounding viable tissue (invasion), and within vessels with or without systemic spread (**Figure 11.1c, d**).

Clinical Findings

The clinical diagnosis of sepsis can be made when clinical symptoms appear and a septic source can be identified. There are several cardinal signs of sepsis which embody both gram-negative and gram-positive involvement (**Table 11.18**). Constant surveillance of these signs can provide adjunctive information concerning the etiologic agent of sepsis. A septic source can be documented via:

- burn wound biopsy with $>10^5$ organism/g tissue and/or histologic evidence of viable tissue invasion;
- positive blood culture;
- urinary tract infection with $>10^5$ organisms/ml urine; and
- pulmonary infection with positive bacteria and white cells on a class III or better sputum specimen.

In addition to the identification of a septic source, at least five or more of the following criteria should be met: tachypnea (>40 breaths/min in adults), prolonged paralytic ileus, hyper- or hypothermia (<36.5° or > 38.5°C), altered mental status, thrombocytopenia (<50 000 platelets/mm^3), leukocytosis or leukopenia (<3.5 or > 15.0 cells/mm^3), unexplained acidosis, or hyperglycemia. Local evidence of invasive wound infection includes black or brown patches of wound discoloration, rapid eschar separation, conversion of wounds to full thickness, spreading periwound erythema, punctate, hemorrhagic subeschar lesions, and violaceous or black lesions in unburned tissue (ecthyma gangrenosum) (**Table 11.17**). When a patient exhibits signs and symptoms of sepsis, immediate institution of antibiotics is obligatory irrespective of the absence of confirmatory cultures. A delay of 3–4 days in patients with major burn wounds results in an inordinately high morbidity. Specific antibiotic treatment should be administered if routine surveillance has identified the predominant organism (**Figures 11.3, 11.4, 11.5, 11.6a,b**).

Table 11.18 Additional cardinal signs of burn wound sepsis*

Gram-negative sepsis
Burn wound biopsy $>10^5$ organisms/g tissue and/or histologic evidence of viable tissue invasion
Rapid onset – well to ill in 8–12 hours
Increased temperature to 100–103°F (38°–39°C) or may remain within normal limits (37°C)
WBC may be increased
Followed by hypothermia – 94°F (34°–35°C) plus a decrease in WBC
Decreased bowel sounds (ileus)
Decreased BP and urinary output
Wounds develop focal gangrene
Satellite lesions away from burn wound
Mental obtundation
Gram-positive sepsis
Burn wound biopsy $>10^5$ organisms/g tissue and/or histologic evidence of viable tissue invasion
Symptoms develop gradually
Increased temperature to 105°F or higher (>40°C)
WBC 20 000–50 000
Decreased hematocrit
Wound macerated in appearance, ropy and tenacious exudate
Anorexic and irrational
Decreased bowel sounds (ileus)
Decreased BP and urinary output

* Five or more signs or symptoms are definitive diagnostic parameters.

Subacute Bacterial Endocarditis

Bacteremia associated with burn wound manipulations as well as such procedures as tooth extraction, endotracheal intubation, and sigmoidoscopy can be transient.[92,93] In healthy patients, transient bacterial showers are of little consequence. However, patients with a prior history of valvular heart disease are prone to the development of valvular vegetations. Burned patients, even those who were young, healthy adults prior to injury, develop a generalized immunosuppression and experience a significant number of invasive procedures which may increase the risk for endocarditis. The incidence of bacterial endocarditis appears to be increasing as we become more adept at treating major burn injuries; however, its development is usually occult and, like suppurative thrombophlebitis, it is frequently not noted until there are persistent positive blood cultures.[94]

Patients whose risk factor is high for the development of bacterial endocarditis are those with repetitive bacteremias, which may occur after continual instrumentation or surgical intervention. These patients should be closely monitored for the development of heart murmurs, and, if found, should undergo echocardiography to determine the presence of vegetations. Blood cultures should be randomly taken for 72 hours; then appropriate broad spectrum antibiotics should be initiated and continued for the next 6 weeks.

Cannula Infections and Suppurative Thrombophlebitis

Infectious complications associated with intravenous and intra-arterial catheters represent a major problem irrespective of the constant attention to aseptic technique for insertion and appropriate maintenance.[94] The burned patient appears to be especially susceptible to this complication. Catheter infection rates have been reported ranging from 8 to 57%.[95,96] Suppurative thrombophlebitis may be confirmed in up to 5% of patients hospitalized for burns over 20% TBSA.[97]

A recent prospective study documented a high correlation between organisms cultured from the catheter tips and the catheter hubs within 48 hours of insertion and the incidence of catheter infection; that correlation was inversely proportional to the distance of the insertion site from the burn wound.[98] It is interesting to note that the bacteria cultured from infected catheters could be traced to the skin in 96% of the cases. These data tend to support the hypothesis that catheter infections primarily arise from burn wound contaminants migrating down the catheter to the tip. Strict aseptic technique for insertion of intravascular catheters, the use of Teflon catheters, and rotation of the catheter site, tubing and apparatus every 72 hours have been associated with a decrease in catheter infection rates.[99–101]

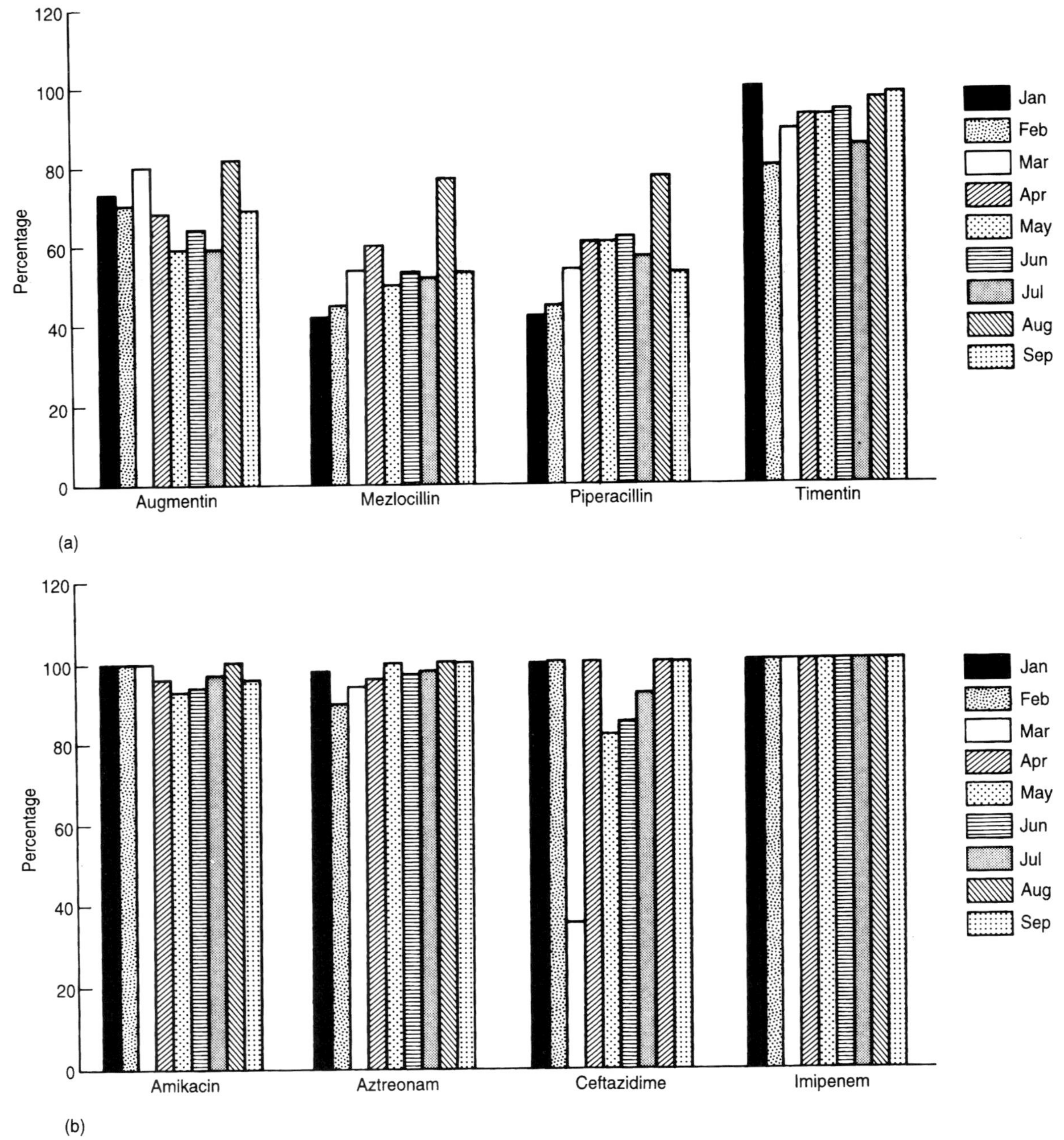

Fig. 11.3 (a) Susceptibility patterns for E. coli *against extended spectrum penicillins and (b) against amikacin and miscellaneous β-lactam antibiotics.*

Suppurative thrombophlebitis should be suspected in those patients who have persistent positive blood cultures without signs of local infection. Often suppuration can occur after the time of catheter removal so cultures at the time of removal may be an unreliable predictor of infection. Gross clinical signs of suppurative thrombophlebitis are frequently not present.[102] Careful records of previously cannulated sites can allow for sequential venotomy and examination for ultraluminal pus along with histologic examination for intimal colonization. Upon confirmation of the diagnosis, immediate operative excision is essential to prevent progressive sepsis. Entire excision of a vein to the port of entry into the central circulation may be required because of the tendency of phlebitis to spring to vein valves and leave an apparently normal vein in between infected foci. The subcutaneous tissue and skin should be packed open where a grossly purulent vein is removed and allowed to granulate and close by secondary intention.

Suppurative Chondritis

Burns to the ear represent a clinical management challenge. Full-thickness injuries can injure the cartilage of the ear, resulting in autoamputation of a part or the entirety of the external auricle. Because of the auricle's comparatively low blood supply, chondritis frequently follows the progression of tissue ischemia. Chondritis is usually seen 3–5 weeks following a burn injury but it may be seen earlier and may occur following partial- and full-thickness injuries. Since the introduction of mafenide acetate, which has become the topical agent of choice for burned cartilaginous surfaces, and subsequent to the proliferation of its use, the incidence of suppurative chondritis has significantly decreased.

Characteristically, the patient complains of dull pain. The ear becomes warm, red, tender, and edematous. Appropriate antibiotics

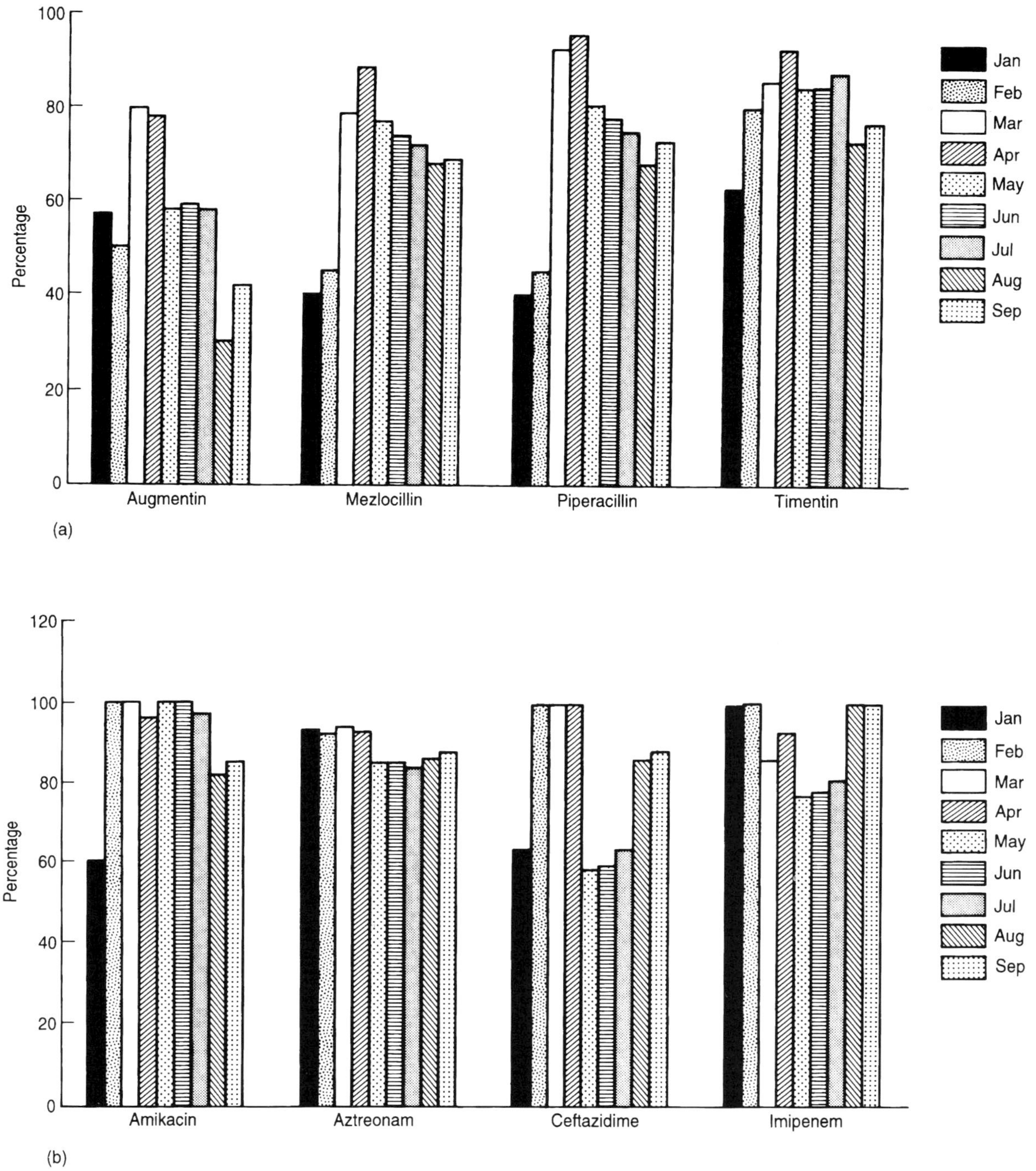

Fig. 11.4 (a) Susceptibility patterns for Kl. pneumoniae *against extended spectrum penicillins and (b) against amikacin and miscellaneous β-lactam antibiotics.*

should be initiated immediately; if there is an identifiable site, immediate incision and drainage of the abscess should be undertaken and culture and sensitivity should be obtained. Should induration and tenderness continue, a more extensive debridement is imperative. Generally the helix is bivalved at the posterior helical margin and all necrotic cartilage is debrided. Difficulty may arise in distinguishing between viable and necrotic tissue; frequently, normal cartilage is sacrificed in order to ensure debridement. Infected cartilage is usually soft, while normal cartilage will feel granular on curettage. If appropriate and adequate excision of the necrotic tissue is not performed, suppurative chondritis can proceed to invade the mastoid bone, thereby creating a potential for intracranial abscess formation.

Suppurative Sinusitis

An infection of the sinuses has become more prevalent recently because of constant long-term transnasal intubation and the use of nasogastric or nasoduodenum tubes for enteral feeding. The diagnosis is usually delayed due to clinically inapparent symptoms; and only after more frequent causes of fever are ruled out does it become evident. Diagnosis is confirmed based on studies. Therapy with broad spectrum antibiotics is initiated; however, surgical drainage of the involved sinuses may be necessary if the infection is unresponsive to the antibiotics. Oral intubation and orogastric feeding may be utilized as a temporary measure; but, if sinusitis becomes complicated and if prolonged

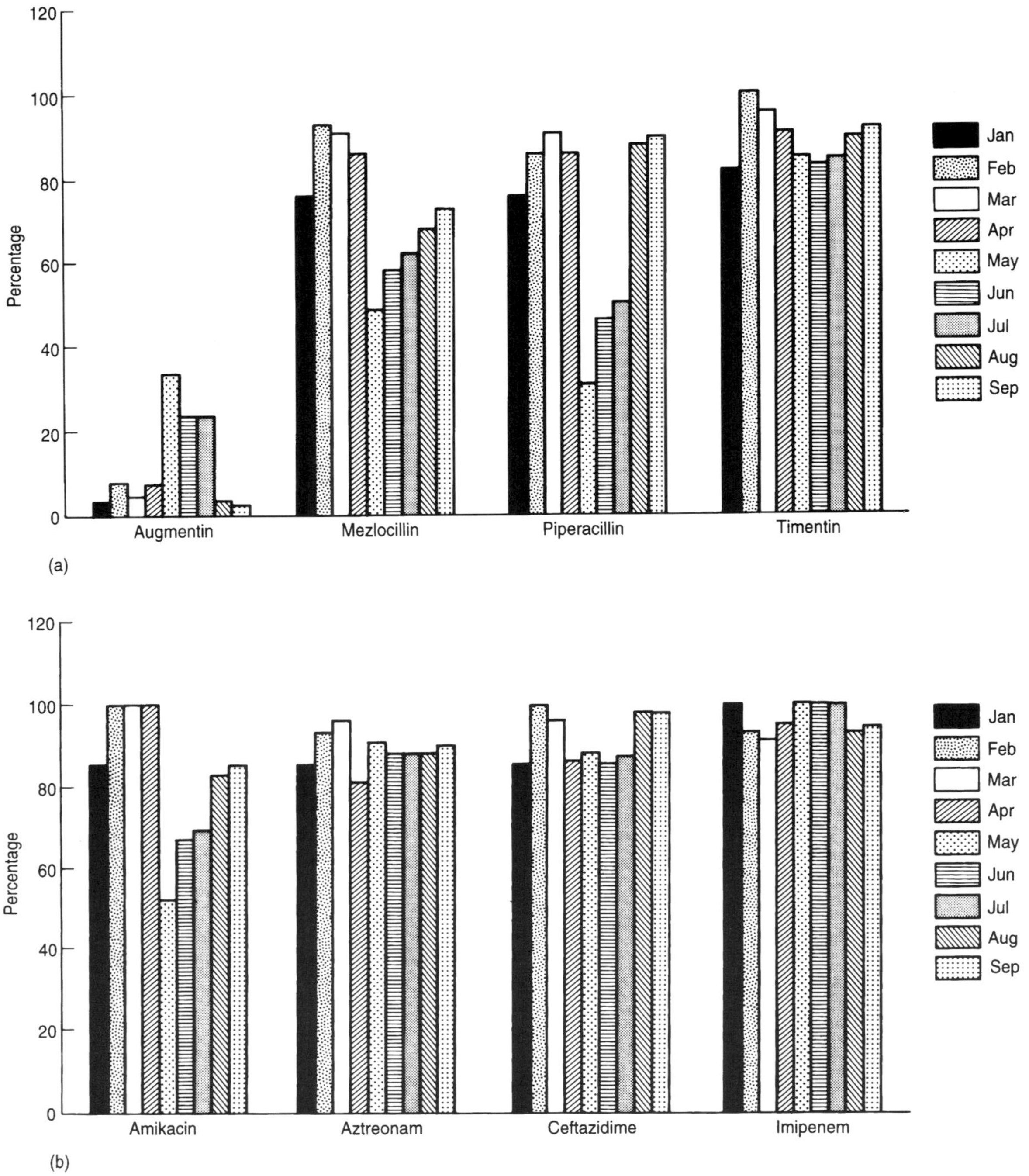

Fig. 11.5 (a) Susceptibility patterns for Ent. cloacae *against extended spectrum penicillins and (b) against amikacin and miscellaneous β-lactam antibiotics.*

treatment is necessary, then a tracheostomy and/or gastrostomy is indicated.

Pneumonia

Pneumonia is the septic complication most frequently encountered in all critically ill patients; and air-borne pneumonia, or bronchopneumonia, is the most common type of pulmonary sepsis. This form of pneumonia occurs relatively early (usually in the second postburn week) and begins as a bronchiolitis secondary to bacterial entry into the tracheobronchial tree with spread of infection to adjacent alveoli in a non-random manner involving the dependent portions of the lung. The causative organisms reflect the flora of the burn wound. Predisposing factors appear to include: burn size; the occurrence of aspiration; the presence of a tracheotomy or nasotracheal tube; the existence of inhalation injury; or the manifestations of other complications such as septicemia and disturbances of fluid and electrolyte balance.[103] Of these factors, physicians have the most control over infections related to tracheostomy and nasotracheal tubes.

The performance of a tracheostomy or the placement of a nasotracheal tube in a burned patient is associated with a high incidence of necrotizing ulcerative tracheobronchitis, with the occurrence rate being greater in the case of tracheostomy. The tracheobronchial infection is a result of both mechanical trauma to the tracheal wall by either the tip of the endotracheal tube or the tube cuff and the flora of the burn wound, which readily gain access to the tracheobronchial tree.

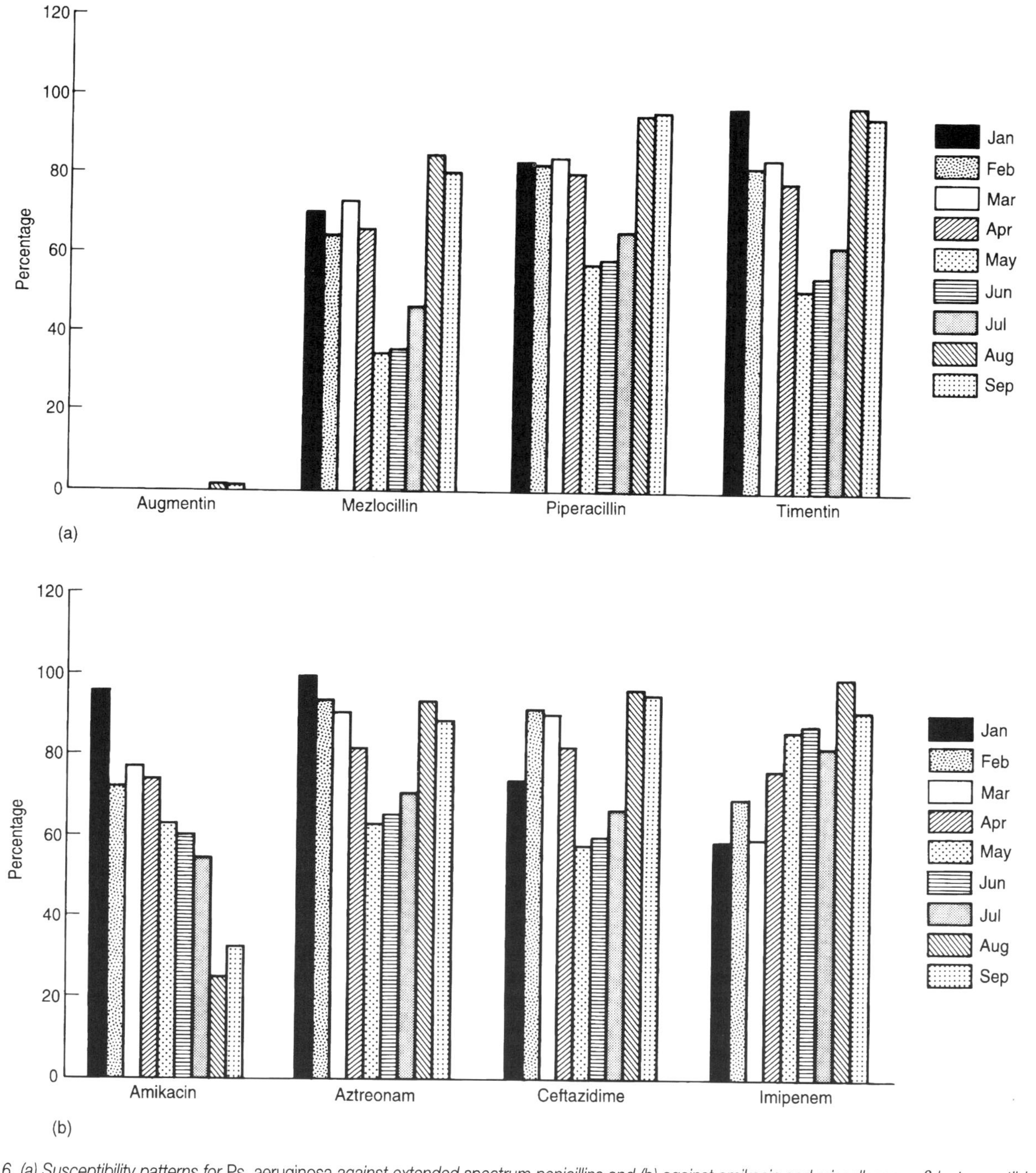

Fig. 11.6 (a) Susceptibility patterns for Ps. aeruginosa *against extended spectrum penicillins and (b) against amikacin and miscellaneous β-lactam antibiotics.*

A mucosal and mural infection may spread distally to involve alveoli and cause bronchopneumonia. Bronchopneumonia is associated with a lower mortality than is hematogenous pneumonia, but in patients dying with this form of pneumonia it is frequently the principal cause of death. This septic complication can be minimized by meticulous aseptic tracheobronchial toilet, by use of effective gastric decompression to prevent emesis and aspiration during periods of ileus, and by limiting endotracheal intubation and the duration of intubation to those patients with specific indications. Lung function should be monitored on a scheduled basis in all patients with extensive burns, particularly those with inhalation injury, and daily roentgenograms of the chest should be obtained. When a pulmonary infiltrate characteristic of bronchopneumonia is identified on a chest roentgenogram, an endobronchial culture should be obtained by the Luken's tube technique. Inhalation therapy should be intensified, and antibiotic therapy should be started with the agent which shows greatest effectiveness against the predominant organism, as determined by a bacterial surveillance program.

A solitary infiltrate occurring relatively late in the postburn course is the usual presenting sign; if the primary infection remains unidentified and untreated, then multiple infiltrates may appear in a random distribution related to the pulmonary vasculature. Late appearing pulmonary infiltrates, particularly a solitary infiltrate, and simultaneous recovery of a positive blood culture necessitate a search for an extrapulmonary site of infection. Sources of hematogenous pneumonia include: a burn wound which has developed invasive infection, previously cannulated veins in which suppurative thrombophlebitis has developed; inapparent perforation of a viscus, such as a posteriorly penetrating

Curling's ulcer; and occult soft tissue infections, such as an injection site abscess. The primary source of infection must be treated; the patient must be given systemic antibiotics to which the causative organism is sensitive; respiratory function should be supported if it is necessary.[10]

Sputum examination

Microscopic examination and culture of expectorated sputum remain the mainstays of the laboratory evaluation of pneumonia. Procurement of expectorated sputum is a noninvasive technique which can be carried out at no risk to the patient, and provides samples of lower respiratory tract secretions for immediate evaluation. In the majority of cases, this allows the clinician to make a presumptive diagnosis. Examination of the sputum should include observation of the color, amount, consistency, and odor of the specimen. Mucopurulent sputum is most commonly found with bacterial pneumonia or bronchitis. Scant or watery sputum is more often noted in cases of viral and other atypical pneumonias. 'Rusty' sputum suggests alveolar involvement and has been most commonly associated with pneumococcal pneumonia. Dark red, mucoid sputum suggests Friedländer's pneumonia caused by encapsulated *Kl. pneumoniae* (**Plate 4**). Foul-smelling sputum is associated with mixed anaerobic infections most commonly seen with aspiration.[11]

In all cases of acute pneumonia, a Gram stain of the sputum should be prepared. In order to maximize the diagnostic yield of the sputum examination, only samples free of oropharyngeal contamination should be reviewed. As a guide, the number of neutrophils and epithelial cells should be quantitated under low power (100×), with further examination reserved for samples containing >25 neutrophils and <10 epithelial cells. Such samples contain minimal oropharyngeal contamination. Samples with more epithelial cells and fewer neutrophils are nondiagnostic and should be discarded. The morphologic and staining characteristics of any bacteria seen should be recorded and an estimate made of the predominant organisms. Where no bacterial predominance exists, this should be noted as well. The sputum Gram stain also is helpful in identifying organisms other than the pneumococcus. Small gram-negative coccobacillary organisms are characteristic of *H. influenzae*. Staphylococci appear as gram-positive cocci in tetrads and grape-like clusters (**Plate 5**). Organisms of mixed morphology are characteristic of anaerobic infection Few bacteria are seen with Legionnaire's disease, mycoplasma pneumonia, and viral pneumonia.

Urinary Tract Infections

Urinary tract infections are usually associated with prolonged and often unnecessary catheterization. It is seldom essential to leave a catheter in place for more than a few days; this device is often misused in cases involving burned patients. Routine monitoring of urine from indwelling catheters should be done by needle aspirates through the rubber catheter with a 25 gauge needle on a regular basis two to three times a week (**Figures 11.7** and **11.8**). It is the practice at SBI-Galveston not to use antimicrobial irrigations to prevent urinary tract infections, because it appears that they are not particularly effective and may lead to infection by antibiotic-resistant organisms. When infections occur, patients should be treated with appropriate systemic antibiotics. Candiduria is often insignificant; but it may reflect an active infection or septicemia, especially when mycelia can be detected. When present, an active infection with *Candida* species usually responds to low doses of amphotericin B or fluconazole.

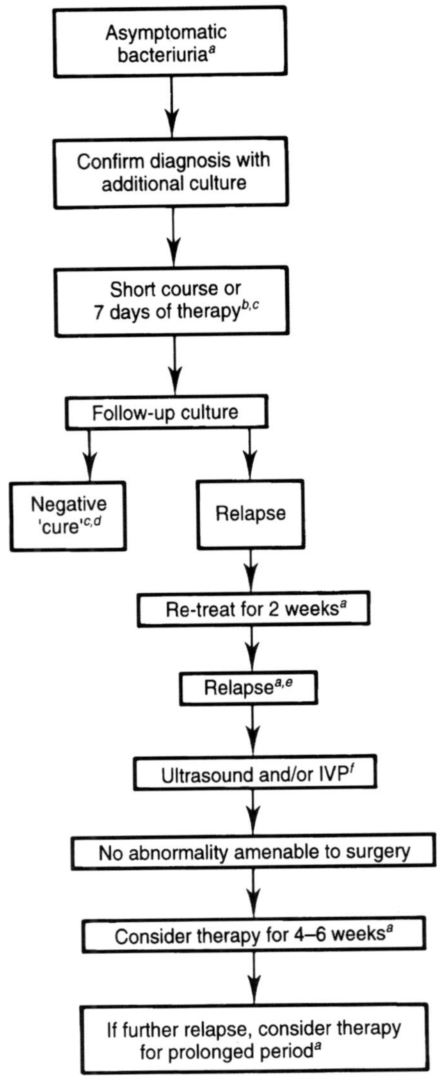

Fig. 11.7 Management of asymptomatic bacteriuria. [a] *Consider no therapy in nonpregnant adults without obstructive uropathy or symptoms of urinary tract infection.* [b] *Consider ultrasound and/or intravenous pyelogram (IVP) in all children and men with correction of significant lesions.* [c] *Follow-up culture required only in pregnancy, in children, and in adults with obstructive uropathy.* [d] *Follow-up cultures monthly in pregnant women and at 6 weeks and 6 months in children.* [e] *Evaluate men for chronic bacterial prostatitis.* [f] *Delay 2 months postpartum in pregnant women.* [g] *Consider ultrasound and/or IVP after three to four reinfections.*

Sources of Intra-abdominal Infections

Regional enteritis

The onset of regional enteritis may be acute, especially in the young, and can mimic acute appendicitis. The correct diagnosis of early regional enteritis can be made only at the time of surgery, which reveals a thickened bowel wall and mesenteric lymph node involvement. The final diagnosis is usually established by contrast radiography. Perforation as the result of an ulcer burrowing through the entire thickness of the bowel wall may occur. Usually the perforation is confined and may result in abscesses or internal fistulas. Rarely does the ulcer perforate freely into the peritoneal cavity. Perianal or perirectal abscesses and fistulas are also common manifestations of regional enteritis. Systemic antibiotics are often of

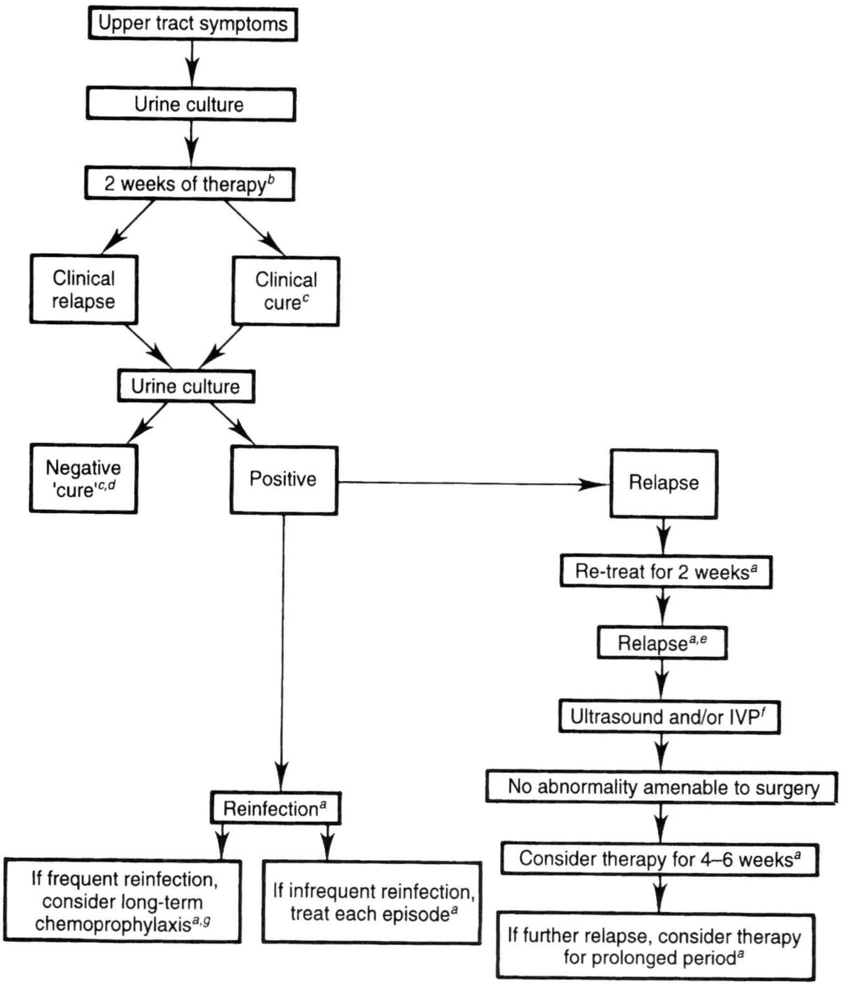

Fig. 11.8 Management of upper urinary tract infections. [a] *Consider no therapy in nonpregnant adults without obstructive uropathy or symptoms of urinary tract infection.* [b] *Consider ultrasound and/or intravenous pyelogram (IVP) in all children and men with correction of significant lesions.* [c] *Follow-up culture required only in pregnancy, in children, and in adults with obstructive uropathy.* [d] *Follow-up cultures monthly in pregnant* women and at 6 weeks and 6 months in children. [e] Evaluate men for chronic bacterial prostatitis. [f] Delay 2 months postpartum in pregnant women. [g] *Consider ultrasound and/or IVP after three to four reinfections.*

value in the management of suppurative complications. Surgery is indicated to drain abdominal abscesses, to correct fistulas, and to treat free perforations. The principal complications of surgery are enterocutaneous fistula, intraperitoneal or wound sepsis, and prolonged postoperative ileus.

Necrotizing enterocolitis in neutropenic patients

Necrotizing enterocolitis occurs in patients who are severely granulocytopenic from any cause. Left upper quadrant abdominal pain is usual. Irritation of the adjacent diaphragm may result in pain referred to the left shoulder. Splenic enlargement and tenderness are often present along with high, spiking temperatures. Radiographic examination may reveal an elevated left hemidiaphragm, basilar pulmonary infiltrates, atelectasis, or a left pleural effusion. Shift of the colon and stomach down and to the right, and extra intestinal gas, either diffusely mottled or producing an air–fluid level in the left upper quadrant, may also be observed. Ultrasonography, computed tomography, and MRI are the preferred diagnostic techniques for the evaluation of suspected splenic abscess. Initial antibiotic therapy should have a broad spectrum of activity. A combination of antibiotics which can act against streptococci as well as both aerobic and anaerobic gram-negative bacilli would be appropriate as initial antimicrobial therapy.

Acute cholecystitis

Acute cholecystitis is usually superimposed on a histologic picture of chronic cholecystitis. Ninety-five percent of all the gallbladders removed for acute cholecystitis exhibit fibrosis, flattening of the mucosa, and clusters of chronic inflammatory cells as sequelae of previous disease. Rokitansky–Aschoff sinuses are present in more than half of the cases. These sinuses represent mucosal herniations presumably related to increased hydrostatic pressure during previous episodes of cystic duct obstruction. The early acute changes may be only edema and venous congestion. These changes are followed by focal necrosis and an influx of neutrophils as secondary bacterial proliferation occurs. Actual gangrene or perforation may also follow (**Figure 11.9**). Immediate surgery is indicated for gangrenous cholecystitis, perforation with peritonitis, and suspected pericholecystic abscess. In these patients, cholecystectomy with intraoperative cholangiography is the procedure of choice.

Initial obstruction of the cystic duct may be accompanied by a mild epigastric pain followed by reflex nausea and vomiting. If the obstruction is transient, these symptoms subside within 1–2 hours.

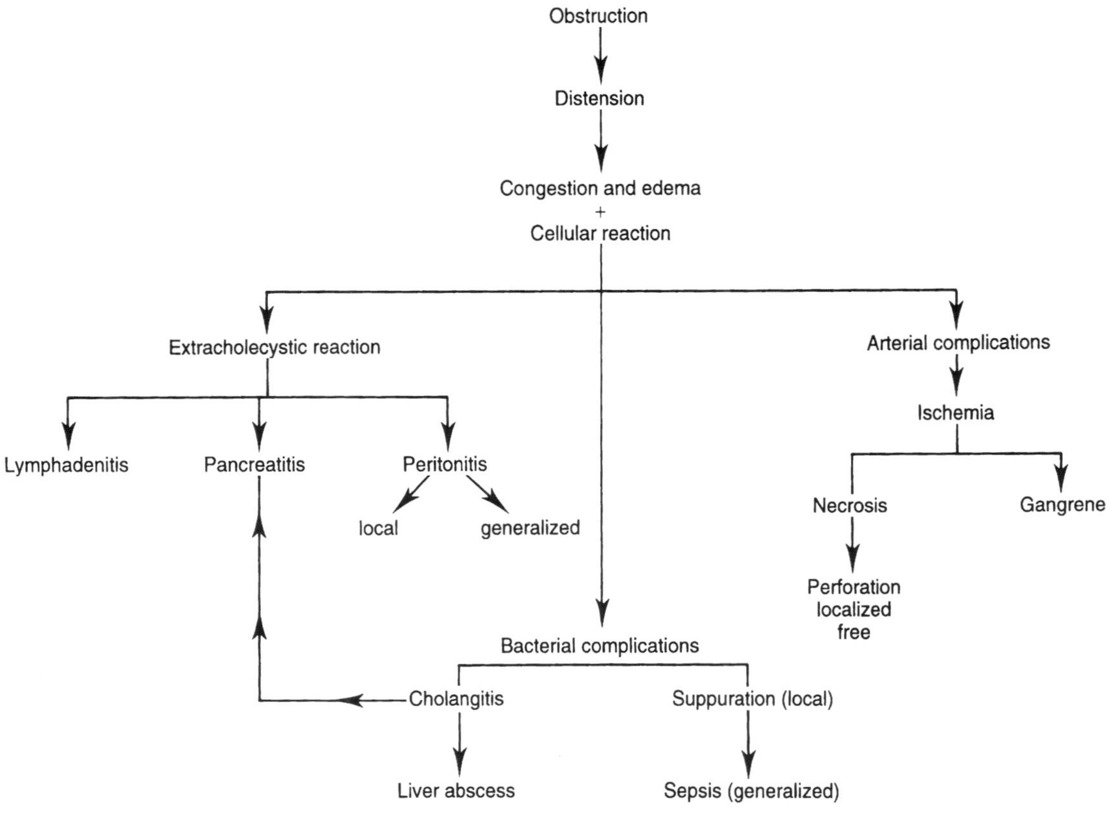

Fig. 11.9 Pathogenesis of acute cholecystitis.

With persistent obstruction, the symptoms of acute cholecystitis evolve. Pain shifts to the right upper quadrant and becomes increasingly severe. Signs of peritoneal irritation may be present and, in a small number of patients, the pain may radiate to the right shoulder or scapula. The gallbladder is palpable in 30–40% of these cases. Moderate temperature elevations and minimal icterus occur in two-thirds of patients. Notably, repeated chills and fever, jaundice, or hypotension could suggest suppurative cholangitis appearing as a consequence of common duct obstruction. Most patients with acute cholecystitis experience a complete remission within 1–4 days. However, approximately 25–30% of patients require surgery or develop some complication.

In the presence of cholecystitis and cholelithiasis, appreciable numbers of various bacteria may be found in the bile and walls of the gallbladder, even in the absence of symptoms. Organisms found in the biliary tract are commonly the same as the normal intestinal flora: namely, the enteric gram-negative bacilli, including *E. coli, Klebsiella/Enterobacter*, and *Proteus* spp. as well as the enterococci. In addition, recent studies have demonstrated the frequent presence of anaerobic organisms including *Bacteroides*, *Clostridium*, and *Fusobacterium* spp. When present, these anaerobes are often involved in polymicrobic infections or mixed with other anaerobes and aerobic gram-negative bacilli.

An appropriate initial antibiotic regimen includes an aminoglycoside (gentamicin or tobramycin) or a cephalosporin in addition to an agent such as clindamycin or metronidazole, to treat for *Bacteroides fragilis*. Available evidence suggests that perioperative antibiotics provide a useful adjunct to surgery as preventative measures for postoperative infectious complications. Because wound infection is thought to be due to contamination of an incision with infected bile at the time of operation, prophylactic antibiotics should be given in a manner which will achieve high blood and tissue concentrations at the time of surgery.

Cholangitis

Cholangitis can be defined to encompass varying degrees of inflammation and/or infection involving hepatic and common bile ducts. Since the mucosa of the gallbladder is contiguous with the common bile duct via the cystic duct, it is not surprising that varying degrees of choledochitis occur as a limited cholangitis with cholecystitis. In fact, specimens of the common duct taken at the time of cholecystectomy for acute cholecystitis usually show localized edema and inflammation. In most cases, cholangitis is indistinguishable from uncomplicated acute cholecystitis.

In a manner similar to that described for cholecystitis, obstruction of the common duct results in increased pressure, edema, congestion, and necrosis of the walls of the biliary tree followed by rapid proliferation of bacteria within the biliary tree. In most instances, obstruction is due to gallstones; however, obstruction may be due to prior biliary tract surgery, tumor, chronic calcific pancreatitis, or parasitic infections. The onset is usually acute, with high fever, chills, and diffuse pain and tenderness over the liver. Jaundice is usually prominent. In some cases, shock and other findings of gram-negative bacteremia may be present. Collectively 85% of the patients fulfill Charcot's triad of fever, chills, and jaundice. There is usually marked leukocytosis with an increase in immature forms. The serum bilirubin level is often higher than 4 mg/dl and the serum alkaline phosphatase level is significantly higher than that encountered in acute cholecystitis. Biochemical and even clinical evidence of disseminated intravascular coagulation may be present.

Recent studies using detailed aerobic and anaerobic culture techniques suggest that the bacteriological findings in cholangitis are similar to those in acute obstructive cholecystitis. Gram-negative enteric bacilli and anaerobic bacteria are the most common isolates. Unlike uncomplicated cholecystitis, bacteremia occurs in approximately 50% of the cases. Bacteremia and shock occur commonly and are included as part of the clinical picture of obstructive cholangitis.

Prompt institution of appropriate antibiotic therapy is mandatory, since these severe infections are frequently complicated by bacteremia and shock. Based on the bacteriological findings described above and on knowledge of *in vitro* susceptibilities of these organisms, an appropriate regimen would consist of clindamycin or metronidazole plus an aminoglycoside or cephalosporin antibiotic. Prompt operative intervention with decompression of the common duct is mandatory in all but those few patients who respond promptly to antibiotics.

Infection Control Programs

The major involvement of local burn wound sites in sepsis suggests that the diagnosis and treatment of such infections should focus primarily on the burn wound. Wound colonization will progress to infection only when the surface bacterial counts exceed a critical level. Accurate quantification of the burned patient's bacterial load is therefore the foundation of infection surveillance. This is achieved through routine cultures of sputum, urine, and wounds. Quantitative cultures obtained on a routine basis will monitor the progress of bacterial colonization, provide guidance in the event empirical antibiotic therapy becomes necessary, and also will allow for prompt intervention against bacterial invasion. Cultures of sputum, urine, and wounds should be obtained three times weekly. At SBI-Galveston, physicians routinely biopsy any adherent eschar and use swab cultures for other open wounds.

It is impractical to define all of the major advances which have been made in controlling the complication of burn wound infection. Evidence of such progress includes a general acceptance that the burn wound serves as the site of primary invasion for the majority of instances of local or generalized infection.[28,87] This is primarily because burned skin has lost its defensive properties. Infection control for burned patients is an enormous task which must be considered as a individual entity and not looked upon simply as the control of burn infections. Major burn wounds usually become infected within 3–5 days after admission, so it is obvious that the infection arises from the patient's own bacterial flora and is not an exogenous occurrence. This controversial concept repeatedly causes conflicts among hospital practitioners of infection control and members of burn care teams.

To promote infection control in a burn patient population, burn wounds must be recognized as sites of microbial colonization which may progress to invasion with systemic dissemination if not restrained. Further recognition that this colonization initially arises from the patient's own resident and transient bacteria is sovereign.[4,28,87,104–106] Although bacteria may not normally be recovered from the skin surface nor from the sweat glands, they can be identified in the hair follicles, particularly near the orifices of sebaceous glands. Bacteria of normal endogenous skin flora are resistant to heat injury to practically the same degree as are the skin cells. The bacteria on the surface are heat killed as are the tissue cells of the surface; and initial swab cultures are usually sterile. However, the bacteria in the hair follicles and sebaceous glands may survive (dependent on the extent of the burn injury); and the quantitative counts of biopsied specimens may show the same numbers of bacteria per gram of tissue (10^3) as found in the tissue prior to burning.[87,103,106] As these bacteria increase in number following the thermal injury and reach levels of greater than 10^5 bacteria per gram of tissue, they will erupt from the hair follicles and sebaceous glands and begin transmigrating through the tissue, invading the dermal–subcutaneous boundary. Perivascular growth is accompanied by thrombosis of vessels and necrosis of any remaining dermal elements, transforming partial-thickness burns to full-thickness burn injuries. Levels of bacterial growth which exceed 10^5 bacteria per gram of tissue constitute localized burn wound infection, and levels greater than 10^8–10^9 bacteria per gram of tissue may be associated with lethal burns.[4,28,87,106,107] As the levels of bacterial growth increase, so does the incidence of septicemia.[4,108]

Maintaining wounds at low contamination levels diminishes the frequency and duration of septic episodes caused by wound flora. This is accomplished by cleansing wounds two to three times per day by either showering or tubbing a patient. Some burn facilities still immerse patients in a tub in order to remove the debris and exudate which has accumulated between dressing changes; however, most burn facilities no longer advocate this cleaning technique because of the potential for seeding surface bacteria to open burn wounds. SBI-Galveston, along with other burn facilities, has exclusively used the shower technique to wash down the debris from patients. It is important to note that wound cleansing can be quite painful and the associated hematogenous seeding can cause a bacteremia. The technique of early excision may prevent these disadvantages. An alternative for treatment for small second degree burns is to use a biological dressing. Biological dressings contain no toxins or bacterial properties; however, they provide a wound environment which prevents desiccation, reduces bacterial proliferation, diminishes or prevents loss of heat, water, protein, and red blood cells, and encourages rapid wound healing. Biological dressings also diminish pain. Some examples of such synthetic skin substitutes include Biobrane, Opsite, and Omiderm.

Daily inspection of wounds is essential. Burn wound biopsies should be taken from any area of a wound which has changed in appearance as described in **Table 11.17**. Bacterial sepsis is often preluded by changes in the color, odor, or amount of exudate from the wound, while fungal invasion is clinically conspicuous by rapidly emerging and spreading dark discolorations. Consequently, burn wounds must be closely assessed for these manifestations. Few histologically demonstrated fungal infections are initially determined by culture; therefore, treatment should be predicated on the identification of invasive hyphae by histologic examination and may subsequently be confirmed by culture.

There is a controversy over the best method to determine the presence of infections, with some burn centers using surface cultures and others preferring contact plates. The area of greatest concern surrounds the identification of specific organisms. SBI-Galveston has found quantitative biopsies to be quite useful. Robson discovered that when colony counts were less than 10^2 graft survival was greater than 90%, but when colony counts were greater than 10^5, only a 60% graft survival rate was observed.[109] At SBI-Galveston, physicians have routinely modified our topical antimicrobial therapy, alternating between silver sulfadiazine and mafenide acetate when colony counts were greater than 10^5 Mafenide acetate is more successful at penetrating the necrotic dermis than is silver sulfadiazine. This technique has been demonstrated to be successful in decreasing wound colony counts; however, early excision and grafting has been more rewarding. Quantitative swabs, smear cultures, and/or contact plates (Rodak®) provide information regarding the presence of potential infectious agents, but quantitative wound biopsies are a better determinant of bacterial loads. Quantitative cultures showing high bacterial counts correlate with histologic evidence of burn wound infection in approximately 80% of cases.[4,87,110] If quantitative biopsies reveal greater than 10^3 organisms/g of tissue, then a change in topical therapy is indicated. If bacterial counts exceed 10^5 organisms/g of tissue, then localized burn wound infection should be considered as a possibility and a histologic examination performed. If histologic evidence of invasion is present, systemic antibiotics which are consistent with the etiologic agent of infection should be administered, and the wound should be excised.[87–89]

Additional measures can be taken to diminish the incidence of burn wound colonization. The microorganisms initially populating a burn wound represent a mixture of endogenous resident flora and exogenous contaminants seeded by contact with the environment and attending personnel. Immunosuppressed burned patients need to be protected from exposure to these environmental contaminants; however, the most elaborate methods of isolation have failed to effectively minimize the incidence of infection, even though they have significantly reduced the incidence of cross-contamination.[111–114] The most effective means of decreasing the exposure of burned patients to exogenous bacteria is strict observation of appropriate hand-washing among the health care providers. Waterproof gowns and gloves should be worn whenever direct contact with body fluids and wound exudates are unavoidable so as to protect both patients and health care providers from inadvertent contamination. All dressing materials should be maintained as patient specific. Intravenous pumps and poles, blood pressure devices, monitoring equipment, bedside tables, and beds should be cleaned on a daily basis with antibacterial solutions. Terminal cleaning, following the discharge of the patient, should include the walls, ceiling, baseboards, and floors. Mattresses should be covered with vinyl and frequently inspected for cracks in their surfaces. Air filters should be repeatedly monitored for bacterial and fungal growth.

Most burn units now house severely burned patients within individual, self-contained isolation rooms. Even within these units, common areas exist, predominantly the bathing or showering facilities. These areas should be conscientiously cleansed between patients with an effective bactericidal agent which is more specifically directed at those bacteria which predominate in each individual unit. Disposable or single-use sterilizable instruments should be used for blunt debridements, and the use of any other type of instrument should be discouraged.

Antimicrobial Therapy

It is evident that the human population is not germ-free; ergo, health is not the absence of bacteria but more like a delicate balance between man and his microbes. The intact skin and the mucous membrane are man's most significant defenses, and any alterations of the integument disturbs these defenses as well as the balance with microbial flora. Infection occurs when the microbes gain access to underlying tissues and achieve a critical number. The major objective of the burn surgeon is to prevent this microbial invasion when and wherever possible and, when contamination occurs, to reduce the microbial levels so that wound healing can proceed unretarded.[110]

Resident and transient microbes of the skin are the etiologic agents of infection, and antimicrobials are designed to eliminate these offenders. With the discovery of antimicrobials, the solution to the abrogation of wound infections seemed to be resolved; however, it soon became evident that, even though the antimicrobials may provide a balance between man and his microbes through their ability to render the microbe ineffective and prevent burn wound infections, the microbes soon overcame this obstacle.

The use of therapeutic antimicrobials can provide precise delivery of a specific agent to eliminate an offending microbe whose sensitivity has already been determined, whereas prophylactic or perioperative antimicrobials cannot be easily selected. Usually the decision is based on the common occurrence of those predominating pathogens found among a burn patient population. While the quality of the surgical outcome can be severely compromised by infection, the actual numbers of these infections have been relatively small.[110,115,116]

Preventing infection in burn patients requires two defensive maneuvers. The first echelon of protection or prophylaxis is the establishment of techniques which will effectively obstruct burn wound contamination.[116–119] The first level of treatment involves three steps:

- total area disinfection with appropriate cleansers must include the wound and encompassing areas;
- exclusion of the potential source of infection by debridement with grafting, provided that the graft bed contains $<10^5$ bacteria per gram of tissue;[110,116,118]
- topical antimicrobial therapy which includes: the appropriate selection of an agent for a specific microbial flora, ascertained via agar well susceptibility assays, and the utilization of appropriate antimicrobials which are necessary for restraining local wound contamination and potential sepsis.[120–122]

The second echelon of this antimicrobial approach also involves three stages:

- Preliminary topical and systemic antimicrobial therapy should be introduced when sepsis is suspected and should be directed against those organisms which are common to burn populations. This approach is based on the microbiology data accumulated from studies on the whole burn population.[120]
- The burn patient's local and general ability to resist microbial burn invasion and resistance should be enhanced through appropriate resuscitative therapies and nutritional therapies.[123]
- Immunological procedures which augment host resistance should be utilized such as administration of cryoprecipitates if appropriate.

The Use of Topical Antimicrobial Compounds and Agents

One of the most effective means of achieving a microbial balance in a colonized or infected wound is via the proper use of prophylactic topical agents. Maintaining wounds at low colonization levels diminishes the frequency and duration of septic episodes caused by wound flora[87] and thus reduces the caloric and fluid demands required by the patient during each septic episode. The introduction of topical antimicrobial agents has resulted in a significant reduction in burn mortality to date.[121,124] Of course, no single agent is thoroughly effective against all organisms and each possesses its own advantages and disadvantages. Almost all currently used topical agents retard wound healing; the application of some increases a patient's metabolic rate. Their effectiveness is measured by their ability to inhibit bacterial growth *in vitro* and reduce wound colony counts *in vivo*. Recent studies have demonstrated that some agents used in the past are no longer effective in inhibiting bacterial growth *in vitro*.[125] Wounds in which the quantitative culture counts remain less than 10^2 organisms/g tissue may remain dressed in the topical agent of choice. On the other hand, should the colony count show an increase beyond that point, then a change in the topical agent is strongly recommended.

Sodium hypochlorite

Currently the most effective topical antibacterial agent for cleansing a wound is sodium hypochlorite (NaOCl).[126] It transcends the topical antimicrobial effects and tissue toxicity of such products as povidone-iodine, acetic acid, and hydrogen peroxide.[65] While povidone-iodine is bactericidal at 1 and 0.5% concentration, it is toxic to fibroblasts; acetic acid at 0.25% is toxic to fibroblasts and not bactericidal. Hydrogen peroxide at 3% and 0.3% is toxic to fibroblasts only; at 3%, it is bactericidal.[27,126]

Studies by Heggers and his coworkers[127] clearly defined the efficacy of NaOCl at a concentration of 0.025% which was found to be bactericidal, nontoxic to fibroblasts, and not inhibiting to wound healing, provided appropriate buffers are used. The NaOCl is only effective over a 24-hour time frame after the buffer (0.3 N NaH_2HPO_4) is added to the NaOCl.[128] NaOCl soaks are most beneficial in reducing the bacterial numbers in a wound.

NaOCl is a broad spectrum antiseptic and is bactericidal for *Ps. aeruginosa*, *S. aureus*, as well as other gram-negative and gram-positive organisms.[66,127] It is effective against MRSA, MRSE, and the enterococci. NaOCl can be used separately or in concert with other antibacterials to control colonization or infection. NaOCl also enhances wound healing and increases wound breaking strength more than mafenide acetate does.[127]

Silver nitrate ($AgNO_3$)

Formerly used as a 10% solution, $AgNO_3$ was found to be toxic at this concentration. It has now been reinstated as a 0.5% solution which is nontoxic. In its current form, it apparently does not injure regenerating epithelium in the wound and is bacteriostatic against *S. aureus*, *E. coli*, and *Ps. aeruginosa*. $AgNO_3$ is most effective when the wound is carefully cleansed of all emollients and other debris and debrided of all dead tissue. Multilayered coarse mesh dressings should be placed over the wound and saturated with the $AgNO_3$ solution. Like silver sulfadiazine, $AgNO_3$ has limited penetration since the ion Ag^+ is rapidly bound to the body's natural chemical substances, such as Cl^-.[120,121,124,129] Since it is hypotonic in nature, it can cause osmolar dilution, resulting in hyponatremia and hypochloremia. Serum electrolytes must be monitored very carefully.

Notable detriments to the use of $AgNO_3$ include that it is expensive, light sensitive, and turns black upon contact with tissues and other Cl^--containing compounds. Further, it also requires special handling; if allowed to dry or if it is covered with an impervious dressing, hyperpyrexia could occur.

Klebsiella species, the *Providencia* species, and other Enterobacteriaceae are not as susceptible to it as are other bacteria. *Ent. cloacae* can cause methemoglobinemia by converting nitrite to nitrate as well as other nitrate-positive organisms.[120,121,124,129]

Silver sulfadiazine

Silver sulfadiazine (Silvadene®, Thermazine®, Flamazine®, SSD®, Burnazine®) is a 1% water-soluble cream combining sulfadiazine with silver (Ag^+). The Ag^+ ion binds with the DNA of an organism and, consequently, releases the sulfonamide which interferes with the intermediary metabolic pathway of the microbe. It is most effective against *Ps. aeruginosa*, the enterics, and equally as effective as any antifungal drug against *Candida albicans*. *S. aureus* and some strains of the *Klebsiella* species have been less effectively controlled. Recently there have been reports of *Ps. aeruginosa* resistance.[130] Silver sulfadiazine can be applied with equal effectiveness using either the closed or open methods. Antimicrobial effectiveness has been observed to last for up to 24 hours. More frequent changes are required if a creamy exudate forms on the wound. Some of the benefits of this topical agent are its ease of use and its ability to reduce pain. It has some tissue penetrating ability, but is limited to the surface epidermal layer.[120,129] It is not associated with the acid–base disturbances or pulmonary fluid overload, as is the case with mafenide acetate.[121,124]

Silver sulfadiazine can be used separately or in combination with other antibacterials or enzymatic escharotomy compounds. It can be combined with nystatin which enhances the antifungal capability of this agent. By itself, silver sulfadiazine has been shown to retard wound healing; however, in conjunction with nystatin or *Aloe vera*, the wound retardant effect is reversed. The breaking strength is not affected; in fact, it may be enhanced when combinations are employed.[131] One disadvantage may be a reported granulocyte reduction; however, this appears to be reversible.[120,121,124,129]

Mafenide acetate

Mafenide acetate (Sulfamylon®) is available both in a 10% water-soluble cream or a 5% solution and has more substantial bacteriological data to support its efficacy than do any of the other topical antimicrobials. Mafenide acetate has been shown to be effective against a broad range of microorganisms, especially against all strains of *Ps. aeruginosa* and *Clostridium*.[121,124,132] After a wound has been cleansed of debris, mafenide acetate is applied to the wound like 'butter'. The treated burn surface is left exposed for maximal antimicrobial potency.[121,124,132] The cream is applied a minimum of twice a day and is reapplied between applications if it is rubbed off.

Advantages of the cream include its ability to control *Ps. aeruginosa* wound infections, its ease of application, and the absence of the need for dressings. Additionally, it has an ability to permeate burn eschar and thereby to circumvent the colonization of a burn. The 5% solution is applied to an eight-ply gauze dressing, to the point of saturation, and then changed every 8 hours. It has been proclaimed to have effective tissue-penetrating ability and appears to be especially effective after the dead tissue is removed from the granulating bed.[121,129,132,133]

Unfortunately, several detrimental aspects are associated with the use of mafenide acetate. Protracted use, with the low environmental pH, favors the growth of *Candida albicans*. Mafenide acetate is converted to *p*-sulfamyl-vanzoic acid by monoamine oxidase, which is a carbonic anhydrase inhibitor; this subsequently causes metabolic acidosis in the patient. In the unburned patient, respiratory alkalosis is present; therefore, an imbalance is not present. On the other hand, if an inhalation injury exists with its concomitant respiratory acidosis and is associated with metabolic acidosis initiated by this drug, the end result can be fatal. This complication can also be seen when treatment with mafenide acetate occurs during septic episodes with metabolic acidosis, or if it is applied over a large area of the body surface.[121,124,132,134] Another detrimental problem encountered with mafenide acetate is that it is painful when applied to superficial partial-thickness burns with intact free nerve endings. This disadvantage is not completely relevant since mafenide acetate was not designed for minor burns and is said not to be painful on large full-thickness injuries. Also, its requirement to remain uncovered for antimicrobial activity may be considered a disadvantage if a dressing is required. The 5% aqueous solution of mafenide acetate can be used in a wet dressing covered by a splint.[121,124,133,134]

It has been shown by others that fatality in major burns can be reduced by 33% with the use of mafenide acetate.[71,72] As with silver sulfadiazine, mafenide acetate can be used individually or in conjunction with other antimicrobials. However, mafenide acetate retards wound healing and reduces the breaking strength of healed wounds.[120]

Povidone–iodine

A 10% ointment of povidone–iodine was designed after the demonstration of its broad spectrum of antimicrobial attributes in liquid form. Although its active antimicrobial component is iodine, there has been no documentation associated with skin hypersensitivity or toxic effects. It has a broad spectrum of antibacterial and antifungal activities.[120,121,124,126,135,136] Povidone–iodine ointment can be employed effectively with both closed and open techniques. Quantitative bacteriological assessments imply that iodine is most efficacious when it is administered every 6 hours. Used in this way, it is effective in controlling and/or preventing colonization.

Some problems are encountered when using this drug. It can cause pain when applied. Recent studies intimate that it may be absorbed more extensively than was previously thought and could cause toxicity and renal failure as well as acidosis Concomitantly, it has been shown to be cytotoxic to fibroblasts as previously described.[120,121,124,126,135,136] In any case, it is a highly effective disinfectant when used on intact skin.

Gentamicin sulfate

Garamycin, or gentamicin sulfate, is available as a 0.1% water-soluble cream and is chemically similar to other aminoglycosides, such as kanamycin and neomycin. It has a broad spectrum of antimicrobial activity. Its use in wounds is based on its microbiocidal capabilities against *Ps. aeruginosa*. Unfortunately, its topical application and abuse have rapidly stimulated gentamicin resistance.[120,121,124,126,135,136]

Bacitracin/polymyxin

Topical *antibiotics*, such as bacitracin/polymyxin, have been unproductive in controlling infection, specifically in grafting procedures. Lowbury made a very astute statement when he said: 'It was gratifying to have a topical chemoprophylactic agent which was not an antibiotic, the use of which would cause the emergence of antibiotic resistance.'[119,137] Many surgeons rely on this topical agent for skin graft coverage because it is nontoxic and is similar to petrolatum gauze dressings which were previously employed as dressings for grafts. These two combined antibiotics have little or no effect on localized burn wound infections.[138]

Nitrofuratonin

The topical antimicrobial, Furacin, was previously used and had questionable value therapeutically. In the past decade, however, researchers have shown that Furacin, or nitrofurantoin, is effective in the treatment of methicillin-resistant *S. aureus* and other methicillin-resistant staphylococci. While Furacin is effective 75% of the time for most gram-negatives other than *Ps. aeruginosa*, bacitracin/polymyxin is only 21% effective.[138,139]

Mupirocin (Bactroban®, Beecham Laboratories)

Mupirocin is one of several antibiotics derived from the fermentation of *Ps. fluorescens* and is also known as pseudomonic acid A. While the antimicrobial activity derived from cultures of *Ps. fluorescens* was first reported over a century and a half ago, this activity could not be adapted as an antimicrobial agent until Fuller *et al.*[140] executed a more complete isolation and purification of pseudomonic acid A. It is this exploration, along with research associating the antimicrobial activity of mupirocin with an inhibition of microbial isoleucyl tRNA synthetase which causes inhibition in protein synthesis, which has made the clinical application of mupirocin possible.[140,141]

In vitro studies have subsequently established that mupirocin has omnipotent inhibitory activity against gram-positive microbes, specifically *S. aureus* and *S. epidermidis*. Mupirocin's efficiency in the treatment of infection or colonization due to *S. aureus*, whether methicillin sensitive or not, has been shown in various clinical settings.[140–142] Rode and coworkers[143] have provided additional data regarding the efficacy of mupirocin in the treatment of established wound infections with *S. aureus* which is resistant to systemic methicillin, as well as topical mafenide acetate and povidone–iodine. Recent *in vitro* and *in vivo* endeavors have shown mupirocin to be equally as efficacious in methicillin-resistant burn wound infections.[138] Mupirocin, while not sanctioned for gram-negative organisms, has been shown to be 75% effective against most enteric organisms and is significantly better than bacitracin/polymyxin.[138]

Table 11.19 presents data on a study which confirms that the antimicrobial effectiveness of several topical agents, as tested via the agar well diffusion technique, were comparable.[138,139] Mafenide acetate and silver sulfadiazine had a comparable antimicrobial activity to that of mupirocin for the gram-negative organisms *Ps. aeruginosa, E. coli* and *Kl. pneumoniae*, along with *S. aureus*. Mupirocin inhibits wound healing when compared to controls by a half-life of 2 days, while the breaking strength is significantly enhanced over controls ($p<0.05$).[131]

Nystatin (Mycostatin®, Squibb, Nilstat®, Lederle)

Nystatin is an antifungal antibiotic produced by *Streptomyces noursei*. Nystatin exerts its antifungal activity by binding to sterols in the fungal cell membrane. The drug is not active against organisms (e.g. bacteria) which do not contain sterols in their cell membranes. As a result of this binding, a membrane is no longer able to function as a selective barrier, and potassium and other cellular constituents are lost. Nystatin has fungistatic or fungicidal activity against a

Table 11.19 Topical antimicrobial susceptibility assays of both gram-positive and gram-negative organisms*

	Mafenide acetate	SSD	Furacin	Bact/Poly†	Mupirocin®(%)≠
No. of isolates	165	165	144	153	153
Susceptibility	145 (87.9‡)	145 (87.9‡)	109 (75.7‡)	33 (21.6)	128 (83.7‡)
Resistance	20 (12.1)	20 (12.1)	35 (24.3%)	120 (78.4)	25 (16.3)

* Modified from reference 138, Strock *et al.* (1990).
† Bacitracin/Polymyxin.
‡ $p < 0.01$.
≠ Bactroban®, Beecham Laboratories.

variety of pathogenic and nonpathogenic yeasts and fungi. *In vitro*, nystatin concentrations of approximately 3 μg/ml inhibit *Candida albicans* and *C. guilliermondii*. Concentrations of 6.25 μg/ml are required to inhibit *C. krusei* and *Candidum lactis*. In general, there is little difference between minimum inhibitory and fungicidal concentrations for a particular organism. Nystatin is not active against bacteria, protozoa, or viruses.

Oral Administration. Nystatin is used orally for the treatment of intestinal candidiasis. In patients with coexisting intestinal candidiasis and vulvovaginal candidiasis, nystatin may be administered orally, in conjunction with intravaginal application of an antifungal agent. While there is limited evidence that, by reducing intestinal candidal colonization, combined oral and intravaginal antifungal therapy may provide some improvement in mycologic response and reduction in recurrence rate of vulvovaginal candidiasis, most evidence suggests that combined therapy does not substantially reduce the risk of recurrence compared with intravaginal therapy alone.

Cutaneous and mucocutaneous infections. For the treatment of cutaneous or mucocutaneous candidal infections, nystatin may be applied topically as a cream, lotion, or ointment to affected areas two to four times daily. The cream or lotion formulations are preferred over the ointment for use in moist, intertriginous areas. In the treatment of candidiasis, conditions which favor growth of yeast and release of its irritating endotoxin, such as the use of occlusive dressings and ointment formulations, should be avoided. Concomitant therapy should include attention to proper hygiene and skin care in order to prevent the spread of infection and reinfection. In addition, the affected areas should be kept dry and exposed to air, if possible. Nystatin may be combined with SSD in order to increase the antimicrobial spectrum.

Discussion

The therapeutic effectiveness of topical antimicrobials can best be monitored by quantitative bacteriological analysis of a burn wound.[4,105,144] Previously, there were no *in vitro* tests available to support a selection of the most effective topical antimicrobial agent for any given organisms which cause burn wound infection. Studies by Nathan and colleagues,[121] as well as by others,[139,145] recently provided evidence of a reproducible susceptibility method for testing pathogenic bacteria against the various topical antimicrobial agents. The bacterial isolates are spread over an agar surface with 6 mm wells cut into the agar; and then the topical antimicrobials are introduced into these wells. Subsequently, the zones of inhibition can predict the agent's capability to provide the equilibrium between patient and bacteria. Recently, Enquay Pharmaceuticals has designed commercialized topical antimicrobials, currently under FDA review. The antimicrobials it assays are bacitracin/polymyxin, mafenide acetate, silver sulfadiazine, nitrofurazone, nystatin, plus a negative control.[139] While current data are generated and new agents discovered, the microbes continue to alter their susceptibility. Thus, no legendary 'topical antimicrobial agent of choice' will likely ever be available therapeutically.[139,145]

Though topical antimicrobial therapy has significantly diminished the occurrence of invasive burn wound sepsis, we must search for other prophylactic and preventative methods to halt burn wound infection. While bacterial control is imperfect at best, all wounds, as well as the patient as a whole, must be scrupulously monitored with adjunctive burn wound biopsies when indicated, with blood and other body fluid cultures, as well as with early excision and grafting to prevent, diagnose, and treat infections in a timely manner.[4,28,108,110,116,117,121]

Mode of Action of Antimicrobials

Prior to the initiation of any antimicrobial therapy, each burn surgeon must consider four major essentials:

- each antimicrobial must be selected based on its effect and its specificity for the microbe present;
- such decisions should be made on the basis of culture and susceptibility data;
- the time, dosage, route of administration, and duration of treatment should be in accordance with what is required in order to make the organism powerless; and
- consideration should be given to local and systemic host resistant factors.

Other factors to be considered are age of patient, type of operation, length of operation, and underlying disease factors, to mention only a few.[120] **Table 11.20** summarizes the mode of action of the classes of antimicrobials.

Table 11.20 The metabolic effects of antimicrobials

Interrupts cell wall synthesis
Aztreonam
Bacitracin
Cephalosporins
Imipenem
Penicillins
Vancomycin
Interrupts cell membrane permeability
Amphotericin B
Nystatin
Polymyxin B
Polymyxin E (colistin)
Interrupts protein synthesis
Amikacin
Chloramphenicol
Erythromycin
Gentamicin
Kanamycin
Lincomycin
Neomycin
Rifampin
Streptomycin
Tobramycin
Interrupts DNA synthesis
Ciprofloxacin
Griseofulvin
Nalidixic acid
Norfloxacin
Novobiacin
Interrupts intermediary metabolism
Mafenide acetate
Nitrofurans
Silver sulfadiazine
Sulfonamides
Trimethoprim

It is essential to fully comprehend the terms 'antibiotic', 'antimicrobial', and 'chemotherapeutic' agents, which have become interchangeable in medicine today.

- *Antibiotic*: a life destructive, biological substance produced by a living microbe with the capacity to inhibit or kill bacteria in dilute concentrations.
- *Antimicrobial*: a substance which suppresses growth or kills bacteria. Compounds possessing this antibacterial activity are usually synthesized in a laboratory, e.g. sulfonamides.
- *Chemotherapeutic*: a life destructive chemical substance or combination of the above, e.g. carbolic acid, phenol, sodium hypochlorite, or acyclovir.[120] The mechanisms of action are mobile. Intermediary inhibition is accomplished by chemical substances which inhibit metabolism, e.g. sulfonamides, which act as analogs of *p*-aminobenzoic acid, and thereby avert a synthesis of folic acid. The action of silver sulfadiazine is primarily due to silver toxicity in a microbe coupled with the action of sulfa. However, some antimicrobials, such as penicillins, require the bacteria to be in an actively metabolizing state and interact between a cell wall and a cell membrane in order to be effective; otherwise, they have little or no effect on a microbe whose cell wall is completely developed. Other antimicrobials, such as colistin or the polymyxins, affect the bacterial membrane. These antibiotics contain both lipophilic and lipophobic chemical molecules, giving them the ability to disrupt the lipid–protein interface which is the foundation of the microbial membrane. This disruption prevents the membrane from freely diffusing nutrients which are necessary for cell survival. Consequently permanent binding of the cytoplasmic membrane by this type of antimicrobial is *biocidal*.

Antibiotic interference, which inhibits protein synthesis, occurs via two major biosynthetic pathways of microbial inhibition. One interferes with transcription, the process by which an encoded message is transferred to a messenger RNA (mRNA). The other occurs when RNA is in the process of protein synthesis. Consequently, protein synthesis may be inhibited by one or both of the above mechanisms. All aminoglycosides bind to the 30S ribosomal subunit, and therefore inhibit peptide bond composition which eventually forms an inactive 70S ribosome. Chloramphenicol binds to the microbe's 50S ribosome, thus preventing the attachment of the active aminoacyl end of the aminoacyl-tRNA. Those antibacterials responsible for DNAse inhibition include nalidixic acid, novobiocin, and the quinolones (i.e. ciprofloxacin), which are variable in their interactions and may interfere with transcription, DNA polymerase, and interaction with purine analogs, respectively[115,120] (**Table 11.20**).

The activities described above against the invading bacteria are not selective for bacteria alone. Those antibiotics which affect membranes, RNA, DNA and the intermediary metabolism of bacteria also attacks a host's metabolic process and, thus, interfere with a host's healing process.

Systemic Antimicrobial Therapy: the Rationale

The employment of systemic antibiotics can be dichotomized into three major approaches: perioperative, prophylactic, and therapeutic. The use of systemic antibiotics is extremely essential in burn surgery, in comparison with other surgical services, so it is essential that we define a few terms related to antibiotics.

- *Perioperative* may be also considered prophylaxis; however, it involves the administration of systemic antibiotics as a protective measure for any type of surgical intervention. The time frame for administration should be short-lived and dosing is usually limited to one to three doses, depending on the operative procedure.
- *Prophylactic* is a precautionary or preventative measure designed to preserve health and prevent the possible spread of disease (e.g. penicillin prophylaxis for 72 hours to prevent streptococcal infections in burns, tetanus toxoid for tetanus).
- *Therapeutic* refers to an administration of antibiotics for the treatment of infection. Depending on the infection, therapy may continue for several days.[120]

As mentioned above, prophylactic penicillin is usually administered to circumvent the emergence of *Str. pyogenes* or group A streptococci, and other β-hemolytic streptococci which are frequently responsible for graft loss, surgical and burn wound sepsis, and other sequelae related to these infections. Cellulitis, resulting from a streptococcal infection, usually resolves under penicillin therapy. One can easily confirm this sequel via a skin scraping of a cellulitic lesion and a Gram stain. The presence of gram-positive cocci in chains is confirmation that the existing cellulitis is caused by streptococci.[4,12,116,120]

Any article dealing with the prevention or treatment of surgical and burn wound infections will inescapably encounter some controversy. Independent of the most conspicuous questions regarding choice of antibiotic, route of administration, timing and duration, and the prophylactic versus perioperative administration of antibiotics are the fundamental concerns which impinge upon such vehemently argued issues as excessive use of a medication, real risks versus potential benefits, and, last but not least, the ascending costs of hospital care.

Krizek and his colleagues published a paper in 1975, and then again in 1985, where they described the fluctuation in use of antimicrobials.[146,147] While major changes were observed for other areas of surgery, there has been little change in the use of antibiotics for burns in general; but there appears to be a significant demarcation when one reviews their use for in-patient burns (**Table 11.21**). The responders in a 1985 survey showed a 16% decrease in their use of prophylactic antimicrobial therapy; this decrease appears somewhat incompatible with current methodologies in burn care (i.e. early excision and grafting). It might also be a reflection of the burn size treated by the surgeon.[92]

The general consensus regarding burn injuries is dependent on the size and the environment in which the incident occurred. A little burn (<10%) caused by scalding water might be considered a clean wound, which would require no antimicrobial coverage. A large flame burn due to a gas heater explosion in a garage should be considered a dirty wound, possibly contaminated or colonized with exogenous microbes present in the garage environment. This complication can be compounded by contaminated devices or

Table 11.21 Antibiotic usage in the treatment of burns

Category	1974 (%)	1984 (%)
All burns	53*	54
In-patient burns	85	69

* Percent responders using antibiotics.

substances in the environment used to extinguish the flames (old blankets, etc.).

Burn size and the circumstances surrounding the event must influence the burn surgeon in his decision to use or not use antibiotics.[146,147] Sasaki *et al.*[92] shows that several burn wound manipulations are responsible for bacteremias; not only do the trauma and tangential excision induce a bacteremia in approximately 50% of cases when compared with other methods of manipulation, but routine instrumentation can also cause bacteremia.[92,148,149] The bigger the size of the initial burn, the greater the increase in the incidence of bacteremia. Those patients with a positive blood culture had an average total body surface area (TBSA) injury of 46.6%, while those with a 25.5% TBSA injury had negative blood cultures.[92]

Further clarification may be sustained via definitions of several terms which are related to the issues involved in determining when and when not to use antimicrobial agents.

- *Bacteremia*: the transient presence of microorganisms in blood (i.e. bacteria in blood after brushing one's teeth or after sigmoidoscopy).[148–150]
- *Septicemia*: the invasion of the blood stream by pathogenic bacteria from a local foci of infection which provides an active multiplication of these bacteria and which is frequently accompanied by hyperthermia, hypothermia, and prostration.[150] This is a clinical diagnosis predicated on any three of the cardinal clinical and laboratory criteria for sepsis.
- *Colonization*: the presence of bacteria demonstrated by bacterial counts less than 10^5 bacteria per gram of tissue with no evidence of invasion, based on histopathologic data.[28,87] This can be monitored by quantitative biopsies and kept in control by the use of topical antibacterials.
- *Burn wound sepsis*: the presence of bacteria: where bacterial biopsy counts exceed 10^5 bacteria per gram of tissue[28,87,88] (see Table 11.18 for additional cardinal signs of sepsis).

Determination on the use of antimicrobial agents must be based on the knowledge of existing microorganisms which are present not only on injured skin, but in the wound which is ready for closure. All wounds which contain β-hemolytic streptococci or have a bacterial count $>10^5$ should be treated with appropriate systemic or topical antimicrobials or both prior to closure.[115,117,118]

ADMINISTRATION OF SYSTEMIC ANTIMICROBIALS

Selecting a suitable antibiotic must be predicated on several factors:

- the possible pathogenic organism which could or can establish a burn wound infection;
- susceptibility patterns of etiologic agents which are characteristic of each hospital environment; and
- the kind of wound, i.e. incisional, traumatic, or burn wound.[110,115]

A plethora of experimental and clinical data compiled over the past 25 years clearly indicates that *in vivo* use of systemic antibiotics, when delivered more than 3–4 hours post-surgery, is totally ineffective.[110,115,120] The risk of burn wound infection directly corresponds to the quantitative number of pathogenic organisms surviving in a wound. Determining the number of viable microbes present in burned tissue, or other biological body fluid, via quantitative analysis, furnishes confirmatory data concerning the extent of contamination or infection.[116,117]

Pharmacokinetics

The precise description of the pharmacokinetics of any drug can be extremely complex, the clinician can benefit considerably from the estimates that are fairly accurate and yet comprehensible. It is the aim of this chapter to be useful in the construction of therapeutic regimens and in the modification of these regimens for individualization of antimicrobial therapy.[151] More extensive discussions of pharmacokinetics can be found in several excellent books.[152–154]

It is important to note here, that in attempting to provide an adequate dosing regimen for a burn patient, the surgeon should take into consideration the hypermetabolic state of the patient. Such hypermetabolism necessitates higher dosages than normal since excretion rates are enhanced.[102,103,111,120]

The time-dependent interactions of antibacterial agents are important to both effectiveness and toxicity. The interactions of drugs and microorganisms depend on achieving antibiotic concentrations immediately adjacent to the bacteria; consequently these levels depend on human drug interactions which include absorption, distribution, metabolism, excretion, and clinical status. Additionally, the serum and tissue concentrations of drugs may correlate with dose-related toxicities. Consequently time-dependent interactions with humans can also be used to construct dosing regimens.

Volume of distribution

The volume of distribution (V_D) of a drug is interpreted as that volume in which the total amount of drug in the body (A) would have to be uniformly divided in order to give an observed plasma concentration (C_P).

$$V_D = \frac{A}{C_P}$$

Consequently if 140 mg of gentamicin were given to a 70 kg patient and the serum concentration was found to be 8 μg/ml (= 8 mg/l), then the volume of distribution would be (140 mg) ± (8 mg/l) = 17.5 liters.

The V_D is often represented in terms of body weight, l/kg. If expressed as l/kg, then the actual V_D is obtained simply by multiplying V_D per kg by the body weight.

If we modify the equation above, the dose (or amount) necessary to produce any desired serum concentration can be calculated with a drug whose V_D is known or the serum concentration that can be expected with any chosen dose. Thus, if the goal is to produce a serum concentration of gentamicin at 10 μg/ml (= 10 mg/l) in a 70 kg man and the V_D is known to be 0.25 l/kg, then the dose must = V_D (C_P) = (0.25 l/kg) (70 kg) (10 mg/l) = 175 mg.

The volume of distribution need not and usually does not correspond to any actual anatomical or physiologic space. It is simply a mathematical tool.

Most antimicrobial agents have a V_D of between 0.15 and 0.40 l/kg. However, a few have larger V_D. The important clinical use of the V_D is that it provides an initial or loading dose that promptly delivers a therapeutic serum concentration. The V_D is also useful, as addressed below, in calculating subsequent or maintenance doses to attain therapeutic and yet safe serum concentrations.

Half-life

The half-life of a drug is interpreted as the time required for the serum concentration to fall to one-half its original concentration as it is being eliminated from the body.

Usually the half-life associated with a drug is the half-life of the predominant phase of drug elimination that absorption of the drug has been completed. It is also given that the fall in the serum concentration is parallel to the fall in the total concentration of drug in the body. The half-life of a drug remains constant over time if there has been no change in the processes of drug elimination, which the surgeon must anticipate when administering antibacterial therapy to a burn patient. During each half-life, 50% of the total amount of drug in the body is eliminated, and the serum concentration falls by 50%. The half-lives of antimicrobial agents are variable. All of the current β-lactam antibiotics except ceftriaxone have very short half-lives (usually < 1.5 hours). The aminoglycosides half-lives are somewhat longer (2–3 hours). Ceftriaxone, flucytosine, sulfisoxazole, and vancomycin have half-lives of 3–6 hours. Sulfamethoxazole, tetracycline, and trimethoprim have half-lives of 6–12 hours. Doxycycline has a relatively long half-life of 20 hours.

Clinically a drug's half-life is prolonged in renal and hepatic dysfunction. The half-life may also be influenced by age with extensions of the half-life in the newborn and the elderly and with shortened half-lives in young children when compared with young adult values. Other drugs administered concomitantly can also alter a drug's half-life. However, it must be kept in mind that one is treating a thermally injured individual who is infected.

Repetitive dosing

With repetitive dosing of a drug at regular intervals, the peak serum concentrations and the trough concentrations rise to a steady state, and after this steady state is reached, the peak and trough serum concentrations remain constant if the dose remains constant and of course if there is no change in the rate of drug elimination. The attainment of a plateau or steady state is also applicable to continuous dosing at a constant rate where the serum concentrations climb until a steady state is reached and remain constant.

The rate at which the steady state is achieved is exclusively a function of the half-life of drug elimination and is dependent on the rate of drug delivery. Consequently giving more per dose or per unit of time ultimately provides a higher concentration at the steady state, but the steady state is still reached at the same time. A useful interpretation is that the steady state is achieved after four half-lives. In actuality, after one half-life the peak and trough of the mean serum concentration is about 50% after three half-lives, 88% after four half-lives, 94% of the ultimate plateau levels. Therefore, when a dosage change is made or when a drug is discontinued, the new steady state is achieved after about four half-lives.

Clearly, the principle of a steady state has greater significance clinically with a half-life of several hours or longer than with a half-life of an hour or less. Generally, in antimicrobial chemotherapy, a loading dose must be considered whenever the half-life of the chosen drug is estimated to be 3 hours or longer. A loading dose should also be considered whenever the half-life of the chosen drug is estimated to be extended beyond 3 hours by hepatic or renal dysfunction.

TREATMENT OF INFECTIONS IN BURNS

The major role of an antibiotic is to eliminate a potential agent of infection in a burned patient. The systemic treatment of an infection is often begun based on empirical knowledge of the most common types of microbial infections seen in burn populations and the antibiotics which are most efficacious in their treatment. These infections can be divided into gram-negative and gram-positive bacterial infections in order to discuss the best antimicrobial therapies to be used in treatment.

Gram-positive Bacterial Infections

The three most common gram-positive organisms responsible for causing burn wound infections are the streptococci, staphylococci, and enteroccocci (see Table 11.5).

Streptococcal infections

Immediately post-admission for a burn wound, patients are prophylactically treated with the natural penicillins for 72 hours in order to prevent the emergence of the β-hemolytic streptococci of group A or B (*Str. pyogenes* or *Str. agalactiae*). Cellulitis may develop due to streptococcal infection, and usually responds to treatment with natural penicillins. The natural penicillins, which consist of penicillin G and penicillin V, are usually bactericidal in action. Like most other β-lactam antibiotics, the antibacterial activity of the drugs results from inhibition of mucopeptide synthesis in the bacterial cell wall. Resistance to these antibiotics is caused by the production of β-lactamases and/or intrinsic resistance. β-Lactamases can inactivate the drugs by hydrolyzing the β-lactam ring of the penicillin antibiotic. Intrinsic resistance can result from the presence of a permeability barrier in the outer membrane of an organism or alteration in the properties of target enzymes (penicillin-binding proteins). Should resistance or tolerance to the penicillins develop, then culture and sensitivity data would be utilized in order to select a therapeutic antibiotic for treating streptococcal infection appropriately.[8,151]

Staphylococcal infections

Staphylococcus aureus and *S. epidermidis* are natural pathogens found on skin and, therefore, are the most common cause of infections in burn populations (see Table 11.1). These microbes generally produce penicillinases which break the penicillin ring and make natural penicillins ineffective against these bacteria. These types of infections are generally treated by penicillinase-resistant penicillins which are termed 'methicillin-sensitive' and by vancomycin for those staphylococcal infections which are termed 'methicillin-resistant'.[4,115]

Penicillinase-resistant penicillins are active against many strains of *S. aureus* and *S. epidermidis* which are resistant to other commercially available penicillins because 60–95% of clinical isolates of *S. aureus* and 10–70% of clinical isolates of *S. epidermidis* produce penicillinases and are resistant to natural penicillins. These antibiotics include parenteral antibiotics (methicillin, nafcillin and oxacillin) as well as oral antibiotics (cloxacillin, dicloxacillin, nafcillin, and oxacillin).[4,115,151]

Nafcillin is the most frequently used intravenously since adverse renal effects have been reported most frequently with patients receiving IV methicillin, and hepatoxicity has been reported most frequently in patients receiving IV oxacillin. Hypersensitivity reactions are among the most frequent adverse reactions to penicillinase-resistant penicillins.[4,115,151]

Dicloxacillin is the penicillinase-resistant penicillin which is most completely absorbed from the GI tract; it is, therefore, the most frequently used oral form of these antibiotics. Dosage adjustments are generally unnecessary when nafcillin or dicloxacillin are used in patients with renal impairment. *In vitro* studies indicate that a synergistic bactericidal effect can occur against penicillinase-producing and non-penicillinase-producing *S. aureus* which are susceptible to penicillinase-resistant penicillins when nafcillin is used in conjunction with gentamicin or tobramycin.[151]

Vancomycin, alone or in conjunction with other anti-infectives, is generally considered the treatment of choice for infections caused by methicillin-resistant staphylococci. In the burn population, wherein methicillin-resistant staphylococci are reported with increasing frequency, initial therapy for suspected staphylococcal infections should include vancomycin. Vancomycin is bactericidal and appears to bind to the bacterial cell wall, causing blockage of glycopeptide polymerization. This effect, which occurs at a site different from that affected by the penicillins, produces immediate inhibition of cell wall synthesis and secondary damage to the cytoplasmic membrane. Vancomycin is administered only by slow intravenous infusion. It is very irritating to tissue and therefore cannot be given intramuscularly. It is also not appreciably absorbed from the GI tract and, therefore, cannot be given orally for the treatment of systemic infections. It must be given slowly over at least 1 hour since rapid IV administration can result in a hypotensive reaction referred to as the 'red man's syndrome' or 'red neck syndrome'. The reaction is characterized by a sudden decrease in blood pressure which can be severe and may be accompanied by flushing and/or a maculopapular or erythematous rash on the face, neck, chest, and upper extremities; the latter manifestation may also occur in the absence of hypotension.[115,151] Vancomycin must be carefully dosed and serum levels of the drug monitored since there is a narrow therapeutic versus toxic serum concentration range for this drug.

A burned patient exhibits an increased creatinine clearance of vancomycin because of his hypermetabolic state after a burn trauma. Because of the wide interpatient variability of vancomycin elimination in a burned patient, the dosage must be individualized in order to provide optimal serum concentrations. The appropriate peak therapeutic blood level is 20–40 μg/ml in the treatment of staphylococcal sepsis with a trough of between 5 and 10 μg/ml. Toxic trough levels higher than 15 μg/ml are thought to be the cause of the nephrotoxicity which may be manifested by transient elevations in the BUN (blood urea nitrogen) or serum creatinine clearance and by the presence of hyaline and granular casts and albumin in the urine. Toxic peak levels of greater than 50 μg/ml are thought to cause ototoxicity. Vancomycin may cause damage to the auditory branch of the eighth cranial nerve. Permanent deafness has occurred as a result. Tinnitis may precede the onset of deafness and necessitates discontinuance of the drug. Deafness may progress despite cessation of vancomycin therapy.[115,151]

Infections caused by MRSA (methicillin-resistant *Staphylococcus aureus*) or methicillin-resistant *S. epidermidis* can be treated with vancomycin in conjunction with rifampin and/or an aminoglycoside. Because of the additive toxicities with the concurrent systemic use of ototoxic or nephrotoxic drugs such as the aminoglycosides, their use should be carefully monitored.[151]

Enterococcal bacterial infections

The enterococcal microbial isolates most frequently isolated from burn wounds at Shriners Burns Institute are *Ec. faecalis* and *Ec. faecium.* Enterococcal bacteria, unlike other gram-positive microorganisms, are not very susceptible to any of the penicillin antibiotics. Presently the only antibiotic that appears to be 98–100% effective against the gram-positive organisms that are methicillin resistant and against the enterococci is vancomycin. The carbapenem antibiotic, imipenem, and the aminoglycoside gentamicin are synergistic against the enterococci; but vancomycin is still the superior agent.

Gram-negative Bacterial Infections

The four most common gram-negative microbial isolates in the burn population at Shriners Burns Institute – Galveston are *Ps. aeruginosa*, *E. coli*, *Kl. pneumoniae*, and *Ent. cloacae*, in that order (see Table 11.13). The antibiotic arsenal used and its efficacy is quite varied based on the individual susceptibility of the microbial isolate to each antibiotic agent singly and in combination with other antibiotics.

Aminoglycosides

The aminoglycosides and, in particular, gentamicin, were historically the antibiotics of choice in the treatment of gram-negative infections. The synergistic activity with penicillinase-resistant penicillins and vancomycin in the treatment of staphylococcal infections further standardized its premier status before the advent of newer extended-spectrum penicillins, the third generation cephalosporins, the monobactams, the carbapenems, and the quinolones[115,151] (see Figures 11.3–11.6).

Aminoglycosides are usually bactericidal in action. Although the exact mechanism has not been fully elucidated, these drugs appear to inhibit protein synthesis in susceptible bacteria by irreversibly binding to 30S ribosomal units. The aminoglycosides consist of amikacin, gentamicin, kanamycin, neomycin, netilmicin, paromomycin, and tobramycin. The aminoglycosides' narrow therapeutic blood serum range is a critical factor in dosing burn populations since their hypermetabolic state makes dosing a function of the patient's blood levels and their creatinine clearance. As with vancomycin, ototoxicity and nephrotoxicity occur most frequently with toxic serum levels and the additive toxicities of their concurrent use should be carefully monitored.[114,115]

Recommended therapeutic trough levels for gentamicin and tobramycin are between 1 and 2 μg/ml, and for amikacin are between 5 and 10 μg/ml. The acceptable peak levels are 4–10 μg/ml for gentamicin and tobramycin and 20–30 μg/ml for amikacin. An increased risk of toxicity occurs in gentamicin and tobramycin with prolonged peak serum concentrations of greater than 10–12 μg/ml and concentrations greater than 30–35 μg/ml for amikacin and/or trough concentrations greater than 2 μg/ml for gentamicin and tobramycin and greater than 10 μg for amikacin. Although gentamicin is used IV or IM extensively in the burn population, resistance due to increased permeability of the bacterial cell wall, alterations in the ribosomal binding site, or the presence of a plasmid-mediated resistance factor which is acquired by conjugation, all led to the increased usage of tobramycin and amikacin. Amikacin is not a suitable substrate for most of the aminoglycoside-modifying enzymes produced by plasmid-mediated resistance. Currently even amikacin appears to be only 70–80% effective against *Ps. aeruginosa* isolates at the Shriners Burns Institute (see Figure 11.6b).

Extended-spectrum penicillins

The advent of the extended-spectrum penicillins, and their reputed synergistic effect with aminoglycosides, brought a new era of antibiotic therapy in burn infections. The extended-spectrum penicillins, which consist of carbenicillin, mezlocillin, piperacillin, and ticarcillin, are more active than other penicillins against gram-negative bacilli because they are more resistant to inactivation by β-lactamases which is produced by gram-negative bacteria and/or because they more readily penetrate the outer membranes of these organisms. Extended-spectrum penicillins reportedly vary in their rates of bactericidal action and in their completeness of this effect. This appears to result partly from differences in drug-induced morphologic effects on susceptible bacteria and subsequent formation of bacterial variants with varying degrees of osmotic stability. The extended-spectrum penicillins should therefore never be used alone in the treatment of gram-negative infections. A synergistic effect between extended-spectrum antibiotics and aminoglycosides are generally unpredictable and should be confirmed with appropriate *in vitro* studies (see Figures 11.3a, 11.4a, 11.5a, 11.6a).

The combination of ticarcillin with clavulanic acid, a β-lactamase inhibitor, results in a synergistic bactericidal effect against many strains of β-lactamases producing bacteria. Clavulanic acid has a high affinity for and irreversibly binds to certain lactamases which can inactivate the extended-spectrum penicillins. The usage of extended-spectrum penicillins in the treatment of gram-negative bacterial infections provides a burn population with a much less toxic antibiotic when compared to the aminoglycosides since the most frequent adverse reactions to extended-spectrum penicillins are hypersensitivity reactions, Gl effects, and local reactions.

Third generation cephalosporins

Third generation cephalosporins were the first antibiotics since aminoglycosides which could be used alone in the treatment of gram-negative infections. The third generation cephalosporins are β-lactam antibiotics which are usually bactericidal; like the penicillins, their activity results from inhibition of mucopeptide synthesis in a cell wall. β-Lactam antibiotics bind to several enzymes, which are involved in cell wall synthesis and cell division. In a bacterial cytoplasmic membrane; this binding results in the formation of defective cell walls and osmotically unstable spheroblasts. The target enzymes have been classified as penicillin-binding proteins (PBPs) and appear to vary substantially among bacterial species. The β-lactam antibiotic spectra of activity is based on an affinity of these antibiotics for different PBPs in susceptible organisms. The third generation cephalosporins (which consist of cefixime, cefoperazone, cefpodoxime, ceftazidime, ceftizoxime, ceftriaxone, and moxalactam), display an expanded spectrum of activity against gram-negative bacteria compared with the first and second generation cephalosporins. Currently, the susceptibility of *E. coli* to ceftazidime is 100%, and the susceptibility of *Ent. cloacae* to cefotaxime ranges from 70% to 100%. The most frequently reported adverse reactions to cephalosporins are hypersensitivity reactions (approximately 5%). Other, less frequent, adverse reactions include hematologic effects, renal and genitourinary effects, hepatic effects, GI effects, and local effects (see Figures 11.3b, 11.4b, 11.5b, 11.6b).

Miscellaneous β-lactam antibiotics

Aztreonam is termed a synthetic monobactam antibiotic because, unlike other β-lactam antibiotics which are bycyclic, it is a monocyclic β-lactam antibiotic. The antibacterial activity of aztreonam results from inhibition of mucopeptide synthesis in the bacterial cell wall; but, in addition, aztreonam has a high affinity for PBP 3.[151] Although aztreonam has a narrow spectrum of activity, it is active *in vivo* against many of the gram-negative bacteria which are most frequently found in burn units, including most Enterobacteriaceae and *Ps. aeruginosa*. At Shriners Burns Institute – Galveston, *Ps. aeruginosa* exhibits a 90–100% susceptibility to aztreonam. Aztreonam has a high degree of stability against hydrolysis by bacterial β-lactamases including both plasmid-mediated and chromosomally mediated enzymes (see Figure 11.6b). Adverse effects reported with aztreonam are similar to those reported with other β-lactam antibiotics, and the drug is generally well tolerated.

Imipenem/cilastatin sodium is a combination of imipenem, a carbapenem antibiotic, with cilastatin sodium, a specific and reversible inhibitor of dehyropeptidase I which inactivates imipenem by hydrolyzing the β-lactam ring. Imipenem is usually bactericidal in action. Like other β-lactam antibiotics, the antibacterial activity of imipenem results from inhibition of mucopeptide synthesis in the bacterial cell wall. Imipenem has an affinity for, and binds to, most penicillin-binding proteins (PBPs) of susceptible organisms. Imipenem is able to penetrate the outer membrane of most Gram negative bacteria and gain access to the PBPs more readily than many other currently available β-lactam antibiotics. *In vitro* studies also indicate that imipenem may have a postantibiotic inhibitory effect against some susceptible organisms such as *S. aureus*, *E. coli*, and *Ps. aeruginosa*. At Shriners Burns Institute – Galveston, *E. coli*, *Kl. pneumoniae*, and *Ent. cloacae* all showed susceptibility of 90–100% to imipenem/cilastatin sodium. *Ps. aeruginosa* showed a susceptibility of 80–100% to imipenem/cilastatin sodium. *In vitro* studies indicate that imipenem is a potent inducer of β-lactamases and can reversibly derepress inducible, chromosomal, mediated β-lactamases in *Ps. aeruginosa*, and Enterobacteriaceae. Although these enzymes inactivate aztreonam and most cephalosporins, adverse effects reported with imipenem and cilastatin are similar to those reported with other β-lactam antibiotics; and the drug is generally well tolerated although adverse central nervous system effects, including seizures and myoclonus, have been reported with IV imipenem and cilastatin sodium (see Figures 11.3b, 11.4b, 11.5b, 11.6b).

Quinolones

The quinolones class of antibiotics includes parenteral antibiotics (ciprofloxacin and ofloxacin) and oral antibiotics (ciprofloxacin, enoxacin, nalidixic acid, norfloxacin and ofloxacin). Ciprofloxacin IV is the most effective quinolone in the treatment of serious gram-negative and gram-positive infections. It is usually bactericidal in action and works by inhibiting DNA synthesis. Susceptibility of *Ent. cloacae* at Shriners Burns Institute to ciprofloxacin was 98.8%. A postantibiotic inhibitory effect can be produced *in vitro* in some organisms (including some strains of the Enterobacteriaceae, *Ps. aeruginosa*, *S. aureus*, and *Ec. faecalis*) by serial passage in the presence of increasing concentrations of the drug. Strains of MRSA, which are resistant to ciprofloxacin, have been reported with increasing frequency, and such strains can emerge at relatively rapid rates. Ciprofloxacin usage is contraindicated in pediatric patients because it causes arthropathy in immature animals. The most frequent adverse effects of the drug involve the GI tract or the CNS.

Antifungals

Amphotericin B

Chemistry. Amphotericin B is an antifungal antibiotic produced by *Streptomyces nodosus*. The drug is an amphoteric polyene macrolide which occurs as a yellow to orange, odorless or practically odorless powder and is insoluble in water and in anhydrous alcohol. Each mg of amphotericin B contains not less than 750 μg of anhydrous drug. Amphotericin B for injection is commercially available as a sterile, buffered, lyophilized yellowish powder which contains sodium desoxycholate as a solubilizing agent.

Fungi. *In vitro*, amphotericin B concentrations of 0.03–1.0 μg/ml usually inhibit *Aspergillus fumigatus*, *Paracoccidioides brasiliensis*, *Coccidioides immitis*, *Cryptococcus neoformans*, *Histoplasma capsulatum*, *Mucor mucedo*, *Rhodotorula* spp., and *Sporothrix schenckii*. *Blastomyces dermatitidis* may require slightly higher drug concentrations for inhibition. The minimum inhibitory concentration (MIC) of amphotericin B for *Candida* varies with species and strains; the MIC for *C. albicans* and *C. guilliermondii* is 0.2–1.9 mg/ml, and for strains of *C. tropicalis* the MIC ranges from 0.2–25 mg/ml. It has been suggested that to successfully treat a systemic fungal infection, serum amphotericin B concentrations should be maintained at twice the *in vitro* MIC for the infecting fungus.

Protozoa. Amphotericin B is active *in vitro* and *in vivo* against *Leishmania braziliensis*. The drug is also active *in vitro* and *in vivo* against *L. mexicana* and *L. donovani*, including antimony-resistant strains of the organisms. *In vitro*, amphotericin B concentrations of 1 mg/ml result in complete elimination of *L. donovani* amastigotes in human monocyte-derived macrophages and *L. donovani* promastogites in cell-free media. The drug is also active *in vitro* against *L. tropica*.

Absorption. Amphotericin B is poorly absorbed from the GI tract and must be given parenterally to treat systemic fungal infections. Immediately after completion of IV infusion of 30 mg of amphotericin B, average peak serum concentrations of 1 mg/ml can be achieved; with a dose of 50 mg, average peak serum concentrations will be approximately 2 mg/ml. Immediately after infusion, no more than 10% of the amphotericin B dose can be accounted for in serum. Average minimum serum concentrations of approximately 0.4 mg/ml have been reported when doses of 30 mg were given daily or when doses of 60 mg were given every other day.

Elimination. The elimination half-life of amphotericin B in patients whose renal function is normal prior to therapy is approximately 24 hours. Then after the first 24 hours, the rate at which amphotericin B elimination decreased. Over a 7-day period, the cumulative urinary excretion of a single dose of amphotericin B is about 40% of the administered drug. Following long-term administration of the drug, the elimination half-life of amphotericin B was 15 days, which suggests that slow release of the drug from the peripheral compartment may have accounted for the long half-life. It has been estimated that only about 3% of a total dose of amphotericin B is excreted in urine unchanged. The drug can be detected in blood for up to 4 weeks and in urine for up to 4–8 weeks after discontinuance of therapy. Amphotericin B is not hemodialyzable.

Adverse Effects. Most patients who receive IV amphotericin B experience several of the following reactions: headache, chills, fever, hypotension, tachypnea, malaise, muscle and joint pain, anorexia, weight loss, dyspepsia, cramping, epigastric pain, and nausea and vomiting. Most of these reactions are considered to be dose related, and they are usually less severe when the drug is administered slowly or on alternate days. Antipyretics, antihistamines, and antiemetics provide some symptomatic relief from many of the adverse effects of amphotericin B. The febrile reaction, which is sometimes accompanied by shaking chills, usually appears 1–3 hours after the start of IV infusion of amphotericin B and thus can be differentiated from chills due to bacterial infection; the febrile reaction usually subsides within 4 hours after discontinuance of the IV infusion.

Other acute reactions (e.g. hypotension, nausea, vomiting, tachypnea) appear 1–3 hours after initiating IV infusion of amphotericin B; the severity of these reactions may decrease with subsequent doses of the drug. IV administration of corticosteroids prior to or during amphotericin B therapy reportedly decreases the severity of febrile reactions.

Nephrotoxicity occurs in about 80% or more of the patients receiving the drug IV. Although nephrotoxicity of amphotericin B involves several mechanisms, including direct vasoconstriction, the drug appears to have a lytic action on cholesterol-rich lysosomal membranes of renal tubular cells.[151,154]

Fluconazole

Chemistry. Fluconazole is a synthetic triazole-derivative antifungal agent. The drug is structurally related to imidazole-derivative antifungal agents (e.g. butoconazole, clotrimazole, ketoconazole, miconazole) since it contains a five-membered azole ring attached by a carbon–nitrogen bond to other aromatic rings. However, imidazoles have two nitrogens in the azole ring and fluconazole and other triazoles (e.g. itraconazole, terconazole) have three nitrogens in the ring.

Spectrum. Fluconazole is active against fungi, including yeasts and dermatophytes. Fluconazole does not appear to have antibacterial activity.

Absorption. The pharmacokinetics of fluconazole are similar following IV or oral administration. The drug is rapidly and almost completely absorbed from the GI tract, and there is no evidence of first-pass metabolism. Oral bioavailability of fluconazole exceeds 90% in healthy, fasting adults; peak serum concentrations of the drug generally are attained within 1–2 hours after oral administration. The rate and extent of GI absorption of fluconazole are not affected by food.

Unlike some imidazole-derivative antifungal agents (e.g. ketoconazole), GI absorption of fluconazole does not appear to be affected by gastric pH. Studies in healthy, fasting adults indicate that peak serum concentrations, areas under the concentration–time curves (AUCs), time to peak serum concentrations, and elimination half-life of fluconazole are not affected substantially by concurrent administration of drugs that increase gastric pH.

In healthy, fasting adults who received a single 1 mg/kg oral dose of fluconazole, peak serum concentrations of the drug averaged 1.4 mg/ml. Following oral administration of a single 400-mg dose of fluconazole in healthy, fasting adults, peak serum concentrations average 6.72 mg/ml (range: 4.12–8.1 mg/ml).

In healthy adults receiving 50 or 100 mg doses of fluconazole given once daily by IV infusion over 30 minutes, serum concentrations of the drug 1 hour after dosing on the sixth or seventh day of therapy range from 2.14 to 2.81 or 3.86 to 4.96 mg/ml, respectively.

Elimination. The serum elimination half-life of fluconazole in adults with normal renal function is approximately 30 hours (range: 20–50 hours). Serum elimination half-life of the drug is 22 hours after the first day of therapy and 23.8 and 28.6 hours after 7 and 26 days of therapy, respectively.

In patients with impaired renal function, plasma concentrations of fluconazole are higher and the half-life prolonged; elimination half-life of the drug is inversely proportional to the patient's creatinine clearance. In addition, there is limited evidence that elimination of the drug may be impaired in geriatric patients. The elimination half-life of fluconazole reportedly is not affected by impaired hepatic function.

Renal clearance of the drug averages 0.27 ml/min per kg in adults with normal renal function. Approximately 60–80% of a single oral or IV dose of fluconazole is excreted in urine unchanged, and about 11% is excreted in urine as metabolites. Small amounts of the drug are excreted in feces.

Fluconazole is removed by hemodialysis and peritoneal dialysis. The amount of the drug removed during hemodialysis depends on several factors (e.g. type of coil used, dialysis flow rate).

Adverse effects. Fluconazole generally is well tolerated. Adverse effects have been reported in about 5–30% of patients receiving fluconazole for 7 days or longer and have been severe enough to require discontinuance of the drug in about 1–2.8% of patients.

Fever, edema, pleural effusion, oliguria, hypotension, arthralgia/myalgia, anaphylaxis, and finger stiffness have been reported rarely in patients receiving fluconazole. Hypokalemia, which required potassium replacement therapy and/or discontinuance of fluconazole, has occurred occasionally, including in several neutropenic patients with acute myeloid leukemia. Increased serum creatinine and BUN concentrations also have been reported.[151,154]

Factors Rendering Antimicrobials Neutralized

The binding of antimicrobials to proteins of tissue has been a subject of major concern for microbiologists and surgeons alike. This binding accounts for the reduced tissue levels which are occasionally noted when therapeutic doses of the aminoglycosides and cephalosporins are administered. Insoluble acid proteins, along with intracellular proteins, such as nucleic acids, are the components responsible for such an event.[115,120,151] Polymyxins bind to the phospholipids of a tissue membrane, while soluble intracellular protein binding occurs with such drugs as penicillin and cephalosporin.[115,120,151] The antimicrobial action of tobramycin and gentamicin is diminished by high calcium and magnesium concentrations.[120] Among other factors which diminish the activity of antimicrobials are included blood flow, intracellular location of bacteria, and pH. Anaerobic and hypercapnic conditions have been shown to render antibacterials, such as aminoglycosides, inactive or less responsive against facultative organisms. Although nonprotein-bound drugs diffuse exceedingly well into locations containing blood clots, such a condition can significantly reduce the antibacterial effect upon staphylococcal organisms which are present at the time of surgery.[120,151] Moreover, inert substances, such as fecal material, can render aminoglycosides inactive or alter the antimicrobial potential.[120,151]

The appearance of antimicrobial-resistant bacteria has been considered to be primarily the result of a predictable process, i.e. the development of a spontaneous mutation of a microbe with an occurrence rate of one organism in 10 million to 1 billion cell divisions and with discriminative proliferation of the resistant organism in the presence of the antibiotic. Even more devastating is the phenomenon called 'infectious drug resistance'. This is a process whereby a genetic marker, called a plasmid, which carries an antibiotic-resistant factor is transferred from a resistant organism to a nonresistant one of the same species or of a different species.[8,120,151]

Lacey[8] has reported on the ecological relationship between staphylococci and humans; and he presents some threatening concerns. Both *S. aureus* and *S. epidermidis* reside in cohabitation on the body surfaces and in nasopharyngeal cavities of humans. It is in the realm of possibility that the reservoir for these resistant plasmids could have originated in *S. epidermidis* which subsequently is then transferred to *S. aureus*. The encoding of plasmid tetracycline resistance in *S. epidermidis* is similar to that in *S. aureus*. The most probable site for transfer occurs on the surface of skin of a host.[9,155]

In a study by Siegel *et al.*[156] on the continuous nontherapeutic use of antimicrobials in food-producing animals, the incidence of drug resistance was monumental. Organisms isolated from the feces of both bovine animals and swine demonstrated a minimum of 50% resistance to dihydrostreptomycin and oxytetracycline, and resistance was as high as 90% in most cases.

The delivery of tetracycline was found by Burton and colleagues[157] to magnify colonization of the intestinal tract of humans by a resistant *E. coli* of bovine origin. The use of this antibacterial subsequently provided a mechanism for these drug-resistant factors to *E. coli* which were resident flora in humans.[156]

Summary

Topical and systemic antibacterials are powerful chemotherapeutic agents. They can not, and will never, render humans germ-free. The incidence of infection in operative procedures has changed little in the decades since the discovery of antimicrobials, and infection is most obviously not the result of visitation from without.[110,116,117] Antimicrobials should be used with therapeutic accuracy, observing that there are many pitfalls.[115,120] In conclusion, physicians should aim to 'SHOOT WITH A RIFLE, NOT A SCATTER GUN'.

Acknowledgements

The author wishes to acknowledge Ms Cassie Maness for her devoted and conscientious efforts in the preparation of this manuscript. I would also like to acknowledge our Graphic Arts Department: Ms Sandra Baxter, our medical illustrator, who provided timely and precise illustrations of the data, and Mr Lewis Milutin Jr, and Ms Tina Garcia for their photographic expertise.

References

1. Robson M C, Heggers J P. Surgical infection. I. Single bacterial species or polymicrobic in origin. *Surgery* 1969; **65:** 608.

2. Balows A, Hausler W J, Jr, Herrmann, K L, Isenberg H D, Shadomy, H J, (eds.) *Manual of Clinical Microbiology*. 5th ed. Washington D.C: American Society for Microbiology, 1991: 1364 pp.

3. Baron S, Jennings P M. *Medical Microbiology*. 3rd ed, New York: Churchill Livingstone, 1991: 1340 pp.

4. Heggers J P, Robson M C eds. *Quantitative Bacteriology: Its Role in the Armamentarium of the Surgeon.* 1st ed. Boca Raton, FL: CRC Press, Inc. 1991: 139 pp.

5. Dowell V R Jr, Lombard G L, Thompson F S M, Armfield A Y. *Media for isolation; Characterization and Identification of Obligately Anaerobic Bacteria.* Washington DC: US Department of Health, Education & Welfare, NCDC, November 1977: 1–46.

6. Holt, J G, Krieg N R, Smeath P H A, Staley J T, Williams S T, eds. *Bergey's Manual of Determinative Bacteriology*. 9th ed. Baltimore: Williams & Wilkin Co, 1994.

7. Gibbs B M, Skinner F A, eds. *Identification Methods for Microbiologists, Part A.* New York: Academic Press, 1966: 204 pp.

8. Lacey R W. Antibiotic resistance plasmids of *Staphylococcus aureus* and their clinical importance. *Bacteriol Rev* 1975; **39:** 1–32.

9. Heggers J P, Phillips L G. Boertman J A, *et al. The Epidemiology of Methicillin-Resistant Stapphylococcus aureus in a Burn Center. J. Burn Care Rehabil* 1988: **9:** 610–12.

10. Ellner P D. *Current Procedures in Clinical Bacteriology*. 2nd ed. Springfield, IL: Charles C Thomas, 1978: 229 pp.

11. Mandell G L, Douglas, R G Jr, Bennett J E eds. *Principles and Practice of Infectious Diseases*. 3rd ed. New York: Churchill Livingstone, 1990; **2:** 2340 pp.

12. Robson, M C, and Heggers, J P. Surgical infection. II. β-hemolytic streptococcus. *J Surg Res* 1969; **9:** 289.

13. Christie R, Atkins N E, Munch–Peterson E. A note on a lytic phenomenon shown by Group B streptococci. *Aust J Exp Biol* 1944; **22:** 197.

14. Gunn B A. SXT & Taxo A disks for presumptive identification of Group A & B streptococci in throat cultures. *J Clin Microbiol* 1976; **4:** 192.

15. Smith L D S, Holderman L V. *The Pathogenic Anaerobic Bacteria*. 2nd ed. Springfield, IL: Charles C Thomas, 1968; 423 pp.

16. Kingsley R F. Selective medium for *Bacillus anthracis*. *J Bacteriol* 1966; **92:** 784.

17. Pennington J E, Gibbons N D, Strobeck J E, *et al.* *Bacillus* species infection in patients with hemotolic neoplasia. *JAMA* 1976; **235:** 1473.

18. Turnball P C B, French T A, Dowsett E G. Severe systemic and pyogenic infections with *Bacillus cereus. BMJ* 1977; **1:** 1628.

19. Turnball P C B, Nottingham J F, Ghosh A C. A severe necrotic enterotoxin produced by certain food, food poisoning and other clinical isolates of *Bacillus cereus. Br J Exp Path* 1977; **58:** 273.

20. McManus W F, Goodwin C W, Mason A D Jr, Pruitt B A Jr. Burn wound infection. *J Trauma* 1981; **21:** 3133–8.

21. Brook I, Randolph J G. Aerobic and anaerobic bacterial flora of burns in children. *J Trauma* 1981; **21:** 558–63.

22. Hartford C E, Ziffren S E. Electrical injury. *J Trauma* 1971; **11:** 331–6.

23. Gorbach S L, Thadepalli H. Isolation of *Clostridium* in human infections: evaluation of 114 cases. *J Infect Dis* 1975; **131**(Suppl): S81–5.

24. Davies D M. Gas gangrene as a complication of burns. *Scand J Plast Reconstr Surg* 1979; **12:** 73–5.

25. Sherman R T. The prevention and treatment of tetanus in the burn patient. *Surg Clin North Am* 1970; **50:** 1277–81.

26. Larkin J M, Moylan J A. Tetanus following a minor burn. *J Trauma* 1975; **15:** 546–8.

27. Artz C P, Moncrief J A. *The Treatment of Burns*. Philadelphia: W B Saunders Co, 1969: 585 pp.

28. Teplitz C. The pathology of burn and fundamentals of burn wound sepsis. In: Artz C P, Moncrief J A, Pruitt B A Jr eds. *Burns: A Team Approach*. Philadelphia: W B Saunders Co, 1979: 45–94.

29. Heggers J P, Barnes S T, Robson M C, *et al.* Microbial flora of orthopaedic war wounds. *Milit Med* 1969; **134:** 602.

30. Speller D C E, Stephens M E, Viant A C. Hospital infection by *Pseudomonas cepacia. Lancet* 1971; **1:** 1798.

31. Bassett D C J, Stokes K J, Thomas W R G. Wound infection with *Pseudomonas multivorans. Lancet* 1970; **1:** 1188.

32. Gilardi G L. *Pseudomonas maltophilia infections* in man. *Am J Clin Pathol* 1969; **51:** 58.

33. Rigney M M, Zilinsky J W, Rouf M A. Pathogenicity of *Aeromonas hydrophila* in red leg disease in frogs. *Curr Microbiol* 1978; **1:** 175–9.

34. Scholz D, Scharmann W, Blobel H. Leucocidic substances from *Aeromonas hydrophila. Zbl Bakt Hyg, I Abt Orig A* 1974; **228:** 312–16.

35. Bernheimer A W, Avigad L S, Avigad G. Interactions between aerolysin, erythrocyte membranes. *Infect Immun* 1975; **11:** 1312–19.

36. von Graevenitz A, Mensch A H. The genus *Aeromonas* in human bacteriology: report of 30 cases and review of the literature. *N Engl J Med* 1968; **278:** 245.

37. D'Alauro F, Ansinelli R. *Aeromonas hydrophila* septicemia in a previously healthy man. *JAMA* 1978; **240:** 1139.

38. Harris R L, Fainstein V, Elting L, Hopfer R L, Bodey G P. Bacteremia caused by *Aeromonas* species in hospitalized cancer patients. *Rev Infect Dis* 1985; **7:** 314–20.

39. Qadri S M H, Gordon L P, Wende R D, Williams R P. Meningitis due to *Aeromonas hydrophila. J Clin Microbiol* 1976; **3:** 102–4.

40. Davis W A, Kane J G, Garagusi V F. Human *Aeromonas* infections. *Medicine* 1978; **57**(3): 267–77.

41. Feaster F T, Nisbet R M, Barber J C. *Aeromonas hydrophila* corneal ulcer. *Am J Ophthalmol* 1978; **85:** 114–17.

42. Salton R, Schick S. *Aeromonas hydrophila* peritonitis. *Cancer Chemother Rep* 1973; **57:** 489–91.

43. Hanson P G, Standridge J, Jarett F, Maki D G. Fresh-water wound infection due to *Aeromonas hydrophila. J Am Med Assoc* 1977; **238:** 1053–4.

44. Fulghum D D, Linton W R Jr, Taplin D. Fatal *Aeromonas hydrophila* infection of the skin. *South Med J* 1978; **71**(6): 739–41.

45. Lawson M A, Burke V, Chang B J. Invasion of HEp-2 cells by fecal isolates of *Aeromonas hydrophila. Infect Immun* 1985; **47:** 680–3.

46. Atkinson H M, Trust T J. Hemagglutination properties and adherence ability of *Aeromonas hydrophila. Infect Immun* 1980; **27:** 938–46.

47. Purdue G F, Hunt J L. *Aeromonas hydrophila* infection in burn patients. *Burns* 1988; **14**(3): 220–1.

48. Edwards P R, Ewing W H. *Identification of Enterobacteriaceae*. 3rd ed. Minneapolis: Burgess Publishing Co, 1972: 362 pp.

49. Johnson W G, Pierce A K, Sanford J P. Changing pharyngeal bacterial flora of hospitalized patients. *N Engl J Med* 1969; **281:** 1137.

50. Selden R, Lee S, Wang W L L, *et al.* Nosocomial *Klebsiella* infections: intestinal colonization as a reservoir. *Ann Intern Med* 1971; **74:** 657.

51. Bizo A. *Serratia marcescens* vescicula tenuissima lactic primo roseo: Dehine rubro repleta. *Bil ital gl legg sc* 1823; **30:** 288.

52. Davis J T, Foltz E, Blakemore W S. *Serratia marcescens:* a pathogen of increasing clinical importance. *JAMA* 1970; **214:** 2190.

53. Heniyoji E Y, Whitson T C, Obashi D K, Allen B C. Bacteremia due to *Serratia marcescens. J Trauma* 1971; **11:** 417.

54. Alexander R H, Reichenbach D D, Merindino K A. *Serratia marcescens* endocarditis. *Arch Surg* 1969; **98:** 287.

55. Quintilani R, Gifford R H. Endocarditis from *Serratia marcescens. JAMA* 1969; **208:** 2055.

56. Hall A, Inguagiato G J, Park C. *Serratia marcescens* septicemia complicating splenectomy in a child. *Virginia Med Month* 1971; **98:** 605.

57. Dutton A A C, Ralston M. Urinary tract infection in a male urological ward with special reference to the mode of infection. *Lancet* 1957; **1:** 115.

58. Middleton J E. The sensitivity in vitro of the *Providencia* group of enteric bacteria to 14 antiobiotics and nitrofurantoin. *J Clin Pathol* 1958; **11:** 270.

59. Solberg C O, Matsen J M. Infection with providence bacilli. A clinical and bacteriologic study. *Am J Med* 1971; **50:** 241.

60. Von Graevenitz A, Strouse A. Isolation of *Erwinia* species from human sources. *Antonie van Leeuwenhoek* 1966; **32:** 429.

61. Von Graevenitz A. *Erwinia* species isolates. *Ann NY Acad Sci* 1970; **174:** 436.

62. Nichols R E, Smith J. Clinical aspects of anaerobic infections in the surgical patient. *Am J Med Technol* 1975; **41:** 87.

63. Felner J M, Dowell V R Jr. Bacteroides bacteremia. *Am J Med* 1971; **50:** 878.

64. Dowell J R Jr, Lombard G L. Presumptive identification of anaerobic nonspore forming gram-negative bacilli. Washington DC: US Department of Health, Education and Welfare, NCDC, 1980: 1–13.

65. Becker W K, Cioffi W G Jr, McManus A T, *et al.* Fungal burn wound infection. A 10 year experience. *Arch Surg* 1991; **126**(1): 44–8.

66. Bruck H M, Nash G, Foley F D, *et al.* Opportunistic fungal infection of the burn wound with phycomycetes and *Aspergillus. Arch Surg* 1971; **102:** 476–82.

67. Desai M H, Herndon D N, Abston S. Candida infection in massively burned patients. *J Trauma* 1981; **21**(3): 237–9.

68. Nash G, Foley F D, Goodwin M N Jr *et al.* Fungal burn wound infection. JAMA 1971; **215:** 1664–6.

69. Spebar M J, Lindberg R B. Fungal infection of the burn wound. *Am J Surg* 1981; **21**(3): 237–9.

70. Spebar M J, Lindberg R B. Fungal infection of the burn wound. *Am J Surg* 1979; **138:** 879–82.

71. Burdge J J, Rea F, Ayers L. Noncandidal, fungal infections of the burn wound. *J Burn Care Rehabil* 1988; **9**(6): 599–601.

72. Pruitt B A Jr. Phycomycotic infections. *Probl Gen Surg* 1984: 664–78.

73. Neame P, Rayner D. Mucormycosis: a report of 22 cases. *Arch Pathol* 1960; **70:** 261–8.

74. Kobayashi K, Mukae N, Matsunaga Y, Motchit M. Diagnostic value of serum antibody to candida in an extensively burned patient. *Burns* 1990; **16**(6): 414–17.

75. Goldstein E, Hoeprich P D. Problems in the diagnosis and treatment of systemic conditions. *J Infect Dis* 1980; **125:** 190–3.

76. Kidson A, Lowbury E J L. Candida infection of burns. *Burns* 1980; **6:** 228–30.

77. Solomkin J S, Simmons R L. Candida infection in surgical patients. *World J Surg* 1980; **4:** 381–94.

78. Prasad J K, Feller I F, Thomson P D. A ten year review of *Candida* sepsis and mortality in burn patients. *Surgery* 1987; **101:** 213–16.

79. Mead J H, Lupton G P, Dillavou C L, *et al.* Cutaneous rhizopus infection. *JAMA* 1979; **242:** 272–4.

80. Del Pelacio Hernandez A. Nosocomial infection by *Rhizomucor pusillus* in a clinical hematology unit. *J Hosp Infect* 1983: **4**(1): 45–9.

81. Gartenberg G, Bottone E J, Keusch F T, *et al.* Hospital acquired mucormycosis (*Rhizopus rhizopodiformis*) of skin and subcutaneous tissue: epidemiology, mycology and treatment. *N Engl J Med* 1978; **299:** 1115–18.

82. Linneman C C Jr, MacMillan B C. Viral infections in pediatric burn patients. *Am J Dis Child* 1983; **135:** 750–3.

83. Deepe G S Jr, MacMillan B C, Linnemann C C Jr. Unexplained fever in burned patients due to cytomegalovirus infection. *JAMA* 1982; **248:** 2299–301.

84. Goodwin C W, McManus W F. Viral infections in burned patients. *Immunology* 1985; **12:** 3–4, 8–9.

85. Edgar P, Kravitz M, Heggers J P, *et al.* Herpes simplex in pediatric burn patients. *Proc Am Burn Assoc* 1990; **22:** 56.

86. Weintraub W H, Lilly A B, Randolph J G. A chickenpox epidemic in a pediatric burn unit. *Surgery* 1974; **76:** 490–4.

87. Teplitz C, Davis D, Mason A D, Moncrief J A. Pseudomonas burn wound sepsis. I. Pathogenesis of experimental pseudomonas burn wound sepsis. *J Surg Res* 1964; **4:** 200–16.

88. Pruitt B A, Foley F D. The use of biopsies in burn patient care. *Surgery* 1973; **73:** 887–97.

89. Parks D H, Linares H A, Thompson P D. Surgical management of burn wound sepsis. *Surg Gynecol Obstet* 1981; **153:** 374–6.

90. Shehan D C Hrapchak B B *Theory and Practice of Histotechnology*. St Louis: C V Mosby, 1980: 146, 162, 232, 245.

91. Milne J A *An Introduction to the Diagnostic Histopathology of the Skin*. Baltimore: Williams and Wilkins Co., 1972: 199 pp.

92. Sasaki T M, Welch G W, Herndon D N, *et al.* Burn wound manipulation induced bacteremia. *J Trauma* 1979; **19**(1): 46–8.

93. Beard C H, Ribeiro C D, Jones D M The bacteremia associated with burns surgery. *Br J Surg* 1975; **62:** 638–41.

94. Hamory B H Nosocomial sepsis related to intravascular access. *Crit Care Nurs Q* 1989; **11**(4): 58–65.

95. Samsoondar W, Freeman J B, Coultish I, *et al.* Colonization of intravascular catheters in the intensive care unit. *Am J Surg* 1985; **149:** 730–2.

96. Maki D G, Jarrett F, Sarafin H W. A semiquantitative culture method for identification of catheter related infection in the burn patient. *J Surg Res* 1977; **22:** 513–20.

97. Stein J M, Pruitt B A Jr. Suppurative thrombophlebitis: a lethal iatrogenic disease. *N Engl J Med* 1970; **282:** 1452–5.

98. Franceschi D, Gerding R L, Phillips G, Fratianne R B. Risk factors associated with intravascular catheter infection in burned patients; a prospective randomized study. *J Trauma* 1989; **29**(6): 811–16.

99. Smallman L, Burdon D W, Alexander-Williams J. The effect of skin preparation and care on the incidence of superficial thrombophlebitis. *Br J Surg* 1980; **67:** 861–2.

100. Sheth N K, Franson T R, Rose H D, *et al.* Colonization of bacteria on polyvinyl chloride and Teflon intravascular catheters in hospitalized patients. *J Clin Microbiol* 1983; **18:** 1061–3.

101. Maki D G, Botticelli J T, LeRoy M L, *et al.* Prospective study of replacing administration sets for intravenous therapy at 48 to 72 hour intervals. *JAMA* 1987; **258:** 177–81.

102. Pruitt B A Jr, Stein J M, Foley F D, *et al.* Intravenous therapy in burn patients: suppurative thrombophebitis and other life threatening complications. *Arch Surg* 1970; **100:** 399–404.

103. Artz C P, Moncrief J A. *The treatment of Burns*. Philadelphia: W B Saunders Co, 1969: 585 pp.

104. Heggers J P, Robson M C, Ko F, *et al.* Transient and resident microflora of burn unit personnel and its influence on burn wound sepsis. *Infect Control* 1982; **3:** 471–4.

105. Pruitt B A Jr, McManus A T. Opportunistic infections in severely burned patients. *Am J Med* 1984; **76:** 146–53.

106. Robson M C Bacterial control in the burn wound. *Clin Plast Surg* 1979; **6**(4): 515–22.

107. Burke J R, Quinby W C, Bondoc C C, *et al.* The contribution of a bacterial isolated environment to the prevention of infection in seriously burned patients. *Ann Surg* 1977; **186:** 377–87.

108. Perez-Cappelano R, Manelli J C, Dalayret D, *et al.* Evaluation of the septicaemic risk by quantitative study of the cutaneous flora in patients with burns. *Burns* 1976; **3:** 42–5.

109. Robson M C, Krizek T S. Predicting skin graft survival. *J Trauma* 1973; **13**(3): 213–17.

110. Robson M C, Krizek T J, Heggers J P. Biology of surgical infection. In: Ravitch M M, ed. *Current Problems in Surgery* Chicago: Yearbook Medical Publishers, 1973: 1–62.

111. Robson M C. Burn sepsis. *Crit Care Clin* 1988; **4**(2):281–98.

112. Levenson S M, Alpert S, DelGuerico L, *et al.* The use of whole and partial body isolators for the care of severely burned patients. *Ann NY Acad Sci* 1968; **150**(3): 1009–11.

113. Lowbury E S L, Babb S R, Ford P M. Protective isolation in a burn unit: the use of plastic isolators and air curtains. *J Hyg* 1971; **69:** 529–46.

114. Nance F C, Lewis V, Bornside G H. Absolute barrier isolation and antibiotics in the treatment of experimental burn wound sepsis. *J Surg Res* 1970; **10:** 33.

115. Heggers J P. The use of antimicrobials agents. In: Krizek T J, Robson M C, eds. *Clinics in Plastic Surgery*. Philadelphia, PA: W B Saunders Co, 1979; **6:** 545–51.

116. Robson, M C. Quantitative bacteriology and the burned patient. In: Heggers J P, Robson M C, eds. *Quantitative Bacteriology: Its Role in the Armamentarium of the Surgeon*. Boca Raton, FL: CRC Press, 1991: 97–108.

117. Robson M C, Duke W F, Krizek T J. Rapid bacterial screening in the treatment of civilian wounds. *J Surg Res* 1973; **14:** 426.

118. Robson M C. Wound healing and wound closure. In: Heggers J P, Robson M C, eds. *Quantitative Bacteriology in the Armamentarium of the Surgeon*. Boca Raton, FL: CRC Press, 1991: 43–53.

119. Lowbury E J L. Wits versus genes: the continuing battle against infection. *J Trauma* 1979; **19:** 33–45.

120. Heggers J P. Antimicrobial agents. In: Heggers J P, Robson M C, eds. *Quantitative Bacteriology: Its Role in the Armamentarium of the Surgeon*. Boca Raton, FL: CRC Press, 1991: 115–25.

121. Moncrief J A. Topical antibacterial treatment of the burn wound. In: Artz C P, Moncrief J A, Pruitt B A Jr, eds. *Burns, a Team Approach*. Philadelphia, PA: W B Saunders Co, 1979: 250–69.

122. Nathan P, Law E J, Murphy D F, McMillan B G. A laboratory method for selection of topical antimicrobial agents to treat infected burn wounds. *Burns* 1979; **4:** 177–187.

123. Piotech J B, Meakins J L. Predicting infection in surgical patients. *Surg Clin North Am* 1979; **59:** 185–97.

124. Moncrief J A, Lindberg R B, Switzer W E, Pruitt B A. The use of a topical sulfonamide in the control of burn wound sepsis. *J Trauma* 1966; **6**(3): 407–19.

125. Holder I A, Schwab M, Jackson L. Eighteen months of routine topical antimicrobial susceptibility testing of isolates from burn patients: results and conclusions. *J Antimicrob Chemother* 1979; **5:** 455–63.

126. Lineweaver W, McMorris S, Soucy D, Howard R. Cellular and bacterial toxicities of topical antimicrobials. *Plast Reconstr Surg* 1985; **75:** 394–6.

127. Heggers J P, Sazy J A, Stenberg B D, *et al.* Bactericidal and wound healing properties of sodium hypochlorite. *J Burn Care Rehabil* 1991; **12:** 420–4.

128. Fader R C, Maurer A, Stein M D, Abston S, Herndon D N. Sodium hypochlorite decontamination of split-thickness cadaveric skin infected with bacteria and yeast with subsequent isolation and growth of basal cells to confluency in tissue culture. *Antimicrob Agents Chemother* 1983; **24:** 181–5.

129. Robson M C. The use of topical agents to control bacteria. In: Dimick A R, ed. *The Burn Wound in Practical Approaches to Burn Management*. Deerfield, IL: Flint Laboratories, Travenol, Inc, 1977: 17–19.

130. Heggers J P, Robson M C. The emergence of silver sulfadiazine resistant *Pseudomonas aeruginosa*. *Burns* 1978; **5:** 184–7.

131. Unpublished data, 1994.

132. Moncrief J A. The status of topical antibacterial therapy in the treatment of burns. *Surgery* 1968; **63:** 862.

133. Kucan J O, Smoot E C. Five percent mafenide acetate solution in the treatment of thermal injuries. *J Burn Care Rehabil* 1993; **14:** 158–3.

134. Lindberg R B, Moncrief J A, Mason Jr A D. Control of experimental and clinical burn wound sepsis by topical application of sulfamylon compounds. *Ann NY Acad Sci* 1968; **150:** 950.

135. Georgiade N G, Harris W A. Open and closed treatment of burns with povidone-iodine. In: Polk H C Jr, Ehrenkranz N J eds. *Therapeutic*

Advances and New Clinical Impressions: Medical and Surgical Antisepsis with Betadine Microbicides. Yonkers NY: Purdue Frederick and Co, 1972: 250–67.

136. Krizek T J, Davis J H, DesPrez J D, *et al*. Topical therapy of burns – experimental evaluation. *Plast Reconstr Surg* 1967; **39:** 248.

137. Livingston D H, Cryer H G, Miller F B, Malangoni M A, Polk H C, Weiner L J. A randomized prospective study of topical antimicrobial agents on skin grafts after thermal injury. *J Plast Reconstr Surg*. In Press.

138. Strock L L, Lee M, Rutan R L, *et al*. Topical Bactroban® (Mupirocin): efficacy in treating MRSA wounds infected with methicillin-resistant staphylococci. *J Burn Care Rehabil* 1990: **11:** 454–9.

139. Heggers J P, Carino, E S, Sazy J A, *et al*. A topical antimicrobial test system (TOPITEST®): Nathan's agar well revisited. *Surg Res Commun* 1990; **8:** 109–16.

140. Fuller A T, Mellows G, Woodford M, *et al*. Pseudomonic acid, an antibiotic produced by *Pseudomonas fluorescens*. *Nature* (*Lond.*) 1971; **234:** 416–17.

141. Buchvald J. An evaluation of topical mupirocin in moderately severe primary and secondary skin infections. *J Int Med Res* 1988; **16:** 66–70.

142. Denning D W, Driffith D H. Eradication of low-level resistant *Staphylococcus aureus* skin colonization with topical mupirocin. *Infect Control Hosp Epidemiol* 1988; **9**(6): 261–3.

143. Rode H, DeWet P M, Shepard G H, *et al*. Bacterial efficacy of mupirocin in multiantibiotic resistant *Stapylococcus aureus* burn wound infection. *J Antimicrob Chemother* 1988; **21:** 589–95.

144. Pruitt B A Jr, Foley F. The use of biopsies in burn patient care. *Surgery* 1973; **73:** 8878–97.

145. Heggers J P, Robson M C, Herndon D N, Desai M H. The efficacy of nystatin combined with topical microbial agents in the treatment of burn wound sepsis. *J Burn Care Rehabil* 1989; **10:** 508–11.

146. Krizek T J, Koss N, Robson M C. The current use of prophylactic antibiotics in plastic and reconstructive surgery. *Plast Reconstr Surg*, 1975; **55:** 21–33.

147. Krizek T J, Gottlieb L J, Koss H, Robson M C. The use of prophylactic antibacterials in plastic surgery: a 1980's update. *Plast Reconstr Surg* 1985; **76:** 953–63.

148. Richards J H. Bacteremia following irritation of foci of infection. *JAMA* 1932; **99:** 1496–7.

149. LeFrock J L, Ellis C A, Turchik, J B, Weinstein L. Transient bacteremia associated with sigmodoscopy. *N. Engl J Med* 1973; **289:** 467–9.

150. Bennington J L ed. *Saunders Dictionary and Encyclopedia of Laboratory Medicine and Technology*. Philadelphia, PA: W B Saunders Co, 1984: 167, 1375.

151. Kucers A, Bennett McK N. *The Use of Antibiotics*. 5th ed. Philadelphia, PA: J B Lippincott Co, 1987: 1–1678.

152. Gladtke E, von Hattingberg H M. *Pharmacokinetics: An Introduction*. New York: Springer-Verlag, 1979.

153. Rowland M, Tozer T N. *Clinical Pharmacokinetics: Concepts and Applications*. Philadelphia: Lea & Febiger, 1980.

154. *Physicians Desk Reference®* PDR, 48th ed. Montvale NJ: Medical Economics Co Inc, 1994: 517–519 and 1095–1096.

155. Shanson D C, Kensit J G, Duke R. Outbreak of hospital infection with a strain of *Staphylococcus aureus* resistant to gentamicin and methicillin. *Lancet* 1976; **2:** 1347.

156. Siegel D, Huber W B, Enloe F. Continuous non-therapeutic use of antibacterial drugs in feed and drug resistance of gram-negative enteric flora of food producing animals. *Antimicrob Agents Chemother* 1974; **6:** 697–706.

157. Burton G C, Hirsh, D C, Blendin D C, *et al*. The effects of tetracycline on the establishment of *Escherichia coli* of animal origin and the *in vivo* transfer of antibiotic resistance in the intestinal tract of man. In: Skinner F A, Carr J E eds. *Normal Microbial Flora on Man*. Symposium #3. New York: Academic Press, 1973: 507–21.

CHAPTER TWELVE

12

Modern Treatment of a Burn Wound

Michael J. Muller, Marc Nicolai, Renee Wiggins, Kirsty MacGill and David N. Herndon

Introduction

The natural action of a full-thickness burn wound is to promote an inflammatory response at the junction of the burned, dead layer, the eschar, and the underlying viable tissue. At this interface, bacterial proliferation in the eschar attracts polymorphonuclear leukocytes (neutrophils) which release large quantities of proteolytic enzymes and inflammatory mediators. Subsequent enzymatic action results in separation of the eschar from the now granulating interface. If a burn is large, then the inflammatory response at the burned site becomes generalized. (This effect is described more fully elsewhere.) Briefly, mediators such as prostanoids, thromboxane, histamine, cytokines, and tumor necrosis factor are all produced and released from a burned site. The serum levels of these mediators become measurable and increase in proportion to increasing size of a burned area. The hypermetabolic response with protein catabolism, increased metabolic rate, increased susceptibility to infection, marked weight loss, and poor wound healing continue until the outpouring of mediators abates. While topical antimicrobial agents such as mafenide acetate and silver sulfadiazine have decreased the frequency and severity of systemic sepsis, these agents prolong eschar separation and, therefore, the hypermetabolic response.

Treatment of full-thickness burns by awaiting spontaneous separation and subsequent skin grafting is a prolonged process associated with much pain and suffering, severe metabolic derangements, multiple septic episodes, and lengthy hospitalization. While this technique may be acceptable for small inconsequential burns, modern burn care is based on operative treatment of burn wounds. This chapter reviews the evidence supporting early excision of full-thickness burn wounds, discusses operating techniques and wound closure, briefly describes the process of skin graft incorporation, and examines the quality of life for those who have survived massive burns.

The colour plates for this chapter appear between pp 264 and 265.

Rationale for Excision

Prompt wound closure has been shown repeatedly to improve survival, decrease length of hospital stay, and curb expenditure for burned patients of all ages. Children particularly have benefited from more aggressive surgical intervention.[1,2] There has been a remarkable increase in the burn size associated with a 50% mortality risk (**Table 12.1**). It is now unusual for a child to succumb to burn injury of any size, even if it is associated with a smoke inhalation injury. Improving nutritional support and control of sepsis have played a part in this achievement; but the major advance has been surgical in nature. Burke[3] reported on results of total excision of full-thickness burns in 1974. He applied homografts (cadaver skin) to seal wounds, controlled rejection by adding immunosuppressives, and cared for his patients in laminar flow chambers. Children with massive burns began surviving their injuries in situations where they had never done so before. Improved mortality, shorter hospital stay, and fewer metabolic complications were noted by others when early excision was retrospectively compared with late excision.[4] In a trial of 32 children, with an average age of

Table 12.1 Mortality and burn size

Age (years)	Burn size of 50% 1942–1952* (%TBSA)	Mortality 1980–1991† (%TBSA)
0–14	49	98
15–44	46	70
45–64	27	46
>65	10	19

%TBSA, percentage of total body surface area burned.
* Bull and Fisher.[1]
† Muller and Herndon.[2]
Adapted from Muller M J, Herndon D N. The challenge of burns. *Lancet* 1994; **343:** 216–20, with permission.

7 years and burn size of 65% total body surface area (TBSA), who either underwent total excision to fascia or serial debridement, mortality, overall blood loss, and cumulative operating time were equivalent.[5] The early excision group had their length of hospital stay almost halved (97 ± 8 days versus 57 ± 5 days). Since that time, hundreds of children with burns >30% TBSA treated with early excision have enjoyed a length of hospital stay less than 1 day per % TBSA burn.[6]

The mortality of adult burned patients at Massachusetts General Hospital declined from 24%, in 1974, to 7%, for 1979–1984, after prompt eschar excision and immediate wound closure was instituted as standard therapy in 1976.[7] Logistical regression analysis showed that this treatment significantly improved survival (p<0.001) Thirty adult patients admitted to the Shriners Burn Institute – Galveston with large burns, ~73% TBSA, were randomized to receive conservative or active excision on admission.[8] In patients with burns greater than 50% TBSA and no inhalation injury, mortality was decreased with early excision, perhaps due to age differences. Total blood requirements were similar between groups, negating an often used argument against excisional therapy. This study was expanded to include 85 patients, aged 17–55 years.[6] Those patients aged 17–30 years without inhalation injury showed significantly decreased mortality if treated by early excision (9%), than if treated conservatively (45%). Patients with a concomitant inhalation injury or aged greater than 30 years derived no survival benefit from early excision.

Older burned patients have been shown to benefit from an early surgical approach. Dietch[9,10] operated upon 114 consecutive patients with an average age of 68 years and showed a reduction of 40% in mean length of hospital stay when compared to national averages; and mortality was less than predicted. Many studies[11–15] show that early excision can be safely performed in the elderly, with clear benefit of a lower duration of hospitalization and number of septic episodes. Saffle[13] showed that the number of preexisting medical conditions had no effect on survival, a salient point when planning treatment. The elderly also benefit from aggressive surgical treatment of their donor site wounds. They very commonly have loose and movable skin. If donor sites or burns are situated on the lower abdomen, the flank, or thigh, then they are amenable to excision and repair in the same manner as a reduction abdominoplasty.[16] This has the effect of reducing the area of open wound and decreasing the metabolic demand placed on their physiology.

Munster[17] and colleagues demonstrated a statistically significant decrease in length of stay which significantly correlated with a decrease in the interval between surgical interventions over a 14-year period at their institution. Other variables such as burn size, inhalation injury and age remained static during this time (**Table 12.2**). The average annual increase of hospital charges for burn care grew at 9.6%, which was substantially lower than the hospital as a whole – 10.8%. Mortality rate decreased significantly, while burn indices remained constant. Aggressive surgical intervention in burn care can be associated with cost containment.

Table 12.2 Hospital stay and interval between surgeries

	LOS (days)	Surgical interval (days)
1979	23	14
1990	14*	6

LOS, length of hospital stay. LOS significantly decreased as the interval between surgical interventions decreased.
Adapted from Munster A M, Smith-Meek M, Sharkey P. Effect of early surgical intervention on mortality and cost effectiveness in burn care. *Burns* 1994; **20:** 61–4, with permission from Elsevier Science Ltd, Oxford.

Partial-thickness Wounds

Janzekovic[18] observed that deep donor sites could be overgrafted with thinner split-thickness skin harvested from another area. She then extended this concept to dermal burns by excising thin layers of burn until living tissue was reached. Split skin grafts were immediately applied. This tangential excision and autografting of dermal burns was a major advance. Prior to this time, only full-thickness burns were excised and this usually occurred as a formal integumentectomy which took subcutaneous fat and lymphatics down to an underlying layer of investing fascia. This process was commonly known as fascial excision. Tangential excision technique was used by Janzekovic in more than 2000 patients and, as a result, hospital stay, pain, and reconstructive procedures were all decreased.[19] Heimbach[20] observed that deep partial thickness burns took many weeks to heal instead of converting to full-thickness because topical antimicrobials controlled infection. These wounds showed persistent blistering, pruritus, hypertrophic scar formation, and poor functional results. These observations promoted prospective trials of early excision and grafting versus nonoperative treatment of burns of indeterminant depth[21] of less than 20% TBSA. Shorter hospitalization, lower cost, less time away from work and greater use of blood products were seen in those treated operatively. Long-term follow-up demonstrated no difference in need for reconstruction, incidence of blisters, incidence of loss of motion, or contour irregularities. Those patients treated nonoperatively required more late grafts for closure and developed more hypertrophic scarring.

Deep partial-thickness burns to the hand are problematic. While full-thickness burns of the hand should be excised and grafted as soon as practicable after diagnosis and if area coverage is not required in patients with massive burns,[22,23] the role of early operation for partial-thickness hand burns is contentious.[24–27] If donor skin is available and the depth of the burn cannot be determined (partial or deep partial) and wound healing will not be complete in 10 days, then excision and grafting is reasonable and certainly indicated if early discharge is advantageous. If wide area coverage is paramount or wounds will heal quickly, other techniques can be used. These include topical antimicrobials covered with dressings or a plastic glove, enclosing the hand in a plastic bag filled with topical antimicrobials, or application of a Biobrane[R] glove.[28]

Hypertrophic scar formation is common. Dark skinned people and children are more prone to its development; however, the most important determinant of hypertrophic scarring is delayed wound healing. Deitch[29] has clearly shown that if wounds take more than 10 days to heal, then the risk is significant; and the risk rises to 80% if healing is delayed beyond 21 days. Surgery is indicated for those with wounds failing to heal promptly.

Operative treatment is also an effective means of limiting the duration of pain which burned patients must endure. The ghastly experience of wound debridement in the tub by picking at the eschar, sometimes for many weeks, is recounted by many as the worst part of burn survivorship. Excisional therapy of the burn wound is humane and lifesaving, offers improved cosmetic and functional results, is cost-effective, and swiftly returns a patient to their normal environment.

Scald Burns

Hot water scald burns of small or moderate size have been shown to be the exception to the general rule of early excision. Young children who had scald burns about 20% TBSA needed less area excised and had smaller blood transfusion requirements if operated upon in the second and third week postburn.[30] Earlier operation resulted in greater blood transfused, while later operation led to much increased hospital stays (**Table 12.3**).

A subsequent prospective trial randomized 24 children to early or late excision if their hot water scald injury had caused burns of clinically indeterminant depth.[31] No patient experienced a significant wound infection or systemic sepsis. Only half of the delayed excision group ultimately required surgical intervention and a significantly smaller area of excision was necessary for the remainder (**Table 12.4**).

Table 12.3 Scald burn excision

Day 1st surgery	0–5	6–10	11–20	>20
n	37	14	19	15
Weight (kg)	12.2±0.4	11.9±0.4	11.1±0.5	11.1±0.8
% TBSA	27±3	20±2	24±3	26±4
Blood loss (ml)	890±150*	400±70	430±140	240±160
Length of stay	24±2	26±2	31±3	51±7‡

Data presented as means±SEM.
* ‡Significantly different to all other groups.
Adapted from Irei M, Aleston S, Bonds E, Ruton T, Desai M, Herndon D N. The optimal time for excision of scald burns in toddlers. *J Burn Care Rehabil* 1986; **7:** 508–10.

Primary tangential excision involves blood loss; this is one of the chief drawbacks of the technique. Decreased blood loss seemed apparent during the first few days postburn.[33] Therefore, 318 children and adolescents with burns >30% TBSA were studied. The average blood loss per surface area excised (ml/cm^2) was compared at various postburn periods of excision (**Figure 12.1**). No operative deaths occurred, and mean operative time was 2.4 ± 0.1 hours. The entire full-thickness burn, with the exception of the face and perineum, was tangentially excised via a hand knife; and contiguous partial-thickness burn was removed to the point of punctate bleeding using serial passes of an electric dermatome. Those whose blood pressure was greater or less than 40% of baseline, whose urine output was less 0.75 ml/kg/h, or who developed pulmonary edema intraoperatively, or whose hematocrit was >48 or <24% were excluded due to inappropriate perioperative resuscitation. Overall mortality was 5% for an average size burn of 60% TBSA. Notably, early excision had no adverse effect on mortality.

Blood loss is greatly reduced if excision is performed very early postburn. Vasoactive metabolites are much elevated during this time, particularly thromboxane – a potent vasoconstrictor.[34] Abundance of these vasoconstrictors, both locally and systemically, explains the clear advantage of day 1 burn wound excision.

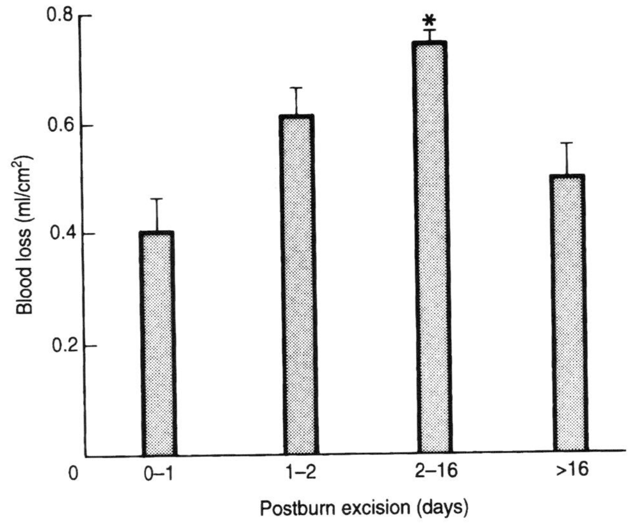

*Fig. 12.1 Blood loss during burn wound excision. Histogram depicting changes in blood loss over time for patients with burns >30% TBSA. *Significantly different ANOVA p<0.01 vs. 0–1 and >16.*
(Adapted from Herndon D N, Broemeling L, Barrow R E, Nichols R J, Ruton R L. Early burn wound excision significantly reduces blood loss. Ann Surg *1990;* **211:** *753–62, with permission.)*

Surgical Techniques and Practices

Perioperative Nursing Role

To more accurately reflect the role and responsibilities of the nurse in surgery, the term perioperative nurse is rapidly replacing terminology such as operating room nurse, theatre nurse, or surgical nurse. This role includes preoperative, intraoperative, and postoperative phases of assessment and care. As defined by the National Association of Theatre Nurses, the role of the perioperative nurse is to:

- act as liaison with ward nurses and others to identify patient/nursing care requirements during the perioperative phase;
- provide planned individual care before, during, and after surgery/anesthesia monitoring;
- evaluate the effectiveness of care delivered;
- work with others to complete operative and other procedures;
- assess and evaluate changing needs and carry out patient care during the perioperative period;

Table 12.4 Early vs. late excision

	n	Age	Burn size (% TBSA)	Postburn day excised	% Excised	Blood loss (TBBT)
Early excision	12	1.8±0.4	28±3	3±1	21±4	1.2±0.3
Late excision	6//12†	1.9±0.5	24±3	16±1	8±2*	0.3±0.1*

Data expressed as means±SEM.
TBBT, total body blood turnover.
* Significantly different compared with early excision.
† Only 6 of 12 underwent excision.
Adapted from Desai M H, Ruton R L, Herndon D N. Conservative treatment of scald burns is superior to early excision. *J Burn Care Rehabil* 1991; **12:** 483.

- ensure patient safety;
- maintain records of nursing care.

There is a process by which the perioperative nurse collects, organizes, and utilizes relevant data in order to develop a care plan with realistic, attainable goals (**Figure 12.2**). Such planning enhances continuity of care which seems to foster trust among the nurse, the patient, and the family of the patient. Consequently, this decreases some of the psychological trauma for a patient and family. Because this expanded role integrates the perioperative nurse into the 'total picture' of patient care, multidisciplinary communication is greatly improved, enabling a nurse to better function as a patient advocate during the intraoperative phase.

The preoperative phase is most appropriately defined as the period of time from admission to an institution to the time a patient is transferred from a unit to an operating room. During this time, a circle of communication must develop around the patient. Direct communication may be limited to a circle encompassing the unit nurse, perioperative nurse, and anesthetist, but may include exchange with extensive ancillary staff such as music therapists, child life specialists, or information psychologists who work to allay fears in an anxious child. Communication of information surrounding the patient and family is the basis of the development of an individualized care plan. Following data collection and analyses, a perioperative nurse is able to formulate nursing diagnoses.

Initial patient assessments are important for determining transport and operating room needs. In addition to routine contents, such as history and physical examination, recent laboratory values, and surgical consents, a nurse reviews a patient's chart for information regarding the nature and extent of a burn injury, need for and type of grafting anticipated, amount of blood/blood products which will be necessary, and any special equipment required. Good communication between nurse and surgeon is crucial in procuring the appropriate type(s) and quantities of graft material(s). Since there are multiple ways in which the same burn injury may be treated, it is imperative that a surgical plan be clearly identified by a burn team. Regardless of the type required, these materials are expensive and usually in limited supply.

Perioperative teaching to a patient/family is essential regardless of age, neurological status, or emergent nature of a case. Teaching is best accomplished by a primary nurse circulator with first-hand knowledge of operating room procedures. Teaching offers a nurse an opportunity to develop a relationship with a patient and family. The perioperative nurse should consult with a unit nurse and review the medical record prior to meeting with a patient and family. Data collected from the history and physical examination consent forms and progress notes as well as a verbal report from a unit nurse will help a perioperative nurse develop a concise teaching plan. In order to provide a patient with age-appropriate information, a perioperative nurse must be familiar with the stages of human growth and development. Ideally, teaching should take place the evening prior to the planned procedure, with this information reinforced prior to the administration of preoperative medications. The entire teaching process must include the family in order to ensure their understanding and gain their cooperation and involvement in the perioperative plan of care.

A perioperative nurse plans the transport of a patient to an operating room. Transport must be well orchestrated and performed by an organized, informed team in order to prevent untimely delays and to insure patient safety. Considerations include maintenance of respiratory and hemodynamic status, thermoregulation, and physical/psychological comfort for a patient. An anesthetist, anesthesia assistant, or respiratory therapist may also be present during transport in order to provide supplemental oxygen or mechanical ventilation. Patency of intravenous catheters are verified and should be sutured in place. Core temperatures are maintained by providing heat reflective or warmed blankets and covering of the scalp. Preoperative medication(s) should be administered so that peak level times will provide maximum sedation and/or anxiolytic effect. A patient with multiple catheters, splints/traction devices, or need for ventilatory assistance is best transported in his/her existing bed. This reduces the risk of displaced catheters and tubes, decreases the amount of time a patient is disconnected from monitors, and eliminates unnecessary transfers which may cause discomfort.

Perioperative nursing responsibilities include nutritional support intraoperatively by continuous enteral feedings. The feeding pump is discontinued only during transport, bronchoscopic procedures, and the insertion of catheters which require a patient to be in the Trendelenburg position. The rate remains unchanged from predetermined calculations unless otherwise determined by an anesthetist in order to compensate for intravenous fluids or blood volume requirements.

Nursing concerns intraoperatively include:

- potential hypothermia related to radiant, contact, and convective heat loss;
- potential fluid/electrolyte imbalance due to surgical intervention and active blood loss;
- the presence of adequate supplies of fluids and blood products;

PREOPERATIVE PHASE
ASSESSMENT
Ø
Unit nurse — Patient charts — Patient/family interview
Ø
Data collection
Ø
NURSING DIAGNOSIS
Ø
Problem identification
Ø
PLAN
Ø
Statements of expected outcomes
Intraoperative nursing intervention
Ø
INTRAOPERATIVE PHASE
IMPLEMENTATION
Ø
Initiate intraoperative nursing interventions
Documentation of actions
Ø
EVALUATION
Ø
Determine and document effectiveness of intraoperative nursing interventions
Ø
POSTOPERATIVE PHASE
Ø
Post-anesthesia recovery for return to nursing unit

Fig. 12.2 The process by which the perioperative nurse collects, organizes, and utilizes relevant data in order to develop a care plan with realistic, attainable goals.

- potential infection due to surgical intervention; and
- preparation and monitoring of a patient.[35]

Thermoregulation of a burned patient is one of the most important and challenging intraoperative tasks for the perioperative nurse. This is especially true in a pediatric population since bradycardia, often a result of hypothermia, may be fatal.[35] Basal metabolic rates which may be as high as 100% above normal, extensive skin integumentary destruction, a high ratio of body surface area to mass, and anesthetic agents which depress the body's shivering response or cause cutaneous vasodilation further abet a potentially rapid decrease in a patient's core temperature. Multiple interventions are employed in an effort to maintain a patient's core temperature intraoperatively. First, an acceptable temperature prior to transfer is maintained. If the core temperature is less than 36.5°C and a patient is not in immediate danger of loss of life or limb, policy is to delay transport until the problem is corrected. In the operating room, heat lamps and heaters assist in warming a patient.

In one institution, a bank of triple high intensity discharge heat lamps combined with a set of 3000 W radiant heaters are permanently installed in the ceiling directly over the surgical table. The radiant heaters are rheostat equipped, allowing heat output to be regulated from 0 to 100%. Initial settings are 50% and are adjusted according to patient need. Both lamps and heaters are turned on well in advance of patient transfer in order to warm drapes and table. The room temperature is increased to a minimum of 29°C with a relative humidity of 50%. Traffic flow is minimized to avoid drafts and loss of room heat. The surgical prep, irrigation, and dressing solutions are warmed to 35–37°C. Blood/blood products and intravenous solutions are administered via a rapid infusion warming unit at 38°C and humidified oxygen or inhalation gases are warmed to 35°C.

Although esophageal or rectal probes are acceptable, indwelling bladder catheter probes seem to be the safest, most accurate and trouble-free method of monitoring patient core temperatures. A digital readout is constantly displayed on overhead monitors and assessed every 30 minutes in conjunction with urine output. Rarely are thermoregulatory complications encountered when these interventions are used. In the event that these measures prove inadequate, nonoperative sites are covered with warm sterile sheets or sterile plastic bags. Warmed bags of IV solutions may be packed next to axilla, groin, and scalp. The circulating nurse must also be attentive to the well-being of the surgical team given the increased ambient temperature.

In order to avoid hypo- or hypervolemia, accurate hemodynamic monitoring in a burned patient is crucial, especially in a pediatric population due to the high ratio of body surface area to mass.[36] Within the first 24 hours postburn, massive edema resulting in hypovolemia and impaired renal function is a potentially fatal problem, further complicated by the possibility of blood loss intraoperatively. A perioperative nurse assists an anesthetist with the preparation of pressure catheters and continues to monitor a patient during their insertion. Indicators which a nurse can monitor are pulse rate, blood pressure waveform, capillary bed refill, and urinary output.[36] These factors are more accurate than blood pressure in determining hemodynamic status since hypotension is a very late indictor of hypovolemia in children.[37]

In most cases, both central venous and arterial pressures are monitored. The subclavian vein is generally used for central venous catheter placement. Femoral or radial arteries are typically used for the arterial catheter placement. As with temperatures, data from both are continuously displayed on overhead monitors. The subclavian catheter allows intermittent monitoring of natural venous pressure, which has limited value as an indicator of hemodynamic status in burned patients.[38] It is important, however, for the early detection of pulmonary edema. The subclavian catheter provides a source for blood gas sampling when arterial catheters are not placed, and provides access to large lumen veins which are less likely to sclerose due to infusions of irritating antibiotics or cardiac medications. The arterial catheter provides continuous monitoring of systolic, diastolic, and mean arterial pressures; it also provides access for frequent blood gas samplings during a case.

The surgical table is prepared with sterile drapes and towels. The occiput is padded; and an appropriate sized shoulder roll is used to provide hyperextension for airway maintenance. A towel is provided which swaddles the wrist and is tucked under the buttocks, while the arm is gently pulled cephalad. This position aids subclavian placement. Several towels are placed under the buttocks in order to thrust the pelvis forward to aid femoral catheter placement. A small sterile backfield is prepared with sterile gauze pads. Povidone–iodine solution is used to prepare insertion site(s). Catheters are sutured in place using number 2–0 silk. Tape or occlusive dressings are unacceptable due to the frequent tubbing and bathing of patients. Following pressure catheter insertion, a flexible bronchoscopic procedure is performed on all flame injuries. A circulating nurse assists an anesthetist in obtaining right and left bronchial washings for Gram stain and quantitative cultures.

Adequate quantities of blood/blood products are ensured, checked, and made available for rapid infusion during a surgical debridement. Anticipated transfusions are based on preoperative laboratory values and expected blood loss. The authors' anesthesia staff use the following formula for blood loss calculations: 0.40 ml/cm^2 of excised area if within 24 hours and, 0.75 ml/cm^2 of excised area 2–16 days postburn. A nurse also assists in evaluating the fluid volume status by monitoring and reporting qualitative and quantitative urinary output at least every 30 minutes. An output of 1.0 ml/kg per hour in children weighing less than 30 kg is expected as a partial indicator of adequate renal and peripheral tissue perfusion. One practice of calculating urine output is to begin surgical debridement with 0 min/0 urine output. Depending upon the surgeon and region of donor site(s) available, the subcutaneous tissue may be injected with 0.45% NaCl or equivalent solution to 'lift' the tissue and ease the harvesting of donor(s). Since this fluid is rapidly absorbed by a patient, the total amount injected must be reported to the anesthetist as soon as possible.

A variety of methods are employed to promote hemostasis. They include: tourniquets, 5–20% topical thrombin spray, topical epinephrine chloride, time and pressure, and electrocautery. Depending upon the severity of bleeding, one or a combination of all five methods may be employed. Tourniquets are obviously limited to extremities and are usually used on excisions beyond 48 hours post burn (**Plate 6**). The other methods are almost always used. With topical thrombin spray in hand, a scrub nurse keeps a vigilant eye as an excision is performed. As a viable capillary bed is reached, he/she literally follows the dermatome or knife with a liberal application of topical thrombin spray. Following complete excision of each region, sponges soaked in epinephrine chloride are applied. The region is then wrapped with elastic pressure dressings. After 5–20 minutes the dressings are removed and active bleeders are cauterized. The dilution ratio of epinephrine chloride should be no less than 1:10 000; its use must be reported to the anesthetist, as hypertension or paroxysmal tachycardia may result.

Surgical preps are performed in an operating room on a customized stainless steel surgical table. Features of this table include a 5 cm high peripheral rim which channels water, blood/body fluids, and tissue into a drainage/maceration system located in the floor. Table height is adjustable, and it can be positioned in the Trendelenburg position for pressure catheter placement and reverse Trendelenburg to facilitate drainage. A built-in digital scale allows accurate weights to be taken pre- and post-surgery in order to facil-

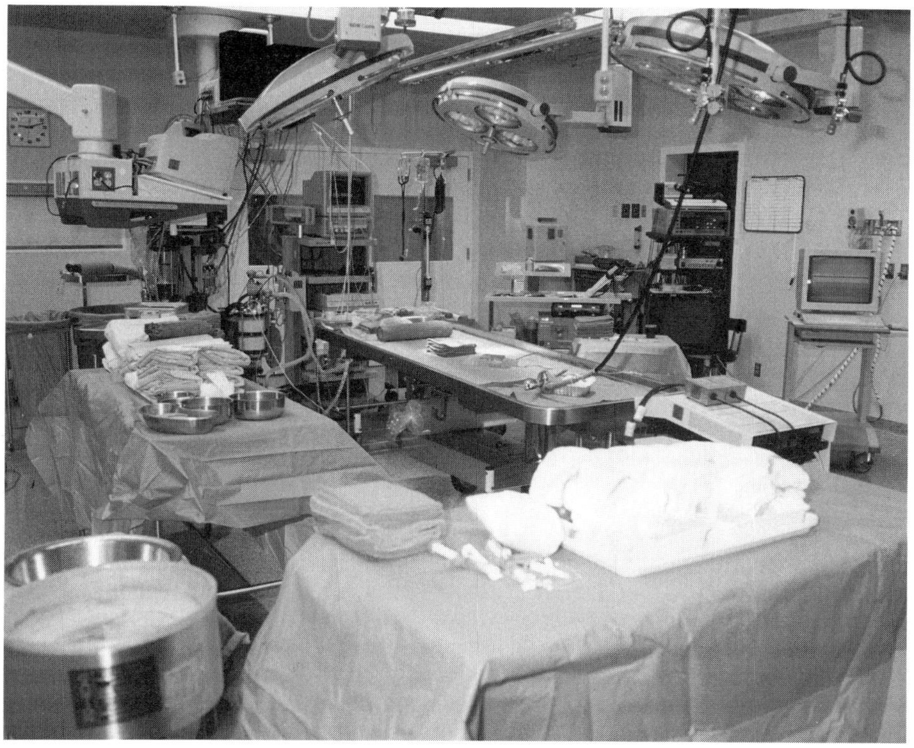

Fig. 12.3 Typical operating room set-up.

itate accurate determination of intravenous fluids, caloric intake, and medications (**Figure 12.3**)

Regardless of percent burn, a total body prep is performed using povidone–iodine scrub solution because of its broad spectrum capabilities against bacteria, fungi, and some viruses. Gentle debridement is performed to remove all loose burned tissue and eschar. If a homograft has been used in previous surgeries and is to be removed, it is usually done at this time. Existing blisters will be opened, cultured, and drained. The indwelling bladder catheter is removed if insertion time exceeds 72 hours. A patient is rinsed with 37°C filtered municipal water provided through a self-retracting overhead hose system. Once prepped, a patient is elevated from the table or log rolled and the soiled drapes are removed and replaced by a dimpled foam pad covered by sterile drapes and new shoulder roll. A new bladder catheter is inserted and a specimen for culture and sensitivity obtained. An appropriate site is selected, and the electrocautery plate is placed at this time.

Autografts are usually harvested prior to debridement. This technique avoids contamination of a surgically clean field and provides time for the scrub team to prepare the grafts. A light film of glycerol or NaCl is applied to a donor sight, allowing the dermatome to glide smoothly. Two scrub nurses are required when enough autograft has been harvested. One remains at the surgical fields assisting with donor site dressings, debridement, etc., while the other prepares the grafts. The graft is placed on a mesher dermal side down and run through. It is then turned dermal side up and placed on fine mesh gauze. Maximum expansion is achieved using a bulb irrigation syringe and NaCl. The edges of the gauze are closely trimmed and grafts are approximated on large metal trays. This allows a surgeon to pick appropriate sized pieces and estimate amounts of additional donor which will be required (**Plates 7** and **8**).

All grafts, except to the face, are covered with a topical antimicrobial using closed technique. Polysporin/mycostatin ointment (Polymyco) is a usual choice. The medication is spread on fine mesh gauze and wounds are dressed with additional bulky gauze dressings applied for further protection. Finally, an elastic compression dressing is applied in a figure eight technique so as to provide even pressure. This is especially important when extremities are involved; when applicable, a nurse checks capillary bed refills before a patient is transferred to a recovery room or unit. Splints are also applied at this time if required. As tissue is excised, a scrub nurse collects it in sterile specimen containers and labels it as to specific site. A small portion of each is sent to microbiology for quantitative culture. The remainder of each is weighed and sent to pathology to be examined for invasive microorganisms. Through cooperative efforts of the nurse and anaesthetist, systemic antibiotics are administered as scheduled. Late or missed doses can be avoided by providing the anesthetist with all required medications and their schedule at the beginning of a case.

Tangential Excision

Tangential excision allows for the removal of denatured tissue while preserving much of the surrounding viable tissue. Body contours are better preserved than with fascial or late excision.[3,18,20,39] Under ketamine anesthesia with oxygen supplementation, usually via mask in children, at 30°C and 100% relative humidity to maintain normal PaO_2 levels, the entire burn wound, with the exception of the face and perineum, is excised. Core temperatures are monitored, often via a probe combined with a urinary catheter, and are kept between 36°C and 38°C by warming the operating environment to between 28 and 30°C and using thermostat controlled radiant heaters. Intravenous fluids, including blood, are administered at a temperature of 38°C using a high-volume fluid warmer. A hand dermatome is used to excise full-thickness wounds except for small areas of the hands and feet which are excised with a blade. Deep partial-thickness wounds are tangentially excised using serial passes of an electric dermatome set at a depth of 0.005–0.01 inch until punctate bleeding is achieved. The perineum and face are left for eschar separation in order to preserve the maximum amount of viable tissue. A Watson knife set at a depth of 0.015–0.025 inch is used for full-thickness injury. The technique is somewhat akin to slicing bread and is aided greatly by traction and countertraction to place the area under tension. To ensure that adequate depth is obtained, the excised tissue can be grasped as it appears from the top of the instrument and traction applied. Healthy fat has a yellow glistening appearance and this must be obtained. Dullness, punctate hemorrhages, discoloration, or thrombosed vessels indicate nonviable tissue upon which grafts will fail. Deeper excision is mandatory in order to ensure graft survival. Partial-thickness injuries are debrided to a white, shiny surface with punctate bleeding which is myriad and copious if a burn depth is superficial and which is less frequent from larger vessels if a burn is a deep partial-thickness one (**Figure 12.4**). Hemostasis is obtained with a combination of thrombin spray, epinephrine 1:400 000 soaked gauze packs, calcium alginate sheets, pressure, electrocoagulation, and suture ligation.

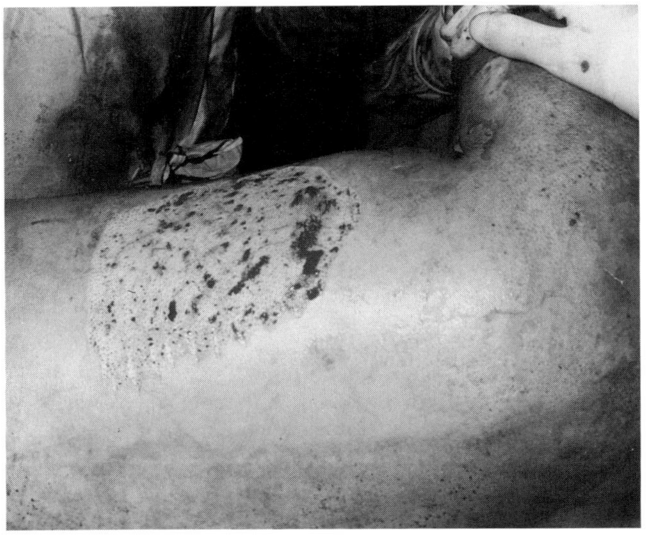

Fig. 12.4 An extensive partial-thickness flame burn extending to deep dermis. The bleeding in the excised area is from larger vessels indicating deeper dermal injury. Healthy white dermis can be seen.

Fascial excision is reserved for those areas where fat or muscle has been burned 'fourth degree'. This involves surgical removal of the full thickness of integument, including all the subcutaneous fat, down to the layer of investing fascia. The advantages of this technique are that grafts take very well to fascia and that blood loss is reduced. Episodes of sepsis lead to ischemic necrosis of subcutaneous fat subsequent to poor peripheral perfusion and microvascular stasis. This becomes problematic in patients with very large burns and leads to late graft loss; moreover, these ischemic areas become portals for invasive wound sepsis. The disadvantages of fascial excision are lymphedema and aesthetic quality. All lymphatics are excised, so lymphedema of dependent parts is often troublesome. The excised fat never regenerates and can give a spindly appearance to the areas excised, while any increase in body fat is deposited in the remaining beds of adipose tissue. Moon faces and thick necks can result. Fascial excision is also indicated for life-threatening invasive wound sepsis, particularly with fungi and yeasts such as *Aspergillus* and *candida*, and for large areas of failure of graft take in a critical patient with massive burns.

Burn Wound Closure

Autologous, partial-thickness skin grafts are the mainstay of wound closure. A graft, by definition, is completely detached from its origin and blood supply; and, therefore, its survival depends on the development of a new blood supply. Skin graft healing is a unique biological process; and the cellular mechanisms and hormonal mediators are still being defined. The process can be arbitrarily divided into the stages of adherence, plasmic imbibition, and revascularization.[40]

Adherence

When a graft is placed on a clean wound, it rapidly adheres because fibrin bonds the graft and a recipient bed. At first the adherence is weak and easily disrupted by shear forces, fluid accumulation, or hematoma formation. After 3 days, fibrovascular ingrowth and then a collagen network stabilize the graft. Fibrin bonding is faster in granulating wounds but adherence is better onto fascia. Adherence is worse in chronic and contaminated wounds because of granulation tissue fragility and bacterial protease enzymes.

Plasmic imbibition

Fluid is absorbed over the first 48 hours with accumulation of osmotically active metabolites with depolymerization of proteoglycans in the intracellular matrix. As a result, graft swelling occurs. It is unknown whether plasmic imbibition contributes to cellular nutrition or perhaps keeps a graft well hydrated with open endothelial channels. Thinner grafts have shorter distances over which diffusion occurs and therefore they tolerate this phase better than thicker grafts.

Revascularization

Morphologic changes are visible and follow the historical changes which occur. At first, a graft is white and depressed. After about 8 hours, a split-thickness graft is usually pink, but a full-thickness graft may appear cyanotic and blue because of stagnant blood. Circulation is restored 4–7 days after grafting. The newly formed vascular connections then differentiate into afferent and efferent vessels and later become reinnervated. Lymphatic circulation is also restored after a week. Historically, fine vascular channels develop in the fibrin network between graft and recipient bed. Direct anastomosis may occur between existing vessels in a graft and these newly formed vascular channels or buds. This is the inosculation theory. Alternatively, the vascular buds may invade a graft and form a new microvascular network, using preexisting channels only occasionally. Of course, both processes may occur simultaneously.

If complications such as a seroma or hematoma occur, graft revascularization is delayed. Careful hemostasis, grafting after 34 hours, quilting sutures, pressure dressings, and perforations in the graft to allow drainage have all been used to reduce the risk of such problems developing. Revascularization can also occur by continued granulation tissue formation and capillary proliferation which then invades a graft. This process is prolonged and is better survived by thinner grafts. Full-thickness grafts revascularize by establishment of flow within the dermal plexus of vessels and can, therefore, survive even if small areas of the bed are avascular, by bridging a blood supply over the defect. Full-thickness grafts tolerate ischemia poorly and may necrose completely or develop epidermal blistering, dermal scarring, and loss of appendages. There is also an increased risk of hypertrophic scarring if graft healing is delayed. Therefore, full-thickness grafts do best in areas with a rich blood supply such as the head, neck, and hands. Split-thickness grafts can survive on relatively poor beds and granulation tissue.

Graft Maturation

Epithelium

The epidermis of a graft thickens in the first few days because of edema. In a split-thickness graft, from the third post-graft day, there is marked mitotic activity in the epidermis; and this proliferation causes epithelial thickening which may persist for several weeks. The epithelial hyperplasia and cell migration to the surface causes scaling and desquamation of the graft. In a full-thickness graft, mitosis of the epithelium is delayed until revascularization has occurred. The epithelial appendages in the graft initially degenerate, but then the transplanted sweat and sebaceous glands regenerate. Until this occurs, patients may complain of dryness of the graft; and in thin grafts, this may be a continuing problem. Sweat gland function also depends on sympathetic reinnervation of the graft and follows the pattern of the recipient, not the donor site.

Hair

The original hair shafts are lost in the first week as a graft desquamates. New hair growth in full-thickness grafts is usually first detectable at 14 days and subsequently develops the same density, orientation and pigmentation as at the donor site. If graft revascularization is delayed, hair growth may be patchy, depigmented, and random so as to indicate deep dermal damage. Thick partial-thickness grafts may grow sparse fine hair, but this is rare as hair follicles are located deep within the dermis and subcutaneous tissue. Potential for later hair growth should be considered when harvesting full-thickness grafts in children.

Pigmentation

Graft color depends on vascularity and melanin production. Partial-thickness grafts from below the umbilicus to the head and neck region tend to develop a yellowish brown hue with time; and if taken from above the clavicle, the color match is better. Full-thickness grafts from head and neck donor sites provide the best color match for facial skin and may also blush.

Nerves

The timing and quality of graft reinnervation depend on a recipient site and graft thickness. Neurohistochemical studies show early ingrowth of nerve fibers into a graft from both the surrounding skin and the graft beds, and the majority of invading nerves enter the evacuated neurolemmal sheaths. Clinical studies show partial-thickness grafts develop sensation early, beginning at 4 weeks. Full-thickness grafts are slower to reinnervate but develop a better quality of sensation. The final sensory pattern in the graft resembles the recipient site. In human skin grafts, the sensory modalities of pain, light touch, and temperature return in that order; and sensation continues to improve for several years.

Contraction

Skin grafts inhibit wound contraction. Full-thickness skin grafts inhibit contraction better than thick split-thickness grafts which are better than thin or meshed grafts. Delayed healing increases the amount of wound contraction. Corps found that the amount of wound contraction depends not on the amount of dermis but the proportion of dermal thickness in the graft. As yet, mechanisms of inhibition of wound contraction by a graft are unclear. An interaction between the dermis and myofibroblast is postulated and a decrease in myofibroblast population under grafts has been found.

Dermis

The fate of dermal collagen in skin grafts is unclear. Graft collagen becomes hyalinized 3–4 days after grafting; hydoxyproline levels, which reflect collagen content, decrease in the first week. An estimated 85% of graft collagen is turned over by 5 months and in split-thickness grafts not all of the lost dermal collagen is replaced. Elastic fibers in the graft degenerate and are then slowly replaced.

Techniques of Wound Closure

If a burn is small and donor sites are plenty, grafts can be applied unmeshed or as 'sheet skin'; however, this technique requires experienced personnel to attend to the graft every few hours for a number of days in order to ensure that seromas and hematomas are controlled and expressed. Another, less labor-intensive, technique is to mesh a graft at a ratio of 1:1 or 1.5:1, but not to expand or stretch the mesh. If performed carefully, blood and seroma will drain away from the wound and an excellent cosmetic appearance will be left. These grafts are best laid perpendicular to the long axis of limbs, particularly across joint flexural creases. This will decrease the degree of contracture if it occurs. The bandages and dressings can be left intact until review.

If burns are huge and donor sites scarce, then areas such as the scalp, scrotum, and axillae may need to be harvested. These are meshed at a ratio of 4:1 and widely expanded. A wound is then sealed by application of unexpanded 2:1 meshed fresh or frozen partial-thickness cadaver skin grafts (homografts). These are applied at 90° to the autograft in a sandwich pattern as described by Alexander[41] (**Figure 12.5**). The cellular immune depression associated with massive burns makes rejection phenomena to the homograft uncommon. Fresh homografts, stored at 2°C in nutrient media, achieve an adherence rate of 95%. The face, neck, and ears are sheet grafted (unmeshed) with thick split skin, if at all possible, as this should give the best cosmetic appearance (**Figures 12.6–12.9**).

Large area donor sites are covered by scarlet red gauze, followed by dry gauze and compression bandages if anatomically possible. Bandages are removed 6 hours later and donor sites exposed. If donor sites fail to dry or develop excess moisture, a 40 W heat lamp is positioned 18 inches (46 cm) away. Heat is applied for 20 minutes each hour until dry. Smaller donor sites can be treated with moist or adherent dressings such as Opsite or Biobrane. These dressings can be applied to larger areas with innovation and effort, but they carry the risk of promoting infection if fluid accumulates beneath the occlusive layer. This can cause conversion to full-thickness wounds. Split-thickness grafts heal

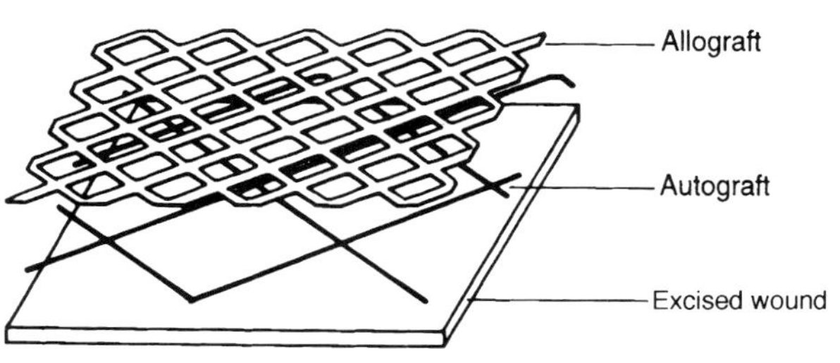

Fig. 12.5 Schematic arrangement of 'Sandwich' technique for wide area coverage. Homograft overlies widely meshed autograft and seals the wound. (From Alexander J W, MacMillan B G, Law E, Kittur D S. Treatment of severe burns with widely meshed skin autografts and meshed skin allograft overlay. J Trauma *1981;* **21:** *434, with permission.)*

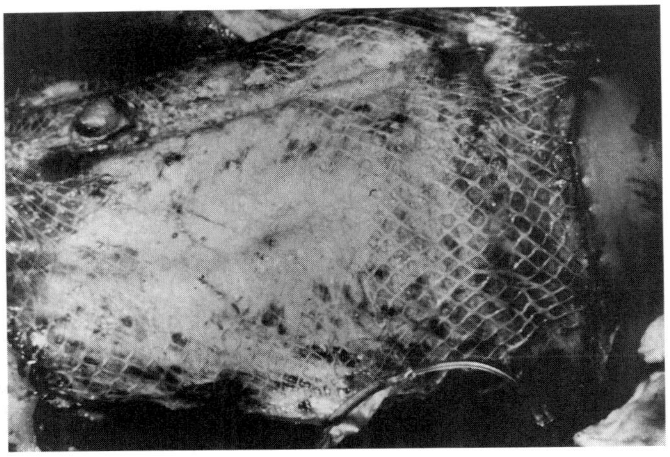

(12.6)

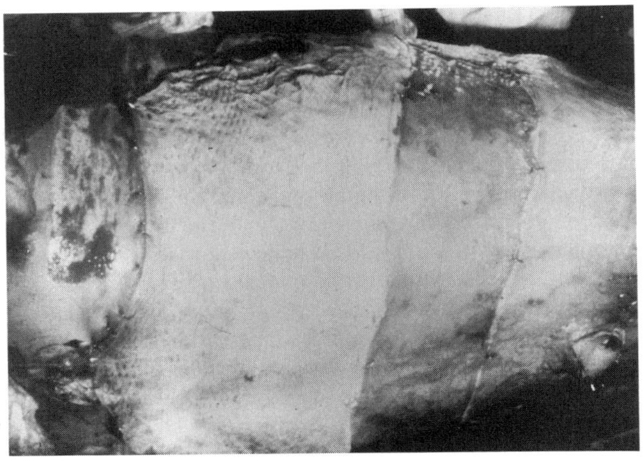

(12.7)

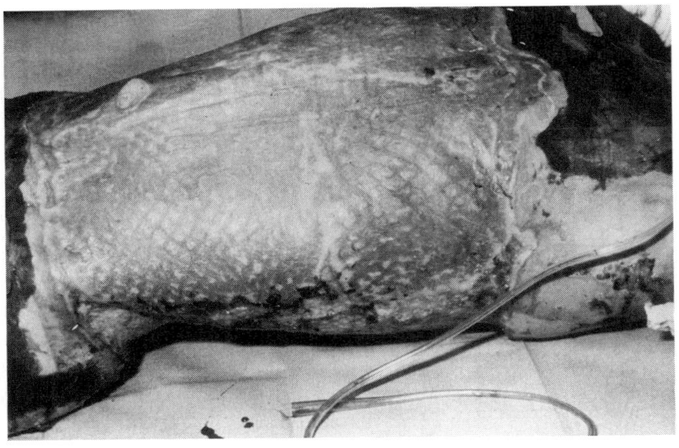

(12.8)

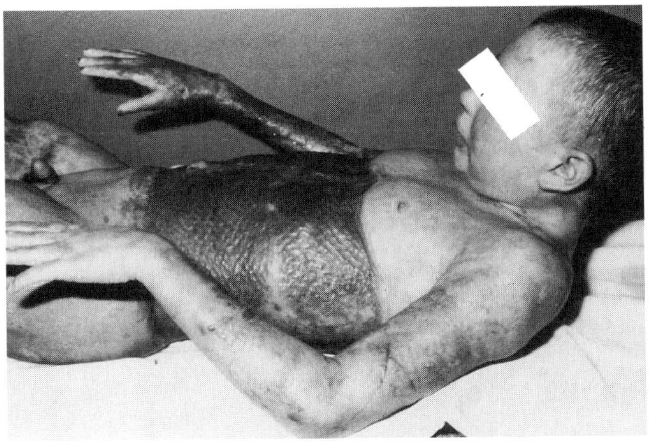

(12.9)

Figs. 12.6–12.9 'Sandwich' technique for closing large burns is shown in stages. (12.6) Initial grafting uses widely meshed (4:1) autograft. (12.7) The widely meshed autograft is overlaid by 2:1 meshed homograft rotated at 90°. (12.8) The interstices epithelialize and the homograft falls off. (12.9) One month after grafting, autograft has fully covered the wound.

primarily by epithelialization from remaining epithelial elements. In a thin split graft, this healing is rapid as the residual hair follicles, sweat glands, and sebaceous glands are close together; but in thicker skin grafts, healing is slower. The time to heal depends on depth of harvest, vascularity of the donor site, wound management, and general patient factors such as age.

The dermis heals with scar formation, and there is no regeneration of harvested dermis. This has implications, particularly in patients who require harvesting of healed donor sites. There is greater risk of hypertrophic scarring after harvesting of deeper grafts. Patients return to the operating room as soon as donor sites are healed for further autografting and replacement of nonadherent homografts, a process which is accelerated remarkably by treatment with recombinant human growth hormone (GH), 0.2 mg/kg per day), injected subcutaneously once daily. Briefly, donor site wound healing is accelerated by 25% even if patients present late, are infected, and are malnourished. There is a transient hyperglycemia in a third of patients which, therefore, require insulin. This is self-limiting due to an increase in endogenous insulin secretion and usually disappears after a few days. GH-treated patients require less infused albumin in order to maintain normal serum levels; this is an indication of a net positive protein balance induced. The effect of GH in these severely and massively burned patients is truly remarkable. The usual hospital stay for a 30 kg patient with a 60% TBSA burn of 42 days is reduced to 32 days. This tremendous decrease in length of hospital stay realizes a net savings of 15% in total costs.

Alternatives in Wound Closure

Massively burned patients can sometime have such limited area which can be used for donor-site harvesting that recropping may have to be performed very often in order to achieve wound closure. Even if harvesting is performed at as shallow a depth as possible, say 0.006–0.008 inch, there is a point at which any subsequent recropping is of largely nonviable epithelium.[42] This loss of the donor sites' regenerative capabilities has drastic implications, not only for the closure of the original burn, but also for the ability to perform reconstructive procedures at some later time. Even though growth factor therapy[43,44] will speed the rate of donor site healing, and thereby result in more rapid wound closure, it is still unclear whether these growth factors alter the character of the healed wound. The finite number of donor harvests which can be performed from any given autologous site can interfere with optimal reconstructive results.

Cultured epithelial autografts and artificial skin substitutes are two techniques which can aid wound closure in those whose burns are so large, >80% TBSA, that autologous donor tissue is severely limited.[45] Simply put, from a small patch of donor skin, larger confluent sheets of epithelial cells are grown *in vitro* on nutrient media. Over a period of 2–4 weeks, surface area coverage from the original donor can be expanded 100 times or more.[46,47] Unfortunately, this process is lengthy and may take over 20 days to grow enough surface area for transplantation. Even then, the finished product is only five or six layers thick, virtually transparent, and extremely pliable. In the interim, wounds are kept sealed with homograft which is replaced if adherence is lost. The cultured skin is best delivered on gauze backing in order to improve handling ability and to provide something which can be stapled. Without gauze backing, the epidermis tears when attempts are made to fix it in place. After placement, the grafted site must be kept completely immobile. Active and passive range of motion exercises are contraindicated for up to 2 weeks after application so as to prevent graft loss.[47] Suspension via skeletal traction pins is sometimes used to enhance graft take.[48]

Cultured skin will usually engraft (take) quite well with 80–90% take commonly being reported.[45] A repeated problem has been the development of many large bullae, as a result of minimal shear forces, even 6 months after application. The fluid from these bullae have been examined for thromboxane and prostaglandin levels.[49] When these levels were compared to routine burn blister fluid, they were found to be markedly *elevated* (**Table 12.5**).

Table 12.5 Comparison of normal blister fluid and CEA blister fluid

	Burn blister fluid	CEA blister fluid
Prostaglandin E_2 (ng/ml)	0.37 ± 0.05	18.6 ± 12.8*
Thromboxane B_2 (ng/ml)	3.75 ± 0.45	24.2 ± 12.3*

Data are presented as means ± SEM.
* $p < 0.05$ compared with burn blister fluid.
From Herndon D N, Ruton R L. Use of dermal plates and cultured cells for permanent skin replacement. *Wound* 1992; **4:** 50–3, with permission.

Elevated levels of thromboxane suggest an ongoing acute inflammatory process. Over time, most of the cultured skin has had to be replaced by autograft due to ongoing graft loss.[50] This is perhaps explained by transmission election micrographs of the cultured epidermal–wound interface revealing a lack of normal anchoring fibril attachments to the type I and type III collagen in the underlying layer. An ongoing inflammatory response occurs which prevents secure adhesion of the cultured epidermis to the wound interface even many months after application. This reduces its clinical utility. Allogeneic dermis, or dermal substitutes, may improve long-term adherence of cultured epidermis. If a cadaveric allograft is found to be vascularized and adherent to the wound bed, the cadaveric epidermis can be removed by dermabrasion or tangential excision at a depth of 0.004–0.006 inch leaving the allogeneic dermis *in situ* to serve as a recipient bed for epidermal grafts.[51]

Skin Substitutes

Burke and Yannas[52] invented an artificial bilaminar skin composed of biodegradable collagen–glycosaminoglycan dermal analog covered by a temporary thin silicone elastomer membrane – Integra™. It was designed to adhere to a wound surface, thereby controlling bacterial invasion and fluid loss inducing cellular and vascular invasion which would synthesize a dermal matrix.[53] The silicone elastomer membrane is removed after 3 weeks and the 'neodermis' can be grafted. This material has been subjected to a multicenter trial involving 139 test sites on 106 patients who were followed for 1 year after grafting. Artificial dermis take was 80% compared with 95% for autograft. Autograft donor thickness was significantly thinner, 0.006 ± 0.002 compared to 0.013 ± 0.018 inches, for graft upon the neodermis. Consequently, the donor sites healed 4 days faster. At the completion of the study, patients preferred the artificial dermis to control sites as less hypertrophic scarring had developed. Improved appearance of wounds was also noted in pigs grafted with a cellular allograft dermis (Alloderm) which was autografted after incorporation.[54]

Other techniques which hold promise include the creation of a bilayered skin using cultured autologous epidermis added to allogenic fibroblast collagen lattice a few days prior to application. Take rates of up to 70% have been reported and cosmetic appearance is good.[55] Another promising skin substitute is Dermagraft, a living tissue analog composed of human neonatal fibroblast grown on a polyglactin acid/Vicryl™ mesh. This dermal replacement is then immediately grafted with meshed split-thickness autologous skin. A take rate of 70–90% was achieved and no evidence of immunological reaction to the allogeneic fibroblast was seen. The concept of a prefabricated skin replacement is most appealing, but we may have to be content with prepackaged dermis or neodermis which is later used as a bed for cultured epidermal autograft. Until these technologies have been perfected, widely meshed autograft with cadaver-graft overlay remains the optimum treatment for those burned less than 90% TBSA.

Aftermath

Once surgery is completed, postoperative procedures and evaluations begin. Postoperative bed/positioning requirements are determined by the areas grafted. Through the collaborative efforts of a surgeon, perioperative nurse, and physical therapist the bed and associated special equipment are prepared prior to the end of surgery and the patient is transferred directly to the bed rather than to a transport stretcher. This practice eliminates unnecessary movement which may cause shearing of grafts or potential pain. Information regarding the patient and surgical procedure is conveyed to a post-anesthesia or intensive care nurse well in advance. The post-anesthesia care nurse must be knowledgable about the medication(s) used to maintain the case during surgery in order to provide appropriate safety and environmental considerations during the emergent phase. Once transferred to the post-anesthesia recovery room or intensive care unit, nursing considerations include airway, alterations in fluid and electrolyte balance, alterations in hemodynamic status, alterations in thermoregulation, alterations in thought processes, and pain. When a patient is stabilized regarding airway, breathing and circulation, and monitoring of vital signs established, blood is drawn for gas analysis and hematology. A chest x-ray is obtained for verification of line placement and the absence of pneumothorax or atelectasis. Urine output is monitored in conjunction with vital signs and is maintained at 0.8 ml/kg/h or greater. Communication with family members is reestablished. Preoperative teaching regarding the surgery, monitoring equipment, dressings, etc. is reinforced, and family are invited to the bedside as soon as possible.

Psychological follow-up of severely burned children and adolescents is heartening.[56–61] Patients and their parents seem to cope very well. Testing 25 children and their parents who have survived injuries of >80% TBSA (via the Child Behavior Checklist, Teacher Report Form, Piers–Harris Children's Self-concept Scale,

Parenting Stress Index, and a questionnaire) at an average of 5 years postburn has shown that the children do better than treatment teams expect.[57] Boys had a higher self-regard in the area of behavior and had higher esteem of their intellectual abilities and physical appearance than a reference group. Visible scars, particularly on the face, are associated with lower scores in psychological testing in the areas of physical appearance, happiness, and satisfaction. In spite of this, these same children gave every impression of adjusting well to their change in body image.

Parental stress was significantly raised, caused partly as a result of burn teams' expectations that the primary care givers ensure compliance with the use of pressure garments and exercises. Parents did report their children as less acceptable, more moody, and less reinforcing to their own sense of self-worth. The stress felt by parents decreased with time. Financial burden was a recurrent theme identified as a stressor. Clearly, the parents of burned children need much support in order to help them cope and adjust. Also, we must be sensitive to the fact that child patients may be superficially well adjusted but may be harboring feelings of self-deprecation. The shy introvert should be followed carefully.

The children say they are glad to be alive. On the whole they cope, live, love, achieve, and are optimistic. They wish they had never been burned. They sometimes hurt deeply. Their process of reconciliation is prolonged, and we are bound to support them and their families during this time. A team approach which includes surgeons, operative nurses, therapists, psychologists, and the families of burned patients seems to be the most effective in producing physical and emotional recovery from traumatizing burn injuries.

References

1. Bull J P, Fisher A J. A study of mortality in a burns unit: a revised estimate. *Ann Surg* 1954; **139:** 269–74.

2. Muller M J, Herndon D N. The challenge of burns. *Lancet* 1994; **343:** 216–20.

3. Burke J F, Bandoc C C, Quinby W C. Primary burn excision and immediate grafting: a method for shortening illness. *J Trauma* 1974; **14:** 389–95.

4. Pietsch J B, Netscher D T, Nagaraj H S, Groff D B. Early excision of major burns in children: effect on morbidity and mortality. *J Pediatr Surg* 1985; **20**(4): 754–7.

5. Herndon D N, Parks D H. Comparison of serial debridement and autografting and early massive excision with cadaver skin overlay in the treatment of large burns in children. *J Trauma* 1986; **26**(2): 149–52.

6. Herndon D N, Barrow R E, Rutan R L, Rutan T C, Desai M H, Abston S. A comparison of conservative versus early excision therapies in severely burned patients. *Ann Surg* 1989; **209:** 547–53.

7. Tompkins R G, Burke J F, Schoenfeld D A, *et al.* Prompt eschar excision: a treatment system contributing to reduced burn mortality. *Ann Surg* 1986; **204**(3): 272–81.

8. Thompson P, Herndon D N, Abston S, Rutan T. Effect of early excision on patients with major thermal injury. *J Trauma* 1987; **27**(2): 205–7.

9. Deitch E A, Clothier J. Burns in the elderly: an early surgical approach. *J Trauma* 1983; **23**(10): 891–4.

10. Deitch E A. A policy of early excision and grafting in elderly burn patients shortens the hospital stay and improves survival. *Burns* 1985; **12:** 109–14.

11. Hara M, Peters W J, Douglas L G, Morris S F. An early surgical approach to burns in the elderly. *J Trauma* 1990; **30**(4): 430–2.

12. Scott-Conner C E H, Love R, Wheeler W. Does rapid wound closure improve survival in older patients with burns. *Ann Surg* 1990; **56:** 57–60.

13. Saffle J R, Larson C M, Sullivan J, Shelby J. The continuing challenge of burn care in the elderly. *Surgery* 1990; **108**(3): 534–43.

14. Hunt J L, Purdue C F. The elderly burn patient. *Am J Surg* 1992; **164:** 472–6.

15. Lewandowski R, Pegg S P, Fortier K, Skimmings A. Burn injuries in the elderly. *Burns* 1993; **19**(6): 513–15.

16. Ikeda J, Sugamata A, Jumbo Y, Yukioka T, Makino K. A new surgical procedure for aged burn victims: applications of dermolipectomy for burn wounds and donor sites. *J Burn Care Rehabil* 1990; **11**(1): 27–31.

17. Munster A M, Smith-Meek M, Sharkey P. The effect of early surgical intervention on mortality and cost-effectiveness in burn care, 1978–91. *Burns* 1994; **20**(1): 61–4.

18. Janzekovic Z. A new concept in the early excision and immediate grafting of burns. *J Trauma* 1970; **10:** 1103–8.

19. Janzekovic Z. The burn wound from the surgical point of view. *J Trauma* 1975; **15:** 42–61.

20. Heimbach D M. Early burn excision and grafting. *Surg Clin North Am* 1987; **67**(1): 93–107.

21. Engrav L H, Heimbach D M, Reus J L, Harnar T J, Marvin J A. Early excision and grafting vs nonoperative treatment of burns of indeterminant depth: a randomised prospective study. *J Trauma* 1983; **23:** 1001–4.

22. Goodwin C, Maguire M S, McManus W F, Pruitt B A. Prospective study of burn wound excision of the hands. *J Trauma* 1983; **23**(6): 510–17.

23. Wang X-W, Sun Y-H, Zhang G-Z, Zhang Z-M. Tangential excision of eschar for deep burns of the hand: analysis of 156 patients collected over 10 years. *Burns* 1984; **11:** 92–8.

24. Levine B A, Sirinek K R, Peterson H D, Pruitt B A. Efficacy of tangential excision and immediate autografting of deep second degree burns of the hand. *J Trauma* 1979; **19**(9): 670–3.

25. Edstrom L E, Robson M C, Macchiaverna J R, Scala A D. Prospective randomised treatments for burned hands: nonoperative vs operative. *Scand J Plast Reconstr Surg* 1979; **13:** 131–5.

26. Salisbur R E, Wright P. Evaluation of early excision of dorsal burns of the hand. *Plast Reconstr Surg* 1982; **69**(4): 670–5.

27. Frist W, Ackroyd F, Burke J, Bondoc C. Long term functional results of selective treatment of hand burns. *Am J Surg* 1985; **149:** 516–21.

28. McHugh T P, Robson M C, Heggars J P, Phillips L G, Smith D J, McCallum M C. Therapeutic efficacy of Biobrane in partial and full thickness thermal injury. *Surgery* 1986; **100**(4): 661–4.

29. Deitch E A, Wheelahan T M, Rose M P, Clothier J, Cotter J. Hypertrophic burn scars: analysis of variables. *J Trauma* 1983; **23**(10): 895–8.

30. Irei M, Abston S, Bonds E, Rutan T, Desai M, Herndon D N. The optimal time for excision of scald burns in toddlers. *J Burn Care Rehabil* 1986; **7**(6): 508–10.

31. Desai M H, Rutan R L, Herndon D N. Conservative treatment of scald burns is superior to early excision. *J Burn Care Rehabil* 1991; **12:** 482–4.

32. Desai M H, Herndon D N, Broemeling L, Barrow R E, Nichols R J Jr, Rutan R L. Early burn wound excision significantly reduces blood loss. *Ann Surg* 1990; **211:** 753–62.

33. Curreri P W. Hard questions on excision. *J Trauma* 1979; **19**(Suppl): 931–3.

34. Herndon D N, Abston S, Stein M D. Increased thromboxane B_2 levels in the plasma of burned and septic burned patients. *Surg Gynecol Obstet* 1984; **159:** 210–13.

35. Chameides L, *et al.* Textbook of Pediatric Advanced Life Support City: Publ. 1988.

36. Zing B M. Managing burns in children, an intraoperative nursing care plan. AORN J 1991; **54**(3): 568–75.

37. Baxter C R. Crystalloid resuscitation of burn shock. 7–32.

38. Demuch M W, Dimick A R, Gillespie R W, *et al.* Advanced Burn Life Support.

39. Heimbach D M, Engrav L E. *Surgical Management of the Burn Wound.* New York: Raven Press, 1984.

40. Barbul A, Regan M C. Biology of wound healing. In: Fisher J E, ed. *Surgical Basic Science.* St Louis: C V Mosby, 1993: 67–89.

41. Alexander J W, MacMillan B G, Law E, Kittur D S. Treatment of severe burns with widely meshed skin autograft and meshed skin allograft overlay. *J Trauma* 1981; **21**(6): 433–8.

42. Huang K F, Linares H A, Evans M J, *et al.* Can donor sites be harvested indefinitely. *Proc Am Burns Assoc* 1992.

43. Sherman S T, Demling R H, Lalonde C, *et al.* Growth hormone enhances reepithelialization of human split thickness skin graft donor sites. *Surg Forum* 1989; **40:** 37–39.

44. Brown G, Curtsinger L, Brightwell J R, *et al.* Enhancement of epidermal regeneration by biosynthetic epidermal growth factor. *J Exp Med* 1986; **163:** 1319–24.

45. Munster A M, Weiner S H, Spence R J. Cultured epidermis for the coverage of massive burn wounds: a single centre experience. *Ann Surg* 1990; **211:** 676–80.

46. Pittkelkow M R, Scott R E. New techniques for the in vitro culture of human skin keratinocytes and perspectives on their use for grafting of patients with extensive burns. *Mayo Clin Proc* 1986; **61:** 771–7.

47. Green H, Kekinde O, Thomas J. Growth of cultured human epidermal cells into multiple epithelia suitable for grafting. *Proc Natl Acad Sci USA* 1979; **76:** 5665–8.

48. Desai M H, Mlcack J M, McCauley R L, *et al.* Lack of long-term durability of cultured keratinocyte burn-wound coverage: a case report. *J Burn Care Rehabil* 1991; **12:** 540–5.

49. Herndon D N, Rutan R L. Use of dermal templates and cultured cells for permanent skin replacement. *Wounds* 1992; **4**(2): 50–3.

50. Herndon D N, Rutan R L. Comparison of cultured epidermal autograft and massive excision with serial autografting plus homograft overlay. *J Burn Care Rehabil* 1992; **13:** 154–7.

51. Cuono C B, Langdon R, Berdall N, *et al.* Composite autologous–allogeneic skin replacement. Development and chemical application. *Plast Reconstr Surg* 1987; **80**(4): 626–37.

52. Heimbach D, Luterman A, Burke J, *et al.* Artificial dermis for major burns. *Ann Surg* 1988; **208:** 313–20.

53. Burke S F, Yannas I V, Quinley W C, *et al.* Successful use of a physiologically acceptable artificial skin in the treatment of extensive burn injury. *Ann Surg* 1981; **194:** 413–428.

54. Livesey A, Nag A, Hollyoak M, Herndon D N, Wainwright D. Transplanted acellular allograft dermal matrix: potential as a template for the reconstitution of viable dermis. *Transplantation* 1995; (in press).

55. Hull B E, Finley R K, Miller S F. Coverage of full-thickness burns with bilayered skin equivalents: a preliminary clinical trial. *Surgery* 1990; **107:** 496–502.

56. Blakeney P, Meyer W, Moore P, *et al.* Social competence and behavioral problems of paediatric survivors of burns. *J Burn Care Rehabil* 1993; **14**(1): 65–72.

57. Blakeney P, Meyer W, Moore P, *et al.* Psychosocial sequelae of pediatric burns involving 80% or greater total body surface area. *J Burn Care Rehabil* 1993; **14**(6): 684–9.

58. Moore P, Blakeney P, Broemeling L, Portman S, Herndon D N, Robson M. Psychological adjustment after childhood burn injuries as predicted by personality traits. *J Burn Care Rehabil* 1993; **14**(1): 80–2.

59. Blakeney P, Moore P, Broemeling L, Hunt R, Herndon D N, Robson M. Parental stress as a cause and effect of pediatric burn injury. *J Burn Care Rehabil* 1993; **14**(1): 73–9.

60. Abdullah A, Blakeney P, Hunt R, *et al.* Visible scars and self-esteem in pediatric patients with burns. *J Burn Care Rehabil* 1994; **15**(2): 164–8.

61. Meyer W J, Blakeney P, Moore P, Murphy L, Robson M, Herndon D N. Parental well-being and behavioral adjustment of pediatric survivors of burns. *J Burn Care Rehabil* 1994; **15**(1): 62–8.

CHAPTER THIRTEEN

13

ANESTHESIA FOR BURNED PATIENTS

WERNER W. LINGNAU, LEE C. WOODSON, RAY J. NICHOLS AND DONALD S. PROUGH

INTRODUCTION

Severe burn injuries, defined as burns exceeding 41% of total body surface area (TBSA), occur in about 20 000 patients annually, or eight patients per 100 000 population per year.[1,2] Anesthetic management of thermally injured patients is challenging. As the surgeon concentrates on surgical diagnosis and therapy, the anesthesiologist must provide anesthesia and preserve vital organ functions. Airway management, circulatory stabilization, and pulmonary support are essential. In about 20–30% of fire victims, smoke inhalation and carbon monoxide intoxication complicate the burn injury. Cardiovascular instability reflects both hypovolemia and, in severely burned patients, cardiac dysfunction. Pulmonary complications may result from inhalation injury, noncardiac pulmonary edema, or sepsis.

Prompt, effective treatment is mandatory at the scene of the accident, in the emergency room, and in the operating room (OR). Detailed knowledge about the pathophysiologic changes that accompany burn injuries facilitates anesthetic management during the three phases of burn injury: early resuscitation, debridement and grafting, and the reconstructive phase. The doses of many drugs must be adjusted. The trauma anesthesiologist,[3] being specially trained in pre-hospital care, transport, resuscitation, and postoperative support, is an important member of the team managing burned patients.

PATHOPHYSIOLOGY

Inhalation Injury

Inhalation injury contributes heavily to morbidity and mortality in burned patients.[4–6] Three distinct injuries – carbon monoxide intoxication, upper airway injury, and pulmonary inhalation injury – may occur individually or concurrently.[7] **Figure 13.1** illustrates sites and mechanisms of injury.

Victims who die at the scene usually do so as a result of hypoxia and carbon monoxide poisoning.[8,9] Victims trapped in burning buildings or vehicles become hypoxic from breathing an oxygen-

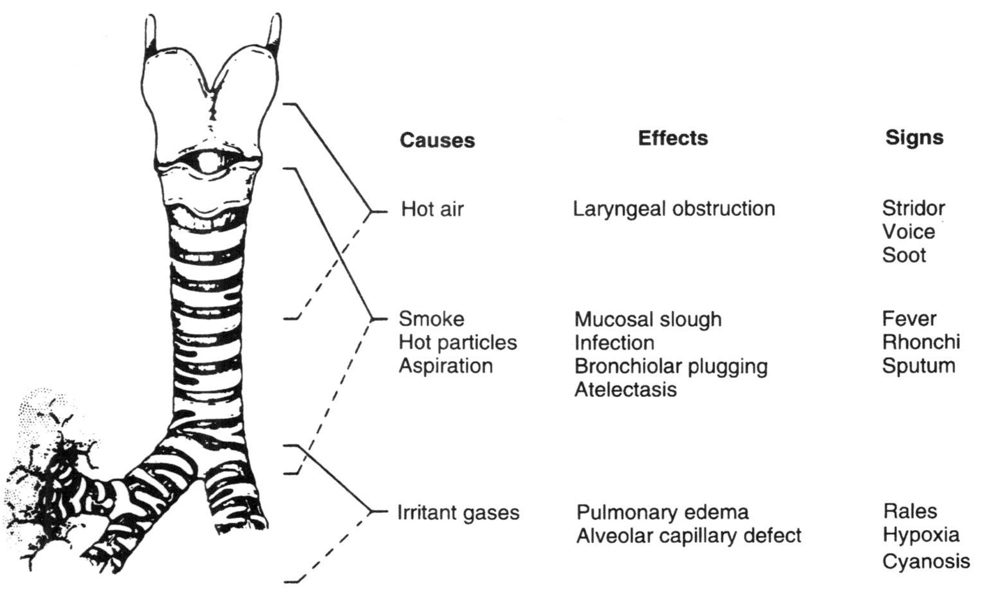

Fig. 13.1 Mechanisms of inhalation injury at various sites within the tracheobronchial tree. (From Quinby W C. Burns. In Burke J C, et al, eds. Trauma Management: Early Management of Visceral, Nervous System and Musculoskeletal Injuries. *St Louis: Mosby Year Book, Inc., 1988.)*

deficient gas mixture that contains carbon monoxide. Carbon monoxide has over 200 times the affinity of oxygen for binding sites on hemoglobin. Carbon monoxide also shifts the oxyhemoglobin dissociation curve to the left, inhibiting the release of oxygen to the tissues (**Figure 13.2**).[10] Transported by blood to the tissues, carbon monoxide binds to the cytochromes in the oxidative phosphorylation cascade.[11] Neurological and cardiac impairment may result from tissue hypoxia.[12]

Symptoms of carbon monoxide intoxication include headache, nausea, angina, dyspnea, irritability, and altered consciousness (**Table 13.1**). Because such patients may have a normal $Pa\text{O}_2$ and show no cyanosis, it is essential to measure the concentrations of oxy- and carboxyhemoglobin by CO-oximetry. Carboxyhemoglobin saturations greater than 15% are toxic; those greater than 50% usually are lethal.[13]

The treatment is displacement of carbon monoxide from hemoglobin by delivering high inspired concentrations of oxygen. As face masks deliver a maximum $F\text{IO}_2$ of only 0.45, intubation often is necessary to achieve a higher $F\text{IO}_2$. The elimination half-life of carbon monoxide can be reduced, by breathing 100% oxygen rather than room air, from 4 hours to 40 minutes.[14,15] Giving 100% oxygen at 2.5 atmospheres in a hyperbaric chamber decreases the half-life to 24 minutes.

Smoke inhalation results in major physiologic changes in the microvasculature of the bronchial and pulmonary circulation[7,16,17] (**Figure 13.2**). Changes in the airway microcirculation appear immediately after smoke inhalation. Fiberoptic bronchoscopy, often performed by the anesthesiologist while the patient is undergoing surgery, may demonstrate evidence of soot particles, hyperemia and edema,[16,18] widely accepted criteria for diagnosing inhalation injury.

After inhalation injury, pulmonary transvascular fluid flux increases.[19,20] Extravascular lung water, as assessed by thermal dilution techniques, gravimetric analysis, or by histology, is elevated.[19–22] Pulmonary artery pressure and pulmonary vascular resistance rise, starting 4–12 hours after inhalation injury.[23–25] The changes in resistance occur because of pulmonary venoconstriction. Pulmonary capillary pressure also rises after smoke inhalation injury.[25,26]

Table 13.1 Clinical manifestations of carbon monoxide poisoning associated with varying levels of blood carboxyhemoglobin

Blood carboxyhemoglobin concentration (%)	Signs and symptoms
0–10	None (angina may be noted in patients with coronary artery disease)
10–20	Slight headache, exercise-induced angina, dyspnea on vigorous exertion
20–30	Throbbing headache, dyspnea on moderate exertion
30–40	Severe headache, nausea and vomiting, weakness, visual disturbance, impaired judgement
40–50	Syncope, tachycardia, tachypnea and dyspnea at rest
50–60	Coma, convulsions, Cheyne–Stokes respiration
60–70	Compromised cardiorespiratory function
70–80	Death

From Grande C M *et al*. Hyperbaric medicine: a trauma perspective. In Stene J K, *et al*., eds. *Trauma Anesthesia*. Baltimore: Williams & Wilkins, 1991.

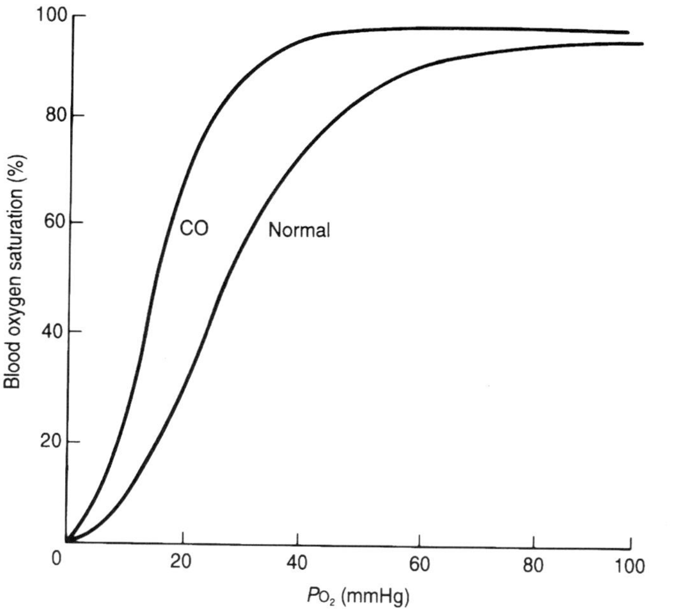

Fig. 13.2 The oxygen–hemoglobin dissociation curve is shifted leftward (i.e. gives up oxygen less readily) as result of carbon monoxide (CO) inhalation. (From Strongin J, et al. Pulmonary disorders in the burn patient. In Martyn J A J, ed. Acute Management of the Burned Patient. *Philadelphia: W B Saunders, Co., 1990.)*

Changes in pulmonary microvascular pressure, however, are not as important as changes in vascular permeability, especially during the first 24 hours after injury.[27] The increase in pulmonary microvascular fluid flux is associated with migration of polymorphonuclear cells into the lung, as evidenced by histology, bronchoalveolar lavage, and detection of mediators (proteases and oxygen free radicals), which are released by polymorphonuclear cells.[20,22,28] Mediators released from damaged tissue increase capillary permeability.[17,29] Inflammatory cells produce oxygen metabolites and release proteolytic enzymes.[20,30] Patients with burns and inhalation injury require more volume for resuscitation than patients who only have burns. The increased fluid requirements cannot be explained by increased extravascular lung water alone.[31]

Hypovolemia

One of the clinical hallmarks of thermal injury is hypovolemia, often evidenced in severely burned patients as hemoconcentration and hypotension. Because more plasma and interstitial fluid than red cell mass is lost, shock is more similar to that seen in crush injuries than to shock due to hemorrhage. Peripheral edema, which in burned patients results from the loss of plasma into the interstitium, usually takes several hours to develop. Hypovolemia may occur unexpectedly in the conscious, extensively burned patient who is hemodynamically stable in the emergency department, only to become frankly hypotensive as fluid sequestration progresses. Local and peripheral edema formation may lead not only to hypovolemia, but to increased interstitial pressures which may impair local tissue perfusion. Poor systemic perfusion ultimately may culminate in vital organ dysfunction; impaired local perfusion can convert viable second degree burns (partial-thickness, i.e. epidermis and some dermis) to third degree burns (full-thickness).

Clinical problems in managing hypovolemia have prompted studies of the microvascular changes that induce the fluid shifts accompanying thermal injury. Up to a sevenfold increase in cutaneous lymph flow occurs almost immediately after thermal injury [29,32–34] and is sustained for approximately 48 hours. The factors responsible for this increased fluid flux involve all the components of the Starling equilibrium:[35,36]

$$Q = kA\,[(P_c - P_i) + \sigma(\pi_i - \pi_c)]$$

where Q is fluid filtration, k is the capillary filtration coefficient (conductivity of water), A is the area of the capillary membrane, P_c is the capillary hydrostatic pressure, P_i is the interstitial hydrostatic pressure, σ is the reflection coefficient for albumin, π_i is the interstitial colloid osmotic pressure, and π_c is the capillary colloid osmotic pressure.

Venular contraction increases P_c[37] as P_i decreases,[38] thereby increasing the hydrostatic pressure gradient for transvascular fluid extravasation. At the same time, σ decreases[37] and the oncotic pressure gradient opposing the hydrostatic pressure gradient is diminished. Resuscitation with crystalloid solutions decreases π_c, while loss of plasma proteins increases π_i.

Large amounts of resuscitation fluids are necessary to maintain intravascular volume and cardiac preload. Pain, fear, and reflex responses to hypovolemia, decreased cardiac output, and hypotension induce release of catecholamines (**Table 13.2**).[39,40] Increased sympathetic tone may maintain arterial blood pressure even though peripheral perfusion is impaired. In addition to producing cardiovascular changes, these neural mediators release interleukin-6,[41,42] a cytokine that stimulates the synthesis of acute phase reactants and reduces the synthesis of albumin.[41,42] Burned patients exhibit an accelerated breakdown of body protein that can also contribute to a delayed fall in plasma proteins, especially albumin.[43,44] These changes may maintain edema. Reduced plasma protein concentrations can enhance edema formation even if the oncotic pressure gradient has been maintained by a reduction in π_i.[45,46] With large burns, edema is formed in organs distant from the burn injury, partly because of hypoproteinemia. Periods of shock and subsequent reperfusion injury after resuscitation may cause secondary tissue injury that contributes to edema formation.

The various formulae that are used to calculate fluid replacement as a function of the extent of the burn injury are discussed elsewhere in this book. However, it cannot be overemphasized that these formulas are only guidelines; treatment must be adjusted individually based on monitored variables. Rapid restoration and maintenance of systemic perfusion are crucial to improving outcome.

Pharmacologic Considerations

Pharmacokinetic and pharmacodynamic changes in burned patients[47] include rapid changes in fluid distribution between plasma volume and interstitial fluid, increased extracellular volume, and changes in hepatic and renal elimination. As distribution is a dynamic process of drug transfer between compartments, an increase in the volume of distribution in burned patients results in the need for larger loading doses to achieve required plasma concentrations. Protein binding of drugs is altered by changes in plasma protein composition, including hypoalbuminemia and increases in acute phase proteins. Exaggerated responses to the normal dose of albumin-bound drugs, e.g. anticonvulsants, sulfonylureas, etc., are likely because the free fraction of these drugs is elevated. On the other hand, the free fraction of drugs, such as lidocaine, propranolol, and muscle relaxants, that are bound by α_1-acid glycoprotein, decreases because the concentration of this acute phase protein is increased in burned patients.[48] Because most clinical chemistry laboratories report total drug concentration rather than the active free fraction,[49] measurement of serum levels of drugs may be misleading.

Muscle Relaxants

Burn injuries profoundly influence responses to both succinylcholine and to nondepolarizing muscle relaxants. In burned patients, sensitization to the muscle relaxant effects of succinylcholine[2] can produce exaggerated hyperkalemic responses severe enough to induce cardiac arrest. In contrast, burned patients are resistant to the effects of nondepolarizing muscle relaxants.[50]

Cardiac arrest in burned patients after succinylcholine was first reported in 1958.[51] It was not until 1967,[52] however, that an exaggerated hyperkalemic effect was identified as the cause of this phenomenon. Several clinical studies have documented exaggerated increases in potassium concentrations after succinylcholine in burned patients.[53–55] However, considerable individual variability exists; only a few patients in these series developed dangerously high potassium levels although the size of the increase was greater after about 3–4 weeks. The earliest exaggerated hyperkalemic response described occurred 9 days after injury[53] although normal responses were observed in the remaining patients in this series for up to 14–20 days. The shortest postburn interval associated with succinylcholine-induced cardiac arrest was 21 days.[56] Controversy surrounds recommendations regarding the safe use of succinylcholine after burn injury. Various authors recommend avoidance of succinylcholine after intervals ranging from 5 to 21 days postburn.

An increase in the numbers of acetylcholine receptors and proliferation of these receptors away from the neuromuscular junction have been suggested as common mechanisms explaining both reduced sensitivity to nondepolarizing relaxants and exaggerated hyperkalemia after succinylcholine administration in burned patients. Under normal conditions, nicotinic acetylcholine receptors are concentrated at the neuromuscular junction; thus the membrane-depolarizing effects of nicotinic cholinergic agonists are restricted to a small fraction of the muscle membrane. Denervation and immobilization increase the number of extrajunctional acetylcholine receptors and enlarge the area sensitive to acetylcholine.[57] As a result of receptor proliferation, the entire membrane becomes sensitive to cholinergic agonists and depolarization can cause release of potassium from a large portion of the muscle cell surface rather than just the motor endplate. The resulting large-scale shift of intracellular potassium can generate life-threatening hyperkalemia. Similar changes have been suspected to occur after burn injuries.

Table 13.2 Hormone concentrations in normal volunteers and in patients with burns

Subjects	Insulin (units/ml)	Glucagon (pg/ml)	Cortisol (ng/ml)	Epinephrine (pg/ml)	Norepinephrine (pg/ml)
Normal volunteers	11.3	143	8	35	184
Patients with burns	19.6	325	32	376	1558

Samples were taken after a fast of 8 hours or more. Data expressed as mean ± standard error. All values in patients are significantly different from normal ($p < .01$).
From Wolfe R R, *et al.* Effect of severe burn injury on substrate cycling by glucose and fatty acids. *N Engl J Med* **317:** 403–8, 1987.

Responses to nondepolarizing relaxants are also altered by burn injury. Three- to fivefold greater doses are required to achieve adequate relaxation.[50] Resistance is apparent by 7 days after injury and peaks by approximately 40 days. Sensitivity returns to normal after approximately 70 days.[58–60] Two reports described slight but measurable resistance to nondepolarizers persisting for more than a year after complete healing of wounds.[58,60] The mechanism of the altered response appears to involve pharmacodynamic rather than pharmacokinetic changes. Burns greater than 25% total body surface area require higher total dose and plasma concentrations of nondepolarizing blockers to achieve a given level of twitch depression.[58,60,61]

Resistance to nondepolarizing muscle relaxants may not be caused by changes in the numbers of acetylcholine receptors. Although Kim *et al.*[62] reported an increase in numbers of acetylcholine receptors in rat diaphragms after scald injuries, Marathe *et al.*[61] were unable to demonstrate increases in either receptor density or the ratio of extrajunctional to junctional receptors at a time when resistance to atracurium was maximal. Thus, although changes in nicotinic receptor density and distribution have been demonstrated after denervation and immobilization,[57] these changes have not always been observed after burn injuries. Therefore, the mechanism of the altered response of burn patients to muscle relaxants has not been established.

Because proliferation of acetylcholine receptors across the muscle membrane has been used to explain both resistance to nondepolarizing muscle relaxants and the exaggerated hyperkalemic response to succinylcholine, the observation of resistance of a patient to metocurine for up to 463 days after burn[60] has been used to suggest that hyperkalemic responses to succinylcholine also could persist for more than a year. However, the theoretical mechanism of the altered drug responses in burned patients is speculative; no pathologic responses to succinylcholine in burned patients have been reported more than 66 days after burns.[58,63]

Sedatives and Analgetics

Thermally injured patients appear to require higher doses of sedatives and analgetics than nonburned, traumatized patients. However, the pharmacokinetics of these drugs do not explain the increased requirements. For example, the clearance of diazepam is prolonged after burns while that of lorazepam is minimally altered. Lorazepam is eliminated by conjugation,[64] which is little affected by age, disease, or concurrent administration of drugs. In contrast, the P-450 cytochrome oxidase system, which plays a part in the elimination of diazepam,[65] is sensitive to those factors. Because of multiple factors influencing responses to drugs, doses must be titrated to desired effects.

Other Drugs

As infections, sepsis, and multiple organ failure are major complications in burned patients, the anesthesiologist must consider the possibility of impaired hepatic and renal clearance. A variety of antibiotics, such as aminoglycosides, tetracycline, polymyxin, and clindamycin, that are used to treat burned patients can potentiate neuromuscular blockade.[66,67]

ANESTHETIC MANAGEMENT

Preanesthetic Evaluation

Although all phases of anesthetic care can be challenging in burned patients, particularly important problems include airway management, vascular access, and fluid resuscitation. The principles applied for the initial management of the burned patient are the ABCs of trauma care.[68] The percentage of the body surface area burned as well as the depth should be estimated and recorded. Volume resuscitation should be started immediately and a bladder catheter inserted to monitor urinary output. Specific information about the accident can suggest additional nonthermal injuries, such as chest trauma, orthopedic injuries or intracranial pathology,[69] which may require emergency surgical care.[68,70] If possible, a history of preexisting diseases, allergies, and current medications should be obtained. Cardiovascular status should be evaluated and evidence of respiratory distress and smoke inhalation assessed.[71,72] Patients with significant full-thickness burns should be treated in a specialized burn center.

Emergency escharotomy, which can be performed at the bedside using sedation and electrocautery, may be required early in circumferential burns to retain limb blood flow and to permit thorax expansion.[73] High-energy electrical burns and severe crush injuries may cause compartment syndromes that require fasciotomy.[74] Prophylactic systemic antibiotics are strongly discouraged as their administration will select out resistant strains.[75]

Monitoring

Intraoperative monitoring is comparable to that of any critically ill patient undergoing major surgery. The minimum standards of the American Society of Anesthesiologists require electrocardiography (EKG), measurement of arterial blood pressure, respiratory rate, and body temperature, and the continuous presence of a trained anesthesiologist or a nurse anesthetist. Standard EKG gel electrodes often do not adhere to eschar, and skin staples and alligator clips can be substituted. Using bioimpedance, the ventilatory frequency can be monitored through the EKG cables. A Doppler flow probe can be used to detect pulses in small children. Pulse oximetry, which monitors both oxygen saturation and heart rate, allows assessment of both oxygenation and peripheral circulation. Systolic blood pressure measured by the return of pulse oximetry during cuff deflation correlates well with values obtained by conventional methods.[76] Capnography monitors carbon dioxide elimination and ventilatory frequency and provides the single best method to rule out esophageal intubation.[77] Capnography may be particularly valuable in adjusting ventilation in these patients whose energy expenditure and carbon dioxide production may greatly exceed normal (**Figure 13.3**). In extensively burned patients, the cheek may be the only site from which to obtain a pulse oximeter recording.

In severely burned patients more invasive monitoring is indicated. Urinary output is an indicator not only of kidney function, but also of overall organ perfusion, as renal blood flow decreases early in circulatory dysfunction. A urinary catheter also can monitor body temperature and suggest additional trauma, which may be manifested as hematuria or myoglobinuria. Discolored urine may provide the first evidence of a hemolytic transfusion reaction.

Rapid blood loss can produce sudden hemodynamic changes that are not detected by intermittent blood pressure recordings. Arterial catheters provide on-line measurement of blood pressure as well as access for sampling arterial blood. During excision of extensive burns, it is useful to obtain regular samples for blood gas analysis and measurements of hematocrit, glucose, sodium, potassium, and calcium. Because calcium metabolism is disturbed in severely burned patients,[78] replacement is often necessary, especially if large volumes of citrated blood or fresh frozen plasma are required.

Central venous and pulmonary artery catheters provide venous access and enhance circulatory assessment. If catheters must be inserted through burned skin, fixation may be difficult. Every arterial

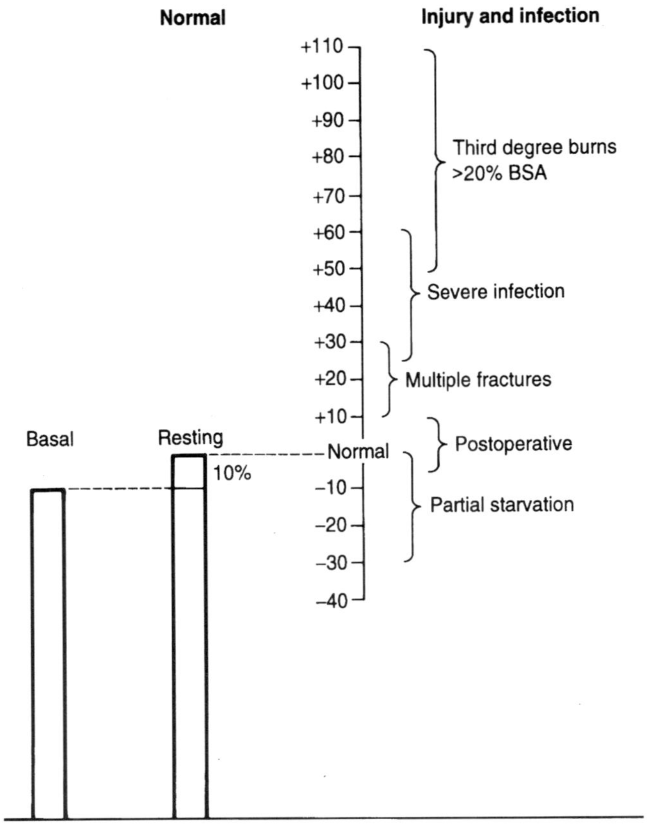

Fig. 13.3 Injury and sepsis increase resting energy expenditures in contrast to either baseline or nutritional depletion. (From Elwyn D H. Nutritional requirements of surgical patients. Crit Care Med **8:** *9–20, 1980.)*

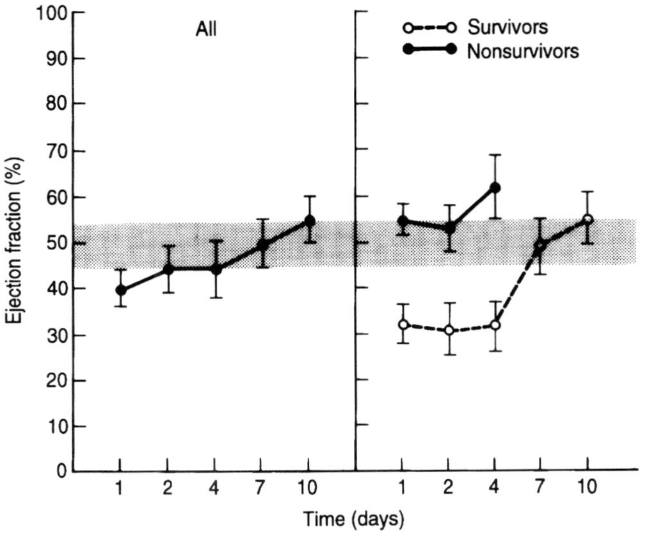

Fig. 13.4 The mean (± SE) ejection fraction plotted versus time for all patients, survivors, and nonsurvivors. The hatched area shows the normal range. (From Parker M M, et al. Profound but reversible myocardial depression in patients with septic shock. Ann Intern Med **100:** *483–90, 1984.)*

and central venous catheter should be secured by sutures, and daily changes of the dressings are mandatory. If inserted through burned skin, catheters should be exchanged at predetermined intervals to decrease the risk of nosocomial infection. In general, a large-lumen cathether is mandatory for volume replacement. The Seldinger technique is a convenient way to insert large catheters after relatively small venipunctures. Recommended sites for central venous catheter placement are, in descending order of desirability, the left subclavian or right internal jugular, right subclavian, and the femoral veins. The subclavian route carries a greater risk of complications (pneumothorax, hemothorax, hydrothorax) than the other techniques. In burned children and in conscious patients, central venous access through the internal jugular vein may be inconvenient and includes the risk of unintended removal. Femoral vein catheters in the inguinal region are associated with a higher incidence of infections and may be a stimulus for deep venous thrombosis.

Pulmonary artery catheters permit estimates of the determinants of heart function (preload, afterload, contractility) and allow the calculation of oxygen delivery and consumption, which correlate inversely with mortality after major trauma.[79] If patients have developed secondary burn sepsis, myocardial performance may be impaired, despite relatively high cardiac output (**Figure 13.4**).[80] Nevertheless, invasive catheterization must be considered in the light of the increased risk of catheter-related infections and endocarditis.[81]

Airway Management

One should consider the possibility of inhalation injury in any patient who gives a history of being burned in a confined space or who demonstrates on physical examination the classic signs, including facial burns, an edematous, injected tongue, sooty oral or nasal secretions, singed nasal hair, bronchorrhea, and hoarseness. When used to predict inhalation injury, each of these signs has a high false-positive rate. For example, 70% of patients with facial burns do not have an inhalation injury.[16,82] Hypoxemia may be absent in up to 80% of patients with inhalation injury at the time they first present.[9] The most severe inhalation injuries are incurred when the fire involves plastic materials.[83–85]

One may suspect cyanide toxicity, a complication of inhalation of the smoke from burned plastics (**Table 13.3**), if unexplained metabolic acidosis persists.[86] The treatment, sodium nitrite or thiosulfate, is usually unnecessary because the liver enzyme rhodanase and endogenous thiosulfate stores remove the compound from the circulation once splanchnic blood flow has been reestablished by volume resuscitation.

Upper airway injury

Upper airway injury includes damage to the oropharynx, the nasopharynx, and the hypopharynx. Tissues that have freely

Table 13.3 Common toxic products of combustion

Substance	Toxic products
Polyvinyl chloride	Hydrogen chloride, phosgene, chlorine
Wood, cotton, paper	Acrolein, acetaldehyde, formaldehyde, acetic acid, formic acid
Petroleum products	Acrolein, acetic acid, formic acid
Nitrocellulose film	Oxides of nitrogen, acetic acid, formic acid
Nitrogen-containing compounds (polyurethane)	Isocyanate, hydrogen cyanide
Polyfluorocarbons (Teflon)	Octafluoroisobutylene
Melamine resins	Ammonia, hydrogen cyanide

(From Strongin J, *et al.* Pulmonary disorders in the burn patient. In Martyn J A J, ed. *Acute Management of the Burned Patient.* Philadelphia: W B Saunders, Co., 1990.)

expandable loose tissue, such as the pharyngeal epiglottic surface and laryngeal ventricles, become edematous. Edema over the false cords, aryepiglottic folds, and arytenoid eminences can be massive enough to prolapse into the airway, causing partial or complete obstruction.[87,88] Airway edema may progress insidiously until sudden, complete airway obstruction occurs. Therefore, in the patient who presents with frank stridor or airway obstruction, intubation is essential, preferably with the largest tube that the larynx can accommodate, as the thick secretions that are produced later may obstruct a smaller tube. Later reintubation may be very difficult because of anatomical distortion by edema. Airway edema usually is maximal between 8 and 12 hours after injury, in parallel with the generalized extravascular fluid accumulation occurring during fluid resuscitation. Patients at risk for airway edema must be observed continuously and assessed at frequent intervals if a secure artificial airway has not been inserted.

An anesthesiologist managing anesthesia for a burned patient undergoing early debridement must consider airway complications when planning airway management. For intubation, fiberoptic bronchoscopy is a useful approach, but requires nasal preparation (i.e. topical application of local anesthetics and vasoconstrictors).[89,90] Phonation and forced expiratory maneuvers may be used to facilitate blind intubation[84,87] in a compliant patient. If the diagnosis of airway compromise is evident, it is prudent to manage the airway as one would a case of acute epiglottitis.

Table 13.4 Intubation criteria for burned patients

General criteria	
	Impaired mucociliary clearance function
	Age ≤16 years: Resp. rate >60 or $Paco_2$>60 mmHg
	Age >16 years: Resp. rate >40 or $Paco_2$>50 mmHg
	Pao_2<60 mmHg or Sao_2<85% (at ambient air)
	in the absence of coronary disease
Upper airway injury	
	Glottis opening <50%
	Presence of airway edema
Carbon monoxide poisoning	
	Carboxyhemoglobin concentration >20%
Associated injuries	
	Unconsciousness (brain injury, drug intoxication)
	Chest trauma, lung contusion
	Hemodynamic instability

Smoke inhalation

The diagnosis of injury below the cords may be made from an appropriate history and clinical examination. Xenon-133 scans or bronchoscopy may be performed for confirmation.[91] Bronchoscopy, by far the most practical method,[89] can be performed by the anesthesiologist during the surgical procedure. Airway injury usually is evident from erythema and edema of the tracheobronchial tree. In the worst cases, the bronchial septa may be blunted and the respiratory mucosa may be ulcerated. Bronchoscopy can be used to irrigate and suction thick mucus plugs and to obtain bronchial washings for cell counts, Gram stains, and cultures. Cultures of the washings can be used to guide antimicrobial therapy. Though fiberoptic bronchoscopy through an endotracheal tube is highly recommended and, in addition, confirms correct tracheal positioning of the endotracheal tube, direct bronchoscopy is sometimes unavoidable, especially in children. If examination of the airway demonstrates no inhalation injury, postoperative recovery from anesthetic drugs can be followed by extubation. In cases involving airway compromise, consideration should be given to keeping the patient intubated to provide a secure airway, and to allow mechanical ventilation and to facilitate pulmonary toilet.

Management of inhalation injuries is supportive. Oxygen-enriched air and, if necessary, mechanical ventilation with positive end-expiratory pressure (PEEP) is the mainstay of therapy,[92] often starting in the OR. **Table 13.4** lists the criteria for intubation of burned patients, based upon pulmonary dysfunction, upper airway injury, carbon monoxide poisoning, or associated injuries. PEEP is believed to work in part by reducing airway hyperemia[93] and by increasing functional residual lung capacity. Because the adverse effects of PEEP on cardiac output and oxygen delivery may occur even when applied to a poorly compliant lung,[94] these must be balanced against the improvement in Pao_2. When PEEP exceeding 10 cmH_2O is used, hemodynamics must be carefully monitored, preload optimized, and inotropic agents used if necessary to maintain cardiac output and oxygen delivery. High-frequency ventilators are reportedly effective but are not in widespread use.[95] Humidification of inspired gases is also helpful in the OR to avoid inspissation of secretions.[96] Steroids have no role in this condition.[97,98]

We try to avoid either prolonged intubation or tracheotomy in our patients. Both are associated with serious sequelae, including death, mediastinitis, tracheomalacia, tracheoesophageal fistula, tracheal stenosis, and vocal cord injury.[99–103] Tracheotomy appears to be more morbid than intubation. First, there is an additional wound. Second, positioning of the shorter tracheostomy tube while avoiding shear forces within the trachea is difficult.

Burned children seem able to sustain the high respiratory rates required to clear increased production of carbon dioxide.[104,105] If children must be intubated, the nose is our preferred route as intubation can be performed on the spontaneously breathing patient with or without the aid of a fiberoptic bronchoscope. It also interferes less in the care of neck burns. In younger children, i.e. ≤ 10 years of age, a cuffless endotracheal tube should be used if sufficient ventilatory pressures can be achieved despite the leak.

Transport to and from the OR

It is wise to intubate before transporting patients in whom consciousness is depressed, who have posterior pharyngeal swelling, or who have full-thickness circumferential nasolabial burns.[106,107] Transport from the emergency room or the intensive care unit to the OR of an intubated patient requires movement from a controlled environment through isolated areas such as elevators. The team accompanying the patient must be able to manage the airway, perform reintubation and provide advanced life support. Special consideration should be given to the extent of pulmonary dysfunction and to the level of ventilatory support necessary before transportation. The amount of oxygen needed during transport should be determined, and equipment should be suitable to continue the level of pulmonary support without interruptions. Three categories of burned patients who require transportation to and from the OR can be distinguished (**Table 13.5**). In any of these conditions, a functioning venous catheter must be available.

Table 13.5 Transport to and from the OR

Patient's condition	Leads to	Patient's monitoring
Weight ≥ 10 kg Hemodynamically stable No artificial airway	⇒	Standard transportation to a prewarmed OR
Weight < 10 kg TBSA burned > 25% < 50% Stable, no artificial airway	⇒	Monitoring: EKG, respiratory rate, SaO_2; accompanied by RN, O_2, mask, hand-bagging device
Weight < 10 kg TBSA burned ≥ 50% Hemodynamically unstable, and/or ventilatory support	⇒	Monitoring: in addition to above, invasive arterial blood pressure, accompanied by anesthesiologist portable ventilator & monitor

Preparation for Anesthesia

The initial task after arriving in the OR is to switch from portable equipment to the breathing circuit and monitoring system in the room. If necessary, additional monitoring should be accomplished and intravascular access should be secured. The importance of large, secure intravenous catheters cannot be overemphasized. Sixteen-gauge catheters allow a maximal flow rate of only 100 ml/min of crystalloid fluids and, according to La Place's law, this rate decreases with the length of a central venous catheter. More viscous fluids (i.e. blood or albumin) flow more slowly. Therefore, a larger bore central venous catheter can be invaluable.

Nonburned areas are preferred for the insertion of vascular lines. Cutdowns are associated with a prohibitively high incidence of suppurative thrombophlebitis. As the venous lines are also needed postoperatively, central placement using the subclavian route is recommended.

Hypovolemia and rapid hemorrhage are common complications of the debridement of burns. To keep pace with rapid blood loss, the anesthesiologist must prepare in advance. Fluid replacement therapy may be difficult because intraoperative estimates of blood loss are often inaccurate. Systems to pressurize blood bags and warm infused blood at high flow rates are helpful. The anesthesiologist should concentrate on the adequacy of fluid resuscitation and on cardiopulmonary and renal function. Renal function is particularly important, not only because it is a good indicator of peripheral perfusion, but because the development of renal failure dramatically increases mortality. Monitoring of urinary output is mandatory in all major burn debridements.

Intraoperatively, changes in the shape of the arterial pressure waveform and frequent hematocrit measurements are useful guides to the adequacy of resuscitation. One can expect roughly 3–4% of the circulating volume to be lost for each 1% of body surface excised.[108] However, blood loss varies with the time since the occurrence of the burn injury and with local infection (**Table 13.6**).

To avoid hypothermia, burned patients should be maintained in a thermoneutral environment, the temperature at which the patient neither gains nor loses heat, as either process increases energy consumption.[109] The patient is fully exposed and the loss of keratinized skin removes the vapor barrier, facilitating the loss of both fluid and heat through evaporation. In addition, anesthetized patients lose the ability to thermoregulate by vasoconstriction since general anesthesia reduces peripheral and central receptor sensitivity to cold, depresses the thermoregulatory center, and produces peripheral vasodilatation.

Table 13.6 Calculation of expected blood loss

Surgical procedure	Predicted blood loss
<24 h since burn injury	0.45 ml/cm² burn area
1–3 days since burn injury	0.70 ml/cm² burn area
>4 days since burn injury	0.90 ml/cm² burn area
in infected burn wounds	1.0–1.25 ml/cm² burn area

$$\frac{\text{Predicted blood loss} \bullet 1.3}{\text{Body weight (kg)}} = \text{Relative blood loss (\%)}$$

Skeletal muscle relaxants eliminate shivering and thereby impede one of the methods of thermogenesis. Room temperature should be maintained at about 30°C and the patient given heated humidified gases to breathe.[110] Body temperature can be monitored in the nasopharynx, rectum, urinary bladder, or by a pulmonary artery catheter.

Heating blankets and radiant heat lamps should be available. Intravenous and topical solutions should be warmed. We find it essential to have a blood warmer that can warm fluid to body temperature despite flow rates of 500 ml/min.

Selection of Anesthetic Agents

Many techniques have been described for the maintenance of anesthesia in burned patients. Intravenous agents offer many advantages (**Table 13.7**). Intravenous ketamine can be used as the primary anesthetic in burned patients at a dose of 0.5–1.5 mg/kg IV. Ketamine also may be continuously infused at a rate of 0.7–5.4 mg/min (adult dosage) (**Table 13.7**). The intramuscular route without venous access should be limited to extreme emergencies. Ketamine preserves hypoxic and hypercapnic ventilatory stimulation and reduces airway resistance. If pulmonary function is adequate, patients anesthetized with ketamine may be allowed to breathe spontaneously without an endotracheal tube. The advantages are that the circulation is not impaired by positive-pressure ventilation and there is no danger of accidental extubation during positioning for the surgical procedure.[111] Moreover, injuries or complications related to endotracheal intubation decrease with its

Table 13.7 Dosage guidelines for the most commonly used intravenous anesthetic infusions

		Infusion rate	
Anesthetic	Loading dose (mg/kg)	Maintenance of anesthesia* (mg/min)	Sedation (mg/min)
Thiopental	2.0–4.0	10–20	1.0–5.0
Methohexital	1.5–3.0	5.0–8.0	0.5–2.5
Midazolam†	0.2–0.4	0.1–1.0	0.035–0.7
Etomidate	0.2–0.4	1.0–2.0	0.5–1.0
Propofol	1.5–2.0	4.0–12.0	2.0–5.0
Ketamine‡	0.5–1.0	0.7–5.4	1.0–2.0

* Adjuvant to other agents (i.e. nitrous oxide, opioids).
† Infusion rate for midazolam is highly variable. Values in the table represent most commonly used doses.
‡ Ketamine is contraindicated in head-injured patients. Its inclusion in this table pertains to use in other injuries.
From Nolan J P. Intravenous agents. In Grande C M, *et al.*, eds. *Textbook of Trauma Anesthesia and Critical Care*. St Louis: Mosby Year Book, Inc., 1993.

reduced duration. On the other hand, aspiration and depressed ventilation represent substantial hazards that are greatly magnified if other intraoperative concerns, such as replacement of rapid blood loss, distract the anesthesiologist from observation of the airway. If any doubt exists, a secure artificial airway should be instituted. Although pharyngeal and laryngeal reflexes are partially retained, ketamine does not prevent aspiration.

In response to ketamine, heart rate, blood pressure and cardiac index increase (**Figure 13.5**). Stimulation of the circulation is attributed to sympathetic activity. A side effect of ketamine is the occurrence of unpleasant hallucinations during the postoperative period. Benzodiazepines (midazolam more than diazepam) reduce the incidence of emergence delirium.

Table 13.8 lists commonly used narcotics. Fentanyl (0.005 mg/kg) provides effective, low-cost analgesia in hemodynamically stable patients who are receiving ventilatory support. To avoid volatile anesthetics, a combination of midazolam (0.1 mg/kg) and fentanyl can serve as a total intravenous technique. Alternatively, a combination of alfentanil and propofol maintenance can be used. After a loading dose of alfentanil 100 μg/kg, the intraoperative requirement was 1.24 ± 0.7 μg/kg/min, and after a propofol induction dose of 2 mg/kg the maintenance rate was 100 μg/kg/min.[112] With this technique, inhalation agents could be avoided and satisfactory postoperative analgesia was present in most patients 2 hours after operation.[112]

An anesthetic technique involving nasotracheal intubation, after mask induction with halothane, nitrous oxide, and oxygen, has been described.[113] The proponents particularly emphasize avoiding the potential problems of the ketamine-based technique.[113] Volatile anesthetics produce dose-dependent cardiac depression and vasodilation, among other cardiovascular effects (**Table 13.9**),[114–116] These agents also tend to abolish hypoxic pulmonary vasoconstriction and thereby affect ventilation/perfusion matching. However, predictable washin and washout avoids concerns about altered pharmacokinetics of intravenous agents (**Figure 13.6**).

Anesthesia and blood transfusions have been demonstrated to impair immune function.[117] Both transfusions and anesthesia (methoxyflurane) were found to increase susceptibility to peritoneal *E. coli* infections in rats although neither altered susceptibility to an intravenous *E. coli* challenge.[117]

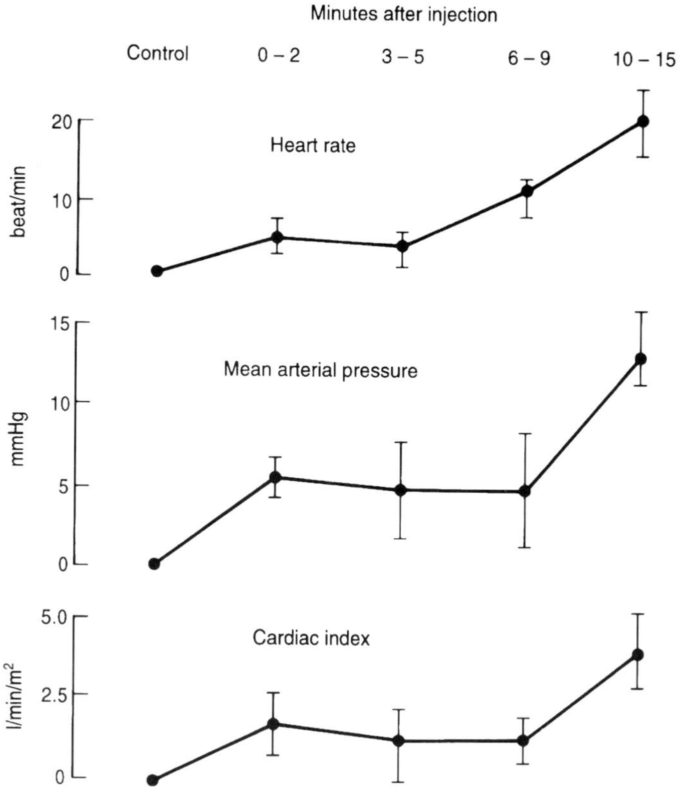

Fig. 13.5 Heart rate, mean arterial pressure, and cardiac index changes during a 15 minute period after administration of ketamine to critically ill patients. (From Nolan J P. Intravenous agents. In Grande C M, et al., eds. Textbook of Trauma Anesthesia and Critical Care. *St Louis: Mosby Year Book, Inc., 1993.)*

SUMMARY

Burned patients, both children and adults, constitute challenges for the anesthesiologist in the emergency room, the OR, and the intensive care unit. Burn injury and inhalation injury cause rapid changes in fluid homeostasis, circulatory stability and res-

Table 13.8 Clinically relevant characteristics of the five most commonly used narcotics

	Morphine	Meperidine	Fentanyl	Sufentanil	Alfentanil
Relative potency	1.0	0.1	100–200	700–1200	30–60
LD_{50} in dogs (mg/kg)	200	700	10	4.0	59.5–87.5
Analgesic dose	70–210 μg/kg	0.7–2.1 mg/kg	1.0–2.0 μg/kg	0.25 μg/kg	4.8 μg/kg
Anesthetic dose*	0.5–3.0 mg/kg	3.0–10 mg/kg	50–100 μg/kg	5.12 μg/kg	100–300 μg/kg loading dose + 25.50 μg/kg/h
MIC_{50}			15 ng/ml		270–400
MIC_{90}			25 ng/ml		
MIC_{95}			30 ng/ml		
Cardiovascular stability	+/–	– –	++++	++++	+++
Histamine release	++	+++	–	–	–
Respiratory depression	++	++	+++	+++	+++
Elimination half-life (h)	3.0	2.5	3.5	2.5	1.5

LD_{50}, the dose that is lethal in 50% of subjects; $MIC_{50,90,95}$, minimum intra-arterial concentration that prevents response to sternotomy incision in 50%, 90%, and 95% of patients; –, no; +, yes.
* Doses used for cardiac surgery. Smaller doses combined with other drugs are sufficient for most trauma patients.
From Capan L M, *et al.* Principles of anesthesia for major trauma victim. In Capan L M, *et al.*, eds. *Trauma Anesthesia and Intensive Care*. Philadelphia: J B Lippincott, Co., 1991.

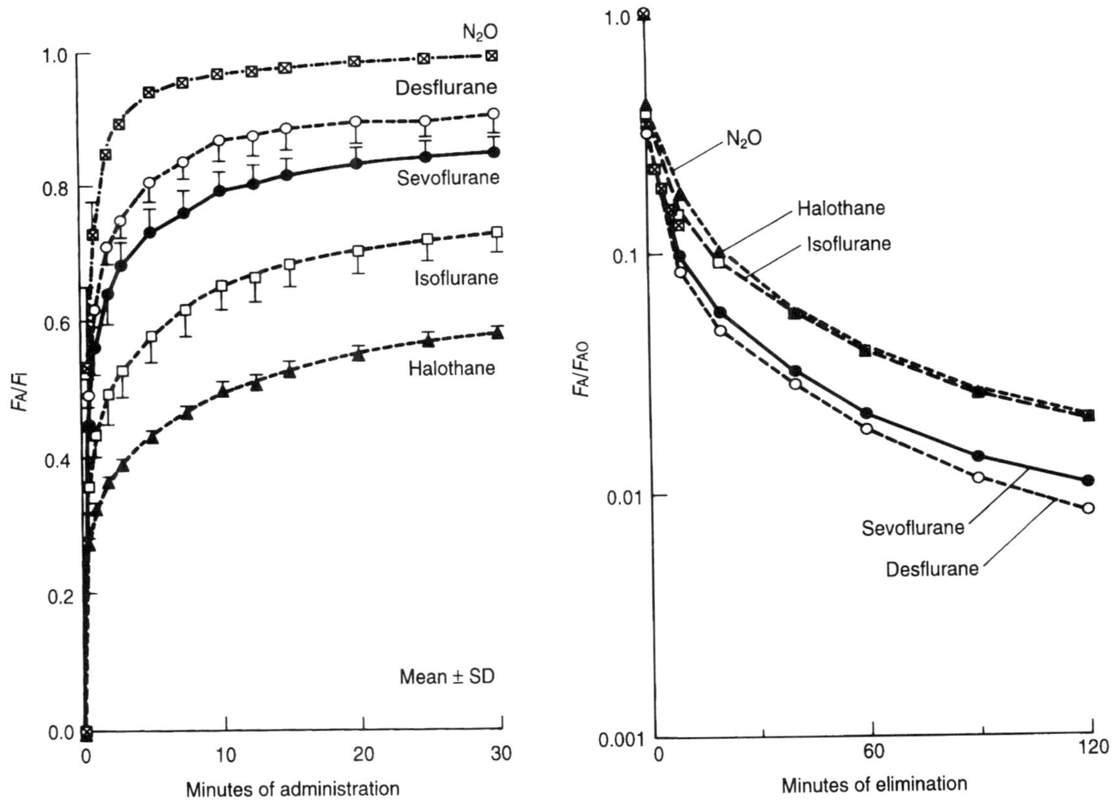

Fig. 13.6 (a) Washin curves of a number of inhalational agents. Consistent with the low blood/gas partition coefficient of desflurane, its ratio of end-tidal anesthetic concentration (FA) to inspired anesthetic concentrations (FI) increases more rapidly than the other volatile agents. (b) Washout curves of a number of inhalational agents. FA, End-tidal anesthetic concentration; FAO, end-tidal anesthetic concentration immediately before beginning of elimination. (From Yasuda N, et al. Comparison of kinetics of sevoflurane and isoflurane in humans. Anesth Analg **72:** *316–24, 1991.)*

Table 13.9 Cardiovascular effects of inhalation agents

Effect	Halothane	Enflurane	Isoflurane
Contractility	↓↓	↓↓	↓
Cardiac output	↓↓	↓↓	↓
Systemic vascular resistance	→↓	↓	↓↓
Mean arterial pressure	↓↓	↓↓	↓↓
Heart rate	↓	↑→	↑↑
Sensitization of myocardium to catecholamines	↑↑↑	↑→	→
Baroreceptor reflexes	↓↓↓	↓↓↓	↓

From Nolan J P. Inhalation agents. In Grande C M, *et al.*, eds. *Textbook of Trauma Anesthesia and Critical Care*. St Louis: Mosby Year Book, Inc., 1993.

piratory function. Venous access with a large intravenous cannula is mandatory to restore intravascular volume. Endotracheal intubation, ventilatory support, and oxygen therapy may be needed in inhalation injury or carbon monoxide poisoning. Knowledge of pharmacokinetic and pharmacodynamic differences in the use of muscle relaxants avoids potential complications. Surgical procedures such as debridement and grafting may have to be done early and repeatedly. As long as the special needs of these critically injured patients are recognized, a variety of anesthetic techniques can produce a good outcome. Both the spontaneously breathing patient as well as the unstable patient under general anesthesia in the OR require vigilant anesthetic management.

REFERENCES

1. Herndon D N, Rutan R L, Rutan T C. Management of the pediatric patient with burns. *J Burn Care Rehabil* 1993; **14:** 3–8.

2. American Burn Association. Hospital and prehospital resources for optimal care of patients with burn injury: guidelines for development and operation of burn centers. *J Burn Care Rehabil* 1990; **11:** 98–104.

3. Grande C M, Stene J K, Barton C R. The trauma anesthesiologist. *Md Med J* 1988; **37:** 531–6.

4. Thompson P B, Herndon D N, Traber D L, Abston S. Effect on mortality of inhalation injury. *J Trauma* 1986; **26:** 163–5.

5. Herndon D N, Gore D, Cole M, *et al.* Determinants of mortality in pediatric patients with greater than 70% full-thickness total body surface area thermal injury treated by early total excision and grafting. *J Trauma* 1987; **27:** 208–12.

6. Shirani K Z, Pruitt B A Jr, Mason A D J. The influence of inhalation injury and pneumonia on burn mortality. *Ann Surg* 1987; **205:** 82–7.

7. Heimbach D M, Waeckerle J F. Inhalation injuries. *Ann Emerg Med* 1988; **17:** 1316–20.

8. Larsen L E. Smoke poisoning. Inhalation injuries from remaining at the scene of a fire. *Ugeskr Laeger* 1989; **151:** 419–22.

9. Heimbach D M, Waeckerle J F. Inhalation injuries. *Ann Emerg Med* 1988; **17:** 1316–20.

10. Goodwin C W, Aulick L H, Becker R A, Wilmore D W. Increased renal perfusion and kidney size in convalescent burn patients. *JAMA* 1980; **244:** 1588–90.

11. Goldbaum L R, Orellano T, Dergal E. Joint Committee on Aviation Pathology: XVI. Studies on the relation between carboxyhemoglobin concentration and toxicity. *Aviat Space Environ Med* 1977; **48:** 969–70.

12. Somogyi E, Balogh I, Rubanyi G, Sotonyi P, Szegedi L. New findings concerning the pathogenesis of acute carbon monoxide (CO) poisoning. *Am J Forensic Med Pathol* 1981; **2:** 31–9.

13. Larkin J M, Brahos G J, Moylan J A. Treatment of carbon monoxide poisoning: prognostic factors. *J Trauma* 1976; **16:** 111–14.

14. Pruitt B A, Erickson D R, Morris A. Progressive pulmonary insufficiency and other pulmonary complications of thermal injury. *J Trauma* 1975; **15:** 369–79.

15. Stone H H, Martin J D, Claydon C T. Management of the pulmonary burn. *Am Surg* 1967; **33:** 616–20.

16. Moylan J P. Inhalation injury: a primary determinant of survival following major burns. *J Burn Care Rehabil* 1981; **2:** 78–84.

17. Traber D L, Herndon D N. Pathophysiology of smoke inhalation. In Haponik E F, Munster A M, eds. *Respiratory Sequelae of Burns*. New York: McGraw Hill, Inc, 1990: 61–73.

18. Robinson L, Miller R H. Smoke inhalation injuries. *Am J Otolaryngol* 1986; **7:** 375–80.

19. Herndon D N, Traber D L, Niehaus G D, Linares H A, Traber L D. The pathophysiology of smoke inhalation injury in a sheep model. *J Trauma* 1984; **24:** 1044–51.

20. Traber D L, Herndon D N, Stein M D, Traber L D, Flynn J T, Niehaus G D. The pulmonary lesion of smoke inhalation in an ovine model. *Circ Shock* 1986; **18:** 311–23.

21. Traber D L, Schlag G, Redl H, Traber L D. Pulmonary edema and compliance changes following smoke inhalation. *J Burn Care Rehabil* 1985; **6:** 490–4.

22. Kimura R, Traber L D, Herndon D N, Linares H A, Lübbesmeyer H J, Traber D L. Increasing duration of smoke exposure induces more severe lung injury in sheep. *J Appl Physiol* 1988; **64:** 1107–13.

23. Sugi K, Theissen J L, Traber L D, Herndon D N, Traber D L. Impact of carbon monoxide on cardiopulmonary dysfunction after smoke inhalation injury. *Circ Res* 1990; **66:** 69–75.

24. Abdi S, Herndon D, Mcguire J, Traber L, Traber D L. Time course of alterations in lung lymph and bronchial blood flows after inhalation injury. *J Burn Care Rehabil* 1990; **11:** 510–15.

25. Isago T, Fujioka K, Traber L D, Herndon D N, Traber D L. Derived pulmonary capillary pressure changes after smoke inhalation in sheep. *Crit Care Med* 1991; **19:** 1407–13.

26. Holloway H, Perry M, Downey J, Parker J, Taylor A. Estimation of effective pulmonary capillary pressure in intact lungs. *J Appl Physiol* 1983; **54**: 846–51.

27. Isago T, Noshima S, Traber L D, Herndon D N, Traber D L. Analysis of pulmonary microvascular permeability after smoke inhalation. *J Appl Physiol* 1991; **71:** 1403–8.

28. Herndon D N, Traber L D, Linares H, *et al.* Etiology of the pulmonary pathophysiology associated with inhalation injury. *Resuscitation* 1986; **14:** 43–59.

29. Montero K, Lübbesmeyer H J, Traber D L, Kimura R, Traber L D, Herndon D N. Inhalation injury increases systemic microvascular permeability. *Surg Forum* 1987; **38:** 303–5.

30. Basadre J O, Sugi K, Traber D L, Traber L D, Niehaus G D, Herndon D N. The effect of leukocyte depletion on smoke inhalation injury in sheep. *Surgery* 1988; **104:** 208–15.

31. Herndon D N, Traber D L, Traber L D. The effect of resuscitation on inhalation injury. *Surgery* 1986; **100:** 248–51.

32. Arturson G. The changes in capillary filtration, diffusion and permeability in experimental burns. *Bibl Anat* 1965; **7:** 453–9.

33. Arturson G. Microvascular permeability to macromolecules in thermal injury. *Acta Physiol Scand Suppl* 1979: 111–22.

34. Arturson G, Soeda S. Changes in transcapillary leakage during healing of experimental burns. *Acta Chir Scand* 1967; **133:** 609–14.

35. Landis E M, Pappenheimer J R. Exchange of substances through the capillary walls. In: Hamilton W F, Dow P, eds. *Handbook of Physiology, Section 2, Vol. 2*. Baltimore, MD: Williams & Wilkins, 1963: 961–1034.

36. Starling E H. On the absorption of fluids from the connective tissue spaces. *J Physiol (Lond)* 1896; **19:** 312–26.

37. Pitt R M, Parker J C, Jurkovich G J, Taylor A E, Curreri P W. Analysis of altered capillary pressure and permeability after thermal injury. *J Surg Res* 1987; **42:** 693–702.

38. Lund T, Wiig H, Reed R K. Acute postburn edema: role of strongly negative interstitial fluid pressure. *Am J Physiol* 1988; **255:** H1069–H1074.

39. Herndon D N, Wilmore D W, Mason A D J, Pruitt B A Jr. Humoral mediators of nontemperature-dependent hypermetabolism in 50% burned adult rats. *Surg Forum* 1977; **28:** 37–9.

40. Wolfe R R, Herndon D N, Peters E J, Jahoor F, Desai M H, Holland O B. Regulation of lipolysis in severely burned children. *Ann Surg* 1987; **206:** 214–21.

41. van Gool J, van Vugt H, Helle M, Aarden L A. The relation among stress, adrenalin, interleukin 6 and acute phase proteins in the rat. *Clin Immunol Immunopathol* 1990; **57:** 200–10.

42. Nijsten M W, Hack C E, Helle M, ten Duis H J, Klasen H J, Aarden L A. Interleukin-6 and its relation to the humoral immune response and clinical parameters in burned patients. *Surgery* 1991; **109:** 761–7.

43. Hartl W, Jauch K W, Herndon D N, Cohnert T U, Wolfe R R, Schildberg F W. Effect of low-dose bradykinin on glucose metabolism and nitrogen balance in surgical patients. *Lancet* 1990; **335:** 69–71.

44. Wilmore D W. Pathophysiology of the hypermetabolic response to burn injury. *J Trauma* 1990; **30:** S4–S6.

45. Harms B A, Kramer G C, Bodai B I, Demling R H. Effect of hypoproteinemia on pulmonary and soft tissue edema formation. *Crit Care Med* 1981; **9:** 503–8.

46. Conhaim R L, Harms B A. A simplified two-pore filtration model explains the effects of hypoproteinemia on lung and soft tissue lymph flux in awake sheep. *Microvasc Res* 1992; **44:** 14–26.

47. Watkins W D, Leslie J B, DeBruijn N P. Pharmacologic principles. In: Miller R D, ed. *Anesthesia*. New York: Churchill Livingstone, 1986: 55–73.

48. Martyn J A, Abernethy D R, Greenblatt D J. Plasma protein binding of drugs after severe burn injury. *Clin Pharmacol Ther* 1984; **35:** 535–9.

49. Zini R, Riant P, Barre J, Tillement J P. Disease-induced variations in plasma protein levels. Implications for drug dosage regimens (Part I). *Clin Pharmacokinet* 1990; **19:** 147–59.

50. Martyn J A J, Szyfelbein S K, Ali H H. Increased *d*-tubocurarine requirement following major thermal injury. *Anesthesiology* 1980; **52:** 352–6.

51. Moncrief J A. Complications of burns. *Ann Surg* 1958; **147:** 443–75.

52. Tolmie J D, Joyce T H, Mitchell G D. Succinylcholine danger in the burned patient. *Anesthesiology* 1967; **28:** 467–70.

53. Viby-Mogensen J, Hanel H K, Hansen E, Graae J. Serum cholinesterase activity in burned patients. II: Anaesthesia, suxamethonium and hyperkalaemia. *Acta Anaesthesiol Scand* 1975; **19:** 169–79.

54. Schaner P J, Brown R L, Kirksey T D, Gunther R C, Ritchey C R, Gronert G A. Succinylcholine-induced hyperkalemia in burned patients. *Anesth Analg* 1969; **48:** 764–70.

55. Birch A A Jr, Mitchell G D, Playford G A, Lang C A. Changes in serum potassium response to succinylcholine following trauma. *JAMA* 1969; **210:** 490–3.

56. McCaughey T J. Hazards of anesthesia for the burned child. *Can Anaesth Soc J* 1962; **9:** 220–33.

57. Fambrough D M. Control of acetylcholine receptors in skeletal muscle. *Physiol Rev* 1979; **59:** 165–227.

58. Yentis S M. Suxamethonium and hyperkalaemia. *Anaesth Intensive Care* 1990; **18:** 92–101.

59. Lorente J A, Garcia Frade L J, Landin L, *et al.* Time course of hemostatic abnormalities in sepsis and its relation to outcome. *Chest* 1993; **103:** 1536–42.

60. Martyn J A, Matteo R S, Szyfelbein S K, Kaplan R F. Unprecedented resistance to neuromuscular blocking effects of metocurine with persistence after complete recovery in a burned patient. *Anesth Analg* 1982; **61:** 614–17.

61. Marathe P H, Haschke R H, Slattery J T, Zucker J R, Pavlin E G. Acetylcholine receptor density and acetylcholinesterase activity in skeletal muscle of rats following thermal injury. *Anesthesiology* 1989; **70:** 654–9.

62. Kim C, Fuke N, Martyn J A. Burn injury to rat increases nicotinic acetylcholine receptors in the diaphragm. *Anesthesiology* 1988; **68:** 401–6.

63. Gronert G A, Theye R A. Pathophysiology of hyperkalemia induced by succinylcholine. *Anesthesiology* 1975; **43:** 89–99.

64. Martyn J, Greenblatt D J. Lorazepam conjugation is unimpaired in burn trauma. *Clin Pharmacol Ther* 1988; **43:** 250–5.

65. Martyn J A, Greenblatt D J, Quinby W C. Diazepam kinetics in patients with severe burns. *Anesth Analg* 1983; **62:** 293–7.

66. Sokoll M D, Gergis S D. Antibiotics and neuromuscular function. *Anesthesiology* 1981; **55:** 148–51.

67. Dupuis J Y, Martin R, Tetrault J P, Atracurium and vecuronium interaction with gentamicin and tobramycin. *Can J Anaesth* 1989; **36:** 407.

68. Grande C M, Stene J K, Bernhard W N. Airway management: considerations in the trauma patient. *Crit Care Clin* 1990; **6:** 37–59.

69. McSwain N E Jr. Mechanisms of injury in blunt trauma. In: McSwain N E Jr, Kerstein M D, eds. *Evaluation and Management of Trauma*. East Norwalk, CT: Appleton-Century-Croft, 1987: 1–24.

70. Purdue G F, Hunt J L. Multiple trauma and the burn patient. *Am J Surg* 1989; **158:** 536–9.

71. Beal D D, Conner G H. Respiratory tract injury: a guide to management following thermal and smoke injury. *Laryngoscope* 1970; **80:** 25–35.

72. Webster J R, McCabe M M, Karp M. Recognition and management of smoke inhalation. *JAMA* 1967; **201:** 287–90.

73. Pruitt B A Jr. The acute burn patient. In: Siegel J H, ed. *Trauma Emergency Surgery and Critical Care*, New York: Churchill Livingstone, 1987: 1099pp.

74. Pruitt B A. The burn patient: I. Initial care. *Curr Probl Surg* 1979; **16:** 1–55.

75. Haburchak D R, Pruitt B A. Use of systemic antibiotics in the burned patient. *Surg Clin North Am* 1978; **58:** 1119–32.

76. Talke P, Nichols R J, Traber D L. Does measurement of systolic blood pressure with a pulse oximeter correlate with conventional methods? *J Clin Monit* 1990; **6:** 5–9.

77. Birmingham P K, Cheney F W, Ward R J. Esophageal intubation: a review of detection techniques. *Anesth Analg* 1986; **65:** 886–90.

78. Szyfelbein S K, Drop L J, Martyn J A. Persistent ionized hypocalcemia in patients during resuscitation and recovery phases of body burns. *Crit Care Med* 1981; **9:** 454–8.

79. Shoemaker W C, Appel P L, Kram H B. Tissue oxygen debt as a determinant of lethal and nonlethal postoperative organ failure. *Crit Care Med* 1988; **16:** 1117–20.

80. Parker M M, Shelhamer J H, Bacharach S L, *et al.* Profound but reversible myocardial depression in patients with septic shock. *Ann Intern Med* 1984; **100:** 483–90.

81. Johnston W E. Complications from the use of pulmonary artery catheters. In: Lumb P D, Bryan-Brown C W, eds. *Complications in Critical Care Medicine*, 1988 Chicago, IL: Year Book Medical Publishers, Inc, 1988.

82. Herndon D N, Langner F, Thompson P, Linares H A, Stein M, Traber D L. Pulmonary injury in burned patients. *Surg Clin North Am* 1987; **67:** 31–46.

83. Herndon D N, Thompson P B, Traber D L. Pulmonary injury in burned patients. In: Cohen B E, ed. *Critical Care Clinics*. Philadelphia: W B Saunders Co, 1985: 79–96.

84. Haponik E F, Crapo R O, Herndon D N, Traber D L, Hudson L, Moylan J. Smoke inhalation. *Am Rev Respir Dis* 1988; **138:** 1060–3.

85. Moritz A R, Henriques F C, McLean R. The effect of inhaled heat on the air passages and lungs: an experimental investigation. *Am J Pathol* 1945; **21:** 311–26.

86. Silverman S H, Purdue G F, Hunt J L, Bost R O. Cyanide toxicity in burned patients. *J Trauma* 1988; **28:** 171–6.

87. Haponik E F, Meyers D A, Munster A M, *et al.* Acute upper airway injury in burn patients. Serial changes of flow-volume curves and nasopharyngoscopy. *Am Rev Respir Dis* 1987, **135:** 360–6.

88. Foley Fd, Moncrief J A, Mason A D Jr. Pathology of the lung in fatally burned patients. *Ann Surg* 1968; **167:** 251–64.

89. Moylan J A, Adib K, Birnbaum M. Fiberoptic bronchoscopy following thermal injury. *Surg Gynecol Obstet* 1975; **140:** 541–3.

90. Hunt J L, Agee R N, Pruitt B A. Fiberoptic bronchoscopy in acute Injury. *J Trauma* 1975; **15:** 641–9.

91. Agee R N, Long J III, Hunt J L, *et al.* Use of 133xenon in early diagnosis of injury. *J Trauma* 1976; **16:** 218–24.

92. Shapiro B A, Cane R D, Harrison R A. Positive end-expiratory pressure therapy in adults with special reference to acute lung injury: a review of the literature and suggested clinical correlations. *Crit Care Med* 1984; **12:** 127–41.

93. Abdi S, Traber L D, Herndon D N, Redl G, Curry B, Traber D L. Bronchial blood flow reduction with positive end-expiratory pressure after acute lung injury in sheep. *Crit Care Med* 1990; **18:** 1152–7.

94. Venus B, Cohen L E, Smith R A. Hemodynamics and intrathoracic pressure transmission during controlled mechanical ventilation and positive end-expiratory pressure in normal and low compliant lungs. *Crit Care Med* 1988; **16:** 686–90.

95. Cioffi W G, Rue L III, Graves T A, McManus W F, Mason A D, Pruitt B A. Prophylactic use of high-frequency percussive ventilation in patients with inhalation injury. *Ann Surg* 1991; **213:** 575–80.

96. Lloyd E L, MacRae W R. Respiratory tract damage in burns. Case reports and review of the literature. *Br J Anaesth* 1971; **43:** 365–79.

97. Levine B A, Petroff P A, Slade C L, Pruitt B A. Prospective trials of dexamethasone and aerosolized gentamicin in the treatment of inhalation injury in the burned patient. *J Trauma* 1978; **18:** 188–93.

98. Robinson N B, Hudson L D, Riem M, *et al.* Steroid therapy following isolated smoke injury. *J Trauma* 1982; **22:** 876–9.

99. Eckhauser F E, Billote J, Burke J F, Quinby W C. Tracheostomy complicating massive burn injury. A plea for conservatism. *Am J Surg* 1974; **127:** 418–23.

100. Hunt J L, Purdue G F, Gunning T. Is tracheostomy warranted in the burn patient? Indications and complications. *J Burn Care Rehabil* 1986; **7:** 492–5.

101. Lund T, Goodwin C W, McManus W F, *et al.* Upper airway sequelae in burn patients requiring endotracheal intubation or tracheostomy. *Ann Surg* 1985; **201:** 374–82.

102. Moylan J A, West J T, Nash G, Bowen J A, Pruitt B A. Tracheostomy in thermally injured patients: a review of five years' experience. *Am Surg* 1972; **38:** 119–23.

103. Calhoun K H, Deskin R W, Garza C, *et al.* Long-term airway sequelae in a pediatric burn population. *Laryngoscope* 1988; **98:** 721–5.

104. Stephenson S F, Esrig B C, Polk H C, Fulton R L. The pathophysiology of smoke injury. *Ann Surg* 1975; **182:** 652–60.

105. Robinson N B, Hudson L D, Robertson H T, Thorning D R, Carrico C J, Heimbach D M. Ventilation and perfusion alterations after smoke injury. *Surgery* 1981; **90:** 352–63.

106. Demling R H. Postgraduate course: respiratory injury. Part III: Pulmonary dysfunction in the burn patient. *J Burn Care Rehabil* 1986; **7:** 277–84.

107. Lamb J D. Anaesthetic considerations for major thermal injury. *Can Anaesth Soc J* 1985; **32:** 84–92.

108. Moran K T, O'Reilly T J, Furman W R. A new algorithm for calculation of blood loss in excisional burn surgery. *Am Surg* 1988; **54:** 207–10.

109. Wilmore D W, Mason A D, Johnson D W, Pruitt B A. Effect of ambient temperature on heat production and heat loss in burn patients. *J Appl Physiol* 1975; **38:** 593–7.

110. Shelly M P, Lloyd G M, Park G R. A review of the mechanisms and methods of humidification of inspired gases. *Intens Care Med* 1988; **14:** 1–9.

111. White P F, Way W L, Trevor A J. Ketamine – its pharmacology and therapeutic uses. *Anesthesiology* 1982; **56:** 119–36.

112. Reyneke C J, James M F, Johnson R. Alfentanil and propofol infusions for surgery in the burned patient. *Br J Anaesth* 1989; **63:** 418–22.

113. Layon A J, Vetter T R, Hanna P G, Bingham H G. An anesthetic technique to fabricate a pressure mask for controlling scar formation from facial burns. *J Burn Care Rehabil* 1991; **12:** 349–52.

114. Brown B R, Crout J R. A comparative study of the effects of five general anesthetics on myocardial contractility. I. Isometric conditions. *Anesthesiology* 1971; **34:** 236–45.

115. Wolf W J, Neal M B, Mathew B P, Bee D E. Comparison of the in vitro myocardial depressant effects of isoflurane and halothane anesthesia. *Anesthesiology* 1988; **69:** 660–6.

116. Sahlman L, Henriksson B A, Martner J, Ricksten S E. Effects of halothane, enflurane, and isoflurane on coronary vascular tone, myocardial performance, and oxygen consumption during controlled changes in aortic and left atrial pressure. Studies on isolated working rat hearts in vitro. *Anesthesiology* 1988; **69:** 1–10.

117. Waymack J P, Miskell P, Gonce S. Alterations in host defense associated with inhalation anesthesia and blood transfusion. *Anesth Analg* 1989; **69:** 163–8.

CHAPTER FOURTEEN

14

THE SKIN BANK

ROBERT L. MCCAULEY

INTRODUCTION

Early excision and coverage of the burn wound has increasingly become the standard of care for burned patients, with primary closure of the burn wound using split-thickness skin grafts being the ultimate goal. In patients with massive thermal injury, temporary coverage with skin donated by another person (allograft or homograft) is essential.[1] Although tissue transplantation was described in the seventeenth century, the development of the US Navy Skin Bank in Bethesda, Maryland in 1949 signified the emergence of modern day skin banking.[2]

HISTORICAL DEVELOPMENT

Transplantation of skin was adopted as a clinical method for wound closure soon after Reverdin's introduction of split-thickness skin grafts in 1869.[3] Girdner reported the first clinical use of allografts in 1881 by harvesting a suicide victim's skin to use for closure of a burn wound. Although a large part of the skin graft initially took, during the second and third weeks, 'erysipelatous inflammation' resulted, probably indicating rejection.[4] Similar investigations were performed simultaneously by Wolfe and Thiersch.[5,6]

In 1938, Bettman reported the successful use of allografts in two children with more than 60% TBSA burn.[7] In 1944, Webster reported that the refrigeration of autograft skin in a vaseline gauze, wrapped in a saline sponge and stored 3 weeks at 4–7°C, still resulted in a successful 'take' of the graft.[8] The routine use of allograft skin did not occur until the early 1950s when Brown and Fryer reported its use in extensive burns as a biological dressing.[9] At that time, allograft was introduced as routine therapy for burn patients at the Brooke Army Medical Center in San Antonio. In 1966, Zaroff reported his 10-year experience with the use of allografts. The benefits listed below are classic and represent the benefits of allograft use as both a physiologic and mechanical barrier:[10]

- reduction in water, electrolyte and protein loss;
- reduction in energy requirements secondary to the attainment of a closed wound;
- reduction in wound infection rates;
- reduction in pain;
- conservation of autografts; and
- improved general welfare and psychological outlook of the patient.

In 1966, Morris *et al.* reported the beneficial effects of allografts in healing infected ulcers and other heavily contaminated wounds as a 'physiologic primary closure'.[11] As a result of those reports, research into the mechanisms of wound healing began in an attempt to elucidate the reasons why allografts were superior to conventional dressings. In 1958, Eade reported reduction in the number of bacteria under biological dressings.[12] Woods *et al.* subsequently reported that phagocytes within a wound used the fibrin network established between the allograft and the wound to trap and phagocytose bacteria without the production of opsonins or antibody.[13] Further investigations by Zarem and O'Donoghue demonstrated that both fresh and preserved skin allograft stimulated neovascularization.[14] Shuck *et al.*, using the Vietnam war experience, extended the use of allografts to difficult nonburn traumatic wounds with great benefit.[15] The effects of allografts in reducing bacteria and promoting healing have proven to be beneficial.

TISSUE PRESERVATION

Clearly, an essential component in the use of allograft is the ability to store the tissue for use at a later time. In 1903, Wentscher experimented with the transplantation of a human skin graft stored in a refrigerator for from 3 to 14 days.[16] Alexis Carrel appears to have been the first investigator to address the problems surrounding storage methods and length of time for storage of human tissues.[17] Although it appears that refrigerated skin grafts were successfully employed in the early 1900s, the routine banking of human tissue was delayed until reliable refrigeration methods became available in the 1930s. The development of the first blood bank at Cook County Hospital in 1937 provided the necessary security for the development and use of banked allograft skin. In 1944, Webster and Mathews reported the successful use of banked allograft skin after 3–8 weeks of refrigeration.[8,18] In 1945, Strumia and Hodge reported the successful use of frozen allograft stored in citrated plasma at −15°C for 1–16 days.[19] Controversy was created when Baxter and Entin demonstrated that skin exposed to dry ice was killed by ice crystal formation.[20] In 1949, Polge *et al.* noted that glycerol in a saline solution allowed frozen sperm to be thawed and remain viable.[21] Several investigators subsequently documented the survival of mammalian skin in the presence of glycerol under freezing conditions.[22] In 1956, Taylor *et al.* documented that glycerol reduced ice crystal formation in tissues with freezing.[23] It was not until 1964 that Lehr *et al.* reported that freezing of rat skin in a glycerol solution led to a successful 'take' when thawed and reapplied.[24] These experimental studies were repeated by Cochrane using a controlled freezing technique with liquid nitrogen storage of rat skin autograft at −100°C in 15% glycerol. A successful 'take' of the autograft was documented after 10 days of freezing with rapid rewarming.[25] In 1968, Cochrane *et al.* reported the first successful clinical use of frozen skin autografts.[26] Subsequently, the burn units at Massachusetts General Hospital and the US Navy Skin Bank established methods for the storage of frozen skin. Although the development of various methods for tissue preservation evolved rapidly, each has specific indications and roles in a skin bank.

Hypothermia

Hypothermia involves the storage of allograft for future use in nutrient media at temperatures of 2–8°C.[27] It is believed that temperature reduction decreases oxygen consumption of viable cells secondary to a slowing of the metabolic rate. Hypothermia is intended for use only on a short-term basis, usually 5–7 days, before the integrity of the allograft is called into question. To date, however, very little information exists as to the reduction in viability of the allograft and subsequent 'take' on patients within a 2-week period. Lehr *et al.* documented the survival of rat autograft skin for 10 days after simple refrigeration.[24]

Cryopreservation

A controlled rate for freezing of allograft is essential when the preservation of cell viability is crucial. Cryopreservation accomplishes this goal by the controlled freezing of tissue, typically 0.5–5.0°C/min in a cryoprotectant solution.[28] This method is usually computer controlled with liquid nitrogen as the coolant. Storage at −196°C in liquid nitrogen is standard for long-term maintenance. May and DeClements have shown that allograft treated with a cryoprotectant and placed in liquid nitrogen will retain 85% viability for 1 year.[29]

Rewarming

There is significant evidence to support the belief that cell viability is affected by the rate at which skin is rewarmed. More specifically, rapid rewarming at a rate of 50–70°C/min is essential to maintain cell viability.[28] Thus, for cryopreserved tissue, temperature changes from −196°C to 0°C must occur in 3–4 minutes. In 1980, May and DeClements provided significant evidence to show that the flat packaging of skin allograft was 10 times more efficient in the rapid rewarming rate when compared to allograft stored in the rolled form.[30] These investigations also pointed out that flat packaging allowed more efficient storage of allograft skin, and, thereby, increased efficiency and decreased liquid nitrogen requirements.

Regional Skin Banks and Their Governance

Regional skin banks have been established throughout the United States as a means to supply the increasing need for allograft skin as well as to provide a mechanism for the donation of cadaveric skin. Most skin banks have evolved into tissue banks with the harvesting of not only skin, but also cornea, various internal organs, heart valves, veins, and bone. Currently there are 250–300 tissue banks in the United States. About 100 of these banks are eye banks only and the remainder provide bone, skin, ligaments, cartilages, tendons, and other musculoskeletal transplants.[31] It is estimated that 30–50 tissue banks procure, process, and distribute skin from cadaveric donors. Although the amount of allograft skin used annually is unknown, May *et al.* estimated 6000 square feet annually among 19 skin banks in 1983.[32] In 1984, the Skin Council of the American Association of Tissue Banks (AATB) estimated the national yearly need for allograft skin to be 32 000 square feet.[33] These tissue banks supply large numbers of allograft tissue to local, regional, and national health care facilities. Consequently, this prompted the establishment of commercial tissue processing organizations. In 1989, the National Organ Transplantation Act (PL98-507) was passed to prohibit the sale of human organs and tissues. Presently, two organizations have emerged as leaders in the field of tissue banking. The AATB and the South Eastern Organ Procurement Foundation (SEOPF) have adopted guidelines and standards for tissue banking to ensure quality control of processed human tissue.[34]

In 1984, the AATB published *Standards for Tissue Banking* to ensure that all activities related to the collection, processing, storage, and distribution of human organs and tissue for medical use are carried out in a safe and professional manner. The standards set by the Skin Council of the AATB specifically outline the necessary protocols required for the establishment of a safe and ethical skin bank. In 1986, AATB developed a program of inspection and accreditation to insure compliance with the processes of retrieval and distribution of human tissue.[35,36]

The SEOPF was founded in 1969 with a primary focus on the transplantation of internal organs, especially kidneys. The SEOPF established the Tissue Banking Committee to provide a means of networking its scarce resources. The subsequent publication of *Guidelines and Standards for Excision, Preparation, Storage and Distribution of Human Tissue Allografts for Transplantation* in 1986 established guidelines for the technical and ethical standards of procurement, storage, and distribution of tissue similar to those designed by the AATB.[36]

More recently the Food and Drug Administration (FDA) issued specific guidelines for quality control of tissue bank specimens which echo previously established guidelines set up by AATB.[37] In 1993, the FDA regulations recognized that although compliance with AATB's standards for the banking of various tissues should provide assurances of safety, the need for improved quality control in the future was apparent. Recently, the AATB has taken these major steps to upgrade its standards and, thus, to monitor compliance by accredited banks:[31]

- more rigid and precise testing requirements for potentially transmissible diseases;
- strengthening of the accreditation program by adding a trained, experienced, full-time staff;
- completion of the AATB Technical Manual to include detailed and responsible avenues for the provision of safe and effective tissue grafts.

Components of a Skin Bank

Since the development of an ability to store allograft skin, thousands of burn victims and patients with nonburn traumatic wounds have benefited. In most parts of the United States, legislation has been passed which enables hospitals to develop a mechanism whereby families of potential donors are informed of their opportunity to donate. According to the Uniform Anatomical Gift Act (UAGA), the recovery of organs and tissues from a deceased individual requires the consent of the next of kin, in order of priority, unless the deceased carries a properly signed and witnessed Uniform Donor Card. The UAGA outlines an order of priority for such a consent as follows: (1) spouse, (2) adult son or daughter, (3) either parent, (4) an adult brother or sister, (5) a guardian of the deceased other than guardian *ad litem*, and (6) any other person authorized or under obligation to dispose of the body.[31] In Philadelphia, the consent rate for requested skin donation from the 7% of acceptable donors was found to be 30%. Thus, skin donations were only obtained from 2% of all deaths screened.[38] The concept of skin donation can be difficult for relatives to understand and requires full explanations in order to alleviate fears of mutilation and disfigurement of the deceased at the time of open casket style funeral services.

Donor Referral

The establishment of a donor referral base is essential for the growth and development of a skin bank. Most hospitals have a centralized referral system for the dispersal of information related to donor procurement. This referral system may operate out of a hospital's emergency room or may be formalized into a decedant affairs department at a particular institution. In many areas, inservices are provided to these institutions by various organ procurement organizations (OPOs) which also serve to coordinate the harvesting of various organs and tissues for later use. Contracts between such OPOs and various hospitals are not uncommon. Consequently, skin banks usually are contacted by the OPO, although contracts between hospitals and skin banks do exist.

Donor Selection

The establishment of a donor referral pattern ultimately necessitates the need for a routine screening process which identifies any disease process which can eliminate a potential donor from being accepted. This is to insure that all procured skin is safe for transplantation. The suitability of any individual for tissue donation is based on medical and social history, clinical status, physical examination, and blood tests.

A general donor criteria worksheet is specifically designed to assess logistical issues such as legal consent for donation, location of the body, and time of death as well as medical history. The United States Public Health Service (USPHS) lists criteria for the exclusion of high risk donors (**Table 14.1**). The USPHS criteria for unsuitable donors include men who have had sex with men since 1977, men and women who had exchanged sex for money or drugs since 1977, past or present intravenous drug abusers, certain hemophiliacs and all sexual partners in the last 12 months of all persons in these categories. Also included are persons who in the past 12 months have had syphilis, gonorrhea or have been exposed to known or potentially HIV-infected blood.[31] To date, more than 3 000 000 tissue transplants have been carried out since the identification of AIDS. AATB records indicate that only two donors' tissues have been associated with documented transmission of the human immunodeficiency virus.[31] Once the basic criteria are met, skin-specific criteria are then utilized to complete the screening process. Potential donors should be between 14 and 75 years of age; however, potential donors above or below this range should be evaluated for size, skin conditions, and state of health. Skin donor specific criteria include the absence of collagen vascular diseases, skin infections, acute burns, dermatitis, toxic exposure to chemicals, tatoos within 3 months or excessive skin trauma, obesity, or malnourishment.

Table 14.1 AATB guidelines for donor exclusion (revised November 1993)

Infection or sepsis by history, physical examination and laboratory testing
History of intravenous drug use
History of neoplasm
History of hepatitis, syphilis, slow virus infection, AIDS, AIDS related complex or high risk of AIDS
History of autoimmune diseases
Positive serologic tests
Toxic substance in potentially toxic amounts in tissues to be collected
Evidence of serious illness of unknown cause
Death from unknown cause

Skin Removal, Processing, and Cryopreservation

The recovery of skin from cadaveric donors is only instituted once donor selection, screening, and proper consent forms have been completed. All necessary arrangements for the time and location of the procurement are made by contacting the appropriate personnel and the procurement site. The tissue bank coordinator usually arranges for a procurement team to perform the recovery. The timing for the retrieval of skin should insure tissue quality and avoid delay of funeral services. Skin from cadaveric donors should be retrieved within 12 hours following the time of death if the donor is unrefrigerated and within 24 hours if the donor is refrigerated. No procedures are utilized which may interfere with investigations of a coroner or medical examiner. All donor skin is procured in an aseptic manner.

The initiation of the skin procurement process begins with an assessment of the donor. This is performed with gloves and protective garb. The body is properly identified and the overall appearance and condition of the body is observed as part of the final step in donor screening. Visual inspection of the skin is completed, and bruises, lacerations, abrasions, tattoos, dermatitis, acne, other skin lesions, or unusual marks are documented. The coordinator then makes a final decision to accept or decline the donation. If the donor is rejected, all of the appropriate personnel are notified. If the donor is accepted, the procedure table is cleansed with alcohol and the body placed onto the table, with the arms positioned such that they do not interface with draping or procurement. A head block is used to elevate the head so as to prevent or decrease periorbital swelling or bleeding. A puncture site is prepped with alcohol and at least 40 ml of blood are obtained from the donor. The femoral vein is the preferred site. The tubes are labeled by a unique donor number, placed in a biohazard zip-lock bag, and packed into an ice cooler.

In order to obtain usable skin donations, a donor must be prepared and the procedure must be carefully followed. The donor's hair is covered with a bouffant head cover and the body rinsed with tap water to remove any debris. Using clean washcloths or lap sponges, the donor is given a chlorhexidine bath and all hair is shaved from the nipple line down to the feet and from one side to the other side down the front of the body. The back is shaved from the shoulders to the feet. All hair and chlorhexidine are rinsed from the body and the table with clean water. The body is then prepped with iodophor from the shoulders on the back, down the trunk and continuing along both legs to the toes. The iodophor is then rinsed with alcohol, in a unidirectional manner and in a caudal direction. The procurement team then washes and dons sterile attire; and the donor is draped in a sterile fashion. The procurement team requires a 'circulator' and one or two 'scrub' technicians. Prior to the removal of skin, each area is moistened with saline sterile dermatome set at 0.010 inches and proper thickness of the skin strip is assessed. The depth gauge is then adjusted as needed. The depth of the cut is continually assessed throughout the procedure as different parts of the body require different settings.

After completely harvesting the skin from one side of the body, all skin strips are rinsed with sterile saline and placed in sterile jars with sterile RPML-1640 media for every 300 ml of skin. The jars are then placed into a cooler. The body is turned over; and the process is repeated. Clean-up includes: the discarding of all used, disposable items, washing of all instruments and donor with clean water, replacement of identification tags, and coverage of the body. Further duties include: completion of on-site retrieval documentation; cleaning of the tables, counters, cabinets, sinks, and floors; removal and proper disposal of all gowns, caps, masks, gloves, shoe covers, etc.; and finally, notification of the facility personnel that the procedure has been completed. Once the procurement team arrives at the skin bank, donor check-in procedures are essential in order to insure proper preservation of skin allograft and disposition of paperwork, serology, and culture laboratory tests. Serum of each donor is tested for anti-HIV-1/2, anti-HCV, anti-HTLV-1, HB_sAg, anti-HB_c and RPR. Under sterile conditions, skin samples are aseptically collected and tested for aerobic and anaerobic bacteria as well as yeast and fungi. Skin and blood samples are then stored in a separate refrigerator for 'UNPROCESSED – NOT CLEAR' tissues. The donor is entered into the donor log and assigned the next consecutive number. Once microbiology surveys and serology tests have cleared, allograft skin is processed and packaged according to AATB Standards and Technical Manual Guidelines.

Tissues are processed and packaged individually so that there is no chance of cross-contamination between donors. Usually, two technicians verify that only one donor is being processed. Only skin from donors with negative serologies and microbiology is processed. Processing is carried out under sterile conditions in a biological safety cabinet. Tissue edges are trimmed and blocked according to preestablished standards in equal measurements of 0.25 sq. ft. If skin is to be meshed, the prepared skin (dermal side down) is placed on 4 inch wide gauze which extends 2 inches beyond each skin edge and folded. Skin must be frozen within 72 hours of procurement using a control rate freezer.

Future Considerations

Skin banking in the United States is in a state of flux. The FDA has issued regulations to strengthen federal oversight of tissue transplantation. The participation of AATB in the congressional considerations of new legislation is crucial. While it is apparent that the FDA requirements will build on AATB standards, AATB continues to strive in upgrading its own standards and requirements for tissue distribution.

Although all major tissue banks are either AATB accredited or pursuing accreditation to date, no program is in place to mandate compulsory registration of tissue banks, nor compliance with accepted donor screening criteria, procurement procedures, or processing methods for that tissue. In addition, the ability to track the distribution of tissue from donor to recipient must form an integral part of any system designed to regulate tissue banking. Uniform inspection procedures and scheduled recertification of tissue banks should address quality assurance issues. Presently, the AATB estimates that 90% skin grafts distributed in the USA last year were produced by AATB accredited banks. However, it appears that only through mandated legislation at a national level will this compliance reach 100%.

References

1. Baxter C R, Marvin J A, Curreri P W. Early management of thermal burns. *Postgrad Med* 1974; **55:** 131.

2. Tier W C, Sell K W. United States Navy skin bank. *Plast Reconstr Surg* 1968; **41:** 543–8.

3. Reverdin J L. *Greffe Epidermique*. Bull de la Sol Imperiale de Chir de Paris. 1869; 493–511.

4. Girdner J H. Skin grafting with grafts from a dead subject. *Med Record NY* 1888; **20:** 119–20.

5. Wolf J R. A new method of performing plastic operation. *BMJ* 1875; **2:** 360–5.

6. Thiersch J C. On skin grafting. *Verhandl 2nd Deutsch Ges Chir* 1886; **15:** 17–20.

7. Bettman A G. Homogenous thiersch grafting as a life saving measure. *Am J Surg* 1938; **39:** 156–62.

8. Webster J P. Refrigerated skin grafts. *Ann Surg* 1944; **120:** 431–49.

9. Brown J B, Fryer M P, Randall P, Lu M. Post mortem homografts as 'biological dressings' for extensive burns and debrided areas. *Ann Surg* 1953; **138:** 618–23.

10. Zaroff L I, Mills W, Duckett J W, Switzer W E, Moncrief J A. *Surgery* 1966; **59:** 368–72.

11. Morris P J, Bondac C, Burke J F. The use of frequently changed skin allografts to promote healing in the non-healing infected ulcer. *Surgery 1966;* **60:** 13–19.

12. Eade G G. The relationship between granulation tissue, bacteria and skin grafts in burn patients. *Plast Reconstr Surg* 1958; **22:** 42–55.

13. Woods W B. Phagocytosis with particular reference to encapsulated bacteria. *Bact Rev* 1960; **224:** 41.

14. O'Donaghue M N, Zarem H A. Stimulation of neurovascularization. Comparative efficacy of fresh and preserved skin grafts in burn patients. *Plast Reconstr Surg* 1958; **22:** 42–55.

15. Shuck J M, Pruitt B A, Moncrief J A. Homograft skin for wound coverage. *Arch Surg* 1969; **98:** 472–8.

16. Perry V P. A review of skin preservation cryobiology. 1966; **3**(2): 109–30.

17. Carrel A. The preservation of tissues and its application to surgery. *JAMA* 1912; **59:** 523–7.

18. Mathews D. Storage of skin for autogenous grafts. *Lancet* 1945; **1:** 775.

19. Strumia M M, Hodge C C. Frozen human skin grafts. *Ann Surg* 1945; **121:** 860–5.

20. Baxter H, Entin M E. Experimental and clinical studies of reduced temperatures in injury and repair in man. III. Direct effect of cooling and freezing on various elements of the human skin. *Plast Reconstr Surg* 1948; **3:** 303–34.

21. Polge C, Smith V A, Parkes A S. Revival of spermatozoa after UV factors and dehydration at low temperatures. *Nature* 1949; **164:** 66.

22. Billingham R E, Medawer P B. The freezing, drying and storage of mammalian skin. *J Exp Biol* 1952; **29:** 454–68.

23. Taylor A C. Survival of rat skin and changes in hair pigmentation following freezing. *J Exp Zool* 1949; **110:** 77–112.

24. Lehr H B, Berggren R B, Lotke P A, Coriell L L. Permanent survival of preserved skin autograft. *Surgery* 1964; **56**(4): 742–96.

25. Bondac C C, Burke J F. Clinical experience with viable frozen human skin and a frozen skin bank. *Ann Surg* 1971; **174**(3): 371–82.

26. Cochrane E T. The low temperature storage of skin. A preliminary report. *Br J Plast Surg* 1966; 118–25.

27. Southard J H, Belzer F O. *Organ Preservation: Principles of Organ Transplantation*. Philadelphia: WB Saunders, 1989; **10:** 195.

28. American Association of Tissue Banks. *Technical Manual for Tissue Banking*. Arlington, VA: AATB, 1987.

29. May S R, DeClement F A. Skin Banking. Part II. Low contamination cadaveric dermal allograft for temporary burn wound coverage. *J Burn Care Rehabil* 1981; **1:** 64–76.

30. May S R, DeClement F A. Skin banking methodology. An evaluation of packaging format, cooling and warming rates and storage efficiency. *Cryobiology* 1980; **17:** 33–45.

31. American Association of Tissue Banks. *Information Alert*. Arlington, VA: AATB, 1993; **3**(6): 1–8.

32. May S R, Still J M, Atkinson W B. Recent developments in skin banking in the clinical uses of cryopreserved skin. *Med Assoc Ga* 1984; **73:** 233–57.

33. Standards Committee of the Skin Council of the American Association of Tissue Banks. Guidelines for the banking of skin tissues. *Am Assoc Tissue Banks Newsletter* 1979; **3:** 5–8.

34. Leslie H W, Bottenfeid S. Donation banking and transplantation of allograft tissues. *Nurs Clin ANM* 1989; **24**(4): 891–905.

35. American Association of Tissue Banks. *Standards for Tissue Banking*. Arlington, Virginia: AATB, 1984.

36. Southeastern Organ Procurement Foundation. *Guidelines and Standards for Excision, Preparation, Storage and Distribution of Human Tissue Allografts for Transplantation*. Richmond, VA: SEOPF, 1988.

37. Real E S and Regulations. *Federal Register* 1993; **58:** 238, 65514–521.

38. May S R, Declements F A. Skin Banking. Part 1. Procurement of transplantable cadaveric allograft for burn wound coverage. *J Burn Care Rehabil* 1981; **2:** 7–23.

CHAPTER FIFTEEN 15

Alternative Wound Coverings

Ronald G. Tompkins and John F. Burke

Serious short-term and long-term problems occur when the epidermal and dermal layers of the skin are destroyed. The short-term problems, which can be life-threatening, include the escape of essential body fluids from the deeper layers of the skin and the invasion of bacteria and other microbes (**Table 15.1**). It is the epidermis, consisting of keratinocytes attached to an underlying basement membrane, which normally provides these very important functions. In serious injuries, these epidermal functions must be replaced very soon after injury by physiologically acceptable wound closures. On the other hand, it is the dermal layer of skin which supports the durable and pliable nature of skin which is so vital to proper skin function and cosmesis in the longer term. Very serious long-term problems with cosmesis and function become important when dermis has been destroyed and not properly replaced. Therefore, dermal function is extremely important in the design of any materials which are intended to permanently replace skin.

When available, the replacement material of choice is the patient's own (autologous) skin as shown in an algorithm describing the decision process to treat acute burns (**Figure 15.1**). In smaller injuries, this can be accomplished by skin grafts without meshing; however, in larger injuries, meshed autologous skin grafts are required. In general, meshed skin grafts should be avoided because of the expected mesh pattern of the scar which comes from the disordered dermal replacement within the interstices of the mesh. Meshing often can be avoided in most injuries which involve less than 30% of the body surface area and in those wounds which do not contain excessive colonization by bacteria and other microbes.

In massive burn injuries with very limited donor skin, both the short-term and long-term problems of skin loss must be solved by alternative wound closure materials. Alternative materials can be used for either wound coverage which will be temporary or for permanent wound closure. Currently, allogenic (cadaver) skin is the most commonly used alternative wound closure material. Many studies are underway, however, to develop materials that would be promptly available as off-the-shelf materials which would substitute for the allografts to provide permanent wound closure. There is increased interest recently to use off-the-shelf alternatives because of the potential risk for viral transmission (e.g. hepatitis, HIV) by the allografts.

Wound *coverage* should be distinguished from wound *closure* (**Table 15.2**). Wound closure materials are biologically accepted by

Table 15.1 Selected functions provided by epidermis and dermis after burn injury

	Short term	Long term
Epidermis	Prevents moisture loss	Prevents moisture loss
	Prevents bacterial, viral, and fungal invasion	Prevents bacterial, viral, and fungal invasion
		Provides pigmentation
Dermis	–	Supports mechanical integrity
	–	Provides cosmetic quality
	–	Provides dermal appendages and nerve complexes

The colour plates for this chapter appear between pp 264 and 265.

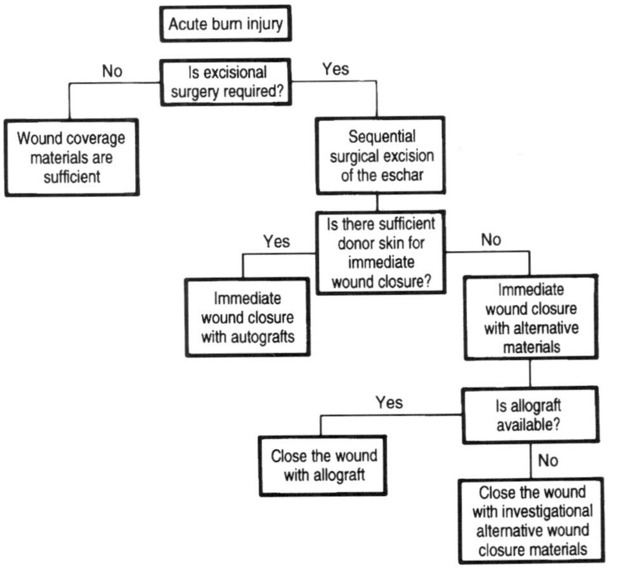

Fig. 15.1. Schematic indicating the role of alternative wound closure materials in the care of acutely burned patients.

Table 15.2 Contrasts of wound coverage vs closure

	Wound coverage	Wound closure
Biologically acceptable to the wound bed	Temporary	Permanently
Incorporates into the healing wound	No†	Yes
Prevents formation of granulation tissue	No	Yes
Biodegrades	No	Yes
Useful in superficial wounds‡	Yes	±
Undergoes transepithelial elimination*	Yes	No

† Incorporates into the wound coagulum and granulation tissue.
‡ Wounds expected to completely heal within 3 weeks.
* The new epidermis migrates beneath the foreign material and eliminates it.

Table 15.3. Design criteria for wound closure materials

Nontoxic, antiseptic, noninflammatory, and nonantigenic barrier to bacteria and other microbes
Normal rates of water and heat conductivity
Immediate, uniform, and intimate adherence to the wound bed
Support for normal local host defense and wound repair mechanisms
Elasticity and long-term durability
Growth potential which is comparable to the patient's own potential in the long term
Long-term mechanical and cosmetic function with wound contracture properties that are comparable to split thickness autografts

the wound bed and become permanently incorporated into the healing wound. On the other hand, wound coverage materials rely upon incorporation into the wound coagulum and ingrowth of granulation tissues for adhesion; this phenomenon is characteristic of many wound coverage materials. These materials in general do not biodegrade and therefore they can only be temporary substitutes and must be replaced with the patient's skin either by reepithelialization or skin grafts. In the case of temporary coverage, the wound should not be colonized with bacteria and it should be sufficiently superficial that it is expected to heal completely within 3 weeks. Epithelial cells from the epidermal appendages grow and replace the destroyed epidermis and gradually the wound coverage material is shed. Therefore, the primary goals for the wound coverage materials in superficial second degree wounds are:

- to limit the microbial invasion of the wound bed (microbial barrier) and thereby to prevent infection;
- to limit the access of air and thereby to minimize pain.

Wound coverage materials have been used temporarily for deep second degree or third degree injuries prior to definitive wound closure with autologous skin in patients with massive burn injuries. Unfortunately, this strategy frequently fails because underlying devitalized burn tissues routinely lead to contained infections when used with these deeper burn injuries. Examples of wound coverage materials include Tegaderm, Biobrane, and porcine skin xenografts.

The best biological approach to alternative wound closure materials that are permanent takes advantage of the host's own cellular and structural recycling processes that are available to all normal tissues. In order that these criteria are met by nonbiological materials, the wound closure materials must biologically interact cooperatively with the host's cellular systems of the wound. They should not remain inert and nonreactive which is characteristic of wound coverage materials.

In distinction to wound coverage material, multiple design properties or requirements should be fulfilled for wound closure materials to successfully mimic normal dermis and epidermis (**Table 15.3**). The material should be composed of materials which do not generate an immune or inflammatory reaction by the host. The material when it degrades cannot release toxic components and it cannot sensitize the host to its antigens or related ones. The material cannot introduce new bacteria, viruses, or fungi into the wound and should actually assist as a barrier to invasion of the wound flora. In major injuries, the wound closure material must assist as an insulator to correct the massive heat and water losses associated with major epidermal damage. The material must immediately and intimately adhere to each and every aspect of the wound to avoid any significant pockets of fluid that can harbor a contained infection. This uniform and intimate adherence facilitates a seamless interface, allowing the normal healing elements to be incorporated into the material, and avoids the development of granulation tissue. The material must be elastic to conform to curvatures, must be durable, and it must have potential to allow growth of the patient.

Three general strategies for alternative wound closure materials have been developed based upon matrix structure and cellular content (**Figure 15.2**). The first strategy uses a noncellular matrix material to mimic the three-dimensional structure and character of dermis and a silastic covering membrane to mimic the physical properties of epidermis. The second strategy uses a combination of matrix and cell culture techniques to create a composite graft material. The third strategy uses an epidermal cell culture method which is intended to replace the epidermis alone. The strategies with noncellular matrix and matrix together with cells both address the problem of dermal replacement whereas the cultured keratinocyte approach is limited to the epidermal component of the soft tissue loss only.

With regard to construction of a dermal matrix device, the first and most extensively evaluated approach clinically was taken by Burke and Yannas[1,2] with the construction of a bilayer, polymeric membrane comprising an upper layer of medical grade silastic (epidermal layer) and a lower layer of highly porous cross-linked collagen and chondroitin 6-sulfate (dermal layer). One example of a composite device is an approach described by Boyce and Hansbrough, and Hansbrough *et al.*[3,4] which is a modification of the collagen–chondroitin 6-sulfate matrix of Burke and Yannas. This composite is a nonporous surface of collagen and glycosaminoglycan which is laminated to the upper layer of the dermal membrane to provide a nonporous and planar surface. The nonporous surface is seeded with cultured, proliferating autologous epidermal cells and the porous dermal collagen–chondroitin 6-sulfate matrix is seeded with proliferating autologous (or potentially allogenic) fibroblasts. The most extensively utilized example of the third strategy involves the culture of the patient's own epidermal cells using methods described by Green *et al.*[5,6]

Dermal Matrix Strategy

The most extensive, prospective, and controlled clinical experience[7] with wound closure materials that are permanent has been

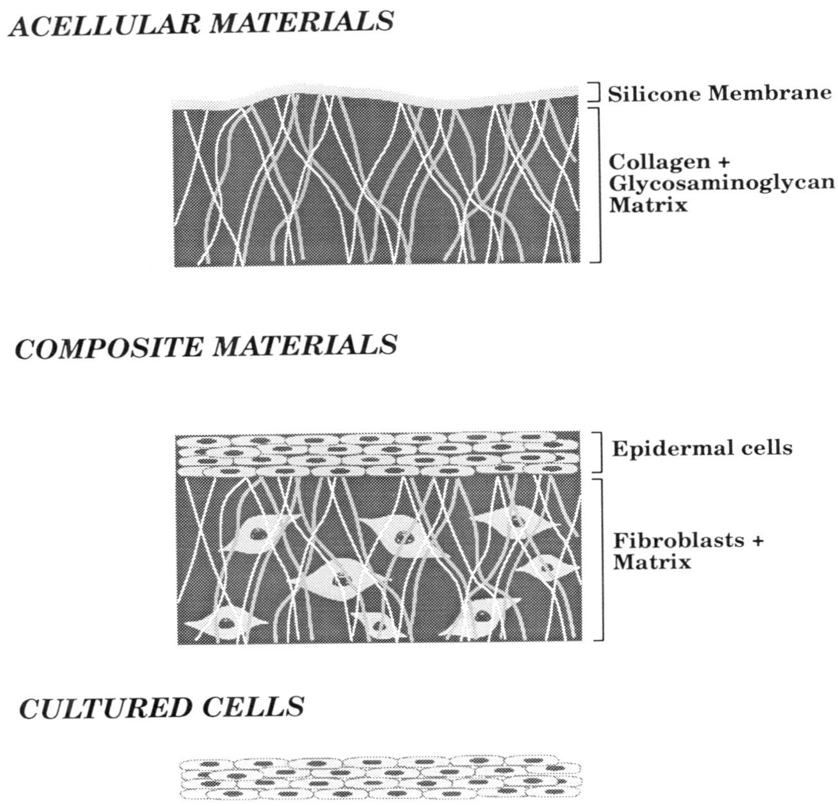

Fig. 15.2. Schematic drawing describing three strategies for alternative wound closure materials.

with the artificial dermis (Integra) that was designed by Yannas and Burke.[8–10] Integra is a totally artificial device which is acellular and is composed of two layers (**Figure 15.3**). The upper layer of silastic has a porosity sufficient to control water loss and to prevent the invasion of microbes. The rate of water vapor loss allowed by the silastic is approximately 5 $mg/cm^2/h$. The lower, highly porous layer is a cross-linked coprecipitate of collagen that is bovine in origin and chondroitin 6-sulfate that comes from shark cartilage. This approach, which does not contain living cells, examines an hypothesis that host cells (endothelial cells and fibroblasts) are abundant in the wound bed and that additional allogenic cells provided by an artificial dermis are unnecessary.

An extremely important design consideration of the material is the creation of an optimal effective pore size (20–125 μm) of the lower dermal layer.[8–10] After extensive study, it was discovered that an optimal pore size allows the migration of the patient's own endothelial cells and fibroblasts into the matrix. A smaller average pore size impairs cellular migration into the matrix, prolongs the apparent interface between the material and the wound bed, and delays or prevents the incorporation of the host's matrix into the wound closure material. Pores that are too large provide insufficient attachment surface area for the invading cells of the host. These host cells provide vascularization and the eventual replacement of the artificial matrix with a new dermal structure or the 'neodermis'. The neodermis is a flat, pink dermis-like surface. Granulation tissue should form only in areas where the wound closure material fails to take properly.

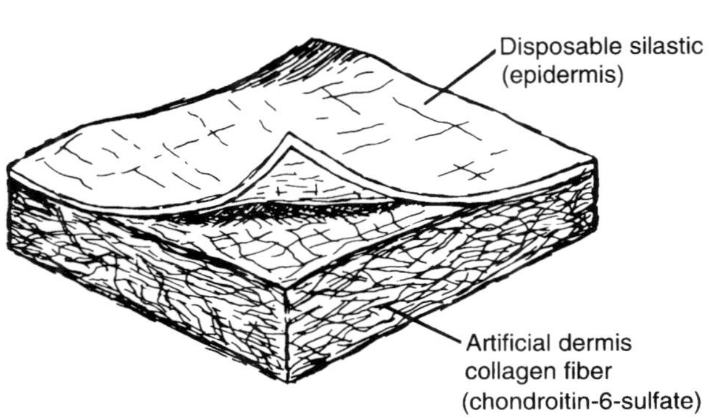

Fig. 15.3. Schematic drawing describing Integra which is composed of a 'dermal' layer and an 'epidermal' layer. (From reference 7, with permission.)

Once the burned tissue has been excised the acellular artificial skin is sutured in place using techniques analogous to those used with autografts (**Figure 15.4**). Once the entire lower layer of the Integra has been populated by host cells, the silastic layer can be removed to provide an excellent vascularized 'neodermal' base. A freshly harvested thin (0.002–0.004 inch) epidermal graft can be used to seed the neodermis with autologous epidermal cells. Since the dermis is provided by the Integra, the dermal portion of the usual split-thickness skin graft need not be included. This neodermal bed could also serve as an excellent surface for cultured epidermal cells and potentially would avoid the creation of a split-thickness donor site although ultra-thin donor sites of approximately 0.003 inch depth are well tolerated. Unfortunately, in massive burns even ultra-thin donor skin is unavailable.

Initial clinical experience with Integra in burn injuries was reported in 10 patients from the Boston Unit of the Shriners Burns Institute and the Sumner Redstone Burn Unit of the Massachusetts General Hospital in 1981[2] and later, long-term results of a total of 21 adult patients at the Massachusetts General Hospital were reported in 1989.[11] In this latter study, a survival benefit with the use of Integra was suggested by an adjusted odds of dying of 0.52 (half the odds of dying as those patients not treated with Integra). As can be appreciated in this later study, the use of Integra had been limited to massive burn injuries (≥ 70% body surface area) in adults whose determinants for survival depend upon many independent parameters in addition to the use of Integra. From this later study, it was estimated that 160 adult massively burned patients would be

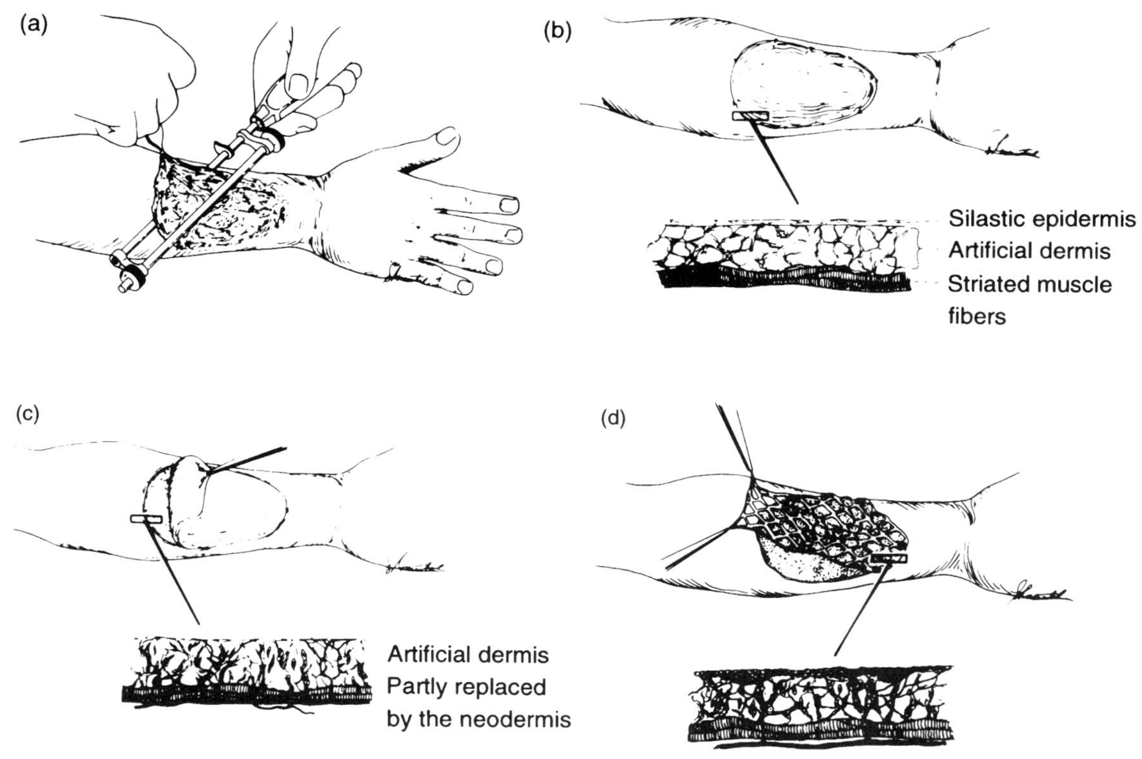

Fig. 15.4. Schematic indicating the clinical application of Integra together with an representation of the host cellular response to Integra. (a) tangential excision of eschar; (b) placement of Integra onto the wound bed; (c) removal of silastic layer; (d) placement of ultrathin epidermal graft. (From reference 2, with permission.)

necessary to demonstrate any potential statistical significance of a survival benefit.

In a report of an 11-center prospectively randomized trial,[7] Integra was used in 149 patients with final long-term evaluations in 82 patients. The 'take' of the Integra was a very acceptable 80% as compared to 95% for meshed autograft. In these patients, donor sites healed an average of 4 days sooner because they were harvested more superficially at an average of 0.006 inch (0.15 mm) as compared to the usual depth of 0.013 inch (0.33 mm) which is commonly used for split-thickness donor skin. At the completion of the study, there was less hypertrophic scarring of the Integra and more patients preferred the areas covered with Integra to the control areas with meshed autograft. The main conclusion of this multicenter trial was that Integra provided a permanent cover that was at least as satisfactory as currently available skin grafting techniques and it allowed donor grafts that were thinner and donor sites that healed more rapidly. Significant technical problems including wrinkles, hematomas, and infections occurred, however, but these problems could be avoided substantially by meshing the Integra in a fashion similar to meshing of autografts.

Long-term evaluation of patients who were engrafted with this material at the Massachusetts General Hospital and the Boston Unit of the Shriners Burns Institute between 1979 and 1990 has recently been reported.[12] Integra became available in September 1979 and has been used in 195 applications in 121 patients. There were 87 patients who survived at least 4 months, mean follow-up of 5.45 years (0.3–10.7 years). The average age was 44 years (range 2–90 years); average burn size was 55% TBSA with 42% TBSA full-thickness. Inhalation injury was present in 63% of the patients. The engraftment rate was 80% overall and 87% in a subgroup which evaluated anatomical site of engraftment. As with other skin graft materials, the posterior arms, shoulder, thigh, back, axilla, groin, and buttock were more difficult to insure engraftment. Hypertrophic scars were absent or minimal in 93% and were moderate in the remaining 7% of the patients. According to the opinions of the patients, although none of the patients felt that Integra appeared identical to normal, 78% felt that it felt and functioned like normal skin and 84% felt that its cosmetic appearance was superior to meshed autograft (**Plate 9**). There was no late contracture formation; it grew normally with the children; and it demonstrated normal healing with minor wounds and normal antibacterial defenses.

The Integra technology has been licensed by Integra Lifesciences Corp. (Plainsboro, NJ). Further clinical studies have not been possible since 1990 because it is not currently available commercially for human usage. It remains under review by the Federal Drug Administration. Additional investigations in animals using this dermal matrix together with the centrifugation of a dermal epidermal cell suspension into the junction between the silastic and dermal matrix (stage II) has resulted in significant improvements in regeneration of the dermis.[13]

Another strategy for dermal matrix replacement has been taken by Lifecell Corp. (The Woodlands, TX) using Alloderm. In this approach, allogenic skin is cryopreserved and dehydrated. This process appears to lethally damage the cells contained within the allograft while maintaining the extracellular matrix structure. The latter structure serves as a template for the host cells that migrate from the wound bed to form a new dermis. Alloderm is currently being evaluated as an allodermal material.

Composite Materials Strategy

One of the earliest reports with a composite material involved transplantation of allograft. After successful 'take' of the allograft, the allogenic epidermal cells were removed and replaced by 'suction blister' autologous keratinocytes.[14] This report stimulated multiple investigators to develop composite materials which include the following methods:

- Transplantation of allograft skin combined with cultured autologous epidermal cells.[15–18]
- Transplantation of gelled collagen seeded with cultured epidermal cells and fibroblasts.[19,20]
- Construction of a modified collagen–GAG matrix with cultured epidermal cells and fibroblasts.[3,4,21]
- Construction of a dermal matrix from fibroblasts on a surgical mesh.[22,23]

The initial experience was rapidly followed by Cuono *et al.*[15,16,18] using cultured autologous keratinocytes and allograft. One advantage of this approach is that the allograft provides wound closure while allowing sufficient time for proliferation of the autologous epidermal cells *in vitro* (~ 3–4 weeks). In this system, presumably the host's own fibroblasts and endothelial cells migrate into the allograft dermal matrix and, by a process of creeping replacement, repopulate the allogenic dermis by autologous tissues. Presumably the donor's dermal cells do not initiate either an immune or inflammatory response.

Another composite approach has been described by Bell *et al.*[20] which is a 'living skin equivalent' (LSE) as shown in **Plate 10**. LSE consists of two layers, the lower layer or dermal equivalent, and the upper layer or epidermis.[20] Both tissue layers in the LSE are made of human allogenic cells derived from neonatal foreskin. The dermal equivalent is composed of bovine collagen and human fibroblasts which are combined before gellation. The dermal equivalent receives an overlay of human epidermal cells to form a stratified, cornified layer of epidermal cells at the air–liquid interface. Properties of the LSE have been investigated in multiple *in vitro* and animal studies. The composite material or Graftskin is being manufactured and tested in a multicenter clinical trial by Organogenesis Inc. (Canton, MA).

As previously mentioned, in 1988 Boyce *et al.*[3] described a modification of the collagen–chondroitin 6-sulfate dermal matrix material described by Yannas and Burke in which a nonporous surface was created on the superficial layer of the dermal matrix with the silastic layer omitted. In this system, autologous fibroblasts were seeded into the dermal portion of the graft and the patient's own epidermal cells were placed upon the nonporous surface. In four patients, Hansbrough *et al.*[4] demonstrated partial success of this composite when applied to limited areas of full-thickness wounds. The 'take' was acceptable with formation of a basement membrane within 9 days of transplantation. In animal studies, the basic collagen–chondroitin 6-sulfate matrix has been further modified to include peptide growth factors[24] and matrix peptides containing the arginine–glycine–aspartic acid (RDG) sequence considered to be required for cell attachment to multiple extracellular matrix molecules.[25]

Composite grafts consisting of collagen–GAG substrates populated with cultured dermal fibroblasts and epidermal keratinocytes were tested by Boyce *et al.* in a pilot study on full-thickness burn wounds of three patients as an alternative to split-thickness skin.[21] Light microscopy and transmission electron microscopy showed regeneration of epidermal and dermal tissue by 2 weeks. Degradation of the collagen–GAG implant was associated with low numbers of leukocytes and new collagen deposition by fibroblasts was seen. Complete basement membrane including anchoring fibrils and anchoring plaques was mature by 3 months and accounted for the absence of blistering of healed epidermis. This cultured skin analog provided an experimental alternative to split-thickness skin graft and developed normal skin anatomy and antigen expression after wound closure.

More recently, another approach for an artificial dermal matrix has been taken in which human fibroblasts are grown on surgical mesh materials as shown in **Figure 15.5**.[22,23] In athymic mice studies[22] a living dermal replacement composed of either polyglycolic acid (PGA) or polyglactin-910 (PGL) mesh containing confluent, cultured human fibroblasts was applied to full-thickness wounds. Expanded mesh human split-thickness skin grafts were placed over the artificial dermal matrix graft. The artificial dermal matrix was intended to provide a dermis for the interstices of the meshed skin. Histologic examination of wounds during a 99-day period after graft placement showed that PGA/PGL-fibroblast grafts vascularized to the wound and the meshed split-thickness skin grafts simultaneously vascularized to the PGA/PGL-fibroblast graft. Epithelialization from the meshed graft bridges proceeded rapidly across the surface of the PGA/PGL-fibroblast grafts. This resulted in an epithelialized layer that covered a densely cellular substratum that resembled dermis. Basement membrane formation at the dermal–epidermal junction of the epithelialized interstices was seen and minimal inflammatory reaction to the PGA/PGL-fibroblast grafts was noted.

In a controlled clinical study[22] with this approach, Hansbrough *et al.* evaluated Dermagraft (Advanced Tissue Sciences, La Jolla, CA), which is composed of human neonatal fibroblasts grown on a PGA Vicryl mesh (Ethicon Inc., Somerville, NJ). The study tested the ability of Dermagraft to function as a dermal replacement when placed beneath meshed, expanded split-thickness skin grafts. Full-thickness burn wounds in 17 patients with burns (mean age, 31 years; range 6–69 years; mean burn size, 23.8% total body surface area) were excised to subcutaneous fat (nine patients), to fascia (three patients), or to a combination of deep dermis and fat (five

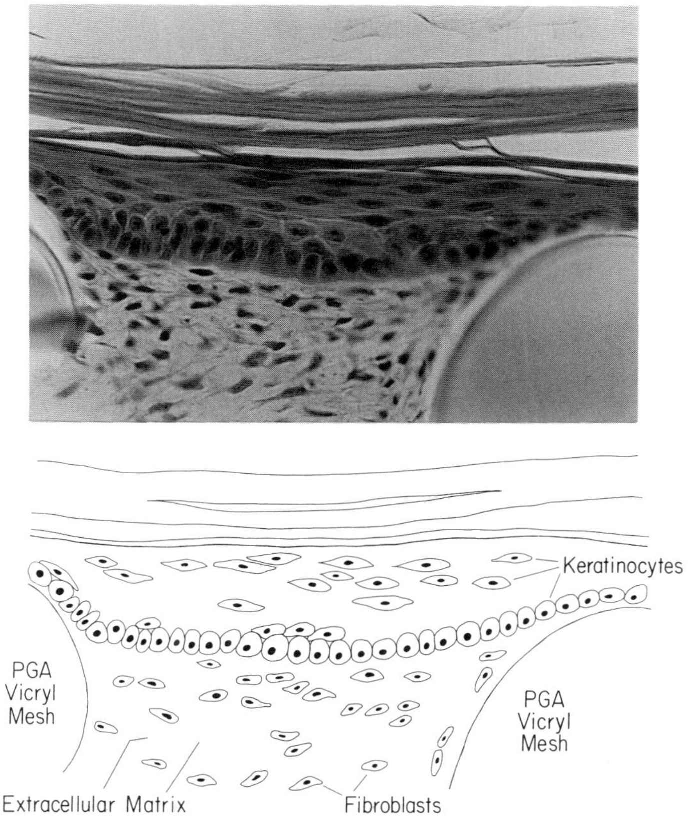

Fig. 15.5. Schematic and photomicrograph of Dermagraft-TC which is composed of human neonatal fibroblasts grown on a polyglycolic acid (Vicryl) mesh with an overlay of allogenic human epidermal cells. In the clinical trials using Dermagraft, Dermagraft has not included the epidermal cell layer. Provided by Advanced Tissue Sciences, Inc.

patients). The results showed that 'take' of skin grafts on control sites was slightly better than take on the Dermagraft; however, the differences were not statistically significant. Mesh interstices epithelialized over the surface of the full-thickness wound in a fashion comparable to the surface of Dermagraft. No evidence of rejection of the allogenic fibroblasts and minimal inflammatory reaction to the Vicryl fibers were seen. The Vicryl was hydrolyzed within the wound over 2–4 weeks although expulsion of the fibers was noted as the healing epithelium advanced to close the interstices. Further clinical trials with Dermagraft are planned.

Cultured Epidermal Cell Strategy

Autologous Cells

Technology to culture the cellular components of skin has been available for fibroblasts and endothelial cells for many years; however, methods to culture epidermal cells were improved by Rheinwald and Green[5] to serially cultivate human epidermal skin cells using a supporting feeder layer of lethally irradiated cells. Further modifications[26] have been sufficient to allow their use in human applications. This serial cultivation technique has allowed the use of the patient's own keratinocytes to assist in the timely closure of their soft tissue wounds. The technique requires a full-thickness skin biopsy consisting of a few square centimeters. After an *in vitro* culture period of 3–4 weeks, the autologous population of keratinocytes has expanded to approximately 1 m^2 of keratinocytes that are available for wound coverage. Investigators have expressed concern with the potential for antigenic cross-reactivity from the persistence of fetal bovine serum proteins which accompany the transplantation of the cultured human autologous epidermal cells.[27,28]

Following the commercialization of this culture method, enthusiastic usage of cultured autologous epidermis (CAE) has taken place. In 1981, the first case report which demonstrated the use of these cells in two patients was published in the *Lancet* by O'Conner *et al.*[29] In 1983–84, this cultured cell method, in addition to other artificial skin technologies, was used in the successful treatment of two patients with massive burn injuries at the Shriners Burns Institute in Boston.[6] Subsequently this cell culture based approach has been evaluated in a wide range of burn centers in North America, Europe, Asia, and Australia.[29–36] The Italian experience was recently reviewed in *Burns*.[37–39]

The largest experience with this approach was recently reported by Rue *et al.* from the US Army Institute of Surgical Research.[40] In their study of 16 patients with an average of 68% TBSA injury, 22 applications of CAEs were used to cover an average of 16% of the patient's body surface area. At the time of the patient's discharge, an average of 4.7% TBSA had been successfully closed using the CAEs. Approximately 64% of the CAEs successfully engrafted initially but this declined to 47% during hospitalization, suggesting a 'delayed' loss of graft. Unfortunately, the patients who might benefit most from this approach showed a lower likelihood of success (**Table 15.4**). In addition to these issues, the cost for these cells in this study when purchased from a private laboratory in the United States ranged from $2000 to $34 000 for each percentage of definitive wound closure at the time of patient discharge.

With wider usage of this new technology, weaknesses in this skin replacement approach have become evident.[41] Although early success of coverage may occur, the cultured autografts can blister and slough. These changes have been associated with elevated levels of inflammatory mediators including prostaglandin E_2 and thromboxane in the blister fluid, suggesting that an ongoing inflammatory process is present.[42]

Table 15.4 Extensively burned patients treated with cultured epidermal autografts – data analysis with respect to patient burn size

	<70% TBSA ($n = 6$)	>70% TBSA ($n = 10$)
Mean age (years)	31.0 ± 5.2 (18–48)	29.0 ± 4.1 (10–56)
Mean burn size (%)	53.5 ± 3.7 (42–64)	77.1 ± 1.4* (70–85)
Mean BSA application (%)	6.6 ± 0.8 (4.0–8.8)	21.5 ± 4.9† (7.4–59–2)
Mean % engraftment		
Initial	72.0 ± 5.5 (10–85)	59.8 ± 7.8 (50–87)
Final	73.5 ± 6.0 (50–88)	30.6 ± 11.1 (0–85)‡
Mean BSA definitive coverage (%)	4.8 ± 0.7 (2.8–7.8)	4.6 ± 1.9 (0–18.6)
Mean patient cost	$16 100 ± $1742 ($9800–$21 350)	$60 270 ± $14 256† ($12 250–$161 000)

* $p < 0.001$; † $p < 0.05$; ‡ $p < 0.001$; ranges given in parentheses; taken from reference 40, with permission.

The shortcomings of the cultured epidermal cell approach for clinical applications have been recognized (**Table 15.5**). Unfortunately the 3–4 weeks that are required for *in vitro* culture allow time for the excised wound to develop granulation tissue even when allografts have generally 'taken' successfully. Therefore, the CAEs are usually placed on granulations or upon wound beds in which the granulation tissue has been freshly excised. Such wound beds are problematic even when meshed autografts are used. Unfortunately also, these wound beds often lead to less optimal long-term cosmetic and functional results irrespective of the type of graft material used. CAE technology does not appear to have corrected this fundamental biological phenomenon.

With regard to cost, this can be minimized if the facilities and expertise to culture autologous epidermal cells is available within an institution. In view of the fact that the technique of cultured human epidermis is costly and arduous, there is a growing consensus that the drawbacks or shortcomings of the cultivation system should be addressed before CAEs can be widely and extensively used in patients who can be satisfactorily treated with other methods.

Controversial issues have arisen using this cultured cell approach including the degree of 'take' of the cultured epidermal autografts (the efficiency in which the cultured cells adhere and persist *in vivo*) and the long-term morphology of the dermal–epidermal junction in the development of normal histological features of this junction. The efficiency of 'take' has been reported to vary

Table 15.5 Shortcomings of the cultured epidermal cell technology

3–4 weeks of culture allowing wound colonization and granulations to develop
Relatively low rate of engraftment or 'take' of each CAE application
Prolonged immobilization of extremities in order to facilitate engraftment
Graft fragility resulting in 'delayed loss'
High cost when purchased commercially

widely between 0 and 85% in burned patients and to be 68% when used purely electively after the excision of congenital hairy nevi.[43]

Important aspects of the durability and storage properties of the cells have been evaluated. Effects of extracellular matrix materials (e.g. fibrin) to serve as glues have also been attempted with limited preliminary success.[44] Optimization for cryopreservation conditions for the cultured cells has been evaluated and beneficial effects of serum were reported.[45] In addition, storage of the cells after detachment from the culture dishes appears to permanently impair the proliferative potential of the CEAs.[46]

A wider difference of opinion arises over the presence and temporal development of normal dermal–epidermal structures including hemidesmosomes and anchoring fibrils which are considered necessary for long-term adherence of the cultured cell grafts to the dermis. Compton reports an 8-year histopathologic study of skin regeneration and wound healing in 22 pediatric patients treated with CEAs grafted to full-thickness burn wounds excised to muscle fascia.[47] Biopsies of CEA have been analysed by light microscopic, immunohistochemical, morphometric, electron microscopic and ultrastructural immunolabeling techniques and compared to controls of meshed split-thickness autograft interstices at comparable times postgrafting. At transplantation, CEAs are undifferentiated and lack both granular and cornified cell layers. By 6 days postgrafting, CEA differentiate all normal epidermal strata but lack rete ridges. *De novo* formation of a confluent basal lamina and mature hemidesmosomes is complete by about 3 weeks. Anchoring fibrils appear sparse and immature (as in the meshed graft interstice controls) compared to normal skin until about 6–12 months. CEAs develop rete ridges and a neodermis with normal stromal and vascular organization at about 6–12 months, whereas meshed graft interstice controls do not. At 4–5 years, elastin expression is also observed in the CEA neodermis, completing the dermal regeneration process. Normal epidermal differentiation is maintained long term. These long-term results indicate that CEAs regenerate a stable normal epidermis and are capable of inducing dermal regeneration from wound bed connective tissue. These findings have been confirmed by others.[37] In an animal study of human keratinocyte transplants in athymic mice by Regauer *et al.*, the type VII collagen constituting the anchoring fibrils was shown to be keratinocyte in origin.[48]

In contrast, Woodley *et al.*[49] examined biopsies from 6 to 153 post-transplantation days in five patients using immunofluorescent staining using antibody probes to connective tissue molecules, by histochemical staining for elastin fibers, and by electron microscopy. The neodermis was found to contain most of the major connective tissue elements early in the post-transplantation period. However, regardless of the time examined, there was a paucity of elastin fibers and poor organization of linking (microthread-like fibers) in the neodermis beneath autografts. In four patients the formation of these same structures remained abnormal[50] and was associated with abnormal keratinocyte differentiation.[51] These observations have also been observed by other investigators.[42] Investigators have recognized that formation of a proper dermal–epidermal junction is not only highly desirable but is likely necessary to develop a pliable and durable long-term result. It was concluded that the perturbations of these connective tissue components in the neodermis may play a role in the poor recoil and elastic properties of burn wounds treated with autografts. Further analysis of studies using this strategy will be necessary to resolve this controversy.

Allogenic Cells

In addition to the application of cultured autologous epidermal cells, in a parallel effort, investigators have transplanted cultured allogenic keratinocytes using methods described by Eisinger *et al.*[26] to accelerate wound healing by repopulating the wound with epidermal cells.[52] In initial studies,[53] acceleration of healing of partial-thickness wound was seen; however, in later studies,[54] essentially no 'take' of these transplanted epidermal cells was found in full-thickness wounds. In later studies in patients with partial-thickness excisions of tattoos[55] and full-thickness wounds in burned patients,[56] the transplanted allogenic cells were not found in the wound beyond the first few weeks post-transplantation by using gender chromosomal analysis of the cells remaining in the wound. These findings have been confirmed by others.[57] Therefore, the beneficial effects of allogenic epidermal cells on the acceleration of partial-thickness wound healing must be dependent upon effects unrelated to the persistence of the transplanted cells within the wound. It is possible that the cultured cells and their associated matrix may provide substances that aid wound healing locally.

Cultured Epidermal Cells and Dermal Matrix

Perhaps the most important clinical issue involved with this approach is the fact that dermis is not replaced by this technology and therefore only a part of the skin replacement problem has been addressed. Considerable interest has developed to combine CAEs with dermal replacement technologies. The potential combinations include CAEs with the following investigational dermal replacement products:

- Integra from Integra Lifesciences Corp., Plainsboro, NJ;
- Dermagraft from Advanced Tissue Sciences, San Diego, CA;
- AlloDerm from LifeCell Corp., The Woodlands, TX;
- Cell-free porcine dermis.[52]

As previously mentioned, it is also possible that the CAEs can be placed directly upon allodermis which has remained intentionally after the allograft's initial closure of the wound. It is expected that the new dermis provided by these approaches may improve the rate of initial engraftment, lower the rate of delayed loss of cells, and improve the long-term cosmetic and functional result.

Given the shortcomings of this very promising technology, consensus regarding the clinical indications for their usage is emerging (**Table 15.6**).[41,42] Certainly the shortcomings of CAEs become more

Table 15.6. Suggested clinical indications for the use of cultured epidermal cell technology

Patients with burn injuries >90% TBSA*	Use of CAEs is recommended because donor sites are extremely limited and the CAEs can contribute to wound closure in a limited but potentially important manner
Patients with burn injuries between 70 and 90% TBSA	Use of CAEs is a matter of clinical judgment which strongly depends upon the quality and location of the available donor site(s). Donor sites involving the face, feet, hands, and genitalia are difficult to harvest and require that dermis remain to provide a cosmetically acceptable and functional result for these essential areas
Patients with burn injuries <70% TBSA	Use of CAEs is not usually necessary when wounds can be closed with standard methods of wound excision and closure using allografts and meshed autografts

* Total body surface area.

acceptable as the extent of injury exceeds 70% TBSA. At the same time, however, the shortcomings of low initial engraftment, delayed graft loss, prolonged immobilization, and cost also increase in importance as the extent of injury increases. At the present time, it would appear that the use of cultured autologous tissue for burn wound closure is in the early stage of its development and application. Continuing research into this extremely important area will likely lead in the long run to more cost-effective and refined methods to effectively treat patients with these life-threatening thermal injuries. In summary, there is general enthusiasm for further efforts to overcome the shortcomings that currently are associated with this very interesting approach.

Summary

In general, results of the relatively few and limited clinical investigations are promising but do not allow a definitive resolution regarding the optimal wound closure material; however, one generality can be made from the available studies. The most successful short-term and long-term results have been achieved only if both dermal and epidermal replacement have been taken into account in a timely fashion. Only with the physiologic replacement of both normal layers of skin can the success criteria previously outlined most likely be achieved. Of the wound closure efforts to date, the most extensively studied and the only approach evaluated by a prospectively randomized clinical trial has been by the creation of an artificial dermal matrix combined with a silastic epidermis such as Integra. Ultimately, the best candidates for permanent wound closure materials will require similar prospectively randomized and controlled clinical trials in order to determine the best approach under defined clinical conditions.

References

1. Yannas I V, Burke J F, Orgill D P, Skrabut E M. Wound tissue can utilize a polymeric template to synthesize a functional extension of skin. *Science* 1982; **215:** 174–6.

2. Burke J F, Bondoc C C, Jung W K, Quinby W C, Yannas I V. Successful use of a physiologically acceptable artificial skin in the treatment of extensive burn injury. *Ann Surg* 1981; **194:** 413–28.

3. Boyce S T, Hansbrough J F. Biologic attachment, growth, and differentiation of cultured human keratinocytes on a graftable collagens and chondroitin-6-sulfate substrate. *Surgery* 1988; **103:** 421–31.

4. Hansbrough J F, Boyce S T, Cooper M L, Foreman T J. Burn wound closure with cultured autologous keratinocytes and fibroblasts attached to a collagen–glycosaminoglycan substrate. *JAMA* 1989; **262:** 2125–30.

5. Rheinwald J G, Green H. Serial cultivation of strains of human epidermal keratinocytes: the formation of keratinizing colonies from single cells. *Cell* 1975; **6:** 331–44.

6. Gallico G G, O'Conner N E, Green H. Permanent coverage of large burn wounds with autologous cultured human epithelium. *N Engl J Med* 1984; **311:** 448–51.

7. Heimbach D, Luterman A, Burke J, *et al.* Artificial dermis for major burns. *Ann Surg* 1988; **208:** 313–20.

8. Yannas I V, Burke J F. Design of an artificial skin. I. Basic design principles. *J Biomed Mater Res* 1980; **14:** 65–81.

9. Yannas I V, Burke J F, Gordon P L. Design of an artificial skin. II. Control of chemical composition. *J Biomed Mater Res* 1980; **14:** 107–31.

10. Yannas I V, Burke J F, Warpehoski M, Design principles and preliminary clinical performance of an artificial skin. In: Cooper S L, Peppas N A, eds. *Advances in Chemistry Series, No. 199. Biomaterials: Interfacial Phenomena and Applications*. Washington, DC: The American Chemistry Society, 1982: 475–81.

11. Tompkins R G, Hilton J F, Burke J F, *et al.* Increased survival after massive thermal injuries in adults: a preliminary report using artificial skin. *Crit Care Med* 1989; **17:** 734–40.

12. Sheridan R L, Hegarty M T, Tompkins R G, Burke J F. Artificial skin in massive burns: results to ten years. *Br J Plast Surg* 1994; **17:** 94–7.

13. Yannas I V, Lee E, Orgill D P, Skrabut E M, Murphy G F. Synthesis and characterization of a model extracellular matrix that induces partial regeneration of adult mammalian skin. *Proc Natl Acad Sci USA* 1989; **86:** 933–7.

14. Heck E L, Bergstresser P R, Baxter C R. Composite skin graft: frozen dermal allografts support the engraftment and expansion of autologous epidermis. *J Trauma* 1985; **25:** 106–12.

15. Cuono C, Langdon R, McGuire J. Use of cultured epidermal autografts and dermal allografts as skin replacement after burn injury. *Lancet* 1986; **1:** 1123–4.

16. Battlebart S, Birchall N, Cuono C B, Langhon R, McGuire J. Composite autologous-allogenic skin replacement: development and clinical application. *Plast Reconstr Surg* 1987; **80:** 626–35.

17. Gao Z R, Hao Z Q, Nie L J, Liu G F. Coverage of full skin thickness burns with allograft inoculated with autogenous epithelial cells. *Burns* 1986; **12:** 220–4.

18. Langdon R C, Cuono C B, Birchall N, *et al.* Reconstitution of structure and cell function in human skin grafts derived from cryopreserved allogeneic dermis and autologous cultured keratinocytes. *J Invest Dermatol* 1988; **91:** 478–85.

19. Bell E, Ehrlich H P, Buttle D J, Nahatsuji T. Living tissue formed *in vitro* and accepted as skin-equivalent tissue of full-thickness. *Science* 1981; **211:** 1052–4.

20. Wilkins L M, Watson S R, Prosky S J, Meunier S F, Parenteau N L. Development of a bilayered living skin construct for clinical applications. *Biotechnol Bioeng* 1994; **43:** 747–56.

21. Boyce S T, Greenhalgh D G, Kagan R J, *et al.* Skin anatomy and antigen expression after burn wound closure with composite grafts of cultured skin cells and biopolymers. *Plast Reconstr Surg* 1993; **91:** 632–41.

22. Hansbrough J F, Cooper M L, Cohen R, *et al.* Evaluation of a biodegradable matrix containing cultured human fibroblasts as a dermal replacement beneath meshed skin grafts on athymic mice. *Surgery* 1992; **111:** 438–46.

23. Hansbrough J F, Dore C, Hansbrough W B. Clinical trials of a living dermal tissue replacement placed beneath meshed, split-thickness skin grafts on excised burn wounds. *J Burn Care Rehabil* 1992; **13:** 519–29.

24. Stompro B E, Hansbrough J F, Boyce S T. Attachment of peptide growth factors to implantable collagen. *J Surg Res* 1989; **46:** 413–21.

25. Cooper M L, Hansbrough J F, Foreman T J. In vitro effects of matrix peptides on a cultured dermal-epidermal skin substitute. *J Surg Res* 1990; **48:** 528–33.

26. Eisenger M, Lee J S, Hefton J M, Darzynkiewicz Z, Chiao J W, de Harven E. Human epidermal cell cultures: growth and differentiation in the absence of dermal components and medium supplements. *Proc Natl Acad Sci USA* 1979; **76:** 5340–4.

27. Johnson L F, deSerres S, Herzog S R, Peterson H D, Meyer A A. Antigenic cross-reactivity between media supplements for cultured keratinocyte grafts. *J Burn Care Rehabil* 1991; **12:** 306–12.

28. Johnson M C, Meyer A A, deSerres S, Herzog S, Peterson H D. Persistence of fetal bovine serum proteins in human keratinocytes. *J Burn Care Rehabil* 1990; **11:** 504–9.

29. O'Connor N E, Mulliken J B, Banks-Schiegel S, Kehinde O, Green H. Grafting of burns with cultured epithelium prepared from autologous epidermal cells. *Lancet* 1981; **1:** 75–8.

30. Clarke J A. Cultured skin for burn injury. *Lancet* 1986; **2:** 809.

31. Eldad E, Burt A, Clarke J A. Cultured epithelium as a skin substitute. *Burns* 1987; **13:** 173–80.

32. Latarjet J, Gangolphe M, Hezez G, *et al.* The grafting of burns with cultured epidermis as autografts in man. *Scand J Plast Reconstr Surg Hand Surg* 1987; **21:** 241–4.

33. Herzog S R, Meyer A, Woodley D, Peterson H D. Wound coverage with cultured autologous keratinocytes: use after burn wound excision including biopsy follow-up. *J Trauma* 1988; **28:** 195–8.

34. Kumagai N, Nishina H, Tanabe H, *et al.* Clinical application of autologous cultured epithelia for the treatment of burn wounds and burn scars. *Plast Reconstr Surg* 1988; **82:** 99–110.

35. Compton C C, Gill J M, Bradford D A, Regauer S, Gallico G G, O'Conner N E. Skin regenerated from cultured epithelial autografts on full-thickness burn wounds from 6 days to 5 years after grafting. *Lab Invest* 1989; **60:** 600–12.

36. Munster A M, Weiner S H, Spence R J. Cultured epidermis for the coverage of massive burn wounds. *Ann Surg* 1990; **211:** 676–9.

37. Franzi A T, D'Anna F, Zicca A, Trabucchi E. Histological evaluation of human cultured epithelium before and after grafting. *Burns* 1992; **18:** S26–S31.

38. Donati L, Magliacani G, Bormioli M, Signorini M, Preis F W. Clinical experiences with keratinocyte grafts. *Burns* 1992; **18:** S19–S26.

39. De Luca M, Bondanza S, Cancedda R, *et al.* Permanent coverage of full skin thickness burns with autologous cultured epidermis and reepithelialization of partial skin thickness lesions induced by allogeneic cultured epidermis: a multicentre study in the treatment of children. *Burns* 1992; **18:** S16–S19.

40. Rue L W, Cioffi W G, McManus W F, Pruitt B A. Wound closure and outcome in extensively burned patients treated with cultured autologous keratinocytes. *J Trauma* 1993; **34:** 662–8.

41. Heimbach D M. A nonuser's questions about cultured epidermal autograft. *J Burn Care Rehabil* 1992; **13:** 127–9.

42. Desai M H, Mlakar J M, McCauley R L, *et al.* Lack of long-term durability of cultured keratinocyte burn-wound coverage: a case report. *J Burn Care Rehabil* 1991; **12:** 540–5.

43. Gallico G G, O'Conner N E, Compton C C, Remensnyder J P, Kehinde O, Green H. Cultured epithelial autografts for giant congenital nevi. *Plast Reconstr Surg* 1989; **84:** 1–9.

44. Ronfard V, Broly H, Mitchell V, *et al.* Use of human keratinocytes cultured on fibrin glue in the treatment of burn wounds. *Burns* 1991; **17:** 181–4.

45. Kearney J N. Cryopreservation of cultured skin cells. *Burns* 1991; **17:** 380–3.

46. Boucher F, Poumay Y, Degen A, Paye M, Leloup R. Utilization of human cultured epidermal keratinocytes: irreversibility of the inhibition of proliferation induced in stored detached cultures. *Burns* 1991; **17:** 205–8.

47. Compton C C. Current concepts in pediatric burn care: the biology of cultured epithelial autografts: an eight-year study in pediatric burn patients. *Eur J Pediatr Surg* 1992; **2:** 216–22.

48. Regauer S, Seiler G R, Barrandon Y, Easley K W, Compton C C. Epithelial origin of cutaneous anchoring fibrils. *J Cell Biol* 1990; **111:** 2109–15.

49. Woodley D T, Peterson H D, Herzog S R, *et al.* Burn wounds resurfaced by cultured epidermal autografts show abnormal reconstitution of anchoring fibrils. *JAMA* 1988; **259:** 2566–71.

50. Woodley D T, Briggaman R A, Herzog S R, Meyers A A, Peterson H D, O'Keefe E J. Characterization of 'neo-dermis' formation beneath cultured human epidermal autografts transplanted on muscle fascia. *J Invest Dermatol* 1990; **95:** 20–6.

51. Peterson M J, Lessane B, Woodley D T. Characterization of cellular elements in healed cultured keratinocyte autografts used to cover burn wounds. *Arch Dermatol* 1990; **126:** 175–80.

52. Fratianne R, Papay F, Housini I, Lang C, Schafer I A. Keratinocyte allografts accelerate healing of split-thickness donor sites: applications for improved treatment of burns. *J Burn Care Rehabil* 1993; **14:** 148–54.

53. Hefton J M, Finkelstein J L, Madden M R, Shires G T. Grafting of burn patients with allografts of cultured epidermal cells. *Lancet* 1983; **2:** 428–30.

54. Madden M R, Finkelstein J L, Staiano-Coico L, *et al.* Grafting of cultured allogeneic epidermis on second- and third-degree burn wounds on 26 patients. *J Trauma* 1986; **26:** 955–62.

55. Brain A, Purkis P, Coates P, Hackett M, Navsaria H, Leigh I. Survival of cultured allogeneic keratinocytes transplanted to deep dermal bed assessed with probe specific for Y chromosome. *BMJ* 1989; **298:** 917–19.

56. Burt A M, Pallett C D, Sloane J P, *et al.* Survival of cultured allografts in patients with burns assessed with probe specific for Y chromosome. *BMJ* 1989; **298:** 915–17.

57. van der Merwe A E, Mattheyse F J, Bedford M, van Helden P D, Rossouw D J. Allografted keratinocytes used to accelerate the treatment of burn wounds are replaced by recipient cells. *Burns* 1990; **16:** 193–7.

58. Tompkins R G, Burke J F. Artificial skin. *Surgical Rounds* 1992; **October:** 881–90.

INHALATION INJURY

CHAPTER SIXTEEN

Pathophysiology of Inhalation Injury

Daniel L. Traber and Valerie Pollard

Introduction

It has been almost a decade since the authors published their first manuscript on inhalation injury.[1,2] In a review article published at that time, it was reported that inhalation injury was a main, if not *the* main, factor responsible for mortality in thermally injured patients.[3,4] That is still true today. Little progress has been made in reducing the mortality associated with inhalation injury.[5] Perhaps, also, some of the developments which have been made in the treatment of inhalation injury are not beneficial. As the pathophysiology of inhalation injury is examined, some rationale for a reevaluation of current treatment regimens may be recommended.

Toxic Smoke Compounds

Approximately 80% of fire-related deaths result not from burn injury but from inhalation of the toxic products of combustion.[6] Many of these compounds may act together, so as to increase mortality. This is especially true of carbon monoxide (CO) and hydrogen cyanide[7,8] where a synergism has been found to increase tissue hypoxia and acidosis[8] and may also decrease cerebral oxygen consumption and metabolism.[9] Victims may be incapacitated by the blinding and irritating effects of smoke as well as the decreasing oxygen concentration that which occurs with combustion and results in progressive hypoxia.

The extent of inhalation damage produced depends on ignition source, temperature, concentration, and solubility of the toxic gases generated. It is thus important to obtain information relative to the source of the fire and the combustion products generated when treating a fire victim (see **Table 16.1**). The more caustic materials, such as acroline and other aldehydes, damage the airway and set off reactions that are inflammatory to the bronchi and parenchyma. On the other hand, carbon monoxide and cyanide rarely damage the airway as they do affect gas exchange. It is also important to know the duration of exposure and the extent to which fire victims were

Table 16.1 Origin of selected toxic compounds other than CO or CO_2

Material	Source	Decomposition products
Cellulose	Wood, paper, cotton, jute	Aldehydes, acrolein
Wool, silk	Clothing, fabric, blankets, furniture	Hydrogen, cyanide, ammonia, hydrogen, sulfide
Rubber	Tires	Sulfur dioxide, hydrogen, sulfide
Polyvinyl chloride	Upholstery, wire/pipe coating, wall, floor, furniture coverings	Hydrogen chloride, phosgene
Polyurethane	Insulation, upholstery material	Hydrogen cyanide, isocyanates, ammonia, acrylonitriles
Polyester	Clothing, fabric	Hydrogen chloride
Polypropylene	Upholstery, carpeting	Acrolein
Polyacrylonitrile	Appliances, engineering, plastics	Hydrogen cyanide
Polyamide	Carpeting, clothing	Hydrogen cyanide, ammonia
Melamine resins	Household and kitchen goods	Hydrogen cyanide, ammonia, formaldehyde
Acrylics	Aircraft windows, textiles, wall coverings	Acrolein

From Prien and Traber.[7]

in an enclosed area since this relates to the dose of toxic materials presented to them. The origins, symptoms, and treatment of some of the more common products of thermal degradation are relevant to further discussion of inhalation injury.

CARBON MONOXIDE TOXICITY

Carbon monoxide toxicity remains one of the most frequent immediate causes of death following smoke-induced inhalation injury; it must be suspected in every fire victim and treated promptly. Inhalation of a 0.1% carbon monoxide mixture may result in generation of a carboxyhemoglobin level as high as 50%. In fact, carbon monoxide has an affinity for hemoglobin which is 200–250 times that of oxygen; therefore, the combined product readily results in a decrease in oxyhemoglobin saturation, leading to anoxia and death. The oxygen-hemoglobin dissociation curve loses its sigmoid shape and is shifted to the left, thus further impairing tissue oxygen availability.[7] Competitive inhibition with cytochrome oxidase enzyme systems, most notably cytochromes *a* and P-450, results in an inability of cellular systems to use oxygen.[10] Lower concentrations of CO may also impair decision-making and psychomotor responses.[11]

Symptoms and Signs

Diagnosis may be difficult and few symptoms generally occur when the carboxyhemoglobin level is less than 10%.[11] Toxic symptoms become manifest at levels greater than 20% and death may occur at levels greater than 60% (see **Table 16.2**).

Diagnosis may be facilitated by use of on-site portable breath analysers or by direct measurement of the carboxyhemoglobin level in a venous or arterial blood sample. High oxygen concentrations are usually administered to a victim in transit to hospital, and there is also some delay from cessation of exposure to measurement of the level, so tests may not reflect the true extent of exposure.[13] A nomogram has been developed which can relate the carboxyhemoglobin levels of a patient to the values which may have been present at the time of smoke inhalation; and this can be used to estimate the true degree of inhalation injury.[14] Blood gas analysis of patients with high carboxyhemoglobin levels will demonstrate a fall in oxygen content (O_2 saturation) but a relatively normal arterial oxygen tension (Pao_2). Evaluation of mixed venous or central venous oxygen tension (Pvo_2) may therefore be more useful in evaluating a therapeutic response.[7] Acid–base balance, plasma lactate levels, and bicarbonate levels should also be measured as an indication of an underlying lactic or metabolic acidosis.

Table 16.2 Symptoms and signs at various concentrations of carboxyhemoglobin (COHb)[11,12]

COHb (%)	Signs and symptoms
0–10	None
10–20	Tightness over forehead, slight headache, dilation of cutaneous blood vessels
20–30	Headache and throbbing in the temples
30–40	Severe headache, weakness, dizziness, dimness of vision, nausea, vomiting, collapse
40–50	As above; greater possibility of collapse, syncope, increased pulse and respiratory rate
50–60	Syncope, increased pulse and respiratory rate, coma, intermittent convulsions, Cheyne–Stokes respirations
60–70	Coma, intermittent convulsions, depressed cardiac and respiratory function, possible death
70–80	Weak pulse, slow respirations, death within hours
80–90	Death in less than 1 hour
90–100	Death within minutes

Treatment

The half-life of carboxyhemoglobin is 250 minutes in room air and 40–60 minutes in a person breathing 100% oxygen; therefore all fire victims should receive 100% oxygen while in transit to a hospital.[15] This allows delivery of an inspired oxygen concentration of 50–60%, which is usually adequate. If, however, loss of consciousness, cyanosis, or an inability to maintain the airway is present, then endotracheal intubation, which allows delivery of 100% oxygen to the patient, may be necessary.

Hyperbaric oxygen therapy has been suggested for CO intoxication if the carboxyhemoglobin level exceeds 25% or if significant clinical toxicity is present. Administration of three atmospheres of pressure will further reduce the carboxyhemoglobin half-life to 30 minutes.[16,17] If neurological impairment persists, this treatment may be repeated.[16] Hyperbaric oxygen treatment has been shown to reverse brain lipid peroxidation produced by CO and the binding of CO to cytochrome oxidase in animal studies.[18,19] It should be noted that the efficacy of this intervention has not been tested in randomized studies and there are some dangers associated with its usage.[20] Most authorities recommend intubation and administration of 100% oxygen instead. Also, only a few hyperbaric centers are sufficiently equipped to aid in treatment. Finally, as many as 10% of survivors may demonstrate a ‘pseudorecovery’ associated with neurological or mental deterioration some months afterward.[11]

Perhaps one of the most deadly problems with CO poisoning is the fact that it induces a disorientation. Thus, an individual exposed to high levels of CO in a fire might not avoid being burned. There have been incidences in which individuals seen leaving a fire accident have later been found dead in the fire area with high CO levels in their blood.

HYDROGEN CYANIDE TOXICITY

Hydrogen cyanide is produced in fires involving nitrogen-containing polymers and may produce a rapid and lethal incapacitation of a victim at the fire source, with death occurring later either from cyanide or carbon monoxide toxicity or from burn-related pathology.[21] Toxicity is produced by inhibition of cellular oxygenation with resultant tissue anoxia which is caused by reversible inhibition of cytochrome oxidase (Fe^{3+}) by cyanide.[13]

Symptoms and Signs

Diagnosis at the fire scene may be difficult and should be suspected in a patient with an underlying lactic acidosis which is not rapidly responsive to oxygen therapy.[14,22] Concentrations greater than 20 ppm are considered dangerous (see **Table 16.3**). A distinctive odor of bitter almonds may initially arouse suspicion of cyanide toxicity in a fire victim. Symptoms may progress rapidly, and include lethargy, nausea, headache, weakness, and coma. Cardiovascular symptoms include acute electrocardiographic S-T segment elevation, which may mimic an acute myocardial infarction.[24] Cyanide increases ventilation through carotid body and peripheral chemore-

Table 16.3 Hydrogen cyanide (HCN) concentrations in air and associated symptoms in humans[11, 23]

HCN concentration (ppm)	Symptoms
0.2–5.0	Threshold of odor
10	(TLV-MAC)
18–36	Slight symptoms (headache) after several hours
45–54	Tolerated for 1/2–1 hour without difficulty
100	Death in 1 hour
110–135	Fatal in 1/2–1 hour
181	Fatal in 10 minutes
280	Immediately fatal

TLV, Total Lung Volume; MAC, Minimum Alveolar Concentration.

ceptor stimulation. Increasing ventilation may augment toxicity in the early stages. Death is later caused by respiratory center paralysis (> 100 ppm). Hydrogen cyanide is found routinely in low levels in the blood of healthy individuals (at levels of 0.02 μg/ml in nonsmokers and 0.04 μg/ml in smokers). Toxicity occurs at a level of 0.1 μg/ml, and at 1.0 μg/ml death is likely.[25]

Treatment

Controversy surrounds the management of hydrogen cyanide poisoning as treatment may in itself be hazardous. Such treatment may, however, be considered in a hypoxic or an unconscious victim. Oxygen therapy has been found beneficial, though hyperbaric oxygen is not recommended.[24,25] Nitrate administration results in oxidation of hemoglobin to methemoglobin, which then competes with cytochrome oxidase for cyanide.[7] Methemoglobin, however, decreases oxygen transport capacity and may thereby worsen the prognosis if administered.[26] Sodium thiosulfate administration, in the presence of the mitochondrial enzyme rhodanase, results in the transfer of sulfur to the cyanide ion, forming thiocyanate. Toxicity is minimal other than an osmotic diuretic action, which in itself may be beneficial. Onset of action, however, is quite slow.[7] Chelating agents, which form a complex with cyanide, thus increasing its renal excretion, may also be administered. Cobalt EDTA is relatively toxic and may cause cardiovascular instability and anaphylaxis; therefore, hydroxycobalamin may be preferable as it is nontoxic apart from causing occasional urticarial reactions.[7,25] In summary, suitable treatment at a fire site involves intravenous administration of sodium thiosulfate (125–250 mg/kg) and hydroxycobalamin (4 g). One hundred percent oxygen should also be given.

Further Toxic Compounds

Other degradation products may also contribute substantially to morbidity and mortality in a burn victim. Hydrogen chloride is produced by polyvinyl chloride degradation and causes severe respiratory tract damage and pulmonary edema. Nitrogen oxides may cause pulmonary edema and a chemical pneumonitis and may contribute to cardiovascular depression and acidosis. Aldehydes, such as acrolein and acetaldehyde, which are found in wood and kerosene, may further contribute towards pulmonary edema and respiratory irritability. The most important aspect of management of acute inhalation toxicology involves the prompt removal of victims from a fire site in order to minimize further exposure to toxic combustion products which may initially 'stun' and render them unable to escape from the fire, and eventually may cause toxicity. Prompt administration of oxygen, maintenance of the basic ABCs (of airway, breathing, and circulation), and rapid hospitalization are then of paramount importance. Finally, a high index of suspicion and a thorough knowledge of the appropriate management of a smoke inhalation victim are essential in assuring a good prognosis.

Injury to the Oropharynx

Much of the pathophysiology that occurs with inhalation injury is related to edema formation, which is the result of an increased transvascular fluid flux. Before a discussion of the changes that follow inhalation injury, a review of the forces responsible for the variables of the Starling–Landis equation[27,28] should be reviewed:

$$J_v = K_f[(P_c - P_{if}) - \sigma(COP_p - COP_{if})]$$

This equation describes the physical forces and physiologic mechanisms which govern fluid transfer between vascular and extravascular compartments. J_v, the transvascular fluid flux, is equal to lymph flow during equilibrium states. As transvascular fluid flux increases, interstitial volume also increases (edema formation) until a new equilibrium with lymph flow occurs. K_f is the filtration coefficient, an index of the total number of pores which are filtering. The number of pores could increase if a larger area of the microcirculation were perfused or if there were more pores per given area of the microcirculation. These pores are the same size as water and electrolytes, as opposed to the larger pores associated with protein. P_c and P_{if} are the hydrostatic pressures in the microcirculation and interstitial space, respectively. *s*, the reflection coefficient, is an index of microvascular permeability to protein. If $s = 1$, the membrane is impermeable to protein; when it is 0, the membrane is completely permeable to protein. COP_p and COP_{if} are the oncotic or colloid osmotic pressures in the plasma and interstitial spaces, respectively.

The damage seen in the oropharynx after inhalation injury is the same as that seen with thermal injury in other areas of the body. The heat denatures protein which, in turn, activates complement.[29,30] Complement activation causes the release of histamine.[30,31] Histamine then causes a formation of xanthine oxidase,[32] an enzyme involved in the breakdown of uric acid to urea. One of the stages in this degradation process is the formation of hypoxanthine from xanthine. During this conversion, oxygen free radicals are released.[33,34] Oxygen free radicals cause edema formation through increasing permeability to protein and increasing the microvascular pressure. The latter is the result of inhibiting the formation of nitric oxide. Eicosanoids are also released,[35,36] which, along with oxygen free radicals, attract polymorphonuclear cells to the area. The attraction then increases the release of oxygen radicals, proteases, and other materials into burned areas.

The massive edema which results in the soft tissue of the oropharynx after burns involves most of the variables in the Starling equation (**Figure 16.1**). There is a large increase in microvascular hydrostatic pressure,[37] a decrease in interstitial hydrostatic pressure,[38] a fall in the reflection coefficient,[37] and an increase in interstitial oncotic pressure.[39,40] The usual treatment for burn resuscitation calls for the administration of large amounts of crystalloid solutions, which have the effect of reducing the plasma oncotic pressure.[41,42] This reduction not only affects the oncotic pressure gradient in the microcirculation but also has been reported to increase the filtration coefficient.[43,44] The result of this almost complete breakdown in control of the microvascular function and the insult of fluid administration is massive edema. This is probably

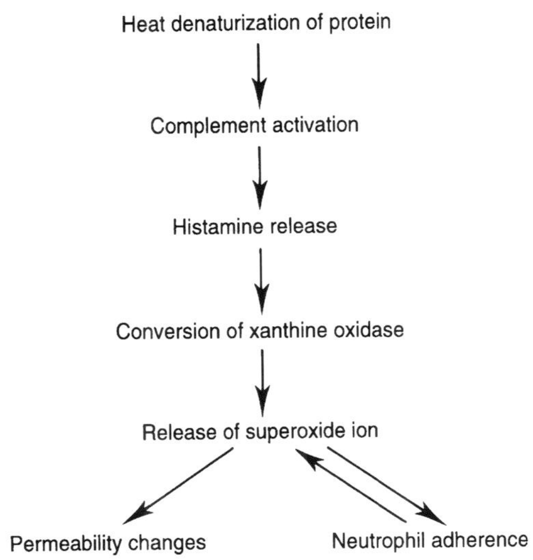

Fig. 16.1 The sequence of changes which occur in the oropharynx as a result of thermal injury to that area.

nowhere more apparent than in the soft tissues of the face and oropharynx. The danger to the patient is extreme. The edema may obstruct the airway, not only making it laborious or impossible to breathe, but also making it difficult for an anesthesiologist to intubate a patient. To avoid this problem, many units prophylactically intubate patients who have evidence of thermal injury to the upper airway on admission. This protocol, however, may present its own problems. The tube may further damage injured areas, especially the larynx.[45] It may be time to reconsider some of these practices. Perhaps some consideration should be given to fluid resuscitation with colloids, which can prevent some of this soft tissue edema and reduce the volume of fluids required for resuscitation.[46,47]

Tracheobronchial Areas

Victims of fire accidents, especially those who are injured in enclosed areas, sustain chemical injury to the respiratory tract as a result of breathing toxic gases associated with the incomplete combustion of burning materials, especially acrolein and formaldehyde.[48–50] Actual thermal injury to the airway is rare. The heat capacity of air is low, and the upper airway is very efficient at warming and cooling the inspiratory gases. Consequently, flames must come almost into direct contact with the airway in order to induce injury.[51] There are some instances in which hot particles might be inhaled. There are also reports of persons with steam inhalation. In these cases, there is direct thermal injury to the airway. In most of these cases, damage to the bronchi and trachea are the result of chemical injury.

With chemical damage to the airway, there are two almost instantaneous happenings: the ciliated epithelial cells separate from the basement membrane,[52–54] and there is an almost immediate dilation of the systemic circulation to the lung and of the bronchial circulation.[55–57] These latter changes appear mainly in the mucosal areas and can be detected by laser Doppler technique.[58] Shortly after this has occurred, edema can be visually detected in the trachea.[1] The edema is also evident histologically[1,59] and by gravimetric techniques.[56,60] The edema is associated with a permeability to larger molecular weight substances.[59,61] The rapid occurrence of these changes to the airway and their universal presence after some insufflation into the bronchial areas should make it relatively easy to diagnose inhalation injury by bronchoscopy.[3,62–64] The degree of airway vasodilatation does not appear to be related to the extent of smoke exposure. Rather, the dilation appears to be an all-or-nothing phenomenon. Longer duration of exposure appears to correlate with more areas of the airway showing a greater dilation. The dilation spreads farther down the bronchial tree with greater duration of exposure to smoke.[60]

The early inflammatory changes that occur in the airway are followed by a period of diffuse exudate formation,[65] which has been demonstrated to occur in copious quantities in both patients[66] and animals subjected to inhalation injury. The protein composition of this material suggests that it is an ultrafiltrate of the lung lymph.[61,65] The transudate can induce a bronchoconstriction. It contains thromboxane (TX) B_2, the stable metabolite of a potent smooth muscle constrictor, TXA_2.[1,67] Thus, the period of airway injury which extends for the following 12–24 hours is associated with bronchoconstriction and an elevation in airway resistance.[68–70] Unlike many other forms of airway inflammatory diseases, inhalation injury also demonstrates narrowing of the large airways. The mucosa of the airway can hold a large amount of edema, which can produce marked narrowing of the airway.

As the time after injury increases, the exudative materials coalesce to form fibrin casts. These materials can induce an almost complete occlusion of the airway[1,71–73] and can obstruct the smallest of the airways. As a result of the destruction of the epithelium and the presence of these airway casts, which function as culture media, there is a greater susceptibility of the airway to infection, often leading to pneumonia, sepsis, and death.

During the recovery period, a pseudomembrane first forms in the airways. This is followed by a squamous cell metaplasia.[74] Healing may take place as late as 18 days after injury.[75] There is a high incidence of permanent airway damage, including airway stenosis and granuloma scar formation of the trachea.[63] It is sometimes difficult to determine whether these long-term effects are the result of the injury or the cure.

Mediation of the Changes in Bronchial Blood Flow

There have been numerous attempts to identify the mediators responsible for the increased bronchial artery blood flow and microvascular permeability which occur with smoke inhalation. Because histamine is associated with vasodilatation and edema formation with burn injury, the effects of H_1 and H_2 histaminergic blockade in inhalation injury in sheep have been studied. Neither the H_1 blocker diphenhydramine nor the H_2 receptor antagonist ranitidine affected the response.[76] In previous studies, prostacyclin (PGI_2) was increased in the blood and lymph after inhalation injury.[65] Because this material is a vasodilator, a compound which blocks the synthesis of PGI_2, the cyclooxygenase inhibitor ibuprofen was investigated to determine if it would affect the bronchial hyperemia which is seen with inhalation injury in sheep. Again, there was no noticeable effect on bronchial artery blood flow after smoke inhalation.[77] Therefore, it appears that neither histamine nor prostanoids are mediators of bronchial hyperemia.

As a result of the inability of antihistamines and antiprostanoids to affect the increase in bronchial blood flow seen with the insufflation of smoke, other possible mediators were evaluated. The most obvious of these was a neural source. Because the vagosympathetic trunk is virtually the only source of innervation of the vasculature of the lung, the first studies performed attempted to determine the effects of blocking this neural trunk with a local anesthetic. These studies were performed in acute preparations. The animals that received the local anesthetic had a markedly reduced response.[78] The majority of motor fibers which innervate the bronchial microvasculature are vasodilatory and parasympathetic and, thus, release acetylcholine. Consequently, the effect of atropine on the elevated bronchial blood flow seen with inhalation injury was evaluated. The sheep that received the anticholinergic compound had an elevation in blood flow which was virtually identical with the untreated animals exposed to smoke. Thus, the increase in blood flow is not mediated by acetylcholine.

Martling *et al.* reported that most of the bronchial circulatory vasodilatation induced by vagal stimulation in a pig was mediated by sensory nerves;[79] these are neuropeptide-containing nerve fibers.[80] The fact that these fibers are capsaicin-sensitive, that is, they could be desensitized by the administration of capsaicin,[81] a material isolated from peppers, led to the determination of how the response to inhalation injury could be affected by capsaicin desensitization. In addition, the bronchial vasodilatation induced by the inhalation of cigarette smoke was prevented by the administration of capsaicin.[79] Lundberg *et al.* also reported that permeability was elevated by cigarette smoke, an effect which was blocked by the administration of capsaicin.[82] Preliminary data demonstrate that the changes in airway blood flow noted with inhalation injury can be reduced by pretreatment with capsaicin.[83]

Some of the bronchial hyperemia which accompanies smoke inhalation may be mediated hematogenously. Experiments were accomplished in which the trachea and right lung were injured with smoke, while the left lung was being ventilated with air. The usual hyperemia and edema were observed in the smoke-insufflated airway.[84] These changes occurred almost immediately as measured by both laser Doppler and radioactive microsphere techniques.[58,85] The air-insufflated lung did not demonstrate a change in bronchial blood flow immediately, but by 24 hours after the contralateral right lung and trachea had been injured, the small airways of the left lung began to show an increase in blood flow. Since the normal sequence of blood flow change in the smoke-injured lung is from trachea down, this hyperemic spread from the small airway up is evidence of a spread of injury from the pulmonary system.[86] The venous drainage of the extrapulmonic airway is into azygous vein.[87,88] Thus, if the extrapulmonic airway is injured, neuropeptides would enter into the azygous vein, and ultimately the pulmonary artery, for distribution to both lungs. The venous drainage of the intrapulmonic airway is directly into the pulmonary microcirculation.[87–89] Thus, injury to the intrapulmonic airway will release mediators into that lung alone. Although hematogenous, the blood flow changes are restricted to the injured lung.

Pulmonary Microvascular Changes

After inhalation injury, microvascular changes occur in the pulmonary microvasculature. There is a profound increase in lung lymph flow.[1,67] Extravascular lung water, as measured by the thermal dilution technique, is elevated.[90] Postmortem histologic and gravimetric analysis of the lung reveals an increased water content.[1,67] These increases in extravascular fluid formation are proportional to the duration of smoke exposure.[91] These changes are obviously related to alterations of the parameters of the Starling equation.

Pulmonary artery pressure and pulmonary vascular resistance increase between 4 and 12 hours after inhalation injury.[57,92,93] Pulmonary capillary pressure, measured by the technique of Holloway *et al.*,[94] also rises approximately 24 hours after smoke inhalation injury.[93] In association with the changes in pressure, there is also an elevation in microvascular resistance. The resistance rises on both sides of the microvasculature but is increased to a greater extent on the venular side of the pulmonary circuit. Simultaneous with these changes in resistance and pressure, permeability to protein was evaluated by measuring the reflection coefficient.[95] This variable was reduced, suggesting a marked elevation in pulmonary microvascular permeability to protein after inhalation injury.[96] These changes in pulmonary microvascular pressure are obviously important in the formation of edema; however, changes in vascular permeability appear to be of much greater importance, especially during the first 24 hours after injury.[96]

Mediation of the Pulmonary Microvascular Changes

There is a change in lung lymph flow after inhalation injury. This phenomenon differs from that seen in the tracheal areas, as it occurs with over a 4-hour latency period after the airway exposure to smoke, suggesting that it is a mediated phenomenon. After inhalation injury there is a marked reduction in the reflection coefficient and an elevation in the filtration coefficient.[96] This demonstrates an elevation in permeability both to proteins and to low molecular weight materials. Further, the relative contributions of permeability and capillary pressure on transvascular fluid flux was determined according to Pitt's method.[37] Capillary permeability was responsible for the majority of the edema found during the first 24 hours. During the next 24 hours, permeability and lung lymph flow began to return toward the baseline value and microvascular pressure appeared to be responsible for most of the lymph flow changes noted at 48 hours after smoke insufflation.[96]

These changes in microvascular fluid flux occur with the elevation of polymorphonuclear cells in the lung, as evidenced by histology and bronchoalveolar lavage and the release of materials associated with polymorphonuclear cells, such as proteases and oxygen free radicals[65,67,91] (**Figure 16.2**). In relation to these latter materials, Demling and LaLonde have reported that one product of lipid peroxidation, conjugated dienes, was more abundant in the pulmonary arterial blood than in the systemic circulation, suggesting a peripheral source for these materials.[97] On the other hand, high concentrations of conjugated dienes have been reported in the lung lymph and pulmonary tissues following inhalation injury, suggesting the lung as a source of these materials.[98–100] The role of the polymorphonuclear cell as the vector of the cytotoxins responsible for pulmonary microvascular permeability changes has likewise been supported by a finding that the proteolytic enzymes, lipid peroxidation, and lung lymph flow changes are markedly reduced

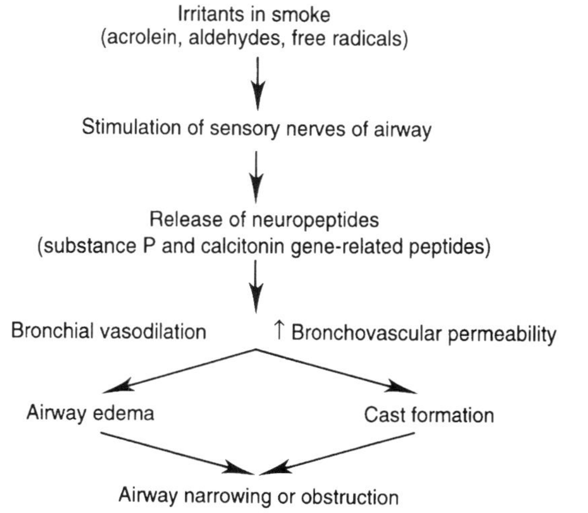

Fig. 16.2 Sequence of events that lead to the airway pathophysiology associated with smoke inhalation.

when the polymorphonuclear cells are depleted using nitrogen mustard.[100] The changes in lung lymph flow seen with smoke inhalation may also be obtunded by administration of antiproteases[101] and oxygen free radical scavengers.[102,103] It has also been reported that the administration of superoxide dismutase prevents the reduction in reflection coefficient which is seen with smoke inhalation.[104] Both proteases and oxygen free radicals have been shown to be released by polymorphonuclear cells.[105,106]

Role of the Bronchial Circulation in Mediating the Pulmonary Parenchymal Injury

The delayed onset of the changes in transvascular fluid flux in the pulmonary bed suggests the release of mediators from other areas. It is certainly difficult to conceive of materials in the smoke traveling from the oral pharynx to the alveoli. Certainly these materials come into contact with the airway circulation. The changes in bronchial blood flow and the denudation of the tracheobronchial basement membrane are phenomena that occur almost instantaneously with smoke insufflation.[53,57] Consequently, this airway injury must in some way guide polymorphonuclear cells to the parenchyma. The mechanisms by which cytokines might reach the pulmonary parenchyma from the airway may be related to the unique anatomy of the bronchial circulation. Systemic drainage from the intrapulmonary bronchi has been demonstrated to drain into the pulmonary circulation at the precapillary level.[87,89] Consequently, chemotactic materials released in the airway could traverse this network and present themselves to the pulmonary microvasculature in order to attract polymorphonuclear cells; this results in adherence to the microvasculature, transepithelial migration, and the release of cytotoxins.

Several experiments physiologically support a bronchopulmonary portal system. Using their dog model with acrolein inhalation injury, Hales and his group demonstrated an elevation in extravascular lung water using both the thermal technique and a gravimetric determination.[59,107] In animals with ligated bronchial arteries, this effect was markedly reduced.[59] In these studies, Hales and his team found histologically that there was edema in the airway and leakage of a high molecular weight dye, monastral blue, from the circulation following inhalation injury. The edema formation and permeability change were not seen when the bronchial circulation was occluded. Similar experiments have been performed in chronically instrumented sheep. The sheep is uniquely different from other animal species, having only a single bronchial artery, which supplies from 50% to 80% of the systemic circulation to the bronchial areas.[108] Occlusion of this vessel with a pneumatic device resulted in a reduction in both lung lymph flow and extravascular lung water, determined by the gravimetric technique.[109]

Recently, a technique to evaluate the role of the bronchial circulation in the parenchymal changes which are induced by inhalation injury has been developed. Pneumatic occluders are placed on the pulmonary arteries and veins of the left lung.[110] When these vessels are occluded, the left lung is isolated from the pulmonary circuit. The blood entering into this lung pouch, then, is the bronchial venous drainage. The flow rate into this pouch is similar to that previously reported for the bronchial blood flow to the left lung. This blood flow into the isolated lung vascular pouch increases markedly with smoke inhalation. The occlusion of the bronchial artery causes a nearly 70% reduction in the blood flow into the pouch. This is in close agreement with previous studies regarding the contribution of the bronchial artery to the total airway blood flow.[56,108] After inhalation injury, there is a marked increase in bronchial blood draining into the pouch. Occlusion of the bronchial artery reduces the blood flow into the pouch by 70% after inhalation injury. This is in agreement with our previous finding after bronchial artery occlusion.[56] These data are consistent with the hypothesis that the bronchial venous drainage enters into the pulmonary circuit. With injury to the airway, mediators would be released into the bronchial venous blood and be delivered directly into the pulmonary microvasculature.

Experiments have also been performed in which one lung was insufflated with smoke while the contralateral lung was insufflated with air. If the smoke exposure was limited to the intrapulmonary airways, the injury was localized to the lung.[98,111] On the other hand, when the smoke damage included the trachea and bronchi (extrapulmonary airway), then the contralateral air-insufflated lung likewise demonstrated injury.[98] The changes in airway blood flow were also investigated using radioactive microspheres. With time, blood flow changes in the lung that was insufflated with smoke showed the greatest intensity in the upper airway, with a gradient down to the smaller airways.[56,60] These changes in blood flow occurred almost instantaneously. On the other hand, the blood flow changes to the air-insufflated lung occurred after a latency period and had greater intensity in the smaller airways.[86] This suggests a hematogenous origin for the mediators of vasodilatation. The venous drainage from the extrapulmonary airway enters into the azygous vein and thus into the right atrium.[87] Mediators, therefore, released from these airways outside the lung would enter into the right heart and be distributed to both lungs. Bronchopulmonary pathophysiology is a fertile area for further investigation (**Figure 16.3**).

Changes in the Systemic Organs Induced by Smoke Inhalation

With burn injury and other forms of trauma, mortality is usually the result of multiple organ system failure.[112,113] The contribution made by acute lung injury to this phenomenon has, in the past, been considered the result of reduced oxygenation. With improved techniques of artificial restoration of arterial oxygenation saturation, it has now become obvious that other factors are involved. It has been

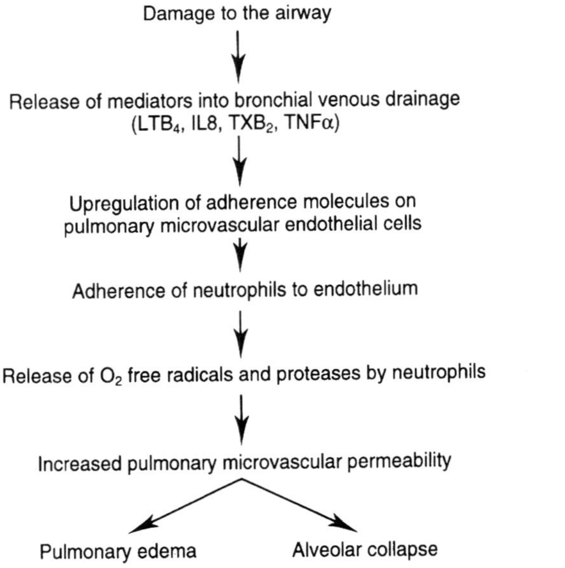

Fig. 16.3 Sequence of events that lead to pathophysiology in the pulmonary microvascular areas. LTB$_4$, leucotriene B$_4$; IL8, interleukin 8; TXB$_2$, thromboxane B$_2$; TNFα, tumor necrosis factor α.

recognized that persons who have suffered combined thermal and smoke inhalation injury require more fluid for resuscitation to non-pathogenic cardiovascular status than individuals with thermal injury alone.[114,115] This phenomenon has been studied by cannulation of a lymphatic which drains the soft tissues of the skin on the lateral surface of sheep.[116] With inhalation injury, there was a twofold increase in the flow from this vessel.[97,117] With thermal injury, this flow was much greater, reaching some three to five times the baseline levels.[117] When smoke inhalation was combined with thermal injury, again, the soft tissue lymphatic showed a severalfold increase in flow. LaLonde *et al.*[118] made a similar finding. These changes in peripheral microvascular fluid flux occur with a concomitant elevation in plasma lipid peroxidation products, suggesting that they may be the result of the release of oxygen free radicals. The etiology of these cytotoxins is unknown.

It has been reported that the lung releases peptidoleukotrienes after inhalation injury.[119] A similar finding has been made by Hales and his group,[120] who reported that a systemic vasoconstriction occurs with inhalation injury and that this systemic vasoconstriction could be reversed by administration of a peptidoleukotriene antagonist. It has also been reported that there is an elevation in systemic vascular resistance with inhalation injury[92] and demonstrated that there is a selective vasoconstriction in the distribution of the cephalic mesenteric artery of sheep after inhalation injury.[121] This vasoconstriction lasts about 4 hours and is followed by reperfusion. Consequently, damage to the systemic circulation may be the result of an ischemia-reperfusion phenomenon. Lung injury is also seen with systemic reperfusion injury.[122] Reperfusion phenomena are mediated by the action of xanthine oxidase.[33] An effect of the xanthine oxidase inhibitor allopurinol on the lung response to smoke inhalation could not be demonstrated.[123] The observation period of our study was limited to 24 hours and it is possible that the reperfusion might have had an effect in later time periods. Further study in this area of investigation is warranted.

In association with these systemic vascular resistance changes, a fall in myocardial contractility has been reported.[92,124] It was natural to assume that this fall in contractility was the result of ischemia reperfusion in the coronary bed as a result of the elevated carbon monoxide levels seen after inhalation injury. The animals with inhalation injury were compared to sheep insufflated with carbon monoxide to an equivalent level of carboxyhemoglobin. The animals given smoke showed a reduction in myocardial contractility but those with CO inhalation showed no such reduction.[92]

Systemic pathophysiology has also been noted with acid aspiration.[125] Aspiration resulted in the disposition of polymorphonuclear cells in the several systemic organs, including the heart. The deposition of these cells was associated with an increase in the wet/dry weight ratio. These results were mediated by leukotrienes and thromboxane.[126] This is in agreement with the results of Quinn, who demonstrated a vasoconstriction and its reversal of systemic vascular resistance changes after insufflating sheep with artificial smoke.[120] It has also been determined that a thromboxane inhibitor will reverse the changes in systemic vascular resistance and myocardial contractility that are seen with smoke inhalation.[127] Additionally, the changes in lung lymph flow in these animals were not as marked. There is, therefore, a great deal of promise in future trials with thromboxane inhibitors.

The basic research that has been performed in the past in the area of inhalation injury has identified a number of possibilities for the intervention of this lethal syndrome. Several clinical studies are underway to evaluate them. In the next decade we expect to see marked progress in the reduction of lethality of this syndrome.

References

1. Herndon D N, Traber D L, Niehaus G D, Linares H A, Traber L D. The pathophysiology of smoke inhalation injury in a sheep model. *J Trauma* 1984; **24:** 1044–51.

2. Herndon D N, Adams T J, Traber L D, Traber D L. Inhalation injury and positive pressure ventilation in a sheep model. *Circ Shock* 1984; **12:** 107–13.

3. Herndon D N, Thompson P B, Traber D L. Pulmonary injury in burned patients. *Crit Care Clin* 1985; **1:** 79–96.

4. Thompson P B, Herndon D N, Traber D L, Abston S. Effect on mortality of inhalation injury. *J Trauma* 1986; **26:** 163–5.

5. Sobel J B, Goldfarb I W, Slater H, Hammell E J. Inhalation injury: a decade without progress. *J Burn Care Rehabil* 1992; **13:** 573–5.

6. Birky M M, Clarke F B. Inhalation of toxic products from fires. *Bull N Y Acad Med* 1981; **57:** 997–1013.

7. Prien T, Traber D L. Toxic smoke compounds and inhalation injury – a review. *Burns Incl Therm Inj* 1988; **14:** 451–60.

8. Moore S J, Ho I K, Hume A S. Severe hypoxia produced by concomitant intoxication with sublethal doses of carbon monoxide and cyanide. *Toxicol Appl Pharmacol* 1991; **109:** 412–20.

9. Pitt B R, Radford E P, Gurtner G H, Traystman R J. Interaction of carbon monoxide and cyanide on cerebral circulation and metabolism. *Arch Environ Health* 1979; **34:** 345–9.

10. Goldbaum L R, Orellano T, Dergal E. Mechanism of the toxic action of carbon monoxide. *Ann Clin Lab Sci* 1976; **6:** 372–6.

11. Einhorn I N. Physiological and toxicological aspects of smoke produced during the combustion of polymeric materials. *Environ Health Perspect* 1975; **11:** 163–89.

12. Schulte J H. Effects of mild carbon monoxide intoxication. *Arch Environ Health* 1963; **7:** 524–30.

13. Charnock E L, Meehan J J. Postburn respiratory injuries in children. *Pediatr Clin North Am* 1980; **27:** 661–76.

14. Clark C J, Campbell D, Reid W H. Blood carboxyhaemoglobin and cyanide levels in fire survivors. *Lancet* 1981; **1:** 1332–5.

15. Crapo R O. Smoke-inhalation injuries. *JAMA* 1981; **246:** 1694–6.

16. Myers R A, Snyder S K, Linberg S, Cowley R A. Value of hyperbaric oxygen in suspected carbon monoxide poisoning. *JAMA* 1981; **246:** 2478–80.

17. Hart G B, Strauss M B, Lennon P A, Whitcraft D III. Treatment of smoke inhalation by hyperbaric oxygen. *J Emerg Med* 1985; **3:** 211–15.

18. Thom S R. Antagonism of carbon monoxide-mediated brain lipid peroxidation by hyperbaric oxygen. *Toxicol Appl Pharmacol* 1990; **105:** 340–4.

19. Brown S D, Piantadosi C A. Reversal of carbon monoxide-cytochrome c oxidase binding by hyperbaric oxygen in vivo. *Adv Exp Med Biol* 1989; **248:** 747–54.

20. Grube B J, Marvin J A, Heimbach D M. Therapeutic hyperbaric oxygen: help or hindrance in burn patients with carbon monoxide poisoning? *J Burn Care Rehabil* 1988; **9:** 249–52.

21. Purser D A, Grimshaw P, Berrill K R. Intoxication by cyanide in fires: a study in monkeys using polyacrylonitrile. *Arch Environ Health* 1984; **39:** 394–400.

22. Baud F J, Barriot P, Toffis V, *et al.* Elevated blood cyanide concentrations in victims of smoke inhalation. *N Engl J Med* 1991; **325:** 1761–6.

23. Kimmerle G. Aspects and methodology for the evaluation of toxicological parameters during fire exposure. In: *Polymer Conference Series: Flammability Characteristics of Materials.* Salt Lake City: University of Utah, 1973.

24. Smith P W, Crane R, Sanders D C, Abbott J K, Endocott B. Effects of exposure to carbon monoxide and hydrogen cyanide. In: *Physiological and Toxological Aspects of Combustion Products.* Washington DC: National Academy of Science, 1976: 75–8.

25. Becker C E. The role of cyanide in fires. *Vet Hum Toxicol* 1985; **27:** 487–90.

26. Moore S J, Norris J C, Walsh D A, Hume A S. Antidotal use of methemoglobin forming cyanide antagonists in concurrent carbon monoxide/cyanide intoxication. *J Pharmacol Exp Ther* 1987; **242:** 70–3.

27. Landis E M, Pappenheimer J R. Exchange of substances through the capillary walls. In: Hamilton W F, Dow P, eds. *Handbook of Physiology, Section 2, Vol. 2*. Baltimore, MD: Williams & Wilkins, 1963: 961–1034.

28. Starling E H. On the absorption of fluids from the connective tissue spaces. *J Physiol (Lond)* 1896; **19:** 312–26.

29. Oldham K T, Guice K S, Till G O, Ward P A. Activation of complement by hydroxyl radical in thermal injury. *Surgery* 1988; **104:** 272–9.

30. Friedl H P, Till G O, Trentz O, Ward P A. Roles of histamine, complement and xanthine oxidase in thermal injury of skin. *Am J Pathol* 1989; **135:** 203–17.

31. Ward P A, Till G O. Pathophysiologic events related to thermal injury of skin. *J Trauma* 1990; **30:** S75–S79.

32. Schlayer H J, Laaff H, Peters T, *et al*. Involvement of tumor necrosis factor in endotoxin-triggered neutrophil adherence to sinusoidal endothelial cells of mouse liver and its modulation in acute phase. *J Hepatol* 1988; **7:** 239–49.

33. Granger D N, McCord J M, Parks D A, Hollwarth M E. Xanthine oxidase inhibitors attenuate ischemia-induced vascular permeability changes in the cat intestine. *Gastroenterology* 1986; **90:** 80–4.

34. Granger D, Rutili G, McCord J. Superoxide radicals in feline intestinal ischemia. *Gastroenterology* 1981; **81:** 22–9.

35. Demling R H, LaLonde C. Topical ibuprofen decreases early postburn edema. *Surgery* 1987; **102:** 857–61.

36. Herndon D N, Abston S, Stein M D. Increased thromboxane B_2 levels in the plasma of burned and septic burned patients. *Surg Gynecol Obstet* 1984; **159:** 210–13.

37. Pitt R M, Parker J C, Jurkovich G J, Taylor A E, Curreri P W. Analysis of altered capillary pressure and permeability after thermal injury. *J Surg Res* 1987; **42:** 693–702.

38. Lund T, Wiig H, Reed R K. Acute postburn edema: role of strongly negative interstitial fluid pressure. *Am J Physiol* 1988; **255:** H1069–H1074.

39. Pitkanen J, Lund T, Aanderud L, Reed R K. Transcapillary colloid osmotic pressures in injured and non-injured skin of seriously burned patients. *Burns Incl Therm Inj* 1987; **13:** 198–203.

40. Lund T, Reed R K. Microvascular fluid exchange following thermal skin injury in the rat: changes in extravascular colloid osmotic pressure, albumin mass, and water content. *Circ Shock* 1986; **20:** 91–104.

41. Onarheim H, Reed R K. Thermal skin injury: effect of fluid therapy on the transcapillary colloid osmotic gradient. *J Surg Res* 1991; **50:** 272–8.

42. Zetterstrom H, Arturson G. Plasma oncotic pressure and plasma protein concentration in patients following thermal injury. *Acta Anaesthesiol Scand* 1980; **24:** 288–94.

43. Sheng Z Y, Tung Y L. Neutrophil chemiluminescence in burned patients. *J Trauma* 1987; **27:** 587–95.

44. Conhaim R L, Harms B A. A simplified two-pore filtration model explains the effects of hypoproteinemia on lung and soft tissue lymph flux in awake sheep. *Microvasc Res* 1992; **44:** 14–26.

45. Calhoun K H, Deskin R W, Garza C, *et al*. Long-term airway sequelae in a pediatric burn population. *Laryngoscope* 1988; **98:** 721–5.

46. Honeycutt D, Traber L, Toole D, Herndon D, Traber D. Colloid resuscitation of *ovine* burn shock. *Circ Shock* 1991; **31:** 72.

47. Demling R H, Kramer G C, Gunther R, Nerlich M. Effect of nonprotein colloid on postburn edema, formation in soft tissues and lung. *Surgery* 1984; **95:** 593–602.

48. Morikawa T. Acrolein, formaldehyde, and volatile fatty acids from smoldering combustion. *J Combust Toxicol* 1976; **3:** 135–51.

49. Zikria B A, Ferrer J M, Floch H F. The chemical factors contributing to pulmonary damage in 'Smoke poisoning'. *Surgery* 1972; **71:** 704–9.

50. Dost F N. Acute toxicology of components of vegetation smoke. *Rev Environ Contam Toxicol* 1991; **119:** 1–46.

51. Moritz A R, Henriques F C, McLean R. The effect of inhaled heat on the air passages and lungs: an experimental investigation. *Am J Pathol* 1945; **21:** 311–26.

52. Hubbard G B, Langlinais P C, Shimazu T, Okerberg C V, Mason A D, Pruitt B A. The morphology of smoke inhalation injury in sheep. *J Trauma* 1991; **31:** 1477–86.

53. Abdi S, Evans M J, Cox R A, Lubbesmeyer H, Herndon D N, Traber D L. Inhalation injury to tracheal epithelium in an ovine model of cotton smoke exposure. Early phase (30 minutes). *Am Rev Respir Dis* 1990; **142:** 1436–9.

54. Barrow R E, Wang C Z, Cox R A, Evans M J. Cellular sequence of tracheal repair in sheep after smoke inhalation injury. *Lung* 1992; **170:** 331–8.

55. Kramer G C, Herndon D N, Linares H A, Traber D L. Effects of inhalation injury on airway blood flow and edema formation. *J Burn Care Rehabil* 1989; **10:** 45–51.

56. Stothert J C Jr, Ashley K D, Kramer G C, *et al*. Intrapulmonary distribution of bronchial blood flow after moderate smoke inhalation. *J Appl Physiol* 1990; **69:** 1734–9.

57. Abdi S, Herndon D, Mcguire J, Traber L, Traber D L. Time course of alterations in lung lymph and bronchial blood flows after inhalation injury. *J Burn Care Rehabil* 1990; **11:** 510–15.

58. Loick H M, Traber L D, Hurst C, Herndon D N, Traber D L. Endoscopic laser flowmetry: a valid method for detection and quantitative analysis of inhalation injury. *J Burn Care Rehabil* 1991; **12:** 313–18.

59. Hales C A, Barkin P, Jung W, Quinn D, Lamborghini D, Burke J. Bronchial artery ligation modifies pulmonary edema after exposure to smoke with acrolein. *J Appl Physiol* 1989; **67:** 1001–6.

60. Ashley K D, Stothert J C Jr, Traber D L, Traber L D, Kramer G, Herndon D. Airway blood flow following light and heavy smoke inhalation injury. *Surg Forum* 1990; **41:** 293–5.

61. Barrow R E, Morris S E, Basadre J O, Herndon D N. Selective permeability changes in the lungs and airways of sheep after toxic smoke inhalation. *J Appl Physiol* 1990; **68:** 2165–70.

62. Pruitt B A, Cioffi W G, Shimazu T, Ikeuchi H, Mason A D. Evaluation and management of patients with inhalation injury. *J Trauma* 1990; **30:** S63–S68.

63. Lund T, Goodwin C W, McManus W F, *et al*. Upper airway sequelae in burn patients requiring endotracheal intubation or tracheostomy. *Ann Surg* 1985; **201:** 374–82.

64. Moylan J A, Adib K, Birnbaum M. Fiberoptic bronchoscopy following thermal injury. *Surg Gynecol Obstet* 1975; **140:** 541–3.

65. Herndon D N, Traber L D, Linares H, *et al*. Etiology of the pulmonary pathophysiology associated with inhalation injury. *Resuscitation* 1986; **14:** 43–59.

66. Mathru M, Venus B, Rao T, Matsuda T. Noncardiac pulmonary edema precipitated by tracheal intubation in patients with injury. *Crit Care Med* 1983; **11:** 804–6.

67. Traber D L, Herndon D N, Stein M D, Traber L D, Flynn J T, Niehaus G D. The pulmonary lesion of smoke inhalation in an ovine model. *Circ Shock* 1986; **8:** 311–23.

68. Prien T, Traber D L, Richardson J A, Traber L D. Early effects of inhalation injury on lung mechanics and pulmonary perfusion. *Intensive Care Med* 1988; **14:** 25–9.

69. Stenton S C, Kelly C A, Walters E H, Hendrick D J. Induction of bronchial hyperresponsiveness following smoke inhalation injury. *Br J Dis Chest* 1988; **82:** 436–8.

70. Petroff P A, Hander E W, Clayton W H, Pruitt B A. Pulmonary function studies after smoke inhalation. *Am J Surg* 1976; **132:** 346–51.

71. Pruitt B A, Erickson D R, Morris A. Progressive pulmonary insufficiency and other pulmonary complications of thermal injury. *J Trauma* 1975; **15:** 369–79.

72. Lippton H, Goff J, Hyman A. Effects of endothelin in the systemic and renal vascular beds in vivo. *Eur J Pharmacol* 1988; **155:** 197–9.

73. Traber D L, Linares H A, Herndon D N, Prien T. The pathophysiology of inhalation injury – a review. *Burns Incl Therm Inj* 1988; **14:** 357–64.

74. Toor A H, Tomashefski J F, Kleinerman J. Respiratory tract pathology in patients with severe burns. *Hum Pathol* 1990; **21:** 1212–20.

75. Wang C Z, Evans M J, Cox R A, *et al*. Morphologic changes in basal cells during repair of tracheal epithelium. *Am J Pathol* 1992; **141:** 753–9.

76. Traber L D, Herndon D N, Abdi S, Traber D L. Histamine does not mediate the increase in bronchial blood flow during inhalation injury. *FASEB J* 1990; **4:** A575 (Abstract).

77. Abdi S, Traber L D, Herndon D N, Traber D L. Ibuprofen does not attenuate the increase in bronchial blood flow after inhalation injury. *Am Rev Respir Dis* 1991; **143:** A785 (Abstract).

78. Abdi S, Maguire J P, Herndon D N, Traber L D, Traber D L. Lidocaine attenuates bronchial artery response to inhalation trauma. *Crit Care Med* 1990; **18:** S200 (Abstract).

79. Martling C R, Matran R, Alving K, Lacroix J S, Lundberg J M. Vagal vasodilatory mechanisms in the pig bronchial circulation preferentially involves sensory nerves. *Neurosci Lett* 1989; **96:** 306–11.

80. Martling C R, Matran R, Alving K, Hokfelt T, Lundberg J M. Innervation of lower airways and neuropeptide effects on bronchial and vascular tone in the pig. *Cell Tissue Res* 1990; **260:** 223–33.

81. Matran R, Alving K, Martling C R, Lacroix J S, Lundberg J M. Effects of neuropeptides and capsaicin on tracheobronchial blood flow of the pig. *Acta Physiol Scand* 1989; **135:** 335–42.

82. Lundberg J M, Martling C R, Saria A, Folkers K, Rosell S. Cigarette smoke-induced airway oedema due to activation of capsaicin-sensitive vagal afferents and substance P release. *Neuroscience* 1983; **10:** 1361–8.

83. Traber L D, Herndon D N, Turner J, Sant Ambrogio G, Traber D L. Peptide mediation of the bronchial blood flow elevation following inhalation injury. *Circ Shock* 1990; **31:** 13 (Abstract).

84. Prien T, Traber L D, Herndon D N, Stothert J C, Jr, Lübbesmeyer H J, Traber D L. Pulmonary edema with smoke inhalation, undetected by indicator-dilution technique. *J Appl Physiol* 1987; **63:** 907–11.

85. Loick H M, Traber L D, Theissen J L, Flynn J, Traber D L. Effect of thromboxane receptor blockade following inhalation injury in sheep. *Anesthesiology* 1991; **75:** A224 (Abstract).

86. Loick H M, Traber L D, Stothert J C Jr, Herndon D N, Traber D L. Smoke inhalation causes an increase in bronchial blood flow and edema in primarly uninjured lung areas. *FASEB J* 1992; **6:** A1818.

87. Charan N B, Turk G M, Dhand R. Gross and subgross anatomy of bronchial circulation in sheep. *J Appl Physiol* 1984; **57:** 658–64.

88. Charan N B, Turk G M, Czartolomny J, Andreazuk T. Systemic arterial blood supply to the trachea and lung in sheep. *J Appl Physiol* 1987; **62:** 2283–7.

89. Lakshminarayan S, Kowalski T F, Kirk W, Graham M M, Butler J. The drainage routes of the bronchial blood flow in anesthetized dogs. *Respir Physiol* 1990; **82:** 65–73.

90. Traber D L, Schlag G, Redl H, Traber L D. Pulmonary edema and compliance changes following smoke inhalation. *J Burn Care Rehabil* 1985; **6:** 490–4.

91. Kimura R, Traber L D, Herndon D N, Linares H A, Lübbesmeyer H J, Traber D L. Increasing duration of smoke exposure induces more severe lung injury in sheep. *J Appl Physiol* 1988; **64:** 1107–13.

92. Sugi K, Theissen J L, Traber L D, Herndon D N, Traber D L. Impact of carbon monoxide on cardiopulmonary dysfunction after smoke inhalation injury. *Circ Res* 1990; **66:** 69–75.

93. Isago T, Fujioka K, Traber L D, Herndon D N, Traber D L. Derived pulmonary capillary pressure changes after smoke inhalation in sheep. *Crit Care Med* 1991; **19:** 1407–13.

94. Holloway H, Perry M, Downey J, Parker J, Taylor A. Estimation of effective pulmonary capillary pressure in intact lungs. *J Appl Physiol* 1983; **54** (3): 846–51.

95. Isago T, Traber L D, Herndon D N, Abdi S, Fujioka K, Traber D L. Determination of pulmonary microvascular reflection coefficient in sheep by venous occlusion. *J Appl Physiol*; **69:** 2311–16.

96. Isago T, Noshima S, Traber L D, Herndon D N, Traber D L. Analysis of pulmonary microvascular permeability after smoke inhalation. *J Appl Physiol* 1991; **71:** 1403–8.

97. Demling R H, LaLonde C. Moderate smoke inhalation produces decreased oxygen delivery, increased oxygen demands, and systemic but not lung parenchymal lipid peroxidation. *Surgery* 1990; **108:** 544–52.

98. Loick H M, Traber L D, Tokyay R, Linares H A, Prien T, Traber D L. Mechanical alteration of blood flow in smoked and unsmoked lung areas after inhalation injury. *J Appl Physiol* 1992; **72:** 1692–700.

99. Isago T, Traber L D, Herndon D N, Traber D L. Pulmonary capillary pressure changes following smoke inhalation in sheep. *Anesthesiology* 1990; **73:** A1234.

100. Basadre J O, Sugi K, Traber D L, Traber L D, Niehaus G D, Herndon D N. The effect of leukocyte depletion on smoke inhalation injury in sheep. *Surgery* 1988; **104:** 208–15.

101. Niehaus G D, Kimura R, Traber L D, Herndon D N, Flynn J T, Traber D L. Administration of a synthetic antiprotease reduces smoke-induced lung injury. *J Appl Physiol* 1990; **69:** 694–9.

102. Brown M, Desai M, Traber L D, Herndon D N, Traber D L. Dimethylsulfoxide with heparin in the treatment of smoke inhalation injury. *J Burn Care Rehabil* 1988; **9:** 22–5.

103. Kimura R, Traber L D, Herndon D N, *et al.* Treatment of smoke-induced pulmonary injury with nebulized dimethylsulfoxide with heparin in the treatment of smoke inhalation injury. *Circ Shock* 1988; **9:** 22–5.

104. Nguyen T T, Herndon D N, Cox C S, *et al.* Effect of manganous superoxide dismutase on lung fluid balance after smoke inhalation injury. *J Appl Physiol* 1995; **78:** 2161–8.

105. Carlin G, Arfors K E. Peroxidation of liposomes promoted by human polymorphonuclear leucocytes. *J Free Radic Biol Med* 1985; **1:** 437–42.

106. Guice K S, Oldham K T, Caty M G, Johnson K J, Ward P A. Neutrophil-dependent, oxygen-radical mediated lung injury associated with acute pancreatitis. *Ann Surg* 1989; **210:** 740–7.

107. Hales C A, Barkin P W, Jung W, *et al.* Synthetic smoke with acrolein but not HCl produces pulmonary edema. *J Appl Physiol* 1988; **64:** 1121–33.

108. Magno M G, Fishman A P. Origin, distribution, and blood flow of bronchial circulation in anesthetized sheep. *J Appl Physiol* 1982; **53:** 272–9.

109. Abdi S, Herndon D N, Traber L D, *et al.* Lung edema formation following inhalation injury: role of the bronchial blood flow. *J Appl Physiol* 1991; **71:** 727–34.

110. Hinder F, Nakazawa H, Matsumoto N, Traber L D, Herndon D N, Traber D L. Separation of the bronchial circulation from the pulmonary in a left lung pouch model. *Am Rev Respir Dis* 1993; **147:** A657.

111. Prien T, Linares H A, Traber L D, Herndon D N, Traber D L. Lack of hematogenous mediated pulmonary injury with smoke inhalation. *J Burn Care Rehabil* 1988; **9:** 462–6.

112. Dinarello C A. The proinflammatory cytokines interleukin-1 and tumor necrosis factor and treatment of the septic shock syndrome. *J Infect Dis* 1991; **163:** 1177–84.

113. Cerra F B. The multiple organ failure syndrome. *Hosp Pract [Off]* 1990; **25:** 169–76.

114. Navar P D, Saffle J R, Warden G D. Effect of inhalation injury on fluid resuscitation requirements after thermal injury. *Am J Surg* 1985; **150:** 716–20.

115. Herndon D N, Barrow R E, Traber D L, Rutan T C, Rutan R L, Abston S. Extravascular lung water changes following smoke inhalation and massive burn injury. *Surgery* 1987; **102:** 341–9.

116. Demling R H, Smith M, Gunther R, Wandzilak T, Pederson N C. Use of a chronic prefemoral lymphatic fistula for monitoring systemic capillary integrity in unanesthetized sheep. *J Surg Res* 1981; **31:** 136–44.

117. Montero K, Lübbesmeyer H J, Traber D L, Kimura R, Traber L D, Herndon D N. Inhalation injury increases systemic microvascular permeability. *Surg Forum* 1987; **38:** 303–5.

118. La Londe C, Knox J, Youn Y K, Demling R. Burn edema is accentuated by a moderate smoke inhalation injury in sheep. *Surgery* 1992; **112:** 908–17.

119. Traber D L, Sugi K, Flynn J T, Traber L D. Leukotrienes and lung response to inhalation injury. *FASEB J* 1989; **3:** A695.

120. Quinn D A, Robinson D, Jung W, Hales C A. Role of sulfidopeptide leukotrienes in synthetic smoke inhalation injury in sheep. *J Appl Physiol* 1990; **68:** 1962–9.

121. Morris S E, Navaratnam N, Townsend C M Jr, Herndon D N. Bacterial translocation and mesenteric blood flow in a large animal model after cutaneous thermal and smoke inhalation injury. *Surg Forum* 1988; **39:** 189–90.

122. Lundberg J M, Saria A. Bronchial smooth muscle contraction induced by stimulation of capsaicin-sensitive sensory neurons. *Acta Physiol Scand* 1982; **116:** 473–6.

123. Ahn S Y, Sugi K, Talke P, *et al.* Effects of allopurinol on smoke inhalation in the ovine model. *J Appl Physiol* 1990; **68:** 228–34.

124. Newald J, Sugi K, Vogl C, Krosl P, Traber D L, Schlag G. Evaluation of heart performance during septic shock in sheep. *Prog Clin Biol Res* 1989; **308:** 237–45.

125. Goldman G, Welbourn R, Kobzik L, Valeri C R, Shepro D, Hechtman H B. Tumor necrosis factor-alpha mediates acid aspiration-induced systemic organ injury. *Ann Surg* 1990; **212:** 513–19.

126. Goldman G, Welbourn R, Kobzik L, Valeri C R, Shepro D, Hechtman H B. Synergism between leukotriene B_4 and thromboxane A_2 in mediating acid-aspiration injury. *Surgery* 1992; **111:** 55–61.

127. Noshima S, Fujioka K, Isago T, Traber L D, Herndon D N, Traber D L. The effect of a thromboxane synthetase inhibitor, OKY-046, on cardiopulmonary function after smoke inhalation injury. *FASEB J* 1991; **5:** A371.

CHAPTER SEVENTEEN

17

Diagnosis and Treatment of Inhalation Injury

JOHN C. FITZPATRICK AND WILLIAM G. CIOFFI, JR

Introduction

The two most critical injuries caused by fires are cutaneous burns and inhalation injury. The multitude of respiratory complications caused by smoke inhalation, cutaneous burns, and their treatment epitomize the clinical challenge which confronts burn care providers today. Of 1256 patients treated at the US Army Institute of Surgical Research from 1985 through 1990, 330 (26%) sustained a significant inhalation injury,[1] with 97 of the 330 patients (29.4%) succumbing to their injuries. Inhalation injury is an acute respiratory tract insult caused by steam or toxic inhalants such as fumes, gases, and mists. Fumes consist of small particles dispersed in air with various irritants or cytotoxic chemicals adherent to the particles. Mists consist of aerosolized irritant or cytotoxic liquids. Smoke consists of a combination of fumes, gases, mists, and hot air. Inhalation injury may occur independently from cutaneous burn injury, although they usually occur together. The injury is notable both for its inhomogenous distribution within a patient and its variable severity between patients. The physicochemical properties of the causative agent, the amount of smoke inhaled, and pre-existing diseases which might decrease the resistance of the recipient to injury determine the site and degree of injury.

Despite increasing clinical interest in the problem of inhalation injury over the past few decades, the pathophysiology of inhalation injury remains poorly understood and few improvements in treatment have occurred. Inhalation injury continues to be one of the most serious associated injuries complicating the care of thermally injured patients today. Early diagnosis of inhalation injury and prevention or treatment of the associated life-threatening complications are necessary in order to decrease the morbidity and mortality related to inhalation injury.

The respiratory tract may be divided into three anatomical regions: the supraglottic, tracheobronchial (major airways), and lung parenchymal regions. Inhalation injury may occur in any region. The site of injury determines the diagnostic and therapeutic needs of the patient. Tracheobronchial and parenchymal injuries constitute the majority of injuries which require prolonged treatment. Supraglottic injuries are caused by both thermal and chemical means and may be so severe that upper airway obstruction occurs quickly. The presence of a supraglottic injury is not a reliable indicator of the presence (or absence) of more distal pulmonary injuries.

Several forms of pulmonary dysfunction may result from the complex pathophysiologic reactions to inhalation injury. Hypoxia, V_A/Q mismatching, increased airway resistance, decreased pulmonary compliance, and increased pulmonary vascular resistance may result from the initial release of vasoactive substances from the damaged epithelium. Immediately after sustaining the inhalation injury, these changes are probably the result of edema formation and release of smooth muscle constrictors such as thromboxane A_2, C3a, and C5a. The tracheobronchial mucociliary apparatus (responsible for clearing foreign material from the respiratory tract) is damaged and nonfunctional. Further epithelial injury results from the toxic inhalants which are present and no longer being removed. Sloughed necrotic epithelium, serous exudate, blood cells and mucus form casts which may cause atelectasis and exacerbate V_A/Q mismatching and hypoxia. Air trapping which occurs distal to obstruction caused by casts may occur, resulting in barotrauma; alternatively, total occlusion of the airways by casts will produce atelectasis and increase the risk of pneumonia.[2]

Frequently patients with inhalation injury develop respiratory failure and require mechanical ventilatory support. Decreased compliance and increased airway resistance may lead to elevated airway pressures and barotrauma, a sometimes unavoidable complication of the use of positive pressure ventilation. Mean airway pressures exceeding the mucosal capillary perfusion pressure may result in ischemia of the already damaged tracheobronchial mucosa, compounding the initial epithelial insult. Overdistension of the normal alveoli leads to alveolar interstitial edema which aggravates the extent of atelectasis, decrement in compliance, and increased V_A/Q mismatch which was caused by the initial injury. Increasing amounts of mucosal slough, interstitial edema and decreasing compliance lead to further elevation in ventilatory pressures and worsening barotrauma, as well as increased likelihood of the development of pneumonia. Multiple organ system failure may develop as a result of perpetuation or exacerbation of the inflammatory process.

Diagnosis

A high index of suspicion for inhalation injury is essential in order to avoid missed injuries. A history of closed space smoke exposure is common among patients with inhalation injury, as is concurrent cutaneous burn injury. Many patients are intoxicated at the time of admission to a hospital and will admit to ethanol or drug use immediately before the time of injury. Most will present with some combination of the symptoms and signs listed in **Table 17.1**.

Table 17.1 Symptoms and signs suggesting possible inhalation injury

Symptoms	Signs
Lacrimation	Conjunctivitis
Severe brassy cough	Carbonaceous sputum
Hoarseness	Facial burns
Shortness of breath	Singed nasal vibrissae
Anxiety	Stridor
Wheezing	Bronchorrhea
	Dyspnea
	Disorientation
	Obtundation
	Coma

The physical findings of inhalation injury causing the greatest concern are hoarseness and stridor. Patients presenting with these findings have partial airway obstruction (usually secondary to edema) and are at substantial risk of complete airway obstruction. This group of patients should be intubated so as to maintain airway patency and avoid catastrophic airway obstruction. Disorientation, obtundation, and coma commonly indicate a significant exposure to carbon monoxide (CO) or the presence of an associated closed head injury. Patients with any suggestion of cranial trauma by history or physical examination will require cervical spine precautions when being moved. Their initial evaluation, as well as the evaluation of patients with initially elevated carboxyhemoglobin levels which do not clinically improve as their carboxyhemoglobin (COHb) levels return to normal, should include both cervical spine films and cranial computed tomography in order to rule out cervical or intracranial trauma.

Carbon monoxide exposure is common among patients with inhalation injury and is responsible for the deaths of most victims found dead at the scene of a fire. The diagnosis is made by direct measurement of the blood carboxyhemoglobin level using a co-oximeter on the admission arterial blood gas. Carbon monoxide displaces oxygen from the four binding sites available on the hemoglobin molecule, and has a much greater affinity for these sites than oxygen. Displacement of oxygen from the binding sites decreases the oxygen carrying capacity of blood in a linear manner and results in inadequate oxygen delivery to the tissues. Measurements of arterial oxygen tension and noninvasive hemoglobin saturation monitoring do not reflect the percentage of carboxyhemoglobin present, and, in fact, may be expected to be normal despite lethal carboxyhemoglobin levels in a fire victim.

Although a majority (56%) of patients with inhalation injury will present with some combination (usually three or more)[3] of history and physical findings indicative of inhalation injury, the specificity (and sometimes sensitivity) of these findings is poor. The inability of clinicians to depend on historical details and physical findings to identify patients with inhalation injury requires the use of fiberoptic bronchoscopy and intravenous xenon-133 ventilation scanning in order to establish the diagnosis. The use of fiberoptic bronchoscopy also allows immediate institution of therapy if severe inhalation injury or impending airway obstruction is diagnosed. Nasotracheal intubation may be conveniently performed under direct visualization over the bronchoscope if the bronchoscope is placed through an appropriately sized endotracheal tube before the procedure.

Fiberoptic bronchoscopy permits a clinician to perform a detailed examination of the supraglottic area and identify patients with marked edema who are at risk for acute airway obstruction and require immediate endotracheal intubation in order to maintain airway patency. Careful examination of the major airways allows the diagnosis of tracheobronchial inhalation injury to be made based on the presence of infraglottic soot or early inflammatory changes (hyperemia, edema, superficial mucosal sloughing, and ulceration) of the tracheal mucosa. These changes often are present before arterial blood gas abnormalities, deteriorating pulmonary function tests, or respiratory failure signal the presence of inhalation injury. The best examination is obtained in patients who are euvolemic and normotensive; hypotensive and hypovolemic patients sometimes do not demonstrate hyperemia and edema, and sloughing or ulceration may not be present in the first few hours after the injury occurs. Under ideal conditions, the accuracy of the examination approaches 100%, while in general use, the accuracy is approximately 87%.[4]

The technique of performing fiberoptic bronchoscopy in patients suspected of having inhalation injury is the same as that used during standard diagnostic bronchoscopy for other diseases. Meticulous attention to the need for good topical anesthesia, both supraglottic and infraglottic, makes the examination tolerable for the patient. When adequate local anesthesia has been achieved in a cooperative patient, intravenous sedation is rarely necessary. Spray bottles of lidocaine or similar agents are particularly useful in anesthetizing the supraglottic area; for anesthesia of the glottis and infraglottic area, 0.5% or 1% injectable plain lidocaine may be instilled through the biopsy channel of the bronchoscope in 3–5 ml aliquots. The use of video endoscopy equipment, especially in teaching institutions, allows observers to learn proper bronchoscopic technique and the gross pathologic appearance of the injury and, in any institution, it allows support personnel to anticipate the needs of the endoscopist, thus directly benefiting the patient.

When experienced personnel perform bronchoscopy in appropriately monitored settings, complications are rare. Excellent large retrospective[5,6] and prospective[7] studies of the risk of bronchoscopy have been published. The risk of major complications, such as death (0.01–0.6%), pneumonia (0.01–0.6%), pneumothorax (0.2–0.4%), hypoxia (0.2%), cardiac arrhythmia (0.6–0.9%) and nausea or vomiting (0.2%), is small. Many of the minor risks of bronchoscopy quoted in these studies, such as hemoptysis, are related to the use of brushes and biopsy forceps, and rarely occur during bronchoscopy for the diagnosis of inhalation injury. The risks of bronchoscopy are sufficiently small in comparison to the risks of delayed treatment for patients with injury, or the risks of iatrogenic complications for patients without injury who might erroneously receive mechanical ventilation, to support the use of bronchoscopy either to confirm or refute the diagnosis in all patients suspected of having inhalation injury.

Intravenous xenon-133 ventilation/perfusion scanning is a means of identifying regions of complete or incomplete small airway obstruction secondary to inhalation injury. After injection of the radionuclide, serial scans demonstrate respiratory exchange and excretion of xenon by the lungs. Areas retaining isotope for more than 90 seconds are presumed to have segmental airway obstruction secondary to inhalation injury. False-positive examinations may occur in patients with a prior history of chronic obstructive pulmonary disease, those who have a chemical tracheobronchitis or pneumonia from aspiration of gastric contents, or those with preexisting respiratory tract infections or pneumonia before smoke exposure. Although not as frequently performed as bronchoscopy, xenon-133 scanning is still useful as a complementary examination, particularly when clinical suspicion is high that inhalation injury has occurred but bronchoscopic examination fails to confirm its presence. The combination of bronchoscopy and xenon-133 scanning is 93% accurate in the diagnosis of smoke inhalation injury.

Pulmonary function tests are useful for the long-term follow-up of inhalation injury. Unfortunately, they are less useful in making an early diagnosis of inhalation injury because they are effort dependent, and it is frequently difficult to obtain reliable and reproducible results in the acute setting. Pain, weakness, dyspnea, or narcotic administration may adversely affect the ability of a patient to comply with testing and, thus, complicate the interpretation of the tests. Despite these concerns, pulmonary function tests are useful for their negative predictive value (94–100%)[8] and low cost when triaging large numbers of victims to identify those who may require additional diagnostic procedures. Normal pulmonary function tests essentially rule out the possibility of significant inhalation injury. The FEV_1/FVC ratio is a sensitive early marker for airway obstruction. In patients able to comply with testing, the magnitude of decrement in this ratio in comparison to the predicted normal value correlates well with the severity of injury. Flow–volume and pressure–volume loops also have utility during long-term follow-up for assessing lung compliance in patients with restrictive fibrosis and changes in chest wall compliance in those with extensive thoracic cage skin grafts.

MANAGEMENT

Although there are many causes of inhalation injury, initial therapy consists of a few commonsense measures to stabilize the patient and confirm the diagnosis; and subsequent treatment (with the exception of specific treatments for poisonings) is supportive. Careful and repeated evaluation of therapeutic interventions is necessary in order to prevent iatrogenic injuries (barotrauma, suction catheter trauma) which perpetuate the inflammatory process and prevent healing. Conservative approaches to the management of inhalation injury stress the use of measures to avoid intubation and positive pressure ventilation; and if ventilatory support is necessary, permissive hypercapnia and borderline adequacy of oxygenation are preferable to attaining arbitrarily 'normal' blood gases at the cost of inflicting barotrauma and volutrauma.

Initial stabilization follows the standard principles of management of trauma and burn patients. First, the patient must be removed from the danger area by persons sufficiently knowledgeable and appropriately equipped to prevent further injury to the patient or to themselves. For patients sustaining both cutaneous burns and inhalation injury, the rescuer must make sure that the burning process has been stopped. A patent airway must be maintained. In most patients, airway obstruction develops gradually; but if obstruction is present when the patient is first seen, it must be relieved immediately by oropharyngeal sweep, oropharyngeal or nasopharyngeal airway, or airway intubation by endotracheal tube, or (rarely) cricothyroidotomy. After adequate ventilation and circulation have been obtained, supplemental 100% oxygen should be administered while the patient is being transported to the nearest appropriate medical treatment facility. Intravenous access should be secured and appropriate fluid resuscitation initiated.

The patient should be assessed for other life-threatening injuries while a pertinent history is obtained and a physical examination is expeditiously performed. Pertinent facts to be obtained are listed in **Table 17.2**. Baseline laboratory studies should be obtained, including arterial blood gases, a chest roentgenogram, and an electrocardiogram. Although the studies may be normal early after sustaining an inhalation injury, they serve as a useful baseline against which subsequent studies may be compared. Direct inspection of the airway by fiberoptic bronchoscopy should be performed if the patient is breathing spontaneously and has a history of smoke exposure and symptoms or signs suggesting possible inhalation injury (see **Table 17.1**), or in any patient requiring ventilatory assistance, to confirm or refute the presence of inhalation injury. Early intubation under semiurgent circumstances in order to protect the airway is preferable to delaying until airway obstruction is so severe that intubation under emergency circumstances is necessary. The natural history of upper airway edema results in maximal edema and peak airway narrowing at approximately 24 hours post-injury. If edema is not present on admission, a period of observation in an intensive care unit is warranted.

Table 17.2 Important injury site characteristics and transport details

Type of materials and fuels ignited
Type of toxic inhalant
Closed space vs. open space exposure
Duration of exposure
Use of supplemental oxygen
Transport time to hospital
Mental status
Evidence of intoxication

Most patients sustaining an inhalation injury will also have sustained a cutaneous thermal injury. The presence of a thermal injury requires appropriate fluid resuscitation to avoid hypovolemic shock, renal failure, and death in the early postburn period. The endpoint of resuscitation is not changed by the presence of an inhalation injury; a urine output of 30–50 ml/h in adults or 0.5–1 ml/kg/h in children weighing 30 kg or less is the best indication at this time that appropriate fluid resuscitation is being administered to the patient. It is common for patients with both inhalation injury and cutaneous thermal injury to require more resuscitation fluid than patients with cutaneous thermal injury alone in order to achieve adequate resuscitation. Several retrospective clinical reviews[9–13] have shown that coexisting inhalation injury increases the fluid resuscitation requirements of patients with cutaneous thermal injury, particularly in the first 24 hours, by 40–75% (range 13.5–110%) in comparison to patients without inhalation injury. A prospective animal study[14] demonstrated that inadequate fluid resuscitation following smoke inhalation injury was detrimental. A group of sheep resuscitated with intravenous fluid infused at a normal maintenance rate following severe smoke inhalation injury experienced significantly increased lung lymph flow, elevated lymph to plasma oncotic pressure, decreased arterial oxygen pressure (Pao_2), decreased cardiac output, and increased mortality (100% versus 30%) in comparison with a group of sheep with an identical smoke inhalation injury resuscitated with intravenous fluid infused at twice the normal maintenance rate. The data indicate that the practice of limiting fluid resuscitation 'to protect the lung' may actually lead to increased extravascular lung water, hypoxia, and decrements in lung function, along with the risks of inadequate tissue perfusion, renal failure, and possible death from hypovolemic shock.

For patients exposed only to simple asphyxiants (carbon dioxide, helium, methane, nitrogen) no evidence of supraglottic or tracheobronchial mucosal injury will be found, and little else can be provided than supportive care. Serial neurological examinations should be performed with all deficits carefully documented so as to allow for objective assessment of the patient's prognosis. If the anoxic period was short and no permanent neurological damage occurred, recovery is to be expected.

For patients with inhalation injury secondary to carbon monoxide exposure, it is important to establish the carboxyhemoglobin level on admission, both to estimate length of treatment for carbon monoxide exposure and for calculation of the peak carboxyhemoglobin level, which in animal models has been shown to correlate with the presence of inhalation injury.[15] It should be noted, however, that a low or normal carboxyhemoglobin level does not rule out the presence of inhalation injury. Patients should receive 100% oxygen until their carboxyhemoglobin level is less than 0%. The elimination half-life ($t_{1/2}$) for carboxyhemoglobin is dependent on oxygen tension. The $t_{1/2}$ for carboxyhemoglobin at sea level is 250 minutes while breathing room air (20.8% oxygen), 40–50 minutes breathing 100% oxygen,[16,17] and 27 minutes breathing 100% oxygen at 2 atmospheres pressure.[18]

There is much controversy regarding the indications for, and efficacy of, hyperbaric oxygen administration. Some proponents recommend the use of hyperbaric oxygen in order to prevent certain neurological complications (blindness, deafness, psychosis, and Parkinson's disease) reputedly due to carbon monoxide poisoning, although the correlation of those changes with carboxyhemoglobin level is poor.[19,20] Physiologic monitoring of patients in hyperbaric chambers is difficult due to the risk of the fire and the effect of pressure on solid state electrical components. Small chambers isolate the patient from physicians and nursing staff; large chambers require exposure of physicians and nursing staff to the risks of 'diving' with the patient. One study reported significant severe complications related to hyperbaric treatment (cardiac arrest, seizures, cardiac arrhythmia) in 7 of 10 patients,[21] leaving open the question of whether the potential benefits outweigh the documented risks associated with hyperbaric oxygen. At this time, except for symptomatic patients (coma, seizures, respiratory failure) with very high carboxyhemoglobin levels for whom the benefits may outweigh the risks of therapy, hyperbaric oxygen should be restricted to randomized prospective trials aimed at determining the efficacy of this therapy for specific groups of patients.

Specific therapy for cyanide poisoning in patients with inhalation injury is also controversial, as there is no consensus on the incidence of clinically important cyanide exposure. Proponents of therapy point out the increased incidence of fires involving polyurethanes, which produce large amounts of hydrogen cyanide (HCN). Opponents cite the lack of correlation between cyanide levels and mortality in fire victims. For adequately resuscitated patients with unexplained severe metabolic acidosis, tachycardia, tachypnea, elevated central venous oxygen content, and normal arterial oxygen content, treatment should be considered. Cyanide uncouples oxidative phosphorylation by binding to mitochondrial cytochrome a–a_3. The goal of therapy is to create a sink of ferric iron which will trap the cyanide until it can be converted to thiocyanate through the actions of the hepatic enzyme rhodanase. The most convenient sink is hemoglobin; administration of amyl and sodium nitrite, which convert the ferrous iron in heme to the ferric form, accelerates the formation of cyanhemoglobin. Both agents are potent vasodilators, however, which limits their use to normotensive or hypertensive patients. Sodium thiosulfate is administered to insure that sufficient sulfur substrate is available to rhodanase for conversion of cyanate (CN) to thiocyanate (SCN), which is excreted by the kidney.

Except for therapy to counteract the effects of specific toxins as described above, the care of patients with inhalation injury is supportive. Despite the lack of specific interventions, assiduous supportive care is essential for decreasing the morbidity and mortality resulting both from complications of the initial injury and iatrogenic injury which is caused by necessary treatment. Treatment algorithms for patients with mild, moderate, and severe inhalation injury are shown in **Table 17.3**. Once the security of the airway has been established and the patient has been placed on supplemental oxygen, priority should be given to minimizing airway edema, maintaining pulmonary toilet, relieving mechanical restriction of chest wall motion, and treating bronchospasm so as to reduce the patient's work of breathing and minimize the need for mechanical ventilation. Elevation of the head of the bed to 30° helps to decrease airway edema and minimizes pressure from abdominal contents which limits diaphragmatic excursion. If the patient has cutaneous burns, appropriate resuscitation must be carried out regardless of the presence of inhalation injury and the possibility that the resulting airway edema may necessitate intubation. Respiratory failure is much easier to treat and much less morbid than persistent hypovolemic shock and renal failure. Circumferential full-thickness burns of the thorax which mechanically limit chest wall excursion require escharotomies to be placed in the anterior axillary lines bilaterally and connected by a transverse incision at the costal margin. These escharotomies may allow some patients to avoid the need for mechanical ventilatory support; in those requiring ventilatory support, escharotomies help minimize pressure generated during ventilator cycles and, thus, avoid iatrogenic barotrauma.

Airway clearance techniques are an essential component of respiratory management of patients with smoke inhalation injury. Therapeutic coughing, chest physiotherapy, early ambulation, airway suctioning, and pharmacologic agents all may be effective in mobilizing and removing retained secretions. Secretions which the

Table 17.3 Treatment algorithms for pathophysiologic events resulting from mild, moderate, and severe inhalation injury

Problem	Diagnostic/treatment	Seen in
Hypoxia	Supplemental oxygen	All injuries
Reactive bronchorrhea, copious secretions	Incentive spirometry, chest physiotherapy, nasotracheal suctioning	All injuries
Inspissated secretions	Humidification, nasotracheal suctioning	Moderate and severe injuries
Wheezing	Diagnostic bronchoscopy to distinguish endobronchial obstruction (plugging) from bronchospasm and edema	Moderate and severe injuries
Plugging (inspissated mucus or mucosal slough)	Humidification, therapeutic bronchoscopy as needed, aerosolized heparin	Moderate and severe injuries
Bronchospasm	Nebulized β_2-agonists; if ineffective, then intravenous aminophylline	Moderate and severe injuries
Respiratory failure	Intubation, mechanical ventilation, permissive hypercapnia, tracheostomy if failure is prolonged (> 14 days)	Severe inhalation injury

patient cannot clear spontaneously may accrete and form life-threatening airway obstructions; they may also cause atelectasis, V_A/Q mismatch, and contribute to the development of pneumonia.

For several reasons (altered mental status, the presence of endotracheal or tracheostomy tubes) the ability to cough may be impaired and stimulation may be necessary for clearance of secretions. Stimulation may be provided by tracheal suctioning or by giving a large tidal volume breath using a manual resuscitation bag and (if possible) providing chest percussion simultaneously. Chest physiotherapy and bronchial drainage may also be useful but frequently are limited by confounding factors such as the location of skin grafts and donor sites. The use of an internal pneumatic percussion device obviates some of these difficulties.

Tracheobronchial suctioning is important for the removal of debris which cannot be cleared by patients with an incapacitated mucociliary apparatus and ineffective cough. Adequate humidification of inspired gas is essential to help limit inspissation of mucus in the injured airways. The patient should be placed in Fowler's position and ventilated with 100% oxygen before suctioning is performed. Suctioning should not be performed for more than 15 seconds (less in children) to minimize the occurrence of transient hypoxia, excessive vagal stimulation, and bradycardia. Adequate preoxygenation and short suctioning times have been shown to decrease or eliminate hypoxic episodes during pulmonary toilet.

Despite adequate humidification, inspissation of secretions still occurs in many patients with severe inhalation injury. In experimental ovine models of inhalation injury, heparin, administered either systemically[22] or by nebulizer;[23] prevented or decreased the formation of tracheobronchial casts. Both methods of treatment produced significant reductions in minute ventilation, peak inspiratory pressure, and positive end-expiratory pressure which should reduce the risk of barotrauma associated with mechanical ventilation. Since heparin delivered by nebulizer has not caused systemic anticoagulation in limited patient trials, that form of administration should remain the treatment of choice if heparin therapy is indicated.

Wheezing may be caused by several different mechanisms, such as endobronchial obstruction from sloughed mucosa, bronchospasm or mucosal edema. The disparate pathophysiologic mechanisms require fundamentally different treatments, and prophylactic therapies (e.g. prophylactic bronchodilator therapy) are of little value. If wheezing occurs and endobronchial obstruction from mucosal slough is ruled out, a trial of standard β_2-agonists may decrease bronchospasm. β_2-Agonists relax bronchial smooth muscle and stimulate mucociliary clearance. If this therapy is not successful, intravenous aminophylline should be instituted and blood levels carefully monitored so as to avoid potential cardiac and central nervous system toxicities. Wheezing from mucosal edema may be minimized by appropriate fluid administration during resuscitation and elevation of the head of the bed. In prospective clinical trials[24,25] steroids have not been shown to be of benefit in altering morbidity or mortality following inhalation injury and may be associated with a higher rate of infection-related complications; therefore, they should be avoided unless the patient was steroid dependent before injury or has persistent bronchospasm unresponsive to other therapy.

When all other techniques fail to remove secretions, the use of fiberoptic bronchoscopy has proven effective. In addition to its diagnostic function, bronchoscopy has important therapeutic applications. Inspissated secretions, particularly when hardened by the presence of blood to form casts, may prove resistant to all simpler methods of removal from the tracheobronchial tree. Bronchoscopy allows instrumentation of the airway under direct vision and enables meticulous pulmonary toilet to be maintained in patients with severe inhalation injury.

Despite all efforts to support unassisted ventilation, patients with moderate or severe inhalation injury may develop respiratory failure and require mechanical ventilatory support. Some patients have preexisting obstructive pulmonary diseases (e.g. emphysema or chronic bronchitis) which make it difficult for them to mobilize adequately the increased volume of secretions caused by the inhalation injury. Others may have cardiovascular insufficiency and be unable to tolerate the volume of fluid required for resuscitation. Some may not be able to achieve and maintain the large minute ventilation required to clear the excess carbon dioxide (CO_2) which is produced by the hypermetabolic response to burn injury. Regardless of the causative mechanism, when tachypnea and recruitment of accessory muscles of respiration are noted by the clinician, the probability of respiratory failure must be considered and plans made to initiate mechanical ventilatory support. Objective data should be collected at this time, not only to document the diagnosis of respiratory failure, but to provide a baseline which can be used for serial assessment of the efficacy of therapy. Common indices which are indicative of respiratory failure include respiratory rate > 30 breaths/min, hypoxemia ($Pa\text{O}_2$<70 mmHg), hypercapnia ($Pa\text{CO}_2$>50 mmHg), vital capacity <4 ml/kg, dead space/tidal volume ventilation ratio (V_D/V_T) > 0.6, and a $Pa\text{O}_2/F\text{IO}_2$ ratio < 200.

The intent of mechanical ventilation is to provide adequate ventilatory support to meet a patient's needs without exacerbating the existing pulmonary lesions or causing barotrauma. Airway resistance is increased in airways narrowed by edema; thus airway pressures must be increased in order to maintain sufficient flow to support minute ventilation. In patients with severe inhalation injury who require mechanical ventilation, it is unnecessary and unwise to ventilate the patient to attain an arbitrarily 'normal' blood gas due to the high mean airway pressures which may be required. High mean airway pressures decrease tracheobronchial mucosal capillary blood flow, resulting in mucosal ischemia. Elevated levels of carbon dioxide are surprisingly well tolerated, provided that the pH can be maintained above 7.25. Thus, the slightly acidic (pH_a = 7.30–7.32) environment associated with permissive hypercapnia can be accepted to minimize the mean airway pressure required for ventilation. Similarly, 'normal' levels of $Pa\text{O}_2$ may require high levels of positive and expiratory pressure, resulting in high mean airway pressures. Oxygen saturations greater than 93% or $Pa\text{O}_2$ > 70 mmHg are sufficient for maintaining adequate oxygen concentration gradient in peripheral tissues. To keep airway pressures to a minimum, ventilator settings may need to be adjusted to slightly higher rates (15–20 breaths min) and small tidal volumes (7–8 ml/kg) with the addition of physiologic PEEP (5 cmH_2O) to prevent small airway closure, alveolar collapse, and resulting high airway and alveolar opening pressures.

Experimental evidence reported by Cioffi *et al.*[26] showed that in a baboon model of moderate smoke inhalation injury, the barotrauma index (rate pressure product) was significantly increased during conventional ventilation in comparison to high-frequency flow interruption ventilation, while both attained adequate ventilation and oxygenation. There was also significantly more parenchymal injury in the group treated with conventional ventilation in comparison to the high-frequency flow interruption group. Data collected in two retrospective studies[1,27] indicate that optimal ventilation and survival in adults may be attained with high-frequency flow interruption ventilation in comparison to conventional (volume-limited) ventilation; significant decreases in the incidence of pneumonia and mortality in patients with inhalation injury have been noted when high-frequency percussive ventilation was used rather than conventional ventilation.

If prolonged ventilatory failure is expected due to severe inhalation injury, preexisting pulmonary disease, or difficulty in maintaining pulmonary toilet (secondary to small airway size or to complications of inhalation injury such as pneumonia), then the risks and benefits of tracheostomy should be considered. Early tracheostomy (performed for airway management rather than endotracheal intubation) has been demonstrated to have a 6% operative complication rate and a 30% long-term complication rate.[25] Long-term endotracheal intubation can cause similar long-term complications and is also uncomfortable for the patient. Endotracheal tubes are limited in size to those which will fit easily through the larynx; in patients with small airways, the small tube size may cause significant resistance to air flow, resulting in increased work of breathing and higher pressure during mechanical ventilatory cycles to achieve adequate air exchange. Pulmonary toilet is also more difficult to maintain through small diameter endotracheal tubes, and residual debris and secretions can cause life-threatening airway obstruction. The multitude of considerations regarding the issue of tracheostomy require that the decision be individualized to each patient. The indiscriminate use of any single rule regarding the type of injury or time of endotracheal intubation is inadequate for selecting patients who will benefit from this procedure.

After a patient's clinical condition has improved to the point where there is sustained improvement in ventilatory indices and decreased bronchorrhea, ventilatory support should be carefully weaned by gradual reductions in inspired oxygen concentration, positive end-expiratory pressure, and ventilator rate until the patient can independently support his own ventilatory needs. Weaning cannot be forced, and patience is important, especially when preexisting disease or prolonged periods of ventilatory assistance and pharmacologic neuromuscular blockade complicate the process. Patients should be capable of supporting their own ventilatory needs when they are hemodynamically stable and no longer tachypneic (respiratory rate < 30 breaths/min), acidotic (pH_a > 7.35), hypoxic (Pao_2>70 with Fio_2<0.40 and Pao_2/Fio_2>300), or weak (vital capacity>10ml/kg and V_D/V_T<0.6). Following weaning and extubation or disconnection of the tracheostomy, the patient should be provided with humidified supplemental oxygen (Fio_2 not greater than 0.4) and carefully observed for evidence of recurrent ventilatory failure necessitating resumption of mechanical ventilatory support.

COMPLICATIONS

Early

Early complications of inhalation injury are usually mechanical or infectious. Rapid recognition of these complications is essential so that appropriate treatment may be started, thus minimizing their potential for morbidity and added mortality. Mechanical complications are usually manifestations of barotrauma or patient care procedures. Barotrauma represents a spectrum of iatrogenic injuries caused by mechanical ventilation and most commonly presents as a pneumothorax, pneumomediastinum, subcutaneous emphysema, or pneumoperitoneum. The type of patient at risk for barotrauma is one who requires high mean airway pressure in order to maintain alveolar recruitment, and thus is also at risk of sustaining persistent tracheobronchial mucosal ischemia. Continued ischemia prevents healing of the already damaged tracheal mucosal injury and may contribute to continued release of inflammatory mediators with potential development of multiple organ system failure, in addition to the continued risk of infectious complications such as tracheobronchitis or pneumonia, which have their own well defined morbidity and mortality.[28] Occasionally barotrauma may occur in unintubated patients as the result of vigorous coughing and usually presents as a spontaneous pneumothorax.

Infectious complications may present as tracheobronchitis or pneumonia. The injured trachea is known to be at risk for infection;[29,30] and respiratory tract infection has been shown to be the most common complication following inhalation injury.[31] The incidence of pneumonia appears to be constant (38%) in patients with inhalation injury as reported in two different patient cohorts from the same institution (1980–1984 and 1985–1990) although the mortality rate in these patients was noted to decrease from 46.6% to 29.4% over the same period.[1] There are many determinants which predispose patients with inhalation injury to develop pulmonary infections; the most significant risk factor (apart from the inhalation injury itself) is colonization of the airway secondary to endotracheal intubation, aspiration, and oropharyngeal colonization with pathogenic organisms.[32] Many of the natural airway defenses which help to prevent infection are bypassed in intubated patients. The source of most pathogenic organisms causing nosocomial infection is the patient; oropharyngeal and burn wound colonization (usually with the patient's own skin and GI tract flora) are the primary repositories of these bacteria. Improvements in outcome in burn patients with pneumonia appear to be related to increased survival in those patients with mild inhalation injury and increased survival in patients placed on high-frequency flow interruption ventilation in comparison to those receiving conventional ventilation.[1]

The diagnosis of tracheobronchitis or pneumonia can be extraordinarily difficult to establish due to the presence of inhalation injury and bacterial colonization of the airway. The diagnosis of tracheobronchitis rests on the presence of fever, leukocytosis, and productive cough as well as organisms and white blood cells on Gram's stain of sputum preparations. In addition, parenchymal infiltrates must be present on the chest roentgenogram in order to make the diagnosis of pneumonia. Inhalation injury itself, without a superimposed infection, is characterized by the presence of white blood cells on Gram's stain sputum preparations, productive cough, fever and leukocytosis (especially if there is an associated cutaneous burn), and patchy perivascular and peribronchial infiltrates on chest roentgenogram. Upper respiratory tract colonization with organisms abnormal for that site, such as gram-negative bacilli and *Staphylococcus aureus*, is also common and, thus, does not support the diagnosis of pneumonia. The diagnosis is best made when the criteria listed above are present (greater than 20 white blood cells and organisms on a Gram's stain sputum preparation) and there has been a substantial change in the quantity and purulence of the patient's sputum, a change in the fever pattern, a need for an increase in the amount of ventilatory support, a change in the pattern of infiltrates on chest roentgenogram, or a decline in the patient's clinical condition without another identifiable source. Unfortunately, techniques such as bronchoalveolar lavage or protected brush specimens have not been helpful in increasing the sensitivity and specificity of the diagnosis of pneumonia.

Treatment consists of empirical intravenous antibiotic therapy based on the results of the Gram's stain sputum preparation and regularly obtained surveillance cultured until the specific sputum culture and antibiotic sensitivity results are available to allow refinement of the antibiotic therapy. Prospective randomized trials of prophylactic antibiotic therapy[24,33] have shown that prophylactic antibiotics do not change the incidence, morbidity, or mortality of pneumonia but do hasten the emergence of resistant flora. Therapy should be administered for an appropriate length of time (usually 10–14 days for common pulmonary pathogens) and both clinical indices and serial Gram's stain sputum preparation result should be followed during treatment so as to verify the clinical effectiveness of administered treatment. When available, serum antibiotic levels should be monitored in order to insure that effective, but not toxic, quantities of antibiotic are being administered. Meticulous pulmonary toilet is also necessary in order to minimize pooling of secretions and prevent atelectasis which may serve as a source of continued infection.

Questions have been posed recently as to whether the incidence of nosocomial pneumonia in thermally injured patients with inhalation injury is affected by the method of stress ulcer prophylaxis being used. In a prospective study[34] of 96 thermally injured patients (49 with inhalation injury), randomized to receive either sucralfate or acid-neutralizing treatment (H_2 blocker and antacid), it was shown that the sputum colonization rate and the overall incidence, type, and time to diagnosis of pneumonia was unaffected by the method of prophylaxis, although a significantly greater number of patients receiving sucralfate developed pneumonia while intubated. The group receiving sucralfate also was noted to have three episodes of clinically apparent upper gastrointestinal bleeding (none in the acid-neutralizing group), but this difference did not reach significance. Thus, in thermally injured patients it appears that the method of stress ulcer prophylaxis does not affect the occurrence of nosocomial pneumonia.

Late

Late complications of inhalation injury may be related to mechanical damage or the consequences of an uncontrolled inflammatory process. These complications are not as easily treated as the early complications of inhalation injury, and prevention is often the only effective therapy. Mechanical complications occur most often as the result of iatrogenic injury from an endotracheal tube or tracheostomy tube cuff. Tube cuffs may cause erosion of the tracheal cartilages, allowing tracheal wall collapse from negative airway pressures during inspiration (tracheomalacia). Injuries to the tracheal epithelium may eventually result in fibrosis and stenosis of the trachea (subglottic stenosis) as the wound contracts. Erosion into adjacent structures (innominate artery or esophagus) may result in exsanguinating hemorrhage or severe mediastinitis. These injuries are difficult to diagnose and often develop slowly; thus, they may not be discovered until after the patient's acute care has been completed and rehabilitation has begun. Tube instability, high cuff pressures (> 20 cmH_2O), and duration of intubation all contribute to airway damage. These injuries are difficult to treat satisfactorily once they occur, emphasizing the importance of prevention (e.g. stabilization of the tube, careful maintenance of the cuff pressure at the minimum required for an appropriate seal [not exceeding 20 cmH_2O], and expedient extubation or conversion to a tracheostomy in patients requiring prolonged ventilatory support) and vigilance as the most important mechanisms to avoid these complications.

Inflammatory complications (bronchiectasis and bronchial stenosis) probably occur as a result of neutrophil activation in the area of airway damaged by inhalation injury. Activated neutrophils produce both proteases and oxygen radicals which may cause severe damage to the already injured bronchial mucosa and extracellular matrix. Although most proteases are produced by neutrophils, other cells to include alveolar macrophages, mast cells, basophils, eosinophils, and fibroblasts all may participate in protease secretion. Oxidants secreted by neutrophils are known to inhibit the function of α_1-antitrypsin, an important inhibitor of proteases such as neutrophil elastase, collagenase, cathepsins, and gelatinase.[35] Normal host defense mechanisms protecting mucosal integrity (antiproteases and antioxidants) have been shown to function poorly after inhalation injury.[36] Uncontrolled degradation of extracellular matrix proteins may lead to acute lung diseases such as adult respiratory distress syndrome (ARDS) and chronic lung diseases such as emphysema and bronchiectasis. Damage of both smoke-injured and normal tissues by proteases and oxidants may lead to persistent escalation of the inflammatory response[37] which prevents healing and worsens pulmonary function, and it may result in inability to ventilate the patient, multisystem organ failure, and death.

Future Directions

Care of the patient with inhalation injury at this time is supportive, with an emphasis on prevention and early recognition of complications. Efforts to minimize barotrauma are important so as to decrease the incidence of the side effects of mechanical ventilation. Further research into the pathogenesis of inhalation injury may lead to the development of specific therapies which can minimize the insult and prevent the exaggerated inflammatory sequelae which can cause considerable morbidity and mortality.

Reduction of Barotrauma

Modification of conventional ventilator therapy to include high-frequency positive pressure ventilation has resulted in favorable trends in the incidence of pneumonia and mortality rates. In a study of patients with severe inhalation injury requiring mechanical ventilation, high-frequency percussive ventilation was found to permit adequate ventilation and oxygenation of patients who had failed conventional ventilation.[2] The utility of this mode of ventilation appears to be its ability to recruit damaged collapsed alveoli and maintain these alveoli in an open state during expiration. Maintaining alveolar recruitment at low mean airway pressures helps to prevent or minimize barotrauma from high airway pressures and overdistension of normal alveoli and allows improved distribution of ventilation. Other methods of ventilation, such as hybrid or total liquid ventilation are being evaluated at present in order to determine their role in the treatment of inhalation injury.

Prospective Therapies

Identification of the pathogenetic mechanisms which amplify the initial mucosal damage caused by smoke exposure and produce pulmonary and systemic dysfunction may permit the development of specific therapies aimed at preventing progressive systemic inflammation. The pathophysiologic responses to inhalation injury are complex, overlapping, and redundant. Almost certainly, control of the inflammatory response will require coordination of several therapies rather than one omnipotent therapy. Current work in the field of lung injury centers on the following areas: mechanisms of neutrophil recruitment and activation, modulation of extracellular proteases and oxygen radicals, the role of deficient surfactant function, prevention of tracheobronchial cast formation, reduction of pulmonary hypertension, and the role of numerous inflammatory mediators (TNF, IL-1, IL-8, prostaglandins and leukotrienes) in propagation of local injury.

Numerous cells residing in the lung can produce chemotactic and activating substances, notably alveolar macrophages (TNF, IL-1, IL-8, platelet-activating factor, platelet-derived growth factor), endothelial cells (IL-1[38] and IL-8[39]), and possibly epithelial cells (IL-8[40] and leukotrienes[41]). Many of these substances are also under investigation for their contributions to the pathogenesis of adult respiratory distress syndrome and multiorgan system failure. Identification of the roles of these substances in amplification of the initial injury response will provide an excellent opportunity to intervene and modulate the inflammatory cascade before injury of normal lung, progression of respiratory dysfunction, and the development of multiorgan system dysfunction occurs.

Extracellular proteases and oxidants are the direct mediators of neutrophil-induced injury. Protease inhibitors such as α_1-antitrypsin and α_2-macroglobulin are the primary antiproteases present in the lung under normal circumstances. Extensive neutrophil activation and release of large amounts of oxidant species result in inactivation of antiproteases. Therapy which increases the quantity of free radical scavengers and functional antiproteases, or controls the synthesis and secretion of oxygen radicals and proteases, may be effective in preventing secondary injury to normal lung. Experimentally, free radical scavengers such as dimethylsulfoxide[23,42] have been shown to improve survival (in one study) and decrease microvascular permeability as measured by lung lymph flow and lung wet to dry weight ratios following inhalation injury in an ovine model. Pentoxifylline[43] has been demonstrated to reduce significantly the degree of leukocytosis, absolute polymorphonuclear cell counts and total protein content of bronchoalveolar lavage fluid, and lung wet to dry weight ratios following inhalation injury. In addition, pulmonary compliance, respiratory index (a measure of oxygenation efficiency), V_A/Q mismatching, pulmonary capillary wedge pressure, and pulmonary vascular resistance were all significantly improved following administration of pentoxifylline. In contrast, a study investigating the effects of nitric oxide[44] insufflation following inhalation injury found improvement in pulmonary vascular resistance without apparent effect on the magnitude of inflammation and little improvement in V_A/Q mismatching or pulmonary gas exchange. In an ovine model of inhalation injury, the administration of a platelet-activating factor antagonist decreased leukocytosis and lipid peroxidation.[45] Clinical studies will be necessary in order to document whether these various agents will favorably influence morbidity and mortality in patients with inhalation injury.

Deficient surfactant function has been demonstrated in many animal models of lung injury as well as in studies of adult respiratory distress syndrome patients.[46] The deficiency results from inactivation of existing surfactant by lipid peroxidation and apoprotein cleavage, as well as from decreased surfactant production by type II pneumocytes. Inactivation of surfactant results in loss of hysteresis in the lung, encourages alveolar collapse, markedly increases peak and mean airway pressure, worsens V_A/Q mismatch, increases extravascular lung water, and greatly decreases ventilatory efficiency.[47] Clinical trials assessing the efficacy of exogenous surfactant administration are ongoing.

In experimental models of inhalation injury, heparin has proved effective, alone[22] and in combination with dimethylsulfoxide,[23,42] in reducing the amount of airway obstruction in damaged airways caused by casts which are formed by sloughed epithelial cells and protein-rich exudate. Significant reductions in minute ventilation, peak inspiratory pressure, and positive end-expiratory pressure were also noted and should reduce the risk of barotrauma during mechanical ventilation.

The first major improvement in the treatment of burn injury came with the recognition of the importance of fluid resuscitation to prevent shock and renal failure. Subsequently, the use of topical antibiotics to control burn wound infection and prevent invasive burn wound sepsis led to the next significant reduction in morbidity and mortality of burn patients. Although progress has been made in the treatment of inhalation injury, the pathophysiology of the injury is still incompletely defined. A better understanding of pathogenetic mechanisms may lead to the development of therapeutic agents and treatment regimens which will modulate the cascades of humoral mediators of organ dysfunction and reduce the morbidity and mortality associated with inhalation injury.

References

1. Rue L W III, Cioffi W G Jr, Mason A D Jr, *et al.* Improved survival of burned patients with inhalation injury. *Arch Surg* 1993; **128:** 772–80.

2. Cioffi W G Jr, Graves T A, McManus W F, *et al.* High-frequency percussive ventilation in patients with inhalation injury. *J Trauma* 1989; **29:** 1350–54.

3. Clark W R, Bonaventural M, Myers W. Smoke inhalation and airway management at a regional burn unit: 1974–1983. Part I: Diagnosis and consequences of smoke inhalation. *J Burn Care Rehabil* 1989; **10:** 52–62.

4. Agee R N, Long J M, Hunt J L, *et al.* Use of ^{133}xenon in early diagnosis of inhalation injury. *J Trauma* 1976; **16:** 218–24.

5. Suratt P M, Smiddy J F, Gruber B. Deaths and complications associated with fiberoptic bronchoscopy. *Chest* 1976; **69:** 747–51.

6. Credle W F Jr, Smiddy J F, Elliott R C. Complications of fiberoptic bronchoscopy. *Am Rev Respir Dis* 1974; **109:** 67–72.

7. Pereira W J Jr, Dovnat D M, Snider G L. A prospective cooperative study of complications following flexible fiberoptic bronchoscopy. *Chest* 1978; **73:** 813–16.

8. Haponik E F. Clinical and functional assessment. In: Haponik E F, Munster A M, eds. *Respiratory Injury: Smoke Inhalation and Burns*. New York: McGraw-Hill, Inc, 1990: 171.

9. Scheulen J J, Munster A M. The Parkland formula in patients with burns and inhalation injury. *J Trauma* 1982; **22:** 869–71.

10. Navar P D, Saffle J R, Warden G D. Effect of inhalation injury on fluid resuscitation requirements after thermal injury. *Am J Surg* 1985; **150:** 716–20.

11. Lu W. clinical analysis of fluid resuscitation in severe burned patients with or without inhalation injury. *Chung-Hua Cheng Hsing Shao Shang Wai Ko Tsa Chih* (*Chinese Journal of Plastic Surgery Burns*) 1992, **8:** 116–18.

12. Hughes K R, Armstrong R F, Brough M D, *et al.* Fluid requirements of patients with burns and inhalation injuries in an intensive care unit. *Intensive Care Med* 1989; **15:** 464–6.

13. Herndon D N, Barrow R E, Linares H A, *et al.* Inhalation injury in burned patients: effects and treatment. *Burns Incl Therm Inj* 1988; **14:** 349–56.

14. Herndon D N, Traber D L, Traber L D. The effect of resuscitation on inhalation injury. *Surgery* 1986; **100:** 248–51.

15. Shimazu T, Yukioka T, Hubbard G B, *et al.* A dose-responsive model of smoke inhalation injury. *Ann Surg* 1988; **206:** 89–98.

16. Fein A, Leff A, Hopewell P C. Pathophysiology and management of the complications resulting from fire and the inhaled products of combustion: review of the literature. *Crit Care Med* 1980; **8:** 94–8.

17. Boutros A R, Hoyt J L. Managment of carbon monoxide poisoning in the absence of hyperbaric oxygen chamber. *Crit Care Med* 1976; **4:** 144–7.

18. Smith G, Ledingham I M, Sharp G R, *et al.* Treatment of coal-gas poisoning with oxygen at 2 atmospheres pressure. *Lancet* 1962; **1:** 816–19.

19. Mathieu D, Nolf M, Durocher A, *et al.* Acute carbon monoxide poisoning: risk of late sequelae and treatment with hyperbaric oxygen. *J Toxicol Clin Toxicol* 1986; **23:** 315–24.

20. Norkool D M, Kirkpatrick J N. Treatment of acute carbon monoxide poisoning with hyperbaric oxygen: a review of 115 cases. *Ann Emerg Med* 1985; **14:** 1168–71.

21. Grube B J, Marvin J A, Heimbach D M. Therapeutic hyperbaric oxygen: help or hindrance in burn patients with carbon monoxide poisoning. *J Burn Care Rehabil* 1988; **9:** 249–52.

22. Cox C S Jr, Zwischenberger J B, Traber D L, *et al.* Heparin improves oxygenation and minimizes barotrauma after severe smoke inhalation in an ovine model. *Surg Gynecol Obstet* 1993; **176:** 339–49.

23. Brown M, Desai M, Traber L D, *et al.* Dimethylsulfoxide with heparin in the treatment of smoke inhalation injury. *J Burn Care Rehabil* 1988; **9:** 22–5.

24. Levine B A, Petroff P A, Slade C L. Prospective trials of dexamethasone and aerosolized gentamicin in the treatment of inhalation injury in the burned patient. *J Trauma* 1978; **18:** 188–93.

25. Moylan J A, Alexander L G Jr. Diagnosis and treatment of inhalation injury. *World J Surg* 1978; **2:** 185–91.

26. Cioffi W G, DeLemos R A, Coalson J J, *et al.* Decreased pulmonary damage in primates with inhalation injury treated with high-frequency ventilation. *Ann Surg* 1993; **218:** 328–37.

27. Cioffi W G Jr, Rue L W III, Graves T A, *et al.* Prophylactic use of high-frequency percussive ventilation in patients with inhalation injury. *Ann Surg* 1991; **213:** 575–82.

28. Shirani K Z, Pruitt B A Jr, Mason A D. The influence of inhalation injury and pneumonia on burn mortality. *Ann Surg* 1987; **205:** 82–7.

29. Demarest G B, Hudson L D, Altman L C. Impaired alveolar macrophage chemotaxis in patients with acute smoke inhalation. *Am Rev Respir Dis* 1979; **119:** 279–86.

30. Loke J, Paul E, Virgulto J A, *et al.* Rabbit lung after acute smoke inhalation: cellular responses and scanning electron microscopy. *Arch Surg* 1984; **119:** 956–9.

31. Pruitt B A Jr, Erickson D R, Morris A. Progressive pulmonary insufficiency and other pulmonary complications of thermal injury. *J Trauma* 1975; **15:** 369–9.

32. Sears S D. Pulmonary infections in the burn patient and their management. In: Haponik E F, Munster A M, eds. *Respiratory Injury: Smoke Inhalation and Burns*. New York: McGraw-Hill, Inc, 1990: 226.

33. Klastersky J, Bogaerts A M, Noteman J, *et al.* Infections caused by Providencia bacilli. *Scand J Infect Dis* 1974; **6:** 153–8.

34. Cioffi W G Jr, McManus A T, Rue L W III, *et al.* Comparison of acid neutralizing and non-acid neutralizing stress ulcer prophylaxis in thermally injured patients. *J Trauma* 1994; **36:** 541–7.

35. Ossanna P J, Test S T, Matheson N R, *et al.* Oxidative regulation of neutrophil elastase alph-1 -protease inhibitor interactions. *J Clin Invest* 1986; **77:** 1939–51.

36. Gadek J E, Fells G A, Zimmerman R L, *et al.* Antielastases of the human alveolar structures. *J Clin Invest* 1981; **68:** 889–98.

37. Henson P M, Johnston R B. Tissue injury in inflammation: oxidants, proteinases and cationic proteins. *J Clin Invest* 1987; **79:** 669–74.

38. Libby P, Ordovas J M, Auger K R, *et al.* Endotoxin and tumor necrosis factor induce interleukin-1 gene expression in adult human vascular endothelial cells. *Am J Pathol* 1986; **124:** 179–85.

39. Strieter R M, Kunkel S L, Showell H J, *et al.* Endothelial cell gene expression of a neutrophil chemotactic factor by TNF-alpha, LPS and IL-1. *Science* 1989; **243:** 1467–9.

40. Standiford T J, Kunkel S L, Basha M A, *et al.* Human alveolar macrophage induced gene expression of neutrophil chemotactic factor/interleukin-1 from pulmonary epithelial cells. *Clin Res* 1990; **38:** 139A.

41. Butler G B, Adler K B, Evan J N, *et al.* Modulation of rabbit airway smooth muscle responsiveness by respiratory epithelium. *Am Rev Respir Dis* 1987; **135:** 1099–104.

42. Kimura R, Traber L D, Herndon D N, *et al.* Treatment of smoke-induced pulmonary injury with nebulized dimethylsulfoxide. *Circ Shock* 1988; **25:** 333–41.

43. Ogura H, Cioffi W G Jr, Okerberg C V, *et al.* The effects of pentoxifylline on pulmonary function following smoke inhalation. *J Surg Res* 1994; **56:** 242–50.

44. Ogura H, Cioffi W G Jr, Jordan B S, *et al.* The effect of inhaled nitric oxide on smoke inhalation injury in an ovine model. *J Trauma* 1994; **37:** 893–8.

45. Ikeuchi H, Sakano T, Sanchez J, *et al.* The effects of platelet-activating factor (PAF) and a PAF antagonist (CV-3988) on smoke inhalation injury in an ovine model. *J Trauma* 1992; **32:** 344–50.

46. Spragg R G, Smith R M. Biology of acute lung injury. In: Crystal R G, West J B, eds. *Lung Injury*. New York: Raven Press Ltd, 1992: 252.

47. Clark W R Jr, Nieman G F. Smoke inhalation. *Burns Incl Therm Inj* 1988; **6:** 473–94.

CHAPTER EIGHTEEN

RESPIRATORY CARE

RONALD P. MLCAK, MANUHBAI H. DESAI AND RAY J. NICHOLS, JR

INTRODUCTION

The multitude of respiratory complications caused by smoke inhalation, thermal burns, and their treatment, epitomize the clinical challenges which confront respiratory care practitioners. Smoke inhalation injury and its sequelae impose demands upon the respiratory care practitioners who play a central role in its clinical management. These demands may range from intubation and resuscitation of victims in the emergency room to assistance with diagnostic bronchoscopies, to performance of pulmonary function studies, monitoring of arterial blood gases, airway maintenance, chest physiotherapy, and mechanical ventilator management.[1] Additional demands are placed upon the respiratory care practitioner in the rehabilitation phase in determining disability or limitations diagnosed by pulmonary function studies or cardiopulmonary stress testing. In some countries outside the United States, the duties of the respiratory care practitioner are augmented by a combination of physicians, nurses, and physiotherapists. It is imperative that a well organized, protocol-driven approach to burn care be utilized so that improvements can be made, and the morbidity and mortality associated with inhalation injury can be reduced. This chapter shall provide an overview of the common hands-on approaches to the treatment of inhalation injury with emphasis on mucociliary clearance techniques, pharmacologic adjuncts, mechanical ventilation, infection control, and the late complications associated with inhalation injury.

BRONCHIAL HYGIENE THERAPY

Airway clearance techniques are an essential component of respiratory management of patients with smoke inhalation. Bronchial hygiene therapy is a term used to describe several of the modalities intended to accomplish this goal. Therapeutic coughing, chest physiotherapy, early ambulation, airway suctioning, therapeutic bronchoscopy and pharmacologic agents have been effective in the removal of retained secretions.

Therapeutic Coughing

Therapeutic coughing functions to promote airway clearance of excess mucus and fibrin cast in the tracheal bronchial tree. The impairment of the cough mechanism will result in retained secretions, bronchial obstruction, atelectasis, and/or pneumonia. A cough may be either a reflex or a voluntary action. The mechanisms of a cough include:

- a deep inspiration;
- the closure of the glottis;
- contraction of the muscles of the chest wall, abdomen, and pelvic floor;
- opening of the glottis; and
- a rapid expulsive exhalation phase.

During a cough, alveolar, pleural, and subglottic pressures may rise as much as 200 cmH_2O. A failure of the cough mechanism may be due to an impairment of any step in the sequences described. When this occurs, it is necessary to perform techniques which are used to improve the cough.

Series of three coughs

The patient is asked to start a small breath and small cough, then a bigger breath and harder cough, and finally a really deep breath and hard cough. This technique is especially effective for postoperative patients who tend to splint from pain.[2]

Tracheal tickle

The therapist places the index and middle finger flat in the sternal notch and gently massages inward in a circular fashion over the trachea. This is most effective in obtunded patients or in patients coming out of anesthesia.[2]

Cough stimulation

Patients with artificial airways cannot cough normally since a tube is either between the vocal cords (endotracheal) or below the cords (tracheostomy). Adequate pressure cannot be built up without approximation of the cords. These patients may have a cough stimulated by inflating the cuff on the tube, giving a large, rapid inspiration by a manual resuscitation bag, holding the breath for 1–2 seconds, and rapidly allowing the bag to release and exhalation to ensue. This technique is normally performed by two persons and is made more effective by one therapist performing vibration and chest compressions from the time of the inspiratory hold, all during exhalation.[2] Coughing and deep breathing is encouraged every hour to aid in removing retained secretions.

Chest Physiotherapy

Chest physiotherapy has come to mean gravity-assisted bronchial drainage with chest percussion and vibrations. Studies have shown that a combination of techniques are effective in secretion removal.[3–6]

Bronchial drainage/positioning

Bronchial drainage/positioning is a therapeutic modality which uses gravity-assisted positioning designed to improve pulmonary hygiene in patients with inhalation injury or retained secretions. There are 12 basic positions in which patients can be placed for postural drainage. Due to skin grafts, donor sites, and the use of air fluid beds, clinical judgment dictates that most of these positions are not practical. In fact, positioning in the Trendelenburg and various other positions may acutely worsen hypoxemia. Evidence has shown that a patient's arterial oxygenation may fall during positioning.[7] To accomplish the same goal it is common practice, in intensive care units, to turn patients side to side every 2 hours so as to aid in mobilizing secretions (**Figure 18.1**).

Percussion

Percussion aids in the removal of secretions from the tracheal bronchial tree. Percussion is done by cupping the hand so as to allow a cushion of air to come between the percussor's hand and the patient. If this is done properly, a popping sound will be heard when the patient is percussed. There should be a towel between the patient and the percussor's hand in order to prevent irritation of the skin.[8] Percussion is applied over the surface landmarks of the bronchial segments which are being drained. The hands rhythmically and alternately strike the chest wall. Incisions, skin grafts, and bony prominences should be avoided during percussion (**Figure 18.2**).

Vibration/shaking

Vibration/shaking is a shaking movement used to move loosened secretions to larger airways so that they can be coughed up or removed by suctioning. Vibration involves rapid shaking of the chest wall during exhalation. The percussor vibrates the thoracic cage by placing both hands over the percussed areas and vibrating into the patient, isometrically contracting or tensing the muscles of their arms and shoulders. Mechanical vibrations have been reported to produce good clinical results. Gentle mechanical vibration may be indicated for patients who cannot tolerate manual percussion. (**Figure 18.3**). Chest physiotherapy techniques should be used every 2–4 hours for patients with retained secretions. Therapy should continue until breath sounds improve.

Early Ambulation

Early ambulation is another effective means of preventing respiratory complications. With appropriate use of analgesics, even patients on continuous ventilatory support can be gotten out of bed and into a chair (**Figure 18.4**). The rocking chair (**Figure 18.5**) has several beneficial effects:

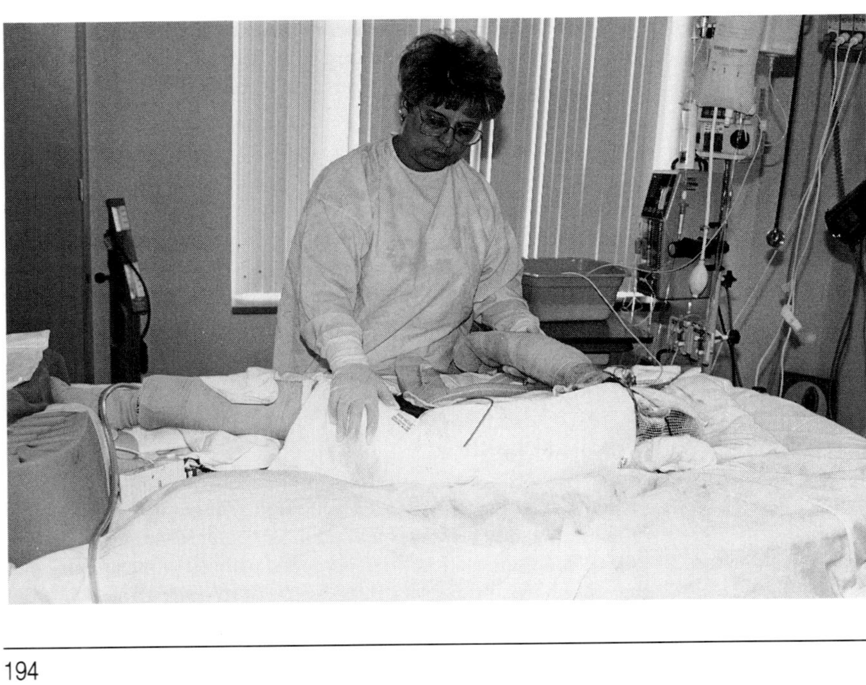

Fig. 18.1 Patient positioning for secretion mobilization.

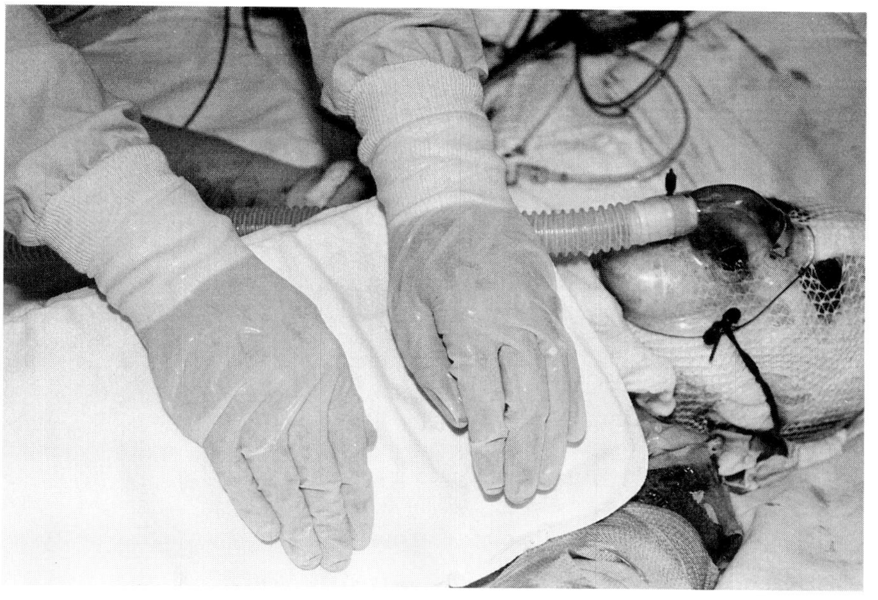

Fig. 18.2 Chest physiotherapy techniques.

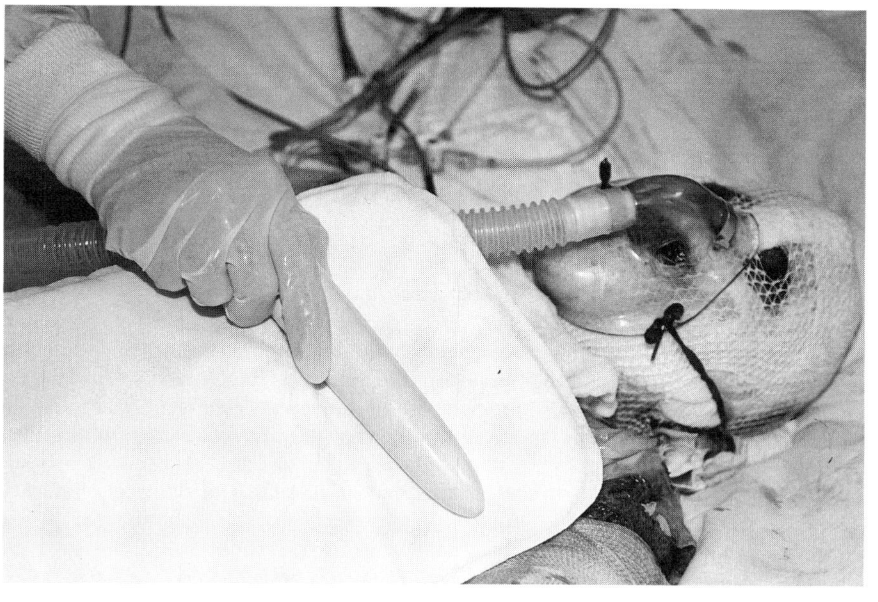

Fig. 18.3 Gentle mechanical chest vibrations.

- the patient can breathe with regions of the lungs which are normally hyperventilated;
- muscular strength and tone are preserved;
- contractions are prevented and exercise tolerance is maintained.[9]

Airway Suctioning

Airway suctioning is another method of clearing an airway. Normal bronchial hygiene is usually accomplished by the mucociliary escalator process. When these methods are not effective in maintaining a clear airway, tracheobronchial suctioning is indicated.[10–13] Nasotracheal suctioning is intended to remove from the trachea accumulated secretions, and other foreign material which cannot be removed by the patient's spontaneous cough or less invasive procedures. Nasotracheal suctioning has been used to avoid intubation which was solely intended for the removal of secretions. Nasotracheal suctioning refers to the insertion of a suction catheter through the nasal passages and pharynx into the trachea in order to aspirate secretions or foreign material. The first step in this process is to hyperoxygenate the patient with 100% oxygen. The patient should be positioned in the Fowler's position and the catheter slowly advanced through the nares to a point just above the larynx. The therapist or nurse then listens for air sounds at the proximal end of the catheter. When airflow is felt to be strongest and respiratory sounds are loudest, the tip of the catheter is immediately above the epiglottis. On inspiration, the catheter is advanced into the trachea. After the vocal cords have been passed, a few deep breaths are allowed and the patient is reoxygenated. Suction is begun while the catheter is slowly withdrawn from the trachea. The patient should not be suctioned for more than 15 seconds without being reoxygenated. Suctioning is not without potential hazards.[14,15] Complications include irritation of the nasotracheal mucosa with bleeding, abrupt drops in PO_2, vagal stimulation, and bradycardia. Preoxygenating and limiting suction time have been shown to decrease or eliminate the fall in the PO_2.[12–14]

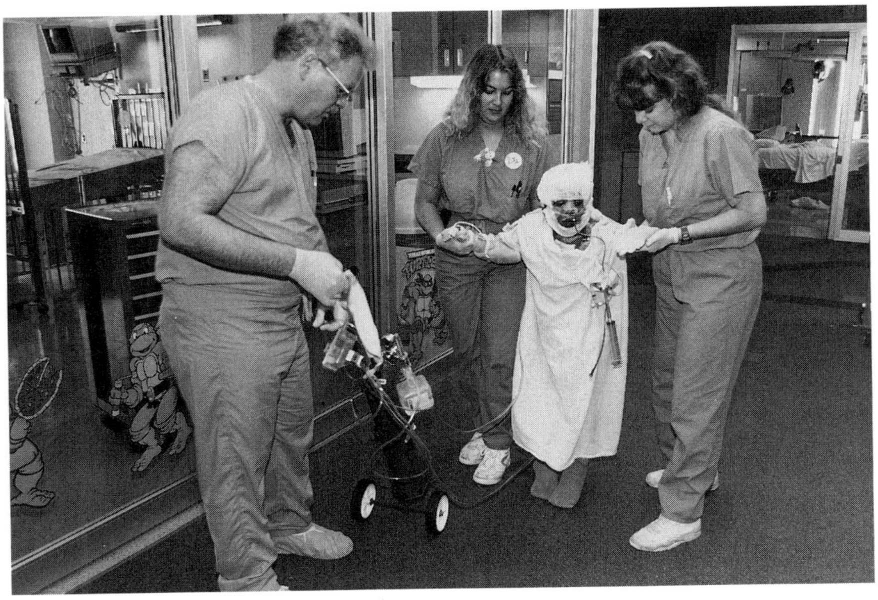

Fig. 18.4 Early ambulation.

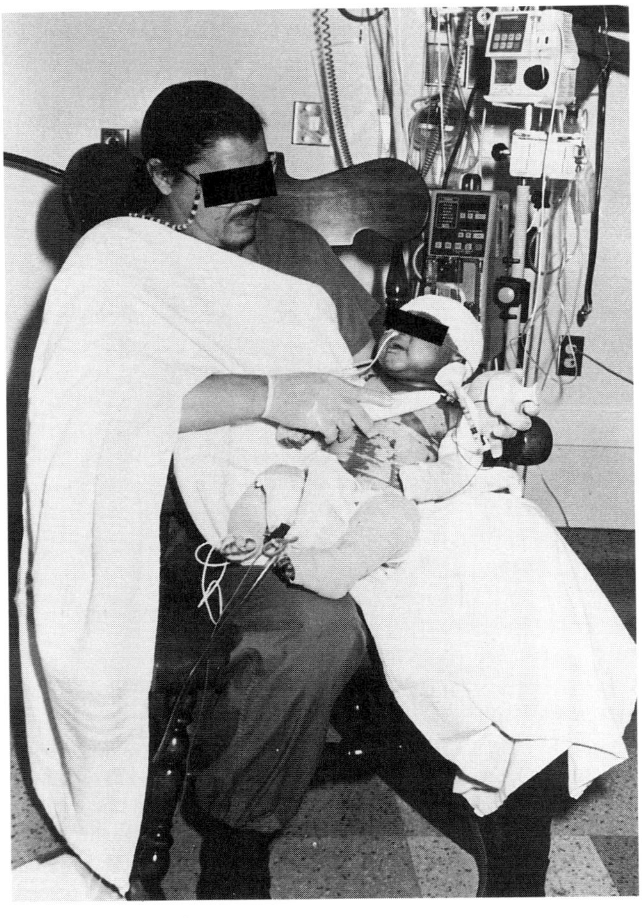

Fig. 18.5 Patient up out of bed, secretions being mobilized by rocking and chest physiotherapy techniques.

Therapeutic Bronchoscopy

When all other techniques fail to remove secretions, the use of the fiberoptic bronchoscope has proven to be of benefit. In addition to its diagnostic functions, bronchoscopy retains important therapeutic applications. Copious secretions encountered in patients with inhalation injury may require repeated bronchoscopic procedures when more conservative methods are unsuccessful. The modern fiberoptic bronchoscope is small in diameter, flexible, and has a steerable tip which can be maneuvered into the fourth or fifth order bronchi for examination or specimen removal.

Pharmacological Adjuncts

Bronchodilators

Bronchodilators can be helpful in some cases. Inhalation injury to the lower airways results in a chemical tracheobronchitis which can produce wheezing and bronchospasms. This is especially true for patients with preexisting reactive airway diseases. Most drugs which are used in the management of bronchospasms are believed to act on the biochemical mechanism which controls bronchial muscle tone. Aerosolized sympathomimetics are effective in two ways: they result in bronchial muscle relaxation and they stimulate mucociliary clearance. The newer bronchodilators are more effective and have fewer side effects than the older generation drugs. Some of the newer compounds which are used in the United States are worthy of note. First, metaproterenol is available in cartridge inhalers, as a liquid to be aerosolized, or as an oral medication in tablets, or as a syrup. The recommended oral dose is 10–20 mg every 6–8 hours or as an inhaled bronchodilator, 1–2 puffs every 3–4 hours. Its duration of action as an inhaled bronchodilator is 1–5 hours.[16]

Albuterol can also be administered orally, parenterally, and by aerosol. Albuterol is available in a metered cartridge inhaler and its standard dose is 1–2 puffs three to four times daily. Aerosolized albuterol has a duration of action of approximately 4–6 hours.[17]

Racemic epinephrine is used as an aerosolized topical vasoconstrictor, bronchodilator, and secretion bond breaker. The vasoconstrictive action of racemic epinephrine is useful in reducing mucosal and submucosal edema within the walls of the pulmonary airways. A secondary bronchodilator action serves to reduce potential spasm of the smooth muscles of the terminal bronchioles. Water, employed as a diluent for racemic epinephrine, serves to lower both adhesive and cohesive forces of the retained endobronchial secretions, thus serving as a bond-breaking vehicle.

Racemic epinephrine has also been used for the treatment of post-extubation stridor.[18] Its mode of action is thought to be related to the vasoconstrictive activity, with the resultant decrease in mucosal edema. Aerosolized treatments may be given every 2 hours as long as the heart rate is not increased.

Hypertonic saline offers a theoretically more effective form of mucokinetic therapy. The deposition of hypertonic droplets on the respiratory mucosa results in the osmotic attraction of fluids from the mucosal blood vessels and tissues into the airway. Thus a 'bronchorrhea' is induced, and the watery solution helps to dilute down the respiratory tract secretions and to increase their bulk, thereby augmenting expectoration. Furthermore, there is evidence that hypertonic saline has a direct effect on the mucoprotein DNA complexes, and by reducing the cohesive intramolecular forces, the salt helps reduce the viscous properties of the mucoid fluid.[19] Excessive use of hypertonic saline is not recommended because irritation can occur in the respiratory tract, absorption can occur, and burn patients who cannot tolerate the sodium load may develop edema.

Finally, aerosolized acetylcysteine is a powerful mucolytic agent in use in respiratory care. Acetylcysteine contains a thiol group; the free sulfhydryl radical of this group is a strong reducing agent which ruptures the disulfide bonds which serve to give stability to the mucoprotein network of molecules in mucus. Agents which break down these disulfide bonds produce the most effective mucolysis.[20] Acetylcysteine is an irritant to the respiratory tract. It can cause mucosal changes, and it may induce bronchospasm. For this reason, patients are evaluated for signs of bronchospasm and a bronchodilator may be added if necessary. Acetylcysteine has proven to be effective in combination with aerosolized heparin for the treatment of inhalation injury in animal studies.[21] Heparin/acetylcysteine combinations have been used as scavengers for the oxygen free radicals produced when alveolar macrophages are activated either directly by chemicals in smoke or by one or more of the compounds in the arachidonic cascade.[22] Animal studies have shown an increased *P/F* ratio, decreased peak inspiratory pressures, and a decreased amount of fibrin cast formation with heparin/acetylcystine combinations.[23] Standard treatment for patients with inhalation injury might include 5000–10 000 units of heparin and 3 ml normal saline nebulized every 4 hours, alternating with 3–5 ml of 20% acetylcysteine for 7 days. This insures that the patient receives an aerosolized treatment every 2 hours. Baseline and daily clotting studies are recommended for the entire length of the aerosolized treatments.

Mechanical Ventilation

Over the past 30 years, and especially over the past decade, there has been an increase in new ventilatory techniques which present alternatives for the treatment of patients with smoke inhalation. Unfortunately, although the number of options available to the clinician has appeared to increase exponentially, well controlled clinical trials defining the specific role for each of the modes of ventilation and comparing them to other modes of ventilation has not been forthcoming. Based upon current available data, the recommendations from the American College of Chest Physicians consensus conference on mechanical ventilation generally serve as guidelines.[24] The general consensus concludes:

- The clinician should choose a ventilator mode that has been shown to be capable of supporting oxygenation and ventilation and that the clinician has experience in using.
- An acceptable oxygen saturation should be targeted.
- Based primarily on animal data, a plateau pressure of greater than 35 cmH_2O is cause for concern. With clinical conditions that are associated with a decreased chest wall compliance, plateau pressures greater than 35 cmH_2O may be acceptable.
- To accomplish the goal of limiting plateau pressures, $P\text{CO}_2$s should be permitted to rise (permissive hypercapnia) unless other contraindications exist that demand a more normal $P\text{CO}_2$ or pH.
- Positive end-expiratory pressure (PEEP) is useful in supporting oxygenation. An appropriate level of PEEP may be helpful in preventing lung damage. The level of PEEP required should be established by empirical trials and reevaluated on a regular basis.
- Large tidal volumes (12–15 ml/kg) with PEEP may be needed to improve oxygenation. Peak flow rates should be adjusted as needed to satisfy patient inspiratory needs.[24]

Modes of Ventilation

In the control mode of ventilation, the ventilator cycles automatically at a rate selected by the operator. The adjustment is usually made by a knob calibrated in breaths/min. The ventilator will cycle regardless of the patient need or desire for a breath, but guarantees a minimum level of minute ventilation in the apneic, sedated or paralysed patient. The control mode of ventilation is often utilized in patients with the adult respiratory distress syndrome due to the high peak pressures needed to achieve adequate chest expansion. The major disadvantage with this mode is that the patient cannot cycle the ventilator and thus the minute ventilation must be set appropriately.

In the assist-control mode of ventilation in which every breath is supported by the ventilator, a backup control rate is set; however, the patient may choose any rate above the set rate. Using this mode of ventilation, the tidal volume, inspiratory flow rate, flow waveform, sensitivity and control rate are set.[25-27]

Advantages are that assist-control ventilation combines the security of controlled ventilation with the possibility of synchronizing the breathing pattern of the patient and ventilator, and it ensures ventilatory support during each breath.

Disadvantages are as follows:

- Excessive patient work occurs in case of inadequate peak flow or sensitivity settings, especially if the ventilator drive of the patient is increased.[25-27]
- It is sometimes poorly tolerated in awake, nonsedated subjects and can require sedation to insure synchrony of patient and machine.
- It can cause respiratory alkalosis.
- It may worsen air trapping with patients with chronic obstructed lung disease.[24]

Synchronized intermittent mandatory ventilation (SIMV)

This mode of ventilation combines a preset number of ventilator-delivered mandatory breaths of preset tidal volume with the facility for intermittent patient-generated spontaneous breaths.[28,29]

Advantages are as follows:

- The patient is able to perform a variable amount of respiratory work and yet there is the security of a preset mandatory level of ventilation.

- SIMV allows for a variation in level of partial ventilatory support from near total ventilatory support to spontaneous breathing.
- It can be used as a weaning tool.

Disadvantages are:

- Hyperventilation with respiratory alkalosis.
- Excessive work of breathing due to the presence of a poorly responsive demand valve, suboptimal ventilatory circuits or inappropriate flow delivery could occur.
- In each case, extra work is imposed on the patient during spontaneous breaths.

Pressure support ventilation (PSV)

Pressure support ventilation (PSV) is a pressure-targeted, flow-cycled, mode of ventilation in which each breath must be patient triggered. It is used both as a mode of ventilation during stable ventilatory support periods and as a weaning method.[30–34] It is primarily designed to assist spontaneous breathing and therefore the patient must have an intact respiratory drive.

Advantages are:

- It is generally regarded as a comfortable mode of ventilation for most patients.
- Pressure support reduces the work of breathing.
- It can be used to overcome the airway resistance caused by the endotracheal tube.
- Pressure support may be useful in patients who are difficult to wean.

Disadvantages are:

- The tidal volume is not controlled and is dependent on respiratory mechanics, cycling frequency, and synchrony between the patient and ventilator.
- Pressure support may be poorly tolerated in some patients with high airway resistances because of the preset high initial flow rates.

Alternate Modes of Ventilation

During the last decade, a new concept has emerged regarding acute lung injury. In severe cases of adult respiratory distress syndrome (ARDS), only a small part of the lung parenchyma remains accessible to gas delivered by mechanical ventilation.[35,36] As a consequence, tidal volumes of 10 ml/kg or more may overexpand and injure the remaining normally aerated lung parenchyma and could worsen the prognosis of severe acute respiratory failure by extending nonspecific alveolar damage. High airway pressures may result in overdistension and local hyperventilation of more compliant parts of the diseased lung. Overdistension of lungs in animals has produced diffuse alveolar damage.[37,38] This is the reason why alternative modes of ventilation, all based on a reduction of end-inspiratory airway pressures and/or tidal volumes delivered to the patient, have been developed and are used by many clinicians caring for patients with severe forms of acute or chronic respiratory failure. Two alternative modes of ventilation, high-frequency ventilation (HFV) and inverse ratio ventilation (IRV) will be discussed.

High-frequency ventilation (HFV)

High-frequency ventilation (HFV) is the administration of small tidal volumes of 1–3 ml/kg at high frequencies of 100–3000 cpm.[39] Because it is a mode of ventilation based on a marked reduction in tidal volumes and airway pressures, it has the greatest potential for reducing pulmonary barotrauma.

There are a number of different types of high-frequency ventilation techniques. The two most common are high-frequency oscillation ventilation (HFOV) and high-frequency jet ventilation (HFJV).

High-frequency jet ventilation is the only high frequency mode routinely used to ventilate patients with ARDS, mainly in Europe.[24] Comparative data concerning the advantages of HFJV over conventional ventilation is limited.

There is no agreement, however, that HFJV is better than conventional mechanical ventilation in ARDS.[40]

High-frequency oscillatory ventilation is a new technique that has shown some promise in the ventilation of patients with inhalation injury.[41,42] Clinical studies indicate that this mode of ventilation may aid in reducing pulmonary barotrauma.[41,42] With this mode of ventilation, subtidal volumes are delivered in a progressive stepwise fashion until a preset oscillatory equilibrium is reached and exhalation is passive.

Clinicians must be familiar with the technique used and its possible limitations. There must be adequate humidification of the respiratory gases or severe necrotizing tracheobronchitis can occur. Special delivery devices for providing adequate humidification during HFV are required.

Inverse ratio ventilation (IRV)

Inverse ratio ventilation (IRV) is the use of an inspiratory/expiratory (I:E) ratio greater than 1:1. The rationale behind this is to maintain a high mean airway pressure and to hold peak alveolar pressure within a safe range. The second theoretical concept underlying IRV is the prolongation of inspiration to allow for recruitment of lung units with a long time constant. Deep sedation and/or paralysis is nearly always required with this mode of ventilation. At this time there is no conclusive scientific data comparing IRV to conventional mechanical ventilation in patients with inhalation injury.

Typical Ventilator Settings Required

Tidal volumes

In volume-cycled ventilation, a machine-delivered tidal volume is set to be consistent with adequate gas exchange and patient comfort. The tidal volume selected for burned patients normally varies between 10 and 15 ml/kg of body weight. Numerous factors, such as lung/thorax compliance, system resistance, compressible volume loss, oxygenation, ventilation and barotrauma, are considered when volumes are selected.[43] Of critical importance is the avoidance of overdistension. This can generally be accomplished by insuring that peak airway and alveolar pressures do not exceed a maximum target. Many would agree that a peak alveolar pressure greater than 35 cmH_2O in adults raises concern regarding the development of barotrauma and ventilator-induced lung injury increases.[44,45] The clinician must always look at the patient to insure adequate chest expansion with the setting of the tidal volume. Expired tidal volumes should be measured for accuracy at the connection between the patient's wye and the artificial airway. This insures that the volume selected reaches the patient and is not lost in the compressible volume of the ventilator tubing.

The range of tidal volumes will vary depending on the disease process, with some diseases requiring maximum tidal volumes and others needing less. Severe interstitial diseases such as pneumonia and ARDS may require a tidal volume of 15 ml/kg to adequately inflate the lungs and improve gas exchange. The acceptable range of 10–15 ml/kg allows the clinician to make more precise adjustments in volume, as needed by the patient.

Respiratory rate

Setting of the mandatory ventilator respiratory rate is dependent on the mode of ventilation selected, the delivered tidal volume, dead space to tidal volume ratio, metabolic rate, targeted $P\text{CO}_2$ levels, and level of spontaneous ventilation.[43] With adults, set mandatory rate normally varies between 4 and 20 breaths/min, with most clinically stable patients requiring mandatory rates in the 8–12 range.[43] In patients with inhalation injury, mandatory rates exceeding 20 per minute may be necessary, depending on the desired expired volume and targeted $P\text{CO}_2$. Along with the $P\text{CO}_2$, pH, and patient comfort, the primary variable controlling the selection of the respiratory rate is the development of air trapping and auto PEEP.[46]

The respiratory rates of children and infants all need to be set substantially higher than those of adults. For pediatrics, the respiratory rate can be set at from 14 to 35 depending on the disease state and the level of targeted $P\text{CO}_2$ one wishes to achieve. Slower respiratory rates are useful in the patient with obstructed airways because slower rates allow more time for exhalation and emptying of hyperinflated areas.

Arterial blood gases should be checked after the patient has been on the ventilator for approximately 20 minutes and the respiratory rate adjusted accordingly.

Flow rates

The selection of peak inspiratory flow rate during volume ventilation is primarily determined by the level of spontaneous inspiratory effort. In patients triggering volume breaths, patient effort, work of breathing, and patient ventilator synchrony depend on the selection of peak inspiratory flow.[26] Peak inspiratory flows should ideally match patient peak inspiratory demands. This normally requires peak flows to be set at 40–100 l/min, depending on expired volume and the inspiratory demand.[24]

Inspiratory/expiratory (I:E) ratio

The time allowed for the inspiratory and expiratory phases of mechanical ventilation is commonly referred to as the inspiratory/expiratory (I:E) ratio. The inspiratory part of the ratio includes the time to deliver the tidal volume before the exhalation valve opens and exhalation begins. The expiratory part of the ratio includes the time necessary for the tidal volume to exit through the exhalation valve before the next inspiration begins. The inspiratory time should be long enough to deliver the tidal volume at flow rates that will not result in turbulence and high peak airway pressures. The usual I:E ratio is 1:2.[47]

In severe lung disease it is acceptable to prolong the inspiratory time to allow for better distribution of gas and enhance oxygen diffusion. When a longer inspiratory time is required, careful attention should be given to sufficient expiration to avoid stacking of breaths and impeding venous return. Prolonged inspiratory time creates a more laminar flow, which helps to keep the peak pressures lower. Fast inspiratory times are tolerated in patients with severe airway obstruction. The fast inspiratory time allows for a longer expiratory phase, which may help to decrease the amount of overinflation.

Inspired oxygen concentration

As a starting point and until the level of hypoxemia is determined, a patient placed on a ventilator should receive an oxygen concentration of 100%. The concentration should be systematically lowered as soon as arterial blood gases dictate. In general, as a result of the concerns regarding the effects of high oxygen concentration on lung injury, the lowest acceptable oxygen level should be selected as soon as possible. In patients who are difficult to oxygenate, oxygen concentrations can be minimized by optimizing PEEP and mean airway pressures and selecting a minimally acceptable oxygen saturation.[48]

Positive end-expiratory pressure (PEEP)

PEEP is applied to recruit lung volumes, elevate mean airway pressure, and improve oxygenation.[49] The level of PEEP used varies with the disease process. PEEP levels should start at 5 cmH_2O and be increased in 2.5 cm increments. Increasing levels of PEEP in conjunction with a prolonged inspiratory time aids in oxygenation and allows for the safe level of oxygen to be used.

Usually a minimum of 5 cmH_2O of PEEP will be indicated for use during mechanical ventilation since tracheal intubation holds the larynx constantly open which leads to alveolar collapse and a reduction in the functional residual capacity.

Optimal PEEP is the level of end-expiratory pressure that results in the lowering of intrapulmonary shunting, significant improvement in arterial oxygenation, and only a small change in cardiac output, arteriovenous oxygen content differences or mixed venous oxygen tension.

Extubation Criteria

Standard extubation criteria include a wide variety of physiologic indices that have been proposed to guide the process of discontinuing ventilatory support. Traditional indices include:

- $Pa\text{O}_2/Fi\text{O}_2$ ratio of greater than 250.
- Maximum inspiratory pressure of greater than 60 cmH_2O.
- Vital capacity of at least 15–20 ml/kg.
- Tidal volume of at least 5–7 ml/kg.
- Maximum voluntary ventilation of at least twice the minute volume.[50,51]

In general these indices evaluate a patient's ability to sustain spontaneous ventilation. They do not assess a patient's ability to protect the upper airway. For this reason, traditional indices often fail to reflect the true clinical picture of a patient with an inhalation injury. For a complete evaluation prior to extubation, bronchoscopic examination will aid in determining if the airway edema has decreased enough to attempt extubation.

Prior to a scheduled extubation it is recommended that reintubation equipment be set up and that the person doing the extubation be experienced in emergency intubations.

If the patient demonstrates signs of inspiratory stridor, the use of racemic epinephrine by aerosol has been effective in reducing the mucosal edema and may prevent the patient from being reintubated.

Infection Control of Respiratory Equipment

Infections are the leading cause of mortality in burned patients. Pneumonia has become one of the most frequent life-threatening infections and is an important determinant of survival.[52] The majority of pneumonias are nosocomial, occurring in the burned patient after 72 hours of hospitalization, and are often associated with either an inhalation injury or endotracheal intubation with exposure to respiratory care equipment, or both.[57–59] One of the most important risk factors predisposing to pneumonia in burned patients is endotracheal intubation.[60–61] The incidence of pneumonia developing is estimated to be five times higher for intubated than nonintubated patients, and tracheostomy increases this risk even higher.[59–62] Exposure to respiratory care equipment adds an increased risk of pneumonia above and beyond the risk associated with endotracheal intubation.[63,64] After the use of nebulization equipment in respiratory care became popular, several epidemics of nosocomial pneumonia were reported.[65] The risk of pneumonia from mechanical ventilators was significant but decreased with a better understanding of the necessity to decontaminate respiratory equipment.[66,67] Intubated patients receiving respiratory care may be at an increased risk of pneumonia because of coincidental exposure to other procedures such as suctioning and bronchoscopy. Respiratory care equipment, if not properly cared for, may provide a source of extraneous organisms that can contaminate the patient's respiratory tract.

The potential role of respiratory care equipment in providing reservoirs for organisms that are capable of infecting the lungs is well established. This problem, particularly pertaining to reservoir devices and medications, has been recognized for a number of years, and effective control strategies have been developed. Most hospitals maintain a bacteriological monitoring system, and significant contamination by this route is not likely.[68] Contamination of the compressed gases used to operate respiratory care devices is uncommon, principally because of the desiccation of gases and the inability of most bacterial species to survive such harsh treatment. Nebulization equipment delivers a fine-particle aerosol and, if contaminated, the aerosol droplets may contain bacteria. Humidification equipment provides water vapor but does not deliver a large quantity of water in particulate form. In fact, humidifiers generally remove bacteria from airstreams, because the bacteria are physically trapped in the fluid phase and are not vaporized.

Bag-mask units have been shown to allow the persistence of infectious organisms and the subsequent infection of other patients on whom the equipment has been later used.[69]

Ventilator circuits are inevitably contaminated by the patient's own respiratory tract flora during exhalation and coughing, and the fluid that collects in this tubing is thereby contaminated. Allowing such a collection of tubing condensate to drain back into a reservoir nebulizer can provide ample time for bacteria multiplication. Towards the end of the changeover time for ventilator circuits, the patient will receive a large inhalation exposure to bacteria.

Table 18.1 Common methods of disinfection and sterilization

Method	Equipment	Advantages	Disadvantages
Autoclaving	Linens, surgical instruments, laryngoscope handles	Inexpensive, fast, nontoxic	Damages heat- and moisture-sensitive equipment
Acid glutaraldehyde	Rubber, plastic, metals	Sterilizes in 1 h, disinfects	Forms toxic residues, in 20 min, lasts 28 days contact dermatitis
recontamination can occur,			
Alkaline glutaraldehyde	Rubber, plastic, metals	Sterilizes in 10 h, disinfects in 10 min, lasts 14 days	Toxic residues, recontamination can occur, contact dermatitis
Gas sterilization	All items moisture or heat sensitive	Effectively sterilizes prewrapped materials	Expensive, time consuming, aeration is needed to remove toxic residues
Boiling	Home care items	Inexpensive, simple	Time-consuming, does not produce sterility, damages sensitive equipment

Table 18.2 Decontamination procedures

Reusable equipment	Change time	Soap and water clean	Disinfectant spray	Liquid disinfectant	ETO	Steam autoclave
Nebulizers	8–12 h	Disassemble	–	–	+	–
Ultrasonic nebulizer	Between patients	Wipe down, clean filters	+	Reusable filter	–	–
Portable spirometers	After PT use	–	Wipe with 70% alcohol	–	+	–
Ventilators	After PT	Fan filters	Cascade and unit	–	–	–
Bag-mask units	After PT use	–	–	–	+	–
Fiberoptic bronchoscopes	After each	+	–	+	+	–

ETO = ethylene oxide, – = non–applicable, + = applicable.

Generally, as long as equipment is sterile when placed in service, changing equipment more often than 24-hour intervals is not necessary.[70] **Table 18.1** demonstrates the time period generally acceptable for equipment changeover as well as the appropriate method of disinfection or sterilization of the product. Whenever possible, disposable respiratory equipment is preferred for use in the burn intensive care unit, since it is frequently contaminated with blood, body fluids and secretions. For hospitals where disposable equipment is not an option, the following types of disinfection of sterilization techniques should be employed (**Table 18.2**).

Disinfection and Sterilizing Techniques

Handwashing

Handwashing is generally considered the single most important procedure for preventing nosocomial infections. Regardless of whatever benefits are accrued by cleaning or sterilization, it is negated if the simple process of handwashing is overlooked. The recommended handwashing procedures depend on the purpose of washing. In most situations, a vigorous brief washing with soap under a strong running water is adequate to remove transient flora. Generally, simple handwashing with soap is performed before and after contact with patients and whenever the hands are soiled.

Antimicrobial handwashing procedures are indicated before all invasive procedures, during the care of patients in strict, respiratory, or enteric isolation, before entering intensive care units. The most commonly used agents are 70% isopropyl alcohol, iodophors, and chlorhexidine. Scrub regimens such as the povidone-iodine surgical scrub are appropriate for these areas.[71] For mechanical removal of microbes, the three key methods are scrubbing, filtration, and sedimentation. In respiratory care, mechanical scrubbing and filtration processes are commonly employed, whereas sedimentation has little current application. The most common nonmechanical physical agent used in the process of sterilization and disinfection is the application of heat.

Scrubbing

Scrubbing is the basic process for disinfection and sterilization. In practice it is both mechanical and chemical. The physical act removes many microbes and is often augmented by soap, water and antimicrobial agents. Unless the microbes are of extreme virulence, contaminated respiratory care equipment is first disassembled and scrubbed so that dirt, debris, and extraneous materials are removed. This step is paramount if the later disinfection or sterilization processes are to be effective.[72]

Filtration

Filtration of bacteria is accomplished by passing a liquid or gas through a material whose pores are small enough to retain the microbes. In that liquid and gases are difficult to disinfect or sterilize, most commonly either is accomplished through the process of filtration.[72] Filters interposed between the ventilator and breathing circuits effectively eliminate contaminants from the driving gas and prevent retrograde contamination. These filters should be changed according to manufacturer's specifications.

Boiling

Boiling is an old method for sanitation and low level disinfection. At sea level, the minimal level of exposure should be 30 minutes, with the time period adjusted upward 5 minutes per 1000 feet elevation above sea level. The efficiency of this process in killing spores can be increased by the addition of sodium bicarbonate sufficient to make a 2% solution or the addition of sodium hydroxide so as to make a 0.1% solution. With the addition of these chemicals, bacterial spores are destroyed in 10–30 minutes.[72]

Pasteurization

Pasteurization is an inexpensive and environmentally safe method of disinfection that has gained popularity for respiratory care equipment. The process employs a mild heat to destroy vegetative pathogens. With the current concerns for environmental safety, pasteurization offers a low-cost, nontoxic alternative to glutaraldehyde or ethylene oxide in areas where disinfection alone is sufficient. Not all respiratory care equipment can be pasteurized; the heat and moisture causes some plastic devices to become deformed, and rubber products such as anesthesia masks and ventilator reservoir bags may deteriorate due to the process.[72]

Autoclaving

Autoclaving is the application of steam and pressure to accomplish sterilization. Steam under 2 atmospheres of pressure has a temperature of 121°C. With this temperature and pressure, virtually all spores are killed within 15 minutes. The moisture enhances the conduction of heat and the rate of killing. With autoclaving the microorganisms are destroyed by disruption of the cell membrane, the coagulation of the cell protoplasm, or both.

Autoclaving is the most commonly used, effective form of sterilization and is preferred unless the material is injured by temperature or pressure. This is problematic for respiratory care, because much of the equipment is rubber or plastic, which cannot withstand the process.

Chemical Agents for Sterilization/Disinfection

Disinfectants act to kill microorganisms by several methods:

- oxidating microbial cells;
- hydrolyzing;
- combining with microbial proteins to form salts;
- coagulating the proteins of microbial cells;
- denaturing enzymes; or
- modifying cell wall permeability.[72]

Aldehydes

Aldehydes contain some of the most commonly used antimicrobials in respiratory care practice. These agents achieve their antimicrobial action through the alkylation of enzymes.

The cidal action of glutaraldehyde is accomplished by disruption of the lipoproteins in the cell membrane and cytoplasm of vegetative bacterial forms. This reaction between the chemical glutaraldehyde and cell proteins is dependent on both time and contact. Items to be disinfected must be free of material that would inhibit contact, and adequate contact time is needed for the chemical reaction to be complete.

Alkaline glutaraldehyde, buffered by a 0.3% bicarbonate agent, is used as a 2% solution. Once activated with the buffering agent, it is fully potent for approximately 14 days. This solution is bactericidal, virucidal, and tuberculocidal within 10 minutes and produces sterilization when applied for 10–20 hours. Equipment disinfected or sterilized with glutaraldehyde should be thoroughly rinsed and dried prior to use, because any residue would be irritating to mucous membranes.

Glutaraldehyde solutions are commonly used for the cold disinfection or sterilization of respiratory care equipment and have a large degree of safety. These solutions can be used to disinfect bronchoscopes as well as many of the current respiratory supplies.

Alcohols

Alcohols, especially ethylene and isopropyl alcohol, are perhaps the most commonly used disinfectants. Alcohols, as a chemical family, have many desirable characteristics needed in disinfectants. They are generally bactericidal and accomplish their bactericidal activity by damaging the cell wall membrane. They also have the ability to denature proteins, particularly enzymes called dehydrogenates. For alcohol to coagulate microbial proteins, water must be present. For this reason, 70% has been considered the critical dilution for alcohol, with a rapid loss of bactericidal activity with dilutions less than 50%. Both ethyl and isopropyl alcohols are rapidly effective against vegetative bacteria and tubercle bacilli but are not sporicidal.

Ethylene oxide

Ethylene oxide is a gas with a broad range of antimicrobial action. It is thought to destroy the microorganism by alkylating cellular constitutes. It kills both spores and bacteria, and has become a very popular method for sterilization much of the heat and moisture sensitive respiratory care equipment. The gas is extremely penetrating and does not require high temperatures for activation. Sterilization of equipment is usually accomplished under conditions of 30–50% relative humidity and at temperatures of 50–60°C.[72]

To avoid contact irritation from ethylene oxide, it is necessary that the residue gas be removed after sterilization is complete. Without the use of an aeration chamber, materials such as neoprene rubber and polyvinyl chloride require extended aeration times up to 7 days.

To be sure that the current infection control practice is effective in each institution, use of random microbiological cultures should be done whenever a problem is suspected or to test the reliability of the disinfection or sterilization techniques.

Late Complications of Inhalation Injury

Tracheal Stenosis

Tracheal complications are commonly seen and consist of tracheitis, tracheal ulcerations, and granuloma formation. The location of the stenosis is almost invariably subglottic and occurs at the site of the cuff of the endotracheal or tracheostomy tube.[73]

Several problems arising after extubation represent sequelae of laryngeal or tracheal injury incurred during the period of intubation. While tracheal stenosis or tracheomalacia are usually mild and asymptomatic, in some patients they can present as severe fixed or dynamic upper airway obstructions. These conditions can require surgical correction. In the management of intubated patients, such complications should be mostly preventable by meticulous attention to the tracheostomy or endotracheal tube cuff. Inflation of the cuff should be to the minimal pressure level consistent with preventing a leak in the ventilator at end inspiration.[45]

Obstructive/Restrictive Disease

Chronic airway disease is a relatively rare reported sequel of inhalation injury and its supportive treatment. Spirometry is a useful screening tool for airway obstruction. Reports in the literature for adults indicate that lung function returns to normal after inhalation injury.[74,75] However, Mlcak *et al.* reported pulmonary function changes following inhalation injury for up to 2.5 years post-injury in children.[76] Fortunately, most pulmonary function abnormalities will persist for only months following lung parenchymal injury. In the great majority of cases eventual resolution of both symptoms and physiological abnormalities will occur. During the resolution phase serial measurement of airflow obstruction should be obtained.[77] Desai *et al.* demonstrated that physiologic insults that occur as a result of thermal injury may limit exercise endurance in children.[78] Data from exercise stress testing showed evidence of a respiratory limitation to exercise. This was confirmed by a decrease in the maximal heart rate, decrease in the maximal oxygen consumption, and increased respiratory rate.

In the cases of persistent severe respiratory symptoms, the severity of the impairment should be documented and the patient evaluated for a pulmonary rehabilitation program.

Conclusion

Inhalation injury and associated major burns provide a challenge for health care workers who provide direct hands on care. The technical and physiologic problems which complicate the respiratory management of these patients require a practical knowledge of the possible sources of nosocomial infections. Patients with inhalation injury frequently require the use of respiratory care equipment that if not properly cared for can aid in the spread of infections. Important priorities for reducing the risk of infections include: an aggressive bronchial hygiene therapy program, the adherence to established infection control practices, the use of universal precautions during procedures and meticulous cleaning of respiratory care equipment, as well as routine epidemiologic surveillance of the established infection control practices within each institution.

References

1. Haponik E. Smoke inhalation injury: some priorities for respiratory care professionals. *Resp Care* 1992; **37:** 609.

2. Frownfelter D. Chicago: Year Book Medical, *Chest Physical Therapy and Pulmonary Rehabilitation*. 2nd ed. 1987: 266 pp.

3. Ivarez S E, Peterson M, Lansford B R. Respiratory treatments of the adult patients with spinal cord injury. *Phys Ther* 1981; **61:** 1738.

4. Chopra S K, Taplin G V, Simmons D H. Effects of hydration and physical therapy on tracheal transport velocity. *Am Rev Respir Dis* 1974; **115:** 1009–14.

5. Marini J J, Person D J, Hudson L D. A prospective comparison of fiberoptic bronchoscopy and respiratory therapy. *Am Rev Respir Dis* 1979; **119:** 971–8.

6. Oldenburg F A, Dolovich M B, Montgomery J M, *et al.* Effects of postural drainage, exercise and cough on mucus clearance in chronic bronchitis. *Am Rev Respir Dis* 1979; **12:** 730–47.

7. Remolina C, Khan A V, Santiago T V. Positional hypoxemia in unilateral lung disease. *N Engl J Med* 1981; **304:** 522–5.

8. Soria C, Walthall W, Price H. *Breathing and Pulmonary Hygiene Techniques: Pulmonary Rehabilitation*. Oxford: Butterworth Publishers, 1984: p. 860.

9. Caldwell S, Sullivan K. *Respiratory Care – A Guide to Clinical Practice*. Philadelphia: J B Lippincott, 1977: p. 91.

10. Albanese A J, Toplitz A D. A hassel free guide to suctioning a tracheostomy. *RN* 1982; **24:** 29.

11. Landa J F, Kwoka M, Chapman G, Bioto M. Effects of suctioning on mucociliary transport. *Chest* 1980; **77:** 202–7.

12. McFadden R. Decreasing respiratory compromise during infant suctioning. *Am J Nurs* 1981; **12:** 2158–61.

13. Wanner A. Nasopharyngeal airway: a facilitated access to the trachea. *Ann Intern Med* 1971; **75:** 592–5.

14. Brandstater B, Maullem M. Atelectasis following trachea suctioning in infants. *Anesthesiology* 1979; **31:** 294–7.

15. Roper P C, Vonwiller J B, Fisk G L, *et al.* Lobar atelectasis after nasotracheal intubation in infants. *Aust Pediat J* 1982; **12:** 272–5.

16. Yee A, Connors G, Cress D. *Pharmacology and the Respiratory Patient, Pulmonary Rehabilitation*. Oxford: Butterworth Publishers, 1984: p 125.

17. Whitbet T L, Manion C V. Cardiac and pulmonary effects of albuteral and isoproterenol. *Chest* 1978; **74:** 251–5.

18. Zimet I. Pharmacology of drugs used in respiratory therapy. *Respiratory Care – A Guide to Clinical Practice*. Philadelphia: J B Lippincott Co, 1977: p 473.

19. Lieberman J, Kurnick N B. Influence of deoxyribonucleic acid content on the proteolysis of sputum and pus. *Nature* 1962; **196:** 988.

20. Hirsh S R, Zastrow J E, Kory R C. Sputum liquification agents: a comprehensive in vitro study. *J Lab Clin Med* 1969; **74:** 346.

21. Brown M, Desai M H, Mlcak R, *et al.* Dimethylsulfoxide with heparin in the treatment of smoke inhalation injury. *J Burn Care Rehabil* 1988; **9**(1): 22.

22. Desai M H, Mlcak R, Brown M. *et al.* Reduction of smoke injury with DMSO and heparin treatment. *Surg Form* 1985; **36:** 103.

23. Desai M H, Brown M, Mlcak R, *et al.* Nebulization treatment of smoke inhalation injury in sheep model with DMSO, heparin combinations and acetylcysteine. *Crit Care Med* 1986; **14:** 321.

24. Slutsky A. American College of Chest Physicians Consensus Conference, Mechanical Ventilation. *Chest* 1993; **104:** 1833–59.

25. Marini J J, Capps J S, Culver B H. The inspiratory work of breathing during assisted mechanical ventilation. *Chest* 1985; **87:** 612–18.

26. Marini J J, Rodriquez R M, Lamb V. The inspiratory workload of patient initiated mechanical ventilation. *Am Rev Respir Dis* 1986; **134:** 902–4.

27. Ward M E, Corbeil C, Gibbons M W, *et al.* Optimilization of respiratory muscle relaxation during mechanical ventilation. *Anesthesiology* 1988; **69:** 29–35.

28. Downs J B, Klein E F, Desautels D, *et al.* Intermittent mandatory ventilation: a new approach to weaning patients. *Chest* 1973; **64:** 331–5.

29. Weisman I H, Rinaldo J E, Rodgers R M, *et al.* Intermittent mandatory ventilation. *Am Rev Respir Dis* 1983; **127:** 641–7.

30. Hirsch C, Kacmareck R M, Stanek K. Work of breathing during CPAP and PSV imposed by the new generation mechanical ventilators. *Resp Care* 1991; **36:** 815–28.

31. Macintyre N R. Respiratory function during pressure support ventilation. *Chest* 1986, **89:** 677–83.

32. Brochard L, Harf A, Lorino H. Inspiratory pressure support prevents diaphragmatic fatique during weaning from mechanical ventilation. *Am Rev Respir Dis* 1989; **139:** 513–21.

33. Fiastro J F, Habib M P, Quan S F. Pressure support compensates for inspiratory work due to endotracheal tubes. *Chest* 1988; **93:** 499–505.

34. Brochard L, Rau F, Lorino H, *et al.* Inspiratory pressure support compensates for the additional work of breathing caused by the endotracheal tube. *Anesthesiology* 1991; **75:** 739–45.

35. Hickling K G. Ventilatory management of ARDS: can it affect outcome? *Intensive Care Med* 1990; **9:** 239–50.

36. Gattinoni L, Pesenti A, Avalli L, *et al.* Pressure volume curve of total respiratory system in acute respiratory failure. *Am Rev Respir Dis* 1987; **136:** 730–60.

37. Dreyfuss D, Soler P, Basset G, *et al.* High inflation pressures, pulmonary edema, respective effects of high airway pressure, high tidal volume and PEEP. *Am Rev Respir Dis* 1988; **137:** 1159–64.

38. Kolobow T, Moretti M P, Fumagalli R, *et al.* Severe impairment of lung function induced by high peak airway pressure during mechanical ventilation. *Am Rev Respir Dis* 1987; **135:** 312–15.

39. Froese A B, Bryan A C, High frequency ventilation. *Am Rev Respir Dis* 1987; **135:** 1363–74.

40. Fusciardi J, Rouby J J, Barakat T, *et al.* Hemodynamic effects of high frequency jet ventilation in patients with and without shock. *Anesthesiology* 1986; **65:** 485–91.

41. Cioffi W, Graves T, McManus W, *et al.* High-frequency percussive ventilation in patients with inhalation injury. *J Trauma* 1989; **29:** 350–4.

42. Cioffi W, Rue L W III, Graves T, *et al.* Prophylactic use of high-frequency percussive ventilation in patients with inhalation injury. *Ann Surg* 1991; **213:** 575–81.

43. Kacmarek R M, Vengas J. Mechanical ventilatory rates and tidal volumes. *Resp Care* 1987; **32:** 466–78.

44. Hickling K G, Henderson S J, Jackson R. Low mortality associated with low volume, pressure limited ventilation with permissive hypercapnia in severe adult respiratory distress syndrom. *Intensive Care Med* 1990; **16:** 372–7.

45. Marini J J. New approaches to the ventilatory management of the adult respiratory distress syndrome. *J Crit Care* 1992; **87:** 256–7.

46. Pepe P E, Marini J J. Occult positive pressure in mechanically ventilated patients with airflow obstruction. *Am Rev Respir Dis* 1982; **126:** 166–70.

47. Kacmarek R M. Management of the patient mechanical ventilator system. In: Pierson D J, Kacmareck R M, eds. *Foundations of Respiratory Care*. New York: Churchill Livingstone Inc, 1992: 973–97.

48. Stroller J K, Kacmareck R M. Ventilatory strategies in the management of the adult respiratory distress syndrom. *Clin Chest Med* 1990; **11:** 755–72.

49. Suter P M, Fairley H B, Isenberg M D. Optimum end-expiratory airway pressure in patients with acute respiratory failure. *N Engl J Med* 1975; **292:** 284–9.

50. Sahn SA, Lakshminarayan S. Bedside criteria for discontinuation of mechanical ventilation. *Chest* 1973; **63:** 1002–5.

51. Tahvanainen J, Salmenpera M, Nikki P. Extubation criteria after weaning from IMV and CPAP. *Crit Care Med* 1983; **11:** 702–7.

52. Herndon D N, Lange F, Thompson P, *et al.* Pulmonary injury in burned patients. *Surg Clin North Am* 1987; **67:** 31.

53. Demling R H. Improved survival after major burns. *J Trauma* 1983; **23:** 179.

54. Luterman A, Dacso C C, Curreri W P. Infections in burned patients. *Am J Med* 1986; **81**(A): 45.

55. Pruitt B A Jr. The diagnosis and treatment of infection in the burned patient. *Burns* 1984; **11:** 79.

56. Pruitt B A Jr, Flemma R J, DiVincenti F C, *et al.* Pulmonary complications in burned patients. *J Thorac Cardiovasc Surg* 1970; **59:** 7.

57. Foley D F, Concrief J A, Mason A D. Pathology of the lungs in fatally burned patients. *Ann Surg* 1968; **167:** 251.

58. Moylan J A, Chan C. Inhalation injury – an increased problem. *Ann Surg* 1978; **188:** 34.

59. Craven D E, Kunches L M, Kilinsky V, *et al.* Risk factors for pneumonia and fatalities in patients receiving controlled mechanical ventilation. *Am Rev Respir Dis* 1986; **133:** 792.

60. Garibaldi R A, Britt M R, Coleman M L, *et al.* Risk factors for postoperative pneumonias. *Am J Med* 1984; **70:** 677.

61. Pennington J E. Hospital acquired pneumonias. In: Wenzel R P, ed. *Prevention and Control of Nosocomial Infections*. Baltimore: Williams & Wilkins, 1987: 321–4.

62w. Centers for Disease Control National Nosocomial Infection Study Report. Annual Summary 1983. *MMWR* 1983; **33**(259): 935.

63. Schwartz S N, Dowling J N, Ben Youic C, *et al.* Sources of Gram-negative bacilli colonizing the trachea of intubated patients. *J Infect Dis* 1978; **138:** 227.

64. Pierce A K, Edmonson E B, McGee G, *et al.* An analysis of factors predisposing to Gram-negative bacillary necrotizing pneumonia. *Am Rev Respir Dis* 1966; **94:** 309.

65. Ringros R E, McKown B, Felton F G, *et al.* A hospital outbreak of *Serratia marcescens* associated with ultrasonic equipment. *Ann Intern Med* 1968; **69:** 719.

66. Simmons B P, Wong E S. CDC guidelines for the prevention and control of nosocomial infections. *Am J Infect Control* 1983; **11:** 230.

67. Rhame F. The inanimate environment. In: Bennett J V, Bracham P S, eds. *Hospital Infections*. Boston: Little, Brown, 1986: 223–50.

68. Cross A S, Roupe B. Role of respiratory assistance devices in endemic nosocomial pneumonia. *Am J Med* 1981; **70:** 681–5.

69. Johanson W G. *Resp Care* 1982; **27:** 445–52.

70. Lareau S C, Ryan K J, Diener C F. The relationship between frequency of ventilator circuit changes and infection hazard. *Am Rev Respir Dis* 1978; **118:** 493–6.

71. Garner J S, Faverno M S. CDC guidelines for the prevention and control of nosocomial infections. *Am J Infect Control* 1986; **14:** 110–29.

72. Edge R S. Infection Control, Respiratory Care Practice. Chicago: Year Book Medical, 1988: 574.

73. Munster A M, Wong L A. *Miscellaneous Pulmonary Complications in Respiratory Injury*, New York: McGraw-Hill, Inc, 1990: p. 326.

74. Demling R H. Smoke inhalation injury. *Postgrad Med* 1987; **82:** 63.

75. Cahalane M, Demling R H. Early respiratory abnormalities from smoke inhalation. *JAMA* 1984; **251:** 771.

76. Mlcak R, Desai M H, Robinson E, *et al.* Pulmonary function changes following thermal injury in children. *Proc Am Burn Assoc* 1990; **22:** 46.

77. Colic G L. Long term respiratory complications of inhalation injury. In: *Respiratory Injury, Smoke Inhalation and Burns*. New York: McGraw-Hill, 1990: p. 342.

78. Desai M H, Mlcak R, Robinson E. Does inhalation injury limit exercise endurance in children convalescing from thermal injury. *J Burn Care Rehabil* 1993; **14:** 16–20.

RESPONSES TO INJURY

CHAPTER NINETEEN

Pathophysiology of the Systemic Inflammatory Response Syndrome

Frank Hinder and Daniel L. Traber

Introduction

Burned patients with or without inhalation injury commonly show pathophysiologic changes which result from inflammatory processes involving the whole organism. The phrase 'systemic inflammatory response syndrome (SIRS)' has recently been introduced to summarize the signs and symptoms of patients suffering from such a condition.[1] SIRS can follow multiple infectious and noninfectious insults. In thermally injured patients, the most common cause of SIRS is the burn itself. Sepsis, SIRS with the presence of infection or bacteremia, is also a common occurrence and a major factor in the high morbidity and mortality seen in themally injured patients. Pathologic alterations of the metabolic, cardiovascular, gastrointestinal, and coagulation systems occur as a result of the hyperactive immune system. These changes can ultimately induce cell damage; in the most severe cases, this damage can cause multiple system organ failure. Both cellular and humoral mechanisms are involved in these disease processes and have been extensively studied in various burn and sepsis models.

Definition of the SIRS

The term SIRS has been recommended by the consensus conference of The American College of Chest Physicians and the Society of Critical Care Medicine since 1991 to describe the general inflammatory process, no matter what has caused it.[1] The proposal was based on a large number of cases in intensive care units with a variety of conditions, both infectious and noninfectious, i.e. burns, sepsis, ischemia, multiple trauma, and pancreatitis. It was also noted that the administration of putative mediators of the inflammatory reaction, such as tumor necrosis factor-alpha (TNFα), induces a similar host response.

For the diagnosis of SIRS to be made, two or more of the following conditions must be present:[2]

- body temperature > 38°C or < 36°C;
- heart rate > 90 beats/min;
- respiratory rate > 20/min or Pa_{CO_2} < 32 mmHg;
- leukocyte count > 12 000/μl, < 4000/μl, or > 10% immature (band) forms.

All of these pathophysiologic changes must occur as an acute alteration from baseline in the absence of other known causes for them such as chemotherapy. This definition is very sensitive, and its clinical and prognostic significance still remains to be demonstrated. The approach to clinically evaluate the above-mentioned alterations as the expression of one pathophysiologic entity represents the current view that different insults can trigger a similar, exaggerated host response. Since SIRS is associated with tissue damage, the syndrome may be stratified by phrases like multiple organ dysfunction syndrome (MODS) and multiple organ system failure (MOSF). The definition of SIRS comprises only the clinical signs of some of the pathophysiologic alterations of systemic inflammation. Nevertheless, the authors will try to convey a more profound picture of the pathophysiology of the systemic inflammatory response.

General Considerations

The crucial pathophysiologic event in systemic inflammation is cell damage. This can occur both as a result of the direct injury to the cell by mediators such as TNFα or oxygen free radicals as well as indirectly by hypoxia due to the mechanisms described below. For analysis of mechanisms and their importance in the development of SIRS, one must consider several factors. The immune system is a complicated network. Soluble mediators secreted by immune and vascular endothelial cells regulate many immune functions and serve as means of communication between different parts of the system. Mediators are involved in the regulation of their own release as well as in the production and secretion of other mediators. Therefore, experimental intervention in order to study the effects of one mediator will necessarily affect the whole network. The existence of a network also explains why administration of a specific mediator might trigger systemic inflammation. Therapeutic intervention at different steps might be successful in the prevention of SIRS if the mediator plays a pivotal role in the development of the systemic inflammatory response. The authors divide the systemic inflammation into four categories in order to define the pathophysiology of systemic inflammation. One must, however, consider that these categories are not entities, but that they are interrelated and that even the same mediators might cause the underlying pathology of different categories. For a complete appraisal of the role of single mediators for all events related to systemic inflammation, the reader is referred to the numerous review articles using this approach to the problem.[3–5]

The Initiating Event

Patients suffering from injuries like sepsis, burns, or multiple trauma demonstrate a state of hypermetabolism; an increase in cellular, endothelial, and epithelial permeability; typical hemodynamic alterations; and often extensive microthrombosis. The exact mechanism by which the different injuries initiate the process which leads to systemic inflammation is not yet fully elucidated. The response might be initiated by the humoral or by the cellular system. Activation of the humoral system has been hypothesized to start the activation cascade after hemorrhagic shock.[6] The complement system which can become activated due to soft tissue injury might interact with the coagulation, fibrinolysis, and kallikrein–kinin systems and trigger the host response. During sepsis and endotoxemia, activation of cells of the reticuloendothelial system might be the first step in the process and subsequently lead to the release of mediators such as TNFα, interleukin-1 (IL-1), IL-6, and IL-8. TNFα[7,8] and IL-1[9,10] can produce most of the systemic inflammatory response independently. The same applies to the platelet-activating factor (PAF),[11] which is secreted by several cell types [macrophages, polymorphonuclear granulocytes (PMN) and platelets] after their activation.

The typical pattern of systemic inflammation can be initiated by the administration of endotoxin. Therefore, endotoxemia can serve as a model of systemic inflammation. Endotoxin is part of the cell wall of gram-negative bacteria and has been used in animal models as well as in healthy volunteers to study different aspects of the systemic inflammation under reproducible conditions. Endotoxin has also been found to be present during states of systemic inflammation in critically ill patients; however, its role in the development of the SIRS is still questioned since plasma levels of endotoxin correlate poorly with outcome. In addition, the administration of anti-endotoxin antibodies to septic patients did not show beneficial effects.[12] Moreover, at least 50% of the cases of sepsis cannot be associated with gram-negative bacteria or endotoxin.[13]

Endotoxin stimulates the cells of the reticuloendothelial system. They are omnipresent in the body, either as tissue-specific macrophages or as their precursors, the monocytes, which circulate in the blood and can enter into organs after stimulation. In addition to other functions important for homeostasis of the organism, these cells phagocytoze and digest foreign material. As mentioned above, monocytes and macrophages synthesize and secrete a wide variety of mediators (cytokines such as TNFα, IL-1, 6, 8, and eicosanoids) which have both effector functions and serve as means of communication for the immune system. Once released, these mediators can act in an autocrine, paracrine, and endocrine fashion and stimulate other cells, most notably PMNs and endothelial cells, which will then undergo typical changes and contribute to systemic inflammation (see below).

The Hemodynamic Response

The full clinical picture of systemic inflammation[21] after thermal injury, multiple trauma, or sepsis includes a hyperdynamic circulation. It is characterized by a low systemic vascular resistance, which requires a high cardiac output to maintain mean arterial pressure. This fall in resistance is not the result of an increase in metabolic rate. The oxygen extraction of the tissues remains the same. Blood is thus flowing to tissues which are not metabolically active. Patients who are not well resuscitated or whose heart function is compromised may not be able to increase their cardiac output to the extent needed in order to maintain arterial pressure during states of extensive vasodilatation and, thus, might go into shock and organ failure. A reduced vascular responsiveness to vasoconstrictors finally prevents successful pharmacologic intervention and patients might die in irreversible shock. It has been hypothesized that the development of the hyperdynamic state might be dependent on the presence of endotoxin or bacteria in the blood. An intravenous bolus injection of 4 ng/kg endotoxin into healthy volunteers mimics some aspects of the hemodynamic response seen in patients.[14,15] The low systemic vascular resistance and the elevated cardiac output can also be induced in animal models by continuous infusion of low-dose endotoxin[16] or bacteria.[17] Studies in conscious sheep revealed that the hemodynamic response to continuous low-dose endotoxin can be divided into three parts.[18] The first two phases might be missed under clinical conditions most of the time due to their short duration (< 3 h).

Phase 1

Systemic vascular resistance and pulmonary vascular resistance increase markedly both upon intermittent administration of endotoxin[19] or during its continuous infusion into conscious sheep.[20] This reaction occurred within 30 min to 1 hour of the endotoxin administration and was attributed to the release of the potent vasoconstrictor thromboxane A_2. Lymph and plasma levels of thromboxane B_2, the stable metabolite of the eicosanoid thromboxane A_2, were found elevated 1 and 4 hours after challenge of sheep with 1 μg/kg endotoxin.[21] Cyclooxygenase[22] and thromboxane synthetase inhibition diminished the hypertensive response.[21] Thromboxane synthetase inhibition was equally effective in preventing the marked pulmonary vasoconstriction after burn injury in pigs.[23] The high pulmonary vascular resistance during phase 1 of endotoxemia has been demonstrated to compromise myocardial function of the right heart in terms of a low ejection fraction and an increase in end-systolic diameter.[24,25] Administration of the thromboxane synthetase inhibitor OKY-046 blocked these early changes in right heart function.[24]

Early systemic vasoconstriction did not occur equally throughout the vasculature. Blood flow through the superior mesenteric artery was particularly reduced.[26] Vasoconstriction of the splanchnic vessels has been associated with the release of so-called myocardial depressant factors[27] and with bacterial translocation.[26] The coincidence of markedly decreased mesenteric blood flow and bacterial translocation has also been demonstrated after burn injury[28] and multiple trauma associated with a state of circulatory shock.[29] Moreover, hypoperfusion, particularly of the ileal mucosa, was still noted during the hyperdynamic phase in a *murine* sepsis model, when blood flow to most of the splanchnic area was not decreased.[30] Bacterial translocation has been hypothesized to be one of the major factors maintaining systemic inflammation. The pathophysiology of gut failure and its role in the development of multiple system organ failure is further discussed in another chapter.

Phase 2

This portion of the response, between 3 and 4 hours after the endotoxin infusion has been started, is characterized more by pulmonary permeability changes (see below) than by hemodynamic alterations. In the hyperdynamic sheep model, the pulmonary artery pressure is mildly elevated and cardiac output demonstrates the lowest values throughout the experiment. The underlying mechanisms of this response are not yet clear. Many mediators of the immune system have been released by that time, including TNFα, IL-6, PAF and peptidoleukotrienes.[31] This might indicate that these mediators are proximal elements of the mediator cascades. Although investigations into the release of many of these cytokines are few as a result of the limitations of respective assays, TNFα has been shown to be increased in both phases 1 and 2 of the response in sheep[32,33] and volunteers.[34,35] Moreover, the vasoconstrictor endothelin is elevated in the chronic sheep model of endotoxemia at that time,[36] as well as the vasodilator atrial natriuretic peptide.[37,38] Endothelin has also been correlated with reductions in cardiac output in septic humans.[39] The hemodynamic changes in phase 2 are most likely the result of the action of the mediator cocktail.

Phase 3

Continuous infusion of endotoxin into sheep and pigs resulted in a hyperdynamic circulation.[20,33,40] In addition to a low systemic vascular resistance and a high cardiac output with a slightly decreased mean arterial pressure, the hyperdynamic response is further characterized by hyporesponsiveness of isolated vessels to vasoconstrictors[41] and an increased pulmonary shunt fraction in the presence of a reduced pulmonary hypoxic vasoconstriction.[20,42,43] The high cardiac output is due to an increase in heart rate in the presence of depressed myocardial contractility.[44,45]

Nitric Oxide

The endothelial-derived relaxing factor, recently identified as nitric oxide (NO), has been implicated as a mediator in this reaction. NO can be synthesized from its precursor L-arginine by two different enzymes. The calcium-dependent constitutive nitric oxide synthase is responsible for the basal release of NO, which seems to play an important role for the regulation of vascular tone under physiologic conditions. *In vitro* data suggest that this enzyme might become inactivated early after administration of endotoxin, thus accounting for some of the vasoconstrictive phenomena seen in phases 1 and 2.[46] Dependent on the species, cells producing the inducible nitric oxide synthase include macrophages, vascular smooth muscle cells, and vascular endothelium upon stimulation by endotoxin, TNFα, interleukin-1 or γ-interferon.[47] On the other hand, it has recently been reported that the human macrophage cannot form NO under these circumstances.[48,49]

NO is a lipophilic gas which can easily enter vascular smooth muscle cells where it stimulates soluble guanylate cyclase[50,51] to synthesize cyclic guanosine monophosphate (cGMP). High levels of cGMP stimulate cells to lower their intracellular Ca^{2+} concentration. This leads to vascular dilatation and hyporesponsiveness to vasoconstrictors. Administration of a nitric oxide synthase (NOS) inhibitor to septic humans[52,53] and to endotoxemic sheep (**Figure 19.1**)[20] increases their vascular resistance and restores their responsiveness to vasoconstrictors. It was assumed that the hemodynamic abnormalities were mediated by NO formed via the inducible NO synthase; however, plasma concentrations of nitrite/nitrate and nitrosylated proteins were not elevated during *ovine* endotoxemia. Species specificity was also indicated by the finding that human macrophages do not produce the inducible form of NO synthase. Yet, the inducible form of the enzyme seems to be present in human hepatocytes. Elevated nitrite levels were reported in one study evaluating septic newborns.[54] There are currently no convincing data available with regard to high nitrite levels in adult humans with SIRS. Ochoa found somewhat elevated nitrite concentrations in some septic patients, but failed to demonstrate them in septic trauma patients.[55] At this point, it can neither be concluded nor can it be excluded that NO is involved in the mediation of the hyperdynamic response during systemic inflammation.

Guanylate Cyclase

The second messenger cGMP appears to play an important role in the vasodilation seen with sepsis. There have been reports of cGMP elevations in plasma of septic patients[56] and endotoxemic rats.[57] cGMP was elevated in tissues removed from animals following a continuous infusion of endotoxin.[58] The guanylate cyclase occurs in a soluble and in a particulate form.[59] The particulate form is activated by atrial natriuretic peptide (ANP).[60,61] The soluble form has a heme group that is activated by NO. This reaction is inhibited by methylene blue and hemoglobin.[62] There is a high probability that ANP is a further source of the stimulation of guanylate cyclase during sepsis and endotoxemia because the cGMP formed in some of the experiments was not inhibited by methylene blue or L-arginine analogs.

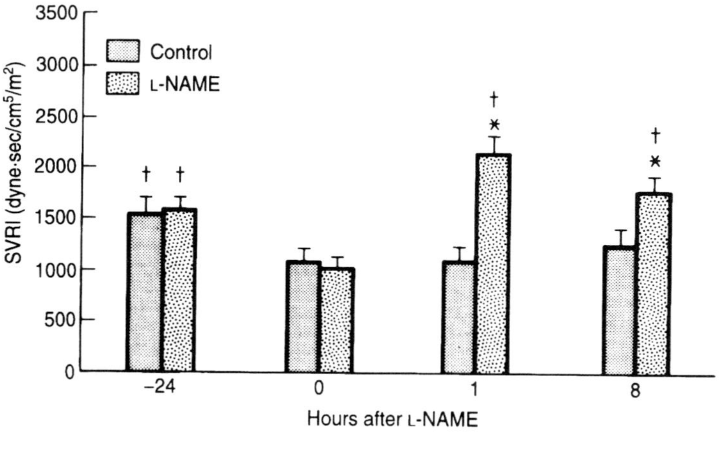

Fig. 19.1 Systemic vascular resistance index (SVRI) in a chronic ovine model of endotoxemia. Sheep received a continuous infusion of E. coli *endotoxin (10 ng/kg/min) for 32 h. The group 'L-NAME' was given a bolus of the nitric oxide synthase inhibitor N^{ω}- nitro L-arginine methylester (L-NAME: 25 mg/kg) at 0 h with a subsequent reversal of the low SVRI, while the control group was injected with the carrier NaCl 0.9%. * $p < 0.05$ vs. control, † $p < 0.05$ vs. 0 h.*

Atrial Natriuretic Peptide

A marked elevation in ANP has also been reported after the injection of endotoxin into sheep.[37,38] It was also found that the increase in plasma levels of ANP was sustained with the continuous infusion of endotoxin (**Figure 19.2**) or bacteria. ANP has been shown to be elevated in septic humans.[56,63] In the rat study reported above, in which the plasma levels of cGMP remained elevated despite administration of a NOS inhibitor, a marked increase in plasma levels of ANP was found.[57] ANP elevates smooth muscle cGMP[64–66] through stimulation of particulate or membrane guanylate cyclase, which is not affected by methylene blue,[59,60] and thereby produces vasodilation. ANP is released from the right atrium and might be the material responsible for the cGMP elevation which was seen in animal models of sepsis and humans with septicemia.

The Kallikrein–Kinin System

The kallikrein–kinin system, which includes several vasoactive substances, has been shown to be activated during endotoxemia in humans[67] and in sheep.[68] Administration of a bradykinin antagonist did not change the cardiovascular or microvascular response to endotoxin in chronically instrumented sheep.[68] Therefore, activation of this mediator cascade seems rather to be an epiphenomenon of endotoxemia.

CHANGES IN PERMEABILITY

Endothelial Permeability

Microvascular permeability is increased both in the systemic[69] and in the pulmonary circulation[70] during endotoxemia. The lung is the organ most commonly compromised during processes which lead to systemic inflammation. Edema formation due to an increase in microvascular permeability is a hallmark of the acute lung injury. The factors which determine the transvascular fluid flux are summarized in the Starling–Landis equation:[71,72]

$$J_v = K_f[(P_{mv} - P_i) - \sigma(\pi_{mv} - \pi_i)]$$

where J_v is the transvascular fluid flux, K_f is the filtration coefficient (measure of the endothelial permeability to small solutes and water as well as of the permeability surface area), P_{mv} is the microvascular hydrostatic pressure, P_i is the interstitial hydrostatic pressure, σ is the osmotic reflection coefficient to protein, π_{mv} is the microvascular oncotic pressure, and π_i is the interstitial oncotic pressure.

A model has been developed in sheep which allows a determination of the variables included in the Starling equation. The lymph flow draining from the efferent vessel of the caudal mediastinal lymph node has been used as a measure of the pulmonary transvascular fluid flux. Using this model, changes in lymph flow and lymph protein flux were evaluated during sepsis and endotoxemia. Again the changes in pulmonary endothelial permeability can be divided into three phases.

Phase 1

Several investigators studied lymph flow and lymph protein flux after administration of bacteria or short time infusion of 1–2 μg/kg of endotoxin in sheep. Two phases of microvascular pathology could be distinguished in these models.[73] During phase 1, there was a high microvascular hydrostatic pressure as defined by the Gaar equation.[74] It was associated with an increase in lung lymph flow, while the lymph protein concentration was low. It was concluded that the high microvascular hydrostatic pressure was responsible for the early increase in transvascular fluid flux. As mentioned above, thromboxane A_2 had been found to be responsible for the vasoconstriction occurring during phase 1 of the response to endotoxin. Therefore, it is not surprising that administration of the thromboxane synthetase inhibitor OKY-046 prevented the rise in lymph flow during phase 1.[21] This effect was also noted after blockage of the cyclooxygenase by ibuprofen.[22] Early edema formation after burns at the site of the injury might be due to a different mechanism. Recent data suggest that a marked fall in interstitial hydrostatic pressure might occur in the injured tissue, which can explain the immediate onset of edema formation after thermal injury.[75,76] These changes might be the result of an inhibition of the fibroblast β_1-integrin attachment to collagen.

Phase 2

During phase 2, lymph flow continues to be high. The lymph protein concentration rises considerably[73] and the pulmonary artery pressure is only mildly elevated. The oncotic pressure gradient between microvasculature and interstitial space is reduced during that period.[77] Together these data suggest that the permeability of the pulmonary endothelium to protein increases in phase 2. In fact, the reflection coefficient for total protein fell from 0.73 to 0.58 with respective changes of the reflection coefficients for albumin (0.66 to 0.5), IgG (0.76 to 0.64) and IgM (0.91 to 0.83) after 4 hours of *E. coli* sepsis in sheep.[78] Confirmation of this hypothesis is still pending in models of endotoxemia, but it has been generally accepted that the changes in pulmonary transvascular fluid flux in phase 2 represent changes in microvascular permeability. The mechanisms of the increased microvascular permeability are still under discussion.

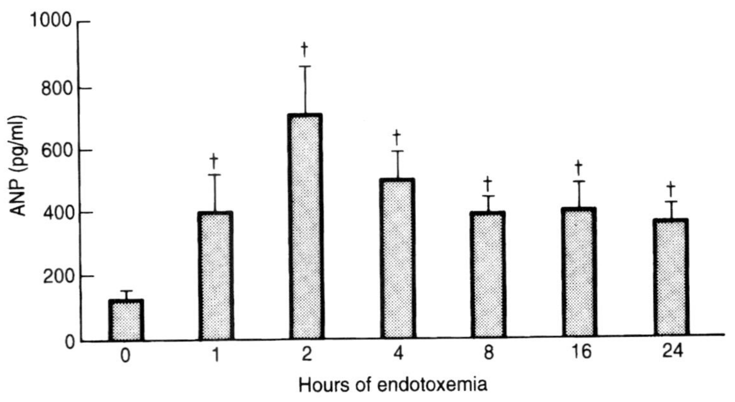

Fig. 19.2 Arterial plasma atrial natriuretic factor (ANP) levels in a chronic ovine model of endotoxemia. Sheep were continuously infused with E. coli endotoxin (10 ng/kg/min) for 24 h. The vasodilator ANP peaked at 2 h, and stayed elevated for the rest of the observation period. †, $P < 0.05$ vs 0 value.

Endothelial cells play an important role in the development of vascular permeability. It has been hypothesized that endothelial cells can contract upon stimulation.[79] As a result, the intercellular gaps might increase in number and/or size, establishing the so-called capillary leak syndrome. The development of the protein-rich high permeability edema can be ameliorated if substances are administered which raise the endothelial cell content of cyclic adenosine or guanosine monophosphate.[80,81] Endothelial cells do not merely serve as targets during systemic inflammation. They actively contribute to the ongoing inflammatory process. Their role in the inflammatory reaction has been estimated so highly that even the term 'endothelial inflammation' has been used to describe it. The endothelial cell can be stimulated by endotoxin, TNFα, or interleukin-1 to express E-selectin, an adhesion molecule.[82] E-selectin on the surface of endothelial cells interacts with the corresponding L-selectin complex on PMNs in order to facilitate the rolling of these cells along the endothelium.[83] Moreover, endothelial cells secrete the proinflammatory cytokine, IL-1,[84] which activates PMNs.

Conflicting data exist regarding the role of PMNs in SIRS. PMNs are usually found at the site of tissue injury, to which they migrate following a concentration gradient of chemotactic stimuli. Stimulation of the endothelial cells causes the PMNs to roll along the vascular endothelial surface and in a further step, after interaction of the PMN, CD11/18 integrin, with its ligand, the intercellular adhesion molecule (ICAM-1) the PMN can emigrate from the vessel into the interstitial space. Antibodies against the common CD18 β chain showed beneficial effects in an animal model of sepsis-induced lung injury.[85] On the other hand, patients who are deficient in CD18 have abundant PMNs in their alveolar spaces. In addition, the monoclonal antibody 60.3 was ineffective in completely blocking the migration of PMNs into the lung in a number of conditions.[86] We have recently reported that in chronic endotoxemia, there were few PMNs in the lung but numerous macrophages.[87] Activated PMNs and macrophages secrete oxygen free radicals and proteases, which is part of their defense mechanism against microorganisms. Administration of oxygen free radical scavengers and antiproteases proved to be useful in diminishing edema accumulation after endotoxin.[88,89] Animals were depleted of their granulocytes by anti-PMN antiserum[90] or by treatment with nitrogen mustard.[91] This did not prevent the changes in microvascular permeability following the administration of endotoxin. Moreover, patients deficient in PMNs would still develop the adult respiratory distress syndrome associated with sepsis.[92,93] On the other hand, treatment of sheep or goats with hydroxyurea, which is another compound used to deplete granulocytes, was effective and diminished the fluid accumulation in the lung.[94] Urea scavenges free radicals, a fact which might explain its efficacy.[95] As the inflammatory response becomes chronic, many mediators have been released; more than one mechanism might be assumed to be responsible for the capillary leak.

Many studies were performed to evaluate the role of metabolites of the arachidonic acid for the increase in permeability. Administration of the thromboxane synthetase inhibitor OKY-046 not only reduced transvascular fluid flux in phase 1, but was also effective in phase 2 after a bolus of endotoxin.[21] Nevertheless, this does not mean that thromboxane A_2 itself had induced the increase in permeability. It has been reported that thromboxane B_2, previously assumed to be an inactive metabolite of thromboxane A_2, might cause lung damage.[96] Moreover, thromboxane synthetase blockage by OKY-046 reduced the plasma conjugated dienes, which are peroxidation products of oxygen free radicals.[21] Granulocyte chemiluminescence was elevated 4 hours after administration of 1.5 μg/kg of endotoxin to chronically instrumented sheep, indicating the production of oxygen free radicals.[97] Oxygen free radicals can increase microvascular permeability both by activation of endothelial cell contraction[98] and by damaging the endothelial cell membrane. OKY-46 has been demonstrated to reverse other forms of oxygen free radical induced lung injury.[99,100] On the other hand, inhibition of the cyclooxygenase did not affect transvascular fluid flux during phase 2, even if thromboxane A_2 is a cyclooxygenase metabolite.[22] This discrepancy is still unexplained. Inhibition of the cyclooxygenase may block both the formation of thromboxane and the salutary eicosanoid prostacyclin. Prostacyclin is elevated after endotoxin administration, and this material has many actions which counter the actions of thromboxane.

Microvascular damage during systemic inflammation might also be regarded as ischemia/reperfusion injury, particularly when it was preceded by a period of intestinal hypoperfusion. Xanthine oxidase-generated oxygen free radicals have been reported to mediate changes in microvascular and epithelial permeability.[101] Endotoxin-induced ileal and cecal permeability was associated with an increased xanthine oxidase activity; inhibition of xanthine oxidase by allopurinol has been shown to reduce intestinal mucosal damage.[102,103] Circulating xanthine oxidase after ischemia/reperfusion injury in rats was associated with pulmonary retention of PMNs and pulmonary capillary leak, which was diminished by pretreatment with allopurinol.[104] Intravenous injection of purified xanthine oxidase, however, induced pulmonary retention of PMNs without increasing microvascular permeability. Therefore, a final evaluation of the role of xanthine oxidase in ischemia/reperfusion induced permeability changes is not yet possible.

TNFα is one of the early mediators in systemic inflammation. It has been reported to be elevated during sepsis and endotoxemia, after hemorrhagic shock or thermal injury. It is considered one of the most important mediators in the cascade, because it has the potential to stimulate or enhance most of the steps of the inflammatory response. Moreover, administration of human recombinant TNFα reproduced most of the effects of endotoxemia, including the alterations in pulmonary microvascular permeability in the chronic sheep model.[105,106] It has been questioned whether the *ovine* response to human TNFα was only related to the cytokine,[81] because contamination of the recombinant material with endotoxin is not uncommon.

TNFα also induces the secretion of PAF, which is a further early mediator of the systemic inflammation. PAF causes an increase in lung lymph flow and permeability to protein when it is infused into conscious sheep.[11] Administration of a PAF antagonist abolished the cardiopulmonary response which occurred during phase 1 and attenuated it during phase 2.[107] PAF had no direct effect on endothelial cells.[11] This suggests that it probably increased microvascular permeability through other mechanisms such as its priming effect on PMNs.[108]

Phase 3

The hyperdynamic cardiovascular response is associated with profound changes in pulmonary transvascular fluid flux in the *ovine* model of continuous endotoxemia.[40,70] These changes in microvascular fluid flux are perhaps more important than those seen in the other phases of sepsis because the late changes are sustained. The lymph protein concentration gradually decreased after phase 2; after 24 hours of endotoxemia the reflection coefficient to protein was at baseline level, while the lymph flow was still high. The microvascular hydrostatic pressure, evaluated by Holloway's technique, was not significantly different from baseline.[109] The elevated transvascular fluid flux was attributed to a high filtration coefficient. An increase in both perfused surface area and pore numbers might have contributed to the change in filtration. On the other hand, repeated injections of endotoxin decreased subsequent lung lymph production in response to endotoxin.[110] Perhaps this may be related to the ability of endotoxin to induce the synthesis of superoxide dismutase.[111]

Since the changes in lung lymph flow produced by endotoxin were associated with elevations in endothelin[36,109] and ANP, these peptides are putative mediators of the elevated pulmonary transvascular fluid flux. Further studies must determine whether these factors affect the pulmonary microvascular changes during the late phases of sepsis and multiple organ failure.

Increased Epithelial Permeability

Permeability changes during systemic inflammation are not restricted to the endothelium. Loss of epithelial barrier function has been noted both in the lung and in the intestine. Administration of 2–4 ng/kg endotoxin to healthy human volunteers increased their alveolar epithelial permeability to the inhaled 492 Da molecule [^{99m}Tc]diethylenetriamine pentaacetate (DTPA) 3 hours after endotoxin had been given.[15] Human volunteers demonstrated a higher intestinal epithelial permeability to mannitol/lactulose.[112] Bacterial translocation occurred during endotoxemia,[26] thermal injury,[23] and multiple trauma with hemorrhagic shock.[113] This might well be interpreted as a loss of intestinal barrier function. Nevertheless, one must bear in mind that epithelial permeability to molecules like lactulose/mannitol and bacterial translocation do not necessarily relate to each other. The epithelium could also be injured by ischemial reperfusion, which occurs in all of these situations.[114]

The Hypercoagulatory Response

Disseminated intravascular coagulation (DIC) is a serious complication of systemic inflammation. During hemorrhagic shock or sepsis widespread activation of the coagulation systems as well as decreased fibrinolysis and levels of inhibitors of the contact and coagulation systems might all contribute to the development of DIC. Endotoxin has been reported to play a decisive role in burn-induced coagulopathy.[6] Endothelial fibrin deposits could be demonstrated in the *ovine* lung ultrastructure *in vivo*, 6 hours after intravenous administration of a bolus of endotoxin. Endotoxin stimulates the production of an endothelium-dependent procoagulant tissue factor (thromboplastin).[115] Thromboplastin is a substrate both for the extrinsic (factor VII) and the intrinsic pathway (factor XII) of blood coagulation. Endotoxin can also damage endothelial cells directly or indirectly by mediators like TNFα, which are released in response to endotoxin. The damaged cells release tissue thromboplastin; in addition, the exposed collagen can then further enhance activation of factor XII. Moreover, endotoxin induces endothelial cell secretion of a fast-acting inhibitor of the plasminogen activator;[116] it decreases the endothelial expression of thrombomodulin,[117] which plays an important role for the activation of the anticoagulatory protein C. In addition to its direct effects, endotoxin can influence the coagulation system by its induction of mediators like TNFα and interleukin-1. Both cytokines have been shown to exert procoagulant activity themselves.[84,118] The resultant principal mediator of coagulation through the different pathways is thrombin. Administration of thrombin-induced intravascular coagulation *in vivo* (sheep and dogs).[119] Moreover, the coagulation cascade seems to interfere with endothelial permeability, because thrombin also increased the pulmonary microvascular permeability to protein.[120,121] So far, multiple coagulation factor abnormalities have already been documented in both septic patients [122] and human volunteers treated with endotoxin.[123] The mechanisms by which the complex failure of the blood coagulation system is initiated are not yet completely understood.

The Two-hit Hypothesis

It has been known in cellular immunology for several years that monocytes and macrophages can undergo several steps during the activation process. For instance, the lymphokine γ-interferon might act as the first signal and prime macrophages. The cells respond with a number of changes, including an increase in the transcription rate of mRNA for TNFα. Nevertheless, no TNFα is produced. If a second stimulus, like endotoxin, is provided in even a small dose, the macrophages are triggered to become fully activated and to secrete large amounts of TNFα. The same effect can be induced if a very high dose of endotoxin is administered. Recently, several studies focusing on organ injury by systemic inflammatory processes indicate that a phenomenon comparable to the cellular events described above can occur and involve the whole body.[124] Dehring *et al.* found a more persistent pulmonary hypertension and an exaggerated hyperdynamic response to bacteremia in sheep when a week-old thermal injury preceded the bacterial challenge.[125] In a rat model of intestinal ischemia/reperfusion injury and endotoxemia, lung albumin leak and mortality rate increased only if both injuries occurred.[126] Combined administration of low doses of endotoxin and TNFα to rats resulted in the similar hypotensive and metabolic effect as a highly lethal dose of either compound.[127] These findings are in keeping with the fact that multiple organ damage usually develops over a prolonged period of time during which several insults might occur. It also emphasizes why it is so important to prevent any subsequent ischemia or host response in general, particularly in patients in whom systemic inflammation is already present.

Summary

Burn injury, a state of hemodynamic shock due to blood loss, the presence of necrotic tissue, or a septic episode might function as the initiating event of SIRS (**Figure 19.3**). The host response to this insult might be a localized inflammation or, if the stimulus surpasses a certain threshold, a systemic inflammatory response might occur. After a limited injury, the local tissue perfusion will increase; mediators released by macrophages and endothelial cells will attract monocytes and polymorphonuclear neutrophils to the area. These cells, as well as the vascular endothelium, are stimulated to express adhesion molecules and their interaction enables the inflammatory cells to leave the vascular lumen and to enter the interstitial space. Once there, activated cells of the immune system will secrete proteolytic enzymes and oxygen radicals, phagocytize and digest bacteria and necrotic tissue, and thereby defend the organism. A side effect of this reaction is that healthy tissue will be affected by the immune attack and will be damaged. As long as the inflammatory response is localized and feedback mechanisms are effective, tissue repair will follow tissue injury as recovery ensues. When the immune system becomes extensively activated and the inflammatory mechanisms escape local control, the whole body can seriously become involved in a systemic inflammatory response. A vicious circle might evolve in which the cytotoxicity of the immune cells might contribute to early organ dysfunction. Widespread increase in microvascular permeability will lead to interstitial edema and thereby impair oxygen diffusion to the tissue. Blood flow also becomes maldistributed due to a loss of vasoregulative function and as a result of widespread microthrombosis. Oxygenated blood does not reach the capillary bed. Moreover, oxygen utilization is impaired. The resultant hypoxic cell damage

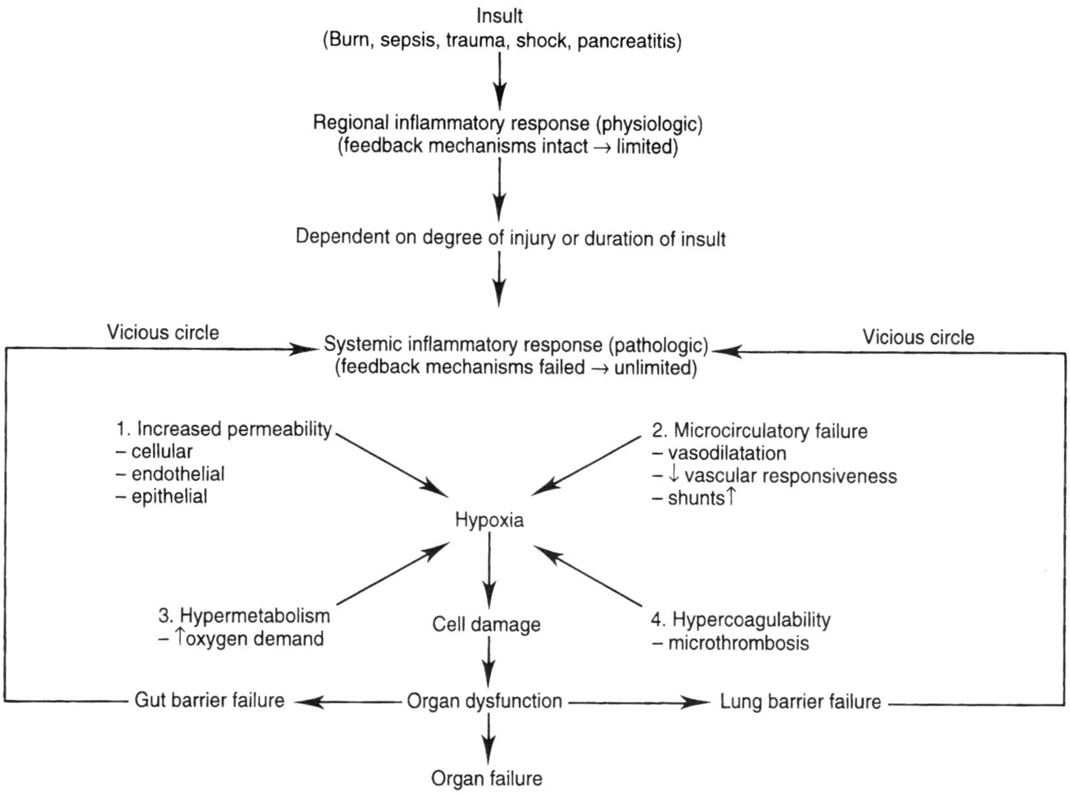

Fig. 19.3 Scheme summarizing the factors that might be involved in the development of organ failure as the final pathway of a wide variety of initiating events. The systemic inflammatory response represents the failure of feedback mechanisms, which usually limit the host response. The inflammatory process might become self-sustaining and comprises several pathophysiologic mechanisms that can all contribute to hypoxic cell damage, which is probably the most important event in the development of organ failure.

further promotes organ dysfunction. One important difference between localized and systemic inflammation is that the early dysfunction of the intestine might itself sustain the inflammatory reaction. Extensive studies have provided evidence that during a state of systemic inflammation, the barrier properties of the intestine seem to fail. Similar changes might also occur in the airway barrier to bacteria. Subsequently, enteral bacteria traverse these barriers in a process called bacterial translocation. These bacteria can be cultured from the blood where they might act as potent stimuli for both the immune system and endothelial cells. Probably dependent on the severity and duration of the inflammatory sequelae, more serious organ damage might result and involve several organ systems up to their failure. Some of the clinical signs of the systemic inflammatory reaction are summarized as the systemic inflammatory response syndrome.

References

1. Bone R C, Balk R A, Cerra F B, *et al.* Definitions for sepsis and organ failure and guidelines for the use of innovative therapies in sepsis. The ACCP/SCCM Consensus Conference Committee. American College of Chest Physicians/Society of Critical Care Medicine. *Chest* 1992; **101:** 1644–55.

2. Bagby G J, Lang C H, Giaimo M E, Spitzer J J. Increased glucose metabolism by epitrochlearis muscle removed from endotoxin-treated rats. *Circ Shock* 1986; **20:** 171–9.

3. Lentz C W, Zeigler S T, Cox C S, Traber L D, Herndon D N, Traber D L. Cytokine response to thermal injury. In: Schlag G, Redl H, Siegel J H, Traber D L, eds. *Shock, Sepsis and Organ Failure. The Second Wiggers Bernard Conference.* New York: Springer–Verlag, 1993: 245–64.

4. Marano M A, Fong Y, Moldawer L L, *et al.* Serum cachectin/tumor necrosis factor in critically ill patients with burns correlates with infection and mortality. *Surg Gynecol Obstet* 1990; **170:** 32–8.

5. Dinarello C A. The proinflammatory cytokines interleukin-1 and tumor necrosis factor and treatment of the septic shock syndrome. *J Infect Dis* 1991; **163:** 1177–84.

6. Schlag G, Redl H, Hallstrom S. The cell in shock: the origin of multiple organ failure. *Resuscitation* 1991; **21:** 137–80.

7. Schirmer W J, Schirmer J M, Fry D E. Recombinant human tumor necrosis factor produces hemodynamic changes characteristic of sepsis and endotoxemia. *Arch Surg* 1989; **124:** 445–8.

8. Tracey K J, Lowry S F, Fahey T, III, *et al.* Cachectin/tumor necrosis factor induces lethal shock and stress hormone responses in the dog. *Surg Gynecol Obstet* 1987; **164:** 415–22.

9. Okusawa S, Gelfand J A, Ikejima T, Connolly R J, Dinarello C A. Interleukin 1 induces a shock-like state in rabbits. Synergism with tumor necrosis factor and the effect of cyclooxygenase inhibition. *J Clin Invest* 1988; **81:** 1162–72.

10. Fischer E, Marano M A, Barber A E, *et al.* Comparison between effects of interleukin-1 alpha administration and sublethal endotoxemia in primates. *Am J Physiol* 1991; **261:** R442–R452.

11. Burhop K E, Garcia J G, Selig W M, *et al.* Platelet-activating factor increases lung vascular permeability to protein. *J Appl Physiol* 1986; **61:** 2210–17.

12. Hoffman W D, Natanson C. Endotoxin in septic shock. *Anesth Analg* 1993; **77:** 613–24.

13. Bone R C. Toward an epidemiology and natural history of SIRS (systemic inflammatory response syndrome). *JAMA* 1992; **268:** 3452–5.

14. Suffredini A F, Fromm R E, Parker M M, *et al.* The cardiovascular response of normal humans to the administration of endotoxin. *N Engl J Med* 1989; **321:** 280–7.

15. Suffredini A F, Shelhamer J H, Neumann R D, Brenner M, Baltaro R J, Parrillo J E. Pulmonary and oxygen transport effects of intravenously administered endotoxin in normal humans. *Am Rev Respir Dis* 1992; **145:** 1398–403.

16. Traber D L, Redl H, Schlag G, *et al.* Cardiopulmonary responses to continuous administration of endotoxin. *Am J Physiol* 1988; **254:** H833–H839.

17. Dehring D, Lingnau W, McGuire R, Traber L D, Traber D L. L-NAME transiently reverses hyperdynamic status during continuous infusion of pseudomonas aeroginosa. *Circ Shock* 1993; **39:** 49 (Abstract).

18. Traber D L. Models of endotoxemia in sheep. In: Schlag G, Redl H, Traber D L, eds. *Pathophysiology of Shock, Sepsis and Organ Failure.* New York: Springer Verlag, 1993: 194–9.

19. Godsoe A, Kimura R, Herndon D, *et al.* Cardiopulmonary changes with intermittent endotoxin administration in sheep. *Circ Shock* 1988; **25:** 61–74.

20. Meyer J, Traber L D, Nelson S, *et al.* Reversal of hyperdynamic response to continuous endotoxin administration by inhibition of NO synthesis. *J Appl Physiol* 1992; **73:** 324–8.

21. Fujioka K, Sugi K, Isago T, *et al.* Thromboxane synthase inhibition and cardiopulmonary function during endotoxemia in sheep. *J Appl Physiol* 1991; **71:** 1376–81.

22. Adams T J, Traber D L. The effects of a prostaglandin synthetase inhibitor, ibuprofen, on the cardiopulmonary response to endotoxin in sheep. *Circ Shock* 1982; **9:** 481–9.

23. Tokyay R, Loick H M, Traber D L, Heggers J P, Herndon D N. Effects of thromboxane synthetase inhibition on postburn mesenteric vascular resistance and the rate of bacterial translocation in a chronic porcine model. *Surg Gynecol Obstet* 1992; **174:** 125–32.

24. Redl G, Abdi S, Nichols R J, *et al.* The effects of a selective thromboxane synthetase inhibitor on the response of the right heart to endotoxin in sheep. *Crit Care Med* 1991; **19:** 1294–302.

25. Redl G, Newald J, Schlag G, Traber L D, Traber D L. Cardiac function in an ovine model of endotoxemia. *Circ Shock* 1991; **35:** 31–6.

26. Navaratnam R L, Morris S E, Traber D L, *et al.* Endotoxin (LPS) increases mesenteric vascular resistance (MVR) and bacterial translocation (BT). *J Trauma* 1990; **30:** 1104–13.

27. Lefer A M. Interaction between myocardial depressant factor and vasoactive mediators with ischemia and shock. *Am J Physiol* 1987; **252:** R193–R205.

28. Morris S E, Navaratnam N, Herndon D N. A comparison of effects of thermal injury and smoke inhalation on bacterial translocation. *J Trauma* 1990; **30:** 639–43.

29. Schlag G, Redl H, Davies J, Dinges H P, Radmore K. Aspects of the mechanisms of bacterial translocation in a hypovolemic-traumatic shock mode in baboons. *Circ Shock* 1991; **34:** 26–7.

30. Xu D, Qi L, Guillory D, Cruz N, Berg R, Deitch E A. Mechanisms of endotoxin-induced intestinal injury in a hyperdynamic model of sepsis. *J Trauma* 1993; **34:** 676–82.

31. Koltai M, Hosford D, Braquet PG. Platelet-activating factor in septic shock. *New Horizons* 1993; **1:** 87–95.

32. Traber D L. Endotoxin: the causative factor of mediator release during sepsis. In: Schlag G, Redl H, eds. *Progress in Clinical and Biological Research.* New York: Alan R Liss, Inc, 1987: 377–92.

33. Sloane P J, Elsasser T H, Spath J A, Albertine K H, Gee M H. Plasma tumor necrosis factor-alpha during long-term endotoxemia in awake sheep. *J Appl Physiol* 1992; **73:** 1831–7.

34. Martich G D, Danner R L, Ceska M, Suffredini A F. Detection of interleukin 8 and tumor necrosis factor in normal humans after intravenous endotoxin: the effect of antiinflammatory agents. *J Exp Med* 1991; **173:** 1021–4.

35. Michie H R, Manogue K R, Spriggs D R, *et al.* Detection of circulating tumor necrosis factor after endotoxin administration. *N Engl J Med* 1988; **318:** 1481–6.

36. Morel D R, Pittet J F, Gunning K, Hemsen A, Lacroix J S, Lundberg J M. Time course of plasma and pulmonary lymph endothelin-like immunoreactivity during sustained endotoxaemia in chronically instrumented sheep. *Clin Sci* 1991; **81:** 357–65.

37. Redl G, Woodson L, Traber L D, *et al.* Mechanism of immunoreactive atrial natriuretic factor release in an ovine model of endotoxemia. *Circ Shock* 1992; **38:** 34–41.

38. Lübbesmeyer H J, Woodson L, Traber L D, Flynn J T, Herndon D N, Traber D L, Immunoreactive atrial natriuretic factor is increased in ovine model of endotoxemia. *Am J Physiol* 1988; **254:** R567–R571.

39. Pittet J F, Morel D R, Hemsen A, *et al.* Elevated plasma endothelin-1 concentrations are associated with the severity of illness in patients with sepsis. *Ann Surg* 1991; **213:** 261–4.

40. Morel D R, Lacroix J S, Hemsen A, Steinig D A, Pittet J F, Lundberg J M. Increased plasma and pulmonary lymph levels of endothelin during endotoxin shock. *Eur J Pharmacol* 1989; **67:** 427–8.

41. Nelson S, Stewart R H, Traber L, Traber D. Endotoxin-induced alterations in contractility of isolated blood vessels from sheep. *Am J Physiol* 1991; **260:** H1790–H1794.

42. Theissen J L, Loick H M, Curry B B, Traber L D, Herndon D N, Traber D L. Time course of hypoxic pulmonary vasoconstriction after endotoxin infusion in unanesthetized sheep. *J Appl Physiol* 1991; **70:** 2120–5.

43. Meyer J, Lentz C W, Stothert J C, Traber L D, Herndon D N, Traber D L. Effects of nitric oxide synthesis inhibition in hyperdynamic endotoxemia. *Crit Care Med* 1993; **22:** 304–12.

44. Sugi K, Newald J, Traber D L, *et al.* Cardiac dysfunction after acute endotoxin administration in conscious sheep. *Am J Physiol* 1991; **260:** H1474–H1481.

45. Noshima S, Noda H, Herndon D N, Traber L D, Traber D L. Left ventricular performance during continuous endotoxin-induced hyperdynamic endotoxemia in sheep. *J Appl Physiol* 1993; **74:** 1528–33.

46. Myers P R, Wright T F, Tanner M A, Adams H R. EDRF and nitric oxide production in cultured endothelial cells: direct inhibition by *E. coli* endotoxin. *Am J Physiol* 1992; **262:** H710–H718.

47. Vallance P, Moncada S. Role of endogenous nitric oxide in septic shock. *New Horizons* 1993; **1:** 77–86.

48. Sakai N, Milstien S. Availability of tetrahydrobiopterin is not a factor in the inability to detect nitric oxide production by human macrophages. *Biochem Biophys Res Commun* 1993; **193:** 378–83.

49. Schneemann M, Schoedon G, Hofer S, Blau N, Guerrero L, Schaffner A. Nitric oxide synthase is not a constituent of the antimicrobial armature of human mononuclear phagocytes. *J Infect Dis* 1993; **167:** 1358–63.

50. Moncada S. The first Robert Furchgott lecture: from endothelium-dependent relaxation to the L-arginine: NO pathway. *Blood Vessels* 1991; **27:** 208–17.

51. Furchgott R F. The 1989 Ulf von Euler lecture. Studies on endothelium-dependent vasodilation and the endothelium-derived relaxing factor. *Acta Physiol Scand* 1991; **139:** 257–70.

52. Petros A, Bennett D, Vallance P. Effect of nitric oxide synthase inhibitors on hypotension in patients with septic shock. *Lancet* 1991; **338:** 1557–8.

53. Geroulanos S, Schilling J, Cakmakci M, Jung H H, Largiader F. Inhibition of NO synthesis in septic shock (Letter). *Lancet* 1992; **339:** 430–5.

54. Shi Y, Li H-Q, Shen C-K, *et al.* Plasma nitric oxide levels in newborn infants with sepsis. *J Pediatr* 1993; **123:** 435–8.

55. Ochoa J B, Udekwu A O, Billiar T R, *et al.* Nitrogen oxide levels in patients after trauma and during sepsis. *Ann Surg* 1991; **214:** 621–6.

56. Schneider F, Lutun P, Couchot A, Bilbault P, Tempe J D. Plasma cyclic guanosine 3′–5′ monophosphate concentrations and low vascular resistance in human septic shock. *Intensive Care Med* 1993; **19:** 99–104.

57. Schuller F, Fleming I, Stoclet J C, Gray G A. Effect of endotoxin on circulating cyclic GMP in the rat. *Eur J Pharmacol* 1992; **212:** 93–6.

58. Nelson S H, Dehring D J, Erhardt J S, Traber L, Traber D. Regional variation in content of c-GMP and associated vascular reactivity in bacteremia. *Circ Shock* 1993; **39:** 54 (Abstract).

59. Martin W, White D G, Henderson A H. Endothelium-derived relaxing factor and atriopeptin II elevate cyclic GMP levels in pig aortic endothelial cells. *Br J Pharmacol* 1988; **93:** 229–39.

60. Cherner J A, Singh G, Naik L. Atrial natriuretic factor activates membrane-bound guanylate cyclase of chief cells. *Life Sci* 1990; **47:** 669–77.

61. Goy M F. Activation of membrane guanylate cyclase by an invertebrate peptide hormone. *J Biol Chem* 1990; **265:** 20220–7.

62. Boulanger C, Schini V B, Moncada S, Vanhoutte P M. Stimulation of cyclic GMP production in cultured endothelial cells of the pig by bradykinin, adenosine diphosphate, calcium ionophore A23187 and nitric oxide. *Br J Pharmacol* 1990; **101:** 152–6.

63. Mitaka C, Nagura T, Sakanishi N, Tsunoda Y, Toyooka H. Plasma alpha-atrial natriuretic peptide concentrations in acute respiratory failure associated with sepsis: preliminary study. *Crit Care Med* 1990; **18:** 1201–3.

64. Leitman D C, Agnost V L, Catalano R M, *et al.* Atrial natriuretic peptide, oxytocin, and vasopressin increase guanosine 3′,5′-monophosphate in

LLC-PK1 kidney epithelial cells. *Endocrinology* 1988; **122:** 1478–85.

65. Gerzer R, Heim J M, Schutte B, Weil J. Cellular mechanisms of action of atrial natriuretic factor. *Klin Wochenschr* 1987; **65** (Suppl 8): 109–14.

66. Garbers D L. The guanylyl cyclase receptor family. *New Biol* 1990; **2:** 499–504.

67. DeLa Cadena R A, Suffredini A F, Page J D, *et al.* Activation of the kallikrein-kinin system after endotoxin administration to normal human volunteers. *Blood* 1993; **81:** 3313–17.

68. Mann R, Woodson L C, Traber L D, Herndon D N, Traber D L. Role of bradykinin in ovine endotoxemia. *Circ Shock* 1991; **34:** 224–30.

69. Matsuda T, Eccleston C A, Rubinstein I, Rennard S I, Joyner W L. Antioxidants attenuate endotoxin-induced microvascular leakage of macromolecules in vivo. *Am J Physiol* 1991; **70:** 1483–9.

70. Nakazawa H, Noda H, Noshima S, *et al.* Pulmonary transvascular fluid flux and cardiovascular function in sheep with chronic sepsis. *J Appl Physiol* 1993; **75:** 2521–8.

71. Landis E M, Pappenheimer J R. Exchange of substances through the capillary walls. In: Hamilton W F, Dow P, eds. *Handbook of Physiology, Section 2, Vol. 2.* Baltimore, MD: Williams & Wilkins, 1963: 961–1034.

72. Starling E H. On the absorption of fluids from the connective tissue spaces. *J Physiol (Lond)* 1896; **19:** 312–26.

73. Brigham K L, Bowers R, Haynes J. Increased sheep lung vascular permeability caused by *Escherichia coli* endotoxin. *Circ Res* 1979; **45:** 292–7.

74. Gaar K A, Taylor A E, Owens L J, Guyton A C. Effect of capillary pressure and plasma protein on development of pulmonary edema. *Am J Physiol* 1967; **213:** 79–82.

75. Lund T, Wiig H, Reed R K, Aukland K. A 'new' mechanism for oedema generation: strongly negative interstitial fluid pressure causes rapid fluid flow into thermally injured skin. *Acta Physiol Scand* 1987; **129:** 433–5.

76. Lund T, Wiig H, Reed R K. Acute postburn edema: role of strongly negative interstitial fluid pressure. *Am J Physiol* 1988; **255:** H1069–H1074.

77. Traber D L, Herndon D N, Fujioka K, Traber L D. Permeability changes during experimental endotoxemia and sepsis. In: Schlag G, Redl H, Siegel J H, Traber D L, eds. *Shock, Sepsis, and Organ Failure: Second Wiggers Bernard Conference.* New York: Springer-Verlag, 1991: 425–47.

78. Smith L, Andreasson S, Thoren Tolling K, Rippe B, Risberg B. Sepsis in sheep reduces pulmonary microvascular sieving capacity. *J Appl Physiol* 1987; **62:** 1422–9.

79. Oliver J A. Endothelium-derived relaxing factor contributes to the regulation of endothelial permeability. *J Cell Physiol* 1992; **151:** 506–11.

80. Farrukh I S, Gurtner G H, Michael J R. Pharmacological modification of pulmonary vascular injury: possible role of cAMP. *J Appl Physiol* 1987; **62:** 47–54.

81. Kurose I, Kubes P, Wolf R, *et al.* Inhibition of nitric oxide production. Mechanisms of vascular albumin leakage. *Circ Res* 1993; **73:** 164–71.

82. Leeuwenberg F M, Jeunhomme T M A, Buurman W A. Induction of an activation antigen on human endothelial cells in vitro. *Eur J Immunol* 1989; **19:** 715–20.

83. Lasky L A. Selectins: interpreters of cell-specific carbohydrate information during inflammation. *Science* 1992; **258:** 964–9.

84. Nawroth P P, Stern D M. Modulation of endothelial cell hemostatic properties by tumor necrosis factor. *J Exp Med* 1986; **163:** 740–5.

85. Walsh C J, Carey D, Cook D J, Bechard D E, Fowler A A, Sugerman H J. Anti-CD 18 antibody attenuates neutropenia and alveolar capillary-membrane injury during gram-negative sepsis. *Surgery* 1991; **110:** 205–12.

86. Doerschuk C M, Winn R K, Coxson H O, Harlan J M. CD18-dependent and independent mechanisms of neutrophil emigration in the pulmonary and systemic microcirculation of rabbits. *J Immunol* 1990; **144:** 2327–33.

87. Wang C Z, Herndon D N, Traber L D, *et al.* Pulmonary inflammatory cell response to sustained endotoxin administration. *J Appl Physiol* 1994; **76:** 516–22.

88. Traber D L. Anti-proteases in endotoxemia. In: Schlag G, Redl H, eds. *Progress in Clinical and Biological Research.* New York: Alan R. Liss, Inc, 1987: 149–57.

89. Seekamp A, LaLonde C, Zhu D G, Demling R. Catalase prevents prostanoid release and lung lipid peroxidation after endotoxemia in sheep. *J Appl Physiol* 1988; **65:** 1210–16.

90. Basadre J O, Singh H, Herndon D N, *et al.* Effect of antibody-mediated neutropenia on the cardiopulmonary response to endotoxemia. *J Surg Res* 1988; **45:** 266–75.

91. Winn R, Maunder R, Chi E, Harlan J. Neutrophil depletion does not prevent lung edema after endotoxin infusion in goats. *J Appl Physiol* 1987; **62:** 116–21.

92. Maunder R J, Hackman R C, Riff E, Albert R K, Springmeyer S C. Occurrence of the adult respiratory distress syndrome in neutropenic patients. *Am Rev Respir Dis* 1986; **133:** 313–16.

93. Laufe M D, Simon R H, Flint A, Keller J B. Adult respiratory distress syndrome in neutropenic patients. *Am J Med* 1986; **80:** 1022–6.

94. Heflin A C J, Brigham K L. Prevention by granulocyte depletion of increased vascular permeability of sheep lung following endotoxemia. *J Clin Invest* 1981; **68:** 1253–6_.

95. Klausner J M, Paterson I S, Goldman G, *et al.* Interleukin-2-induced lung injury is mediated by oxygen free radicals. *Surgery* 1991; **109:** 169–75.

96. Goldman G, Welbourn R, Klausner J M, Valeri C R, Shepro D, Hechtman H B. Thromboxane mediates diapedesis after ischemia by activation of neutrophil adhesion receptors interacting with basally expressed intercellular adhesion molecule-1. *Circ Res* 1991; **68:** 1013–19.

97. Traber D L, Schlag G, Redl H, Strohmair W, Traber L D. Pulmonary microvascular changes during hyperdynamic sepsis in an ovine model. *Circ Shock* 1987; **22:** 185–93.

98. Miller F N, Sims D E. Contractile elements in the regulation of macromolecular permeability. *Fed Proc* 1986; **45:** 84–8.

99. Paterson I S, Klausner J M, Goldman G, *et al.* Thromboxane mediates the ischemia-induced neutrophil oxidative burst. *Surgery* 1989; **106:** 224–9.

100. Turker R K, Aksulu H E, Ercan Z S, Aslan S. Thromboxane A_2 inhibitors and iloprost prevent angiotensin II-induced oedema in the isolated perfused rat lung. *Arch Int Pharmacodyn Ther* 1987; **287:** 323–9.

101. Deitch E A, Taylor M, Grisham M, Ma L, Bridges W, Berg R. Endotoxin induces bacterial translocation, and increases xanthine oxidase activity. *J Trauma* 1989; **29:** 1679–83.

102. Deitch E A, Ma L, Ma W J, *et al.* Inhibition of endotoxin-induced bacterial translocation, in mice. *J Clin Invest* 1989; **84:** 36–42.

103. Deitch E A, Specian R D, Berg R D. Endotoxin-induced bacterial translocation and mucosal permeability: role of xanthine oxidase, complement activation, and macrophage products. *Crit Care Med* 1991; **19:** 785–91.

104. Terada L S, Dormish J J, Shanley P F, Leff J A, Anderson B O, Repine J E. Circulating xanthine oxidase mediates lung neutrophil sequestration after intestinal ischemia-reperfusion. *Am J Physiol* 1992; **263:** L394–L401.

105. Redl H, Schlag G, Lamche H. TNF- and LPS-induced changes of lung vascular permeability: studies in unanesthetised sheep. *Circ Shock* 1990; **31:** 183–92.

106. Johnson J, Meyrick B, Jesmok G, Brigham K L. Human recombinant tumor necrosis factor alpha infusion mimics endotoxemia in awake sheep. *J Appl Physiol* 1989; **66:** 1448–54.

107. Sessler C N, Glauser F L, Davis D, Fowler A A. Effects of platelet-activating factor antagonist SRI 63–441 on endotoxemia in sheep. *J Appl Physiol* 1988; **65:** 2624–31.

108. Vercellotti G M, Yin H Q, Gustavson K S, Nelson R D, Jacob H S. Platelet activating factor primes neutrophil responses to agonists: role in promoting neutrophil-mediated endothelial damage. *Blood* 1988; **71:** 1100–7.

109. Holloway H, Perry M Downey J, Parker J, Taylor A. Estimation of effective pulmonary capillary pressure in intact lungs. *J Appl Physiol* 1983; **54(3):** 846–51.

110. Mann R, Traber L D, Herndon D N, Traber D L. Prior infusion of endotoxin dininishes the pulmonary response to bolus administration of lipopolysaccharide (LPS). *Int J Radiat Oncol Biol Phys* 1988; **20:** 138 (Abstract).

111. Shiki Y, Meyrick B O, Brigham K L, Burr I M. Endotoxin increases superoxide dismutase in cultured bovine pulmonary endothelial cells. *Am J Physiol* 1987; **252:** C436–C440.

112. O'Dwyer S T, Michie H R, Ziegler T R, Revhaug A, Smith R J, Wilmore D W. A single dose of endotoxin increases intestinal permeability in healthy humans. *Arch Surg* 1988; **123:** 1459–64.

113. Roumen R M, Hendriks T, Wevers R A, Goris J A. Intestinal permeability after severe trauma and hemorrhagic shock is increased without relation to septic complications. *Arch Surg* 1993; **128:** 453–7.

114. Zeigler S T, Traber D L, Herndon D N. Bacterial translocation in burns. In: Schlag G, Redl H, eds. *Pathophysiology of Shock, Sepsis, and Organ Failure*, New York: Springer-Verlag, 1993: 300–13.

115. Schorer A E, Rick P D, Swaim W R, Moldow C F. Structural features of endotoxin required for stimulation of endothelial cell tissue factor production. Exposure of preformed tissue factor after oxidant-mediated endothelial cell injury. *J Lab Clin Med* 1985; **106:** 38–42.

116. Colluci M, Paramo J A, Collen D. Generation in plasma of a fast-acting inhibitor of plasminogen activator in response to endotoxin stimulation. *J Clin Invest* 1985; **75:** 818–24.

117. Moore K L, Andreoli S P, Esmon N L, Esmon C T, Bang N U. Endotoxin enhances tissue factor and suppresses thrombomodulin expression of human vascular endothelium in vitro. *J Clin Invest* 1987; **79:** 124–30.

118. Beutler B, Cerami A. Cachectin: more than a tumor necrosis factor. *N Engl J Med* 1987; **316:** 379–85.

119. Malik A B, Horgan M J. Mechanisms of thrombin-induced lung vascular injury and edema. *Am Rev Respir Dis* 1987; **136:** 467–70.

120. Lo S K, Perlman M B, Niehaus G D, Malik A B. Thrombin-induced alterations in lung fluid balance in awake sheep. *J Appl Physiol* 1985; **58:** 1421–7.

121. Malik A B, Lo S K, Bizios R. Thrombin-induced alterations in endothelial permeability. *Ann N Y Acad Sci* 1986; **485:** 293–309.

122. Bone R C. Modulators of coagulation. A critical appraisal of their role in sepsis. *Arch Intern Med* 1992; **152:** 1381–9.

123. Martich G D, Boujoukos A J, Suffredini A F. Response of man to endotoxin. *Immunobiology* 1993; **187:** 403–16.

124. Anderson B O, Harken A H. Multiple organ failure: inflammatory priming and activation sequences promote autologous tissue injury. *J Trauma* 1990; **30:** S44–S49.

125. Dehring D J, Lubbesmeyer H J, Fader R C, Traber L D, Traber D L. Exaggerated cardiopulmonary response after bacteremia in sheep with week-old thermal injury. *Crit Care Med* 1993; **21:** 888–93.

126. Koike K, Moore F A, Moore E E, Poggetti R S, Tuder R M, Banerjee A. Endotoxin after gut ischemia/reperfusion causes irreversible lung injury. *J Surg Res* 1992; **52:** 656–62.

127. Ciancio M J, Hunt J, Jones S B, Filkins J P. Comparative and interactive in vivo effects of tumor necrosis factor alpha and endotoxin. *Circ Shock* 1991; **33:** 108–20.

CHAPTER TWENTY

Metabolic Responses to Burn Injury: Nutritional Implications

Robert R. Wolfe

Injuries as severe as a third degree burn over 10% of the body surface have minimal effect on metabolic regulation or food intake. Consequently, while such injuries may be extremely painful and require skilled medical care for optimal recovery, they do not present a significant nutritional problem. On the other hand, severe burn injury over 30% of the body surface or more results in a pronounced metabolic response which has prolonged nutritional implications. The understanding of the nature of this response and the consequent changes in nutritional requirements is important, not only for the optimal treatment of such patients, but also because many aspects of the response to burn injury can be seen in terms of a more general model of the so-called 'stress response'. This is because the extent of injury is quantifiable and the state of critical illness is maintained for a long enough time (often weeks) to enable nutritional and metabolic studies.

Resting Energy Expenditure

Mechanisms of Hypermetabolism

Resting energy expenditure (REE) after burn injury can be as much as 100% above that predicted from standard tables for size, age, sex, and weight. Although some debate persists regarding some aspects of the genesis of this phenomenon, increased heat loss from the burn wound and increased β-adrenergic activity are probably both important factors. Burned skin loses its effectiveness as a barrier to water loss, leading to increased evaporative heat loss via the wound.[1] In addition, radiation heat loss is increased from burn wounds,[2] presumably due to high blood flow to the burn wound.[3] Occlusive dressings can significantly lower the radiation heat loss from burn wounds, but evaporative heat loss is not reduced significantly.[1] Consequently, patients with large burns which are treated with occlusive dressings will nonetheless have a high rate of water turnover,[4] meaning that fluid and electrolyte requirements are likely to be high in order to maintain normal urine output and plasma concentrations of electrolytes. Despite persistent increased evaporative loss via the wound, occlusive dressings can greatly minimize heat loss. Also, maintenance of a high room temperature (approximately 90° F; 32.2°C) and humidity will further minimize heat loss and thus energy expenditure. Within this context of clinical care, the metabolic response of burned patients becomes similar to that of patients with other forms of critical illness.

The role of adrenergic stimulation in causing burn hypermetabolism is more controversial than the role of increased heat loss. It has been observed that β-blockade in burned children who are treated with excisional therapy and occlusive dressings have not been found to reduce energy expenditure.[5] It therefore seems unlikely that adrenergic blockade can play a significant role in minimizing caloric requirements in patients treated with modern techniques.

Prediction of REE in Burned Patients

A large body of data has enabled the development of predictive equations to estimate REE. For example, in a study incorporating 127 observations in 56 burned children, it was found that predicted basal energy expenditure (PBEE) obtained from the Harris–Benedict equation, body surface area and body weight correlated significantly with REE.[6] On the other hand, neither the days postburn nor burn size was significantly correlated with REE in that or other studies of patients treated with excisional therapy and occlusive dressings.[7] In an uncomplicated recovery from an injury, one would anticipate a progressive decrease of REE over time until the PBEE is reached. In burn injury, this is rarely the case because periods of severe critical illness can occur as much as weeks after injury, thereby disrupting a direct relation between days post-injury and REE. With regard to the lack of relation between burn size and REE, it is important to realize that a relation has never been shown to exist at burn sizes greater than 40%. Even the Brooke Army Base studies, widely referred to as the basis for formulas for caloric requirements,[6] showed no relationship between burn size and REE if smaller burns were excluded from data analysis. Thus, equations predicted to burn size overestimate caloric requirements in patients with large burns.[8] These are precisely the patients least able to tolerate caloric excess.

The single most powerful predictor of REE in burned patients is PBEE. In the paper of Curreri *et al.*,[6] it was found that in fed patients, on average, REE = 1.29 × PBEE; however, there is considerable variation about this average relation. Only 75% of the predictions were with ± 30% of the measured value, and 10% of the measured values varied by more than 45% from the predicted value. Thus, an accurate determination of REE can only be obtained in any given individual patient by direct measurement.

The extensive studies of REE, performed at the Brooke Army Base in the 1970s,[9] led to the conclusion that REE in adults might be 200–300% greater than predicted basal values. These patients were treated with neither early excision of burned tissue nor occlusive dressings. Studies performed in adults treated with early excision and occlusive dressings have consistently found lower values in adult patients than those reported from the Brooke studies. Although the data base in adults treated with early excision and occlusive dressings is not extensive, the same general observations have been made as in children:[7] the PBEE is the most important predictor of REE; and burn size is not related to REE. The average REE (in the fed state) is about 1.3 times greater than PBEE, and there is a large individual variability between PBEE and REE. In virtually all studies of children and adult patients, REE was lower than 2 × PBEE.

Relationship of Total Energy Expenditure (TEE) to REE

Knowledge of the relationship between TEE and REE is essential if FEE measurements are to have any value in predicting caloric requirements. This relationship was documented in a recent study in 15 burned children in whom TEE was determined by the doubly labeled water technique, and REE was determined by indirect calorimetry.[4] TEE was 1.33 ± 0.27 times PBEE, and 1.18 ± 0.17 times REE in the fed state. Importantly, TEE was significantly correlated with measured REE ($r^2 = 0.92$), but not with PBEE. If the average activity factor, calculated as the difference between TEE and REE, was incorporated into a predictive equation based on the measured value of REE cited above, then it was found that the average energy requirement to maintain energy balance was 1.55 × PBEE. This value is significantly lower than those commonly used for patients with large burns. The caloric intake required to insure that 95% of patients achieved energy balance was approximately equal to 2 × PBEE. Expressed differently, 2 × PBEE provided excess caloric intake to all but 5% of patients; and in some patients the excess may have been 70% or more above actual requirement. It is therefore reasonable to aim for the average energy intake (1.5 × PBEE), and to adjust that rate either up or down as dictated by tolerance in terms of blood glucose and triglyceride concentrations, as well as body weight changes over time. Although the above data were generated in children, they are very similar to the value for predicted TEE in adults described earlier.[8] The need to monitor individual tolerance is particularly important in critically ill patients, who may be intolerant of average maintenance levels of energy intake.

Substrate Metabolism

Appropriate nutritional support of burned patients requires knowledge of total caloric requirements, and the nature of alterations in the oxidation of specific substrates. In that context, two aspects of metabolic regulation are fundamental: the intracellular capacity for substrate oxidation, and the availability of energy substrates. Thus, factors regulating the availability of endogenous substrates will be discussed. Second, intracellular oxidation will be discussed both in the context of endogenous as well as exogenous substrates.

Glucose Production

Glucose is produced in the liver from the process of glycogenolysis or gluconeogenesis. Glycogenolysis is the breakdown of glucose stored when intake exceeds requirements for oxidation. Thus, breakdown of glycogen involves essentially no 'net' loss of the lean body, but in a sense represents oxidation of ingested glucose which has simply been physiologically delayed in its metabolism. Gluconeogenesis, on the other hand, involves the production of new glucose. It is a complex reaction sequence of many intermediate steps; it involves some reactions of glycolysis in reverse and some additional reactions which overcome the energy barriers preventing a direct reversal of glycolysis. A variety of substrates can serve as gluconeogenic precursors; but, under most circumstances, lactate is the most important.

Because most lactate is derived from plasma glucose via glycolysis, the resynthesis of glucose from lactate is a cyclic reaction, originally described by Cori,[10] and is commonly called the Cori cycle. When the ability of a tissue to completely catabolize glucose to carbon dioxide and water is limited because of a lack of sufficient oxygen, the Cori cycle maintains a supply of fuel (glucose) which can provide a certain amount of energy anaerobically. The 'net' glucose formation does not increase via the Cori cycle; in that sense, it may be considered a waste of energy, because energy is required to resynthesize the glucose derived from fat oxidation in the liver[11] so that the Cori cycle results in a energy transfer from adipose tissue to muscle, with glucose and lactate serving as the 'currency' in situations in which the muscle is unable to fully rely on fat oxidation. The resting rate of Cori cycle activity in a normal human has been determined to account for approximately 10–15% of the total glucose production in fasting.[12] Because of a great excess of lactate in burn patients due to altered peripheral metabolism of glucose (see below), the Cori cycle is of increased quantitative importance in burn injury.[13]

Glycerol is potentially an excellent gluconeogenic substrate, in that it enters the gluconeogenic pathway closer to glucose than any other substrate. The extent to which glycerol is converted to glucose is primarily a function of its availability, because the conversion of glycerol to glucose is the major route by which glycerol is cleared from the blood. Glycerol contributes only about 3% of the total glucose produced during a short fast in a normal, lean subject. When there is stimulus for fat mobilization, such as during a long fast[14] or severe burn injury,[15] glycerol can contribute as much as 20% of the total glucose production.

Alanine and glutamine account for 50–60% of the total amino acids released from muscle. In nonacidotic conditions, little glutamine is taken up by the kidney; rather, it is taken up by the mucosal cells of the small intestine and converted to alanine.[16] Thus, alanine is the major amino acid precursor for gluconeogenesis. Alanine is released from muscle in far greater quantities than it is present in muscle protein, but its origin is controversial. It has been suggested that pyruvate, resulting from the glycolytic catabolism of glucose, is transaminated and the resulting alanine is released into the bloodstream, where it travels to the liver for reincorporation into glucose.[17] According to this proposal, alanine functions in a metabolic cycle analogous to the Cori cycle in that no new 'net' glucose is produced. The nitrogen required for the transamination of pyruvate is derived from the amino acids which are oxidized by muscle, including the branched-chain amino acids, valine, leucine, and isoleucine, as well as aspartate and glutamate. The role of this process has been proposed to be the transfer of ammonia from muscle to liver in the nontoxic form of alanine.

Glucose Production in Critical Illness

Glucose production is elevated in almost all critically ill patients, including those with severe burn injury.[13] Studies have particularly focused on the response in burn patients, because their relatively stable (yet critical) condition allows reproducible experimental conditions. In a large variety of critical illnesses, it seems likely that the regulation of glucose production is similar in most patients. Gluconeogenesis, particularly from alanine,[18] is elevated; glycogenolysis is also stimulated subsequent to carbohydrate intake. The increased gluconeogenesis from amino acids renders these amino acids unavailable for reincorporation into body protein. Rather, the nitrogen is excreted, primarily in urea, thereby contributing to the progressive depletion of body protein stores.

Relationship Between Muscle Amino Acid Release and Gluconeogenesis

The rate of protein breakdown in critical illness is increased when compared with the rate in normal individuals who are fed comparable levels of protein and calories.[19] This results in an increased efflux of amino acids from the muscle, including gluconeogenic amino acids. Alanine, in particular, is released at an increased rate[18] and seems to be a systemic response to injury, because the release was found to be elevated not only from the burned legs, but also from the unburned legs of patients with burns elsewhere.[20] The increased alanine released into the plasma is cleared in the liver and converted to glucose at an increased rate. It has been proposed that the rate of glucose production is directly influenced by the availability of alanine.[21] When alanine was infused into normal volunteers, contrary to the previous theory, increased alanine delivery to the liver did not stimulate the total rate of glucose production.[22] In contrast, infusing glucose increased alanine release from muscle, indicating that pyruvate availability is rate-limiting for the peripheral formation of alanine. Thus, the increase in total glucose production in critical illness cannot be attributed to an increased rate of alanine delivery to the liver. Rather, the high rate of glucose production and thus glucose uptake (see below) drives the rate of peripheral release of alanine. This general notion is further supported by the fact that plasma amino acid concentrations, including gluconeogenic amino acids, are generally below normal in burn patients. It is unclear how low concentrations of amino acids could be the driving force for gluconeogenesis in the liver. Thus, it can be concluded that factors directly stimulating glucose production at the liver are more important than changes in peripheral metabolism in dictating the rate of glucose production.

Responsiveness of Glucose Production to Glucose and Insulin

Plasma insulin levels are usually normal or elevated in burn patients.[13] The fact that the basal rate of glucose production is elevated, despite a normal or elevated plasma insulin level, can be defined as hepatic insulin resistance, since normally the elevated insulin concentration would lower the rate of glucose production. Furthermore, the plasma glucose concentration is also frequently increased, which would normally directly inhibit glucose production.[23] When glucose is infused into patients, glucose production is suppressed to some extent; but at all glucose infusion rates tested, the residual endogenous glucose production is higher than would be expected in normal volunteers[12] because of this hepatic 'insulin' and 'glucose' resistance. The failure of glucose production to respond to altered substrate delivery, and the sustained glucose production in the face of elevated insulin and glucose levels, argue for a potent hepatic stimulation of glucose production in critically ill patients. Studies in burned patients indicate this stimulation is hormonal.

The best way in which to determine if a hormone is exerting an effect is to lower, pharmacologically, that hormone concentration acutely, or block its action, and observe the response in order to deduce the preblockade action of the hormone. When this approach is used to study the role of the catecholamines by giving adrenergic-blocking agents, the stimulation of glucose production in burn injury cannot be explained by increased catecholamine activity. In fact, when adrenergic blockade was administered to burned guinea-pigs, glucose production increased, as opposed to the decrease which would have been expected had preexistent catecholamine activity been stimulating glucose production.[24] This unexpected increase in glucose production was subsequently explained on the basis of the effect of blockade on fatty acid metabolism.[25]

In contrast to the situation with the catecholamines, blocking glucagon secretion has a pronounced effect on glucose production in burn patients.[18] In a recent study, patients were infused with somatostatin, which inhibits the secretion of glucagon and insulin, and insulin was replaced in order to maintain the preexistent basal concentration. When glucagon was lowered to the normal concentration, glucose production decreased and remained depressed throughout the infusion.[18] This study proved the role of glucagon as the preeminent stimulator of glucose production in burn patients. The role of cortisol and other hormones as simulators of glucose production in burn injury has not been assessed in the same manner as glucagon and the catecholamines; however, the results of hormone infusion experiments indicate that cortisol may play an important role by enhancing and prolonging the effectiveness of glucagon.

Regulation of Lipolysis

In normal humans, lipids constitute more than 80% of the stored fuel reserve. Additionally, fat stores, along with very small carbohydrate stores, can be almost completely depleted without detriment to the individual. Conversely, the use of protein reserves is limited, because even moderate depletion can adversely affect an organism exposed to stress.[22] Consequently, when an individual must rely on endogenous fuel supplies for energy, lipids are physiologically the most desirable source. Most tissues can readily use fatty acids as substrates for energy metabolism. The use of fatty acids by these tissues preserves the limited carbohydrate stores for use by central nervous tissue and red blood cells. Additionally, the brain can partially adapt to use ketone bodies (β-hydroxybutyrate and acetoacetate) as an energy substrate. Thus, it seems reasonable that a theoretically optimal 'stress' response would involve the mobilization and use of fat. The pattern of hormonal response generally associated with varieties of stress, i.e. increased epinephrine, cortisol, glucagon levels, and low insulin levels, as well as increased sympathetic nervous system activity, would be expected to favor the mobilization of lipid from storage depots. Other factors may be simultaneously operative which would tend to suppress the mobilization or use of fat. For example, elevations in the lactate concentration resulting from the stimulation of muscle glycolysis (another catecholamine effect) stimulates reesterification within the adipose cell,[26] meaning that even though lipolysis may be stimulated, the amount of fatty acids released into the plasma may not reflect that stimulation. A decrease in pH inhibits lipolysis;[26] hyperglycemia may both inhibit lipolysis directly[27] and stimulate reesterification by leading to an increased rate of formation of α-glycerophosphate, which forms the backbone to which fatty acids attach to form triglycerols. In addition, adequate blood flow through fat is necessary for an increased lipolytic rate to be reflected to enhanced fatty acid mobilization.[28] Because sympathetic stimulation decreased fat blood flow, this is another potential impediment to the mobilization of fat in injury and sepsis. In summary, although the generalized 'stress response' would seem to favor the mobilization of fat from adipose tissues to the readily usable form of plasma free fatty acids (FFAs), many factors interact to determine if that response actually occurs.

Given all of these potentially interacting variables, it is interesting that, in any form of stress, a stimulation of lipolysis is a fundamental metabolic response. The principal mediator of this response is increased adrenergic activity,[15,29] because β-adrenergic blockade in patients will acutely reduce the rate of release of FFA to the normal range. There is a tachyphylaxis to the repetitive administration of β-blockade, such that chronic blockade in patients does not diminish the FFA level.[30] There are, consequently, other factors in patients which can also stimulate lipolysis if adrenergic activity wanes, or is blocked.

FFA are released at a rate well in excess of the requirement of tissues for FFA as an energy substrate. In severely burned patients, over 70% of released fatty acids are not oxidized, but rather reesterified into triglyceride (TG). Because the rate of release of fatty acids is markedly elevated, the total rate of reesterification is also greatly elevated in patients. The major site of clearance and reesterification of plasma FFA is the liver; the major determinant of TG synthesis is the rate of delivery of FFA to the liver. Under normal conditions, even a high rate of hepatic fatty acid uptake can be accommodated by a proportionate synthesis of TG and secretion into the plasma as VLDL-TG. This plasma TG is returned to the adipose tissue for storage, thereby forming a cycle between TG and FFA.[31] In critically ill patients, there may be a limit to the amount of TG which can be exported from the liver, perhaps reflecting impaired apo-B protein synthesis, which is necessary for the formation of the VLDL-TG before secretion. In this case, fat will accumulate in the liver, even in the absence of a significant amount of hepatic fatty acid synthesis. This response could possibly be antagonized by a large dose of glucose which would stimulate hepatic fatty acid synthesis. On the other hand, insulin and glucose suppress the peripheral mobilization of FFA, and thus the delivery of FFA to the liver. Therefore, during glucose ingestion, the suppressive effect of hyperinsulinemia on FFA release may actually result in a decrease in hepatic TG production, even though glucose uptake may be markedly greater than in the basal state.[31] The clinical observation that the amount of fat in the liver in seriously ill patients is directly related to the severity of illness, and unrelated to the nature of the nutritional support,[32] is predicted from the physiologic basis of the production of hepatic TG.

Glucose Utilization

The glucose concentration in the blood is normally regulated within narrow limits, but the rate of glucose uptake and oxidation can vary greatly. Following a high carbohydrate meal, or during a high-dose glucose infusion, glucose is the major fuel for the body: after several hours of fasting, only about 25% of total carbon dioxide production is from glucose oxidation.[12] Certain tissues, most notably the brain and erythrocytes, depend on glucose for energy and have a relatively constant rate of glucose uptake under most conditions. Therefore, even though the brain and erythrocytes may account for more than 50% of the glucose uptake during fasting, they probably do not play an important role in the observed fluctuations in the rate of glucose oxidation in different physiologic and pathologic states. The liver can play a role in the disposition of a glucose load,[33] but because most of this glucose uptake is not oxidized, the liver is not a site where the rate of glucose oxidation varies much either. The muscle mass, on the other hand, exerts a profound influence on an individual's overall rate of glucose use. Because muscle constitutes approximately 40% of the body mass, any change in the rate of glucose uptake by muscle will significantly affect the overall rate of glucose uptake by the individual. In the resting post-absorptive state, it is debatable whether the muscle takes up any glucose at all;[34] but in the individual with hyperglycemia or exercising, the rate of glucose use by the muscle can increase severalfold. Because of the important role of changes in muscle glucose metabolism in overall energy metabolism, considerable attention has been focused on the regulation of glucose use by muscle.

In normal volunteers, the rate of muscle glucose uptake and use are influenced strongly by the physical state. Muscle glucose uptake and use increase significantly during exercise, and bed rest caused decreased forearm glucose uptake during glucose infusion.[35] The latter response is only evident during glucose infusion, because in the resting state without glucose infusion, the muscle takes up little glucose. The implications of the role of the physical state on glucose clearance is obvious in relation to critically ill patients, because such patients usually are recumbent and perform little exercise.

It is generally accepted that insulin regulates muscle glucose use by controlling the rate of glucose entry. In stress, the ability of insulin to stimulate glucose uptake peripherally is diminished. This insulin resistance is evident at submaximal doses of insulin in all circumstances.[13,36] With uncomplicated (by infection) injury, the resistance can be essentially overcome with a pharmacologic amount of insulin. In contrast, even the maximal effectiveness of insulin on glucose uptake is diminished in septic patients. A variety of indirect lines of evidence have been used to deduce that an impaired ability to oxidize glucose is responsible for the peripheral insulin resistance in patients. For example, plasma lactate concentration is often high, particularly during glucose infusion, even with adequate tissue oxygenation. Until recently, a direct determination of the ability to oxidize pyruvate had not been made. Using stable isotope methodology, we labeled the intracellular pyruvate pool of severely burned patients to quantify both the total rate of production and oxidation of pyruvate. Results indicate that not only is pyruvate oxidation unimpaired, the total rate of oxidation is significantly increased, both in the basal state and during glucose infusion.[37] Thus, high lactate concentrations result in these patients simply from a mass-action effect secondary to a high rate of pyruvate production, and thus do not necessarily reflect any impairment in pyruvate oxidation.

The lack of a significant role of an impairment in glucose oxidation on the overall metabolic response in critically ill patients is further substantiated by the results of a recent experiment in which we stimulated the rate of glucose oxidation in septic patients with dichloroacetate (DCA), a specific stimulator of pyruvate dehydrogenase. The experiment was performed under conditions in which the insulin and glucose concentrations were clamped experimentally at constant values. DCA significantly stimulated glucose oxidation in septic patients, as expected; but this had no effect on leucine oxidation.[38] Leucine flux was also not affected, meaning that the alterations in amino acid oxidation and protein kinetics in patients are not directly related to the rate of glucose oxidation.

Implications for Nutritional Support

The mix of endogenous substrates (glucose, fatty acids) oxidized for energy in critically ill patients is largely determined by their relative availability. In particular, the rate of glucose oxidation is directly related to the availability of plasma glucose, because there appears to be no impairment in its oxidation. The oxidation of fatty acids could be considered to make up the balance between energy requirement and availability of glucose. Fatty acids are released well in excess of their oxidation rate, meaning that, in patients, as much as 70% of FFA is reesterified into triglyceride in the liver, potentially contributing to the development of fatty infiltration of the liver. The extent of reesterification of fatty acids, as opposed to their oxidation, is largely determined by the availability of glucose, in that an abundance of glucose will decrease FFA oxidation and stimulate reesterification.

These observations with regard to the metabolism of endogenous substrates can generally be extrapolated to the metabolism of exogenous substrate given as nutritional support. Carbohydrate intake generally dictates the rate of glucose oxidation, and, by deduction, fat oxidation. Thus, when given at rates below caloric requirement (thereby preventing fat synthesis from glucose), exogenous glucose is an optimal energy substrate. Whereas fat may be used to some extent, if sufficient glucose is given simultaneously, the rate of fat oxidation is usually minimal.

There has been considerable recent activity assessing the optimal form of carbohydrate and fat. Thus, both xylitol and fructose have been proposed as alternative carbohydrates, but little compelling evidence has been obtained supporting an advantage of these compounds over glucose, given that both xylitol and fructose must first be converted to glucose in the liver before peripheral metabolism is possible. A wide variety of fats have been recently advocated, including fish oil, medium-chain triglycerides, 'structured lipids' in which medium- and long-chain fatty acids are incorporated into the same triglyceride molecule, and triacetin. Future research will be necessary to determine if any of these forms of fat offer distinct advantages over long-chain fatty acids.

Protein Requirements

Major trauma, burns, and sepsis have in common a rapid net catabolism of body protein, as well as a redistribution of the nitrogen pool within the body. Muscle protein breakdown is accelerated, whereas certain rapidly produced so-called 'acute-phase' proteins are produced at an increased rate in the liver, wound repair requires amino acids for protein synthesis, and increased immunological activity may also require accelerated protein synthesis. The magnitude of the net catabolism of muscle may be so pronounced that maintenance of lean body mass is an unreasonable goal in a critically ill patient. Nonetheless, provision of dietary protein and/or amino acids is essential for minimizing net protein catabolism. Furthermore, it seems likely that a higher-than-normal intake of protein may be useful. Even the mild stress of simple bed rest increased the protein requirement to maintain N balance.[39] It is also clear that there is a limit to the extent to which increased protein intake can ameliorate net protein catabolism in a previously well nourished critically ill patient. Protein intake more than 1.5 g protein/kg per day has not been shown to provide any advantage[40] and can result in increased concentrations of urea and ammonia. Consequently, it is reasonable that protein be provided to adults at a rate between 1.2 and 1.5 g protein/kg per day. Data quantifying protein requirements in injured children are lacking; however, because they would normally require more protein than adults in order to support growth, it is reasonable to assume that a higher protein intake might be useful. Thus, it is not uncommon to give as much as 3 g protein/kg per day to burned pediatric patients. Nonetheless, at this time, there is no compelling evidence that there is any advantage to providing more than 2 g protein/kg per day. Protein containing a well balanced mixture of amino acids would seem to be the most advantageous for both adults and children. Formulations enriched with branched-chain amino acids have been promoted; but clinical trials have failed to show a significant advantage in most critically ill patients, particularly when concentrations of their amino acids in the unbalanced formulation become rate-limiting for protein synthesis. More recently, research has focused on the importance of glutamine intake in critically ill patients. Because both oral and enteral formulations have omitted glutamine entirely, it is not surprising that some beneficial effects have been found with the addition of glutamine, particularly in terms of improving N balance (which may reflect repletion of the free intracellular glutamine pools). It has been proposed that intracellular glutamine concentration is a key regulator of protein synthesis, but it is not yet clear if administering glutamine in an amount in excess of its normal contribution to protein composition results in the stimulation of protein synthesis. Other specific amino acids, such as arginine and histidine, have also been promoted as having specific, unique 'pharmacologic' effects, but convincing experimental evidence in humans supporting these claims is not yet available.

References

1. Caldwell F T, Bowser G H, Crabtree, J H. The effect of occlusive dressings on the energy metabolism of severely burned children. *Ann Surg* 1981; **193:** 579–91.

2. Caldwell F T, Hammell H T, Dolan F. A calorimeter for simultaneous determination of heat production and heat loss. *J Appl Physiol* 1966; **21:** 1665–71.

3. Aulick L H, Wilmore D H, Mason A D, *et al.* Influences of the burn wound on peripheral circulation in thermally injured patients. *Am J Physiol* 1972; **233:** H520–H526.

4. Goran M I, Peters E J, Herndon D N, *et al.* Total energy expenditure in burned children using the doubly labeled water technique. *Am J Physiol* 1990; **259:** E576–E585.

5. Herndon D N, Barrow R E, Rutan T C, *et al.* Effect of propranolol administration on hemodynamic and metabolic responses of burned pediatric patients. *Ann Surg* 1988; **208:** 484–90.

6. Curreri P W, Richmond D, Marvin J, *et al.* Dietary requirements of patients with major burns. *J Ann Diet Assoc* 1974; **65:** 415–17.

7. Goran M I, Broemeling L, Herndon D N, *et al.* Estimating energy requirements in burned children: a new approach derived from measurements of resting energy expenditure. *Am J Clin Nutr* 1991; **54:** 35–40.

8. Wolfe R R. Caloric requirements of the burned patients. *J Trauma* 1981; **21:** 712–14.

9. Wilmore D W, Long J M, Mason A D, *et al.* Catecholamines: mediators of hypermetabolic response to thermal injury. *Ann Surg* 1974; **180:** 653–68.

10. Cori C F U. Mammalian carbohydrate metabolism. *Physiol Rev* 1931; **11:** 143–285.

11. Exton J H. Gluconeogenesis. *Metabolism* 1975; **21:** 945–90.

12. Wolfe R R, Allsop J R, Burke J F. Glucose metabolism in man: responses to intravenous glucose infusion. *Metabolism* 1979; **28:** 210–20.

13. Wolfe R R, Durkot M J, Allsop J R, *et al.* Glucose metabolism in severely burned patients. *Metabolism* 1979; **28:** 1031–9.

14. Bortz W M, Paul P, Haff A G, *et al.* Glycerol turnover and oxidation in man. *J Clin Invest* 1972; **51:** 1537–46.

15. Wolfe R R, Herndon D N, Peters E J, *et al.* Regulation of lipolysis in severely burned children. *Ann Surg* 1987; **206:** 214–21.

16. Wildmeuller H G, Spaeth A E. Intestinal metabolism of glutamine and glutamate from the lumen as compared to glutamine from the blood. *Arch Biochem Biophys* 1975; **171:** 662–77.

17. Felig P. The glucose-alanine cycle. *Metabolism* 1973; **22:** 179.

18. Jahoor F, Herndon D N, Wolfe R R. Role of insulin and glucagon in the response of glucose and alanine kinetics in burn-injured patients. *J Clin Invest* 1986; **78:** 807–14.

19. Wolfe R R, Goodenough R D, Burke J F, *et al.* Response of protein and urea kinetics in burn patients to different levels of protein intake. *Ann Surg* 1983; **197:** 163–71.

20. Aulick L H, Wilmore D W. Increased peripheral amino acid release following burn injury. *Surgery* 1979; **85:** 560–5.

21. Blackburn G L, Maini B S, Pierce E C. Nutrition in the critically ill patient. *Anesthesiology* 1977; **47:** 181–94.

22. Wolfe R R, Jahoor F, Herndon D N, *et al.* The glucose alanine cycle: origin of control. *J Parent Enteral Nutr* 1985; **9:** 107 (Abstract).

23. Wolfe R R, Shaw J H, Jahoor F, *et al.* Response to glucose infusion in humans: role of the changes in insulin concentration. *Am J Physiol* 1986; **250:** E306–E311.

24. Durkot N J, Wolfe R R. Effects of adrenergic blockade on glucose kinetics in septic and burned guinea pigs. *Am J Physiol* 1984; **241:** R222–R227.

25. Wolfe R R, Shaw J H. Inhibitory effect of plasma free fatty acids on glucose production in the conscious dog. *Am J Physiol* 1984; **246:** E181–E186.

26. Fredholm B B. The effect of lactate in canine subcutaneous adipose tissue in situ. *Acta Physiol Scand* 1971; **81:** 110–13.

27. Schulman G I, Williams P E, Liljenquist J E, *et al.* Effect of hyperglycemia independent of changes in insulin or glucagon on lipolysis in the conscious dog. *Metabolism* 1980; **29:** 317–20.

28. Kavach A G C, Rossell S, Sandor P. Blood flow, oxygen consumption and free fatty acid release in subcutaneous adipose tissue during hemorrhagic shock in control and phenoxybenzamine-treated dogs. *Circ Res* 1970; **26:** 733–48.

29. Wolfe R R, Herndon D N, Jahoor F, *et al.* Effect of severe burn injury on substrate cycling by glucose and fatty acids. *N Engl J Med* 1987; **317:** 403–8.

30. Herndon D N, Barrow R E, Rutan T C, *et al.* Effect of propranolol administration on hemodynamic and metabolic responses of burned pediatric patients. *Ann Surg* 1988; **208:** 484–92.

31. Wolfe R R, Shaw J H, Durkot M J. Effect of sepsis on VLDL kinetics: responses in basal state and during glucose infusion. *Am J Physiol* 1985; **248:** E732–E740.

32. Wolfe B M, Walker B K, Shaul D B, *et al.* Effect of total parenteral nutrition on hepatic histology. *Arch Surg* 1988; **123:** 1084–90.

33. Felig F, Wahren J. Influence of endogenous insulin secretion on splanchnic glucose and amino acid metabolism in man. *J Clin Invest* 1971; **59:** 1702–11.

34. Andres R, Cader G, Zierler K L. The quantitatively minor role of carbohydrate in oxidative metabolism of skeletal muscle in intact man in the basal state. Measurements of oxygen and glucose uptake and carbon dioxide and lactate production in the forearm. *J Clin Invest* 1956; **35:** 671.

35. Lipman R L, Raskin P, Love T. Glucose intolerance during decreased physical activity in man. *Diabetes* 1972; **21:** 101–7.

36. Black P R, Brooks D C, Bessey P Q, *et al.* Mechanisms of insulin resistance following injury. *Ann Surg* 1982: **196:** 420–35.

37. Wolfe R R, Jahoor F, Herndon DN, *et al.* Isotopic evaluation of the metabolism of pyruvate and related substrates in normal adult volunteers and severely burned children: effect of dichloroacetate and glucose infusion. *Surgery* 1991; **110:** 54–67.

38. Jahoor F, Shangraw R E, Miyoshi H, *et al.* Role of insulin and glucose oxidation in mediating the protein catabolism of burns and sepsis. *Am J Physiol* 1989; **257:** E323–E331.

39. Stuart C A, Shangraw R E, Prince M J, *et al.* Bed-rest induced insulin resistance occurs primarily in muscle. *Metabolism* 1988; **37:** 802–6.

40. Wolfe R R, Goodenough R D, Burke J F, *et al.* Response of protein and urea kinetics in burn patients to different levels of protein intake. *Ann Surg* 1983; **197:** 163–71.

CHAPTER TWENTY-ONE

MODULATION OF WOUND HEALING AND THE POSTBURN RESPONSE

MICHAEL J. MULLER, DAVID A. GILPIN AND DAVID N. HERNDON

Extensive full-thickness thermal injury is an especially severe form of trauma causing a substantial cutaneous wound and multiple systemic physiologic derangements. The hormonal and metabolic response to burn injury leads to hypermetabolism, progressive weight loss, increased susceptibility to infection, and poor wound healing. These changes caused by the burn wound can be altered by environmental, nutritional, and pharmacologic means. This chapter will review these techniques with special emphasis on recombinant growth factors and wound repair.

ENVIRONMENTAL FACTORS

Metabolic rate is increased after burn injury up to about 150% of normal levels[1] when burn size is greater than 20–30% TBSA. This figure may be greater if burn wound sepsis is present. If burn size is greater than 40% TBSA, Wilmore showed that hypermetabolism can be attenuated by increasing the ambient temperature from 25°C to 33°C.[2] Mean metabolic rate decreased from 72.0±1 kcal/m^2/h to 65.8±1.7 kcal/m^2/h ($p<0.001$) (normal 49 kcal/m^2/h) in a group of severely burned men cared for by the exposure method. It was further noted that those who failed to respond to lower environmental temperatures by increased metabolic rate and increased catecholamine production were more likely to succumb later to their injuries. When allowed to select their own environmental temperature, they chose ambient temperatures of 31.5±0.7 °C.[3] This is the same range that minimizes the metabolic expenditure required to maintain their above normal core temperatures, consistently 1–2°C higher than nonburned controls.[4] Clearly, patients treated by closed techniques with dressings and bandages tolerate lower ambient temperatures, probably about 26°C. Shivering evokes an enormous increase in energy expenditure and should be avoided. Blockade of evaporative water loss with water impermeable membranes does not ablate hypermetabolism;[5] however, exposure which allows evaporative water loss should be accompanied by environmental heating so as to minimize hypermetabolism.[6] The heat of water evaporation is 0.576 kcal/ml, and water loss can be as high as 200 ml/m^2 body surface area burn/hour; and if the energy of evaporation does not come from the environment, it must be produced by the patient.[7] This most simple but very important means of modulating postburn hypermetabolism can be derived with patient-controlled temperature regulation of their air supply or even regulation of infrared heaters[3] altered at the patient's behest.[8,9] It must be remembered that although increased ambient temperature will attenuate hypermetabolism and increase patient comfort, the underlying altered metabolic state with thermogenic futile substrate cycling will continue and needs additional nutritional support.

NUTRITIONAL MODULATION

Weight loss of 30% has often been observed in patients with moderate sized burns, in spite of maximal oral intake. Wound healing is limited and mortality increased when weight loss exceeds greater than 20% of preburn values. Further, tissue breakdown may liberate as much as 30 g/day of nitrogen.[10] This can be limited by provision of adequate dietary carbohydrate.[2] A patient's appetite seldom exceeds preburn levels and voluntary eating from the hospital tray almost never meets protein or calorie requirements in any but those with small burns. This observation led to a period when most burned patients were given parenteral supplementation of nutrition. This was shown first not to improve mortality or indices of immunity[11] and then to be associated with increased mortality.[12] This may well be the result of a negative effect on the immune system by parenteral nutrition.[13] Immediate enteral nutrition can be safely administered and may limit postburn hypermetabolism[14,15] by preserving intestinal mucosal integrity, thereby limiting bacterial translocation.[16–18]

When the protein metabolic response after burn injury was assessed using stable isotope infusions of leucine, valine, lysine, and urea in the acute, flow, convalescent, and recovery phases, increased protein breakdown was found to be present during the acute, flow, and convalescent phases. The rate of urea production (R_q urea), an indirect measure of net protein catabolism, was significantly increased during the flow phase only, suggesting that protein breakdown was adequately counteracted in the acute and convalescent phases by elevations in protein synthesis but not in the flow phase[19] (**Figure 21.1**). The switch from net protein catabolism to net protein anabolism in convalescence occurs in spite of an elevated protein breakdown rate.

Attempts to modulate protein dynamics have included increased provision of protein, supplementation of branched-chain amino acids, and supplementation of arginine. When children with very large burns (60% TBSA) were fed either 16.5% or 23% of desired calorie intake, neither group achieved the desired level of calories with the higher protein group taking significantly fewer calories (87% vs. 77%), the higher protein group received less intravenous hyperalimentation and fewer glucose infusions. As well, the higher protein group showed better indices of immunity,[6] higher protein levels, fewer bacteremic days, and improved survival.[20] Severely burned adults (70% TBSA) have also been studied with differential protein intake and stable isotope infusions of leucine, α-ketoisocaproic acid, and urea. Protein intake of 1.4 g/kg/day showed balance between protein synthesis and catabolism. When protein intake was increased to 2.2 g protein/kg/day, the isotopic methods did not indicate a further benefit in net protein synthesis, although the absolute rates of protein synthesis and catabolism were stimulated. Urinary nitrogen losses, on the other hand, indicated a significant improvement in net protein synthesis with higher protein intake. Further, the underlying alterations in protein metabolism consequent to the burn injury persisted, regardless of the level of protein intake[21] as the levels of protein intake had no effect on endogenous leucine production or intracellular leucine oxidation. Nutrition alone cannot fully optimize a burned patient's metabolic status.

Branched-chain amino acid enriched nutritional therapy was shown not to alter leucine kinetics when compared to conventional intact protein formulation in severely burned adults in a crossover study using stable isotope infusions of leucine. Nitrogen balance measurements were not statistically different between the study periods and the major consequences of increased intake of leucine from the branched-chain amino acid formula was an enhanced rate of leucine oxidation. Although evidence suggests benefit for surgical patients, branched-chain amino acid formulas appear to not offer any advantages over intact protein.[22] Intact protein was also shown to enhance nitrogen retention and maintain body weight better than free amino acids when fed enterally to burned guinea-pigs.[23]

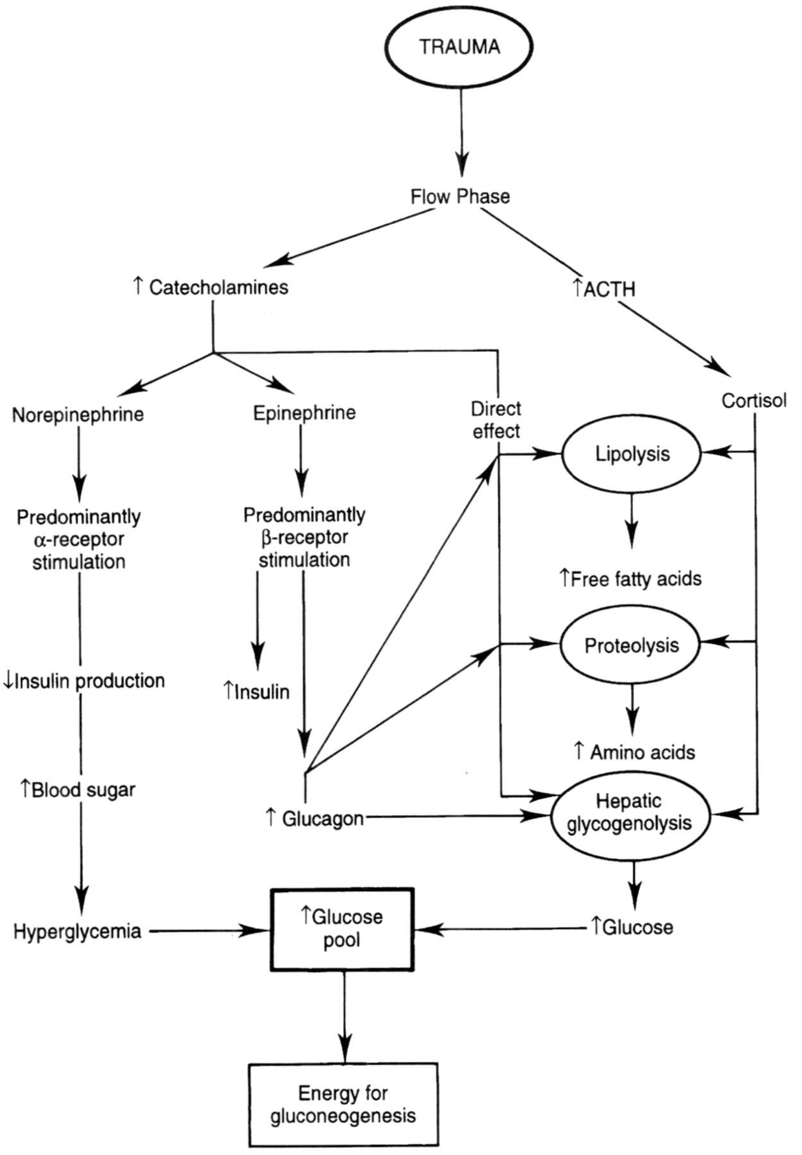

Fig. 21.1 Summary of some of the hormonal changes which occur following trauma. Reprinted with permission from Springer Verlag, from Wilmore D W, Carpenter W A (eds) Metabolic Support of the Critically Ill: Update in Intensive and Emergency Medicine. Enhancing Wound Healing, *1993, pp. 235–51.*

Arginine supplementation appears to provide benefit. It stimulated T-cell immunity in a rat model of sepsis[24] and in a guinea-pig burn model.[25] In human studies, supplemental arginine increased mean CD4 phenotype and mean T-lymphocyte stimulation in both healthy and postoperative cancer patients,[26,27] both wound healing and immune function were stimulated in the elderly.[28] The optimum level of arginine may be 2% of total protein.[29] Arginine appears to achieve most of its stimulatory action secondarily via the hypothalamopituitary axis as a secretagogue of insulin, glucagon, prolactin, and growth hormone because these effects are absent in hypophysectomized rats.

Omega-3 (Ω-3) fatty acids, such as are found in fish oil, lead to the production of prostaglandin E_3 (PGE_3), an immuno-inert substance. Most dietary fats in enteral feeding formulas are linoleic acids, which lead to production of immunodepressive PGE_6. Recently, a linoleic acid restricted, tube feeding formulation of high protein, enriched with Ω-3 fatty acids, arginine, cysteine, histidine, vitamin A, zinc, and ascorbic acid, was compared to two other standard formulations. Trends towards decreased wound infection, shorter length of hospital stay, reduced incidence of diarrhea, lower serum triglycerides, reduced numbers of infectious episodes, and improved preservation of muscle mass were apparent. Increased patient numbers with adjustment for burn size and age in the analysis will almost certainly demonstrate this formulation to be effective in modulating the immune response to burn injury.[30] It has also been shown that postoperative enteral nutrition with supplemental arginine, RNA, and Ω-3 fatty acids significantly improved immunological, metabolic, and clinical outcomes in patients with upper abdominal malignancies who were undergoing major elective surgery.[31]

Enteral feeding, applied as soon as possible, consisting of about 20% protein, 50% carbohydrate with the remainder as low linoleic fats, will help prevent weight loss. Polymeric diets are preferable to the more expensive elemental diets. Quantities required can be estimated by the feeding formulas described elsewhere. It must be stressed that if expense or availability preclude the use of more sophisticated feeds, cows' milk has been used extensively to good effect.

Hormonal Modulation

Following burn injury, the control of metabolic rate shifts from the thyroid axis to that of the sympathetic adrenal axis. Free thyronine (T_4) and free 3,5,3′-triidothyramine (T_3) serum levels decrease while reverse T_3, an inactive metabolite, increases.[32] Plasma norepinephrine and epinephrine are correlated negatively with T_3 while plasma catechol levels are correlated positively with T_3 levels. This syndrome of hypermetabolic, low triiodothyronine of burn injury is similar to other states of critical illness and is also known as the sick euthyroid syndrome.[33] The thyroid remains responsive to TSH, whose levels are also diminished.

Animal studies have revealed that adrenalectomy limits the increase in metabolic rate after burns, but that thyroidectomy does not[34] (**Table 21.1**).

Table 21.1

	Oxygen consumption (mg/g/h)		
	Nonburned	Burned	Increase
Control	0.84±0.10	1.16±0.02*	38%
Thyroidectomized	0.54±0.10	0.80±0.08*	48%
Adrenalectomized	0.85±0.20	0.98±0.02	15%

* 500 g rats with 50% TBSA scald burn; data presented as mean±SEM.

Antiprostaglandins were also shown to limit postburn hypermetabolism to about 15%. Pinealectomy performed before a burn in hamsters did not prevent liver-induced depression of serum T_4 or testosterone.[35] Neither T_3 treatment in burn patients nor T_4 treatment in trauma patients improved survival and may well be disadvantageous by inhibiting T_4 secretion,[36–38] a notion supported by decreased survival in an animal model of sepsis.[39]

While thyroid hormone therapy has not been shown to improve survival and absence of a thyroid does not prevent postburn hypermetabolism, thyroxine therapy may improve wound healing following burn injury. Guinea-pigs were thyroidectomized prior to a 50% TBSA scald burn and treated with different doses of thyroxine. Oxygen consumption, as an index of metabolic rate, was measured at 32°C. Wound healing was significantly improved at an intermediate dose but was retarded at a higher dose[40] (**Table 21.2**).

Table 21.2 Thyroidectomized guinea-pigs treated with T4 postburn

	Dose (μg/kg)	O_2 consumption Burn/control (%)	Wound healing (days)
Nonthyroidectomized	0	53	93
Thyroidectomized	15	44	86
	30	34	63*
	60	41	105
	120	32	138

The quality of scar was improved by T_3 treatment of rats with deep dermal burns. Histologic examination showed better organized collagen bundles, fewer retraction spaces, and smoother scars in the T_3 treated group.[41] Thyroid hormone modulation of the postburn response may improve the quality of survival by limiting unsightly scars.

Growth Factors

Cytokines, particularly interleukin-1 (IL-1), interleukin-6 (IL-6) and tumor necrosis factor (TNF), are the principal chemical messengers which are responsible for many of the events occurring at both the wound and systemically in distal tissues. Cytokines were originally considered to be regulatory chemicals secreted by cells of the immune system, and growth factors were seen as chemicals originating from inflammatory and reparative tissues. Now, the differences between growth factors, peptide hormones, and cytokines are no longer distinct. In this chapter, growth factors and cytokines are considered together and may be defined as any naturally occurring substance having a combination of mitogenic, angiogenic, activating, or chemotactic properties on the cell of origin and/or on other cells.[42] Many of these growth factors are released from damaged tissues at the wound site where they exert local and systemic effects.

Disruption of the vascular endothelium by wounding exposes blood cells to collagen which precipitates a cascade of events ultimately leading to blood clotting, inflammation, and repair. Platelet degranulation, endothelial damage, and leukocytes contribute to a pool of growth factors at the wound site which subsequently regulate enzymatic degradation, phagocytosis, chemotaxis, angiogenesis, and reepithelialization.[43] Reepithelialization, the migration of proliferating epithelial cells from the wound edges, provides a protective roof over the wound under which repair can proceed away from abrasive forces, dehydration and the risk of infection. The wound site contains factors from multiple sources. Growth factors produced locally at the wound site spill over into the circulation where they are carried to distal organs or tissues. The distal tissues are induced to produce more secreted growth factors which in turn are disseminated by the circulation from where they have a 'knock on' effect on yet more target tissues (**Figure 21.2**).

Growth factors bind to specific cell surface receptors which in turn transmit messages to the cell nucleus directing it to upregulate or downregulate synthesis of a specific secretory protein. Typically these receptors consist of three domains: an extracellular, a transmembrane, and an intracellular domain. The union of the extracellular domain with its ligand produces a conformational change in the extracellular domain with subsequent transmembrane activation (**Figure 21.3**). The activation of each receptor is unique; for example, some receptors require the binding of two sites on the same ligand molecule before transmembrane activation occurs. Other receptors require interaction between two neighboring receptor/ligand complexes before transmembrane transmission occurs. Another feature is cross-reactivity between growth factors for a given receptor due to structural homology between adjacent ligand proteins. This feature of sharing exists between the receptors of many factors. Although each receptor/ligand reaction is unique, there are many common features; the growth hormone receptor and its ligand is a good example.

The Growth Hormone/Growth Hormone Binding Protein Complex

Growth hormone (GH) binds to specific receptor molecules on the cell surface. The nature of this binding is rather different from the classical ligand/receptor binding of antibodies to antigens.[44] Antibody molecules acquire their individual specificities by amino acid changes within the hypervariable region of the V domain. The structural integrity of the antibody molecule changes relatively little between antibodies of widely differing antigenic specificity. Recent studies suggest that the binding of growth factors to their receptors occurs as a result of conformational diversity with relatively little change in the amino acid sequence.[44] The GH peptide is an asymmetrical molecule of 191 amino acids containing four helices and supporting *two* receptor binding sites. Topographical examination shows that the shapes of these binding sites on the hormone molecule are quite different.[44] Growth hormone binds two separate surface receptors so as to form a dimeric complex GH–$GHBP_2$. The extracellular portion of the GH receptor which is involved with binding consists of cysteine-rich areas, each region having two antiparallel sheets.[44,45] The receptor also has an area of molecular flexibility allowing it to unite more efficiently to GH. Only after the first receptor is bound to the GH molecule is the second capable of joining the complex. Within the complex, binding of the second receptor causes extra stabilization resulting from interaction between the extracellular domains.[44] Unlike the binding sites on the GH molecule, the amino acid sequences of the receptor sites are largely the same; their structures are also similar. It is noteworthy that there are marked similarities in the structure of the GH receptor extracellular domain and those of several other growth factors.[46] Cytokine/growth factor receptors may be divided into two classes, 1 and 2, on the basis of homology between their extracellular domains. Members of the class 1 receptor family include GH, prolactin, erythropoietin, IL-3, IL-6, IL-7, IL-4, and the granulocyte and granulocyte-macrophage colony stimulating factors (G-CSF, GM-CSF).[46–48] These receptors share structural features to which a sheet arrangement and cysteine-rich area contribute. Several of the receptors have similar molecular troughs within their tertiary structures which may accommodate a particular group of growth factors.[46,47]

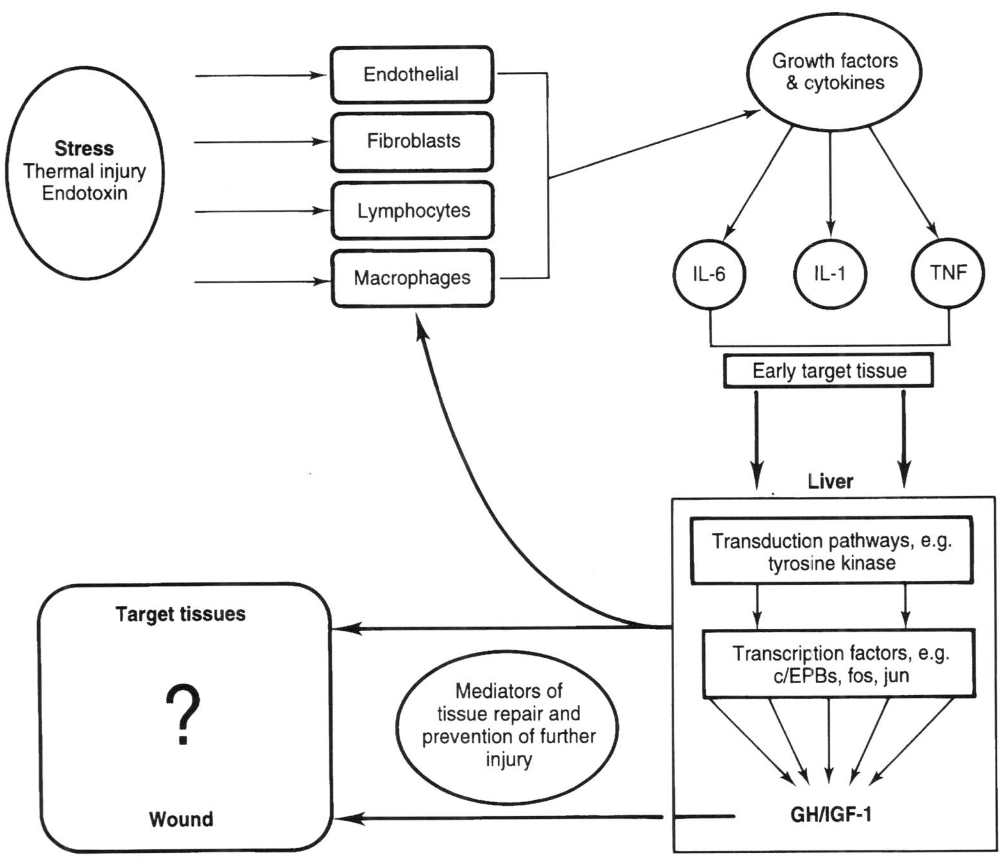

Fig. 21.2 Stress induces the release of inflammatory mediators from cells such as macrophages, lymphocytes, fibroblasts, and endothelial cells. These mediators are thought to be disseminated via the circulation to distal tissues, such as the liver, where they induce families of stress response genes. The protein products of these genes (e.g. growth hormone (GH) and insulin-like growth factor-1 (IGF-1) regulate the processes of wound repair and prevention of further injury in target tissues, such as the wound and other organs.

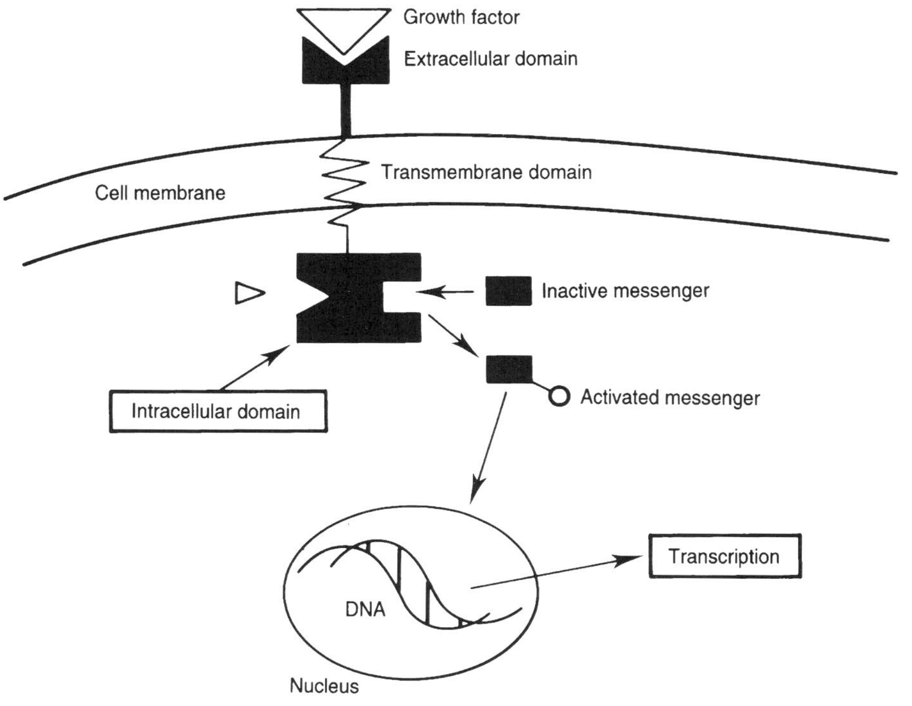

Fig. 21.3 Many growth factors and cytokines produce cell activation by binding to specific cell surface receptors. In doing this, the signal from the cytokine is passed via an intercellular cascade in order to reach the nucleus where protein synthesis is initiated. Reprinted with permission from Herndon D N, Hayward P G, Rutan R L, Barrow R E. Growth hormones and factors in surgical patients. In: Cameron J L, ed. Advances in Surgery, *Vol. 25, Chicago: Mosby Yearbook, Inc., 1991, pp. 65–97.*

The cytokine/growth factor molecules IL-6, GH, prolactin, erythropoietin, G-CSF and myelomonocyte growth factor (MGF), which bind to class 1 receptors, share many architectural similarities, including the presence of four helices in their secondary structures. Although the amino acid sequences of these factors are dissimilar, the positions of the helices within the primary structure of the differing growth factors are similar. The arrangement of helices within the cytokine molecule creates an environment which allows a specific helix to bind to the receptor. A stronger ligand/receptor union may then be created by the interaction of accessory proteins which only bind to specific sites on the ligand. Therefore, cytokines which differ in their primary structure but have similarities in secondary structure may be able to bind to several different cell surface receptors. For example, human GH may bind to prolactin receptors. Perhaps weak binding may, if the growth factor is present in sufficient concentration, have an intracellular effect. More permanent and high affinity binding would only occur if the accessory protein recognizes specific features on the ligand. There may be an 'evolutionary conserved interaction between homologous receptors and structurally similar cytokines'.[46] The structure of the GH–GHBP$_2$ complex is known and is easy to relate to the proposed model. The precise nature of many ligand/receptor binding complexes remains unknown, but it seems reasonable to suggest that the GH complex would have many similarities to those of other cytokines. Growth hormone can bind to both prolactin and GH receptors, indicating a degree of cross-reactivity between some members of the hematopoietic superfamily.[49] The ability of GH to bind to both prolactin and GH receptors may be altered by changing certain amino acid residues in specific areas of the GH molecule.[50] These facts help to provide further evidence for links within the cytokine/growth factor family. The significance of these structural similarities between different peptide ligands and the extracellular receptor domains is that a single growth factor may elicit several different responses, inhibitory or stimulatory, depending upon interactions with other factors and the cellular environment into which it is released. In addition, the phases of phagocytosis, reepithelialization, and angiogenesis are timed and regulated by the factors which predominate at any particular time as well as on the presence and intensity of surface receptors on the target tissues which, in turn, will vary with the state of cellular differentiation. Four growth factors are of particular importance in wound healing: platelet-derived growth factor, fibroblast growth factor, transforming growth factors, and epidermal growth factor.

Platelet-Derived Growth Factor (PDGF)

Platelet-derived growth factor is a glycoprotein dimer consisting of two chains, α and β, which have a 60% homology between their amino acid sequences. The PDGF dimer can exist in one of three forms AA (α, α), BB (β, β) and AB (α,β).[51] The dimers exert their effect by binding to specific surface receptors. There are two types of receptor, α and β. All three dimeric PDGF molecules bind to the α-receptor, but only PDGF (BB) binds to the β-receptor. Platelet-derived growth factor and the factors epidermal growth factor, transforming growth factor and fibroblast growth factor, all activate the same signal transduction pathway, starting with the enzyme tyrosine kinase, within the cytoplasm in order to convey messages to the nucleus.[52] Sources of PDGF include degranulated platelets (from which it derives its name), vascular endothelium and macrophages.[53] PDGF is thought to play a role in regulating other factors. For example, PDGF can induce the production of KC, the rodent homolog of human melanocyte growth stimulatory activity (MGSA)[54] a member of the IL-8 family of autocrine cytokines. MGSA is known to downregulate collagen synthesis in tissue culture and to have chemotactic qualities, which are features of obvious importance in wound healing. Platelet-derived growth factor is itself chemotactic for fibroblasts and inflammatory cells. Clinical studies using topically applied PDGF show enhanced healing of chronic ulcers and nonhealing wounds.[55] Collagen synthesis is also affected by PDGF. The mechanism of action at membrane, cytoplasmic, and nuclear levels, as well as which isoform is optimal, are questions which are still to be determined.

Fibroblast Growth Factor (FGF)

The fibroblast growth factor family consists of seven proteins, all with some degree of structural homology.[56,57] The proteins each have their own cell surface receptors; but as with PDGF, there is cross-reactivity between factors. One receptor binds several FGF factors, but with differing affinities for each. The FGF family helps to control angiogenesis through its stimulatory action on vascular endothelium. FGF-2, from damaged endothelium and macrophages, is thought to have an autocrine feedback upon the vascular lining;[57] this stimulates growth of the endothelial cells. Fibroblast growth factors are also mitogenic for fibroblasts and keratinocytes.[56]

Transforming Growth Factors (TGFα and β)

Transforming growth factor β exists in three forms, TGFβ (1, 2 and 3), and is located within platelet granules.[58,59] TGFβ(1) is a dimer of two identical chains and remains in an inactive complex while linked to a glycoprotein, TGF binding protein. Release and activation of TGFs occur upon exposure of the complex to extremes of physiologic pH, which are conditions found in wounds. *In vivo* animal studies confirm the usefulness of TGF at enhancing wound healing and tensile strength.[60]

TGF and Epidermal Growth Factor (EGF)

Transforming growth factor and epidermal growth factor share a 30% amino acid sequence homology.[61,62] Both factors have been found in wounds. *In vivo* animal studies indicate that EGF is necessary for collagen formation, epithelialization and granulation tissue formation; this suggests that it has an effect on epithelial and fibroblast cells. Clinical studies in which TGF and EGF were topically applied to burn wounds, independently, showed an enhancement in epithelialization, TGF being more effective than EGF.[43] Epidermal growth factor has also been shown to be of benefit in other areas of wound healing, including venous stasis and corneal ulcers.[63,64]

Topical Growth Factors

There is diversity and cross-reactivity between growth factors regarding structure, receptors, and subsequent actions. Clinical studies suggest the benefit of topical factors; however, many obstacles surround such a course, not least of which are the methods used in assessing the efficiency of the factor. Unintentional biosis and the subjective nature of many assessment techniques makes comparisons between studies and factors difficult. The massive production of proteolytic enzymes by neutrophils in wounds may inactivate growth factors. The degree to which this occurs depends on the number and activity of the leukocytes present. The effect of growth factors is entirely dependent on the variable state of receptivity of the wound itself.

An ideal growth factor would be tremendously valuable in the field of burn surgery where large wounds must be closed and kept free of infection. Unfortunately, these two simple aims create a dilemma. Wounds heal best if kept moist, warm, and undisturbed, yet burn wounds contain multiple endogenous bacteria which may flourish under certain conditions, and which may, either by becoming pathogenic themselves or by creating conditions, through local pH changes, favor the growth of other pathogens. Obviously this sequence of events is undesirable and can result in wound infection and systemic sepsis. The application of topical antibacterial agents, frequent dressing changes, improved resuscitation, and early wound excision have vastly reduced infective complications and mortality. Unfortunately, the requirements for prevention of infection and those optimal for wound healing do not completely coincide. Dressing changes abrade epithelializing surfaces and soak up tissue fluid rich in the very growth factors desired for healing. In addition, some topical antimicrobial agents inhibit reepithelialization. The incorporation of growth factors along with topical antibiotics is a possibility as is the direct application of a growth 'cocktail' (possibly of PDGF, FGF, and EGF) onto a skin grafted area. This 'ideal' growth factor should have the qualities listed in **Table 21.3**. It should be nontoxic both locally at the wound site in terms of allergy and systemically if absorbed. Second, there should be no potential drug interactions between the growth factor or its carrier and constituents of dressing materials or topical agents used for wound debridement. No systemically administered drug should cross-react, or interact, with the factor. The growth factor should be inexpensive, readily available, and in a form easy to prepare, apply, and, if necessary, remove (water soluble) without lengthy preparation. The half-life of the agent at the wound site must be sufficiently long for it to have histologic benefit. Burn wounds produce considerable tissue fluid. Even after grafting, tissue fluid loss is substantial. Topical factor preparations should be of physiologic pH with no tendency to create osmotic gradients and electrolyte disturbances, a feature of particular importance in young children. Substantial tissue fluid production at the wound site can dilute topical growth factors and carry them into absorbent dressings, thereby reducing their effectiveness. Tissue fluid can also interfere with wound penetration by the factor. Any topical agent should be stable so that the number of applications required to maintain a therapeutic range are kept to a minimum. Unfortunately maintenance of uniform rates of diffusion, and, therefore, concentration are virtually impossible to standardize. Growth factors interact with one another and the results of patterns established in tissue culture systems must be interpreted with caution as they do not always coincide with the *in vivo* situation. Although sporadic studies are very encouraging in this area, we still have a great many difficulties to overcome in achieving uniformity for assessing 'wound healing' and in standardizing regimens for topical agents.

Table 21.3 Qualities for the ideal growth factor

Nontoxic
Inexpensive
Easily applied and removed if needed
Long half-life when in contact with the wound
Wide therapeutic range
Good tissue penetration
Long shelf life
No interactions with dressing materials

Systemic Growth Factors

Growth hormone and IGF-1 levels are often decreased following burn injury.[65–67] These decreased levels of anabolic growth factors may play a role in the recently reported deficit in transmembrane amino acid transport observed in burned patients. The principal cause of net protein catabolism during flow phase postburn is an accelerated rate of breakdown with a concomitant failure to increase synthesis sufficiently to compensate.[68–71] A variation in transport rates could limit the availability of intracellular amino acids for synthesis. It is well established that growth hormone is a potent anabolic agent and can induce stimulation of net protein synthesis directly or indirectly through the action of IGF-1[70–74] and growth hormone; IGF-1 has been shown to increase transmembrane amino acid transport *in vitro*.[75] Growth hormone's effects include increased appetite, decreased nitrogen losses, increased retention of nitrogen and potassium, weight gain, more rapid wound healing, increased oxygen utilization, and decreased respiratory quotient.[76,77] These effects are in addition to its well known linear growth promoting effect.

GH promotes protein synthesis by increasing the cellular uptake of amino acids and accelerating nucleic acid translation and transcription, thereby enhancing cell proliferation. Fatty acids are released from the hydrolysis of fat for conversion to acetyl-CoA, an essential energy producing molecule for the tricarboxylic acid cycle. Through the preferential use of adipose tissue for energy production, there is a decrease in body fat with the result that protein is spared from catabolism.[78] GH treatment of obese dieters allowed lean body mass conservation at the expense of adipose stores.[79] GH also decreases cellular uptake of glucose, thereby exacerbating or precipitating hyperglycemia, which then triggers insulin release.[80] There is decreased sensitivity to insulin at the cellular level; this causes increased insulin resistance and hyperglycemia.

Growth hormone, when given to GH-deficient children, promotes active growth and rapidly improves nitrogen balance and increases muscle mass.[81] When a rat diaphragm is exposed to pharmacologic doses of GH, the rates of both amino acid transport and protein synthesis increase.[82] GH seems to have a more marked anabolic action in those whose protein balance is catabolic. No improvement in muscle mass or strength was detected in young adults undergoing exercise training, while nontrained subjects showed improve net protein balance through an increased rate of whole-body protein synthesis with no change in protein degradation.[83] Furthermore, the protein catabolic effect of prednisone, a glucocorticoid, was prevented by the concomitant administration of GH.[84]

GH anabolic action appears to be primarily mediated by an increase of protein synthesis. Brachial artery infusion of GH in both normal and postoperative patients revealed a direct effect of GH on skeletal muscle.[85,86] GH also acts to stimulate insulin-like growth factor synthesis. GH administration increases IGF-1 blood concentration via increased IGF-1 production by the liver.[87] GH also increases IGF-1 production in other tissues, such as skeletal muscle and cartilage, where IGF-1 may exert an autocrine/paracrine action.

Growth Hormone in Burn Injury

While the beneficial metabolic effects of growth hormone in burn injury have been known for some time,[88–91] the wound healing potential of GH has only recently been investigated. An extensive prospective randomized, double-blinded clinical trial has examined the basic mechanisms of protein anabolism, hyperglycemia and wound healing in massively burned children and adolescents.

GH (0.2 mg/kg/day) increased protein turnover with elevation of both protein synthesis and breakdown, but with synthesis exceeding breakdown in a group of severely burned (≈ 70% TBSA) hypermetabolic adolescents.[92] This resulted in a net reduction in protein loss of 50% compared to controls. Whole body and isolated limb assessments were performed using [^{15}N]lysine stable isotope technique. GH treatment raised leg blood flow significantly. This increase in peripheral blood flow did not cause an increase in cardiac index which was raised equally in both groups to twice the normal range. Urinary nitrogen excretion was also decreased. A hyperinsulinemic, euglycemic, eukalemic clamp showed a decrease in net protein breakdown in control groups but no further benefit in the GH group. Further, 30-fold increase in GH and a threefold increase in IGF-1 serum levels were noted with no change in insulin, glucagon or cortisol levels.

GH causes hyperglycemia in burned patients by induction of insulin resistance and inhibition of glucose uptake relative to the availability of insulin. This was examined in a group of severely burned adolescents receiving GH (0.2 mg/kg/day) or placebo in blinded fashion.[93] All were hypermetabolic at 140% predicted resting energy expenditure. A euglycemic hyperinsulinemic clamp was performed. Growth hormone administration was also shown to significantly reduce glucose uptake and inhibit glucose oxidation compared to the placebo patients. Glucose utilization (percentage glucose uptake oxidized) in both patient groups remained similar. This implies that GH induces an insulin resistance by inhibiting glucose transport. As counter-regulation, plasma levels of insulin then increase to maintain euglycemia. Clinically, about one-third of patients treated with GH require therapeutic insulin for 2–3 days, after which time borderline hyperglycemia persists but not at a level requiring insulin.

Further examination of this effect revealed increases in levels of stress hormones in a group of severely burned older children who had early morning blood samples collected during their hyperdynamic, hypermetabolic postburn phase[94] (**Tables 21.4, 21.5**).

Table 21.4 Patient characteristics

	n	Age (years)	TBSA (%)	REE/predicted	Heart rate (beats/min)
Placebo	8	11 ± 1	67 ± 6	1.3 ± 0.2	136 ± 7
GH	6	9 ± 2	71 ± 9	1.3 ± 0.1	149 ± 7

Table 21.5 Hormonal and metabolic parameters with GH treatment

	Controls $n = 8$	GH $n = 6$
GH (normal: < 8 mg/ml)	2.3 ± 0.3	30.4 ± 19.9*
IGF-1 (normal: 22–138 U/ml)	56 ± 15	168 ± 24*
Free fatty acids (normal: 0.19–0.90 mEq/l)	0.59 ± 0.04	0.74 ± 0.01*
Glucose (normal: 60–115 mg/dl)	129 ± 13	133 ± 16
Insulin (normal: 5–25 μU/ml)	25 ± 3	33 ± 3*
Total catecholamines (normal: 120–450 pg/ml)	1117 ± 137	1817 ± 177*
Glucagon (normal: 50–200 pg/ml)	158 ± 22	215 ± 18*
Cortisol (normal: 7–27 mg/dl)	21.3 ± 1.6	28.4 ± 5.4

Data presented as mean ± SEM
* Significantly different $p < 0.05$.[94]

GH significantly elevated plasma levels of catecholamines, glucagon and insulin above the already elevated levels found in severely burned patients. Catecholamines and glucagon are typically considered to be catabolic hormones and mediators of the postburn catabolic response. An increase in these mediators might have been expected to increase the hypermetabolic response and its associated protein catabolism; however, as has already been shown, protein anabolism, not catabolism, is induced by GH in burn injury. As insulin infusion has been shown to significantly increase plasma catecholamine levels, it was felt that GH-induced insulin resistance led to hyperinsulinemia and then to subsequent elevation of catecholamine levels.[95] In turn, glucagon release can be stimulated by catecholamines or growth hormone or both, even though they are not the primary stimulus for glucagon release.[96] The reversal of the insulin: glucagon ratio, typically seen in burned patients, was maintained in the GH-treated group. The increase in free fatty acid levels was not surprising, as both catecholamines and GH serve to stimulate lipolysis and release free fatty acids into the circulation. It is significant that metabolic rate/resting energy expenditure was not increased by these hormonal changes as would be expected if the increases in the stress hormone levels were clinically significant.

Wound Healing Effects of GH

Skin is a target tissue for GH, either indirectly via circulating insulin-like growth factor-1 (IGF-1) or directly by GH interaction with specific receptors on the surface of epidermal and dermal cells.[97, 98] Direct effects of GH on cultured human skin fibroblasts have been demonstrated and include increased IGF-1 and IGF binding protein production and increased thymidine uptake.[99,100] Animal studies have shown that biosynthetic GH increased the collagen content and the tensile strength of skin and granulation tissue.[101–103] A significant increase in skin thickness was noted when 12 healthy men, aged 61–81 years, who had subnormal IGF-1 levels, were treated with subcutaneous injections of biosynthetic growth hormone three times per week.[104] Incisional wounds in the skin of rats show increased strength after biosynthetic growth hormone treatment, even if malnourished.[105–107]

GH treatment of the severely burned improves wound healing dramatically if the dose is sufficient. A pilot study showed no protein anabolic benefit at 0.03 mg/kg/day or 0.06 mg/kg/day in adult burned patients.[108] GH at a dose of 0.1 mg/kg/day did not raise serum levels sufficiently, or for a long enough time, to improve wound healing in severely burned children (**Figure 21.4**). Using a dose of 0.2 mg/kg/day, a prospective, randomized, placebo-controlled trial has shown accelerated skin graft donor site wound healing by 25% in children with a mean burn size of 60% of their total body surface area. The significance of these results was that these massively burned children could be taken to the operating room for further skin grafting about 2 days earlier if treated with GH. The use of GH resulted in a significant decrease in the overall time to totally close the burn wound. GH was shown to reduce the healing times of the initial donor site compared to the placebo group, as well as that of the second and third donor site; however, the patient numbers for the third donor site group were small. When adjusted for percentage of total body surface area burned (% TBSA), the treated group took 0.54 ± 0.04 days/% TBSA (mean ± SD) and the placebo group took 0.80 ± 0.09 days/% TBSA to achieve total wound closure. This decreased total wound closure time for a patient with the average burn size in the study group of 60% TBSA from 46 to 32 days[109] (**Table 21.6**).

No antibodies to recombinant human GH (rhGH) were exhibited during treatment. Insulin given therapeutically, and, therefore, the

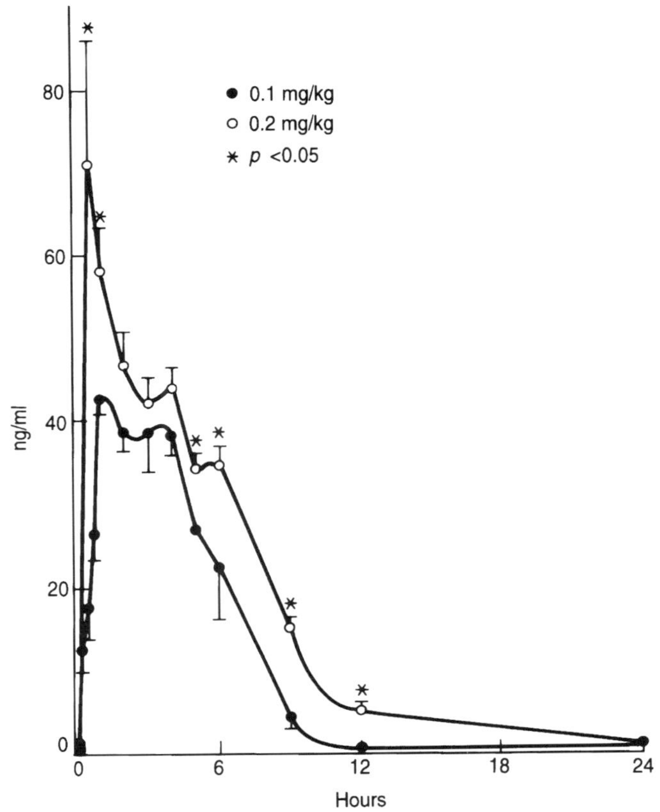

Fig. 21.4 Dose–response curve following parenteral administration of recombinant human growth hormone. Reprinted with permission from Herndon et al. *Effects of recombinant human growth hormone on donor site healing in severely burned children.* Annals of Surgery *1990;* **212***(4): 424–31.*[109]

Table 21.6 Donor site healing times (days)

	First harvest	Second harvest	Third harvest
Placebo	9.0±0.4	9.0±0.7	8.0±1.0
GH (0.2mg/kg/day)	7.0±0.5*	6.0±0.4*	6.0±1.0

* Data presented as mean ± SEM.[109]

hyperglycemia for which it was given, did not affect the rate of healing. Over 100 children have now been treated with rhGH, including a number who were not included in the prospective trial due to extremes of age or late presentation. Infants younger than 2 years of age showed the same beneficial effects of rhGH as those who are older, without adverse effect. Patients presenting 2 or 3 weeks after injury, who were all in poor condition and looked cachectic from sepsis, hypermetabolism, or inadequate nutrition, were noted to have donor site healing times of about 7 days (**Table 21.7**). This is remarkable in patients so nutritionally and metabolically disadvantaged.[110]

Table 21.7 Donor site healing times of infants and late presenters

	n	Age (years)	TBSA burn (%)	Healing time (days)
GH <2 years	9	1.4±0.2	56±5	6.0±0.4*
GH late	6	5.2±1.2	57±7	6.0±0.7*
Control	26	8.4±0.9	67±3	8.5±0.5

* Data presented as mean ± SEM.[110]

Burned adults, when treated with rhGH in a double-blind, randomized study, also showed a 2-day decrease in the length of time for split-thickness donor sites to heal.[111] The effect of GH on burned patients is profound and beneficial. Insulin resistance is induced, but glucose utilization does not change. Protein anabolism is induced in spite of further elevation of the levels of catabolic hormones. Improved donor site wound healing is so marked that it is visible (**Figure 21.5**).

Another postburn response in children is growth retardation. Severe delays in both height and weight growth have been demonstrated in pediatric patients who had sustained greater than a 40% TBSA burn. This growth delay persisted for as long as 3 years postinjury without any 'catch-up' growth experienced.[112] Major illnesses have been demonstrated to produce a profound change in growth. Growth changes can be transient, disappearing with the resolution of the illness, or permanent, such as with intrinsic defects of endocrine function or with pathologic states, like chronic renal failure. In other serious medical conditions, once resolution is achieved, the patient experiences a period of explosive growth and is able to return to comparable peer-group growth patterns. This 'catch-up' growth spurt has been observed in other severe trauma conditions.[113] This does not occur in pediatric burned patients who do not exhibit such a growth spurt. Nail and hair growth are attenuated during the catabolic phase of burn response and evidence is mounting that a bony lesion exists which is of an aplastic nature.[114,115] The exact mechanism of this growth retardation is unknown. Adequate nutrition is required for normal growth. It may be that these patients continue to expend energy stores on the damaged integument, thus leaving few resources for growth. Short-term GH use during the acute phase of injury does not prevent this condition.

Growth hormone has many uses in patients who are catabolic, malnourished, or have received severe trauma such as burning.[116,117] Its more widespread availability and application will benefit many[118] and ultimately reduce costs. Growth hormone use in an American pediatric burn center with bed costs of US $1600 per day has achieved an 18% cost saving for severely burned (≈60% TBSA) children.[119]

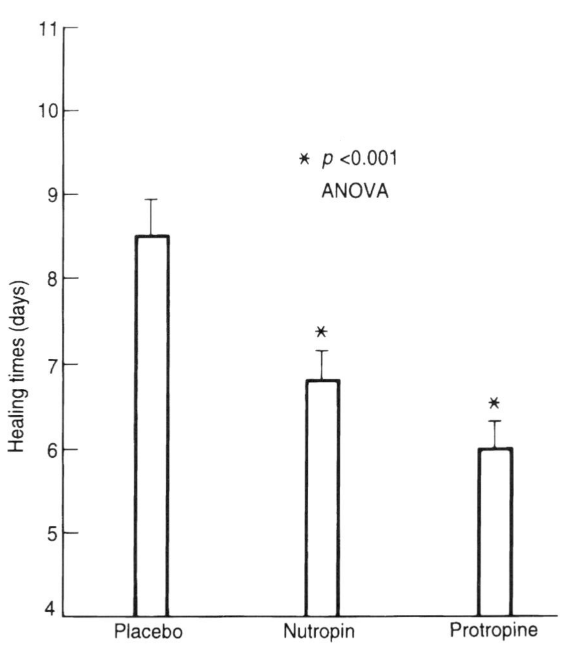

Fig. 21.5 Differences in donor site healing time following treatment with Protropin, Nutropin, and placebo. Reprinted with permission from Gilpin et al. Recombinant human growth hormone accelerates wound healing in children with large cutaneous burns. Annals of Surgery, *1994;* **220***(1): 23.*

INSULIN-LIKE GROWTH FACTOR-1

Growth hormone acts both directly and indirectly via IGF-1 production in the liver and elsewhere.[120,121] IGF-1 serum levels are decreased in burned patients.[122] This is consistent with the observation that hepatic IGF-1 secretion is directly impaired despite normal pituitary GH secretion in many disease states and that simultaneous use of GH and IGF-1 gives enhanced anabolic effects in normal humans.[123]

Growth hormone given to septic patients failed to increase IGF-1 levels. Also, the IGF-1 response to GH treatment is attenuated with increasing severity of trauma or burn.[124,125] These facts have led to speculation that IGF alone or in combination with GH, may achieve better results in malnourished, septic burned patients. Early animal work has been most encouraging.

When 1 mg/day of IGF-1 was administered via osmotic pumps implanted subcutaneously to 50% scald-burned rats, circulating IGF-1 levels were significantly decreased in untreated animals compared to unburned controls, while recombinant human IGF-1 (rhIGF-1) treated animals showed IGF-1 levels which were restored to levels similar to unburned controls.[126] The metabolic rates (estimated by oxygen consumption) of burned animals treated with IGF-1 were comparable to those of the unburned control group, while placebo-treated burned rats had significantly elevated metabolic rates. That is, postburn hypermetabolism was completely obviated. Using the same model, small intestinal mucosal DNA and protein content, gut mucosal weight, splenic weight, and body weight were increased with 3 mg/kg/day IGF-1. Additionally, the IGF-1 treated rats had a decrease in the usual postburn hyperglycemia, a positive nitrogen balance, and increased weight gain for 5 days. The incidence of bacterial translocation to the mesenteric lymph nodes was reduced from 90% to 30% as gut mucosal function was improved.[127] IGF-1 (3 mg/g/day) given by continuous infusion to 50% scald-burned rats attenuated body weight loss, corrected the burn-induced decrease in hepatic adenosine triphosphate concentration, prevented burn-induced decrease in hepatic ketone body levels, and prevented the fever-induced impairment in hepatic redox potential.[128] Inhaled, aerosolized barrier IGF-1 accelerated epithelial repair of smoke-injured trachea in sheep.[129]

Early experience with IGF-1 in burned adults has shown short-term (2–3 days) induction of protein anabolism. Further treatment induces increased binding protein production so that levels of free IGF-1 fall. IGF-1 alone has not produced any improvement in wound healing at a dose of 10 mg/kg/h when given for 7 days. Growth hormone, 0.2 mg/kg/day, did accelerate donor site wound healing by about 25%. The addition of IGF-1 to GH gave only a marginal further benefit in wound healing (unpublished results).

β-ADRENERGIC RECEPTOR AGENTS

The hyperdynamic circulatory response to burn injury, stimulated by 10-fold increases in catecholamines, plays a significant role in increasing energy expenditure. Tachycardia of 120–150 beats/minute is often sustained for many weeks in massively burned patients. Cardiac dysfunction commonly contributes to mortality with myocarditis, cardiomyopathy, and focal myocardia increases often found at autopsy.[130,131] These findings are similar to those found in patients who succumb to other catechol excess states such as pheochromocytoma. Adrenergic blockade had been used with success in pathologic hypercatecholamine states and thyrotoxicosis by decreasing myocardial work load, whole-body irritability, and tremulousness.[132] Total catecholamine absence in 60% burned rats, induced by either adrenalectomy or chronic reserpine administration, certainly decreased hypermetabolism but also increased mortality.[133]

Catecholamines also stimulate lipolysis in burned patients.[134,135] Acute administration of β-blocking agents precipitously decreases the rate of release or appearance of free fatty acids (FFA) in plasma, indicating the important role which preexisting sympathetic activity plays in the mobilization of FFA. Chronic catecholamine blockade could, therefore, indirectly increase protein catabolism, since FFA is the primary endogenous energy substrate. The concern that adrenergic blockade could have a detrimental metabolic effect has been amplified by the notion that catecholamines may have a direct protein anabolic effect.[136–138] Wilmore examined adrenergic blockade in exposed patients with α-, β-, and combined α- and β-blockade.[2] α-Blockade alone did not change metabolic rate; however, significant decreases were seen with combined α- and β-blockade and with β-blockade alone. The decrease in metabolic rate was associated with a decrease in pulse rate, blood pressure, minute ventilation, and free fatty acids. Larger than normal doses were required to obtain adequate blockade. In the same study, a significant correlation between increasing urinary catecholamine excretion and an increasing metabolic rate was induced by cold stress. Four nonresponders to cold stress who showed a paradoxical decrease in metabolic rate later succumbed. Consequently, adrenergic blockade which interferes with cold stress response (catecholamine-induced calorigenic response), would seem best avoided.

A number of more recent and extensive studies have shown that limited β-blockade can be safely used in severely burned patients. Propranolol, 2 mg/kg/day was given intravenously to 18 patients for 5 days with burns of 70 ± 30% TBSA.[139] Heart rate was decreased by 20%, left ventricular work index by 22%, and rate pressure product by 36%. Plasma glucose, free fatty acids, triglyceride, and insulin levels remained unchanged. Propranolol concentrations were approximately ten times the blood levels normally required for effective β-blockade at 700 ± 500 mg/ml. Catecholamine levels were not affected by nonselective β-blockade; however, blood urea nitrogen was elevated in the treated group. Stable isotope infusions of urea were performed in both the fed and fasted state. Rate of urea production (R_a) was increased one- to fivefold in the treated group. This led to speculation that blockade of the skeletal muscle cell β_2-adrenoreceptor was preventing normal agonist activity of evaluating catecholamines with acceleration in net protein balance to further catabolism. Burned patients have an increase in both protein synthesis and protein breakdown, both possibly as a result of catecholamine excretion.

A group of six septic patients, age 17 ± 3 years, with burns 82 ± 11% TBSA, were given propranolol under continuous hemodynamic monitoring with a Swan–Ganz catheter.[140] Pressure–work index and rate pressure product were significantly decreased with both 0.5 and 1.0 mg/kg. Cardiac index, oxygen delivery index, and oxygen consumption were improved without adversely affecting overall oxygen delivery or total body oxygen consumption. The ability of patients treated with propranolol at this dose, 1–2 mg/kg/day, necessary to achieve the desired 25% decrease in heart rate, to respond appropriately to cold stress and isoproterenol challenge was undiminished.[141]

β_1-Selective blockade with metoprolol has been compared with β_1, β_2 nonselective blockade using propranolol. At a dose of 0.5 mg/kg/day, metoprolol decreased heart rate by 18% and rate pressure product by 15%. Equivalent effects were achieved by adjusting the dose of propranolol. Stable isotope infusions of leucine, urea, and glycerol were used to assess protein and lipid metabolism. Metoprolol had no effect on protein or lipid metabolism, while propranolol showed a decrease in lipolysis (Ra Glycerol) and no change in urea production.[142]

Selective β_1-blockade is a metabolically inert, cardiovascularly safe means of limiting the postburn hyperdynamic cardiovascular response. Therefore, metoprolol would appear to be the drug of choice for the often encountered problem of burn-induced hypertension.[143] Tremulousness, irritability, and marked tachycardia are almost universal among those with large burns; and β-blockade is indicated for these patients.

Selective β_2-adrenergic receptor agonists have known protein anabolic effects. Clenbuterol, a totally selective β_2-agonist, has structural similarities to epinephrine and is well known to promote protein anabolism in normal animals via β_2-adrenergic receptor activation.[144] Post-surgical rats and burned rats showed increased muscle mass and body weight with clenbuterol, and showed evidence that hypermetabolism was also increased.[145,146]

In 30% burned rats given a dorsal incision and clenbuterol, 2 mg/kg/day, by continuous infusion, muscle and body mass were increased after both 14 and 21 days.[147] Nontemperature-dependent hypermetabolism occurred which was not aggravated by clenbuterol. Increased wound breaking strength was induced by clenbuterol in a free-feeding group. This effect was obviated by nutritional matching (pair feeding) indicating that substrate availability is essential for clenbuterol to show effect. β-Blockade with metoprolol combined with selective β_2-stimulation with clenbuterol or salbutamol may offer stressed patients induction of protein anabolism, enhanced wound healing and decreased myocardial strain at reasonable cost.

Modulators of Inflammation

The result of the inflammatory response to skin burn is the release of mediators such as cytokines, histamine, and thromboxane which produce distant organ inflammation as a result of lipid peroxidation. Oxidants are produced by activated neutrophils, free metal ions, increased cell xanthine oxidase activity, and increased arachidonic acid metabolism. Allopurinol, a xanthine oxidase inhibitor, has prevented lipid peroxidation and attenuated burn edema in a sheep burn model.[148] Ibuprofen, a cyclooxygenase inhibitor, also inhibits oxidant release from neutrophils and decreases lipid peroxidation in the lungs after burn.[149] Ibuprofen also decreased hypermetabolism in a 50% rat burn model.[133] Flurbiprofen, a topical anti-inflammatory agent, similarly prevents O_2 radical release from neutrophils. When applied to a skin burn in a sheep model, flurbiprofen attenuated the postburn hypermetabolic state to as similar an extent as that seen with total excision and complete wound closure.[150] In the same sheep burn model, it decreased total fluid requirements and decreased oxidation changes. Human trials are clearly indicated.

Summary

Wound healing is regulated and coordinated by growth factors produced locally at the wound site and distally in central tissues such as the liver. These factors interact with one another and with specific surface receptors. Binding of a growth factor ligand to its receptor starts a cascade of intracellular events in which a chemical messenger stimulates specific genes within the nucleus. In this way, growth factors (including PDGF, FGF, TGF, and EGF) regulate and coordinate important processes in wound healing: phagocytosis, angiogenesis, collagen deposition, and epithelialization.

Complete healing of the cutaneous wound curtails the hypermetabolic response which follows burn injury. The degree of hypermetabolism which develops prior to complete wound closure can be limited by environmental warming, avoidance of infection, and, in the future, by topical or systemic agents which affect O_2 radical release and inflammatory cascades. The effects of the hypermetabolic response can be limited by immediate, adequate enteral nutrition supplemented with extra protein, Ω-3 fatty acids, arginine, and glutamine. Growth factors and β-adrenoreceptor agents actually speed wound closure, as well as reversing protein catabolism. If these modalities are combined with active surgical treatment of the burn wound, then mortality, morbidity, and hospitalization can be significantly decreased.

References

1. Rutan T, Herndon D N, Van Osten T, Abston S. Metabolic rate alterations in early excision and grafting versus conservative treatment. *J. Trauma* 1986; **26**(2): 140–2.

2. Wilmore D W, Long J M, Mason A D, Skreen R W, Pruitt B A. Catecholamines: mediator of the hypermetabolic response to thermal injury. *Ann Surg* 1974; **180:** 653–69.

3. Wilmore D W, Lang J M, Skreen R W, *et al.* Studies of the effect of variations of temperature and humidity on energy demands of the burned soldier in a controlled metabolic room. *Annual Report 1973*. Ft Sam Houston, US Army Institute of Surgical Research. Symbol MEDDH-288 (R).

4. Aulich L H, Hander E H, Wilmore D W, Mason P A, Pruitt B A. The relative significance of thermal and metabolic demands on burn hypermetabolism. *J Trauma* 1979; **19**(8): 559–66.

5. Zawacki B E, Spitzer K W, Mason A D Jr. Does increased evaporative water loss cause hypermetabolism in burn patients. *Ann Surg* 1970; **171:** 236–40.

6. Neely A W, Petra A B, Holloman G H, Rustitan F W, Turner M D, Hardy J D. Researches on the cause of burn hypermetabolism. *Ann Surg* 1974; **179**(3): 291–94.

7. Barr P O, Birke G, Liljedahl S O, *et al.* Oxygen consumption and water loss during treatment of burns with warm dry air. *Lancet* 1968; **1:** 164–8.

8. Wilmore D W, Mason A D Jr, Johnson D W, *et al.* Effect of ambient temperature on heat production and heat loss in burn patients. *J Appl Physiol* 1975; **38:** 593–7.

9. Danielsson U. Arturson G, Wennberg L. The elimination of hypermetabolism in burned patients. *Burns* 1976; **2**(2): 110–14.

10. Sonhoff H S, Pearson E, Artz C P. An estimation of nitrogen requirements for equilibrium in burn patients. *Surg Gynecol Obstet* 1961; **112:** 159.

11. Herndon D N, Stein M D, Rutan T C, Abston S, Linares H. Failure of TPN supplementation to improve liver function, immunity, and mortality in thermally injured patients. *J Trauma* 1987; **27:** 195–204.

12. Herndon D N, Barrow R E, Stein M, *et al.* Increased mortality with intravenous supplemental feeding in severely burned patients. *J Burn Care Rehabil* 1989; **10:** 309–13.

13. Moore F A, Feliciano D V, Andrassy R J, *et al.* Early enteral feeding, compared with parenteral, reduces post operative septic complications: the results of a meta-analysis. *Ann Surg* 1992; **216:** 172–83.

14. McDonald W S, Sharp C W, Deitch E A. Immediate enteral feeding in burn patients is safe and effective. *Ann Surg* 1991; **213**(2): 177–83.

15. Mochizuki H, Trocki O, Dominioni L, *et al.* Mechanism of prevention of postburn hypermetabolism and catabolism by early enteral feeding. *Ann Surg* 1984; **200:** 297–310.

16. Mochizuki H, Trocki O, Dominioni L, *et al.* Reduction of postburn hypermetabolism by early enteral feedings. *Curr Surg* 1985; **42:** 121–5.

17. Herndon D N, Ziegler S T. Bacterial translocation after thermal injury. *Crit Care Med* 1993; **21**(2): S50–S54.

18. Saito H, Trocki O, Alexander J W, Kopcha R, Heyd T, Joffe S N. The effect of route of nutrient administration on the nutritional state, catabolic hormone secretion, and gut mucosal integrity after burn injury. *J Parenter Enteral Nutr* 1987; **11:** 1–7.

19. Jahoor F, Desai M, Herndon D N, Wolfe R R. Dynamics of the protein metabolic response to a burn injury. *Metabolism* 1988; **37**(4): 330–7.

20. Alexander, J W, MacMillan B G, Stinnett J D, *et al.* Beneficial effects of aggressive protein feeding in severely burned children. *Ann Surg* 1980; **192:** 505–17.

21. Wolfe R R, Goodenough R D, Burke J F, Wolfe M H. Response of protein and urea kinetics in burn patients to different levels of protein intake. *Ann Surg* 1983; **197:** 163–71.

22. Yu Y-M, Wagner D A, Walesreswski J C, Burke S F, Young V R. A kinetic study of leucine metabolism in severely burned patients: comparison between a conventional and branched chain amino acid-enriched nutritional therapy. *Ann Surg* 1988; **207**(4): 421–9.

23. Trocki O, Mochizuri H, Dominioni L, Alexander J W. Intact protein versus free amino acids in the nutritional support of thermally injured animals. *J Parenter Enteral Nutr* 1986; **10**(2): 139–45.

24. Madden H P, Breslin R J, Wasserkrug H L, Efron G, Barboh A. Stimulation of T cell immunity by arginine enhances survival in peritonitis. *J Surg Res* 1988; **44:** 658–63.

25. Saito H, Trocki O, Wang S L, Gonce S S, Joffe S N, Alexander J W. Metabolic and immune effects of dietary arginine supplementation after burn. *Arch Surg* 1987; **122:** 784–9.

26. Barbul A, Sisto D A, Waserkrug H L, Efron G. Arginine stimulates lymphocyte immune response in healthy human beings. *Surgery* 1981; **90**(2): 244–51.

27. Daly J M, Reynolds J, Thoun A, *et al.* Immune and metabolic effects of arginine in the surgical patient. *Ann Surg* 1988; **208**(4): 512–23.

28. Kirk S J, Hurson M, Regan M C, Host D R, Wasserkrug H L, Barbul A. Arginine stimulates wound healing and immune function in elderly human beings. *Surgery* 1993; **114**(2): 155–60.

29. Alexander J W, Gottschlich M M. Nutritional immunomodulation in burn patients. *Crit Care Med* 1990; **18**(2): S149–S153.

30. Gottschlich M M, Jenkins M, Warden G D, *et al.* Differential effects of three enteral dietary regimens on selected outcome variables in burn patients *J Parenter Enternal Nutr* 1990; **14**(3): 225–36.

31. Daly J M, Lieberman M D, Goudfine J, *et al.* Enteral nutrition with supplemental arginine, RNA, and omega-3 fatty acids in patients after operation: immunologic, metabolic, and clinical outcome. *Surgery* 1992; **112:** 56–67.

32. Becker R A, Vaughan G M, Goodwin C W, *et al.* Interactions of thyroid hormones and catecholamines in severely burned patients. *Rev Infect Des* 1983; **5**(Suppl 5): S908–S913.

33. Aun F, Medeiros-Neto G A, Younes R N, Birogini D, Ramos de Oliveira M. The effect of major trauma on the pathways of thyroid hormone metabolism. *J Trauma* 1983; **23**(12): 1048–50.

34. Herndon D N, Wilmore D W, Mason A D, Pruitt B A. Humoral mediators of non-temperature dependent hypermetabolism in 50% burned adult rats. *Surg Forum* 1977; **28:** 37–9.

35. Vaughan G M, Shirani K Z, Vaugnology M K, Pruitt B A, Mason A D. Hormonal changes in burned hamsters. *Endocrinology* 1985; **117**(3): 1090–5.

36. Brent G A, Hershman J M. Thyroxine therapy in patients with severe non thyroidal illnesses and low serum thyroidine concentration. *J Clin Endocrinol Metab* 1986; **63**(1): 1–8.

37. Becker R A, Vaughan G M, Ziegler M G, *et al.* Hypermetabolic low tricoelathyronine syndrome of burn injury. *Crit Care Med* 1982; **10**(12): 870–5.

38. Becker R A, Vaughan G M, Goodwin C W, *et al.* Plasma norepinephrine, epinephrine and thyroid hormone interactions in severely burned patients. *Arch Surg* 1980; **115:** 439–43.

39. Little S. Effect of thyroid hormone supplementation on survival after bacterial infection. *Endocrinology* 1985; **117**(4): 1431–5.

40. Herndon D N, Wilmore D W, Mason A D, Curreri P W. Increased rates of wound healing in burned guinea pigs treated with Triiodo thyronine. *Surg Forum* 1979; **30:** 95–7.

41. Mehregan A H, Zamick P. The effect of trioela thyronine in healing of deep chemical burns and marginal scars of skin grafts. A histologic study. *J Cutan Pathol* 1974; **1:** 113–16.

42. Herndon D N, Nguyen T T, Gilpin D A. Growth factors: local and systemic. *Arch Surg* 1993; **128**(11) 1227–33.

43. Martin P M, Wooley J H, McCluskey J. Growth factors and cutaneous wound repair. *Prog Growth Factor Res* 1992; **4:** 25–44.

44. Vos A M, Ultsch M, Kossiakoff A A. Human growth hormone and extracellular domain of its receptor: crystal structure of the complex. *Science* 1992; **255:** 306–12.

45. Fuh G, Mulkerrin M G, Bass S, *et al.* The human growth hormone receptor. *J Biol Chem* 1990; **265**(6): 3111–15.

46. Bazan J F. Haemopoietic receptors and helical cytokines. *Immunol Today* 1990; **11**(10): 350–4.

47. Bazan J F. A novel family of growth factor receptors: a common binding domain in the growth hormone, prolactin, erythropoietin and IL-6, receptors and the p751 L-2 receptor-chain. *Biochem Biophys Res Commun* 1989; **164**(2): 788–95.

48. Bazan J F. Structural design and molecular evolution of a cytokine receptor superfamily. *Proc Natl Acad Sci USA* 1990; **87:** 6934–8.

49. Leung D W, Spencer S A, Cachianes G, *et al.* Growth hormone receptor and serum binding protein: purification, cloning and expression. *Nature* 1987; **330:** 537–43.

50. Cunningham B C, Wells J A. Rational design of receptor-specific variants of human growth hormone. *Proc Natl Acad Sci USA* 1991; **88:** 3407–11.

51. Hammacher A, Hellman U, Johnson A, *et al.* A major part of PDGF purified from human platelets is a heterodimer of one A chain and one B chain. *J Biol Chem* 1986; **263:** 16493–8.

52. Ullrich A, Schlessinger J. Signal transduction by receptors with tyrosine kinase activity. *Cell* 1990; **61:** 203–12.

53. Ross R, Glomset J A, Kariya B, Harker L. A platelet dependent serum factor that stimulates the proliferation of arterial smooth muscle cells in vitro. *Proc Natl Acad Sci USA* 1974; **71:** 1207–10.

54. Kawahara R S, Deng Z-W, Deuel T F. Glucocorticoids inhibit the transcriptional induction of JE, a platelet derived growth factor inducible gene. *J Biol Chem* 1991; **266:** 13261–6.

55. Robson M C, Phillips L G, Thomason A, Robson L E, Pierce G F. Platelet derived growth factor BB for the treatment of chronic pressure ulcers. *Lancet* 1992; **339:** 23–5.

56. Schweigerer L, Neufield G, Friedman J, *et al.* Capillary endothelial cells express basic fibroblast growth factor, a mitogen that promoted their own growth. *Nature* 1987; **325:** 257–9.

57. Folkman J, Klagsbrun M. Angiogenic factors. *Science* 1987; **235:** 442–7.

58. Assoian R K, Sporn M B. Type-beta transforming growth factor in human platelets: release during platelet degranulation and action on vascular smooth muscle cells. *J Biol Chem* 1986; **102:** 1217–23.

59. Mustoe T A, Pierce G F, Thomason A, Gramates P, Sporn M B, Deuel T F. Accelerated healing of incisional wounds in rats induced by transforming growth factor. *Science* 1987; **237:** 1333–6.

60. Quaglino D, Nanney L B, Ditesheim J A, Davidson J M. Transforming growth factor beta stimulates wound healing and modulates extracellular matrix gene expression in pig skin: incisional wound model. *J Invest Dermatol* 1991; **97:** 34–42.

61. Derynk R. Transforming growth factor. *Cell* 1988; **54:** 593–5.

62. McGrath M H. Peptide growth factors and wound healing. *Clin Plast Surg* 1990; **17:** 421–32.

63. Falanga V, Eaglstein W H, Bucalo B, Katz M H, Harris B, Carson P. Topical use of human recombinant epidermal growth factor (h-EGF) in venous ulcers. *J Dermatol Surg Oncol* 1992; **18:** 604–6.

64. Brown G L, Curtsinger L, Jurkiewicz, *et al.* Stimulation of healing of chronic wounds by epidermal growth factors. (See comments). *Plast Reconstr Surg* 1991; **88:** 189–94.

65. Jeffries M K, Vance M L. Growth hormone and cortisol secretion in patients with burn injury. *J Burn Care Rehabil* 1992; **13:** 391–5.

66. Abribat T, Brazeau P, Davignon I, Garrel D R. Insulin-like growth factor-1 blood levels in severely burned patients: effects of time post injury, age of patient and severity of burn. *Clin Endocrinol* 1993; **39:** 583–9.

67. Moller S, Jensen M, Svensson P, Skakkebaek H. Insulin-like growth factor-1 (IGF-1) in burn patients. *Burns* 1991; **17**(4): 279–81.

68. Tessari P, Inchiostro S, Biolo G, *et al.* Differential effects of hyperinsulinemia and hyperaminoacidemia on leucine-carbon metabolism in vivo. *J Clin Invest* 1987; **79:** 1062–9.

69. Gelfand R A, Glichman M G, Castellino P, Louard R J, DeFronzo R A. Measurement of L-^{14}C-leucine kinetics in splanchnic and leg tissues in humans. *Diabetes* 1988; **37:** 1365–72.

70. Wolfe R R, Jahoor F, Hartl W H. Protein and amino acid metabolism after injury. *Diabetes Metab Rev* 1989; **5:** 149–64.

71. Finkelstein J W, Roffward H P, Boyer R M, Kream J, Hellman L. Age-related change in the twenty-four hour spontaneous secretion of growth hormone. *J Clin Endocrinol Metab* 1972; **35**(5): 665–70.

72. Soroff H S, Rozin R R, Mooty J, *et al.* Role of human growth hormone in the response to trauma: metabolic effects following burns. *Ann Surg* 1967; **166**(5): 739–52.

73. Liljadahl S O, Gemzell C A, Plantin L O, Birke G. Effect of human growth hormone in patients with severe burns. *Acta Chir Scand* 1961; **122:** 1–4.

74. McManson J M, Smith R J, Wilmore D W. Growth hormone stimulates protein synthesis during hypocaloric parenteral nutrition. *Ann Surg* 1988; **208:** 136–49.

75. Shorwell M A, Kilbeg M S, Oxender D L. The regulation of neutral amino acid transport in mammalian cells. *Biochem Biophys Acta* 1983; **737:** 267–84.

76. Roe C F, Kinky J. The influence of human growth hormone on energy sources in convalescence. *Surg Forum* 1962; **13:** 369–71.

77. MacGorman L R, Rizza R, Gerich J E. Physiological concentrations of growth hormone exert insulin like and insulin antagonistic effect on both hepatic and extra hepatic tissues in man. *J Clin Endocrinol Metab* 1981; **53:** 556–9.

78. vanVliet G, Bosson D, Craen M, *et al.* Comparative study of the lipolytic potencies of pituitary-derived and biosynthetic human growth hormone in hypopituitary children. *J Clin Endocrinol Metab* 1987; **65:** 876.

79. Clemmons D R, Snyder D K, Williams R, et al. Growth hormone administration conserves lean body mass during dietary restriction in obese subjects. *J Clin Endocrinol Metab* 1987; **64:** 878.

80. Young F G. Insulin and insulin antagonists. *Endocrinology* 1963; **73:** 654.

81. Tanner J M, Hughes C P R, Whitehouse R H. Comparative rapidity of response of height, limb muscle and limb fat to treatment with human growth hormone in patients with and without growth hormone deficiency. *Acta Endocrinol* 1977; **84:** 681–96.

82. Kostyo J L. Rapid effects of growth hormone on amino acid transport and protein synthesis. *Ann NY Acad Sci* 1968; **148:** 389–407.

83. Yarasheski K E, Campbell J A, Rennie M K, *et al.* Effect of strength training and growth hormone administration on whole-body and skeletal muscle leucine metabolism. *Med Sci Sports Exerc* 1990; **22:** 505A.

84. Horber F F, Haymond M W. Human growth hormone prevents the protein catabolic side effects of prednisone in humans. *J Clin Invest* 1990; **86:** 265–72.

85. Fryburg D A, Gelfand R A, Barrett E J. Growth hormone acutely stimulates forearm muscle protein synthesis in normal humans. *Am J Physiol* 1991; **260** (*Endocrinol Metab* **23**): E499–E504.

86. Mjaawand M, Unneberg K, Larsson J, Nilsson L, Revhaug A. Growth hormone after abdominal surgery attenuated forearm glutamine, alanine, 3-methyhistidine and total amino acid effluse in patients receiving total parenteral nutrition. *Ann Surg* 1993; **271**(4): 413–22.

87. Daughaday W H, Hall K, Salmon W D Jr, *et al.* Letter to the editor. On the nomenclature of the somatomedins and insulin-like growth factors. *J Clin Endocrinol Metab* 1987; **65:** 1075–6.

88. Soroff H S, Rozin R R, Mooty J, *et al.* Role of human growth hormone in the response to trauma: metabolic effects following burns. *Ann Surg* 1967; **166:** 739–52.

89. Liljadahl S O, Gemzell C A, Plantin L O, *et al.* Effect of human growth hormone in patients with severe burns. *Acta Chir Scand* 1961; **122:** 1–4.

90. Wilmore D W, Moyland J A Jr, Bristow B F, Mason A D, Pruitt B A. Anabolic effects of growth hormone and high caloric feedings following thermal injury. *Surg Gynecol Obstet* 1974; **138:** 875–84.

91. Soroff H S, Pearson E, Green N L, Artz C P. The effect of growth hormone on nitrogen balance at various levels of intake in burned patients. *Surg Gynecol Obstet* 1960; **111**(3): 259–73.

92. Gore D C, Honeycutt D, Jahoor F, Wolfe R, Herndon D N. Effect of exogenous growth hormone on whole-body and isolated limb protein kinetics in burned patients. *Arch Surg* 1991; **126:** 38–43.

93. Gore D C, Honeycutt D, Jahoor F, Rutan T, Wolfe R R, Herndon D N. Effect of exogenous growth hormone on glucose utilization in burn patients. *J Surg Res* 1991; **51:** 518–23.

94. Fleming R Y D, Rutan R I, Jahoor F, Barrow R E, Wolfe R R, Herndon D N. Effect of recombinant human growth hormone on catabolic hormones and free fatty acids following thermal injury. *J Trauma* 1992; **32:** 698–703.

95. Rowe J W, Young J B, Minaker K L, *et al.* Effect of insulin and glucose infusions on sympathetic nervous system activity in normal man. *Diabetes* 1981; **30:** 219–25.

96. Thompson, J C, Marx M. Gastrointestinal hormones. *Curr Probl Surg* 1984; **21**(6): 1–80.

97. Gabrilove J L, Schwartz A, Churg J. Effect of hormones on the skin in endocrinologic disorders. *J Clin Endocrinol Metab* 1962; **22:** 688–92.

98. Tavakkol A, Elder J T, Griffiths C E M, *et al.* Expression of growth hormone receptor, insulin-like growth factor 1 (IGF-1) and IGF-1 receptor mRNA and proteins in human skin. *J Invest Dermatol* 1992; **99:** 343–9.

99. Conover C A, Liu F, Powell D, *et al.* Insulin-like growth factor binding proteins from cultured human fibroblasts. Characterization and hormonal regulation. *J Clin Invest* 1989; **83:** 852–9.

100. Cook J J, Haynes K M, Werther G A. Mitogenic effects of growth hormone in cultured human fibroblasts. Evidence for action via local insulin-like growth factor I production. *J Clin Invest* 1988; **81:** 206–12.

101. Jorgensen P H, Andreassen T T, Jorgensen K D. Growth hormone influences collagen deposition and mechanical strength of intact rat skin. A dose-response study. *Acta Endocrinol (Copenh)* 1989; **120:** 767–72.

102. Jorgensen P H, Andreassen T T. A dose-response study of the effects of biosynthetic human growth hormone on formation and strength of granulation tissue. *Endocrinology* 1987; **121:** 1637–41.

103. Jorgensen P H, Andreassen T T. The influence of biosynthetic human growth hormone on biomechanical properties and collagen formation in granulation tissue. *Horm Metab Res* 1988; **20:** 490–3.

104. Rudman A, Feller A G, Nagraj H S. Effect of human growth hormone in men over 60 years old. *N Engl J Med* 1990; **323:** 1–6.

105. Jorgensen P H, Andreassen T T. The influence of biosynthetic human growth hormone on biomechanical properties of rat skin incisional wounds. *Acta Chir Scand* 1988; **154:** 623–6.

106. Zaizen Y, Ford E G, Costin G, Atkinson J B. The effect of perioperative exogenous growth hormone on wound bursting strength in normal and malnourished rats. *J Pediatr Surg* 1990; **25:** 70–4.

107. Atkinson J B, Kosi M, Srikanth M S, *et al.* Growth hormone reverses impaired wound healing in protein-malnourished rats treated with corticosteroids. *J Pediatr Surg* 1992; **27:** 1026–8.

108. Belcher H J C R, Mercer D, Judkins K C, *et al.* Biosynthetic growth hormone in burned patients: a pilot study. *Burns* 1989; **15:** 99–107.

109. Herndon D N, Barrow R E, Kunkel K R, Broemeling L, Rutan R L. Effects of recombinant human growth hormone on donor-site healing in severely burned children. *Ann Surg* 1990; **212**(4): 424–31.

110. Gilpin D A, Barrow R E, Rutan R L, Broemeling B S N, Herndon D N. Recombinant human growth hormone accelerates wound healing in children with large cutaneous burns. *Ann Surg* 1994; **220**(1): 19–24.

111. Sherman S K, Demling R H, Lalonde C, *et al.* Growth hormone enhances re-epithelialization of human split thickness skin graft donor sites. *Surg Forum* 1989; **40:** 37–9.

112. Rutan R I, Herndon D N. Growth delay in postburn pediatric patients. *Arch Surg* 1990; **125**(3): 392–5.

113. Prader A. Catch-up growth. *Postgrad Med J* 1978; **54**(suppl): 133–46.

114. Bruno L P, Stern P J, Wyrick J D. Skeletal changes after burn injuries in an animal model. *J Burn Care Rehabil* 1988; **9:** 148–51.

115. Klein G L, Herndon D N, Rutan T C, *et al.* Bone disease in burn patients. *J Bone Miner Res* 1993; **8:** 337–45.

116. Voerman H J, Strack R V S, Groeneveld A B J, *et al.* Effects of recombinant human growth hormone in patients with severe sepsis. *Ann Surg* 1992; **216**(6): 648–55.

117. Byrne T A, Morrissey T B, Gatzen C, *et al.* Anabolic therapy with growth hormone accelerates protein gain in surgical patients requiring nutritional rehabilitation. *Ann Surg* 1993; **218**(4): 400–18.

118. Muller M J, Gilpin D A, Biolo G, Herndon D N. Biosynthetic human growth hormone: current and potential applications in amino acids. In: Latifi R, Landers R G, eds. *Amino Acids in Cancer and Critical Illness*, 1994.

119. Rutan R, Herndon D N. Justification for the use of growth hormone in a pediatric burn center. *Proceedings of the American Burn Association*, Orlando, FL, 1994.

120. Chwans W J, Bistrian B R. Role of exogenous growth hormone and insulin-like growth factor 1 in malnutrition and acute metabolic stress: a hypothesis. *Crit Care Med* 1991; **19**(10): 1317–22.

121. Boulivare S D, Tamborlane W V, Matthews L S, Sherwin R S. Diverse effects of insulin-like growth factor 1 on glucose lipid and amino acid metabolism. *Am J Physiol* 1992; **262** (*Endocrinol Metab* **25**): E130–E133.

122. Moller S, Jensen M, Svensson P, Skakkeback N E. Insulin-like growth-factor-1 (IGF-1) in burn patients. *Burns* 1991; **17**(4): 279–81.

123. Kupfer S R, Underwood L E, Baxter R C, Clemmons D R. Enhancement of the anabolic effects of growth hormone and insulin-like growth factor 1 by use of both agents simultaneously. *J Clin Invest* 1993; **91:** 391–6.

124. Dahn M S, Lange M P, Jacobs L A. Insulin-like growth factor-1 production is inhibited in human sepsis. *Arch Surg* 1988; **123:** 1409–14.

125. Kimbrough T D, Shernan S, Ziegler T R, *et al.* Insulin-growth factor-1 response is comparable following intravenous and subcutaneous administration of growth hormone. *J Surg Res* 1991; **51:** 472–6.

126. Strock L L, Singh H, Abdullah A, *et al.* The effect of insulin-like growth factor-1 on postburn hypermetabolism. *Surgery* 1990; **108**(2): 161–4.

127. Huang K F, Chung D H, Herndon D N. Insulin-like growth factor-1 (IGF-1) reduces gut atrophy and bacterial translocation after severe burn injury. *Arch Surg* 1993; **128:** 47–54.

128. Dong Y-L, Huang K F, Xia Z F, *et al.* Impact of erogenous insulin-like growth factor-1 on hepatic energy metabolism in burn injury. *Arch Surg* 1993; **128**(6): 703–8.

129. Barrow R E, Wang C Z, Evans M J, Herndon D N. Growth factors accelerate epithelial repair in sheep trachea. *Lung* 1993; **171**(6): 335–44.

130. Linares H A. Autopsy findings in burned children. In: Carvajal H F, Parks D H, eds. *Pediatric Burn Management. Burns in Children*. Chicago, IL: Yearbook Medical Publishers, Inc, 1988: 298–9.

131. Joshi W. Effects of burns on the heart. *JAMA* 1970; **211**(13): 2130–4.

132. Gelfand R A, Hutchinson-Williams K A, Bonde A A, *et al.* Catabolic effects of thyroid hormone excess: the contribution of adrenergic activity to hypermetabolism and protein breakdown. *Metabolism* 1987; **36**(6): 562–9.

133. Herndon D N. Mediators of metabolism. *J Trauma* 1981; **21:** 701–5.

134. Wolfe R R, Herndon D N, Peters E J, *et al.* Regulation of lipolysis in severely burned children. *Ann Surg* 1987; **290**(2): 214–21.

135. Wolfe R R, Durkot M J. Evaluation of the role of the sympathetic nervous system in the response of substrate kinetics and oxidation to burn injury. *Circ Shock* 1982; **9:** 395–406.

136. Garber A J, Karl I E, Kipnis D M. Alanine and glutamine synthesis and release from skeletal muscle. IV. β-adrenergic inhibition of amino acid release. *J Biol Chem* 1976; **251:** 851–7.

137. Miles J M, Nissen S L, Gerich J E, Haymond M W. Effects of epinephrine infusion on leucine and alanine kinetics in humans. *Am J Physiol* 1984; **247:** E166–72.

138. Keller U, Kraenzlin W, Stauffacher W, Arnaud M. β-adrenergic stimulation results in diminished protein breakdown, decreased amino acid oxidation and increased protein synthesis in man. *J Parenter Enteral Nutr* 1987; **11** (suppl): 7S (Abstract).

139. Herndon D N, Barrow R E, Rutan T C, Minifee P, Jahoor F, Wolfe K R. Effect of propranolol administration on hemodynamic and metabolic responses of burned pediatric patients. *Ann Surg* 1988; **208:** 484–92.

140. Minifee P K, Barrow R E, Abston S, Desai M, Herndon D N. Improved myocardial oxygen utilization following propranolol infusion in adolescents with postburn hypermetabolism. *J Pediatr Surg* 1989; **24:** 806–11.

141. Honeycutt D, Barrow R. Herndon D N. Cold stress response in patients with severe burns after beta-blockade. *J Burn Care Rehabil* 1992; **13**(2): 181–6.

142. Herndon D N, Nguyen T T, Wolfe R R *et al.* Lipolysis in burned patients is stimulated by the Beta 2-receptor for catecholomines. *Arch Surg* 1994; **129:** 1301–5.

143. Popp M B, Silverstein E B, Srivastaver L S, Laggie J M H, Knowles H C, MacMillan B G. A pathophysiologic study of the hypertension associated with burn injury in children. *Ann Surg* 1981; **193**(6): 817–24.

144. Choo J J, Horan M A, Little R A, *et al.* Anabolic effects of clenbuterol on skeletal muscle are mediated by beta-2 adrenoreceptor activation. *Am J Physiol* 1992; **263** (*Endocrinol Metab* **26**): E50–E56.

145. Carter W J, Dang A S Q, Faas F G, *et al.* Effects of clenbuterol on skeletal mass, body composition and recovery from surgical stress in senescent rats. *Metabolism* 1991; **40:** 855–60.

146. Chance W T, Von Allmen D, Benson D, *et al.* Clenbuterol decreases catabolism and increases hypermetabolism in burned rats. *J Trauma* 1991; **31:** 365–70.

147. Hollyoak M A, Muller M J, Meyers N A, Williams W G, Barrow R E, Herndon D N. Beneficial wound healing at metabolic effects of clenbuterol in burned and non-burned rats. *J Burn Care Rehabil* 1995; in press.

148. Demling R H, Lalonde C. Early postburn lipid perioxidation: effect of ibuprofen and allopurinol. *Surgery* 1990; **107:** 85–93.

149. Jin L J, Lalonde C, Demling R H. Lung dysfunction after thermal injury in relation to prostanoid and oxygen radical release. *J Appl Physiol* 1986; **61:** 103–12.

150. Demling R H, Lalonde C. Identification and modifications of the pulmonary and systemic inflammatory and biochemical changes caused by a skin burn. *J Trauma* 1990; **30:** S57–S62.

CHAPTER TWENTY-TWO

Nutritional Support of the Burned Patient

Marsha Hildreth and Michele Gottschlich

Introduction

This chapter is devoted to assessing the nutritional needs of a thermally injured patient and describing how to provide the nutritional support needed to minimize the devasting effects of hypermetabolism and the subsequent catabolism. Metabolic rates of patients with burns of 40% or greater total body surface area (TSBA) are 100–150% greater than basal. Failure to meet these increased energy and protein requirements results in impaired wound healing, cellular dysfunction and decreased resistance to infection.

Just as with other areas of treatment in burn cases, nutritional management has undergone several pendulum swings in recent years. Prior to 1940, the amount of nutrition required to maintain weight was not realized; therefore, huge weight loss resulted in patients with burns over 30% TSBA. As more information was obtained concerning the effect of nutrition on wound healing, immunity, and outcome, nutrition became a priority and in some cases overfeeding resulted. In the 1970s, total parenteral nutrition (TPN) was thought to be the answer to the protein-calorie wasting which occurred in burned patients. TPN was used extensively in patients with burns so as to offset the devasting effects of hypermetabolism. Studies conducted since that time have shown that TPN offers no nutritional advantage over enterally administered calories in most cases and may be associated with metabolic and immunological complications.[1–3] Currently the use of TPN in burn patients is limited to supporting those patients with gastrointestinal dysfunction. Enteral feeding increases gut blood flow, preserves gastrointestinal function, minimizes bacterial translocation from the gut as a result of decreased gut mucosal atrophy, and has proven to be the preferred route of nutritional supplementation.[4,5]

The hypermetabolism and negative nitrogen balance associated with thermal injures was recognized by Cutherbertson[6,7] over 60 years ago. Since that time, much has been learned concerning therapies to minimize the hypermetabolic response of a burned patient including: maintaining patients in a warm environment, providing pain control, achieving early closure of the burn wound, using biological and synthetic wound dressings, and preventing serious wound infection. Most patients with greater than a 20% total body surface burn exhibit an elevated resting energy expenditure (REE).[8] These patients are at risk of not achieving nutritional goals due to ileus and other complications associated with thermal injury and the treatment required for wound closure. Routine daily monitoring of these patients is required in order to provide optimal nutritional support and improve outcome. The dietitian is the center of this monitoring, but the entire burn team must realize the importance of the nutritional support and must be vigilant in assuring its success. The burn team must include not only all medical, nursing, and paramedical personnel, but also the patient and the patient's family. In order for the dietary nutritional support to be achieved, especially with so many disciplines involved, there must be an established nutritional protocol which standardizes the assessment, initiation, and monitoring of the nutritional support.

Initial Nutritional Assessment

The goal of the initial assessment is to determine the caloric and protein needs of a patient immediately upon admission. It has been shown that early enteral feedings within the first 24 hours post-injury decreases hypermetabolism, decreases the level of catabolic hormones, improves nitrogen balance, maintains gut mucosal integrity, decreases the incidence of diarrhea, and decreases the length of hospital stay.[9–11] In its nutritional protocol, a hospital will have to determine what means of assessing energy needs is appropriate for its patients. For the initial assessment, a formula estimating caloric needs should be implemented. A number of formulas have been developed for this purpose. Some are very specific and identify a certain population, normally according to age. Only the most commonly used in each age group will be reviewed.

A dietitian as well as a physician should be active in assessing the nutritional status of a patient. The accuracy of the height and weight obtained on admission should be verified with the preburn height and weight and by plotting the admission indices on a growth chart. The distribution of the burns and their cause must be assessed along with how these will affect the nutritional management of the patient. Those children injured by possible abuse must be carefully assessed for signs of malnutrition. Other information obtained from the nutritional history which may be significant is as follows:

- Personal background.
- Chronic conditions or disease states which might interfere with good nutritional status.
- Any hypermetabolic condition which might result in inadequate food intake.
- Any physical conditions which might result in inadequate food intake.
- Any predisposing factors such as chemotherapy, radiation therapy, or alcoholism.
- Any recent weight loss or gain during a short time.
- Food preferences and allergies.

Indirect Calorimetry

If indirect calorimetry is available to an institution caring for burned patients, it should be utilized on admission and at least once a week until the patient is healed. Indirect calorimetry by means of a metabolic chart can measure energy expenditure and can be used in the nutritional assessment of the burned patient. Resting energy expenditure (REE) is determined from oxygen (O_2) consumption and carbon dioxide (CO_2) production during respiratory gas exchange in a relationship as defined by the Weir equation.[12] Indirect calorimetry measures energy needs and allows determinations of the respiratory quotient (RQ) defined by the ratio of CO_2 production to O_2 consumption. An increase in the RQ from the normal fasting ratio of 0.70–0.85 towards 1.0 suggests a net increase in CO_2 production, a byproduct of carbohydrate metabolism, usually as a result of delivery of additional calories. A low RQ may indicate an inadequate calorie intake just as an RQ between 0.85 and 1.0 may suggest adequate intake when considered with other nutritional assessment parameters.

There are several disadvantages to using indirect calorimetry. The measurements are accurate for only the immediate time frame; therefore, several measurements must be done at varying times during the day to best approximate the energy needs of a patient. Factors which increase daily energy requirements above resting conditions such as tubbings and dressing changes, infection, and physical therapy must be considered in assessing daily needs. A common practice is to multiply the REE by a stress factor of 1.2–1.5 in order to achieve weight maintenance.

Factors Affecting Metabolic Rate

Kilocalorie and protein intake should be calculated daily and compared to the estimated energy and protein requirements. Inadequate intake may indicate that some manipulation in the dietary regimen is required in order to increase the intake. A more thorough look at a patient is required in order to determine if the present feeding regimen is being tolerated. If not, then the problem must be addressed.

There are a number of factors which affect the stress response and increase metabolic rate in burned patients. These include pain, anxiety, fear, and cold stress. The environmental temperature on a burn unit should be kept warm (33°C), and the humidity should be low. Frightening and painful procedures should be kept to a minimum. Occlusive dressings are utilized in order to decrease evaporative water loss, and dressing changes are performed quickly and efficiently to avoid intermittent hypothermia resulting in 'cold stress'. In some instances, only one extremity should be exposed at a time.

Calorie Needs

Pediatric Formulas

The nutritional needs of children are quite different from those of adults and vary significantly during childhood as the requirements for growth, development, and activity levels change with age. Children usually have proportionally less body fat and a smaller muscle mass than adults. These considerations put burned children in an especially high-risk population with a greater chance for rapid development of protein–calorie malnutrition.

Table 22.1 shows some of the most commonly used formulas for determining energy requirements in pediatric burned patients. Since children generally have a high body surface area in relation to their weight, a formula based on body surface area is beneficial in determining the caloric needs of this population. The SBI–Galveston formula has proven to be one such formula even though it has been determined that, as it was originally described, it overestimates the caloric needs of burned children.[13] It is utilized in patients with large burns who will be subjected to numerous surgeries and/or studies which require nothing by mouth for several hours. The revised SBI–Galveston formula was derived after studying 102 patients

Table 22.1 Formulas for determining energy needs for pediatric burned patients

	Age	Daily requirements
Galveston Infant[14]	0–12 mo.	2100 kcal/m^2 + 1000 kcal/m^2 burn
1982[15]	All	1800 kcal/m^2 + 2200 kcal/m^2 burn
Revised[13]	1–11 y	1800 kcal/m^2 + 1300 kcal/m^2 burn
Adolescent[16]	12 y + above	1500 kcal/m^2 + 1500 kcal/m^2 burn
Curreri, Junior[17]	0–1	BMR + 15 kcal/% burn
	1–3	BMR + 25 kcal/% burn
	4–15	BMR + 40 kcal/% burn
RDA[18]	0.0–0.5	kg × 115 (kcal)
	0.5–1.0	kg × 105 (kcal)
	1–3	kg × 100 (kcal)
	4–10	kg × 85 (kcal)
	M: 11–14	kg × 60 (kcal)
	F: 11–14	kg × 48 (kcal)

Children's Hospital Medical Center, Akron, Ohio

Normal requirements for height–age (RDA)[18] + added needs for burn hypermetabolism:[19]

Weight (kg)	kcal/% burn
0–9	15
10–13	20
14–18 (burns > 40%)	20
14 (all other burns)	30

BMR, Basal metabolic rate; M, male; F, female.

under the age of 12 years, and it was determined that fewer calories were required for weight maintenance at a rate of 900 kcal/m^2 burned.[13] This formula reflects the amount of calories which need to be delivered throughout the entire hospitalization.

It was found through other studies that the calorie requirement formulas for infants and adolescents needed to be more specific for these age groups. Therefore, other formulas were derived (**Table 22.1**). All of the SBI – Galveston formulas are based on body surface area (m^2) and burn surface area. Therefore, an accurate height and weight is essential, as well as the % TBSA of burns.

Adult Formulas

Again, many formulas have been devised for adult burned patients; however, according to Williamson in a 1989 survey,[20] the Curreri or modified Curreri formulas were most often utilized with the Harris–Benedict basal energy expenditure (BEE) equation with various adjustment factors also being popular (**Table 22.2**).

Elderly Formula

The Curreri Senior (for patients more than 60 years old) formula for determining calorie requirements of elderly burned patients takes into account lower basal requirements.[26] That formula is: basal + 65 kcals/% burn.

Nutritional Needs of Special Patients

Toxic epidermal necrolysis

Toxic epidermal necrolysis (TEN) or Stevens–Johnson syndrome is characterized by epidermal sloughing, mucosal inflammation, and ulceration. Nutritional support is included in the recommended treatment for TEN. This support, at times, may be difficult due to gastrointestinal ulceration. Generally the use of total parenteral nutrition is limited due to the risk of sepsis, but in the most severe cases it may be indicated. A nasogastric or duodenal feeding tube is inserted upon admission and the patient is fed with milk or a soy-based formula enterally. A study of six TEN patients indicated that calorie goals based on the latest surface area formulas for the age group were adequate to maintain weight in a pediatric population.[27] These patients should be slowly progressed to solid foods as tolerated. They should be watched carefully for wound healing and their calories reduced to normal requirements as soon as skin coverage is obtained. Heimbach reporting on adult patients with TEN found measurements of oxygen consumption and carbon dioxide production to be in the high-normal range.[28] Weight stability and positive nitrogen balance were achieved in these patients by providing approximately 2500 kcal/day.

Electrical injuries

Calorie and protein requirements of patients with electrical injuries are calculated as those for patients with thermal injuries. A nasogastric tube is inserted and the gut gastric contents are monitored for pH, occult and overt blood, and evidence of dysfunction. Gastrointestinal involvement may include paralytic illeus, nausea or vomiting, GI bleeding, perforation, or direct damage to viscera. Feedings are started as soon as tolerated.

Protein Needs

Protein requirements in burn patients are increased due to the increased demands for wound healing and nitrogen losses through wound exudate and urine. It has been reported that the period for greatest nitrogen loss is between the 5th and 10th postburn days.[25] Protein requirements are currently recommended based on either a percentage of total kilocalories or grams of protein per kilogram of ideal body weight and per percent burn. Recommendation is for calorie:nitrogen ratios from 100:1 to 200:1.[29,30] One such protocol is as follows:

- Birth to 0.5 years – 4.4 g/kg
- 0.5 years to 2.0 years – 4.0 g/kg
- 1.0 years to adult 120:1 (kcal:N)

Matsuda and colleagues[31] and Alexander *et al.*[32] determined that, for burns over 10% TBSA, 20% of the kilocalories should be provided from protein in order to optimize nitrogen retention and replenish protein lost through the burn wound. The nonprotein kilocalorie to nitrogen ratio recommended is 100:1. Another guideline for protein administration in children under 1 year of age is 3–4 g/kg[33] because of the inability of infants to tolerate high renal solute loads.[34]

Table 22.2 Commonly utilized formulas for adult burned patients

Curreri[16,21,22]	Age 16–59 y	Basal (approx. 25 kcal/kg + 40 kcal/% burn)
	Age > 60 y	Basal (approx. 20 kcal/kg + 65 kcal/% burn)
Modified Harris–Benedict[22–24]	All ages	Calculated or measured RMR × M where M ranges from 1.3 to 2.0

Long's Modified Harris–Benedict:[25]

Males: BMR = (66.47+13.75W+5.OH – 6.76A) × (activity factor) × (injury factor)

Females: BMR = (55.10+9.56W+1.85H – 4.68A) × (activity factor) × (injury factor)

activity factor:	confined to bed	1.2
	out of bed	1.3
injury factor:	severe thermal burn	2.10
	skeletal trauma	1.35
	major sepsis	1.60
	minor operation	1.20

RMR, resting metabolic rate; M, modifier; W, weight; H, height; A, age.

Davies and Liljedahl[35] have suggested the following formula for determining protein administration for children:

- 3 g/kg + 1 g/% BSAB

They recommended the following for adults:

- 1 g/kg + 3 g/% BSAB

Diets providing high calorie to nitrogen ratios are necessary for maintaining a positive nitrogen balance in patients with large burns and result in improved immune function and increased survival rates. On the other hand, excessive administration of protein may be harmful. Large protein loads have been shown to cause increased calciuresis and may contribute to the increased incidence of renal stones in burn patients.[36,37]

Albumin

One of the primary functions of albumin is the maintenance of colloid oncotic pressure. Hypoalbuminemia results in significant intestinal mucosal edema which can impair intestinal absorption and result in diarrhea.[38] Gottschlich *et al.* failed to show a correlation between hypoalbuminemia and the occurrence of diarrhea in a study of tube-fed burn patients.[39] Serum albumin is monitored daily in critical burned patients. If the level drops below 2.5 g/dl in patients with more than a 40% TBSA burn or a 30% TBSA third degree burn, albumin is administered. The rate of administration is generally 6.25 g for patients under 2 years, 12.5 g for those under 11 years and 25 g for those over 11 years.

Arginine

Recently, there have been a number of studies conducted to determine the efficiency of the use of specific amino acids in the diets of burned patients to improve their immune function. Barbul and associates found in normal healthy volunteers an improvement in delayed hypersensitivity responses with arginine supplementation.[40] A study in animals by Saito and colleagues showed that optimal immune function and survival were achieved when 2% of the total dietary energy intake was in the form of arginine.[41] Therefore, the protein in the diet of a burned patient should contain supplemental arginine up to approximately 2% of the total calories.

Glutamine

Glutamine supplementation has proven to be beneficial in patients maintained on prolonged intravenous hyperalimentation.[42] It may also be important in other trauma or septic patients; however, the benefits of glutamine in burn patients have not been determined. If patients are receiving adequate diets, glutamine supplementation seems to provide only minimal benefits.

Carbohydrates

Adequate carbohydrate intake is the first priority of energy provision to a burned patient. Large amounts of this nutrient must be supplied in order to avoid excessive protein catabolism. The diet of the burned patient should contain approximately 50% of calories as carbohydrate.[43]

Data from parenteral nutrition studies suggest that an optimal glucose infusion rate of approximately 5 mg/kg/min is necessary to maximize protein sparing but avoid side effects.[44] In pediatric patients, dextrose can be initiated at 7–8 mg/kg/min and advanced as needed to a maximum of 20% dextrose solution.[33] In infants, an infusion of dextrose should be started at a rate of 5 mg/kg/min and advanced to 15 mg/kg/min over a 2-day period.[33]

Excessive carbohydrate intake can have adverse consequences. Some of these problems are the result of the conversion of carbohydrate to fat. Some of the fat is deposited in the liver and results in altered liver function. Also lipogenesis from carbohydrate results in increased CO_2 production and increased respiratory demands.

Fat

Several aspects of lipid metabolism are significantly changed in burned patients. In general, the adult burned patient needs approximately 25–30% of his total calories from fat. Fat serves as a high-density source of calories, a carrier of fat-soluble vitamins, and a source of essential fatty acids without which burned patients (especially infants) may develop essential fatty acid deficiency syndrome. Generally, recommendations are that fat comprise between 30% and 40% of total dietary calories for the older pediatric patient[45] and up to 50% of total dietary calories for patients younger than 1 year of age.[33]

It has been suggested that by replacing the omega-6 (ω-6) fatty acids which are obtained from vegetable and animal acids with omega-3 (ω-3) fatty acids, postburn immunosuppression might be avoided. This was supported by the results of a burned guinea-pig model study.[5] In another animal study, mice were administered a diet high in ω-3 fatty acids and infected, and they had a higher mortality rate than those fed a diet containing ω-6 fatty acids.[46] Therefore, the ideal fat composition of the diet of the burned patient has yet to be identified.

Fatty acids should be given at least twice a week when TPN is used as the only nutritional source so as to prevent a fatty acid deficiency, but they can be increased in amounts and used as a calorie source. Normally, they should not exceed more than 30–40% of the total nonprotein calories.[47] In pediatric patients the essential fatty acid deficiency requirements are met by providing 0.5–1.0 g/kg/day.[33] To provide a calorie source, the recommendations are to start at 0.5–1.0 g/kg/day and to advance to a maximum of 3 g/kg/day.[48]

Nutrient Administration Techniques

Enteral

After the nutrient needs are determined, another important consideration is the route of nutrition support since this appears to influence postburn outcome. Small burns (<25% surface area) not complicated by facial injury, psychological difficulties including possible abuse, inhalation injury, or preburn malnutrition can usually be maintained by a high calorie, high protein oral diet. In these cases, the dietitian must provide daily evaluation of menu selection and food consumption. Patients with larger surface area burns generally cannot meet their nutrient requirements by oral intake alone. Although both tube feedings and central venous hyperalimentation are commonly used in patients with burns in excess of 25% body surface area, enteral access is recommended whenever possible.[49]

Burn patients are normally fed nasogastrically or nasoenterically. The severity of the burn and the frequency of surgeries are among the factors that determine which enteral route is indicated. In general, the stomach is appropriate in alert patients with an intact gag reflex and a functional gastrointestinal tract. Continuous infusions using a tube feeding pump are recommended, with hourly monitoring of gastric residuals.

Gastric ileus, which limits the use of the stomach for nutrition support, is common in the more centrally injured burned patient.

Small bowel usually maintains normal motility and absorption, making it a practical feeding route. Gastric ileus is characteristic of the ebb phase, but often resurfaces during operative procedures, septic episodes, or other complicating events. Therefore, some clinicians routinely pass a feeding tube beyond the pylorus into the duodenum or jejunum. Transpyloric feeding significantly reduces the risk of tube feeding aspiration and can be a safe route of alimentation even during critical periods such as resuscitation, surgery, anesthesia for major dressing changes and tubbings or septic ileus.[50–52] The feeding tube must remain in the small bowel. To ensure this placement, the outside portion of the feeding tube should be measured from the nares to the end of the tube once enteric placement is verified and then this measurement should be repeated at frequent intervals. Accidental displacement of the feeding tube can be avoided by securing it with staples or suture. To maintain gastric decompression a nasogastric tube can be connected to suction and maintained until bowel sounds have returned.

Timing

The optimal time for initiating a tube feeding program is another consideration. Traditionally, enteral support was not a major component of the early management of the burned patient. In fact, it was common for enteral nutrition to be delayed for 3–10 days, depending on the severity of the injury and the resolution of gastric ileus. During this time, patients would typically receive 5% dextrose intravenously, which contains only 170 kcal/l and no protein.

Currently it is thought that enteral nutrition support should be implemented as soon as it is clinically feasible postburn.[39, 50, 51, 53] A significant nutrient deficit can develop when alimentation is delayed following thermal injury. This, then, can have a direct bearing on subsequent morbidity and mortality. In addition, it is widely believed that enteral delivery of nutrients significantly reduces subsequent septic complications, presumably by preserving gut barriers and host defenses.[5,52]

Most tube feeding products can be started at full strength. The tube feeding can begin at approximately half the final desired volume and can be increased by 5 ml/h in the child and 10 ml/h in the older child and adult as tolerated until the final hourly rate is achieved. The patient can be gradually weaned from the tube feeding regimen as oral intake improves and nutrient needs decrease. During convalescence, the tube feeding can be held 1–2 hours before mealtime in order to stimulate appetite. Once the patient demonstrates the ability to orally consume approximately 25–50% of caloric needs, tube feeding can be reduced to nocturnal delivery. Eventually, when the patient is able to eat 80–90% of his or her caloric needs, tube feedings can be discontinued.

Composition

The composition of enteral feeding should take into account the unique metabolic and age-related alterations in nutrient utilization which accompany an extensive burn injury. Suggested regimens are described for infants less than or equal to 1 year and for patients older than 1 year, including adults.

Infants It is extremely important to meet energy and nutrient requirements during infancy in order to facilitate burn recovery as well as permit the process of growth and development. This is a challenging age group in which to accomplish dietary goals for nutritional requirements are higher per kilogram of body weight than at any other period of life. At the same time, stomach capacity is limited and some organ systems are immature, so food substrates must be tailored according to age limitations and to provide for the conditionally essential and/or increased nutrient needs in response to burns.

Few studies have examined what constitutes optimal nutritional support modalities for the burned infant. Consequently, enteral protocols are generally conservative, typically relying on commercial infant formulas. The normal dilution of infant formula is 20 kcal/ounce (0.66 kcal/ml). Gradually advancing the concentration to 24 kcal/ounce is routinely safe. Further progression to 27 or 30 kcal/ounce to meet infants' caloric needs must be monitored carefully due to the resulting increased renal solute load.

The protein content of infant formulas range from 9 to 12% of total kcal. This level is sometimes insufficient in babies with large surface area burns. The addition of a protein module to the infant formula may be indicated in such cases if, once again, the patient is carefully monitored. Infant formulas derived from soy protein should not be used unless casein or whey intolerance has been confirmed because the biological value of soy is less than that of animal protein. Nutrition support regimens containing significantly reduced fat content are likewise not routinely recommended during infancy since fat is an extremely important nutrient during central nervous system maturation.

Older Children and Adults Tube feedings for patients over 1 year of age generally are selected from formularies established for adults. The coincident fluid needs and energy requirements normally result in utilizing a 1 kcal/ml tube feeding product. Burned patients usually have adequate digestive and absorptive capabilities; therefore, formulas containing intact protein should be utilized.[54] Since protein allowances established for burned patients are between 20 and 23% of calories,[32,52] a high protein solution is advocated. Modular tube feedings have evolved, which not only take into consideration energy and protein guidelines, but also offer means of tailoring the fat, amino acid, vitamin, and mineral contents as well.[32,39,55,56]

Parenteral

Due to the mechanical and metabolic complications associated with parenteral hyperalimentation and the added risks of immunocompromise and infection, TPN should be reserved for only those burned patients with prolonged alimentary tract dysfunction.[1,57,58] Herndon and colleagues[1] have recently described a syndrome of iatrogenic immunosuppression and increased mortality in patients with burns exceeding 50% body surface area randomized to receive intravenous supplementation of enteral calories when compared to a control group receiving enteral calories alone.

Routine Monitoring of Nutritional Indicators

The evaluation of nutritional status and development of a nutrition intervention plan needs to be established within 24 hours of admission for patients with burns exceeding 25%. Appropriateness of the prescribed diet therapy must be continuously monitored in order to insure the safety and efficacy of the current program, to determine when adjustments in the feeding regimen are required to meet the burn patient's changing needs, and lastly, to identify and correct any observed complications related to nutritional or metabolic support. The assessment of energy requirements and the ability to meet these needs are perhaps the most important aspects of the nutrition evaluation. Fairly accurate determination of the extent of hypermetabolism as well as actual calorie and protein intake (oral, enteral and parenteral) are crucial, since both overfeeding and underfeeding have been associated with serious complications. The nutritional assessment should also include serum and urinary proteins, immune function and body composition. Suggested guidelines for clinical, laboratory and diagnostic monitoring are reviewed in Tables 22.3 and 22.4. The rationale for a comprehensive, dynamic assessment and monitoring program in burns as well as guidelines for interpretation have been reviewed extensively elsewhere.[59–61]

COMPLICATIONS

Both parenteral and enteral support are associated with a number of gastrointestinal, infectious, technical, and metabolic complications. Many of these complications are predictable, and incidence can be minimized by strict monitoring procedures.

Gastrointestinal

Gastrointestinal complications observed in burned patients from enteral feeding include nausea, vomiting, abdominal distension, aspiration, and more frequently, diarrhea and constipation. Nausea and vomiting may occur for a variety of reasons, including tube migration, poor gastric emptying, medications, anxiety, or being fed too rapidly. Diarrhea, a frequently cited complication, may result from various causes: a deficiency or use of antacids, potassium, or phosphorus supplements.[39,62] Tube feeding, hyperosmolality or a low serum albumin level does not appear to adversely affect intestinal absorption in burn patients.[39] Early enteral support can minimize the incidence of diarrhea.[39]

Tube feedings can usually be continued in spite of the occurrence of diarrhea, and it is not necessary to dilute a nutritional product unless additional fluids are required. Antidiarrheal medications such as Imodium, Diasorb, Lomotil or Kaopectate can be mixed with the tube feeding in order to remedy the situation. The use of a bulking agent may help to normalize stool consistency.

Constipation may occur and should be monitored and treated so as to facilitate tolerance of enteral nutrition. Constipation can be alleviated by providing adequate fluids, administering bulking agents, and encouraging increased physical activity. A laxative may be administered to help promote elimination, and in some instances enemas may be required.

Aspiration of tube feedings is the most serious and life-threatening complication from enteral support. The risk of aspiration during gastric feedings can be lessened by ensuring adequate bowel sounds, avoiding excessive filling of the stomach by using continuous drip feedings, and frequently checking gastric residuals. The patient's head should also be elevated at least 30 degrees. Positioning the feeding tube beyond the pylorus can further reduce the incidence of aspiration in the severely injured patient.

Gastrointestinal side effects from parenteral feedings are obviously quite different from enteral support. Morphologic and functional changes occur in the small and large intestine when nutrition is maintained exclusively by vein. A significant reduction in the mass of the small and large intestine occurs, and there is a marked decrease in mucosal enzyme activity.[63–66]

Table 22.3 Clinical monitoring protocol and indicators of care

Initial assessment
- Acute patients should be assessed within 24 hours of admission
- Determine energy needs to maintain preburn weight
- Determine protein needs to achieve nitrogen balance or to minimize loss (20–23% of caloric needs)
- Determine fluid and micronutrient needs
- Recommend vitamin/mineral supplementation
- Nutritional assessments should meet departmental standards (i.e. assessments should address nutritional requirements
- individualized for age, % burn, GI tolerance, drug and nutrient intake and pertinent laboratory data)
- Select feeding modality(ies) that will insure adequate intake of nutrient needs (oral, enteral, parenteral or combination)
- Initiate tube feeding or parenteral nutrition support within 72 hours postburn for patients with burns exceeding 25% TBSA

Evaluation of tolerance and effects of nutritional therapy
- Compare present weight to preburn weight
- Assess swallowing ability and oral feeding tolerance
- Conduct nutrient analysis and record daily and cumulative intake for calories and protein until condition stabilizes.
- Determine percent compliance with established goals.
- Diet order for tube feeding or parenteral nutrition should meet the calculated oral intake deficit within ± 10%
- Monitor patient's ability to tolerate advances in nutrition regimen if applicable
  1. Episodes of diarrhea, constipation or emesis should be evaluated and treated appropriately
- Monitor timing and frequency of surgical procedures, dressing changes, physical and hydrotherapy, and other treatments and adjust feeding schedule accordingly
- Follow reports of skin graft adherence, healing progress or percent open wound
- Monitor for occurrence of sepsis
- Compare discharge weight to preburn weight
  1. Discharge weight should be within ± 10% of preburn weight (exception: patients with amputations)

Adapted from Gottschlich M M. Assessment and nutritional management of the burn patient. In: Winkler M F, Lysen C, eds. Suggested Guidelines for Nutrition and Metabolic Management of Adult Patients Receiving Nutrition Support. Chicago, IL: The American Dietetic Association, 1993.

Infectious

Care must be taken during the preparation and delivery of tube feeding products to avoid bacterial contamination. Most manufacturers recommend that the formula sit at room temperature for no longer than 8 hours. The most serious complication of TPN is catheter-related sepsis. It is not surprising that catheter placement through a burn wound is associated with a higher infection rate.[10] Certainly the adherence to strict protocols of infection control and catheter care will minimize the occurrence of infection in the burn patient already heavily colonized with bacteria and thus very susceptible to infection. In addition, the central venous catheter should be avoided for hemodynamic monitoring, infusion of blood products, blood draws, or the administration of drugs.

Metabolic

A number of metabolic complications have been associated with certain nutrition support practices following burns. The provision of excessive calories or a large carbohydrate load, for example, can result in undesirable increases in carbon dioxide production and ventilatory requirements. This could precipitate or compound respiratory distress in severely burned patients.[67–69]

Hyperglycemia is commonly observed following a major burn,[70] particularly when a patient is elderly, septic, or following the institution of TPN or growth hormone. Pronounced hyperglycemia leads to glycosuria and osmotic diuresis, resulting in dehydration and hyperosmolarity. This syndrome can usually be prevented in the enterally fed patient by administration of exogenous insulin by sliding scale or continuous infusion along with careful monitoring. It is almost never necessary to decrease the volume of tube feeding in order to control hyperglycemia. Hyperglycemia following the

Table 22.4 Laboratory data and diagnostic tests

Parameter	Frequency	Comments
Serum measurements		
Electrolytes	Daily until stable	Frequent determinations of serum sodium, potassium, chloride, calcium, phosphorus and magnesium are the best clinical guides to intravenous electrolyte replacement
Blood urea nitrogen and creatinine	Daily until stable, then twice weekly	If azotemia develops, increase the delivery of free water and/or decrease protein content of nutrient substrate
Liver Profile	Three times/week	
Glucose	Daily until stable	Some patients with previously normal glucose tolerance prior to injury may require sliding scale insulin therapy during aggressive nutritional support following burns
Albumin, transferrin, prealbumin or retinol-binding protein	Weekly	Indicative of extent of depletion of visceral proteins. Delivery of a large quantity of blood products or the long half-life of certain secretory proteins can complicate interpretation. In burn patients, prealbumin seems to be a particularly good indicator of nutritional status
Delayed hypersensitivity skin testing, total lymphocyte count, C3, or IgG	Weekly	Suboptimal nutritional status can cause deficits in immune function. Recommend including at least one parameter of host defense in a nutrition assessment workup
Prognostic inflammatory and nutrition index	Weekly	A multiparameter index may be more sensitive and specific than individual nutrition assessment parameters
Urine measurements		
Urea (for nitrogen balance)	Daily	Nitrogen balance adjusted for nitrogen loss contained in burn wound exudate indicates whether nitrogen intake is exceeding body mass breakdown. Conditions favoring optimal wound healing and anabolism include nitrogen balance determinations exceeding (+)5 g N
Creatinine (for creatinine height index)	Daily	Used to assess lean body mass in patients with normal renal function
Indirect calorimetry		
Resting energy expenditure	One time per week minimum	Valuable indicator of severity of hypermetabolism as well as diminished energy needs with convalescence. Nutrition intake goal = REE × 1.3
Respiratory quotient (RQ)	Three times/week	Way to check accuracy of nutrition support in terms of over or underfeeding. If > 1.0, reduce caloric intake. If < 0.80, increase feedings

Data from references 1–8, 18, 28. 30–32, 52, 59–61, 68, 70–73.

institution of TPN is treated with exogenous insulin, a reduction in the rate of glucose administration, or both.

Metabolic complications resulting from derangements in protein, fat, fluid, electrolytes, and micronutrient metabolism are also possible following burns. Inability to tolerate the nutrient load, deficiencies in essential nutrients, and toxicities have all been described despite increased knowledge of and improvements in the composition of enteral and parenteral solutions. Therefore, it is important that the clinician be aware of these metabolic disturbances and recognize their signs and symptoms in order to make appropriate adjustments in the nutrition support regimen.

Summary

The aftermath of a burn injury evokes numerous nutritional aberrations. It is recognized that among these deviations are effects on nutrient kinetics, requirements, and tolerances. Consequently, considerable attention must be focused on the nutrition care plan. For some, provision of proper nutrition can reduce complications such as poor wound recovery and sepsis. For others, particularly the severely injured, aggressive nutritional support can make the difference between survival and death.

At present, the precise nutrient requirements of burned patients are not clear, although it is widely accepted that maintenance of energy balance and replacement of large protein losses remain of paramount importance. It appears prudent to minimize fat intake. In addition, vitamin and mineral supplementation are suggested, particularly vitamins A and C, and zinc. Enteral feeding programs are preferred due to their cost-, immunologic- and risk benefit ratios. Adherence to sound principles of early implementation of a high quality enteral feeding regimen, whenever possible, along with individual balancing and continuous monitoring will most often result in beneficial effects with minimal complications.

The future regarding nutrition support in burns requires an

expansion of our knowledge of the actions of specific nutrients such as arginine, glutamine, the ω-3 series of lipids, as well as key vitamins and minerals which are involved in immunologic, hematologic, and reparative processes. In addition, the interaction of nutrients with hormones and growth factors needs further elucidation. As we better define the effects of nutrition on the host following burns, we will be able to use nutrients as pharmacologic agents rather than simply as subtrates for one treatment of burn-induced catabolism and the minimization of malnutrition. This aside, current state of the art diet therapy practices represent, without a doubt, an integral component of the burn care program.

References

1. Herndon D N, Barrow R E, Stein M, Linares H, Rutan R, Abston S. Increased mortality with intravenous supplemental feeding in severely burned patients. *J Burn Care Rehabil* 1989; **10:** 309–13.

2. Derganc M. Parenteral nutrition in severely burned children. *Scand J Plast Reconstr Surg* 1979; **13:** 195–200.

3. Popp M B, Law E J, MacMillan B G. Parenteral nutrition in the burned child: a study of twenty-six patients. *Ann Surg* 1974; **179:** 219–25.

4. Alexander J W. Immunological responses in the burned patient. *J Trauma* 1979; **19:** 887–9.

5. Alexander J W, Gottschlich M M. Nutritional immunomodulation in burn patients. *Crit Care Med* 1990; **18:** S149–53.

6. Cutherbertson D P. The disturbance of metabolism produced by bony and nonbony injury with notes of certain abnormal conditions of bone. *Biochem J* 1930; **24:** 1244–63.

7. Cutherbertson D P, Zagreb H C. The metabolic response to injury and its nutritional implications: retrospect and prospect. *J Parenter Enteral Nutr* 1979; **3:** 108–29.

8. Curreri P W. Assessing nutritional needs for the burned patient. *J Trauma* (Suppl) 1990; **30**(12): S20–3.

9. Chiarelli A, Enzi G, Casadei A, Baggio B, Valerio A, Mazzoleni F. Very early nutrition supplementation in burned patients. *Am J Clin Nutr* 1990; **51:** 1035–9.

10. Saito H, Trocki O, Alexander J W, Kopcha R, Heyd T, Joffe S N. The effect of route of nutrient administration on the nutritional state, catabolic hormone secretion and gut mucosal integrity after burn injury. *J Parenter Enteral Nutr* 1987; **11:** 1–7.

11. Mochizuki H, Trocki O, Dominioni L, Brackett K A, Joffe S N, Alexander J W. Mechanism of prevention of postburn hypermetabolism and catabolism by early enteral feeding. *Ann Surg* 1984; **200:** 297–308.

12. Weir J W. New methods for calculating metabolic rate with special reference to protein metabolism. *J Physiol* 1949; **109:** 1–9.

13. Hildreth, M A, Herndon D N, Desai M H, Broemeling L D. Current treatment reduces calories required to maintain weight in pediatric patients with burns. *J Burn Care Rehabil* 1990; **11:** 405–9.

14. Hildreth M A, Herndon D N, Desai M H, Broemeling L D. Caloric requirements of patients with burns under one year of age. *J Burn Care Rehabil* 1993; **14:** 108–12.

15. Hildreth M A, Carvejal H F. Caloric requirements in burned children: a simple formula to estimate daily caloric requirements. *J Burn Care Rehabil* 1982; **3:** 78–80.

16. Hildreth M A, Herndon D N, Desai M H, Duke M A. Caloric needs of adolescent patients with burns. *J Burn Care Rehabil* 1989; **10:** 523–6.

17. Day T, Dean P, Adams M C, Luterman A, Ramenofsky M L, Curreri P W. Nutritional requirements of the burned child: the Curreri Junior formula. *Proc Am Burn Assoc* 1986; **18:** 86.

18. Food and Nutrition Board. *National Research Council Recommended Dietary Allowances*. 9th ed. Washington, DC: National Academy of Science, 1980.

19. O'Neil C E, Hutsler D, Hildreth M A. Basic nutritional guidelines for pediatric burn patients. *J Burn Care Rehabil* 1989; **10:** 278–84.

20. Williamson J. Actual burn nutrition care practices: a national survey (part II). *J Burn Care Rehabil* 1989; **10:** 185–94.

21. Curreri P W, Richmond D, Marvin J, Baxter C R. Dietary requirements of patients with major burns. *J Am Diet Assoc* 1974; **65:** 415–17.

22. Pasulka P S, Wachtel T L. Nutritional considerations for the burned patient. *Surg Clin North Am* 1987; **67:** 109–31.

23. Baxter C R. Metabolism and nutrition in burned patients. *Compr Ther* 1987; **13:** 36–42.

24. Cunningham J J, Hegarty M T, Burke J F. Measured and predicted calorie requirements of adults during recovery from severe burn trauma. *Am J Nutr* 1989; **49:** 404–8.

25. Long C L. Energy expenditure of major burns: *J Trauma* 1979; **19:** 904–6.

26. Adams M R, Kelly C H, Luterman A, Curreri P W. Nutritional requirements of the burned senior citizen: the Curreri Senior formula. *Proc Am Burn Assoc* 1987; **19:** 83.

27. Hildreth M A. Calorie needs of pediatric patients with toxic epidermal necrolysis. *Proc Am Diet Assoc.* 1990; 90A–99.

28. Heimbach D M. Toxic epidermal necrolysis pathophysiology. *Symposium: Electrical, Non-thermal Injuries, and Pain Management*. 22nd Annual Meeting American Burn Association. 1990; **92–110.**

29. Sutherland A B. Nitrogen balance and nutritional requirements in the burn patient: a reappraisal. *Burns* 1976; **2:** 238–44.

30. Kagan R J, Matsuda T, Hanumadass M, Castillo B, Jonasson O. The effect of burn wound size on ureagenesis and nitrogen balance. *Ann Surg* 1982; **195:** 70–4.

31. Matsuda T, Kagan R J, Hanumadass M, *et al.* The importance of burn wound size in determining the optimal calorie: nitrogen ratio. *Surgery* 1983; **94:** 562–8.

32. Alexander J W, MacMillan B G, Stinnett J D, *et al.* Beneficial effects of aggressive protein feeding in severely burned children. *Ann Surg* 1980; **192:** 505–17.

33. American Academy of Pediatrics Committee on Nutrition. *Pediatric Nutrition Handbook*. Elk Grove Village, IL: The Academy, 1985.

34. Gottschlich M M. Acute thermal injury. In: Lang C E, ed. *Nutritional Support in Critical Care*. Rockeville, MD: Aspen Publishers, 1987: 159–81.

35. Davies J W L, Liljedahl S L. Metabolic consequences of an extensive burn. In: Polk H C, Stone H H, eds. *Contemporary Burn Management*. Boston: Little, Brown and Company, 1971; 151–69.

36. November-Dusansky A, Moylan J A, Linkswiler H, Elson C. Calciuretic response to protein loading in burn patients. *Burns* 1980; **6:** 198–201.

37. Waymack, J P, Warden G D, Tweddell J S. Renal calculi in the burned child. *Burns* 1987; 13: 190–3.

38. Brinson R R, Kolts B E. Hypoalbuminemia as on indicator of diarrheal incidence in critically ill patients. *Crit Care Med* 1987; **15:** 506–9.

39. Gottschlich M M, Warden G D, Michel M, *et al.* Diarrhea in tube-fed burn patients: incidence, etiology, nutritional impact, and prevention. *J Parenter Enteral Nutr* 1988; **12:** 338–45.

40. Barbul A, Siato D A, Wasserkrug H L, Efron G. Arginine stimulates lymphocyte immune response in healthy human beings. *Surgery* 1981; **90:** 244–51.

41. Saito H, Trocki O, Wang S L, Gonce S J, Joffe S N, Alexander J W. Metabolic and immune effects of dietary arginine supplementation after burn. *Arch Surg* 1987; **122:** 784–9.

42. Hwang T L, O'Dwyer S T, Smith R J, Wilmore D W. Preservation of small bowel mucosa using glutamine enriched parenteral nutrition. *Surg Forum* 1980; **37:** 56–8.

43. Waymack J P, Herndon D N. Nutritional support of the burned patient. *World Journal of Surgery* 1992; **16:** 80–6.

44. Burke J F, Wolfe R R, Mullany C J, *et al.* Glucose requirements following burn injury: Parameters of optimal glucose infusion and possible hepatic and respiratory abnormalities following excessive glucose intake. *Ann Surg* 1979; **190:** 274–85.

45. Kennedy-Caldwell C, Caldwell M O. Pediatric enteral nutrition. In: Rombeau J L, Caldwell M O, eds. *Enteral and Tube Feeding*. Philadelphia: WB Saunders, 1984: 442.

46. Peck M D, Alexander J W, Ogle C K, Babcock G F. The effect of dietary fatty acids on response to *Pseudomonas* infection in burned mice. *J Trauma* 1990; **30:** 445–52.

47. Barton R D, Cerra F B. Metabolic and nutritional support. In: Moore E E, Mattox K L, Feliciano D V, eds. *Trauma*. Norwalk, CT: Appleton and Lange, 1991: 965–96.

48. Kernes J A. Fat requirements. In: Kernes J A, ed. *Manual of Pediatric Parenteral Nutrition*. New York: John Wiley, 1983: 103–27.

49. A.S.P.E.N Board of Directors. Guidelines for the use of parenteral and enteral nutrition in adult and pediatric patients. *J Parenter Enteral Nutr* 1993; **17:** 1SA–52SA.

50. Jenkins M, Gottschlich M M, Mayes T, Khoury J, Warden G. Enteral feeding during operative procedures. *J Burn Care Rehabil*, 1994; **15:** 199–205.

51. Jenkins M, Gottschlich M M, Alexander J W, Warden G D. Enteral alimentation in the early postburn phase. In: Blackburn G L, Bell S J, Mullen J, eds. *Nutritional Medicine: a case Management Approach*. Philadelphia, PA: WB Saunders Co, 1989: 1–5.

52. Gottschlich M M, Alexander J W, Bower R H. Enteral nutrition in patients with burns or trauma. In: Rombeau J L, Caldwell M D, eds. *Enteral and Tube Feeding*. Philadelphia: WB Saunders Co, 1984: 306–24.

53. Jenkins M, Gottschlich M M, Alexander J W, Warden G D. Effect of immediate enteral feeding on the hypermetabolic response following severe burn injury. *J Parenter Enteral Nutr* 1989: **13:** 12(5).

54. Trocki O, Mochizuki H, Dominioni L, Alexander J W. Intact protein versus free amino acids in the nutritional support of thermally injured animals. *J Parenter Enteral Nutr*. 1986; **10:** 139–45.

55. Gottschlich M M, Jenkins M, Warden G D, *et al*. Differential effects of three enteral dietary regimens on selected outcome variables in burn patients. *J Parenter Enteral Nutr* 1990; **14:** 225–36.

56. Bell S J, Molnar J A, Carey M. Adequacy of a modular tube feeding diet for burned patients. *J Am Diet Assoc* 1986; **86:** 1386–91.

57. Gottschlich M M, Warden G D. Parenteral nutrition in the burned patient. In: Fischer J E, ed *Total Parenteral Nutrition*. 2nd ed. Boston: Little, Brown and Co, 1991: 279–98.

58. Goodwin C W. Parenteral nutrition in thermal injuries. In: Rombeau J L, Caldwel M D, eds. *Clinical Nutrition: Parenteral Nutrition*. 2nd ed. Philadelphia: WB Saunders, 1993: 566–84.

59. Gottschlich M M. Assessment and nutritional management of the burn patient. In: Winkler M F, Lysen C, eds. *Suggested Guidelines for Nutrition and Metabolic Management of Adult Patients Receiving Nutrition Support*. Chigaco IL: The American Dietetic Association, 1993: 64–70.

60. Morath M A, Miller S F, Finley R K, Jones L M. Interpretation of nutritional parameters in burn patients. *J Burn Care Rehabil* 1983; **4:** 361–6.

61. Kagan R J, Gottschlich M M, Jenkins M E. Nutritional support in the burned patient. In: Robin A P, ed. *Probl Gen Surg* 1991; **8:** 57–75.

62. Guenter P A, Settler R G, Perlmutter S, Marino P L, DeSimone G A, Rolandelli R H. Tube feeding-related diarrhea in acutely ill patients. *J Parenter Enteral Nutr* 1991; **15:** 277–80.

63. Johnson L R, Copeland E M, Dudrick S J, Lichtenberger L M, Castro S A. Structural and hormonal alterations in the gastrointestinal tract of parenterally fed rats. *Gastroenterology* 1975; **68:** 1177–83.

64. Thompson J S, Vaughan W P, Forst C F, Jacobs D L, Weekly J S, Rikkers L F. The effect of the route of nutrient delivery on gut structure and diamine oxidase levels. *J Parenter Enteral Nutr* 1987; **11:** 28–32.

65. Spitz J, Gandhi S, Hecht G, Alverdy J. The effects of total parenteral nutrition on gastrointestinal function. *Clin Nutr* 1993; **12:** (suppl 1): S33–S37.

66. Levine G M, Deren J J, Skiger E, Zinno R. Role of oral intake in maintenance of gut mass and disaccharide activity. *Gastroenterology* 1974; **67:** 975–82.

67. Askanazi J, Rosenbaum S H, Hyman A I, Silverberg P A, Milic-Emili J, Kinney J M. Respiratory changes induced by the large glucose loads of total parenteral nutrition. *JAMA* 1980; **243:** 1444–7.

68. Talpers S S, Romberger D J, Bunce S B, Pingleton S K. Nutritionally associated increased carbon dioxide production. Excess total calories vs. high proportion of carbohydrate calories. *Chest* 1992; **102:** 551–5.

69. Ireton-Jones C S, Borman K R, Turner W W. Nutrition considerations in the management of ventilator dependent patients. *Nutr Clin Pract* 1993; **8:** 60–4.

70. Gottschlich M M, Baumer T, Jenkins M, Khoury J, Warden G D. The prognostic value of nutritional and inflammatory indices in burn patients. *J Burn Care Rehabil* 1992; **13:** 105–13.

71. Mancusi-Ungaro H R, VanWay C W, McCool C. Caloric and nitrogen balances as predictors of nutritional outcome in patients with burns. *J Burn Care Rehabil* 1992; **13:** 695–702.

72. Murphy M, Bell S J. Assessment of nutritional status in burn patients. *J Burn Care Rehabil* 1988; **9:** 432–3.

73. Waxman K, Rebello T, Pinderski L, *et al*. Protein loss across burn wounds. *J Trauma* 1987; **27:** 136–40.

CHAPTER TWENTY-THREE

EFFECTS OF BURN INJURY ON BONE AND MINERAL METABOLISM

GORDON L. KLEIN

The effects of burn injury on homeostasis of three critical minerals (calcium, phosphorus, and magnesium) have not been studied in great detail. These three minerals play key roles in metabolism and also are stored in bone, a tissue which may be significantly affected by burn injury. This chapter covers the roles of calcium, phosphorus, and magnesium in normal body metabolism, the homeostasis of these elements, what is known of the alterations in calcium, phosphorus, and magnesium homeostasis by burn injury with suggestions for corrective therapy, and what is known about the effects of burn injury on bone growth and remodeling.

METABOLIC FUNCTIONS OF CALCIUM, PHOSPHORUS, AND MAGNESIUM

All three of these minerals play important roles in intracellular and extracellular metabolism.

Calcium

Calcium plays a major role in neuromuscular impulse propagation and membrane depolarization and, consequently, in muscle contractility. Calcium may also serve as a second messenger, mediating the secretory release of peptides such as amylase, insulin, and aldosterone via intracellular pathways utilizing calmodulin, an intracellular calcium receptor protein, or protein kinase C. From the standpoint of extracellular metabolism, calcium serves as a cofactor in blood coagulation, specifically in the conversion of prothrombin to thrombin and the activation of several factors in the coagulation cascade. Calcium also contributes to plasma membrane stability by binding to phospholipids.[1-4]

Phosphorus

Phosphorus plays major roles in intracellular energy metabolism. Phosphorus, in the form of phosphate esters, is a constituent of purine nucleotides, an important source of intracellular energy. Phosphorylation of various metabolic intermediate products is also the means of intracellular energy transfer. In the form of phospholipids, phosphorus is also a major structural component of cell membranes.[1]

Magnesium

Magnesium, primarily stored in mitochondria, is a vital co-factor for the function of enzymes involved in the transfer of phosphate groups; and thus, it is important for all reactions which require adenosine triphosphate (ATP) and in reactions involving replication, transcription, and translation of nucleic acids.[1] Extracellular magnesium is important in plasma membrane excitability.

HOMEOSTASIS OF CALCIUM, PHOSPHORUS, AND MAGNESIUM

Calcium

Absorption of calcium is generally well regulated by the body. With high calcium intake, absorption can be as low as 20%, while with low calcium intake, absorption can reach 70%.[4,5] The mechanism for this regulation is shown in **Figure 23.1**. With high calcium intake, there is a transient hypercalcemia followed by a suppression of parathyroid hormone secretion, and consequently a suppression of parathyroid hormone stimulation of renal conversion of 25-hydroxyvitamin D, the chief circulating form of vitamin D, to calcitriol, or 1,25-dihydroxyvitamin D. With low calcium intake, the reverse occurs. There is a transient reduction of serum calcium concentration, followed by a rapid, within 5 minutes, rise in parathyroid hormone secretion. Parathyroid hormone will under normal circumstances stimulate bone resorption and increase renal tubular calcium reabsorption in order to raise serum calcium concentration. Furthermore, it stimulates the renal enzyme 25-hydroxyvitamin D-1-α-hydroxylase to convert 25-hydroxyvitamin D to calcitriol. Calcitriol then binds to intestinal epithelial cells and increases transcellular calcium absorption by altering cell membrane phospholipid and by facilitating the intracellular passage of the absorbed calcium by stimulating the cellular synthesis of calcium

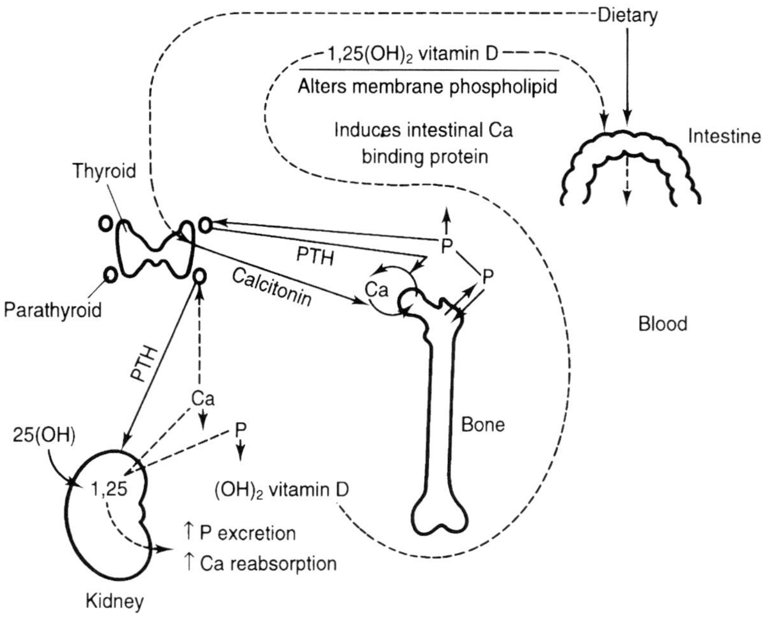

Fig. 23.1 Diagram of actions involved in calcium homeostasis.

binding proteins. Thus, the efficiency of calcium absorption is improved. Calcium, given intravenously, bypasses the intestinal control mechanism and suppresses parathyroid hormone production as well as production of calcitriol by the kidney. The bone stores 99% of the body's calcium.[1]

Phosphorus

In contrast to calcium, the intestine plays no significant regulatory role in phosphorus absorption. Approximately 80% of dietary phosphate is absorbed. Homeostatic control appears to rest primarily within the kidney.[6,7] The regulatory mechanisms are unknown, but they are most likely independent of parathyroid hormone.[6,7] Thus, the renal excretory rate of phosphate will primarily regulate the serum phosphorus concentration and maintain it within a normal range. The bone stores approximately 90% of the body's phosphate.[1]

Magnesium

Approximately 60% of the body's magnesium is stored in the skeleton.[8] Magnesium absorption, like phosphorus, varies directly with dietary intake with about 40% of an average daily load being absorbed.[8] The relationship between calcium and magnesium absorption is described as inverse, but the mechanism of this is not clear.[9] Renal excretion is the main route for magnesium elimination from the body, and it may vary with serum magnesium concentration. Thus, hypermagnesemia and hypercalcemia inhibit renal tubular reabsorption of magnesium while hypomagnesemia and parathyroid hormone increase magnesium reabsorption.[10]

Effect of Burn Injury on Calcium, Phosphorus, and Magnesium Homeostasis

The effects of burn injury on mineral homeostasis have not been studied in great detail. Data from the studies at the University of Texas Medical Branch and the Shriners Burns Institute in Galveston are used to supplement the available literature. In data collected from 11 adult patients in the burn unit between December, 1989 and January, 1992[11] low serum concentrations of ionized calcium, phosphorus, and magnesium were far more common than high serum levels of these minerals. Six patients had low serum concentrations of ionized calcium, three of them manifested hypocalcemia during the first 48 hours postburn, and five demonstrated this finding by the 11th postburn day. Hypocalcemia was most prevalent on day 4 postburn. Four of these patients were hypophosphatemic; this was most prevalent on day 7 postburn. Five of the patients were hypomagnesemic, with this finding most likely to be present on day 3 postburn. In contrast only one patient demonstrated hypercalcemia, and one hyperphosphatemia. No one was hypermagnesemic. In each case, the elevated serum level of either ionized calcium or phosphorus was transient. It must be pointed out that these data are not comprehensive and were not collected for the purpose of pinpointing the day of diagnosis or the maximum degree of abnormality in serum levels of calcium, phosphorus or magnesium. Therefore, these data can be interpreted as only approximations. However, in our patients, hypocalcemia occurred despite the administration of at least 3 grams a day of calcium by enteral infusion of milk.

These data are consistent with the existing literature, which states that hypocalcemia can occur up to at least 7 weeks postburn,[12-14] while hypophosphatemia has been described mainly in the first postburn week.[14] Hypomagnesemia is less consistently described and seemed to occur in one study only on postburn day.[1] The explanations for these occurrences are not certain. Hypocalcemia cannot be diagnosed from determinations of total serum calcium concentration, due to the variability of serum albumin concentration postburn. Determination of serum ionized calcium concentration should be encouraged, if available, for a more accurate diagnosis. Several possible mechanisms for hypocalcemia have been proposed. One is the shift of calcium from extracellular to intracellular compartments, as has been suggested by the accumulation of calcium in the erythrocyte of the postburn patient,[15] a manifestation of what is termed the 'sick cell syndrome'. Alternative hypotheses include the possibility of increased urinary calcium excretion, not observed in severely burned adults, especially when corrected for creatinine.[11] Losses of calcium in tissue exudate could theoretically contribute to hypocalcemia. While it has been argued that the amount of calcium in wound exudate is probably insufficient to entirely account for postburn hypocalcemia,[16] there are not enough studies which actually measure the calcium content of the burn wound exudate.

While fecal calcium losses can be high in burn patients[16] and the large amount of corticosteroids produced by burn injury may impair intestinal calcium absorption,[17] there is no evidence to suggest that hypocalcemia is caused by corticosteroid-induced impairment of intestinal reabsorption of calcium secreted into the intestinal lumen. Other proposed mechanisms include diminished bone resorption. Although recently published data from severely burned adults noted a reduced osteoclastic surface on iliac crest bone biopsies,[11] this measurement is the least sensitive on analysis of bone histomorphometry since the resorptive surface normally constitutes only about 6% of the total bone surface.[11,18] Possible explanations for postburn hypophosphatemia include intracellular accumulation of phosphate, inadequate phosphate intake, excessive urinary phosphate excretion, or phosphate loss into the extravascular fluid. In a recent review of the subject, Dolecek[16] found increased urinary phosphate excretion only during the third and fourth weeks postburn while hypophosphatemia was documented to occur earlier.[14,16] Thus, it is possible that the increased urinary phosphate excretion, seen later postburn, is more a function of increased tissue breakdown and filtered load than of inappropriate or excessive urinary phosphate losses. There is little documentation of inadequate phosphate intake following burns. Our patients were taking in 1.6 grams of phosphate per day in their enteral milk infusions alone.[11] Loss of significant phosphate in the extravascular fluid, excessive secretion of phosphate into the intestine with failure to reabsorb, and intracellular accumulation are all theoretically possible but remain unproven. Similarly, the cause of hypomagnesemia occurring postburn is unknown although excessive urinary and fecal losses have been reported.[16,19]

Rationale for Therapy

Because of their importance in the maintenance of bodily metabolic processes, low serum levels of ionized calcium, phosphorus, and magnesium should be treated (**Figures 23.2**). Hypocalcemia, especially in the immediate postburn period during the resuscitation effort, can potentiate the abnormalities of cardiac muscle produced by hyperkalemia[20] and cause unresponsiveness to repletion in shock.[20] If a patient is not hypocalcemic, there is insufficient evidence of benefit following provision of parenteral calcium during resuscitation,[21-23] unless the patient has hyperkalemia, hypomagnesemia, or calcium channel blocker toxicity.[24] Similarly, while caution should be exercised during massive transfusion with citrate-containing blood, calcium therapy may not be necessary[20,25] if the patient is normocalcemic and if hepatic and renal function are only minimally impaired. The liver will clear citrate, which may transiently chelate calcium, at a rate of 1 unit of blood transfused every 5 minutes.[25] Only when clinical and electrocardiographic evidence suggests hypocalcemia should treatment be initiated. Calcium infusions, when given, should be administered slowly, since rapid replacement of calcium has resulted in cardiac arrhythmias.[20,25]

Hypophosphatemia may result in tissue hypoxemia due to increased hemoglobin affinity for oxygen and decreased tissue ATP, metabolic, encephalopathy, possible hemolysis, shortened platelet survival time, myalgias, weakness, and possible impairment of myocardial contractility.[26] Hypomagnesemia blunts the effect of parathyroid hormone secreted in response to hypocalcemia, on target organs. Thus, hypocalcemic tetany may occur in the presence of hypomagnesemia,[27] as can generalized convulsions, muscle tremors, and weakness.[27]

Recommended Treatment

Hypocalcemia

Acute symptomatic hypocalcemia should be treated with intravenous calcium. In adults, 90–180 mg of elemental calcium over 5–10 minutes is given so as to reverse twitching. In infants or children, calcium chloride in a 20 mg/kg/dose or calcium gluconate in a 200–500 mg/kg/dose in four divided doses is suggested.[28,29] Caution should attend the use of parenteral chloride since it may cause phlebitis and/or acidosis. While hypocalcemia is asymptomatic and patients can tolerate enteral feedings, milk, as is given at our medical center, can provide adults with as much as 3 g/day of bioavailable calcium.[11] If, as we and others have found, hypocalcemia can occur despite the enteral provision of such a large quantity of calcium, intermittent parenteral administration of calcium salts will be necessary.

Symptomatic hypophosphatemia requires parenteral treatment, with a starting dose of 2 mg/kg infused over 6 hours and treatment continued until serum phosphorus concentrations exceed 1.0 mg/dl (0.3 mmol/l).[26] Infants and children with symptomatic hypophosphatemia should receive 5–10 mg/kg infused over 6 hours followed by 15–45 mg/kg given by infusion over 24 hours or until the serum phosphorus concentration rises above 2.0 mg/dl (0.6 mmol/l).[30]

Our adult patients who were given enteral milk infusions took on an average 1.6 grams a day of phosphate; this should be sufficient to treat asymptomatic hypophosphatemia as long as enteral feedings are tolerated.[11] Hypophosphatemia has not been reported to be

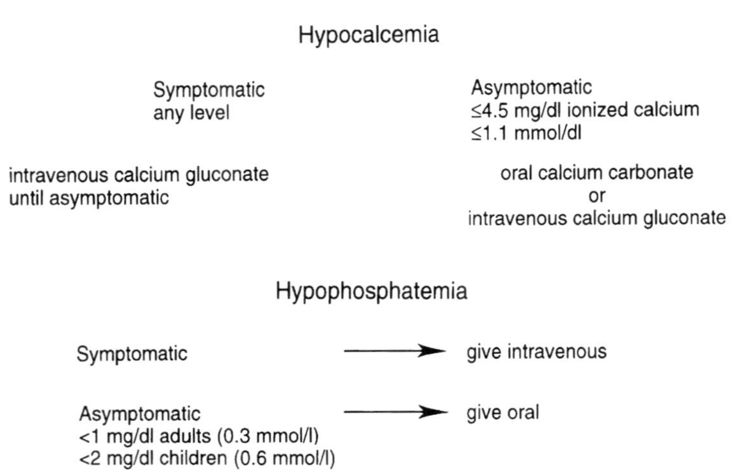

Fig. 23.2 Algorithm for the management of low levels of ionized calcium, phosphorus or magnesium that may occur post burn.

prolonged in adult burn patients and there appear to be few instances where parenteral phosphate supplements are needed. Should hypophosphatemia persist or recur despite the large amount of phosphate given enterally, a parenteral supplement would, of course, become necessary.

Adults who have signs or symptoms of magnesium deficiency with serum magnesium concentration below 1.5 mEq/l (1.8 mg/dl) or 0.8 mmol/l) usually require parenteral therapy. A 24-hour infusion of 48 mEq/l (58 mg/dl or 24 mmol/l) may be the treatment of choice.[27] For those who have convulsions or arrhythmias in association with hypomagnesemia, intravenous administration of 8–16 mEq (10–19 mg, 4–8 mmol) over 5–10 minutes may be necessary. This bolus would then be followed by the parenteral infusion mentioned above. For children, magnesium sulfate can be given parenterally for symptomatic hypomagnesemia 20–40 mEq (25–50 mg, 10–20 mmol) per dose followed by a 24-hour infusion of 25–50 mEq (30–60 mg, 12–25 mmol)/kg not exceeding 830 mEq (1 g, 450 mmol) per 24 hours.[30] If there is any impairment of renal function, the dose of magnesium should be reduced by 50%. While milk infusion should serve to maintain normal serum magnesium concentration, if patients cannot tolerate enteral feedings, parenteral administration of 8 mEq (10 mg, 4 mmol) magnesium should be given daily to adults and the 24-hour infusion of magnesium sulfate as stated above should be given to children in order to maintain normal serum magnesium levels.[27,30] This dose can be adjusted according to those levels.

Bone

The main storage depot of the body for calcium, phosphorus, and magnesium is bone. Both linear growth and bone remodeling appear to be adversely affected by burn injury. Linear growth at the epiphysis of long bones usually occurs by means of proliferation of cartilage cells with production of extracellular matrix; these cartilage cells and matrix undergo a series of biochemical changes which lead to the appearance of ossification centers, which appear as single expanding foci. As these ossifications expand, cartilaginous tissue is replaced by bone in a vascular supply system which provides for the delivery of nutrients, hormones, and growth factors.

It has been reported by Rutan and Herndon[31] that linear growth velocity is retarded for up to 3 years in children with severe burns. The mechanism for this effect of burn injury is unknown, but it has been established that the rate of growth does return to normal.[31] The effects of burn injury on bone remodeling are profound. In a study of 12 adult patients with burns of greater than 50% total body surface area, there was a marked reduction in bone formation.[11] Children suffering burns of 40% or greater total body surface area have reduced bone mass, which appears to be of long duration.[32] To put these findings in perspective, it is necessary to discuss the normal process of bone remodeling.

Bone remodeling is a continuous process of breakdown of calcified bone matrix by osteoclasts and formation of new bone matrix by osteoblasts, and the mineralization of that matrix by calcium and phosphate forming a mature crystal lattice of calcium phosphate hydroxyapatite. Bone resorption and formation are normally biochemically linked. All the details of this linkage are not known, but as an example, parathyroid hormone receptors have been identified on osteoblasts but have so far not been identified on osteoclasts.[33] Thus, parathyroid hormone can increase the number of osteoblasts on bone surfaces in both humans[34] and animals.[35] Therefore, osteoblasts, which are bone forming cells, must serve as an intermediary in the process of parathyroid hormone-mediated bone resorption.

What has been found in burn patients who underwent iliac crest bone biopsy from 9 weeks to 9 months following burn injury of 50% or greater of total body surface area is a *dissociation* of formation from resorption.[11] By administering tetracycline to the patients in two doses separated by 2 weeks, we found that the newly mineralized bone surface taking up tetracycline was markedly reduced in burned patients when compared to age- and sex-matched ambulatory controls.[11] In contrast, the distance between the two tetracycline labels in the bone was not significantly reduced.[11] Inasmuch as tetracycline is taken up at the bone surface by newly mineralized bone and forms a band which can be seen under a fluorescent microscope, the distance between the two bands of tetracycline divided by the interval between doses gives the *mineral apposition rate*, a measure of osteoblast function. The length of bone surface taking up tetracycline is an indirect measure of the number of osteoblasts present on the bone surface[36] and the *bone formation rate* is a product of the mineral apposition rate and length of bone surface taking up tetracycline. Thus, it was found that the bone formation rate in burn patients was reduced, while the mineral apposition rate was not significantly different from controls. Also consistent with these findings is the reduced amount of osteoid, or unmineralized bone matrix, in burned patients.[11] This is the product of osteoblasts. Therefore, all evidence indicates a decrease in the number of osteoblasts in burned patients, possibly through a recruitment defect in the marrow, although those osteoblasts which are present in bone appear to function normally. The net effect of the reduction in bone formation is a dissociation of formation from resorption, possibly setting up the patient for bone loss.

There are several potential contributing factors to this pathology including the production of cytokines which potentially resorb bone, such as interleukins-1 and 6,[37–39] immobilization, which reduces bone formation and increases resorption,[40,41] and increased corticosteroid production, which may have direct toxicity to osteoblasts[33] and also increases bone resorption.[17] Another possible contributing factor is aluminum loading, which can cause reduced bone formation in uremic patients[42] and in those receiving total parenteral nutrition.[43] Aluminum loading in adult burn patients would be most significant in the sources which bypass the intestinal, pulmonary, and cutaneous barriers to aluminum entry into the blood. The main sources would be albumin[44,45] and calcium gluconate;[45–47] however, it is highly unlikely that aluminum loading constitutes the primary cause of this pathology in adults because similar histomorphometric abnormalities were found in the bone biopsies of adult burn patients without detectable bone aluminum.[11] The long-term significance of this uncoupling of bone formation and resorption has yet to be determined. Similarly, a method for preventing its occurrence has yet to be developed.

References

1. Broadus A E. Physiologic functions of calcium, magnesium, and phosphorus. In: Favus M J, ed. *Primer on the Metabolic Bone Diseases and Disorders of Mineral Metabolism*. Kelseyville, CA: American Society for Bone and Mineral Research, 1990: 29–30.
2. Joff G A, Rosenberg R B. Physiology of hemostasis the fluid phase. In: Nathan D G, Oski F A, eds *Hematology of Infancy and Childhood*. Philadelphia, PA: W B Saunders, 1993: 1534–60.
3. Rasmussen H. The calcium messenger system. *N Engl J Med* 1986; **314:** 1094–101.
4. Rasmussen H. The calcium messenger system. *N Engl J Med* 1986; **314:** 1164–70.
5. Neer R M. Calcium and inorganic phosphate homeostasis. In: DeGroot L J, ed. *Endocrinology*. Philadelphia, PA: W B Saunders, 1989: 927–53.
6. Klein G L, Coburn J W. Parenteral nutrition: effect on bone and mineral homeostasis. *Annu Rev Nutr* 1991; **11:** 93–119.

7. Portale A A, Hallorain B P, Murphy M M, Morriss R C Jr. Oral intake of phosphorus can determine the serum concentration of 1,25-dihydroxyvitamin D by determining production rate in humans. *J Clin Invest* 1986; **77:** 7–12.

8. Silverberg S J. The distribution and balance of calcium, magnesium and phosphorus. In: Favus M J, ed. *Primer on the Metabolic Bone Diseases and Disorders of Mineral Metabolism.* Kelseyville, CA: American Society for Bone and Mineral Research, 1990: 30–2.

9. Lemann J Jr. Intestinal absorption of calcium, magnesium and phosphorus. In: Favus M J, ed. *Primer on the Metabolic Bone Diseases and Disorders of Mineral Metabolism.* Kelseyville, CA: American Society for Bone and Mineral Research, 1990: 32–6.

10. Lemann J Jr. The urinary excretion of calcium, magnesium and phosphorus. In: Favus M J, ed. *Primer on the Metabolic Bone Diseases and Disorders of Mineral Metabolism.* Kelseyville, CA: American Society for Bone and Mineral Research, 1990: 36–9.

11. Klein G L, Herndon D N, Rutan T C, *et al.* Bone disease in burn patients. *J Bone Miner Res* 1993; **8:** 337–45.

12. Pruitt B A. Complications of thermal injury. *Clin Plast Surg* 1974; **1:** 667–91.

13. Lennquist S, Lindell B, Nordstrom H, Sjoberg H E. Hypophosphatemia in severe burns. *Acta Chir Scard* 1979; **145:** 1–6.

14. Szyfelbein, S K, Drop L J, Martyn J A. Persistent ionized hypocalcemia in patients during resuscitation and recovery periods of body burn. *Crit Care Med* 1981; **9:** 454–458.

15. Baar S. The effect of thermal injury on the loss of calcium from calcium loaded cells: its relationship to red cell function and patient survival. *Clin Chem Acta* 1982; **126:** 25–39.

16. Dolecek R. Calcium-active hormones and postburn low-calcium syndrome. In: Dolecek R, Brizio-Moltens L, Moltens A, Traber D, eds. *Endocrinology of Thermal Trauma: Pathophysiologic Mechanism and Clinical Interpretation.* Philadelphia, PA: Lea and Febiger, 1990: 216–37.

17. Hahn T J, Halstead L R, Teitelbaum S I, Hahn B H. Altered mineral metabolism in glucocorticoid induced osteopenia: Effect of 25-hydroxyvitamin D administration. *J Clin Invest* 1979; **64:** 655–65.

18. Sherrard D J, Baylink D J, Wergedal J A, Maloney N A. Quantitative histological studies on the pathogenesis of uremic bone disease. *J Clin Endocrinol Metab* 1974; **39:** 119–35.

19. Heath H, III. Biogenic amines and secretion of parathyroid hormone and calcitonin. *Endocr Rev* 1980; **1:** 319–338.

20. British Committee for Standardization in Haematology Blood Transfusion Task Force. Guidelines for transfusion for massive blood loss. *Clin Lab Haematol* 1988; **10:** 265–73.

21. Stueven H, Thompson B M, Aprahamian C, *et al.* Use of calcium in pre-hospital cardiac arrest. *Ann Emerg Med* 1983; **12:** 136–139.

22. Stueven H A, Thompson B M, Aprahamian C, Tonsfeldt D J. Calcium chloride, reassessment of use in asystole. *Ann Emerg Med* 1984; **13:** 820–822.

23. Harrison E E, Amey B D. Use of calcium in electromechanical dissociation. *Ann Emerg Med* 1984; **13:** 844–845.

24. Harinan R J, Mangiardi L M, McAllister R G, Surawicz B, Shabetal R, Kishida H. Reversal of the cardiovascular effects of verapamil by calcium and sodium. Differences between electrophysiologic and hemodynamic response. *Circulation* 1979; **59:** 797–804.

25. Dzik W H, Kirkley S A. Citrate toxicity during massive blood transfusion. *Transfusion Med Rev* 1988; **2:** 76–94.

26. Gupta A, Hruska K A. Hyperphosphatemia and hypophosphatemia. In: Favus M J, ed. *Primer on the Metabolic Bone Diseases and Disorders of Mineral Metabolism.* Kelseyville, CA: American Society for Bone and Mineral Research, 1990: 143–7.

27. Rude R K. Magnesium deficiency and hypermagnesemia. In: Favus M J, ed. *Primer on the Metabolic Bone Diseases and Disorders of Mineral Metabolism.* Kelseyville, CA: American Society for Bone and Mineral Research, 1990: 141–3.

28. Weinstein R S. Hypocalcemia in acute illnesses. In Favus M J, ed. *Primer on the Metabolic Bone Diseases and Disorders of Mineral Metabolism.* Kelseyville, CA: American Society for Bone and Mineral Research, 1990: 138–9.

29. Carpenter T O. Neonatal hypocalcemia. In: Favus M J, ed. *Primer on the Metabolic Bone Diseases and Disorders of Mineral Metabolism.* Kelseyville, CA: American Society for Bone and Mineral Research, 1990: 139–41.

30. Greene M G. In: *The Harriet Lane Handbook.* St Louis, MO: Mosby-Yearbook, 1991: 150–244.

31. Rutan R L, Herndon D N. Growth delay in postburn pediatric patients. *Arch Surg* 1990; **125:** 392–5.

32. Klein G L, Herndon D N, Langman C B, *et al.* Long term reduction in bone mass after severe burn injury in children. *J Pediatr* 1995; **126:** 252–6.

33. Simmons D J, Seitz P K, Kidder L S, *et al.* Partial characterization of rat marrow stromal cells. *Calcif Tissue Int* 1991; **48:** 326–34.

34. Parisien M, Charhon S A, Arlot M, *et al.* Evidence for a toxic effect of aluminum or osteoblasts: a histomorphometric study in hemodialysis patients with aplastic bone disease. *J Bone Miner Res* 1988; **259–67.**

35. Rodriguez M, Felsenfeld A J, Llach F. Aluminum administration in the rat separately affects the osteoblast and bone mineralization. *J Bone Miner Res* 1990; **5:** 59–67.

36. Parfitt A M, Drezner M K, Glorieux F H, *et al.* Bone histomorphometry: standardization of nomenclature symbols and units. Report of the ASBMR Histomorphometry Nomenclature Committee. *J Bone Miner Res* 1987; **2:** 595–610.

37. Kupper T J, Deitch E A, Baker C C, Wong W. The human burn wound as a primary source of interleukin-1 activity. *Surgery* 1986; **100:** 409–15.

38. Guo Y, Dickerson C, Chrest E J, *et al.* Increased levels of circulatory interleukin-6 in burn patients. *Clin Immunol Immunopathol* 1990; **54:** 361–71.

39. Ishimi Y, Miyausa C, Jin C H, *et al.* IL-6 is produced by osteoblasts and induces bone resorption. *J Immunol* 1990; **145:** 3297–303.

40. Arnaud S B, Sherrard D J, Maloney N A, *et al.* Effects of one-week head-down tilt bed rest on bone formation with calcium endocrine system. *Aviat Space Environ Med* 1992; **63:** 14–20.

41. Leukens S, Arnaud S, Taylor A K, Baylink D J. Immobilization causes an acute and sustained increase in markers of bone resorption. (Abstract). *Clin Res* 1990; **38:** 123A.

42. Ott S M, Maloney N A, Coburn J W, Alfrey A C, Sherrard D J. The prevalence of bone aluminum deposition in renal osteodystrophy and its relation to the response to calcitriol therapy. *N Engl J Med* 1982; **307:** 709–13.

43. Ott S M, Maloney N A, Klein G L, *et al.* Aluminum is associated with low bone formation in patient receiving chronic parenteral nutrition. *Ann Intern Med* 1983; **98:** 910–14.

44. Milliner D S, Shinaberger J H, Shuman P, Coburn J W. Inadvertent aluminum administration during plasma exchange due to aluminum contamination of albumin replacement solutions. *N Engl J Med* 1985; **312:** 165–7.

45. Sedman A B, Klein G L, Merritt RJ, *et al.* Evidence of aluminum loading in infants receiving intravenous therapy. *N Engl J Med* 1985; **312:** 1337–43.

46. Koo W W K, Kaplan L A, Horn J, *et al.* Aluminum in parenteral nutrition solutions – sources and possible alternatives. *J Parenter Enteral Nutr* 1986; **10:** 591–5.

47. Klein G L, Herndon D N, Rutan T C, Barnett J L, Miller N L, Alfrey A C. Risk of aluminum loading in burn patients and ways to reduce it. *J Burn Care Rehabil* 1994; **15:** 354–8.

CHAPTER TWENTY-FOUR

Vitamin and Trace Element Homeostasis following Burn Injury

Alison J. Manning, Nicholas Meyer and Gordon L. Klein

Introduction

Guidelines for vitamin and trace element intake following burn injury have no documented basis.[1,2] Recommendations for micronutrient intake and supplementation are based on observations of increased nutrient losses through urine and burn wounds, or findings of low levels of micronutrients in blood or tissues. Conditions which cause varying micronutrient requirements are common in surgical patients. These include active growth, malabsorption and intestinal parasitism,[3] drug-nutrient interactions,[4] and hypermetabolism induced by injury or infection.[5] Furthermore, the needs and metabolic changes of a burned patient complicate the task of supplying micronutrient requirements, since protein and energy are less efficiently utilized without proper micronutrient intake.

It is often difficult to evaluate clinical vitamin and micronutrient deficiencies in burned patients. While clinical manifestation of vitamin and micronutrient deficiencies are listed in **Table 24.1**, cutaneous signs of deficiency may be entirely obscured by the burn wound. Metabolic changes following burn injury may obscure other deficiencies. For example, insulin resistance in burn patients may obscure glucose intolerance seen with chromium deficiency. Therefore, in the absence of diagnostic signs on physical examination and with the limited means to measure vitamin and micronutrient levels in blood or tissue in many parts of the world, the rationale for provision of adequate amounts of vitamins and micronutrients for burn-injured patients must remain pragmatic. We have selected certain vitamins and minerals which have been documented to play roles in energy and protein metabolism, wound healing, inflammatory responses and antioxidant action. These nutrients should be considered for supplementation in the burn-injured patient.

Vitamins

Vitamin A – Wound Healing

The specific function of vitamin A in wound healing is not completely understood. Supplemental vitamin A enhanced fibroplasia and collagen accumulation in wounds in an *in vitro* study to determine the mechanism of effects of the vitamin. Additionally, fibroblast differentiation and collagen synthesis were stimulated.[6] Vitamin A is also required for an adequate inflammatory response in wound healing.[7]

There are decreased serum vitamin A levels in burn victims, possibly due to the reduced level of retinol binding protein (RBP) which transports vitamin A from the liver to other tissues.[8,9] Other situations associated with lower plasma vitamin A levels and common to burned patients include diarrhea[10] and giardiasis.[11] Growth hormone may play a role in the synthesis or secretion of the RBP–vitamin A complex from the liver.[12,13] Neomycin decreases absorption of vitamin A. Toxicity occurs with high dosing 20–30 times the recommended dietary allowance (RDA) over a short period. While toxicity has not been reported in burned patients, one needs to be aware of the physical finding of vitamin A toxicity (**Table 24.1**).

Thiamin – Energy and Protein Metabolism and Wound Healing

Thiamin functions as a co-factor in the conversion of pyruvate to acetyl-CoA and α-ketoglutarate to succinyl-CoA in the Krebs cycle and to transketolase in the hexose monophosphate shunt for the oxidation of glucose. Thiamin needs are related to energy intake. Thiamin may also be an important factor in wound healing since it is necessary for lysyl oxidase function in collagen formation.[7] Oral requirements for normal adults are 0.5 mg/1000 kcal (or 1.4 mg/day).[14] Evidence of elevated thiamin requirements exists in burn injury.[15] Burned patients exhibited low urinary thiamin excretion levels in both a fasting state and after injection of the vitamin. The extent of the abnormalities paralleled the severity of the burn. Doses of 10–20 mg of thiamin per day may be necessary in severely burned patients.

Riboflavin – Energy and Protein Metabolism and Wound Healing

Riboflavin functions as part of the coenzymes flavin mononucleotide (FMN) and flavin adenine dinucleotide (FAD) in oxida-

Table 24.1 Physical signs possibly related to vitamin and trace element nutrition

		Physical findings in possible:	
Nutrient	Organ system	Deficiency	Excess
Vitamin A	Skin	Follicular hyperkeratosis	Sunburn-like erythematous eruption; dry rough scaling
	Hair	Broken, coiled swan-neck hairs, thin, sparse	Loss of body hair
	Gums		Bleeding, red, swollen, reddened gingiva
	Tongue	Diminished taste sensation	Fissures on tongue
	Eyes	Dry conjunctiva, keratomalacia, Bitot's spots	Papilledema, possible complaints of headache, diplopia and dizziness
	Hematologic		Slow clotting time, increased serum alkaline phosphatase
Carotene	Skin	Yellow pigmentation sparing sclerae	
Vitamin E	Neurological	Ophthalmoplegia, foot drop. Ataxia, sensory loss, motor weakness, loss of vibratory sense, deep tendon reflexes	
Vitamin D	Neuromuscular	Generalized weakness. Tetany	
	Skeletal	Rickets, osteomalacia	
	Hematologic	Decreased Ca^{2+} & PO_4, increased alkaline phosphatase	Increased Ca^{2+}, PO_4 & cholesterol, decreased Mg
Vitamin K	Skin	Subcutaneous ecchymoses in response to minor trauma	
	Hematologic	Hypoprothrombinemia	Transient hyperprothrombinemia
Thiamin	Cardiovascular	Tachycardia, cardiomegaly, congestive heart failure	
	Muscular	Generalized weakness	
	Neurological	Ataxia, sensory loss, motor weakness, loss of vibratory sense, deep tendon reflexes, peripheral neuropathy, ophthalmoplegia, foot drop	
Riboflavin	Skin	Scrotal, vulval dermatitis	
	Tongue	Pebbly or granular dorsum; erythematous, purplish red/magenta colored	
	Eyes	Circumcorneal injection angular palpebritis, photophobia	
	Lips	Inflammation, cheilosis/ vertical fissuring, angular stomatitis, later complicated by redness, swelling & ulceration	
	Neurological	Peripheral neuropathy	
Niacin	Skin	Symmetrical dermatitis of skin exposed to sunlight, thickened pressure points, hyperkeratosis, hyperpigmentation,	

Table 24.1 Physical signs possibly related to vitamin and trace element nutrition – *contd*

		Physical findings in possible:	
Nutrient	Organ system	Deficiency	Excess
Niacin – *contd*		photosensitization, stomatitis, cracking, desquamation	
	Tongue	Surface partially to completely bald, smooth and beefy red, fissuring, edema	
	Gastrointestinal	Diarrhea, constipation, achlorhydria	
	Neurological	Tremors	
Pyridoxine	Skin	Seborrheic inflammation accompanied by fine scaling and itching – involving face and intertriginous areas	
	Tongue	Scaling sensation succeeded by reddening and hypertrophy of filiform papillae	
	Eyes	Scleral icterus, mild	
	Hematologic	Anemia	
	Neuropsychiatric	Personality changes manifested by irritability and depression	
Vitamin B_{12}	Skin	Hyperpigmentation	
	Gums	Inflammation with generalized stomatitis and ulceration	
	Tongue	Filiform papillary atrophy	
	Neurological	Ataxia, sensory loss	
		Peripheral neuropathy	
Folic acid	Skin	Hyperpigmentation	
	Gums	Inflammation with generalized stomatitis and ulceration	
	Tongue	Lobulated with filiform papillary atrophy	
	Eyes	Pallor of everted lower eyelids, desquamation	
Biotin	Skin	Generalized dermatitis	
	Hair	Broken, coiled, swan-neck hairs, thin, sparse	
Pantothenic acid	Muscular	Generalized weakness	
	Neurological	Peripheral neuropathy	
Vitamin C	Skin	Subcutaneous ecchymoses in response to minor trauma, delayed wound healing, decubitus ulcers	
	Nails	Splinter-type hemorrhages under the nails	
	Hairs	Broken, coiled, swan-neck hairs, thin, sparse	
	Gums	Bleeding, red, swollen, reddened gingiva. Generalized stomatitis and ulceration	
	Cardiovascular	Capillary fragility	
	Muscular	Generalized weakness	
Iron	Skin		Slate gray/hemosiderosis

Table 24.1 Physical signs possibly related to vitamin and trace element nutrition – *contd*

		Physical findings in possible:	
Nutrient	Organ system	Deficiency	Excess
Iron – *contd*	Nails	Spoon-shaped koilonychia	
	Lips	Pallor	
	Tongue	Filiform papillary atrophy	
	Eyes	Pallor of conjunctivae	
Zinc	Skin	Generalized dermatitis, delayed wound healing, decubitus ulcers	
	Nails	White-spotting	
	Hair	Broken, coiled, swan-neck hairs, thin, sparse	
	Tongue	Diminished taste sensation	
	Eyes	Photophobia	
	Endocrine	Impaired growth, hypogonadism	
Iodine	Endocrine	Hypothyrodism	Goiter
Selenium	Cardiovascular	Cardiomyopathy	
	Muscular	Muscle pain, weakness	
Chromium	Endocrine	Glucose intolerance	
Copper	Skin	Hypopigmentation	
	Gastrointestinal	Anorexia, nausea, vomiting	
	Hair	Kinky, steely hair	
	Hematologic	Neutropenia, serum lipid changes (cholesterol), anemia (sideroblastic)	
	Neurological	Intention tremor and psychoses	
	Skeletal	Bone abnormalities resembling scurvy	
Manganese	Hematologic	Abnormal clotting not corrected by vitamin K	
Magnesium	Neuromuscular	Spontaneous generalized muscle spasm, tremor, convulsions	

Information combined using references 29, 48, 68, 69.

tion–reduction reactions involving the electron transport chain, fatty acid synthesis and oxidation and amino acid oxidation. Riboflavin converts pyridoxine and folate to their active forms, and is required for the synthesis of niacin from tryptophan. An increased need for this nutrient has been documented in burn-injured patients.[15] Riboflavin may also play a role in wound healing as dietary deficiency can slow this process.[16] Urinary excretion of riboflavin in burned patients increases with the severity of the burn. Patients with minor or superficial burns did not show these changes unless a complicating factor was present such as low intake of food, preexisting deficiency, or serious infection. It is recommended that 10–20 mg of riboflavin be given daily to severely burned patients and doses might need to be continued for long periods.

Psychological sequelae following burn injury sometimes prompt the use of psychotropic drugs in these patients. There is evidence of interference with riboflavin metabolism using chlorpromazine, imipramine, and amitriptyline. In age-, sex-matched pair-fed control rats, the conversion of the vitamin to its coenzyme derivatives was inhibited after chlorpromazine administration despite intake levels above the recommended daily allowance (RDA) in a 7-week period.[17] Marginal and subclinical riboflavin deficiency will result in significant deterioration of personality.

Niacin – Energy and Protein Metabolism

Niacin is an essential component of the enzyme cosubstrates, nicotinamide adenine dinucleotide (NAD) and nicotinamide adenine dinucleotide phosphate (NADP). These are central electron transport carriers for cells in more than 200 reactions in anaerobic glycolysis, the Krebs cycle, and fatty acid synthesis and oxidation. Niacin can be synthesized from the indispensable amino acid, tryptophan, in healthy adults. Tryptophan deficiency in the diet may contribute to niacin deficiency. In considering the adequacy of niacin in the diet, the dietary content of tryptophan and niacin must be quantitated in terms of niacin equivalents. Generally, 60 mg of tryptophan are equivalent to 1 mg of niacin. The dependence of tryptophan on pyridoxine (vitamin B_6) also impacts niacin deficiency. A lack of vitamin B_6 will reduce the formation of niacin from tryptophan, as it is required for this conversion. In addition, niacin deficiency is accompanied by decreased pyridoxine. Excess leucine, a branched-chain amino acid, may antagonize niacin synthesis and precipitate pellagra.[18] Niacin requirements are related to energy intake with the RDA established at 6.6 niacin equivalents needed per 1000 kcal.

Pyridoxine (vitamin B_6) – Energy and Protein Metabolism

Pyridoxine serves as a coenzyme in reactions involved in amino acid biosynthesis and catabolism including: transamination, deamination, decarboxylation, and desulfhydration. Vitamin B_6 enzymes are important in the degradation pathways for tryptophan, methionine, and glycine. Vitamin B_6 functions in the synthesis of epinephrine, norepinephrine, histamine, and porphyrin precursors to heme. Pyridoxine appears to have a role as a modulator of steroid hormone receptors.[19] There have been observations of the occurrence of a pyridoxine-responsive glucose intolerance in some individuals.[20] Pyridoxine deficiency can be produced in humans within 1 week on a deficient diet. Low pyridoxine levels have been observed in children with burns.[21] Requirements are increased with increased protein intake.

Folic Acid – Energy and Protein Metabolism

Folate functions as an enzyme cosubstrate involving methyl donor reactions. Deficiencies result in impaired synthesis of DNA and RNA. Inadequate supplies of vitamin B_{12} and the indispensable amino acid, methionine, impair folate utilization. Thus, a deficiency of either of these nutrients can produce signs of folate deficiency. Indiscriminate use of folate may mask the neurological lesions of pernicious anemia associated with vitamin B_{12} deficiency while correcting the megaloblastic anemia seen in folate deficiency. While sodium bicarbonate can impair folic acid absorption,[22,23] no clinical proof exists that folate deficiency, with or without anemia, can occur with the use of antacids or histamine receptor antagonists.

Vitamin B_{12} – Energy and Protein Metabolism

Vitamin B_{12} functions as a coenzyme to maintain normal folic acid metabolism and plays a role in catabolism of odd-chain-length fatty acids. Deficiency appears to result in a loss of tissue carnitine. Reduction of carnitine reduces β-oxidation of fatty acids.[24] In vitamin B_{12} deficiency, the fatty acid carrier, propionyl carnitine, builds up in the cell and is excreted in the urine since the forward reaction in the pathway is blocked. Marginal carnitine deficiency in animals results in fatty liver, but is relieved by carnitine intake.[24] Little is written on vitamin B_{12} deficiency and burns. Its role with carnitine has not been studied in the burned patient. Requirements for vitamin B_{12} are increased with parasites and increased hematopoiesis.

Vitamin C (Ascorbic Acid) – Antioxidant Properties and Wound Healing

Burns result in increased microvascular permeability and require significant fluid volume resuscitation in the first 24 hours after injury. Inflammatory mediators have been studied regarding their role in this process. Some researchers have suggested that oxygen free radicals such as superoxide, hydroxyl, peroxide, and the transition metals iron and copper, may cause increased postburn vascular permeability.[25,26] Thus, administration of vitamin C, a free radical scavenger, during fluid resuscitation, may benefit these patients. Recent studies have found that high-dose vitamin C administration during 24-hour resuscitation reduced required fluid volume;[27] and high-dose vitamin C must be given until 8 hours after burn injury in order to maintain these results.[28]

Ascorbic acid can act as an antioxidant with superoxide anion ($.O_2^-$), hydroxyl radical (OH^-), and toxic forms of oxygen as possible reactants. It appears, in aerobic systems, that the efficiency of radical quenching of ascorbate is inversely related to the concentration of the vitamin.[29] In its function as a pro-oxidant, vitamin C may also improve circulating levels of vitamin E[30] since the reduced form of vitamin C can donate electrons to regenerate vitamin E from tocopherol free radicals.

Vitamin C is an essential co-factor for proline and lysine hydroxylase enzymes in collagen biosynthesis. If vitamin C is absent, an improper sequence of amino acids is produced, and the remaining steps of synthesis cannot proceed. Capillary fragility ensues. New wounds do not heal adequately, and old wounds may fall apart due to a loss of tensile strength and degeneration of the extracellular matrix. Administration of vitamin C rapidly restores the healing process to normal.[31] There is evidence *in vitro* of increased utilization of vitamin C during phagocytosis.[32] Ascorbic acid may increase the activation of leukocytes and macrophages at the injured site.[33] These are initial steps in the wound healing phase.

Vitamin E (α-Tocopherol) – Antioxidant Properties

In cell membranes α-tocopherol functions as a scavenger for lipid peroxyl radicals (LOO·) terminating lipid peroxidation chain reactions. In an animal study[34] where thermal injury to skin resulted in acute lung injury and the appearance of lipid peroxidation products in plasma and tissues, various treatments were evaluated.[34] The study demonstrated that treatment of the thermally injured animals with vitamin E or iron chelators afforded protection from lung injury. In 14 burn patients analysed for lipid peroxides and antioxidants in plasma, significantly lower mean α-tocopherol levels in plasma compared to controls were observed.[35,36] A report on administration of antioxidants tocopherol, ascorbic acid, superoxide dismutase, and catalase in burned mice had no effect on mortality.[37] Tocopherol given in high doses of at least 25 IU/kg preceding injury and continued thereafter for 2 days did improve survival, but this benefit was not seen if tocopherol was not started until after injury.

Other Vitamins

Pantothenic acid deficiency is associated with decreased wound strength probably because of an effect on cell replication.[38] Vitamin K has no direct role in wound healing but is required for coagulation which precedes wound healing.

MICRONUTRIENTS

Manganese – Energy and Protein Metabolism

Manganese is associated with various enzymes in the Krebs cycle, pentose phosphate shunt, and glycolysis. Deficiency is uncommon as magnesium can substitute for manganese in many enzyme reactions.[39] There is no practical method for assessing manganese status. Requirements in burn injury are not known. Attention to manganese status after burn injury is of interest with slow growth reported during manganese deficiency[40] and after burn injury,[41] and slow growth, skeletal abnormalities, and defects in lipid and carbohydrate metabolism reported from animal studies.[42]

Copper – Role in Inflammation and Antioxidant Properties

In a burned patient, the presence of copper is important for wound healing and immunity. Induced copper deficiency in animals increased susceptibility to infection. The mechanism is likely related to copper's role in superoxide dismutase and the cytochrome *c* oxidase system.[43] Following a burn, serum copper initially rises and then falls below normal after 10 days post-injury, with the degree of hypocupremia being directly related to total burn size.[44,45] These changes are thought to be related to the fate of its plasma binding protein, ceruloplasmin. Interleukin-1 stimulates the liver to produce ceruloplasmin, among other acute phase reactants, as part of the stress response to injury; its concentration initially rises and then falls, presumably by leakage into the interstitium and through the wound, taking copper with it.[44] In addition, the elevation of hydrocortisone during the stress response promotes biliary excretion of copper.[46] Elevated plasma silver levels associated with the use of silver sulfadiazine have also been shown to diminish plasma ceruloplasmin levels and possibly antagonize copper directly.[47]

Superoxide dismutase, a free radical scavenger in the cytosol, contains zinc and copper. In a study of 12 burn patients randomized to receive polyethylene glycol-conjugated superoxide dismutase (PEG-SOD),[48] patients received either 500 or 1000 units of PEG-SOD per kilogram of body weight intravenously within 6 hours of injury. Conjugated dienes, a marker of oxygen radical-mediated tissue injury, were near control levels in the 1000 units/kg group for up to 200 hours after injury. Diene levels increased after 72 hours in the 500 units/kg group. Researchers concluded that PEG-SOD prevented conjugated diene formation from oxygen free radicals, with 1000 units/kg being more effective than 500 units/kg.

Zinc – Wound Healing, Role in Inflammation, and Antioxidant Properties

Zinc is necessary for the synthesis of RBP in the liver. This link to vitamin A metabolism potentially connects zinc availability to vitamin A functions. Zinc is a co-factor in ubiquitous metalloenzymes involved in deoxyribonucleic acid (DNA), ribonucleic acid (RNA) and protein synthesis, and is therefore important in wound healing. Zinc deficiency has adverse effects on the healing process[13] including: reduced epithelialization, reduced gain of wound strength, and decreased collagen strength. Supplemental zinc therapy has been shown to be beneficial in wound healing.[49] However, these results became inconsistent with later findings as more attention was paid to initial zinc status. The overall conclusion from the literature to date is that patients with initially normal serum levels of zinc do not experience a beneficial effect from zinc supplementation.[50,51] Zinc toxicity occurs with prolonged high dosing, including reduced absorption of copper.[52] Soy formulas have low bioavailability of zinc and decreased zinc absorption due to their high phytate content.[53]

Zinc is involved in immune function,[54,55] collagen metabolism, and synthesis of nucleic acids and proteins.[56–58] Burn patients are at risk for zinc deficiency. The hypermetabolic state present after major burn injury induces hyperzincuria reaching five times normal excretion.[56,59] Following tissue injury, a redistribution of zinc occurs. Zinc uptake is increased in the wound, liver, spleen, and lung while zinc levels decrease in plasma and skin.[56,60,61] Like copper, zinc is also a component of superoxide dismutase, and, therefore, also plays a role in supporting free radical scavenging activities.

Iron – Role in Inflammation

Serum iron concentration falls in response to injury or infection. Inflammation is associated with reduced intestinal iron absorption, a primary increase in ferritin synthesis, and a decreased rate of iron release from reticuloendothelial and parenchymal storage sites producing a state of low serum iron concentration and accumulation of iron in cellular ferritin stores.[62] The true significance of this effect is unclear. Microorganisms require iron to multiply, and some argue that hypoferremia is a protective response in an attempt to limit infection.[63] Neutrophils from iron deficient patients have impaired bactericidal action which can be restored with iron therapy; and cell-mediated immunity is also diminished in states of hypoferremia. Iron excess has also been shown to impair lymphocyte and neutrophil function. Optimal iron therapy remains undefined.[62]

Selenium

Glutathione peroxidase contains selenium at its active site and is dependent on adequate supplies of that element for its synthesis. This is the only known selenium-containing enzyme in humans. Its role is to protect cellular components from oxidative damage. Selenium also appears to affect metabolism and toxicity of a variety of drugs and chemicals and protects against the toxicity of silver, cadmium, and mercury.[64]

In an effort to elucidate the mechanism of protection of the cell from oxidative damage, plasma selenium, lipid peroxide and glutathione peroxidase (GSH-Px) activities were measured in thermally injured young pigs for 30 days.[65] Immediately postburn, mean lipid peroxide and GSH-Px activity decreased, while selenium concentration increased. After 3 weeks, lipid peroxide levels peaked, whereas GSH-Px and selenium were below levels noted at the beginning of the study. Selenium concentration directly correlated with GSH-Px activity and correlated inversely with lipid peroxide levels.

Therapeutic Implications

As mentioned at the beginning of the chapter, there are insufficient data to support guidelines for vitamin and trace element intake after burn injury.[1,2] While antioxidant status in burn injury appears to be relevant, the importance and specific needs for vitamin C and E, zinc, copper and selenium in the burn patient remain to be clarified. A survey of burn centers in the United States reported on vitamin supplementation practices.[66] Among the findings were that 87% of respondents routinely prescribed vitamins with 97% of those using a multivitamin preparation. Fifty-eight percent of multivitamin dosages exceeded 100% of the RDA. Most facilities also considered burn size, nutritional status prior to admission, and dietary intake in the decision to supplement. Ascorbic acid was prescribed in addition to multivitamin preparations in 72% of respondents. Additional vitamin A was given by 10% of respondents. Those who did not provide 100% of RDAs were believed to be providing enteral support which covered additional vitamin needs. Another separate survey of burn centers in North America was done regarding trace element supplementation practices.[67] Ninety percent of respondents prescribe or recommend trace elements for their burned patients. Criteria of 'higher risk', meaning burn size greater than 40% total body surface area (TBSA), use of total parenteral nutrition (TPN), advanced age, infancy, sepsis, ethanol abuse, or renal problems were cited as reasons why trace elements were supplemented. Trace elements most often supplemented were zinc, iron, copper, and, manganese. The report concluded that present guidelines for trace element supplementation are inadequate.

A proposed vitamin/trace element protocol is shown in **Table 24.2**; however, the interactions among nutrients and between drugs and nutrients require elucidation in burn-injured patients. Cognizance of physical signs of nutrient deficiency and excess is important but may not directly apply to evaluation of acutely burned patients (**Table 24.1**). When more traditional causes of symptoms of nutrient deficiency or excess are ruled out, nutritional status must be considered and investigated with appropriate nutritional laboratory tests. Burn centers need to evaluate how their overall treatment impacts on vitamin and trace element needs following burn injury.

Table 24.2 Proposed vitamin and mineral supplementation

Younger than 12 years
- Polyvisol 1 ml q.d. or chewable multivitamin 1 tablet q.d.
- Ascorbic acid 250 mg q.d.
- Folic acid 1 mg q.m.w.f.
- Vitamin A
  - < 2 years, 2500 IU
  - 2–12 years 5000 IU
- Zinc sulfate
  - < 2 years, 55 mg
  - 2–12 years, 110 mg
- Vitamin E 5 mg

Older than 12 years
- Vi-Daylin 10 ml q.d. or Theragran Multivitamin 1 tablet q.d.
- Ascorbic acid 500 mg q.d.
- Folic acid 1 mg q.m.w.f.
- Vitamin A 10 000 IU
- Zinc sulfate 200 mg
- Vitamin E 10 mg

REFERENCES

1. Gottschlich M M, Warden G D. Vitamin supplementation in the patient with burns. *J Burn Care Rehabil* 1990; **11**(3): 275–9.

2. Carvajal H F. Energy and protein metabolism in the pediatric burn patient. In: Suskind R M, LeWinter-Suskind L, eds. *Textbook of Pediatric Nutrition*. New York: Raven Press Ltd, 1993: 217–23.

3. Solomons N W, Keusch G T. Nutritional implications of parasitic infections. *Nutr Rev* 1981; **39:** 149–61.

4. Caldwell M D, Kennedy-Caldwell C, Winkler M F. Micronutrients and enteral nutrition. In: Rombeau J L, Caldwell M D, (eds). *Enteral and Tube Feeding*. 2nd ed. Philadelphia: W B Saunders Co, 1990: 73–117.

5. Cerra F B, Hypermetabolism, organ failure, and metabolic support. *Surgery* 1987; **101:** 1–14.

6. Demetriou A A, Levenson S M, Retture G, Seifter E. Vitamin A and retinoic acid: induced fibroblast differentiation in vitro. *Surgery* 1985; **98:** 931–34.

7. Goodson W H, Hunt T K. Wound healing. In: Kinney J M, Jeejeebhoy K N, Hill G L, Owen O E eds. *Nutrition and Metabolism in Patient Care*. Philadelphia: W B Saunders, 1988: 635–42.

8. Rai D, Courtemanche A D. Vitamin A assay in burned patients. *J. Trauma* 1975; **15:** 419–424.

9. Szenbeni A, Negyesi G, Fever L. Vitamin A levels in the serum of burned patients. *Burns* 1980; **7:** 313–18.

10. Gottschlich, M M, Warden G D, Michel M A, *et al.* Diarrhea in tube-fed burn patients: incidence, etiology, nutritional impact and prevention. *J Parenter Enteral Nutr* 1988; **12:** 338–45.

11. Mahalanabis D, Simpson T W, Chakraborty M L, Ganguli C, Bhattacharjee A K, Mukherjee K L. Malabsorption of water miscible vitamin A in children with giardiasis and ascariasis. *Am J Clin Nutr* 1979; **32:** 313–18.

12. Ahluwalia G S, Kaul L, Ahluwalia B S. Evidence of facilitory effect of growth hormone on tissue vitamin A uptake in rats. *J Nutr* 1980; **110:** 1185–93.

13. Effect of growth hormone on vitamin A storage and release (Experimental Nutrition). *Nutr Rev* 1981; **39:** 139–40.

14. Food and Nutrition Board. *Recommended Dietary Allowances*. 10th ed. Washington DC: National Academy Press, 1989.

15. Lund C C, Levenson S M, Green R W, *et al.* Ascorbic acid, thiamin, riboflavin and nicotinic acid in relation to acute burns in man. *Arch Surg* 1947; **55:** 557–83.

16. Cooperman J M Riboflavin. In: Machlin L J, ed. *Handbook of Vitamins: Nutritional Biochemical, and Clinical Aspects*. New York: Marcel Dekker Inc, 1984: 299–327

17. Pinto J, Huang Y P, Rivlin R S. Inhibition of riboflavin metabolism in rat tissues by chlorpromazine, imipramine, and amitriptyline. *J Clin Invest* 1981; **67:** 1500–06.

18. Belavady B, Strikantia S G, Gopalan C. The effect of the oral administration of leucine on the metabolism of tryptophan. *Biochem J* 1963; **87:** 652–5.

19. Compton M M, Cidlowski J A. Vitamin B and glucocorticoid action. *Endocr Rev* 1986; **7:** 140–8.

20. Linder M C. Nutrition and metabolism of vitamins. In: Linder M C, ed. *Nutritional Biochemistry and Metabolism with Clinical Applications*. 2nd ed. New York: Elsevier, 1991: 111–89.

21. Barlow G B, Wilkinson A W. Plasma pyridoxal phosphate levels and tryptophan metabolism in children with burns and scalds. *Clin Chim Acta* 1975; **64:** 79–82.

22. Benn A, Swan C H J, Cooke W T, Blair J A, Matty A J, Smith M E. Effect of intraluminal pH on the absorption of pteroylmonoglutamic acid. *BMJ* 1971; **1:** 148–50.

23. Mackenzie J F, Russell R I. The effect of pH on folic acid absorption in man. *Clin Sci Mol Med* 1976; **51:** 363–8.

24. Broquist H P, Borum P R. Carnitine biosynthesis; nutritional implications. *Adv Nutr Res* 1982; **4:** 181–204.

25. Demling R H, Katz A, Lalonde C, Ryan P, Tin L-J. The immediate effect of burn wound excision on pulmonary function in sheep: the role of prostanoids, oxygen radicals and chemoattractants. *Surgery* 1987; **101:** 44–5.

26. Till G O, Guilds L S, Mahrougui M, Friedl H P, Trentz O, Ward P A. Role of xanthine oxidase in thermal injury of skin. *Am J Pathol* 1989; **135:** 195–202.

27. Matsuda T, Tanaka H, Shimazaki S, *et al.* High dose vitamin C therapy for extensive deep dermal burns. *Burns* 1992; **18:** 127–31.

28. Tanaka H, Broaderick P, Shimazaki S, *et al.* How long do we need to give antioxidant therapy during resuscitation when its administration is delayed for two hours? *J Burn Care Rehabil* 1992; **13:** 567–72.

29. Combs G F. The Vitamins: Fundamental Aspects in Nutrition and Health. San Diego: Academic Press, Inc, 1992: 223–50.

30. Machlin L J, Langseth L. Vitamin–vitamin Interactions. In: Bodwell C E, Erdmand J W, eds. *Nutrient Interactions*. New York: Marcel Dekker, Inc, 1988: 287–312.

31. Ruberg R L. Role of nutrition in wound healing. *Surg Clin North Am* 1984; **64:** 705–14.

32. Shilotri P G. Glycolytic, hexose monophosphate shunt and bactericidal activities of leukocytes in ascorbic acid deficient guinea pigs. *J Nutr* 1977; **107:** 507–12.

33. Leibovitz B, Siegel B V. Ascorbic acid, neutrophil function and the immune response. *Int J Vitam Nutr Res* 1978; **48:** 159–64.

34. Till G O, Hatherill J R, Tourtellotte W W, Lutz M J, Ward P A. Lipid peroxidation and acute lung injury after thermal trauma to skin. Evidence of a role for hydroxyl radical. *Am J Pathol* 1985; **119:** 376–84.

35. Gasser H, Paul E, Redl H, *et al.* Loss of plasma antioxidants after burn injury. *Circ Shock* 1991; **34:** 13.

36. Redl H, Gasser H, Schlag G, Marzi I. Involvement of oxygen radicals in shock related cell injury. *B M J* 1993; **49:** 556–65.

37. Fang C H, Peck M D, Alexander J W, Babcock G F, Warden G D. The effect of free radical scavenger on outcome after infection in burned mice. *J Trauma* 1990; **30:** 453–6.

38. Grenier J F, Aprahamian M, Genot C, Dentinger A. Pantothenic acid (vitamin B_5) efficiency on wound healing. *Acta Vitaminol Enzymol* 1982; **4:** 81–5.

39. Pike R L, Brown M L. Minerals and water. *Nutrition: An Integrated Approach* 3rd ed. New York: Macmillan, 1984: 167–98.

40. Linder M C. Nutrition and metabolism of the trace elements. In: Linder M C, ed. *Nutritional Biochemistry and Metabolism with Clinical Applications.* 2nd ed. New York: Elsevier, 1991: 215–76.

41. Rutan R L, Herndon D N. Growth delay in post burn pediatric patients *Arch Surg* 1990; **125:** 392–5.

42. Underwood E J. *Trace Elements in Human and Animal Nutrition.* 3rd ed. New York: Academic Press, 1971.

43. Meydani S N, Hayek M, Coleman L. Influence of vitamins E and B_6 on immune response. *Ann NY Acad Sci* 1992; **669:** 125–40.

44. Brian J E, Caldwell F T, Wood R C. Hypocupremia in a major burn. *J Trauma* 1987; **27:** 335–6.

45. Boosalis M G, McCall I T, Solem L D. Serum copper and ceruloplasmin levels and urine copper excretion in thermal injury. *Am J Clin Nutr* 1986; **44:** 899–906.

46. Karcioglu Z A, Sarper R M, eds. *Zinc and Copper in Medicine.* Springfield, I L: Charles C Thomas, 1980.

47. Hill C H, Starcher B, Matrone G. Mercury and silver interrelationship with copper. *J Nutr* 1977; **107:** 1889–95.

48. Gottschlich M M. Micronutrients. In: Skipper A, ed. *Dietitian's Handbook of Enteral and Parenteral Nutrition.* Rockville: Aspen Publishers, Inc, 1989: 163–203.

49. Pories W J, Henzel J H, Rob C G, Strain W H. Acceleration of wound healing in man with zinc sulphate given by mouth. *Lancet* 1967; **1:** 121–4.

50. Barcia P J. Lack of acceleration of healing with zinc sulphate. *Ann Surg* 1970; **172:** 1048–50.

51. Husain S L, Fell B S, Scott R. Zinc and healing. *Lancet* 1970; **2:** 1361–2.

52. Mills C F. Dietary interactions involving the trace elements. *Ann Rev Nutr* 1985; **5:** 173–93.

53. Lonnerdal B, Bell J G, Hendrickx A G, Burns R A, Keen C L. Effect of phytate removal on zinc absorption from soy formula *Am J Clin Nutr* 1988; **48:** 1301–6.

54. Fraker P J, Haas S M, Luecke R W. Effect of zinc deficiency on the immune response of the young adult A/J mouse. *J Nutr* 1977; **107:** 1889–95.

55. Prasad A S. Clinical endocrinological and biochemical effects of zinc deficiency. *Clin Endocrinol Metab* 1986; **3:** 567–89.

56. Ronaghy H A. The role of zinc in human nutrition. *World Rev Nutr Diet* 1987; **54:** 237–254.

57. Prasad A S. Clinical endocrinological and biochemical effects of zinc deficiency. *Clin Endocrinol Metab* 1986; **3:** 567–89.

58. Liszewski R F. The effect of zinc on wound healing: a collective review. *J Am Osteopath Assoc* 1981; **81:** 104.

59. Prasad A S. Zinc in growth and development and spectrum of human zinc deficiency. *J Am Coll Nutr* 1988; **7:** 377–84.

60. Henzel J H, DeWesse M S, Lichti E L. Zinc concentrations within healing wounds. Significance of post operative zincuria on availability and requirements during tissue repair. *Arch Surg* 1970; **100:** 349–57.

61. Okada A, Takgi Nezu R, Lee S. Zinc in clinical surgery – a research review. *Jpn J Surg* 1990; **20:** 635–44.

62. Peto T E A, Hershko C. Iron and infection. *Bailliere's Clin Haematol* 1989; **20:** 435–55.

63. Weinberg E D. Infection and iron metabolism. *Am J Clin Nutr* 1977; **30:** 1485–90.

64. Levander O A, Cheng L. *Micronutrient Interactions: Vitamins Minerals and Hazardous Elements.* New York: Academy of Sciences, 1980: 335–72.

65. Bienkowski W, Gromadzinska J, Powowicz Z, *et al.* Concentrations of selenium and lipid peroxides and glutathione peroxidase activities in plasma of thermally injured pigs. *Acta Chir Plast* 1991; **33:** 126–32.

66. King N, Goodwin W. Use of vitamin supplements for burned patients: a national survey. *J Am Diet Assoc* 1984; **84:** 923–925.

67. Shippee R L, Wilson S W, King N. Trace mineral supplementation of burn patients: a national survey. *J Am Diet Assoc* 1987; **87:** 300–3.

68. Kight M A. The nutrition physical examination. New York: Council on Renal Nutrition Quarterly (*CRN Q*) 1987; **11**(3): 9–12.

69. Figueroa-Colon R. Clinical and laboratory assessment of the malnourished child. In: Suskind R M, Lewinter-Suskind L, eds. *Textbook of Pediatric Nutrition* New York: Raven Press Ltd, 1993: 195.

CHAPTER TWENTY-FIVE

HYPOPHOSPHATEMIA*

DAVID W. MOZINGO AND ARTHUR D. MASON, JR

Certain humoral and metabolic responses to thermal and mechanical trauma which maintain homeostasis and prevent cellular dysfunction also produce alterations in electrolyte balance. An example of such an alteration involves renal retention of sodium during the resuscitative phase of burn injury, which alters sodium balance in the course of preserving intravascular volume. Despite the markedly increased cardiac output and renal plasma flow which occur in the subsequent flow phase, a decrease in blood volume persists and results in sustained elevation of plasma renin activity, secretion of antidiuretic hormone, and sodium retention.[1]

Conversely, the severe hypophosphatemia which often follows major injury occurs concomitantly with a 50–100% increase in resting energy expenditure, leading to a possible deficiency in the high energy phosphate compounds essential for cellular metabolism. Thermal injury induces a precipitous decrease in serum phosphate concentration which reaches its nadir between the second and fifth postburn days. This phenomenon has been recognized for quite some time[2] and was recently confirmed by the authors in a large series of burned patients.[3] Despite aggressive phosphorus supplementation, normal levels of serum phosphorus are rarely reached prior to the tenth postburn day (**Figure 25.1**). Of 550 patients studied, 175 had serum phosphorus concentrations below 2.0 mg/dl, and of these 49 were below 1.0 mg/dl, with the lower limit of normal serum phosphorus being 3.0 mg/dl. Such hypophosphatemia is not exclusive to thermal injury, having been described following multiple trauma[4] and elective surgery.[5] The exact mechanism by which thermal injury or severe stress induces hypophosphatemia is unknown. Several events associated with burn injury, however, affect phosphorus metabolism, and these may combine to produce hypophosphatemia.

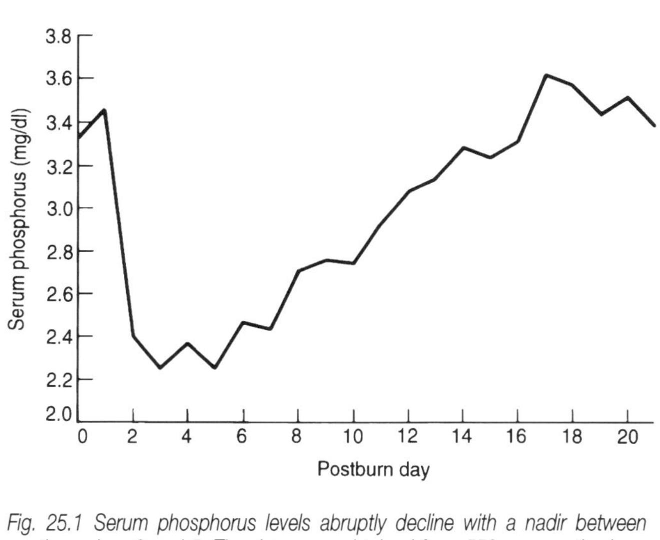

Fig. 25.1 Serum phosphorus levels abruptly decline with a nadir between postburn days 2 and 5. The data were obtained from 550 consecutive burn patients admitted to the US Army Institute of Surgical Research.

* From the US Army Institute of Surgical Research, Fort Sam Houston, Texas, USA. The opinions or assertions contained herein are the private views of the authors and are not to be construed as official or as reflecting the views of the Department of the Army or the Department of Defense.

ETIOLOGY OF POSTBURN HYPOPHOSPHATEMIA

Many of the pathophysiologic changes and therapeutic interventions which occur during the first postburn week influence serum phosphorus concentration (**Table 25.1**). Hypophosphatemia does not necessarily imply phosphorus depletion. In the case of burn injury, most patients are healthy prior to injury and presumably have normal phosphorus stores. Nor do simple calculations of phosphate balance explain the dramatic decrease in serum levels; simultaneous reduction of urinary phosphate excretion is observed, suggesting an extrarenal mechanism. The fractional excretion of phosphate, however, increases during the early period of diuresis following burn injury (postburn days 2–4), potentially contributing to the decline in serum levels. The pathophysiologic events and therapeutic interventions discussed below are associated with hypophosphatemia in other disease states and in certain experimental animal models; but the extent of their contributions to the postburn decrease in serum phosphorus has not been critically evaluated and is, at present, undefined.

Table 25.1 Possible causes of postburn hypophosphatemia

Fluid resuscitation	
	Volume loading
	Lactate administration
Carbohydrate administration	
	Enteral alimentation
	Parenteral hyperalimentation
	5% Dextrose
Elevated catecholamines	
Phosphate-binding antacids/sucralfate	
Acid–base disturbance	
Electrolyte imbalance	
	Hypokalemia
	Hypomagnesemia
	Hypocalcemia
Carbonic anhydrase inhibition (mafenide acetate)	

Stress Response

In the early postburn period, the classic 'fight or flight' response occurs, with elevation of plasma catecholamines, glucose, glucagon, and cortisol. Exogenous epinephrine administration has been associated with the development of hypophosphatemia and the profound catecholamine release accompanying thermal injury may contribute to the early decrease in serum phosphorus. The mechanism by which this occurs is uncertain but may be a consequence of the accompanying hyperglycemia resulting in a redistribution of phosphorus from the extracellular to the intracellular compartment. In acute clinical states of glucagon excess, tubular reabsorption of phosphate is impaired in both the proximal and distal nephron, leading one to expect renal phosphate wastage.[6] Since urinary excretion of phosphate is usually decreased in the early post-injury period, the importance of hyperglucagonemia remains uncertain. Administration of pharmacologic doses of glucocorticoids enhances phosphorus excretion and impairs phosphate absorption by the gut and reabsorption by the kidney. Whether or not the adrenocortical response significantly contributes to the hypophosphatemia following burn injury is not known.

Resuscitation and Topical Therapy

Administration of large doses of sodium lactate for initial burn resuscitation may decrease the serum phosphorus concentration by several mechanisms.[7] Lactate is converted to glucose in the liver, a process requiring high energy phosphate availability. Additionally, though it does not usually occur clinically, metabolic alkalosis induced by lactate infusion may result in depression of serum phosphorus concentration. Alkalosis is associated with an increase in glycolysis which promotes transfer of phosphorus to the intracellular space. During resuscitation, alkalemia is uncommon and patients are more likely to manifest a mild metabolic acidosis which is compensated by hyperventilation, resulting in a normal or mildly alkaline blood pH. Acidosis markedly inhibits renal phosphate reabsorption, resulting in phosphaturia. The contribution of this mechanism to postburn hypophosphatemia is probably minor; early renal phosphate wastage is not observed, perhaps being obscured by diminished glomerular filtration early in burn injury. In addition, the *p*-carboxy metabolite of mafenide acetate strongly inhibits carbonic anhydrase. Such inhibition diminishes proximal tubular reabsorption of phosphate and probably occurs following topical burn wound treatment with mafenide, but the magnitude of the effect is unknown.

Expansion of the extracellular fluid volume is also associated with inhibition of proximal tubular phosphate reabsorption. A tight coupling exists between sodium and phosphate transport across the renal epithelial cell. In patients with burns, mobilization and excretion of the large edema volume usually begins by the second postburn day and continues throughout the next week to 10 days. In contrast to the relative paucity of phosphate excretion during the first 24 hours following injury when glomerular filtration is markedly reduced, a modest loss of phosphate may occur with diuresis of the edema fluid. In fact, the diuretic phase is associated with an increase in the fractional excretion of phosphate despite a concomitant reduction in the serum phosphate concentration.[8] Phosphorus excretion during the natriuretic phase of early burn injury is consistent with the tight coupling observed in other diuretic states.

Ulcer Prophylaxis

Effective prophylaxis against Curling's ulcers with H_2 antagonists and antacid buffering has been a mainstay of burn care for the past two decades. Significant degrees of hypophosphatemia and phosphate depletion occur during continuous or chronic administration of phosphate-binding agents containing magnesium, calcium, and aluminum. These agents bind not only dietary phosphate, but also phosphate secreted into the intestinal lumen, often resulting in a net negative phosphate balance. The severity of such hypophosphatemia clearly depends on the dose of phosphate-binding agents, dietary phosphorus intake, and preexisting phosphate balance. To reduce alimentary scavenging of dietary and secreted phosphate, buffering with antacids containing aluminum phosphate salts ($AlPO_4$), which do not bind any additional phosphate, may be utilized. Sucralfate, which is also effective in preventing upper gastrointestinal stress ulceration following thermal injury, is not a buffering agent, but as a complex salt of aluminum hydroxide, it is capable of binding phosphate. Its administration has also been associated with the development of hypophosphatemia in critically ill patients.[9]

Hyperventilation

Respiratory alkalosis is often present during the first week postburn and may be enhanced by anxiety or pain, and even by the inhibition of carbonic anhydrase induced by mafenide acetate burn cream. As fluid resuscitation progresses, respiratory rate and tidal volume progressively increase, resulting in a minute ventilation which may be twice normal. Mild hyperventilation induces only a slight decline of serum phosphorus levels; prolonged, intense hyperventilation, however, may result in serum phosphorus values less than 1.0 mg/dl.[10] During respiratory alkalosis, phosphorus virtually disappears from the urine, eliminating renal losses as the causative mechanism. Respiratory alkalosis induces a rapid movement of carbon dioxide from the intracellular to the extracellular space. Intracellular pH increases, activating glycolysis and increasing the formation of intracellular phosphorylated carbohydrate compounds. The readily diffusible inorganic phosphate pool supplies the required phosphorus; serum phosphorus concentrations consequently fall abruptly. The extent to which this mechanism contributes to postburn hypophosphatemia is also uncertain.

Metabolic Support

Administration of carbohydrates may play a major role in the development of postburn hypophosphatemia. Infusion of glucose solutions or oral intake of carbohydrates produces mild hypophosphatemia in healthy individuals. This decrease in serum phosphate is associated with an increase of inorganic phosphate, ATP, and glucose 6-phosphate in muscle cells. The mechanism by which such carbohydrate administration induces hypophosphatemia is somewhat speculative. Experience with phosphate-deficient total parenteral nutrition and subsequent development of hypophosphatemia has provided some insight into the etiology.[11,12] As carbohydrates are absorbed, insulin secretion increases, shifting phosphorus from the extracellular to the intracellular space. If phosphate reserve is low, ATP is poorly regenerated since hypophosphatemia inhibits glucose 3-phosphate dehydrogenase. Inorganic phosphates in the intracellular pool become further diminished because of incorporation, initially as newly synthesized ATP, but eventually as triose phosphates when the ATP is consumed in the hexokinase reaction. Glucose utilization by red blood cells requires ATP at the hexokinase and phosphofructokinase steps, but regeneration of ATP does not occur during phosphate deficiency or acute hypophosphatemia due to a block at the glucose 3-phosphate dehydrogenase step. In states of phosphate depletion, the scant phosphate which enters the red blood cell is incorporated into 1,3-diphosphoglycerate, but most is diverted to 2,3-diphosphoglycerate, also preventing complete glycolysis to regain the ATP consumed.

In thermally injured patients, infusion of dextrose-containing solutions usually begins 24 hours postburn; enteral nutrition, in which most of the calories are supplied as carbohydrates, is initiated within several days of injury. These interventions are temporally correlated with the rapid descent of serum phosphorus concentrations. In other clinical states, severe hypophosphatemia following the initiation of enteral or parenteral nutrition is most commonly associated with the feeding of patients with advanced protein-calorie malnutrition. When total body phosphorus is depleted by starvation, serum phosphorus levels usually remain normal, but carbohydrate administration produces a rapid marked decline in serum phosphorus concentration. If untreated, this may result in multisystem organ dysfunction, respiratory and cardiac failure, or death. Thermally injured patients are usually well nourished prior to burn injury; the clinical scenario of refeeding hypophosphatemia may not apply to them. Similar findings, however, have been recently described in previously well nourished surgical intensive care unit patients in whom the initiation of isotonic enteral feedings resulted in a decrease of serum phosphorus from normal levels to approximately 1 mg/dl, a level which is considered to be dangerously low and requires prompt supplementation.[13] In addition, the authors have recently reported that hypophosphatemia in thermally injured patients is exacerbated by the initiation of enteral feeding and occurs regardless of the postburn day when feeding is initiated.[3] This further reduction of serum phosphorus during the first postburn week, when levels are already low, may be particularly hazardous and speaks for aggressive phosphorus supplementation prior to and during the initiation of enteral alimentation.

Wound Healing

In patients recovering from thermal injury, the burn wound itself may act as a significant phosphorus sink. Despite the overall catabolism accompanying major injury and loss of lean body mass, healing burn wounds and skin grafts are anabolic and require phosphorus for normal repair. In addition, the continued loss of fluid and protein through the burn wound surface is a potential source of unquantified phosphorus loss and may contribute to hypophosphatemia.

Other Electrolytes

Disorders of electrolyte balance may also contribute to the development of hypophosphatemia. Experimental magnesium deficiency in animals may lead to phosphaturia and phosphorus deficiency, but intentional magnesium deficiency in man results in no change or a slight rise in serum phosphate.[14,15] In chronic alcoholics, however, hypomagnesemia and hypophosphatemia are coexistent. Hypokalemia, which is also exacerbated by magnesium deficiency, may result in phosphate wasting and hypophosphatemia. The mechanism is uncertain, but it may be related to coexistent metabolic alkalosis, diuretic use, or an underlying illness. Changes in calcium and phosphate homeostasis, and in the regulating hormones, calcitonin and parathyroid hormone, have been described following thermal injury.[16] Coincident with the early depression of serum phosphorus, the fraction of ionized calcium was shown to decrease and remain low, but within the normal range, for the 14 postburn days studied. Urinary calcium output was low, about 4.5 mmol/day, and urinary phosphate output was as high as 30 mmol/day, despite a low serum phosphorus. Serum calcitonin levels were significantly elevated for up to 2 weeks post injury, whereas parathyroid hormone remained within the normal range. The magnitude of the contribution of the classic regulating hormones of calcium and phosphorus homeostasis to the observed decrease in serum phosphorus following severe injury is not known with certainty. Catecholamines and glucagon are known to induce an increase in calcitonin secretion, and the administration of pharmacologic doses of calcitonin results in phosphaturia. A direct effect of calcitonin on phosphate transport in the nephron has been demonstrated. In those burned patients, it was notable that ionized calcium decreased slightly, though still within the normal range, despite very high levels of calcitonin and normal parathyroid hormone concentrations. A slight, though statistically significant, increase in parathyroid hormone was observed around the fourth postburn day and may be related, albeit indirectly through calcium regulation, to the observed postburn decrease in serum phosphorus concentration.

Summary

Clearly, multiple factors influence the serum phosphorus level following burn injury. Fluid resuscitation and subsequent mobilization of interstitial edema fluids, catecholamine excess, respiratory alkalosis, the use of phosphate-binding antacids or sucralfate, hypokalemia, hypomagnesemia, and the initiation of enteral nutrition have all been associated with hypophosphatemia in other illnesses and experimental models. All or most of these factors may be encountered in the early treatment of burned patients and the contribution and relative importance of individual factors to the depression of serum phosphorus is difficult to analyse. Most likely, carbohydrate administration, respiratory alkalosis, and diuresis of edema fluid are the more important etiologic factors contributing to hypophosphatemia in the early postburn course.

Consequences of Hypophosphatemia

The clinical manifestations of hypophosphatemia (**Figure 25.2**) are mainly those of organ system hypofunction. These responses have been defined through clinical observation and laboratory studies in circumstances in which hypophosphatemia occurred as a relatively isolated event. Phosphorus supplementation has been reported to reverse these abnormalities, suggesting a cause and effect relationship. Hypofunction of organ systems associated with phosphorus

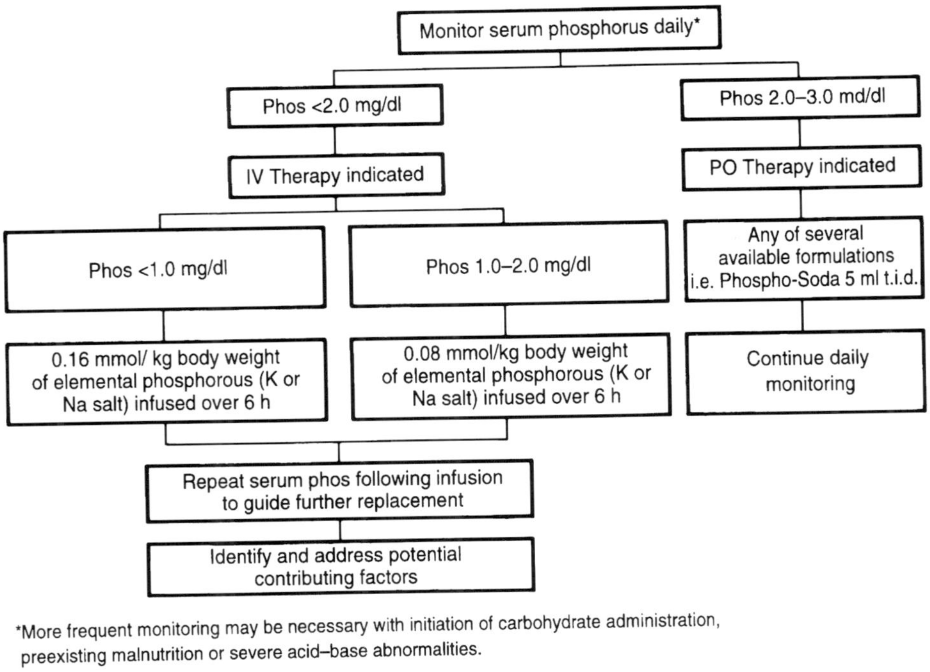

Fig. 25.2 The use of this algorithm permits prompt detection and timely correction of hypophosphatemia following burn injury.

depletion has been attributed to a lack of available inorganic phosphate for synthesis of high energy phosphorus compounds, so breakdown of stored ATP occurs, and the inorganic phosphate is diverted to other intracellular pathways.

Organ system dysfunction following thermal injury is characterized by early hypofunction and later hyperfunction of most organ systems. Whether hypophosphatemia contributes significantly to the early postburn depression of function which occurs in multiple organs is not known. Clearly, some of the clinical manifestations enumerated in **Table 25.2** are commonly observed in thermally injured patients, while others are not usually associated with such injury. Most patients reported to have had complications of hypophosphatemia have also had a coexistent severe illness. It is important to remember that prior cellular injury has been a prerequisite in most instances in which hypophosphatemia has been implicated as a cause of organ system dysfunction. The following discussions of organ system abnormalities should be interpreted in the light of the specific circumstances under which the observations were made.

Table 25.2 Clinical manifestations of hypophosphatemia

CNS
Lethargy, malaise, neuropathy, seizures, coma
Cardiovascular
Impaired cardiovascular contractility
Decreased response to pressor agents
Hypotension
Acute cardiac decompensation
Pulmonary
Tachypnea
Decreased vital capacity
Respiratory failure
Gastrointestinal
Anorexia, dysphagia
Renal
Glycosuria, calciuria, magnesuria, renal tubular, acidosis
Musculoskeletal
Weakness, myalgia, arthralgia, rhabdomyolysis

Cardiac Dysfunction

Although the early depression of cardiac function following burn injury has been attributed to an initial decrease in circulating blood volume, the search for intrinsic myocardial depression following burn injury and for mediators of such depression continues. In experimental studies and in clinical material, a correlation between hypophosphatemia and cardiac decompensation has been reported. Cardiac output, measured by bolus thermodilution, was impaired in seven critically ill hypophosphatemic patients and improved significantly with phosphorus supplementation.[4] In one experimental study, myocardial contractility was impaired by phosphorus deficiency and reversed by phosphorus repletion, suggesting that phosphorus deficiency may be a cause of heart failure in certain clinical conditions.[17] Despite these reports, there appears to be little evidence that hypophosphatemic cardiomyopathy is a frequently encountered clinical entity; most patients in whom this mechanism is invoked have already had a number of other causes for myocardial dysfunction.[18]

Neuromuscular Dysfunction

Varying degrees of areflexic paralysis, paresthesias, sensory loss, weakness, and respiratory insufficiency have been reported to be associated with acute hypophosphatemia, usually induced with feeding malnourished patients.[11] A reduction in available ATP to support respiratory muscle contraction has been suggested as a mechanism for acute respiratory failure, and diaphragmatic contractility has been reported to improve with phosphorus repletion in mechanically ventilated hypophosphatemic patients.[19] Profound generalized muscle weakness associated with isolated phosphorus depletion has been observed in both clinical and laboratory studies.[20,21] In a study of hypophosphatemia and muscle phosphate metabolism in patients with burns or mechanical trauma, no direct correlation was demonstrated between the serum phosphorus concentration and the high energy phosphate content of muscle cells; however, all these patients were receiving phosphorus supplementation during the study.[22] If acute hypophosphatemia is superimposed on preexisting cellular injury, potentially reversible muscle cell dysfunction may extend to irreversible necrosis.[23] Several authors have reported severe rhabdomyolysis associated with severe hypophosphatemia following burns and major trauma.[24,25] This spectacular clinical event is rare but may occur to a lesser, subclinical, extent in critically ill patients.[23,26] Hypophosphatemia as the underlying etiology may often be dismissed since muscle cell destruction results in release of phosphate and elevation of serum phosphorus. In the absence of significant hemochromogenuria, the diagnosis may not even be suspected. Further investigation is required to determine whether this 'asymptomatic' rhabdomyolysis is, in fact, an important clinical entity, or merely an obligate manifestation of critical illness.

Hematologic Dysfunction

When untreated, severe hypophosphatemia may lead to red blood cell dysfunction by alterations in cell shape, survival, and physiologic function. Lack of high energy phosphate results in a decrease in erythrocyte 2,3-diphosphoglycerate and a subsequent leftward shift of the dissociation curve, with a consequent risk of tissue hypoxia.[6] Clinical hypophosphatemia, with or without previous phosphate depletion, results in reduced production of 2,3-diphosphoglycerate, erythrocyte ATP, and other phosphorylated intermediates of red blood cell glycolysis. In a variety of experimental and clinical situations, including burn injury and mechanical trauma, red blood cell 2,3-diphosphoglycerate has been shown to be reduced in the presence of hypophosphatemia.[27,28] In thermally injured patients, it has been demonstrated that postburn disturbance of red cell phosphate metabolism may be prevented by administration of phosphorus in the early postburn course.[28] Hypophosphatemia has also been associated with decreased red cell survival and decreased red cell deformability, and with impaired capillary transit and the potential for further deficiency of tissue oxygenation.

White blood cell dysfunction has also been observed as a result of hypophosphatemia induced by the initiation of phosphate-free parenteral nutrition and was associated with depressed chemotactic, phagocytic, and bactericidal activity of granulocytes.[29] A reduction in granulocyte ATP content was also documented, and amelioration of these white blood cell abnormalities was coincident with phosphorus repletion. Any correlation between these observations and an increased risk of infection remains speculative for hypophosphatemic patients in general and burn patients in particular.

Summary

Though it is clear that organ system dysfunction may be a manifestation of severe untreated hypophosphatemia, the relationship between these specific abnormalities and those observed in either the hypodynamic or the hyperdynamic phases of burn injury remains unclear. Clinical experience dictates that even when severe hypophosphatemia is avoided, the scenario of early organ system hypofunction and later hyperfunction persists. This is not to say that the marked hypophosphatemia observed following burn injury is part and parcel to the disease process, without bearing on the postburn physiologic response, but that, thus far, the pathophysiologic milieu following thermal injury has not permitted definition of the contribution of hypophosphatemia to the overall postburn response. Until cause and effect relationships are defined through ongoing research, aggressive phosphorus repletion should be approached cautiously following thermal injury. Such therapy does, however, clearly ameliorate red blood cell 2,3-diphosphoglycerate depletion which, in and of itself, supports treatment.

Prevention and Treatment of Hypophosphatemia

An unequivocal recommendation to treat hypophosphatemia in thermally injured patients should be supported by evidence that the treatment is of benefit. Such evidence is somewhat lacking in thermally injured patients, but in many analogous instances of hypophosphatemia from other causes, a direct benefit has been ascribed to repletion.

Serum phosphorus levels should be measured daily during the early phase of burn care and intravenous phosphate repletion should be initiated when levels drop below 2.0 mg/dl (**Figure 25.2**). Most of the severe adverse effects of hypophosphatemia occur with concentrations below 1.0 mg/dl, and this replacement strategy should prevent the development of clinically significant hypophosphatemia. Correction of severe hypophosphatemia with serum phosphorus levels less than 1.0 mg/dl requires intravenous replacement, usually with solutions of sodium or potassium phosphate containing 0.16 mmol/kg body weight (5 mg/kg body weight) of elemental phosphorus over 6 hours. The dose may be halved for patients with serum phosphorus levels between 1.0 and 2.0 mg/dl. Following completion of the infusion, a repeat serum phosphorus determination should be obtained, and further treatment should be based on the post-infusion plasma concentration. A potential hazard associated with intravenous administration of phosphate salts is hyperphosphatemia, which may induce metastatic deposition of calcium phosphate salts and hypocalcemia. Additionally, when potassium phosphate salts are used, care must be taken to avoid excessive or too rapid administration of potassium. Phosphorus replacement should be carefully monitored and should proceed with great caution in patients with impaired renal function or evidence of soft tissue injury or necrosis.

Prevention of hypophosphatemia may be facilitated by beginning oral phosphorus replacement prior to interventions such as the initiation of either enteral or parenteral carbohydrate administration, gastric acid neutralization with phosphate binding antacids or sucralfate, and the administration of diuretics. The nadir of serum phosphorus concentration typically occurs between 3 and 5 days postburn, during the period of edema mobilization; the need to initiate phosphorus supplementation should be anticipated in this interval. Additionally, to temper the gastrointestinal losses due to administration of phosphate-binding antacids, substitution of, or alternation with, antacids containing aluminum phosphate should be considered.

For mild asymptomatic hypophosphatemia or for prophylaxis when worsening of hypophosphatemia is expected, oral supplementation with any of several available formulations is recommended. Five milliliters of Phospho-Soda, containing 4.2 mmol/ml of elemental phosphorus, is commonly administered three times daily. Correction of other electrolyte abnormalities, most notably hypomagnesemia, hypocalcemia, and hypokalemia, as well as maintenance of acid–base normality, may prevent further renal phosphate losses and maintain the extracellular phosphate pool. After the tenth postburn day, the phosphorus delivered in standard liquid enteral formulas and hospital diets is usually sufficient to maintain serum phosphorus levels above 3.0 mg/dl.

SUMMARY

Thermal injury induces a precipitous decrease in serum phosphate concentration which reaches its nadir between the second and fifth postburn days. This phenomenon has been recognized for some time, but interest in the problem has been limited. The organ system dysfunctions induced by hypophosphatemia are in many ways similar to certain of the pathophysiologic changes observed following burn injury. The contribution of hypophosphatemia to these manifestations remains undefined. Wound fluid losses, increased circulating catecholamines, intracellular phosphate redistribution, and increased fractional excretion of urinary phosphate, as well as iatrogenic induction of hypophosphatemia through various therapeutic interventions, have been implicated as contributing to postburn hypophosphatemia. Frequent serum phosphate measurement and prompt phosphorus replacement when hypophosphatemia is recognized should minimize any sequelae of this potentially deleterious electrolyte deficiency.

REFERENCES

1. Cioffi W G, Vaughan G M, Heironimus J D, Jordan B S, Mason A D Jr, Pruitt B A Jr. Dissociation of blood volume and flow in regulation of salt and water balance in burn patients. *Ann Surg* 1991; **214**(3): 213–18.

2. Nordstrom H, Lennquist S, Lindell B, Sjoberg H E. Hypophosphataemia in severe burns. *Acta Chir Scand* 1977; **143:** 395–9.

3. Mozingo D W, Cioffi W G, Mason A D Jr, Milner E A, McManus W F, Pruitt B A Jr. Initiation of continuous enteral feeding induces hypophosphatemia in thermally injured patients. *Proceedings of the 35th World Congress of Surgery/International Society of Surgery/International Surgical Week.* 22–27 August 1993.

4. O'Connor L R, Weeler W S, Bethune J E. Effects of hypophosphatemia on myocardial performance in man. *N Engl J Med* 1977; **297:** 901.

5. England P C, Duari M, Tweedle D E T, Jones A, Gowland E. Postoperative hypophosphatemia. *Br J Surg* 1979; **66:** 340.

6. Lau K. Phosphate disorders. In: Kokko J P, Tannen R L, eds. *Fluids and Electrolytes.* Philadelphia, PA: WB Saunders Company, 1986: 398–471.

7. Knochel J P. The pathophysiology and clinical characteristics of severe hypophosphatemia. *Arch Intern Med* 1977; **137:** 203–20.

8. Lennquist S, Lindell B, Nordstrom H, Sjoberg H E. Hypophosphatemia in severe burns: a prospective study. *Acta Chir Scand* 1979; **145:** 1–6.

9. Miller S J, Simpson J. Medication–nutrient interactions: hypophosphatemia associated with sucralfate in the intensive care unit. *Nutr Clin Pract* 1991; **6:** 199–201.

10. Mostellar M E, Tuttle E P Jr. The effects of alkylosis on plasma concentration and urinary excretion of inorganic phosphate in man. *J Clin Invest.* 1964; **43:** 138–49.

11. Solomon S M, Kirby D F. The refeeding syndrome: a review. *J Parenter Enteral Nutr* 1990; **14**(1): 90–7.

12. Sheldon G F, Grzyb S. Phosphate depletion and repletion: relation to parenteral nutrition and oxygen transport. *Ann Surg* 1975; **182**(6): 683–9.

13. Hayek M E, Eisenberg P G. Severe hypophosphatemia following the institution of enteral feedings. *Arch Surg* 1989; **124:** 1325–8.

14. Whang R, Welt L G. Observations in experimental magnesium depletion. *J Clin Invest* 1963; **42:** 305–13.

15. Shils M E. Experimental human magnesium depletion. *Medicine* 1969; **48:** 61–82.

16. Loven L, Nordstrom H, Lennquist S. Changes in calcium and phosphate and their regulating hormones in patients with severe burn injuries. *Scand J Plast Reconstr Surg* 1984; **18:** 49–53.

17. Fuller T J, Nichols W W, Brenner B J, Peterson J C. Reversible depression in myocardial performance in dogs with experimental phosphorus deficiency. *J Clin Invest* 1978; **62:** 1194–2000.

18. Knochel J P. The clinical status of hypophosphatemia. *N Engl J Med* 1985; **313**(7): 447–9.

19. Aubier M, Murciano D, Lecocguic Y, *et al.* Effect of hypophosphatemia on diaphragmatic contractility in patients with acute respiratory failure. *N Engl J Med* 1985; **313:** 420–4.

20. Lotz M, Nay R, Bartter F C. Osteomalacia and debility resulting from phosphorus depletion. *Trans Assoc Am Physicians* 1964; **77:** 281–95.

21. Lotz M, Zisman E, Bartter F C. Evidence for a phosphorus depletion syndrome in man. *N Engl J Med* 1968; **278:** 409.

22. Loven L, Lennquist S, Liljedahl S O. Hypophosphataemia and muscle phosphate metabolism in severely injured patients. *Acta Chir Scand* 1983; **149:** 743–9.

23. Knochel J P, Barcenas C, Cotton J R, Fuller T J, Haller R, Carter N W. Hypophosphatemia and rhabdomyolysis. *J Clin Invest* 1978; **62:** 1240–6.

24. Guechot J, Cynober L, Lioret N, Betourne C, Saizy R, Giboudeau J. Rhabdomyolysis and, acute renal failure in a patient with thermal injury. *Intensive Care Med* 1986; **12:** 159–60.

25. Pfeifer P M. Acute rhabdomyolysis following surgery for burns. *Anaesthesia* 1986; **41:** 614–19.

26. Singhal P C, Kumar A, Desroches L, Gibbons N, Mattana J. Prevalence and predictors of rhabdomyolysis in patients with hypophosphatemia. *Am J Med* 1992; **92:** 458–64.

27. Loven L, Anderson E, Larsson J, Lennquist S. Muscular high-energy phosphates and red-cell 2.3-DPG in post-traumatic hypophosphataemia. *Acta Chir Scand* 1983: **149:** 735–41.

28. Loven L, Larsson L, Nordstrom H, Lennquist S. Serum phosphate and 2, 3-diphosphoglycerate in severely burned patients after phosphate supplementation. *J Trauma* 1986; **26**(4): 348–52.

29. Craddock P R, Yawata Y, VanSanten L, Gilberstadt S, Silvis S, Jacob H S. Acquired phagocyte dysfunction a complication of the hypophosphatemia of parenteral hyperalimentation. *N Engl J Med* 1974; **290**(25): 1403–7.

(a)

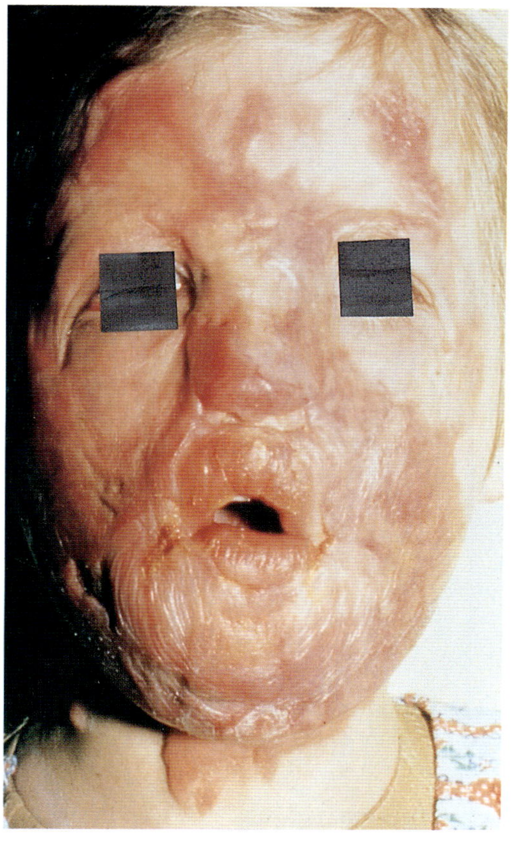

(b)

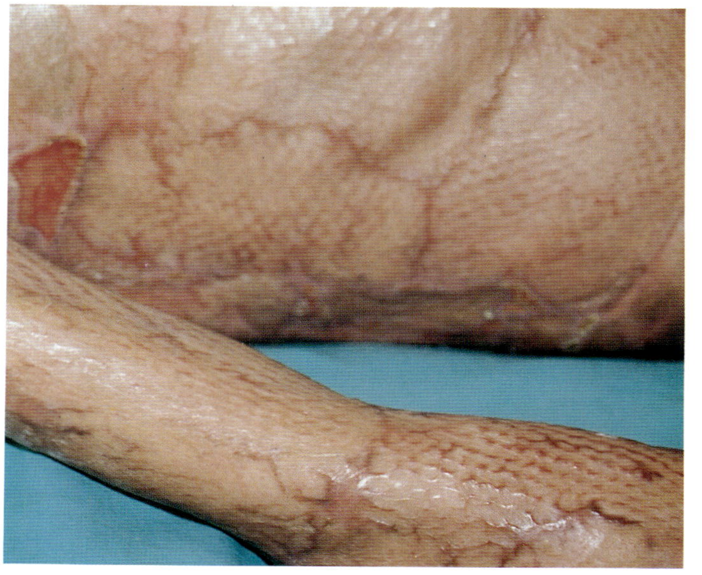

Plate 1: (**a**) Hypertrophic scar in a spontaneously healed deep dermal burn. (**b**) Showing the scar hypertrophy at the perimeter and in the interstices of meshed, expanded skin grafts.

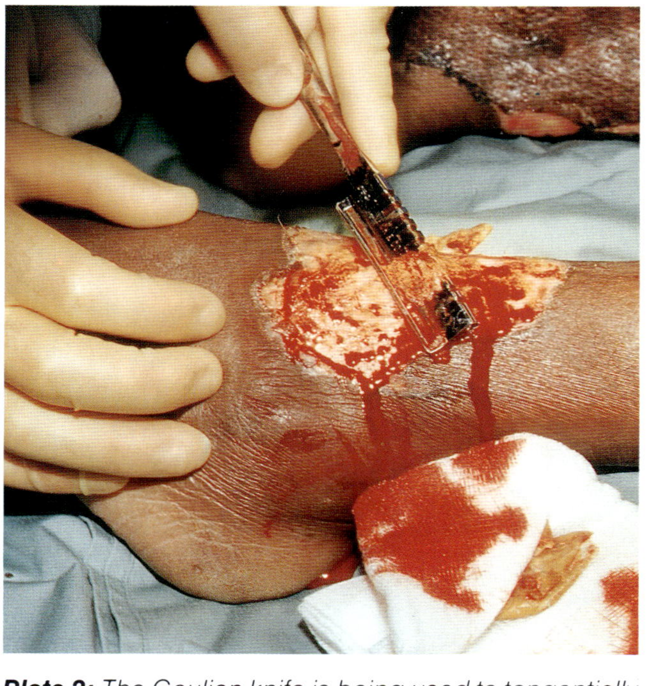

Plate 2: The Goulian knife is being used to tangentially excise a deep burn.

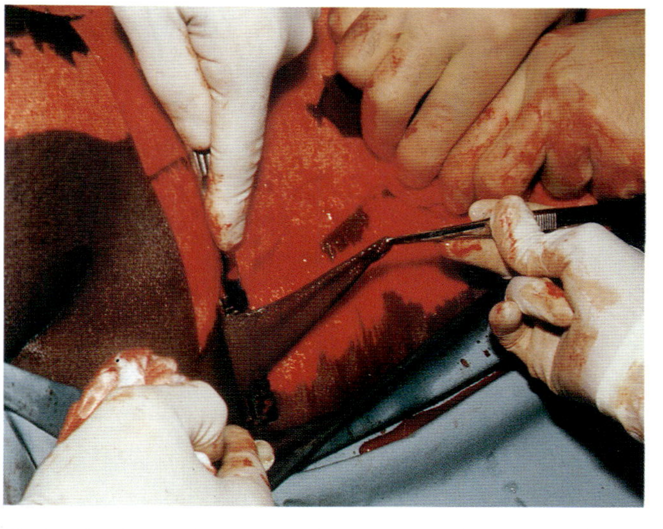

Plate 3: Split-thickness skin grafts being cut with the Goulian knife from the lateral side of the chest. The anterior axillary fold is at the left.

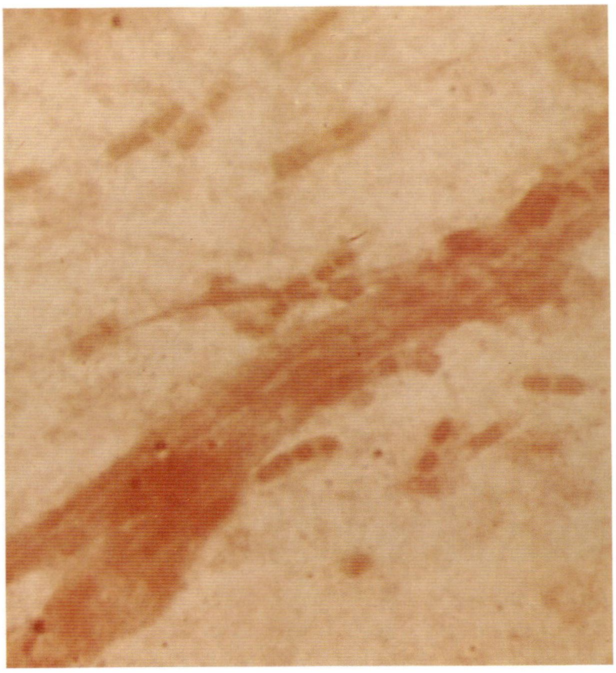

Plate 4: *Gram stain of sputum containing* Kl. pneumoniae.

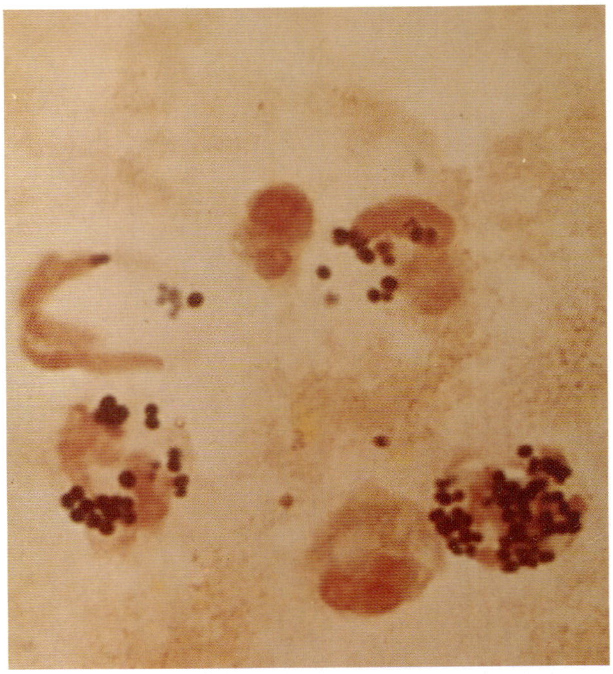

Plate 5: *Gram stain of class III sputum with gram-positive cocci (consistent with staphylococcal pneumonia).*

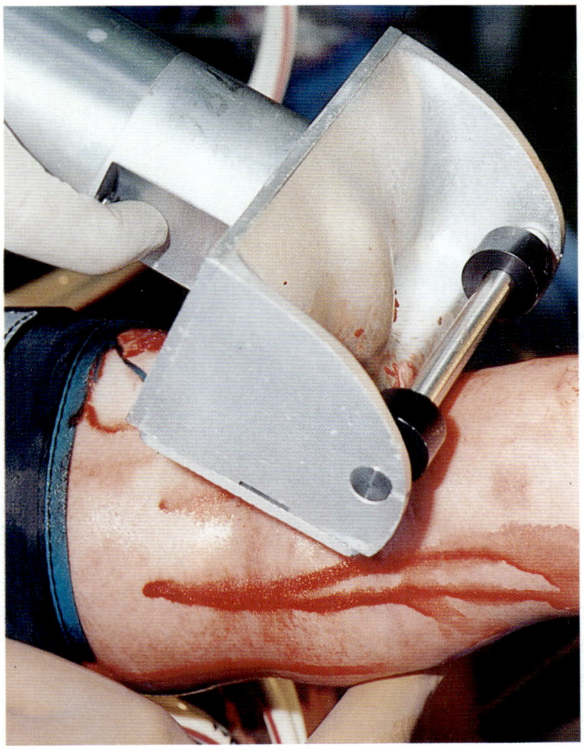

Plate 6: *Excision of burned tissue utilizing tourniquets.*

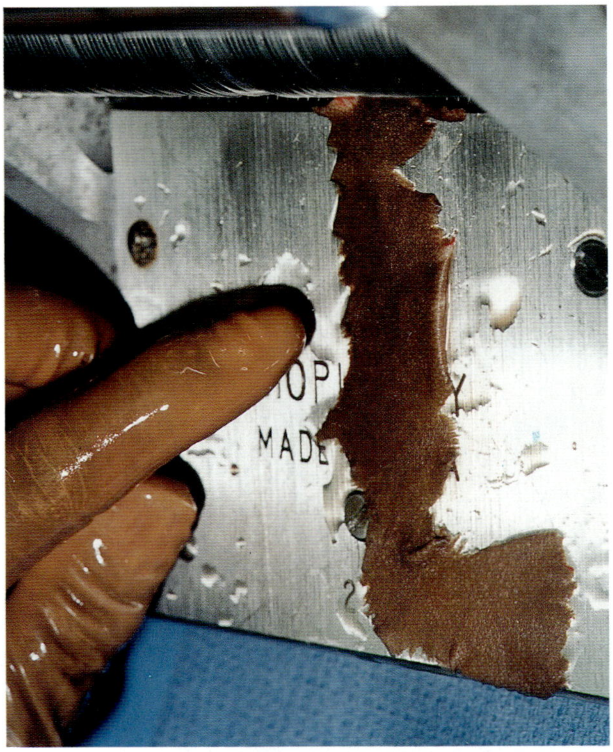

Plate 7: *Meshing of autograft using bioplasty 2:1 mesher.*

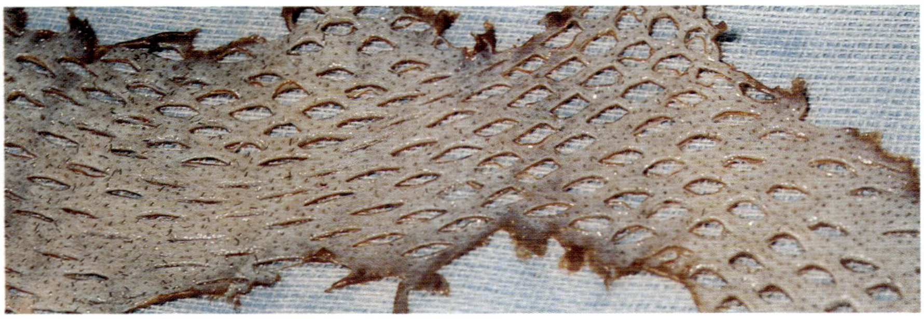

Plate 8: *Meshed 2:1 autograft on fine mesh gauze ready for application.*

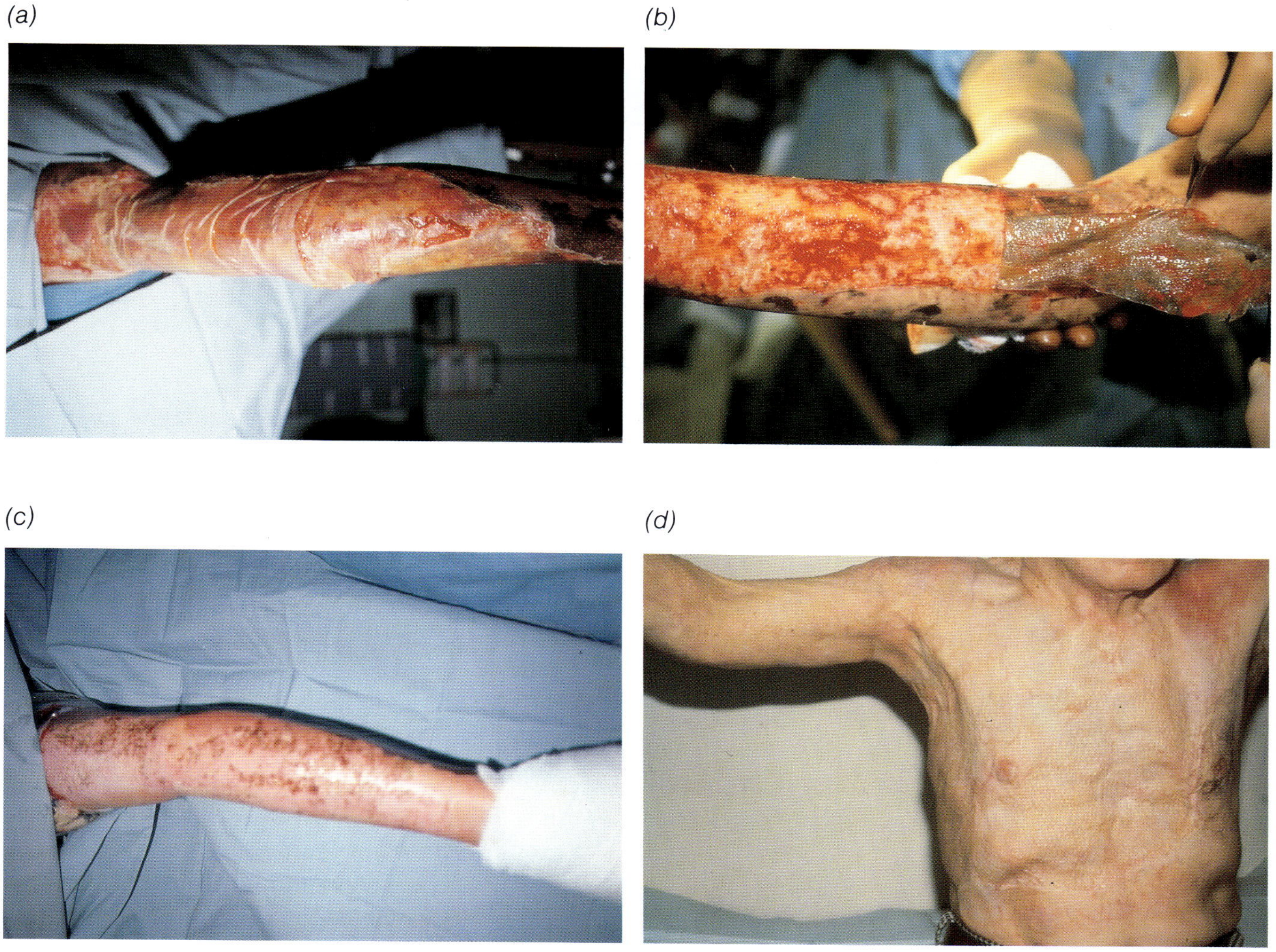

Plate 9: *Photographs of a patient who had right arm, forearm, axilla and chest covered with Integra (Integra Lifesciences Corp., Plainsboro, NJ). (**a**) Operating room photograph of Integra in position a few weeks after placement directly upon fascia. (**b**) Silastic layer being removed before replacement with ultrathin epidermal meshed graft. (**c,d**) Patient two years following engraftment demonstrating the pliability and natural texture of the healed Integra.*

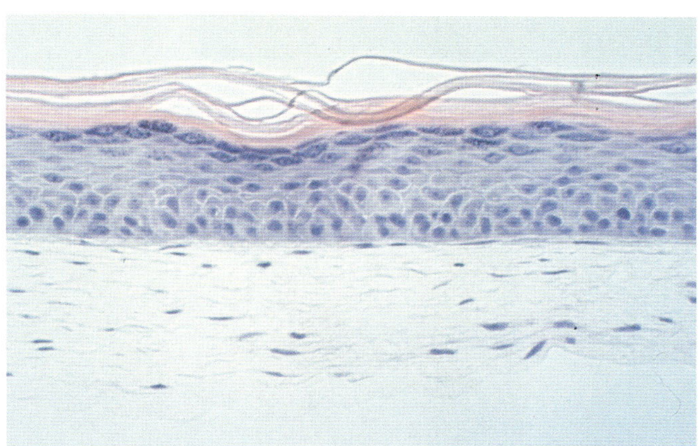

Plate 10: *Photomicrograph of 'living skin equivalent'. The upper layer consists of stratified allogenic human epidermal cells with cornification; the lower layer consists of condensed collagen matrix with allogenic human fibroblasts. (Material provided by Organogenesis, Inc., Canton, MA.)*

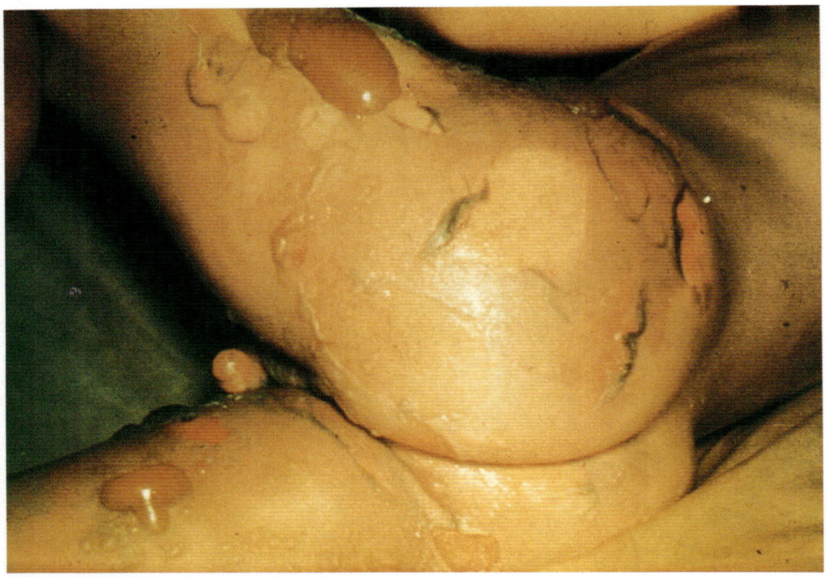

Plate 11: *Skin changes following contact with petrol, showing erythema and blistering. Complete healing occurred in 2 weeks.*

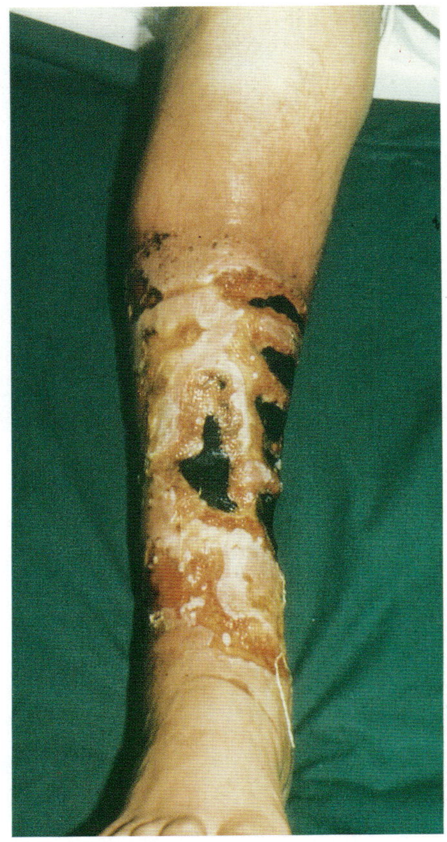

Plate 13: *Sulfuric acid injury from a car battery showing the black discoloration and underlying ulceration.*

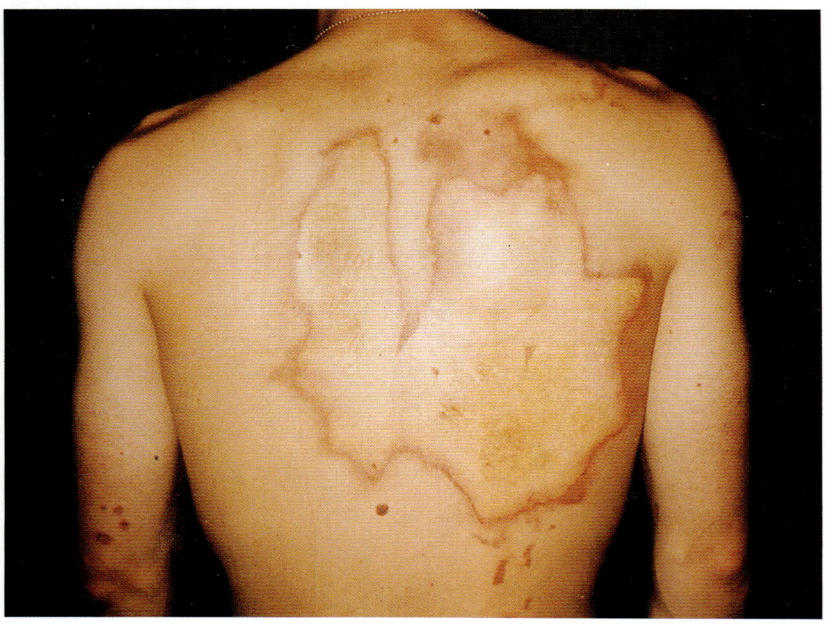

Plate 12: *Phosphorus burn during the Gulf War.*

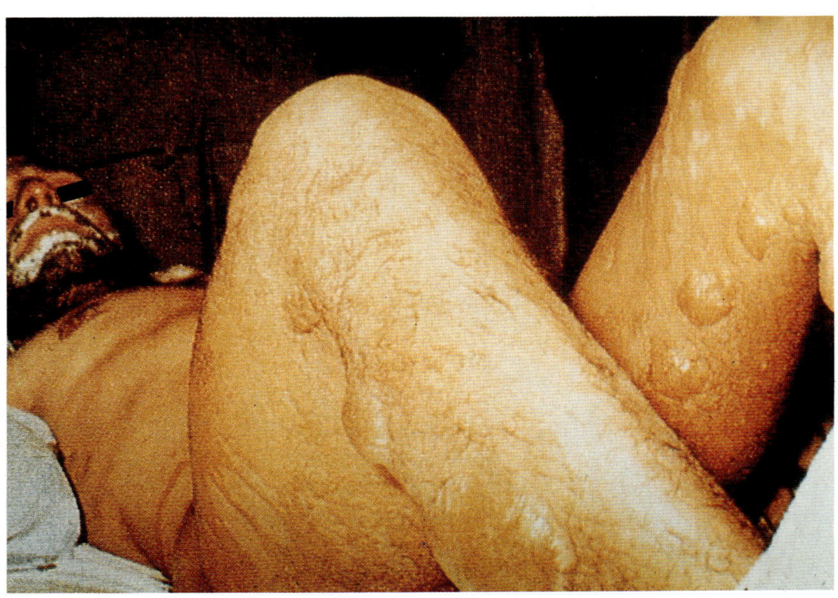

Plate 14: *Blistering following exposure to mustard.*

CHAPTER TWENTY-SIX

MUSCULOSKELETAL CHANGES SECONDARY TO THERMAL BURNS

E. BURKE EVANS

Among trauma states the burn is alone in the ability and tendency of its wound, even as it heals, to create major musculoskeletal deformity. In addition, the protracted burn illness which accompanies severe burns may result in other skeletal change. **Table 26.1** presents a classification of musculoskeletal changes secondary to burns; from that, the most commonly occurring and clinically significant alterations have been selected for discussion in detail.

CHANGES CONFINED TO BONE

Osteoporosis

Osteoporosis is the most frequently occurring postburn change involving the bone. In Shiele's radiographic study of patients with burns confined to the upper extremities, osteoporosis was found in 24 of 70 patients.[9] Klein's ongoing studies suggest that, among persons with serious burns, reduction of bone mass density is pervasive.[10] Stated causes of osteoporosis in thermal burns are bed confinement, immobilization, hyperemia,[11] reflex vasomotor phenomena,[12] and adrenocortical hyperactivity.[13] In Chapter 23 of this book, Klein thoroughly reviews the effects of burn injury on bone metabolism.[10,14] In this section only what is clinically apparent will be discussed.

The more extensive the burn and the greater the number of complications, the longer the patient will be bed confined and relatively immobile. It is easy to understand that the onset of osteoporosis might be accelerated and its intensity more marked in the burn illness which features a hypermetabolic state. If a single extremity of an otherwise normal person is immobilized for a long period of time because of local trauma, as with a fracture, the bones of that extremity will lose mineral to a degree that loss of density can be easily seen in a plain radiograph. So with burns isolated to the extremities, the bones of the affected extremities become osteoporotic; and, in persons with generalized burns, the bones of deeply burned extremities may show more profound mineral loss than is observed in nonburned extremities or in the axial skeleton (**Figure 26.1**). Van Der Wiel *et al.*[15] found in an x-ray absorptiometry study of 16 adults with fractures of one tibia that there was eventual loss of bone mineral density in the contralateral femur and in the lumbar spine, but to a lesser degree than in the ipsilateral femur. These findings, though not strictly analogous to those observed in burns, nevertheless point to the

Table 26.1 Classification of musculoskeletal changes secondary to burns

Alterations limited to bone
- Osteoporosis
- Periosteal new bone formation[1]
- Irregular ossification[1]
- Diaphyseal exostosis[1]
- Acromutilation of fingers[2]
- Pathologic fracture
- Osteomyelitis
- Necrosis and tangential sequestration

Alterations involving pericapsular structures
- Pericapsular calcification
- Heterotopic para-articular ossification
- Osteophyte formation

Alterations involving the joint proper
- Dislocation
- Chondrolysis[3]
- Septic arthritis
- Spontaneous dissolution[4–6]
- Ankylosis

Alterations involving muscles and tendons
- Desiccation of tendons[7]
- Fibrosis of muscles[8]

Alterations secondary to soft tissue
- Muscle and joint contractures
- Malposition of joints
- Scoliosis

Soft tissue injury
- Compartment syndrome
- Nerve injury

Abnormalities of growth
- Acceleration and retardation
- Destruction of growth plate

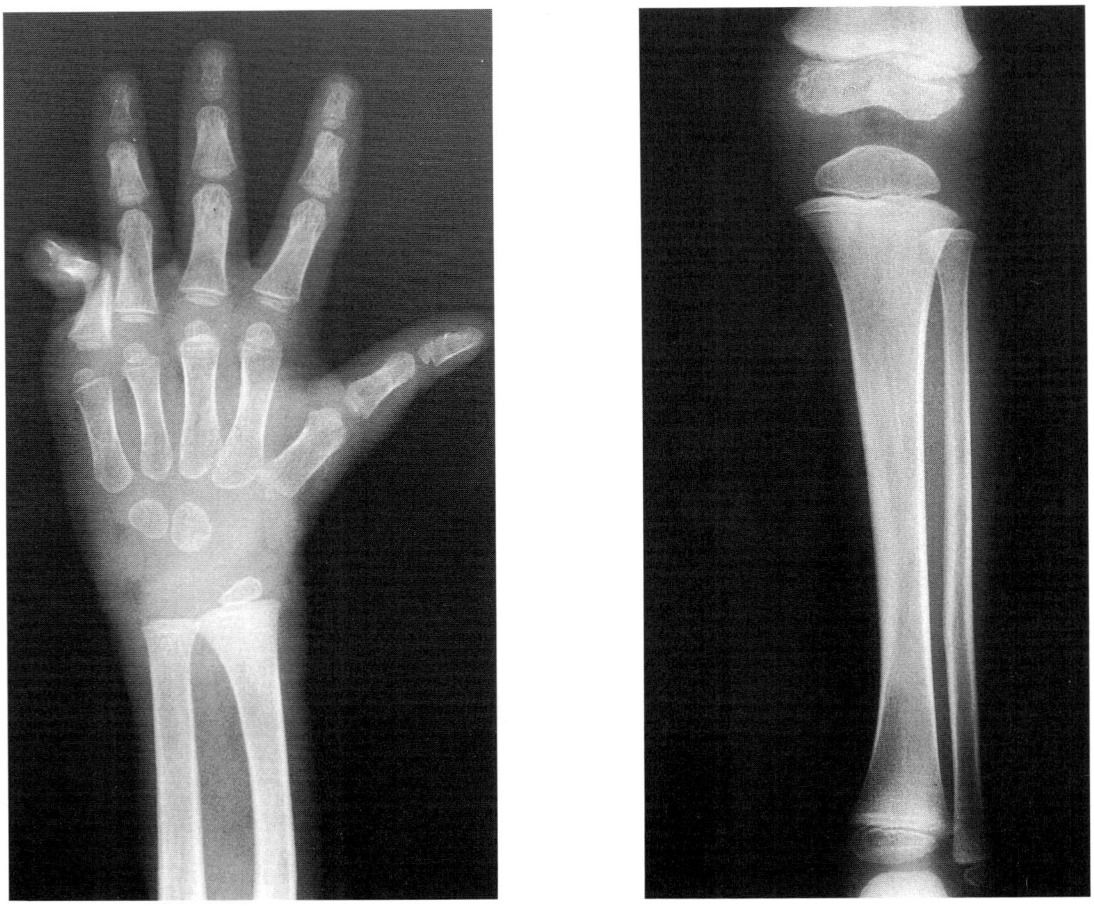

(a) (b)

Fig. 26.1 (a) Six months after injury there is the coarsened trabeculation of marked osteoporosis of bones of left hand and forearm of a 4-year-old male whose 70% full-thickness burn involved head, chest, and both upper extremities. (b) A roentgenogram of the left tibia and fibula obtained the same date as that of the hand shows minimal atrophy.

occurrence of generalized osteoporosis in other trauma states and the difference in loss of bone density relative to local factors. In fractures or in burns, impaired mobility and local hyperemia could account for this difference.

Another characteristic of the osteoporosis of burns that seems to set it apart is its persistence, not just until restoration of the anabolic state, but for months and years after the burn has healed (**Figure 26.2**). This phenomenon may be most clearly observed in patients who have survived 90% burns, but Klein records less than normal bone among even moderately burned children as long as 17 months after injury.[10] It seems obvious that muscle atrophy and/or the failure or inability of the person to return to the preburn level of physical activity surely account in part for this protracted state of reduced bone mineralization.

Probably there is no way to prevent osteoporosis in any patient whose burn is of such severity as to require an extended period of bed confinement. On the other hand, the advance of bone atrophy can at least be favorably modified even among patients with large burns if mobilization and active exercise are initiated soon after the burn. The bones of the axial skeleton, the pelvis, and the lower extremities are most efficiently stressed by weight bearing. Thus, standing is a priority measure. Muscle contraction alone may help to forestall bone atrophy and bone is better stressed if the contraction is resisted. Incrementally increasing resistance during motion or at the termination of an arc of motion or to muscle contraction in an extremity which may not be moved can be supplied by anyone who attends the patient. Isometric muscle contraction can be exacted from even seriously burned patients and is important for bone stress, for maintaining muscle tone and bulk, and for the patient's continuing ready identification of the affected extremity. Passive motion has little or no effect on bone, and, thus, does not figure in the prevention of osteoporosis. Other preventive measures, e.g. closure of the wound and maintenance of nutrition, are routine in critical burn care. Treatment of established osteoporosis involves the more aggressive employment of measures for prevention. There are no long-term studies, however, which measure the effectiveness of exercise, diet, medication, or modality in the treatment of osteoporosis in any state.

Fig. 26.2 (a) Advanced osteoporosis in the hands of a 14-year-old male 9 months after 100% total body surface burn. All growth plates are open. (b) Twenty-four months after injury, osteoporosis persists and there is irregular closure of metacarpal and phalangeal growth plates. (c) Eight months after injury, growth plates of distal tibiae and fibulae remain open. (d) Twenty-four months after injury, distal growth plates of tibiae and fibulae are closed. Other major growth plates remain open. Osteoporosis is unchanged.

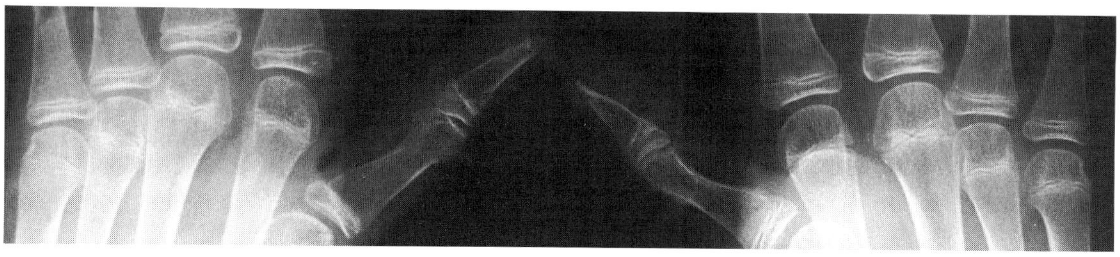
(a)

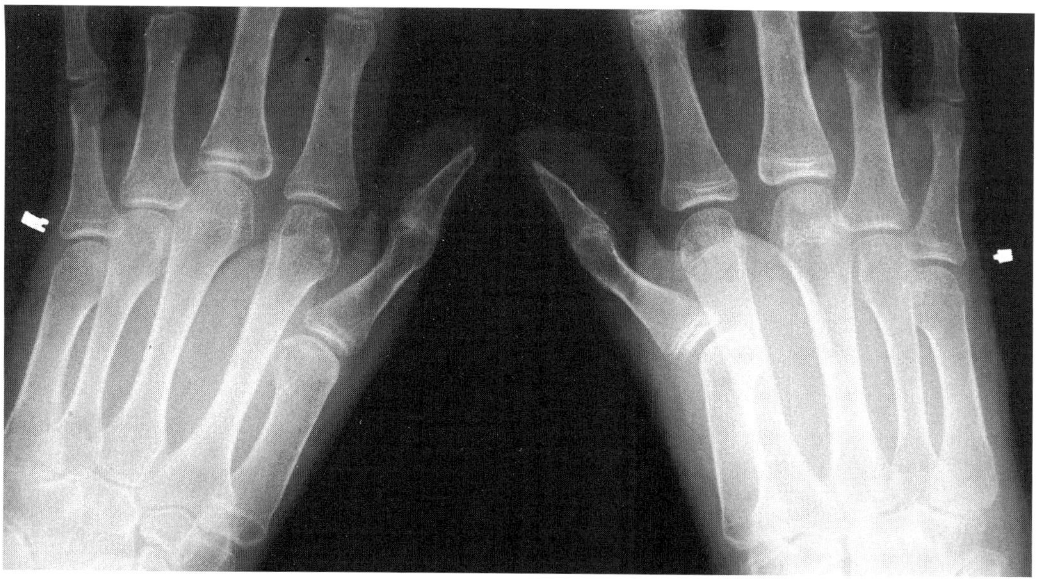
(b)

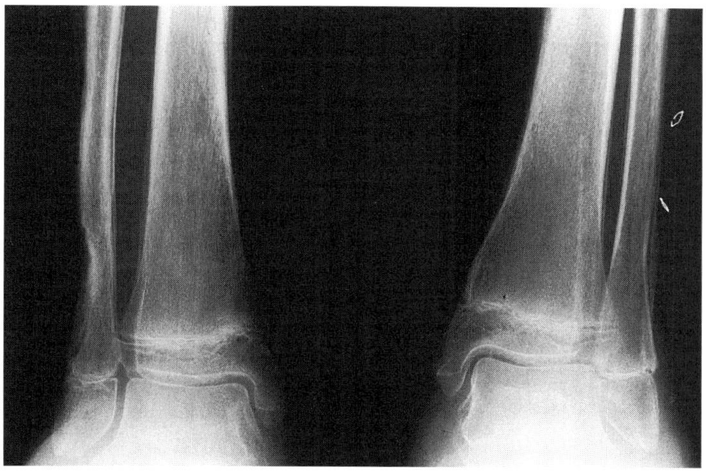
(c)

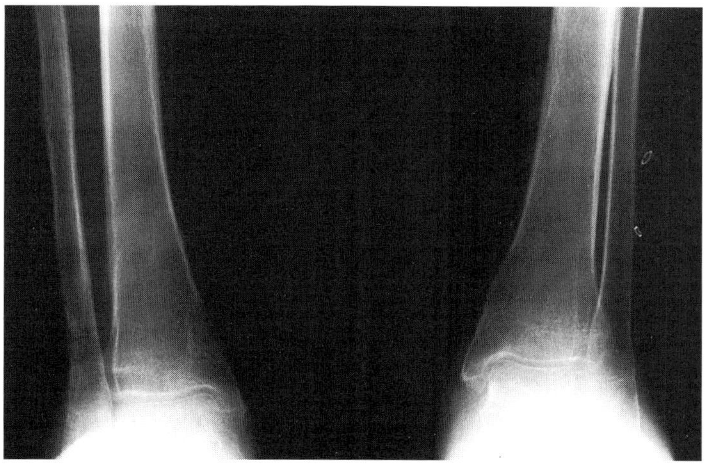
(d)

Osteomyelitis

In burns, bones can become infected by exposure of bone by the burn; by an open fracture accompanying the burn; by extension of infection from a septic joint, introduction of organisms along traction pins, internal fracture fixation devices; or by blood-borne organisms of bacteremia. Considering the apparent great liability of seriously burned patients for developing osteomyelitis, it is surprising that it does not regularly occur. As it turns out, clinically significant osteomyelitis in burned patients is rare. Antibiotics given for the general state may prevent seeding of the bone or may repress any small focus of bone infection.

The cortex of long bones is a good barrier to surface organisms. Even exposure of cortex will have little adverse effect if the blood supply of the bone remains intact. Prolonged exposure will kill the outer layer of the cortex which will in time sequestrate, separating at a well defined cleft between dead and living bone. With minor or moderate exposure, the bone will usually survive long enough for bordering granulation tissue to cover it. For larger defects, it is a common practice to drill closely spaced holes through the exposed cortex so as to encourage buds of granulation tissue to emerge from the still vascular medullary canal. With this practice, there seems to be little risk of infecting the bone, no matter how contaminated the rest of the limb. It may be that there is sufficient centripetal pressure to discourage the invasion of organisms when the holes are fresh and that the holes are rapidly sealed by blood clot and advancing tissue. There are no reports of deep bone infection related to cortex drilling.

With open fractures which remain at the base of or are part of a major soft tissue burn wound, bone infection is probably inevitable. Even so, the infection tends to remain at the fracture site and not to involve the rest of the bone, so that local debridement and stabilization of the soft tissue wound are all that are required for treatment. Dowling reported osteomyelitis of the tibia related to an open bimalleolar fracture in an extensively burned extremity.[16] On the other hand, osteomyelitis developed in neither of the two open fractures reported separately by Choctaw[17] and Wang.[18] Three patients have been treated in whom open fractures of the femur complicated thigh burns. Each case required aggressive and repeated debridement. One fracture was treated in traction, while the other two were treated with external fixators. In one of the patients who was admitted 8 months after acute burn, there was established osteomyelitis of the femur in relation to the exposed fracture. Osteomyelitis did not develop in either of the other patients; in the end, all three had sound femurs.

When traction pins are directed through burned skin for the treatment of fractures or for suspension of a burned extremity, the factors favoring development of infection along the pin track and the formation of cigarette sequestra are:

- the introduction or migration of organisms from the burn wound;
- linear pressure of the traction pin;
- prolonged traction;
- excessive movement of the extremity leading to loosening of the pin;
- sealing of the pin sites.

For traction or suspension, pins may be inserted through acutely burned skin, through eschar, through granulation tissue, or later through ischemic burn scar which may be colonized with uncommon and antibiotic-resistant organisms. No amount of local cleaning is likely to sterilize the surface through which the pin must pass, yet it seems that organisms in sufficient numbers to colonize are rarely introduced in this manner.

Local low-grade infections usually resolve when pins are removed if the pin sites are vigorously curetted of granulation tissue. In one case in which a four-pin custom external fixator was used in the treatment of an open infection of the elbow, there resulted diffuse osteomyelitis of humerus and radius. The infection was controlled with antibiotics and without surgery after the pins were removed. In experience with the use of the Ilizarov system for correction of skeletal deformity in burns, one patient developed a pin track infection of such severity as to require removal of the pin, curettage, and intravenous antibiotics for control of methicillin-resistant staphylococcus.[19]

Hematogenous osteomyelitis and that due to spread from an infected joint are rare. The literature entertains no report of the occurrence of either entity in association with burns. Were bone infection of this sort to be recognized, effective treatment would depend upon the identification of the offending organisms for organism-specific antibiotic regimen.

Fractures

Pathologic fractures were at one time common in burn management because of the practices of delayed excision of eschar and of keeping patients in bed until wounds were completely covered. During that time, fractures occurred because of bone collapse when patients first stood or walked after a prolonged period of bed confinement or when stiff joints were manipulated[20] (**Figure 26.3**). The

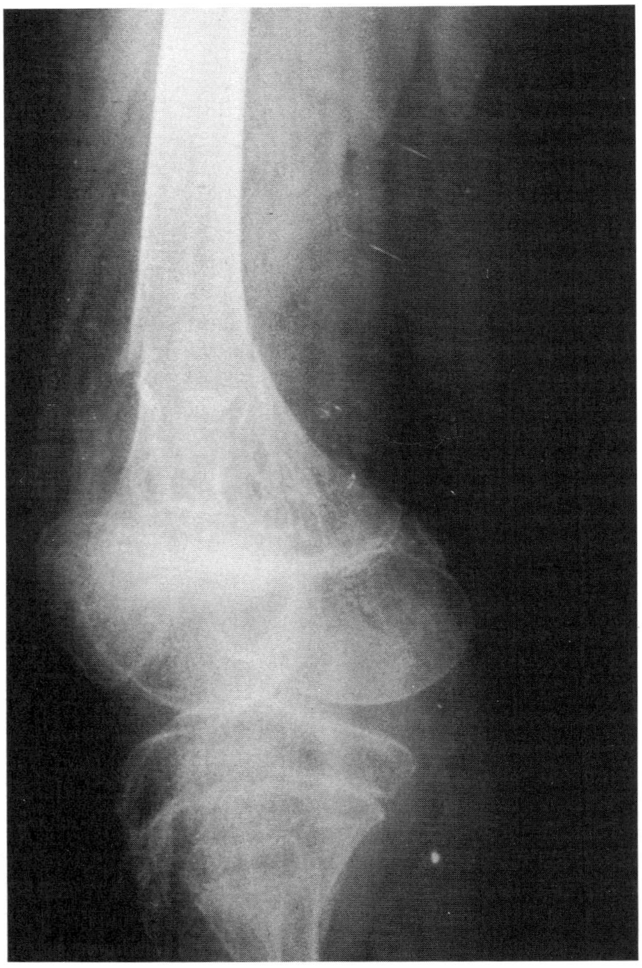

Fig. 26.3 Pathologic fracture of the osteoporotic femur of a 9-year-old girl sustained on the first day she stood after 5 weeks of confinement for 40% total body surface burn.

bones most commonly affected were the femur at its distal metaphysis and the tibia at its proximal one. The only treatment required was support of the extremity until the fracture consolidated, usually in 4–6 weeks. Children were more often affected than adults and the fractures usually compressed one cortex, producing an angular deformity which rapidly corrected with growth. More currently, Klein's study strongly suggests that fractures occur more frequently in burned children than in a matched normal population even months after the acute burn. Now, however, in acute burn management the most frequently seen fractures are those occurring at the time of, or in association with, the burn injury. Falls or violent trauma account for many of the fractures, and the sites are

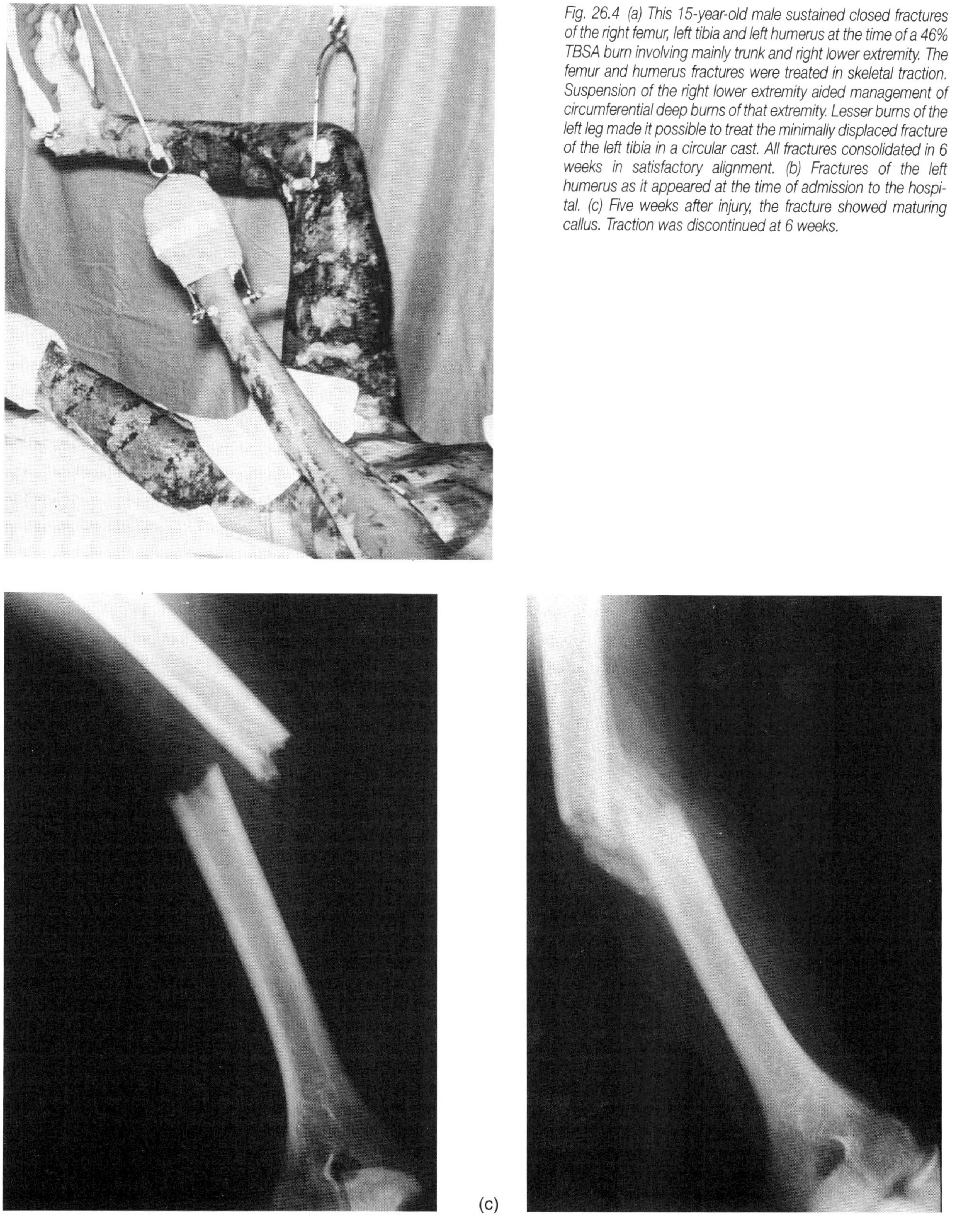
(a)
(b)
(c)

Fig. 26.4 (a) This 15-year-old male sustained closed fractures of the right femur, left tibia and left humerus at the time of a 46% TBSA burn involving mainly trunk and right lower extremity. The femur and humerus fractures were treated in skeletal traction. Suspension of the right lower extremity aided management of circumferential deep burns of that extremity. Lesser burns of the left leg made it possible to treat the minimally displaced fracture of the left tibia in a circular cast. All fractures consolidated in 6 weeks in satisfactory alignment. (b) Fractures of the left humerus as it appeared at the time of admission to the hospital. (c) Five weeks after injury, the fracture showed maturing callus. Traction was discontinued at 6 weeks.

those common to the causes, bearing no relation to the burn itself. Reports indicate that fractures associated with burns occur in all bones of the axial and appendicular skeleton.

Although fractures complicate burn treatment and occasionally delay mobilization of patients, their management need not be complex. Fractures in extremities not burned can be treated in a routine manner by manipulative reduction and plaster immobilization, by open reduction and internal fixation, with an external fixator, or with skeletal traction (**Figure 26.4**). Fractures in extremities with first degree or superficial second degree burns can be managed in the same way. Deep second degree and third degree burns present a different problem only with respect to the early bacterial colonization of third degree burns and the degradation of deep second degree burns to full-thickness burns which will, in turn, become colonized. There is, thus, a precious window of time when fractures requiring open reduction and internal fixation can be definitively treated without increased risk of infecting the bone; however, fracture reduction and stabilization are so important in the functional management of a severely burned patient that the risk of bone infection should be acknowledged and shouldered at any postburn stage. Skeletal traction can often be the management choice, particularly in children and adolescents, even if the treatment protocol requires that the patient be moved from bed for tubbing, dressing change, or additional surgery. The disadvantages of skeletal traction are the confinement to bed and the imposed relatively fixed position of the affected extremity. External fixators, now in common use, have made it possible to align and stabilize fractures in burned extremities without open operation. In fact, external fixation may be the treatment of choice for open fractures in burns, as it often is for open fractures not associated with burns. There is the added functional advantage of patient mobility. Brooker's extensive favorable experience supports this concept.[21] With both skeletal traction and external fixation, there is an added risk of bone infection because of the path from surface to bone provided by the pins. This is a risk worth taking, and it is minimized by scrupulous pin site care and by removal and replacement of any loosening pin.

When casts are used for stabilization of fractures in burned extremities, the wound is made inaccessible and there is an abiding fear that the unattended wound will seriously degrade or at best not improve. Those fears may be well founded; however, Wang[18] showed that a bivalved circular cast could be used effectively for an open comminuted fracture of a proximal tibia with overlying deep burns, and Choctaw[17] reported successful use of a cast for immobilization of an open comminuted fracture after immediate postburn grafting of the affected extremity. Common sense should dictate which fractures can be treated with circular or bivalved casts or with splints. If a reduced or moderately displaced but aligned fracture is so stable as to require external support only for maintenance of alignment, then cast or splint immobilization should be all that is needed. On the other hand, if a fracture, because of instability, requires, for maintenance of reduction, three-point pressure or molding of the cast material, then it will be better treated by other means.

Dowling[16] reported osteomyelitis resulting from open bimalleolar fracture in an extremity with extensive deep burns. In neither of the cases reported by Wang and Choctaw did the bone become infected. There were also no infections among Saffle's 42 fractures, 9 of which were treated by open reduction and internal fixation.[22] With two fractures of the femur, each of which was exposed at the base of a deep chronic burn, aggressive debridement of the wounds and the fracture ends was followed by treatment with skeletal traction in one and by external fixation with the Ilizarov system in the other. Both fractures healed without further complication.

Fractures in burned patients heal quickly. There is no recorded experience which suggests that healing is delayed by the burn. Neither is there any record of failure of union. Callus formation may be abundant.

Among severely burned patients, nondisplaced or minimally displaced fractures may not be detected until unusual local pain in an affected extremity prompts roentgenographic examination or when a roentgenogram obtained for other reason reveals the fracture as an incidental finding. These fractures are usually of no functional significance. Modest angular deformity near a joint may be a problem in adults, though not in children. On the other hand, undetected transphyseal fractures in children can be a major functional threat.

Changes Involving Pericapsular Structures

Heterotopic Bone

Heterotopic bone formation is a rare but functionally important complication of thermal burns. The incidence in a general burn population is reported to be somewhere between 1 and 3%.[1,23–26] In select populations, the incidence may be higher as it will be if patients with periarticular calcification are included in the statistics. For example, Tepperman *et al.* reported a 35.3% incidence among patients referred to a tertiary care center for rehabilitation.[27] Jackson made the observation that the incidence of heterotopic bone could be expected to be less in institutions which admit patients with minor burns.[28] Munster's[29] roentgenographic survey of 88 adult and teenage patients with 160 burned upper extremities yielded a 16% incidence of pericapsular calcification; and the 23% incidence reported by Schiele *et al.*[9] included both heterotopic ossification and calcification. In the early routine roentgenographic study reported by Evans[20] periarticular calcification which did not progress to heterotopic bone was excluded from the final calculation of an incidence of 2%. The 3.3% incidence recorded by Kolar and Vrabec[30] included patients with pericapsular calcification. Even if heterotopic bone occurs infrequently in thermal burns, it remains that once it develops, it often compromises joint motion and is difficult to treat. In addition, its pathogenesis is still incompletely understood; and, thus, protocols for prevention may in fact miss the mark.

Pathogenesis

The metabolic changes occurring after thermal burn are increased metabolic rate; protein catabolism; ureagenesis; fat mobilization; glucogenolysis; gluconeogenesis; elevated glucose flow, and eventual total body weight loss.[31,32] There is an accompanying suppression of the immune system which favors wound infection, but, at the same time, favors survival of skin allografts. Infection, failure of skin graft take or anything which delays closure of a burn wound will extend the altered metabolic state. Though it might be assumed that there occurs, along with the metabolic upheaval, an adverse change in connective tissue milieu, the exact nature of such a change is not known. It is also not known what the metabolic changes have to do with the development of heterotopic bone, but it is clear that the burn disease is necessary to its formation. Other factors to be considered in the genesis of heterotopic bone are percentage of burn, location of burn, period of confinement, osteoporosis, superimposed trauma and genetic predisposition. These factors, though identifiable, are not easy to implicate.

Percentage of burn

Most reported cases of heterotopic bone have had a 20% or greater total body surface burn; however, heterotopic bone has been found in patients with as little as 10% third degree burn.[20] Peterson *et al.*,[5] Munster *et al.*,[29] and Elledge *et al.*[25] have reported affected patients with total body surface burns of 8%, 14%, and 12% respectively. In addition, with the now extensive experience with salvage of patients with 80% or greater burns, it is clear that heterotopic bone occurs no more frequently among these patients at the other end of the percentage spectrum than in the general burn population. It cannot be said, thus, that the percentage of burn is a determining factor.

Location of burn

A high percentage, but by no means all, of the reported heterotopic bone has occurred in joints with overlying deep burn. In their initial report, Evans and Smith described heterotopic bone occurring a distance from any third degree burn involvment.[1] Johnston, in his early report, noted that in one of his three patients, the skin overlying one affected joint was not even superficially burned.[33] If it be assumed that degradation of connective tissue milieu in burns is a total body phenomenon, it follows that heterotopic bone formation need not be burn site dependent. Thus, the location of the burn cannot alone be a determining factor.

Period of confinement

Evans and Smith expressed the belief that length of bed confinement was perhaps the most important factor in the development of heterotopic bone.[1] At the time of that report, patients with even moderate burns might be kept in bed for several weeks. The consequences of prolonged confinement were loss of active range of joint motion and bone demineralization; it was thought that each of these adverse changes might contribute to the formation of heterotopic bone. Thus, any maloccurrence which necessitated longer confinement could be a factor in the pathogenesis. Kolar implicated wound sepsis as such an independent factor along with the length of confinement.[30] Other investigators have not addressed the period of confinement as specifically as Kolar, and there have been no studies of comparative groups of confined and nonconfined patients. Thus, it may never be determined whether or not current aggressive practice of early mobilization of patients will have an effect on the incidence of heterotopic bone.

Osteoporosis

Only Schiele *et al.* have reported a relationship between heterotopic bone formation and osteoporosis.[9] We have noted previously that among their group of 70 adults with burns confined to the upper extremities, 11 of the 16 who developed heterotopic bone had roentgenographically identifiable osteoporosis. In their series of patients, there were 24 who had osteoporosis. Thus, fewer than one-half of these developed heterotopic bone and there were two in the group that developed heterotopic bone who did not have osteoporosis. If the findings in that study are not altogether persuasive, the matter is further confused by the knowledge that the survivors of extensive total body surface burns who may develop profound osteoporosis seem to have no greater liability to the formation of heterotopic bone than the general burn population.

Superimposed trauma

In one of the patients reported by Evans and Smith, the elbow of the more often used and minimallly burned right upper extremity developed heterotopic bone, whereas the elbow of the less used but more seriously burned left upper extremity did not.[1] In the same patient, the right hip spontaneously dislocated. After reduction, that hip developed extensive heterotopic bone in the planes of the rectus femoris and iliopsoas, the muscles stressed by the posterior displacement. The opposite hip developed only a small spicule of heterotopic bone anteriorly at the joint line. Experience with this one patient reinforced the authors' belief that there occurred with burns a general compromise of connective tissue which rendered it particularly susceptible to superimposed trauma and that it was this liability to injury which accounted for the appearance of heterotopic bone at sites of repeated stretching of soft tissue, as at the minimally burned elbow or at sites of recognized abrupt excessive stretching as at the dislocated hip. According to all reports, the elbow is the most common site of heterotopic bone formation in adults and children.[25,26,30,34] Perhaps it is the regular use of this joint which accounts for that orientation. Jackson has pointed out that the elbows are subjected to pressure posteriorly and medially when they are used for leverage or are simply in contact with the bed.[28] He suggests with this observation that external pressure is a factor in the orientation of heterotopic bone to the elbow. There may be other factors as well that favor the elbow. Commonly, the elbow is splinted in extension to prevent flexion contracture. If flexion range is lost, passive stretch and encouragement of active flexion are part of the rehabilitation effort. The posterior structures most affected by this effort are those attached to the olecranon. Thus, it is not surprising that heterotopic bone develops medially in line with and deep to the medial fibers of the triceps. If a flexion contracture develops, the heterotopic bone is commonly in the line of brachialis or biceps attachments to coronoid process and biceps tubercle. And if there is loss of pronation and supination range, stretching may cause heterotopic bone to form in line with the proximal radioulnar ligaments and interosseous membrane. There is an implication here that both the quality and timing of postburn exercise may be important. Gentle passive and active motion should cause less tissue disruption than abrupt passive or active or even chronically repeated motion, and the effect of any mobilization effort must vary with the relative stiffness of the joint and the intrinsic resistance of soft tissue. Thus, the longer a joint is limited in its motion, the stiffer it will become and the greater will be the soft tissue damage with any forced manipulation.

The concept of superimposed trauma as a cause of heterotopic bone is supported by the experimental work of Evans[35] and of Michelsson and Rauschning.[36] Evans found that all burned and nonburned rabbits given a single necrotizing injection of alcohol in one quadriceps muscle readily healed the lesions, whereas rabbits, burned or nonburned, which were given a second same-site injection 7 days after the first, uniformly developed well defined and histologically identifiable ossicles of heterotopic bone. In this experiment, it was clear that, in susceptible animals, it was not the burn which made the difference, but the chronicity of the wound. Michelsson and Rauschning determined that forceful or regular active remobilization of rabbit knees, which had been immobilized for 1–5 weeks, resulted in the development of heterotopic calcification and ossification in the muscles which were stretched. The response was more consistent in the quadriceps of the knees immobilized in extension than in the hamstrings of those immobilized in flexion. The longer the period of immobilization and the more vigorous the remobilization, the greater the response. Muscle necrosis was a prominent histologic finding.

Superimposed trauma is implicated in the development of

heterotopic bone in head-injured patients or those with post-traumatic or infectious transverse myelitis.[37–39] In these patients, it is assumed that tissue media are altered by injury to the central nervous system. The secondary injury, as in burns, is periarticular. In post-traumatic myositis ossificans, the development of heterotopic bone depends upon persistence of the muscle lesion and local necrosis and, thus, at least by inference, upon repeated insults to the affected muscle.

The development of heterotopic bone in burns has been associated with the agitation of patients and their resistance to physical therapy.[1,40] Two affected adults and one affected child in a 10-year study resisted physical therapy programming.[35] One adult refused to move and the other was extremely apprehensive. The child was likewise apprehensive and refused to cooperate with the therapist. The development in all three of posterior heterotopic bone in both elbows could have been ascribed both to the difficulty encountered in mobilizing the elbows and to the continual pressure on the elbows in bed.

Genetic predisposition

It is difficult to explain the low incidence of heterotopic bone among great numbers of patients similarly burned except on the basis of some, as yet unidentified, inherited factor. It is known that persons with proliferative noninflammatory arthritis of the hip are more likely to develop heterotopic bone after total hip replacement than persons who have hips replaced for other reasons. In this instance, the predisposing inherited abnormality is identifiable. Though heterotopic bone formation may occur more regularly among spinal cord-injured and head-injured patients than among burned ones, by no means do all persons with head and spinal cord injuries develop heterotopic bone. The total burn experience at the University of Texas Medical Branch has yielded only two similarly affected siblings. Twin brothers who had 19% and 20% total body surface burns and who were mobile throughout much of their treatment and recovery period developed near identical heterotopic bone of both elbows.[41] There is, however, no scientific proof that genetic predisposition has anything to do with the formation of heterotopic bone in burns. Nor is there any literature to support the idea that a person who develops heterotopic bone when burned will be liable to develop it if he or she sustains head or spinal cord injury.

Characteristics and Behavior

Heterotopic bone associated with burns has been reported to occur about all major joints. The joints most commonly affected are elbow, shoulder, and hip, in that order of frequency. The early manifestations are joint swelling and tenderness not unlike any acute inflammatory process. The patient may call attention to the process by a reluctance to move the affected joint. Onset may be as early as 1 month and as late as 3 months or more after the burn, but it is more likely to be associated with the acute recovery phase of treatment than later. Crawford *et al.* reported that the clinical diagnosis was made in advance of roentgenographic changes in 9 of his 12 patients.[34] Tepperman *et al.*[27] and Peterson *et al.*[26] found that bone scans could help to make a diagnosis before there were roentgenographic changes. The earliest roentgenographic alteration is local periarticular increase in soft tissue density. There follows diffuse stippled calcification in the same distribution in or about the capsule of the joint. It is at this point that the process may reverse itself, perhaps due to the improved state of the patient. Because of this change in course, there may be many patients whose periarticular calcification is never detected. If the calcification persists, it may be assumed that bone will develop by either the intramembranous or the enchondral route or both as it does in animal models.

The flecks of calcification appear roentgenographically to lie within the capsule, whereas heterotopic bone may involve not only capsular structures but may extend as well into the planes of muscles and tendons. At each major joint there is a more or less characteristic distribution of heterotopic bone which is similar to that associated with patients with head and spinal cord injury. At the elbow, posteriorly, disposed bone extends from the olecranon to the medial epicondylar ridge of the humerus in line with the medial border of the triceps muscle (**Figure 26.5a,b**). At the joint, it may extend medially to bridge the ulnar groove.[3,42] The medial, rather than lateral, orientation of the heterotopic bone may be related to the medial position of the olecranon and the greater tension on soft tissue on that side. As Jackson points out, the contact area of the elbow is medial, and continual pressure in this area may have something to do with the orientation.[28] Heterotopic bone on the anterior surface of the elbow develops in the planes of the brachialis and biceps muscles extending from humerus to coronoid process or biceps tubercle. Occasionally, a bridge of heterotopic bone develops between the radius and ulna just distal to the joint. More rarely, bone has been found to fill the olecranon fossa and even to ensheath the entire joint. At the shoulder, bone has been found to extend from the acromion to the humerus in the line of the rotator muscles or deep to the deltoid (**Figure 26.5c**), to lie anteriorly in the plane of the pectoralis major, and, more deeply, to parallel the subscapularis. Hoffer *et al.*[43] reported that heterotopic bone at the shoulder lay anteriorly in the plane of the capsule. At the hip heterotopic bone may extend from pelvis to femur in the planes of rectus or iliopsoas anteriorly or in the plane of the gluteal muscles laterally. Jackson has reported heterotopic bone in the plane of the quadratus femoris.[28] Like the shoulder, the hip may be ensheathed anteriorly with heterotopic bone which appears to originate in the capsule.

When heterotopic bone bridges a joint, it becomes part of the skeleton and may, if loaded, increase in dimension as fully developed ossicles with mature cortex and medullary cavity. If the bone does not bridge a joint, it will, in children, gradually disappear when the burn wound has healed and the child is healthy. In recovering adults, nonbridging bone will, in time, diminish in size, but it may never completely disappear. The same tendency for heterotopic bone to regress after resolution of disease was noted by Lorber, who reported on two patients with paraplegia secondary to tuberculosis in whom deposits of heterotopic bone diminished in size, after return of motor function.[37] Bottu and Van Noyen[44] reported a similar experience with a patient who had transient viral meningoencephalitis, and Jacobs reported almost complete resorption of large bilateral deposits of heterotopic bone in a patient who recovered from paralytic measles encephalomyelitis.[38]

Serum levels of calcium, phosphorus, and alkaline phosphatase have been reported by most authors to be normal or, at best, insignificantly higher in burned patients who have developed heterotopic bone.[1,23,29,45,46] In addition, there is no convincing evidence that calcium intake affects heterotopic bone formation one way or the other. Evans' and Smith's limited routine studies of affected and unaffected patients led the authors to believe that the values of serum calcium, phosphorus, and alkaline phosphatase were so consistently normal as to make further investigation unnecessary.[1] One interesting observation was that of Koepke, whose early, but incomplete, studies suggested that those patients who were susceptible had elevation of serum alkaline phosphatase before development of heterotopic bone, but not afterwards.[24]

Prevention and Treatment

The incidence of heterotopic bone in burns is so low as to make it impractical to administer aspirin or indomethacin or other nonsteroidal anti-inflammatory drugs which are currently used for

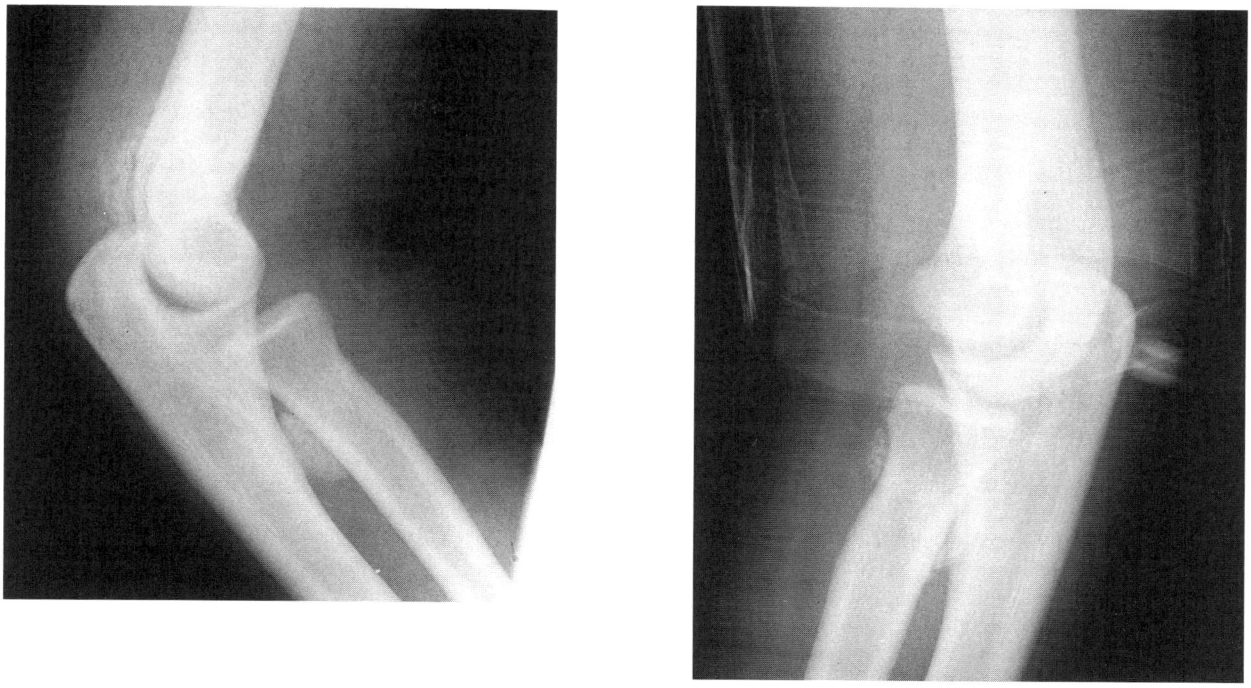

(a)

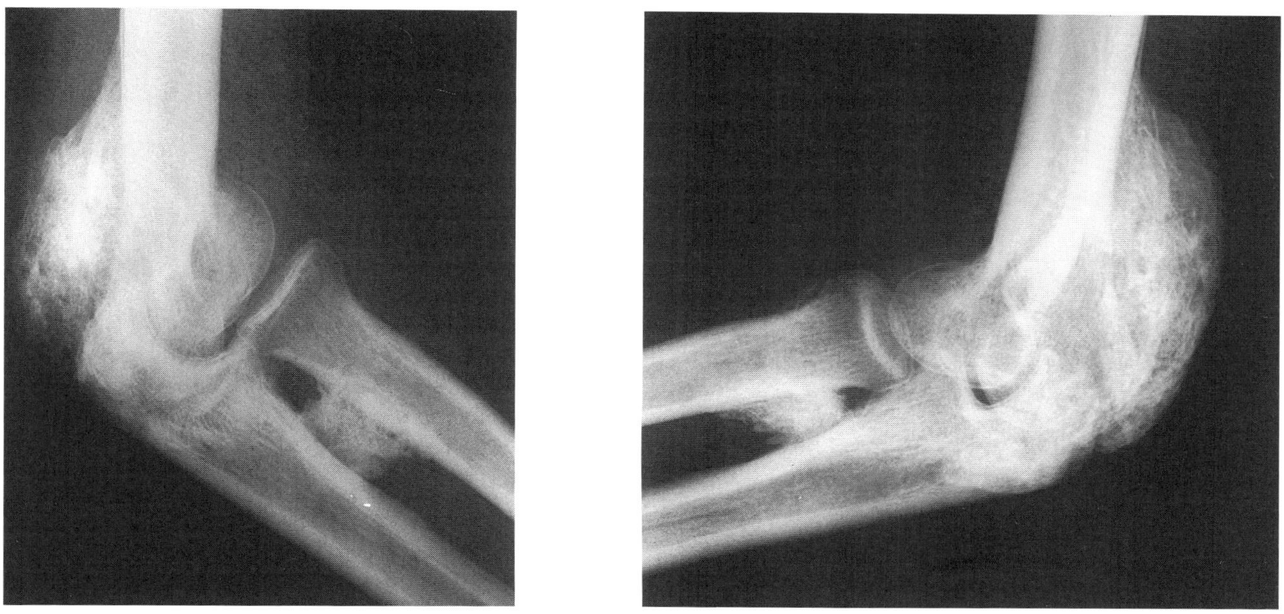

(b)

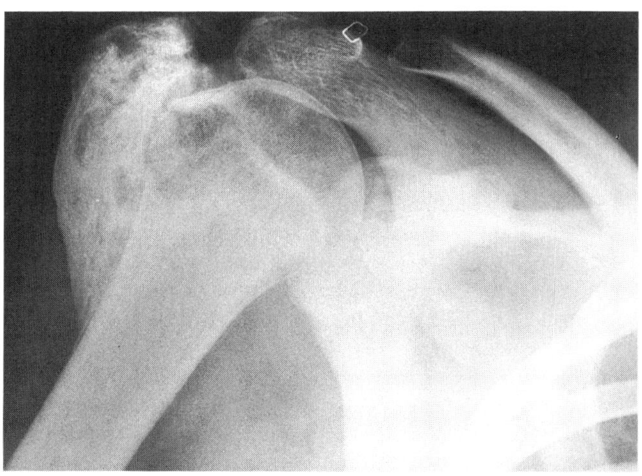

(c)

Fig. 26.5 (a) Three months after 94% TBSA burn of a 16-year-old male, resistance to motion, local swelling, and pain of both elbows prompted obtaining roentgenograms, each of which showed spotty linear soft tissue calcification and ossification along the distal humerus and between the radius and ulna at the level of the biceps tubercle. (b) Six months after burn, elbow flexion and extension were reduced to 10 degrees on the left and to less than 5 degrees on the right. Bridges of immature heterotopic bone extended from the medial epicondylar ridges to the olecranons. Forearm rotation was 0% due to interosseous bridges of heterotopic bone at the level of the bicipital tuberosities. Prognosis for restoring functional range of motion in the elbows is poor. (c) At six months postburn gleno-humeral motion on the right was limited to a few degrees by heterotopic bone underlying the deltoid. At the same time, a lesser deposit of hetero-topic at the left hip did not limit motion.

patients at risk for development of heterotopic bone after major hip surgery. Rather, the thrust in prevention should be toward reducing the period of bed confinement and the duration of the postburn hypermetabolic state. The now prevailing practice of early wound excision and grafting may, in fact, address both of these problems as nearly as it is possible to do so. Even patients with extensive total body surface burns may be out of bed and walking within the first postburn week. Extremity motion is begun as soon as graft and wound stability permit. With this programming, the incidence and intensity of osteoporosis should be reduced as well.

If certain patients are predisposed to the development of heterotopic bone, then the quality and timing of joint mobilization for those patients may be critical. Stretching edematous pericapsular structures in the early postburn period may very well be hazardous if additional tissue damage is the result; however, maintenance of joint motion and muscle function is part of the early excision and grafting program, and it is certain that the longer joint motion is restricted the more likely it is that pericapsular structures will be damaged by stretching. We should like to think that any secondary injury to soft tissue could be avoided by controlled and assisted active motion, gentle terminal stretch, and terminal resistance.

When a patient is reluctant to move a joint previously moved with relative ease, and certainly when there is evidence of unusual swelling about the joint, roentgenograms should be obtained to determine if there is pericapsular calcification or ossification. Once heterotopic bone or calcification is recognized, joint exercise should be restricted to gentle passive and assisted active motion only. Crawford *et al.*[34] observed that ossification progressed to complete ankylosis in all patients who persisted in moving an affected joint beyond the pain-free range. They concluded that active range of motion exercises and stretching were contraindicated if heterotopic bone or calcification was suspected, but that active range of motion could be safely resumed within pain-free range once the diagnosis had been confirmed. In the series of Peterson *et al.*,[26] 18 patients suspected of having heterotopic bone had active range of motion exercises only. Ten regained functional range of motion and eight developed ankylosis.

Surgical excision of heterotopic bone is indicated when joint motion is lost or significantly compromised by bridging bone or exostoses. Evans has suggested that surgery be postponed until the burn wound has healed, scars are soft and associated with no inflammatory response, the patient is healthy, and the offensive bone is roentgenographiclly mature, i.e. well defined and not increasing in dimension[20] (**Figure 26.6**). This position makes sense considering the behavior of heterotopic bone, i.e. proliferation while there are open burn wounds or active scars and regression with wound healing and scar softening. For removal of heterotopic bone, surgical exposures should be planned with extensible incisions so as to facilitate total excision. When there is a bridge of bone, each end of the bridge should be slightly excavated. When there is attachment at only one end, the cartilaginous or fibrous extension should be removed along with the bone. Capsular sheets of bone should be removed completely. If bridging heterotopic bone is incompletely excised, the bridge is likely to recur. When a joint is bridged by bone in only one plane, removal of the offending bone will usually restore functional motion and the likelihood of recurrence of the bridge is small. When a joint is bridged in more than one plane, recurrence is more likely and the chance for restoration of functional range of motion is correspondingly diminished. When the local inflammatory process has caused intra-articular synovial proliferation and cartilage destruction, the joint is most likely destined for ankylosis. Removal of the heterotopic bone about a joint so affected may allow more functional positioning of the joint, but it is not likely to arrest the process. On the other hand, extra-articular arthrodesis by a bridge of heterotopic bone may preserve the joint. This is particularly the case at the elbow when there is only one posterior bridge of bone from olecranon to medial epicondylar ridge of the humerus. In this situation, the olecranon is fixed in the trochlea, but the radiocapitellar and radioulnar joints remain functional. In Evans' experience with removal of single bridges at the elbow, joint cartilage was found to be healthy as long as 5 years after ankylosis. Preservation of pronation and supination was credited with maintaining the synovial bath to provide nutrition for the humeroulnar cartilage. Indeed, when pronation and supination additionally are blocked by bridging bone, cartilage degradation is certain. Evans' further experience with long-term survival of glenohumeral cartilage after ankylosis by bridging bone from acromion to humerus is not as easily explained.

Reported experience with excision of heterotopic bone in burns has not been uniformly favorable. Dias,[46] Hoffer *et al.*,[43] and Peterson *et al.*[26] reported restoration of functional range of motion in most of their patients with timely excision of heterotopic bone. Other surgeons have reported less satisfactory results. In our own experience, results have varied, as anticipated, with severity of affliction. We have learned that if heterotopic bone recurs after excision, it is worthwhile to excise again if the joint affected remains structurally identifiable. For the most part, however, attempts to improve joint function with second operations have failed. We believe that ultimate failure can be predicted at the time of initial surgery; we are convinced that the single most important factor in successful initial excision is in timing surgery to coincide with the patient's return to good health.

Changes Involving the Joint

Dislocation

Luxations and subluxations of joints in burned patients may occur as a result of direct destruction by the burn of ligaments and capsules, loss of articular cartilage due to infection, faulty positioning, and eventually scar contracture. In all phases of management, but particularly in the acute phase, positioning is of prime importance in the prevention of joint deformity. The preferred positions, listed in **Table 26.2**, serve as a guide for the prevention of dislocation of joints and of malposition secondary to scar contracture.

The joints most liable to structural compromise due to exposure by the burn and loss of soft tissue support are knee, elbow, proximal interphalangeal joints of the hand, and metacarpophalangeal joints. These hinge joints have in common a subcutaneous dorsal surface, accounting for their ready exposure.

The elbow, for its trochlear architecture, is more intrinsically stable than the other joints in this group. It requires loss of collateral support to render it easily displaceable. The knee, on the other hand, is immediately in danger of subluxation if there is loss of continuity of its central slip, the patellar tendon, even if the retinacula remain intact. In this circumstance, gravity alone will displace the tibia posteriorly in relation to the femur if the patient is recumbent. The hamstring muscles contribute to the displacement force regardless of the position of the extremity. Loss of collateral ligaments compounds the problem, but loss of collateral ligament stability in the presence of an intact patellar tendon and functioning quadriceps constitutes far less a threat than loss of patellar tendon. For the lower extremity, persistent posterior translation of the tibia beneath the femur with inefficient quadriceps pull is potentially a functional disaster.

For both the elbow and the knee the protecting position is extension. These two joints are rarely at risk for articular displacement from contracture alone and, if there is no ligament or tendon loss, extension resting splints will give adequate positional support.

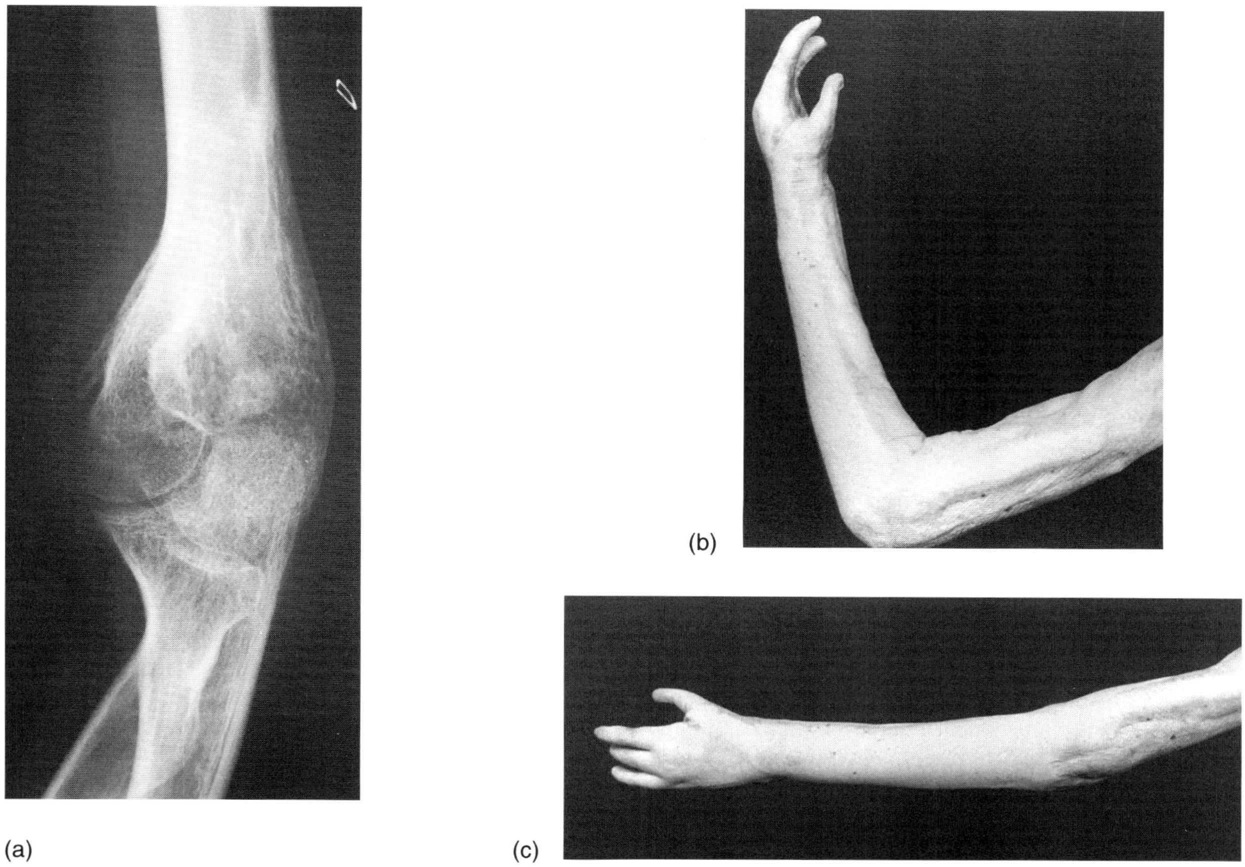

Fig. 26.6 (a) A mature sheet of heterotopic bone extends from humerus to olecranon, obliterating the olecranon fossa 11 months after 53% TBSA burn in a 13-year-old female. Elbow flexion and extension range was less than 10%. Pronation and supination were near normal range. (b) and (c) Three months after excision of heterotopic bone, the patient had attained 90 degrees of elbow motion and a continuing increase to functional (hand to mouth) range was predicted. Now the patient can extend and bend the elbow to 90 degrees.

Table 26.2 Preferred positions for major joints

Joint	Preferred position
Neck	Midline in neutral or slight extension
Shoulders	Scapulothoracic retraction and depression, 85 degrees of glenohumeral elevation with 20–25 degrees of horizontal flexion
Elbows	Extension
Wrists	Slight extension
Metacarpophalangeal joints 2 through 5	80–90 degrees of flexion
Fingers	Proximal and distal interphalangeal extension
Thumbs	Carpometacarpal flexion and abduction, metacarpophalangeal flexion 5–10 degrees, interphalangeal extension
Spine	Extension with no lateral deviation
Hips	Extension and slight external rotation in 15 degrees of symmetric abduction
Knees	Extension
Ankles	Neutral
Feet	Neutral

When there is soft tissue disruption, splinting may not adequately protect either joint. An external fixator with two pin, four cortex fixation above and below the joint will provide stability and will permit access to the wound. For the elbow, it allows fine adjustment to the normal carrying angle as well. If the knee is accurately reducible at the time of application of the fixator, there is a good possibility that the reduction can be maintained. If the tibia cannot be brought forward completely by manual manipulation, it may be necessary to suspend the tibia through a transverse pin at the level of the tibial tubercle. For static vertical traction, the extremity must be elevated from the bed. For dynamic traction, enough weight must be used to accomplish the same elevation. If the tibia can be brought forward by this means, an external fixator will likely hold the reduction. For the knee to remain stable with the tibia forward, the patellar tendon must be reattached and quadriceps integrity reestablished; otherwise, when the fixator is removed, the tibia will once again begin an incremental posterior shift toward its own point of stability. No amount of external splinting or bracing is likely to prevent that shift.

The proximal interphalangeal joints of the hands are more frequently exposed by burn than any others. If the central extensor slip remains intact, there is less risk of subluxation of the joint. Even if there is loss of continuity of the central slip but preservation of the lateral bands, subluxation is easily prevented if the joint is maintained in extension while soft tissue cover is being achieved. It is with loss of the support of lateral bands and collateral ligaments that the joints become liable to dislocation. With the metacarpophalangeal joints, the tendency to displacement or subluxation may be greater because these joints are functionally multiplaner, while the interphalangeal joints are uniplaner. Happily, the metacarpophalangeal joints are less often exposed than the interphalangeal ones.

The protecting position for the proximal interphalangeal joints is full extension. If only the central slip is lost, the position may be held with an external splint. In states of greater instability it may be necessary to use intramedullary transarticular Kirschner wires to hold the position. The wires, though reasonably efficient, do not control rotation, and they carry with them a risk of post-treatment joint stiffness. Pin traction through the distal phalanges in a skeletally stabilized metal splint is another method for maintaining extension of threatened digital joints.[47,48] It has the advantages of patient comfort and mobility, secure positioning of hand and upper extremity, easy maintenance of elevation, and easy access for dressings, for additional surgery, and for exercise of lesser affected joints. The system likewise makes it possible to keep digits separated, thus facilitating local care. Traction should not be used if collateral ligaments are not intact. By whatever means attained, the corrected position must be maintained until the joint is covered with graft. Protection should continue with a standard splint or brace until the joint is sound.

The two joints most likely to dislocate because of faulty positioning are the shoulder and the hip. These two ball and socket multiplaner joints sacrifice stability in favor of mobility. This is particularly true of the shoulder, where the shallow glenoid contains at any one time only one-third of the head of the humerus. In burns, the head of the humerus may begin to subluxate forward if, during prone positioning for management of back and buttock wounds, the arms are maintained in full abduction in the coronal plane. In this position the arms are in at least 15–20 degrees of extension from the more secure neutral position in line with the scapulae and the humeral heads are forced forward against the anterior capsule. Even when the patient is supine, full abduction and extension of the arms should be avoided. For short-term management, particularly when the patient gets out of bed every day, this position probably does not threaten the joint. But if the patient is to be bed confined and the position unrelieved for days or weeks, the head of the humerus may begin to subluxate forward. In the extreme situation, the head of the humerus will dislocate to a medial subcoracoid position. In patients with deep burns extending from chin to axillae to chest, the common posture of elevation and protraction of the scapulae may be associated with upward subluxation of the humeral heads. With one patient in whom the right clavicle was sacrificed distally because of the depth of the burn, the head of the right humerus moved forward and then upward because of loss of anterior stabilizers.

The head of the humerus is most secure in the glenoid fossa when the arm is adducted to neutral and internally rotated – a position which is incompatible with wound management of burns of the trunk, neck, and upper extremities. The protecting position which accommodates the need for abduction for axillary burns is elevation of the arms in line with the scapulae. The arm is then approximately 20 degrees forward of the coronal plane or in 20 degrees of horizontal flexion. When the patient is prone, the protecting position can be gained only if the chest is supported on a chest width mattress or foam rubber pad, either of which will allow the arms to drop forward. When the patient is positioned this way, whether supine or prone, the forearms will be pronated and the arms will be in sufficient internal rotation to favor seating of the head of the humerus in the glenoid.

The hip will tend to subluxate posteriorly if the thigh is persistently allowed to remain flexed, adducted and internally rotated during the acute burn phase. For the most part, however, the protecting position of extension to neutral or 180 degrees and 15–20 degrees of symmetric abduction is easy to attain and maintain and is, in fact, the most desirable position for wound management.

If dislocation of the head of humerus or femur is undetected or if reduction is delayed for other reason, open reduction will likely be required. Reduction of a chronically displaced head of humerus in one seriously burned patient using the Ilizarov technique was hampered by the fragility of the bone. Another head of humerus that had been dislocated anteriorly for several weeks was found at the time of open reduction to have extensive erosion of the articular cartilage.

Infection of a joint may result in its subluxation or dislocation. Hip displacement because of apparent spontaneous dissolution has been described by Evans and Smith.[1] Eszter and Istvan[6] and Cristallo and Dell'Orto[4] reported similar cases. In none of these cases, however, could it be determined that the joint destruction was due to infection.

Septic Arthritis

A joint exposed by a burn or by removal of burn eschar is presumed to be infected. The joints most frequently exposed are the knee, the elbow, the proximal interphalangeal joints of the hand, and the metacarpophalangeal joints, all on the subcutaneous dorsal surfaces. Wrist and ankle are less often affected and other joints rarely. Treatment requires stable positioning of the joint for maximum reduction of wound size so as to facilitate soft tissue closure or grafting and to allow aggressive daily lavage. The position for all of the joints listed except the ankle is extension. The ankle is positioned in neutral. External fixation, intramedullary pinning, or skeletal traction may be required in order to secure the position. To maintain ankle position it is sometimes appropriate to insert a large vertical Steinmann pin through calcaneus and talus into the tibia. The position should be maintained until the exposed joint is covered with epithelialized granulation tissue or skin graft. Exposed adjacent bone can be shaved or drilled so as to encourage surface granulation. Drilling is particularly useful at the elbow where the olecranon is regularly exposed. Often, however, granulation tissue will quickly extend the wound margins and effectively close the wound so as to allow split-thickness skin grafting. If the burn is isolated to the joint or if the extremity is not otherwise seriously burned, a local muscle, skin or compound flap may be used to close the joint. Free vascularized flaps are useful and should always be considered if it is anticipated that nerve graft or tendon graft or transfer at the site will be required in the future. Incremental remobilization of the joint may proceed when wound closure is sound. Culture of material from an exposed joint will likely yield a variety of organisms consistent with those of the general burn wound, requiring, thus, broad spectrum antibiotic management.

The incidence of hematogenous septic arthritis is obscured by its frequent association with severe burns and because there are rarely separable clinical signs such as local heat and swelling, elevation of temperature, and elevation of sedimentation rate. Local tenderness and greater than usual pain with motion may focus attention on the affected joint. Aspiration of the joint will confirm a diagnosis. A roentgenogram is helpful, but in the early phases of infection will show only local cellulitis as increased periarticular soft tissue density. If a patient has been receiving broad spectrum antibiotics, material aspirated from the affected joint may not grow an organism in culture. Clearly, without organism identification and sensitivity determinations, specific antibiotic therapy cannot be initiated.

We have been of the opinion that debridement and exteriorization of the joint and regular vigorous lavage are as important as antibiotics in the treatment of closed infected joints. We believe now that arthroscopic debridement and closed irrigation should be considered as an alternative method of management whether or not skin over the affected joint is burned. Rarely in burns, a joint may become infected from adjacent metaphyseal osteomyelitis. In this situation joint preservation is the treatment priority, and measures are the same as for septic arthritis of strictly hematogenous origin.[41] In children most infected joints can be salvaged. Adult joints are less resilient. Persistent joint infection will destroy cartilage and lead to ankylosis.[5,49] All chronically infected joints are liable to dislocation because of surface destruction and capsular laxity.

Amputations

In burns, major amputations are most often performed because of non-viability of the extremity or because a surviving extremity is rendered useless by scar, deformity or insensitivity. Occasionally, in an extensive burn, a severely burned extremity which might be salvaged in part is sacrificed to reduce the extent of the burn or as a lifesaving measure.

In thermal burns, the level of extremity amputation is determined by the viability of muscles and tendons. The more distal the site the better, and it is important to retain joints even if motion will be restricted. For example, if a forearm or leg must be sacrificed, the elbow or knee should be spared if the more proximal muscles controlling that joint are intact, if the bone bleeds, and if there is the possibility that the remaining tissue of the stump has sufficient blood supply to produce granulations for grafting. Aside from affording a better functional prospect, sparing the joint will provide the surgeon opportunity at a later time to choose an appropriate revision level if the joint does not function. The patient will at that time be healthier and stump closure will be routine. Jackson suggests that it may be technically feasible to cover even nonviable bone with a free flap in order to maintain extremity length.[28]

Prostheses can be easily fitted over stumps covered with split-thickness grafts. Ridges of hypertrophic scar will break down if there is friction within the socket of the prosthesis. A scar often softens and flattens because of the constant even pressure of a well fitted socket; prostheses fitted early over grafted stumps may prevent scar thickening. Breakdown may occur at points where the graft is adherent to bone. This problem may necessitate surgical freeing of the adherent graft and reshaping of the bone. Minor hip and knee flexion contractures complicate the fitting and function of a prosthesis; thus, every effort should be made to maintain full extension of these joints. Late revisions of amputations in children are required when the bone overgrows in length and when offensive terminal exostoses develop. The overgrowing bone can be shortened and the exostoses removed.

It is important, in the early management of upper extremity amputations in infants and young children, to supply temporary prosthetic extensions. This provides functional orientation to a prosthesis, maintains muscle bulk and tone, and encourages continuing bimanual activity at normal extremity length until a prosthesis with appropriate terminal device can be applied. Children quickly acquire prehension and transfer skills if they have an opposable stump and they may reject prostheses if they are not applied early. It is equally important to restore bipedal function as soon as possible. If delay of healing or ulceration of a lower extremity stump prevents early prosthetic fitting, an ischial weight-bearing device which suspends the stump will permit the child to walk in advance of prosthetic fitting. Inflatable plastic air bags provide both even pressure and accurate fit for weight bearing in container sockets. Early prosthetic fitting is desirable in teenagers and adults as well, but is not as critical as it is in children. As in non-burned persons, an upper extremity prosthesis may be rejected at any age if the opposite extremity is fully functional.[50]

Alterations in Growth

In 1959, Evans and Smith reported that a patient who was 24 years of age when burned had a subsequent 1½ inch increase in height. It was suggested that one explanation for this growth spurt might be local change in hemodynamics with stasis, passive hyperemia, and chronic inflammation. We have not since documented height changes in burned adults, but we have observed children whose growth after burn has seemed to be retarded. The study of Rutan and Herndon confirms growth delay in seriously burned children, particularly in the first postburn year. If growth plates remain open, it is difficult to explain overall growth retardation except on an endocrine or humoral basis. It is easy, however, to explain extremity length differences on the basis of premature closure of growth plates due to direct involvement of the bone or to severity of overlying burn. Frantz reported lower limb length discrepancy in four patients with foot and ankle burns.[51] Growth plates closed prematurely in only two of the cases. Jackson described two patients with digital and lower extremity deformity respectively due to partial closure of growth plates.[28] In Ritsila's case, contracture alone was apparently the cause of growth retardation in an upper extremity.[52] It seems reasonable, though hard to prove, that growth in a severely burned extremity would be retarded because of functional impairment. One patient, a 3-year-old boy with 80% total body surface burn and sufficiently deep burns of the right upper extremity to require mid-humerus amputation, demonstrated, 4 years after the burn, failure of development of the right shoulder girdle. The factors operant in this case could be premature closure of growth plates of scapula and clavicle, restrictive scar, and disuse atrophy.

There is yet another confusing aspect of premature closure of growth plates in that within an extremity with total full-thickness burn, only a few of the growth plates will close prematurely. The explanation for this capricious selectivity is at best obscure. Evans and Calhoun recorded an example of spotty closure of growth plates in a 14-year-old male with 90% total body surface burn.[19] There was complete closure of distal tibial and fibular epiphyses 1 year after burn together with closure of all digital epiphyses in the feet and of several digital epiphyses in the hands. Other major epiphyses were spared (**Figure 26.2**).

In early experience, abnormal growth plate closure was observed in a 6-year-old girl with 50% third degree burn which did not involve legs or ankles.[53] Rapidly destructive septic arthritis of one ankle resulted in closure of the adjacent tibial growth plate.

Only occasionally can growth changes be anticipated because of obvious affection of the bone. More often the changes are subtle. It seems clear, thus, that among seriously burned children, regular height and extremity length measurements must be part of ongoing postburn assessment until it is determined that the extremities and trunk are developing on schedule. Extremity and trunk alignment must likewise be part of the assessment as subtle angular deformity can occur because of partial closure of a growth plate. Jackson's report addresses this problem.[28]

So-called growth arrest lines seen in the roentgenograms of non-burned children, who have serious illness or major trauma other than burns, are commonly observed in burned children. In burns, as in other conditions, these transverse markers of relatively increased mineralization represent normal recovery from an insult to enchondral bone formation due to serious stress. They are of no clinical or functional significance. They are more related to total burn than to involvement of select burned extremities as all major long bones are affected. There is no evidence that growth arrest lines *per se* have any effect on growth.

REFERENCES

1. Evans E B Smith J R. Bone and joint changes following burn. *J Bone Joint Surg, [Am]* 1959; **41:** 785.

2. Rabinov D. Acromutilation of the fingers following severe burns. *Radiology* 1961; **77:** 968–73.

3. Peters W J. Heterotopic ossification: can early surgery be performed, with a positive bone scan? *J Burn Care Rehabil* 1978; **11**(4): 318.

4. Cristallo V, Dell'Orto R. Pathological dislocation of the hip. *Arch Ortop* 1966; **79:** 57–61.

5. Evans E B, Larson D L, Abston S, Willis B. Prevention and correction of deformity after severe burns. *Surg Clin North Am* 1970; **50:** 1361–75.

6. Eszter V, Istvan S. Atipusos septicus arthritisek spontan luxatiok egesi serulteken. *Orv Hetil* 1972; **113:** 48.

7. Jozsa L, Reffy A, Menesi L. Thermal injuries of human tendons. *Acta Chir Hung* 1985; **26:** 113–18.

8. Salisbury R E, McKeel D W, Mason A D. Ischemic necrosis of the intrinsic muscles of the hand after thermal injuries. *J Bone Joint Surg [Am]* 1974; **56:** 1701–7.

9. Schiele H P, Hubbard R B, Bruck H M. Radiographic changes in burns of the upper extremity. *Diagn Radiol* 1972; **104:** 13–17.

10. Klein G, Herndon H, Rutan T, *et al.* Long term reduction in bone mass and increased fracture risk in children following severe burns. *J Pediatr.* In press.

11. Owens N. Osteoporosis following burns. *Br J Plast Surg* 1949; **1:** 245–56.

12. Colson P, Stagnara P, Houot H. L-osteoporose chez les brules des membres. *Lyon Chir* 1953; **48:** 950–6.

13. Artz C P, Reiss E. *The Treatment of Burns.* 1st ed. Philadelphia: WB Saunders, 1957.

14. Klein G, Herndon D, Rutan T, *et al.* Bone disease in burn patients. *J. Bone Miner Res* 1993; **8**(3): 337–45.

15. Van Der Wiel H, Lips P, Naura J, Patka C, Harma J, Teule G. Loss of bone in the proximal part of the femur following unstable fractures of the leg. *J Bone Joint Surg [Am]* 1994; **76:** 230–6.

16. Dowling J A, Omer E, Moncrief J A. Treatment of fractures in burn patients. *J Trauma* 1968; **8:** 465–74.

17. Choctaw W T, Zawacki B E, Dorr L. Primary excision and grafting of burns located over an open fracture. *Arch Surg* 1979; **114:** 1141–2.

18. Wang Xue-wei, Zhang Zhong-ning. The successful treatment of a patient with extensive deep burns and an open comminuted fracture of a lower extremity. *Burns* 1984; **10:** 339–43.

19. Evans E B, Calhoun J H. Musculoskeletal changes complicating burns. In: Epps C H Jr, ed. *Complications in Orthopaedic Surgery.* Vol. 2. Philadelphia: JB Lippincott Co, 1994: 1239–78.

20. Evans E B. Orthopaedic measures in the treatment of severe burns. *J Bone Joint Surg [Am]* 1966; **48:** 643.

21. Brooker A F. The use of external fixation in the treatment of burn patients with fractures. In: Brooker A F, Edwards C C, eds. *Fracture Fixation: The Current State of the Art. J of Pediatrics* 1995; **126**, 2: 252–56.

22. Saffle J R, Schnelby A, Hoffmann A, Warden G: The management of fracture in thermally injured patients. *J Trauma* 1983; **23:** 902–10.

23. Boyd B M, Robers W M, Miller G R. Periarticular ossification following burns. *South Med J* 1959; **52:** 1048.

24. Koepke G D. Personal communication, 1964.

25. Elledge E S, Smith A A, McManus W F, Pruitt B A. Heterotopic bone formation in burned patients. *J Trauma* 1988; **28:** 684–7.

26. Peterson S I, Mani M M, Crawford C M, Neff J R, Hiebert J M. Postburn heterotopic ossification: insights for management decision making. *J Trauma* 1989; **29:** 365.

27. Tepperman P S, Hilbert L, Peters W J, Pritzker K P H. Heterotopic ossification in burns. *J Burn Care Rehabil* 1984; **5:** 283.

28. Jackson D MacG. Destructive burns: some orthopaedic complications. *Burns* 1979; **7:** 105–22.

29. Munster A M, Bruck H M, John L A, Von Prince K, Kirkman E J, Remig R L. Heterotopic calcification following burns: a prospective study. *J Trauma* 1972; **12:** 1071–4.

30. Kolar J, Vrabec R. Periarticular soft-tissue changes as a late consequence of burns. *J Bone Joint Surg [Am]* 1959; **41:** 103–11.

31. Heggers J P, Heggers R, Robson M C. Biochemical abnormalities in the thermally injured. *J Am Med Technol* 1981; **43:** 333.

32. Herndon D. Mediators of metabolism. *J Trauma* 1981; **12:** 701.

33. Johnston J T H. Atypical myositis ossificans. *J Bone Joint Surg [Am]* 1957; **39:** 189–94.

34. Crawford C M, Varghese G, Mani M M, Neff J R. Heterotopic ossification: are range of motion exercises contraindicated. *J Burn Care Rehail* 1986; **7:** 323.

35. Evans E B. Heterotopic bone formation in thermal burns. *Clin Orthop* 1991; **263:** 94–101.

36. Michelsson J E, Rauschning W. Pathogenesis of experimental heterotopic bone formation following temporary forcible exercising of immobilized limbs. *Clin Orthop Rel Res* 1983; **176:** 265–72.

37. Lorber J. Ectopic ossification in tuberculous meningitis. *Arch Dis Child* 1953; **28:** 98.

38. Jacobs P. Reversible ectopic soft tissue ossification following measles encephalomyelitis. *Arch Dis Child* 1962; **37:** 90.

39. Garland D E, Blum C E, Waters R L. Periarticular heterotopic ossification in head-injured adults. *J Bone Joint Surg [Am]* 1985; **62:** 1261.

40. VanLaeken N, Snelling C T, Meek R N, Warren R J, Foley B. Heterotopic bone formation in the patient with burn injuries. A retrospective assessment of contributing factors and methods of investigation. *J Burn Care Rehabil* 1989; **10:** 331.

41. Evans E B. Musculoskeletal changes complicating burns. In: Epps C H Jr, ed. *Complications in Orthopaedic Surgery.* Vol 2. Philadelphia: JB Lippincott Co, 1978: 1133–58.

42. Cope R. Heterotopic ossification. *South Med J* 1990; **83**(9): 1058.

43. Hoffer M, Brody G, Ferlic F. Excision of heterotopic ossification about elbows in patients with thermal injury. *J Trauma* 1978; **18:** 667–70.

44. Bottu Y, VanNoyen G. Un cas d'ossification reversible des tissus mous chez une petite patiente paraplegique. *Acta Paediatr Belg* 1963; **17:** 223.

45. Proulz R, Dupuis M. Ossifications et calcifications para-articulaires à la suite de brulures: revue de la literature et présentation de 3 cas. *Union Med Can* 1972; **101:** 282–93.

46. Dias D. Heterotopic para-articular ossification of the elbow with soft tissue contracture in burns. *Burns* 1982; **9:** 128–34.

47. Harnar T, Engrav L, Heimbach D, Marvin J. Experience with skeletal immobilization after excision and grafting of the severely burned hands. *J Trauma* 1985; **25:** 299–302.

48. Youel L, Evans E, Heare T C, Herndon D N, Larson D L, Abston S. Skeletal suspension in the management of severe burns in children. *J Bone Joint Surg [Am]* 1986; **68:** 1375–9.

49. Jackson D MacG. Burns into joints. *Burns* 1976; **2:** 90–106.

50. Malone J M, Fleming L L, Roberson J, *et al.* Immediate, early and late postsurgicial management of upper-lumb amputation. *J Rehabil Res Dev* 1984; **21:** 33–41.

51. Frantz C H, Delgado S. Limb-length discrepancy after third-degree burns about the foot and ankle. *J Bone Joint Surg [Am]* 1966; 48: 443–50.

52. Ritsila V, Sundell B, Alhopura S. Severe growth retardation of the upper extremity resulting from burn contracture and its full recovery after release of the contracture. *Br J Plast Surg* 1976; **29:** 53–5.

53. Evans E B, Larson L, Yates S. Preservation and restoration of joint function in patients with severe burns. *JAMA* 1968; **204:** 843–8.

CHAPTER TWENTY-SEVEN

THE IMMUNOLOGICAL RESPONSE AND STRATEGIES FOR INTERVENTION

ANDREW M. MUNSTER

INTRODUCTION AND OVERVIEW

The heightened susceptibility of burn patients to infection has been noted for over 30 years. By the mid-1960s, in both burned humans and experimental animals, alterations in immunoglobulin kinetics, phagocytic function, neutrophil function, and in the humoral response to primary and recall antigens has been documented. Skin testing for delayed hypersensitivity had been performed and prolongation of allograft survival demonstrated. These early historical developments and original work are described in a number of early reviews.[1,2] A review published in the mid-1970s on this subject already contained over 200 references.[3] More recently, extensive new reviews of work in the areas of mechanisms of immunological suppression, the role of inflammatory mediators, and the influence of hormonal milieu have become available.[4–7]

It is widely recognized that the immunological status of the burned patient has a measurable impact on outcome in terms of survival, death, and major morbidity. This can be documented using almost any *in vivo* or *in vitro* test of immune function which happens to be convenient; many of them correlate very well with prognosis (references 8,9, reviewed in reference 10). Nutritional support of the burned patient is considered in detail in Chapter 22 of this work, but nutritional support is clearly essential for adequate immune function. This evolving field is well reviewed in a recent publication in which three papers are particularly recommended for overview.[11–13]

The story of cutaneous burn toxin has been with us for 40 years, and throughout, toxin has had its champions and its detractors. Most recently, using modern immunological techniques, it has been shown that the biological effects of cutaneous burn toxin are indeed separable from endotoxin and affect the cytokine cascade.[14,15] Nevertheless, the precise biological role of burn toxin remains elusive. By contrast, there is now little disagreement that the burn wound remains a serious source of suppressive activity and that early removal of the burned tissue and wound coverage is an essential part of the immunological care of the burned patient.[16–18]

Perhaps the greatest difficulty in attempting to decipher the body's response to injury is the complex interrelationship of the cytokine cascade, the arachidonic acid cascade, and the neuroendocrine axis. The multiple feedback loops and regulatory systems are only just now beginning to be elucidated and the very complexity of the system has defeated the optimism of many workers for the early achievement of simple interventions. These networks have been recently reviewed[19–21] and make interesting reading for individuals wishing to delve into the subject more deeply.

Terminology is evolving rapidly. To help with the reading of this chapter, an algorithm follows (**Table 27.1**) and a short glossary of important cytokine and receptor nomenclature (**Table 27.2**).

THE HOST RESPONSE TO THERMAL INJURY

The Arachidonic Acid Cascade

The major product of the arachidonic acid cascade following thermal injury is prostaglandin E_2 (PGE_2). Originally, because of

Table 27.1 Major time-related responses to injury

Initial (1–2 h)	Subsequent (48 h)	Late
Cytokine induction	Coagulation changes	Sepsis
Activation of AA cascade	Substrate utilization changes	MSOF
Hormonal changes	Lymphocyte, macrophage and neutrophil alterations	Toxic metabolite release
Translocation		

Table 27.2 Some key cytokines and membrane receptors

Name	*Function* (partial list)
Interleukin 1 (IL-1)	Mitogenic, stimulates granulocytes, T & B cell proliferation, fever, acute phase proteins
Interleukin 2 (IL-2)	Mitogenic, activates macrophages, T & B cell activation, fever
Tumor necrosis factor (TNF)	Mitogenic, activates macrophages, stimulates granulocytes, T-cells, fever
Interleukin 6 (IL-6)	Mitogenic, stimulates T & B cells, induces acute phase response
Interleukin 8 (IL-8)	Granulocyte activation and migration
Transforming growth factor β (TGF-β)	Mitogenic, inhibits T & B cells, stimulates cell growth and angiogenesis
CD4	T-cell marker, MHC Class II coreceptor
CD8	T-cell marker, non-NK suppressor cells
CD11	Adhesion molecule (many subtypes)
CD14	Myeloid differentiation antigen, LPB-LPS complex binding
CD18	β chain of epithelial cell receptor
CD21	Complement receptor
CD23	B-cell activation marker
CD25	NK, T & B cell activation marker
CD69	Early B & T cell activation marker
CD71	Ubiquitous leucocyte activation marker

evidence that endotoxin-mediated immunosuppression could be blocked by indomethacin, it was thought that the induction of prostaglandin E_2 production by macrophages was mediated by endotoxin.[22] While this has been partially substantiated, there is also evidence that PGE_2 exerts its suppressive effect principally by inhibition of lymphocyte IL-2 production and T-cell activation.[23] In addition, PGE_2 appears to downregulate IL-6 secretion.[24] The induction of the arachidonic acid cascade itself is complex, apparently dependent on at least two pathways, one calcium channel dependent and one calcium independent.[25] There are massive increases of another arachidonic acid derivative, thromboxane B_2, in the plasma of burned patients, particularly immediately postburn and during septic episode.[26] 6-Keto-prostaglandin-$F_{1\alpha}$ levels are unchanged following burn injury, this being a stable metabolite of prostacyclin (PGI_2), suggesting that there is a postburn alteration in the arachidonic acid pathway in favor of the PGE_2 series and thromboxane B_2. In view of the immunosuppressive effects of PGE_2, and the physiologic actions of thromboxane B_2, which include vasoconstriction, leukocyte and platelet aggregation, and membrane destabilization, these two products must be considered key in the immediate effects of thermal injury. Leukotriene B_4, another arachidonic acid product (see **Table 27.1**), is a potent neutrophil chemotactic factor, and is produced following thermal injury.

The Cytokine Cascade

Following injury, induction of a number of cytokines rapidly occurs, the best studies of these being tumor necrosis factor, interleukin-1, and interleukin-6. Burned patients are no different from other injured patients in the timetable of induction of the cytokines. Tumor necrosis factor-α (TNFα) is detectable early during the period of burn shock; at that time, the levels cannot be correlated with prognosis. By contrast, the maximum TNFα level over the whole clinical course is of prognostic significance.[27] Because endotoxin injuries have very comparable abilities to induce a cytokine cascade, considerable effort has been made to attempt to separate these two mechanisms. Both TNF and endotoxin can cause neutrophil activation, but the pathways appear to be different in that anti-TNF antibody blocks TNF-mediated neutrophil activation but does not inhibit endotoxin-mediated neutrophil activation.[28] Patients with high TNF levels (over 540 pg/ml) have a very poor prognosis, although the absolute level of TNF does not correlate with burn size.[29]

There are further intriguing physiologic actions of TNF which are only now being fully researched. Repeated exposure to endotoxin results in progressively reduced secretions of TNF, and thereby provides a possible mode for endotoxin tolerance. A similar effect is seen if experimental endotoxin-sensitive mice are first treated with dexamethasone.[30,31] Further, it appears that the peak production of TNFα in monocytes occurs concomitantly with massive production of prostaglandin E_2.[32]

Because the physiologic effects of TNF are almost indistinguishable from endotoxin, the induction of TNF has been held responsible for the clinical effects of endotoxemia; the induction and secretion of TNF has become a reasonable target for interventional modalities for sepsis. This will be considered later in this chapter.

Much of the work on the interleukins has been done in trauma rather than burned patients, and some of the data need to be extrapolated. Specifically with regard to interleukin-1 (IL-1), after the initial induction of IL-1, synthesis is significantly impaired for several days after injury.[33] By contrast, there appears to be an upregulated local production of IL-1 and IL-6 in inflammatory sites, thus inducing polymorphonuclear neutrophil chemoattraction.[34]

Interleukin-2 (IL-2) has been identified as a key cytokine in the mediation of the cellular immune response. In a series of burned patients, initial IL-1 production was initially significantly elevated and then returned to normal, but patients with large burns had significantly suppressed production of IL-2 which correlated with the length of time from injury.[35] The kinetics of IL-2 secretion are interesting and of potential importance in postburn immunosuppression. Following lymphocyte activation, there is increased expression of IL-2 receptors (IL-2R) on the surface of the T cell which is then rapidly shed into the serum, resulting in elevated serum IL-2R levels following burn injury. This phenomenon could have two implications: either the free IL-2R now competes with ligands which would activate cell surface IL-2R, or diminished receptor expression on the surface, following a burst of lymphocyte activity, renders the cell relatively inactive and reduces further IL-2 secretion.[36-40]

Investigations of interleukin-8 (IL-8) following burn injury are in their infancy, but because of the importance of pulmonary production of IL-8 following adult respiratory distress syndrome (ARDS), it is an interleukin of potential importance in burned patients.[41]

Interleukin-6 (IL-6) is an interesting cytokine which is probably the most studied of all the immunoregulatory cytokines following injury and stress. It is a ubiquitous cytokine which is produced by a variety of cells and is detected in increased concentrations in blood or tissues following disturbances in physiologic homeostasis of any kind, including psychological stressors.[42] Presumably the most important role of IL-6 following burn injury is the induction of phase reactants, some of which include antibacterial products such as fibronectin.[43] The induction of IL-6 in burn patients is very rapid, is followed by induction of acute phase proteins,[44] and can be closely correlated with prognosis in severe burns.[45] Interestingly, although the induction of prostaglandin E_2 production parallels that of IL-6 induction in the macrophage, and PGE_2 downregulates IL-1 production, it has no effect on blocking the induction of IL-6.[46] Experimentally, the synthesis of acute phase proteins will persist for several days following induction even after the removal of the original stimulant.[47] In addition to the correlation of IL-6 levels with acute phase reactants, these levels can also be correlated with the clinical parameters of inflammation and injury.[48] It has been known for some time that cell activation can be inhibited by high levels of interleukin-6, and that TGFβ elevates macrophage PGE_2 production.[49] Recently evidence has been produced that the immunosuppressive activity of high concentrations of IL-6 are mediated by the activation of TGFβ.[50]

CELL-MEDIATED IMMUNITY

T Cells

Early observations of suppression on cell-mediated immunity using technology available in the 1960s and 1970s documented delays in allograft rejection, impairment in mitogenic and antigenic responsiveness of lymphocytes, burn size related suppression of graft versus host reactivity, suppression of delayed cutaneous sensitivity tests, and diminution in both peripheral lymphocyte numbers and thoracic duct lymphocyte concentration (see reviews quoted earlier). The introduction of immunofluorescent labeling and the characterization of lymphocyte subpopulations led to the description of alterations in the various populations of lymphocytes in peripheral blood and tissue. Currently, there is general agreement that the functional capacity of thymic-dependent lymphocytes (T cells) to perform their normal physiologic responses is impaired; there is enormous controversy as to whether this failure is due to an intracellular defect related to thermal injury, the result of 'overuse', or indirectly the result of downregulation by the cytokine cascade or other products of the inflammatory reaction.

Initially, it was suggested that the immunosuppression of burn injury may be related to an imbalance between suppressor and helper cells.[51] Analysis of peripheral blood in the hands of several groups appeared to show support for this hypothesis.[52-54] More recent evidence supports the theory that, rather than an absolute reduction in CD4 and an increase in CD8 cells, there may be a redistribution of lymphocyte traffic. Suppression in the numbers of the total lymphocyte population is the only consistent overall change.[55-57] Further, not only is there lymphocyte traffic between central lymphocyte stores and the peripheral blood following thermal injury but the responsiveness of these lymphocyte populations also varies according to site; for example, splenic lymphocytes of experimentally burned animals remain most profoundly depressed in response to antigenic stimulation compared with the peripheral blood and other organs.[58] In addition, in peripheral blood, the appearance of 'activation' antigens on CD4 and CD8 cells (HLA-DR, IL-2R and transferrin receptor) is significantly depressed as early as one day postburn.[59] This finding has not been universally confirmed, since other workers have reported an increase in activation receptors CD25, CD69, and CD71 in the peripheral blood of adult burned patients.[60]

Addition of recombinant IL-2 does not appear to reverse the suppression of the appearance of surface markers such as IL-2R in burned patients,[61] although it does not improve the response of NK cells to stimulation.[62] The appearance of free IL-2R in serum has already been alluded to.[32] Another intriguing observation is that peripheral lymphocyte membrane fluidity, usually affected in the stressed state by increased cortisol levels in the blood, is altered in burned patients, which could be part of the explanation of postburn immune suppression.[63] Perhaps the most convincing evidence of T-cell failure following a high level of activation is the temporal coexistence in the same samples of high serum IL-2 levels, low cellular expression of IL-2Rα, and high free soluble IL-2R levels.[64]

In summary, following major thermal injury, there is a partition of lymphocyte compartments with an overall suppression of the total lymphocyte population and strong activation of helper T cells. Following continued activation, and perhaps because of some other still not completely understood physiologic alteration in intracellular or membrane physiology, there is sustained failure of responsiveness of T cells to normal physiologic stimuli which is of clinical consequence. It is also worth mentioning that these findings, although heightened in burn patients, are not unique, but can be brought on by any form of stress, even mental and psychosocial.[65,66] In experimental preparations, at least some of the observed suppression can be alleviated by early removal of the burn wound,[67] thereby creating one further argument for the prompt closure of the burn wound.

Macrophages

Suppression of the ability of the reticuloendothelial system to take up particulate material was among the original observations of burn immunology made in the 1960s (see review in reference 1) and has been recently confirmed.[68] In the more recent report, however, there was a differentially increased uptake of colloid in alveolar macrophages compared with other organs, perhaps indicating alveolar macrophage activation. Macrophages and monocytes appear to be activated in a fashion similar to lymphocytes following thermal injury. A popular way of measuring macrophage activation is the serum neopterin level, which is increased following thermal injury.[69,70] This activation is confirmed by increased expression of the monocyte cell surface antigen C3b and iC3b.[71] At the same time, there is a reduction of HLA-DR, HLA-DQ, and HLA-DP expression by monocytes, and these class II antigens are obligatory for many cell-mediated immunological processes, thereby implying a possible loss of monocyte function following thermal injury.[72] Not only does macrophage function appear to be altered, but products of macrophages are capable of suppressing mitogenic responsiveness in normal lymphocytes[73] and the macrophage/monocyte is among the principal cell types which secrete immunoregulatory cytokines.

C3 production by burned patients' macrophages is suppressed, but the synthetic ability for key cytokines such as IL-6 which, as mentioned,[45] is massively increased, is difficult to assess because so many other cells produce cytokines.[74] In multiple injury and septic patients, elevation of neopterin secretion is accompanied by severe impairment of IL-1 and IL-8 synthesis, but IL-6 synthesis remains high. It is likely that a similar set of circumstances prevails in the burned patient as well.[33] In experimental septic preparations, to which burned patients and burned animals usually bear a striking similarity, there is specific activation of alveolar macrophages which produce superoxide anions, A-glucuronidase, and arachidonic metabolites directly leading to lung injury.[75]

In summary, the macrophage/monocyte axis, which is biologically much more multi-faceted than the lymphocyte, undergoes activation following thermal injury. This activation is differentiated both by product and by site. Proinflammatory cytokines are produced as a short burst, probably inhibited by a feedback loop, at which time there is a decreased receptor expression. The activation includes lung, and may provide the background for the development of the adult respiratory distress syndrome (ARDS) seen in burned patients.

B Cells

The function of bone marrow derived thymocytes or B cells following thermal injury is less well documented than that of macrophages or T cells and particularly confusing because the B cell population is subject to many messenger and environmental influences which are altered as a result of thermal injury. When B cells endocytose and degrade foreign antigens, the fragments of that antigen are expressed on the B cell surface in noncovalent association with class II major histocompatibility complex (MHC) molecules, which serve as recognition complex for CD4 helper T cells. As has been already mentioned[72] the expression of this MHC complex is impaired and, therefore, some diminution of B cell function can be expected as a result of diminished recognition of antigenic presentation.[76] Under the influence of stress-induced corticosteroid circulation, there is a relative increase of circulating B cells compared with T cells in peripheral blood.[77] Spontaneous and cytokine (IL-4 and IL-2)-induced expression of the activation antigen CD23 is significantly reduced during the second to fifth week postburn.[78] At the same time, the release of the proteolytic cleavage product, sCD23, which represents B cell growth and differentiation, is also reduced.[79] On the other hand, interleukin-6 is a polyclonal B cell activator and, therefore, could be expected to induce widespread B cell activation following thermal injury.[80]

If the products of B cell activation, namely the immunoglobulins, are measured *in vivo*, the results are somewhat difficult to interpret because of the increased catabolism of protein and the leakage through the burn wound. This will be discussed later.

In summary, the B cell population is subject to the same nonspecific activation as the rest of the lymphocyte population, and in addition, the products are quickly degraded by other mechanisms to where overall physiologic function is seriously impaired.

Neutrophils

Work on neutrophil dysfunction following thermal injury has been reviewed in previous references,[1–3] as well as in a more recent review of neutrophil disorders following injury.[81] Fc receptor expression is decreased,[82] intracellular killing capacity is depressed (this is a differential suppression, more for some organisms than others),[83] and this is accompanied by a brief increase in neutrophil respiratory burst response.[59] This dysfunction seems to be related to a failure of initial alkalization of the phagolysosome,[84] and subsequent kinetics of acidification are also altered.[85] This is an oxygen-independent bactericidal mechanism, depression of which would impair the capacity of the neutrophil for intracellular killing following thermal injury. Some of this impairment may result from the external environment, as with other immunocytes, because it has been shown that prostaglandin E elevates intracellular cyclic 3′,5′ adenosine monophosphate (cAMP) content in polymorphonuclear cells which can be restored by cyclooxygenase blockade.[86] Expression of CD16 (FcR, Fc IgG receptor) and CD11 (adhesion molecule) on neutrophils is impaired following major injury; and this reduction appears to be directly related to the appearance of bacteremia or pneumonia.[87] These changes in adhesion molecule expression, which is closely related to chemotaxis,[88] may play a part in the failure of delivery of neutrophils in adequate numbers to the local site of a burn.[89] Recently, it has also been found that there is a defect in actin polymerization in burn patients' neutrophils, a basic mechanism of chemotaxis, which may also contribute to a failure of motility.[90]

There is an impairment in leukotriene generation (LTB_4, 20-OH-LTB_4, 20-COOH-LTB_4 from the polymorphs of severely burned patients.[91] This appears to be based on the availability, or lack of availability, of the metabolizable substrate-free arachidonic acid. Because leukotriene B_4 is also a potent neutrophil chemotactic agent, this may further contribute to the failure of neutrophil function.

Basophil granulocytes participate in the dysfunction of other immunologically active cells. Anti-IgE induced basophil histamine release in burned patients is reduced immediately, while the calcium-ionosphere release of histamine does not fail until the second day postburn.[92] As with other cells, the baseline granulocyte oxidative activity in burn neutrophils is increased.[93] Induction of neutrophil activation probably takes several different stimulants, but it is known that tumor necrosis factor and endotoxin can both activate neutrophils;[28] IL-6 is also a potent inducer of superoxide production by the neutrophil.[94]

The Neuroendocrine Axis and Postburn Immunity

The role of opioids in immunity has recently been reviewed.[95] The induction of opioid-induced suppression has been defined for natural killer cells, CD4 and CD8 cells, and the receptor types have been characterized.[96] Clearly, the interrelationship of the neuroendocrine axis and the immune system is key in the stressed burned patient, but the full implications of this axis are only now beginning to be explored. It has been reported that plasma β-endorphins return to normal rapidly after 36 hours postburn. Morphine stimulates neutrophil oxygen consumption.[98] The relationship between opioids and immune changes following thermal injury remains a fertile field for further research.

Endotoxin

Complete discussion of the biological effects of endotoxin is beyond the scope of this chapter, but because the pathophysiology of endotoxemia is interwoven with the immunological response of the burned patient and, in particular, with the cytokine cascade, a brief consideration of endotoxemia is necessary. In this discussion, the terms 'endotoxin' and 'lipopolysaccharide' (LPS) will be used interchangeably.

Endotoxemia in the burned patient has two principal sources: translocation from the gastrointestinal tract and the burn wound. Of course, any septic focus can give rise to endotoxemia. It is well documented that thermal injury increases intestinal permeability, leading to translocation in both experimental animals and man.[99–101] Because endotoxin itself increases intestinal permeability,[102] a vicious cycle may well be set up. Endotoxemia is related to burn size[103] and, further in the postburn course, the level of endotoxin in the plasma is related to prognosis.[104]

The response of cytokine gene regulation to endotoxin is both dose and time independent. Extremely low concentrations of endotoxin (0.001 ng/ml) will induce IL-8 mRNA. With concentrations of 0.01 ng/ml, IL-1β and TNFα mRNA are activated. The cytokine mRNA for IL-1α, IL-6, and GM-CSF are activated only with higher doses of endotoxin and after a longer exposure time.[105] Human monocytes treated with bacterial lipopolysaccharide also release prostaglandin E_2 and thromboxane B_2.[106] Hematologic changes which follow endotoxemia are probably mediated by TNF and IL-1, and include lymphopenia and neutrophilia.[107] Endotoxin induces a polymorphonuclear leucocyte infiltration factor in human macrophages.[108] *Pseudomonas* causes induction of histamines and leukotrienes from mast cells and granulocytes.[109] Interferon-γ is induced, a reaction dependent on the presence of macrophages and IL-2.[110] Different types of endotoxins from different organisms have a different potency and a different timetable in the induction of cytokines.[111] The exact correlation between the clinical action of the lipopolysaccharides and the induction of cytokines is controversial. There are many differences in the induction kinetics in various experimental settings; and it is likely that lipopolysaccharides produce a number of effects independent of the cytokine cascade, more particularly TNF.[112]

Complicating the effect of the endotoxin-induced arachidonic acid and cytokine cascade is the fact that there are a number of natural host antagonists to endotoxin in blood and in the tissues, the best studied of which is lipopolysaccharide-binding protein (LBP).[113] In addition to lipoprotein-binding factor, there are a number of other polysaccharide LPS binders in plasma, complement, tissue factor, endothelial-produced agents such as ELAM and ICAM, and the products of coagulation which can all interfere with the measurable level of endotoxin in plasma.[114] Much attention has been paid recently to the CD14 receptor of monocytes and macrophages. CD14 is the receptor for the LPS–LPS binding protein complex which activates the response to endotoxin, although there is recent evidence that a second receptor may be involved.[115] In burn patients, the same induction followed by activity, receptor expression, and soluble receptor shedding seems to happen for CD14 as it does for IL-2R. It has been reported that soluble CD14 serum levels are observed in conjunction with clinical signs of septicemia.[116] In addition to the appearance of CD14 on macrophages, this receptor is also found on neutrophils and activation of the binding site can induce neutrophils without the need for other cytokines.[117] The injection of lipopolysaccharides into normal human subjects manifests the same alterations in lymphocyte traffic and behavior which has often been documented in burn patients, principally marked by a severe lymphopenia[118] and suppression of lymphocyte proliferation in response to PHA and PWM, apparently a macrophage-dependent effect, but no suppression and PGE_2 or TXB_2 production.[119] Whether the endotoxin (or thermal injury) induced immunosuppression of lymphocytes is mediated by suppressor cells, as yet unidentified suppressor factors, cytokine or PGE_2, is not yet clear.

Experimentally, in the absence of postburn complications or interventions, translocation-generated endotoxemia is cleared by 96 hours postburn.[120] If for any reason endotoxemia persists, the much studied clinical effects of endotoxin can begin to be seen; this includes the cardiovascular response[121] as well as the overwhelming of the Kupffer cell sequestration of LPS in the liver with a resultant spill over to the lung,[122] where surfactant synthesis will be suppressed[123] and alveolar macrophages and neutrophils induced.[124] There is evidence that the mechanism of pulmonary failure in acute endotoxemia and chronic endotoxemia may be different, with chronic endotoxemia leading to activation of the arachidonic acid cascade locally in the lung.[125] The exact contribution to pulmonary failure by the burn injury itself and by the subsequent endotoxemia is not clear, but they may be supplementing each other.[126]

LPS is also capable of inducing opiate production.[127] An important recent addition to our knowledge of endotoxemia has been the observation that different types of antibiotics result in different quantities of endotoxin released from Gram-negative organisms. This may well be relevant to burned patients because of the frequency of broad spectrum antibiotic therapy for these patients. On this point, much more information will be needed.[128]

Humoral Immunity

Original investigations into humoral immunity following thermal injury can be found in previously referenced reviews. Briefly, there is marked diminution of serum IgG concentration, total and all subclasses, and these levels return to normal between 10 and 14 days postburn. Extremely low levels of IgG on admission (300–400 mg%) are predictors of a poor prognosis. IgM and IgA levels appear to be relatively unaffected. There are also perturbations of complement metabolism, including depletion of various serum components. Most of these changes have been ascribed to a combination of leakage through the burn wound, protein catabolism, and a relative diminution in synthesis.

There is a mild impairment of C3 production and release by burned patients' macrophages *in vitro*.[74] Both the classical and the alternative pathways are depleted, but the alternative pathway is more profoundly perturbed.[129] Complement inactivation by heat appears to ameliorate cell-mediated immunosuppression (CMI), suggesting that at least in part some of the impairment of the CMI postburn may be due to a complement-associated mechanism.[130] The results of investigations of immunoglobulin production by cultured B cells have been controversial. Following blunt trauma, there is some suppression of immunoglobulin production, but the suppression can be restored by a variety of lymphokines, suggesting that there is not a basic decrease in B-lymphocyte function.[131, 132] By contrast, in thermal injury, immunoglobulin synthesis may be normal to supernormal[133] or vary depending on the origin of the cells.[134] In summary, it would seem that the defective immunoglobulin production following major injury, including thermal injury, is probably a factor of macrophage/lymphocyte interaction rather than a failure of intrinsic activity by B cells.[135, 136]

An additional group of humoral factors which have been investigated following thermal injury are those concerned with granulopoiesis which will be considered more fully in another chapter.

In brief, there seems to be an impairment of the production of granulocyte colony stimulating factor (GCSF) and of granulocyte macrophage colony stimulating factor (GM-CSF).[137] A number of plasma components which can be considered nutritional in nature have been investigated for their effect on immunity after thermal injury, and one in particular, glutamine, has been reported to make a major contribution to immune reactivity after thermal injury. Diminished glutamine concentrations in blood suppress lymphocyte transformation and, by implication, lymphocyte function.[138]

Finally, mention must be made of unidentified or partially identified immunosuppressive factors in burn serum and in burn subeschar tissue fluid. Mention has already been made of cutaneous burn toxin and the current status of research in this area.[15] A small molecular weight immunosuppressive peptide has been found in blood which is capable of suppressing neutrophil chemotaxis and T-cell blastogenesis, and, to a lesser extent, B-cell blastogenesis.[139,140] Immunosuppressive material exists in subeschar tissue fluid, perhaps by seepage from the serum.[141] There are undoubtedly other products following thermal injury as a result of breakdown, polymerization or other biological processes which are immunosuppressive and which remain unidentified.

Toxic Metabolites

A discussion of toxic intracellular metabolites, such as superoxide anion and hydroxyl ion generation, are beyond the scope of this chapter and are more fully discussed in other chapters in this volume. The subject is mentioned only because the generation of toxic metabolites in cells have a dual importance following thermal injury: first, as the final common pathway for cell damage induced by both the cytokine pathway and by endotoxemia, and second, as the active mode of destruction of microorganisms by phagocytic cells. In this respect, it is worth mentioning that there is a suppression of superoxide anion production in polymorphs following thermal injury.[142] It would also appear that the generation of superoxide anion in some tissues, particularly the liver, following endotoxemia, is an earlier event than was previously thought.[143]

Autoimmune Phenomena

Burned patients produce autoimmune antibodies to a large variety of tissues, which have been extensively investigated.[144,145] At one time, it was thought that the presence of autoantibodies was significant in the induction of suppressive phenomena following thermal injury. Indeed, the control of endotoxemia with polymyxin B, which reduces the effect of suppressor T cells following burns, results in a modest increase in detectable autoimmune antibodies to various tissues.[146] Neither in burned patients nor in controls does actual titer of autoantibodies reach levels regarded as clinically significant, and no clinical correlation between postburn pathology and autoimmunity has ever been convincingly demonstrated. There are several 'downregulatory' mechanisms in place following thermal injury, including anti-idiotype mechanisms, the suppressor cell network, and prostaglandins; so it is possible that the presence of autoantibodies play some part in the induction of downregulatory response.[147]

Intervention

Overview

Search for enhancement of the host defense is as old as research in burn immunology itself. It has been appropriately termed 'Search for the Holy Grail'.[148] The subject has been recently reviewed;[149] indeed, an entire symposium was devoted to the topic recently.[150] It is appropriate to point out, before going into detail, that improvements in the general surgical care of the burned patient have played a major role improving the immunological status of the host, similar to other surgical patients.[151] In particular, early excision of the burn wound with wound coverage,[152–154] plasma exchange therapy,[155] improvements in resuscitation and oxygen delivery,[156] and advances in nutrition[157,158] have played a major role in immunological support of the burned patient. As with all recent advances, a degree of caution is appropriate: for instance, overnutrition can do damage.[159]

The difficulties in evaluating new agents for intervention are enormous. The clinical picture of inflammation and of sepsis is very similar, as it should be, considering that the two induce similar biological cascades. The mortality of thermal injury is rapidly reaching an almost irreducible minimum such that the mortality rate, as an endpoint, will be difficult to influence further, and, therefore, secondary endpoints will have to be used in clinical trials. These and other difficulties have been well outlined in an excellent recent review.[160] We would recommend enthusiastically to future investigators who desire to use intervention for the improvement of the immunological status of burn patients to develop or use one of the detailed scales available for measurement of the septic response.[161]

Active and Passive Vaccination

Early attempts at active and passive vaccination of burned patients (Feller, 1964; Sachs, 1970; Alexander, 1969–74; Jones, 1973, 1977, 1978) have been summarized in a recent review.[162] These attempts were based on the dominance of *Pseudomonas* as a burn pathogen at the time, against which, because of the low number of immunotypes, it is relatively easy to prepare vaccines. With the advent of other gram-negative organisms and finally gram-positive organisms as pathogens, specific vaccination became more difficult. Other studies were beset by difficulties of inadequate or retrospective controls, concurrent advances in other areas on burn therapy, over which there was not adequate control, and the increasing cost of developing human vaccines. Even polyvalent *Pseudomonas* vaccine appears to produce an inadequate IgG_1 and IgG_2 subclass response in patients with thermal injury, throwing some doubts on the possible benefits of active immunization.[163]

The advent of commercial preparations of intravenous immunoglobulin produced an era of renewed enthusiasm for passive vaccination, since older studies[1] have clearly shown that low immunoglobulin concentration postburn, particularly that of IgG, is of poor prognostic significance. Unfortunately, none of the human trials of intravenous immunoglobulin in burned patients was able to demonstrate improvement in survival although there were occasional improvements in *in vitro* findings.[164–167]

There is currently a federal hyperimmune immunological trial (FHIT) in progress, the results of which are not yet available at this time of writing, which may shed further light on the potential utility of passive vaccination.[168] Decrease of serum fibronectin concentration in burned patients has also been documented, and it parallels a decrease in serum opsonizing function.[169] Although definitive studies in burned patients are not available, in severe trauma patients with septic complications the passive administration of fibronectin has failed to improve outcome.[170] While the results of these trials are disappointing, they are not surprising when one considers the multifactorial defects in the host defense. Basically, it is unlikely that any therapy which solely improves antibody concentration would be effective if phagocytic defects, intracellular killing defects, alterations in antigenic recognition and presentation, and cellular chemotaxis and migration, went untreated.

Cell-mediated Immunity and Neutrophils

Use of immunostimulants to treat human disease began with the use of Coley's toxin, a group of mixed bacterial toxins used to treat cancer early in the century. Cancer research has provided most of the data on immunostimulation of host resistance, but research on infection, trauma and burns has benefited from this work as well. The source of the stimulatory substances can be classified roughly into four categories:

1. fungal glycans – which enhance macrophage microbiocidal activity and induce monokine release (an example of this is glucan);
2. detoxified forms of endotoxin which will be dealt with further in this chapter;
3. active components of the mycobacterial cell wall such as used in Freund's adjuvant, the most recent example of this being MDP or muramyl dipeptide; and
4. a number of other agents which stimulate interferon induction and natural killer cells.

In addition, maturation products of normal T cells such as thymic extracts have also provided active substances. Further products have become available thanks to recombinant technology. Currently, there are several such products licensed for use not only in both Europe and the United States but also in Japan. Thymic extracts are actively used in Europe, in both cancer and infection control. Thymic peptide, thymopentin (TP-5) is licenced for use in Italy and Germany at this time of writing. These adjuvants work by their ability to activate one of the two CD4 T-cell populations, either TH1 or TH2 which controls the major features of specific immune responses.[171,172]

A number of these agents have been investigated in human or animal burn settings. Thymopentin (TP-5) has been most extensively examined in experimental animal models in the United

States and in clinical situations in Europe, both in burns and in trauma.[173–178] Reported improvements include an improvement in antigen cocktail induced lymphocyte proliferation, improved DCH responses, opsonization, improved peripheral lymphocyte traffic, and improved survival. In experimental situations, TP-5 decreases prostaglandin E_2 production, and this may be its mode of action. At this time, there are no large prospective randomized studies available which suggest that TP-5 should be added to the routine armamentarium in the management of major burns. The same statement may be applied to all other adjuvants or immunomodulators which have been licenced to this point.

Granulocyte colony stimulating factor has been explored in burned patients and appears to have beneficial effects in burned and burn-infected animals. Clinical trials are currently ongoing both with granulocyte colony stimulating factor and granulocyte macrophage colony stimulating factor in burned patients; the results are awaited with interest.[179,180]

An intriguing approach to downregulate tissue destruction by neutrophils is by interference with the β_2-integrin system by recombinant antibodies. The oxidative burst of neutrophils is an adherence dependent phenomenon which can be blocked by antibodies directed against the α- or β-chain of the MAC-1 integrin. While this has not been attempted in burns, there are preclinical studies available in the treatment of septic shock.[181]

Arachidonic Acid Cascade, Cytokine Cascade

A discussion of interventions aimed at modulation of the arachidonic cascade and cytokine cascade must necessarily extend outside the area of thermal injury, for most of the experimental work in this area is in the treatment of sepsis and trauma rather than pure burn models.

Administration of ibuprofen to block prostanoid production in septic animals has been generally beneficial. In dogs, ibuprofen prevents TNF-mediated septic responses.[182] In an unanesthetized sheep model, ibuprofen improves lung microvascular permeability and the systemic vascular response.[183] In a septic porcine model, ibuprofen improves lung compliance and parameters of pulmonary function.[184] In burn models, however, the contribution of prostanoid blockade has been somewhat less convincing. Decreased bacterial translocation following burns can be achieved by prostaglandin analogs (misoprostol, enisoprost) which improves survival.[185] Other workers were unable to reverse the postburn suppression of murine lymphocyte and neutrophil function with prostaglandin blockade by either indomethacin or ibuprofen.[186] In a septic mouse model, prostanoid blockade actually increased mortality.[187]

There is currently an extensive multicenter ibuprofen trial in progress for extensive care patients. Preliminary results indicate that urinary thromboxane B_2 dimer excretion can be successfully reduced by ibuprofen administration, and that prostanoid blockade has some impact on the clinical sepsis syndrome;[188] final data from this trial are not available at this time of writing.

Much research has been done in the field of tumor necrosis factor blockade; unfortunately, almost none of this work has been published in the burn field. There were early reports showing that recombinant human tumor necrosis factor protects animals against death in a septic model.[189,190] Antibodies against tumor necrosis factor reduce IL-1 and IL-6 induction;[191] in experimental models, suppression of TNF production by a TNF inhibitor (pentoxifylline, PTX) results in a decrease in LPS toxicity.[192] Antibody to TNF also prevents hemorrhage-induced suppression of Kupffer cell function[193] and endotoxin-induced shock and lethality in a rat model.[190] TNFα can also be antagonized by a TNFR immunoadhesin[194] and by the passive administration of soluble human TNF receptor, presumably by competitive inhibition and receptor blockade of macrophage induction.[195] In a baboon model, humanized anti-TNFα antibody protected against the lethal effect of *E. coli* induced shock.[196]

Although this early work looks most encouraging, the lack of information in the burn model will mandate that a great deal more work be done before suppression of TNF production can be accepted as a valid therapeutic modality.

Interleukin-1 blockade is currently undergoing clinical trials with some promising early results in phase III trials.[197,198] In a murine burn wound sepsis model, interleukin-1 administration resulted in improved survival and diminished positive blood cultures.[199] Intervention using other cytokines and cytokine blockades remains controversial. Interferon-γ showed some promise in a prospective trial in the reduction of major septic complications.[200] There is also evidence that suppression of interferon-γ production as well as IL-6 production is of benefit in the septic response.[201–203] There is evidence, by contrast, that IL-6 may be a marker of inflammation rather than an inductive part of the inflammatory cascade, for recombinant IL-6 has strong anti-inflammatory effects.[204] In experimental endotoxin shock in the rat, a leukotriene antagonist has been shown to be of value;[205] in burned patients, the impaired expression of the IL-2 receptor can be reversed by exogenous recombinant IL-2.[206] Interleukin-10 is a strong anti-inflammatory cytokine which downregulates IL-1, IL-6, and TNFα *in vitro* and can protect mice against lethal intraperitoneal injection of endotoxin.[207]

Nonspecific immunoenhancement by lymphocyte culture products, either human or animal, have been shown to be beneficial in *Pseudomonas* challenged animal models in several older reports.[208,209] Unfortunately, the precise nature of the stimulants has not been identified, nor have the data using whole lymphocyte extracts been precisely reproduced in any model of cytokine administration. Platelet-activating factor (PAF) receptor antagonist can also improve survival and downregulate prostaglandin B_2 and PGE_2 release.[210] Finally, the interaction of the neuroendocrine–cytokine axis has been addressed in preliminary fashion. In both septic and burn models, naloxone, a morphine antagonist, appears to attenuate some of the immunosuppressive effects of burn and sepsis.[211,212]

Endotoxin

Production and administration of lipopolysaccharide antagonists is the oldest and most popular experimental technique to modulate the effects of gram-negative sepsis and to support the host. An excellent recent review is recommended for detailed analysis of the structure of lipopolysaccharide and the preparation of antagonists.[213] Anti-LPS agents can be classified into several categories. Chemical compounds which inhibit the biological actions of LPS include polymyxin B, a polycationic antibiotic which stoichiometrically neutralizes the effects of LPS both *in vitro* and *in vivo* by binding directly to the anionic lipid A portion of LPS. Next, there are the structurally based lipid A antagonists which either bind to some portion of the lipopolysaccharide molecule or its precursors such as lipid X, or provide competitive inhibition by blocking a receptor site or sites. Constitutive serum proteins such as lipopolysaccharide-binding protein can be administered.

Bacterial/permeability-increasing protein antagonizes LPS. All *in vitro* test systems for the effects of such neutralizing agents show either decreased expression of membrane receptors, such as CD18 or CD14, or, alternatively, downregulation of cytokine production induced by LPS. For instance, HA-1A antibody, *in vitro*, reduces the production of tumor necrosis factor and IL-6.[214]

In vivo evaluation of these substances is far more difficult. Currently, several clinical trials are in progress for the testing of monoclonal anti-endotoxin antibodies. E5 antibody administration improved patients with clinical signs of organ failure.[215] Animal experiments have been somewhat more controversial, including actual decrease of survival in a recently published canine model.[216] In human trials, successful treatment of gram-negative bacteremia and septic shock have been reported;[217] but the methodology of these clinical studies has been questioned.[218] The mechanism of action of anti-endotoxin antibodies is not known. Anti-LPS monoclonal antibodies inhibit the synthesis of TNF messenger RNA *in vitro*,[219] enhance bacterial and endotoxin clearance,[220] and bind to specific epitopes within the deep core region of LPS.[221] Monoclonal antibodies also reduce endotoxin-induced vascular permeability.[222] In one report, reduction in septic shock and death was obtained by use of an anti-endotoxin core glycolipid preparation.[223] In a more recent report, however, core-lipopolysaccharide hyperimmune globulin was not effective in reducing the incidence of gram-negative systemic complications, while intravenous immunoglobulin was.[224] Another study of surgical patients with and without septic shock noted that patients in septic shock and patients who died showed serum levels of anti-lipopolysaccharide antibody.[225]

Polymyxin B has been quite a popular experimental drug in controlling endotoxemia, and has had both animal and clinical trials following thermal injury. Polymyxin B can act by extracorporeal absorption, by hemoperfusion and fiber absorption, or by direct administration.[226–229] Polymyxin B administered intravenously to burn patients has been reported to reverse the unfavorable T4:T8 ratio, improve natural killer cell function and its responsiveness to exogenous IL-2, and reduce serum endotoxin concentration.[230] Recently, intravenous polymyxin was used to reduce translocational endotoxemia in a group of burned patients with successful reduction of serum endotoxin concentrations; however, in the early postburn stage, no downregulation of cytokine induction and no reduction in clinical septic parameters was seen.[231] Absorption of gram-negative bacteria and their products, attempted and abandoned in the past, is being revisited.[232] Other techniques under current experimental trial include the use of LPS-binding protein,[233] human growth hormone,[234] leumedin and bradykinin antagonists[235] and the use of cytokine downregulation using radical spin trapping.[236]

Toxic Metabolites

There is a dearth of information on the effect of intervention in the prevention of injury by toxic metabolites following thermal injury. The generation of toxic metabolites as a final common pathway to tissue injury has been recently reviewed[237] and this section will merely update some research of particular interest and note what work is available in thermal injury models.

Polymyxin B, in addition to having the anti-endotoxin effect just discussed, is also capable of inhibiting superoxide anion release in polymorphs by inhibition of protein kinase C.[238] Nitric oxide has recently become of interest as a superoxide quencher.[239] One of the mechanisms of cell damage in immunocytes is apparent upregulation of calcium transport across membranes, with an increased intracellular calcium concentration. Calcium channel blockers have been shown to have immunoprotective effects with preservation of antigen presentation function and IL-1 synthesis after hemorrhage.[240] As mentioned previously, some attention has been given to the effect of cyclic nitrones as antioxidants following endotoxemia. Synthetic antioxidants can now be manufactured which are of greater potency than α-phenyl *N-tert*-butyl nitrone (PBN).[241]

Lipid peroxidation has been studied in some detail in the burn model. Lipid peroxidation persists for 3–5 days post-injury in the presence of a sterile burn wound.[242] Fluid resuscitation with deferoxamine, an iron chelator, prevents hydroxyl radical release and prevents systemic burn-induced oxidant injury in the sheep burn model.[243] Intraperitoneal injection of lipid peroxidiation products from burned rats enhances humoral immunity.[244] Two practical difficulties lie in the way of effective intervention using antagonists to toxic radicals following burn injury. First is the extremely short half-life of most standard superoxide scavengers. Second, the apparent evidence that, although toxic radical release does not occur reasonably early following the cause of injury, biologically significant release is a preterminal event which would be difficult to reverse. Clearly, much more research on this subject is needed before the final conclusions are reached.

Combination Therapy

Most workers agree that combination therapy has to be the wave of the future, given the extraordinary complexity of the response to endotoxin, the cytokine cascade, and the feedback loops of the cytokine network. In nonburned patients, several combinations have been attempted. Cytokine therapy in combination with ibuprofen[245] in cancer patients, the combination of indomethacin and thymopentin in major surgical patients,[246] and the combination of antibiotics with cytokines in hemorrhagic shock and infection rat models,[247] appear to provide enhanced effectiveness.

In burn models, the combination of interleukin-1 with indomethacin has shown increased survival[248] as well as IL-2 activated LAK cells, although this is not truly 'combination therapy'.[249] G-CSF and gentamicin have been combined.[250] Experience with the combination of antibiotics and immunoglobulin or anti-endotoxin therapy is mixed. In one recent report, antibiotic therapy with passive immunization with IV Ig resulted in a reduction of mortality and a reduction of hospitalization time[251] but in another study the combination of IgG and T_4 showed no improvement,[252] nor did the combination of polymyxin B with IgG.[253] Perhaps the recent discovery of IL-10 and IL-4 interaction in sepsis will open new approaches to the problem.[254]

Conclusions

Immunology has come of age to the point where a reasonably clear understanding of the timetable of immunological alterations now exists. Following injury, there is immediate activation of the arachidonic acid cascade and the cytokine cascade, together with early translocation of bacteria and endotoxin. Major metabolic, hormonal, and cellular alterations begin within 24–48 hours. After 3–4 days, there is a second peak of endotoxemia which appears to reinduce the cytokine and arachidonic acid cascade. The triggering of toxic metabolites occurs early but is probably not of biological significance until several days after the injury, following the induction of earlier changes. It is clear that there will be no single agent which can alter this course of events; rather, a combination of two to three agents aimed at the interruption of several of the sequences described above at various points in time will be indicated. The influence of intervention in the inflammatory cascade on wound healing and ephithelialization is not known, and needs to be urgently investigated.

In summary, the difficulties of performing excellent clinical studies has only recently become appreciated. It should be re-emphasized that thermal injury has reached a relatively low mortality in most developed countries. Death of the patient as an endpoint for interventions, although obviously essential, becomes a statistical nightmare unless very large multicenter trials involving thousands of patients are recruited. Therefore, investigators must look at secondary endpoints, and pay closer attention to the evaluation of septic complications on some kind of precise quantifiable scale, length of stay, cost of therapy, and similar outcomes. Finally, many of the therapies discussed in this chapter are extremely costly. Cost-effectiveness studies must be conducted in parallel with safety and efficacy studies if new proposed regimens are to take their place successfully in the armamentarium of burn therapy.

Summary

Much progress has been made in the last 20 years in our understanding of the intricacies of the host defect created by thermal injury. The arachidonic acid cascade is triggered early, as is the induction of the inflammatory cytokine cascade. Alterations occur in the function of lymphocytes, macrophages, and neutrophils. Bacteria and bacterial products translocate. The net result of these complex changes following thermal injury is twofold: first, they interfere with the biological efficiency of the host in fighting invading pathogens, and second, there is a cell damage and death from the inflammatory cascade itself, probably by the way of the formation of toxic intracellular metabolites as the final common pathway.

Because of the complexity of these changes, which are only now beginning to be understood, early optimism for successful intervention has not been borne out. There are a number of promising leads for therapy, but it has become apparent that therapeutic modalities will have to be developed which address each of the major immunological alterations following thermal injury, and that there will not be a single accent which can reverse the observed changes for the benefit of the host.

References

1. Munster A M. Alterations of the host defense mechanism in burns. *Surg Clin North Am* 1970; **50:** 1217–25.

2. Rapaport F T, Miligram F, Kano K, *et al.* Immunologic sequelae of thermal injury. *Ann NY Acad Sci* 1968; **150:** 1004–8.

3. Munster A M. Immune response in burns and injuries. In: Seligson D, ed. *Handbook of Clinical Laboratory Science.* Boca Raton: CRC Press 1978: 375–93.

4. Calvano, S E. Hormonal mediation of immune dysfunction following thermal and traumatic injury. In: Gullinard J I, Fauci A S, eds. *Advances in Host Defense Mechanisms.* Vol 6. New York: Raven Press, 1986.

5. Alexander J W. Mechanism of immunologic suppression in burn injury. *J Trauma* 1990; **30:** S70–5.

6. Konig W, Schluter B, Scheffer J, Koller M. Microbial pathogenicity and host defense in burned patients – the role of inflammatory mediators. *Infection* 1992; **2:** S128–34.

7. Heideman M, Bengtsson A. The immunologic response to thermal injury. *World J Surg*, 1992; **16**(1): 53–6.

8. Imhoff M, Gahr R H, Hoffman P. Delayed cutaneous hypersensitivity after multiple injury and severe burn. *Ann Ital Chir* 1990; **61**(5): 525–8.

9. Munster A M, Winchurch R A, Birmingham W J, Keeling P. Longitudinal assay of lymphocyte responsiveness in patients with major burns. *Ann Surg* 1980; **192:** 772–5.

10. Peck M D, Alexander J W. The use of immunologic tests to predict outcome in surgical patients. *Nutrition* 1990; **6:** 16–19.

11. Bach F H. Cell-mediated immunity. Its basis and analysis. *Nutrition* 1990; **6:** 2–4.

12. Wells C L, Jechorek R P, Erlandsen S L, *et al.* The effect of dietary glutamine and dietary RNA on ileal flora, histology, and bacterial translocation in mice. *Nutrition* 1990; **6:** 70–5.

13. Kinsella J E, Lokesh B, Broughton S, Whelan J. Dietary polyunsaturated fatty acids and eicosanoids: Potential effects on the modulation of inflammatory and immune cells: an overview. *Nutrition* 1990; **6:** 24–44.

14. Monge G, Sparkes B G, Allgower M, Schoenenberger G A. Influence of burn-induced lipid-protein complex on IL1 secretion by PBMC in vitro. *Burns* 1991; **17**(4): 269–75.

15. Sparkes B G, Gyorkos J W, Gorczynski R M, Brock A J. Comparison of endotoxins and cutaneous burn toxin as immunosuppressants. *Burns* 1990; **16:** 123–6.

16. Deitch E A, Lu Q, Xu D Z, Special R D. Effect of local and systemic burn microenvironment on neutrophil activation as assessed by complement receptor expression and morphology. *J Trauma* 1990; **30**(3): 259–68.

17. Stratta R J, Saffle J R, Ninnemann J L, *et al.* The effect of surgical excision and grafting procedures on postburn lymphocyte suppression. *J Trauma* 1985; **25:** 46–52.

18. Lazarou S A, Barbul A, Wasserkrug H L, Efron G. The wound is a possible source of posttraumatic immunosuppression. *Arch Surg* 1989; **124:** 1429–31.

19. Wilmore D. Hypermetabolic response to burn injury. *J Trauma* 1990; **30:** S4–S6.

20. Fong Y, Moldawer L L, Shires G T, Lowry S F. The biologic characteristics of cytokines and their implication in surgical injury. *Surg Gynecol Obstet* 1990; **170:** 363–78.

21. Santos A A, Schltinga M R, Lynch E, *et al.* Elaboration of interleukin-1 receptor antagonism is not attenuated by glucocorticoids after endotoxemia. *Arch Surg* 1993; **128:** 138–44.

22. Ninnemann J L, Stockland A E, Condie J T. Induction of prostaglandin synthesis-dependent suppressor cells with endotoxin: occurrence in patients with thermal injuries. *J Clin Immunol* 1983; **3**(2): 42–50.

23. Grbic J T, Mannick J A, Gough D B, Rodrick M L. The role of prostaglandin E_2 in immune suppression following injury. *Ann Surg* 1991; **214:** 253–63.

24. Callery M P, Kamei T, Mangino M J, Flye M W. Interleukin-6 (IL-6) production by endotoxin (LPS)-stimulated Kupffer cells is regulated by prostaglandin E_2. *J Surg Res* 1990; **48**(6): 523–7.

25. Hoffman T, Lizzio E F, Suissa J, *et al.* Dual stimulation of phospholipase activity in human monocytes: Role of calcium-dependent and calcium-independent pathways in arachidonic acid release and eicosanoid formation. *J Immunol* 1988; **140:** 3912–18.

26. Herndon D N, Abston S, Stein M D. Increased thromboxane B_2 levels in the plasma of burned and septic burned patients. *Surg Gynecol Obstet* 1984; **159:** 210–13.

27. Endo S, Inada K, Yamada Y, *et al.* Plasma tumor necrosis factor-α (TNF-α) levels in patients with burns. *Burns* 1993; **19:** 124–7.

28. Moore F D, Socher S H, Davis C. Tumor necrosis factor and endotoxin can cause neutrophil activation through separate pathways. *Arch Surg* 1991, **126:** 70–3.

29. Marano M A, Fong Y, Moldawer L L, *et al.* Serum cachectin/tumor necrosis factor in critically ill patients with burns correlates with infection and mortality. *Surg Gynecol Obstet* 1990; **170:** 32–8.

30. Sanchez–Cantu L, Rode H N, Christou N V. Endotoxin tolerance is associated with reduced secretion of tumor necrosis factor. *Arch Surg* 1989; **124:** 1432–6.

31. Beutler B, Krochin N, Milsark I W, *et al.* Control of cachectin (tumor necrosis factor) synthesis: mechanisms of endotoxin resistance. *Science* 1986; **232:** 977–80.

32. Takayama T K, Miller C, Szabo G. Elevated tumor necrosis factor production concomitant to elevated prostaglandin E_2 production by trauma patients' monocytes. *Arch Surg* 1990; **125:** 29–35.

33. Faist E, Storck M, Hultner L, *et al.* Functional analysis of monocyte activity through synthesis patterns of proinflammatory cytokines and neopterin in patients in surgical intensive care. *Surgery* 1992; **112:** 562–72.

34. Tellado J M, Christou N V. Increased polymorphonuclear neutrophil delivery to inflammatory lesions in anergic patients is medicated via interleukin-1 and interleukin-6. *Surg Forum* 1990; **41:** 99–100.

35. Wood J J, Rodrick M L, O'Mahony J B, *et al.* Inadequate interleukin 2 production: A fundamental immunological deficiency in patients with major burns. *Ann Surg* 1984; **200:** 311–20.

36. Teodorczyk-Injeyan J A, Sparkes B G, Mills G B, Peters W J. Soluble interleukin 2-receptor alpha secretion is related to altered interleukin 2 production in thermally injured patients. *Burns* 1991; **17**(4): 290–5.

37. Teodorczyk-Injeyan J A, Sparkes B G, Peters W J. Serum interleukin-

2 receptor as a possible mediator of immunosuppression after burn injury. *J Burn Care Rehabil* 1989; **10**(2): 112–18.

38. Teodorczyk-Injeyan J A, Sparkes B G, Lalani S, *et al.* IL-2 regulation of soluble IL-2 receptor levels following thermal injury. *Clin Exp Immunol* 1992; **90**(1): 36–42.

39. Teodorczyk-Injeyan J A, Sparkes B G, Mills G B, *et al.* Increase of serum interleukin 2 receptor level in thermally injured patients. *Clin Exp Immunol* 1989; **51**(2): 202–15.

40. Xiao, G-X, Chopra R K, Adler W H, Munster A M, Winchurch R A. Altered expression of lymphocyte IL-2 receptors in burned patients. *J Trauma* 1992; **33:** 74–82.

41. Rodriguez J L, Miller C G, De Forge L E, Kelty *et al.* Local production of interleukin-8 is associated with nosocomial pneumonia. *J Trauma* 1992; **33:** 74–82.

42. Zhou D, Kusnecov A, Shurin M, *et al.* Exposure to physical and psychological stressors elevates plasma levels of IL-6: relationship to the activation of hypothalamic-pituitary-adrenal axis. *Endocrinology* 1993; **133**(6): 2523–30.

43. Lanser M E, Brown G E. Control of hepatocyte fibronectin secretion by interleukin-6. *Surg Res Commun* 1989; **5:** 32.

44. Nijsten M W N, DeGroot, E R, TenDuis H J, *et al.* Serum levels of interleukin-6 and acute phase responses. *Lancet* 1987; **2:** 921.

45. Zhou D, Munster A M, Winchurch R A. Inhibitory effects of interleukin 6 on immunity: possible implications in burn patients. *Arch Surg* 1992; **127:** 65–9.

46. Miller C, Szabo G, Kodys K. Elevated IL-6 production by immunosuppressed trauma patients' monocytes (MO). *J Leuk Biol* 1989; **46:** 323.

47. Mazuski J E, Ortiz, Towle H C, Cerra F B. Withdrawal of inflammatory mediator does not abrogate a sustained hepatic acute phase response. Presented at the meeting of the Surgical Infection Society, Denver, 1989.

48. Nijsten M W, Hack C E, Helle M, *et al.* Interleukin-6 and its relation to the humoral immune response and clinical parameters in burned patients. *Surgery* 1991; **109**(6): 761–7.

49. Miller-Graziano C L, Szabo G, Griffey K, *et al.* Role of elevated monocyte transforming growth factor beta (TNF-β) production in posttrauma immunosuppression. *J Clin Immunol* 1991; **11:** 95–102.

50. Zhou D, Munster A, Winchurch R A. Pathologic concentrations of interleukin 6 inhibit T cell responses via induction of activation of TGF-β. *FASEB J* 1991; **5:** 2582–5.

51. Munster A M. Post-traumatic immunosuppression is due to activation of suppressor T-cells. *Lancet* 1976; **1:** 1329–30.

52. Kupper T S, Green D R. Immunoregulation after thermal injury: sequential appearance of I-J+, LY-1, T suppressor inducer cells and LY-2 T suppressor effector cells following thermal trauma in mice. *J Immunol* 1984; **133:** 3047–53.

53. Hansbrough J F, Bender E M, Zapata-Sirvent R, Anderson J. Altered helper and suppressor lymphocyte populations in surgical patients: a measure of postoperative immunosuppression. *Am J Surg* 1984; **148:** 303–7.

54. Rioja L F, Alonso P, de Haro J, de la Cruz J. Prognostic value of the CD4/CD8 lymphocyte ratio in moderately burned patients. *Burns* 1993; **19**(3): 198–201.

55. O'Mahony J B, Wood J, Rodrick M L, Mannick J A. Changes in T lymphocyte subsets following injury: assessment by flow cytometry and relationship to sepsis. *Ann Surg* 1985; **202:** 580–6.

56. Burleson D G, Mason A D, Pruitt B A. Lymphoid subpopulation changes after thermal injury and thermal injury with infection in an experimental model. *Ann Surg* 1988; **207:** 208–12.

57. Organ B C, Antonacci A C, Chiao J, *et al.* Changes in lymphocyte number and phenotype in seven lymphoid compartments after thermal injury. *Ann Surg* 1988; **210:** 78–89.

58. Deitch E A, Xu D, Qi L. Different lymphocyte compartments respond differently to mitogenic stimulation after thermal injury. *Ann Surg* 1990; **211:** 72–7.

59. Maldonado M D, Venturoli A, Franco A, Nunez–Roldan A. Specific changes in peripheral blood lymphocyte phenotype from burn patients: probable origin of the thermal injury-related lymphocytopenia. *Burns* 1991; **17:** 188–92.

60. Zapata-Sirvent R L, Hansbrough J F. Temporal analysis of human leukocyte surface antigen expression and neutrophil respiratory burst activity after thermal injury. *Burns* 1993; **19**(1): 5–11.

61. Gadd M A, Hansbrough J F, Hoyt D B, Ozkan N. Defective T-cell surface antigen expression after mitogen stimulation: an index of lymphocyte dysfunction after controlled murine injury. *Ann Surg* 1989; **29:** 112–18.

62. Bender B S, Winchurch R A, Thupari J N, *et al.* Depressed natural killer cell function in thermally injured adults: Successful in vivo and in vitro immunomodulation and the role of endotoxin. *Clin Exp Immunol* 1988; **71:** 120–5.

63. Tolentino M V, Sarasua M M, Hill O A, *et al.* Peripheral lymphocyte membrane fluidity after thermal injury. *J Burn Care Rehabil* 1991; **12**(6): 498–504.

64. Teodorczyk-Injeyan J A, Sparkes B G, Mills G B, Peters W J. Immunosuppression follows systemic T lymphocyte activation in the burn patient. *Clin Exp Immunol* 1991; **85**(3): 515–18.

65. Marsland A L, Graham R E, Bachen E A, *et al.* Fitness as a predictor of cellular immune response to mental stress. Presented at the meeting for Research Perspectives in Psychoneuroimmunology IV, Boulder, Colorado 1993.

66. Shelby J, Sullivan J, Groussman M, Gray R, Saffle J. Severe burn injury: effects on psychologic and immunologic function in noninjured close relatives. *J Burn Care Rehabil* 1992; **13**(1): 58–63.

67. Hansbrough J F, Zapata-Sirvent R, Hoyt D. Postburn immune suppression: an inflammatory response to the burn wound? *J Trauma* 1990; **30:** 671–5.

68. Trop M, Schiffrin E J, Carter E A. Role of skin in the burn-induced reduction of reticuloendothelial phagocytic activity in rats. *Burns* 1990; **16:** 57–9.

69. Cooper K D, Oberhelman L, Hamilton T A, *et al.* Neopterin as parameter of cell-mediated immunity response in thermally injured patients. *Burns* 1992; **18**(2): 113–16.

70. Balogh D, Lammer H, Kornberger E, *et al.* Neopterin plasma levels in burn patients. *Burns* 1992; **18**(3): 185–8.

71. Moore F D Jr, Davis C F. Monocyte activation after burns and endotoxemia. *J Surg Res* 1989; **46**(4): 350–4.

72. Gibbons R A, Martinez O M, Lim R C, *et al.* Reduction in HLA-DR, HLA-DQ and HLA-DP expression by Leu-M3 + cells. *Clin Exp Immunol* 1989; **75**(3): 371–5.

73. Yang L, Hsu B. The roles of macrophage (M phi) and PGE-2 in postburn immunosuppression. *Burns* 1992; **18**(2): 132–6.

74. Ogle C K, Johnson C, Guo X, *et al.* Production and release of C3 cultured monocytes/macrophages isolated from burned, trauma, and septic patients. *J Trauma* 1989; **29:** 189–94.

75. Tomomochi G, Masayoshi A, Hidehiko S, Motomichi T. Characteristics of alveolar macrophages in experimental septic lung. *J Leukoc Biol* 1992; **52:** 236–43.

76. Noelle R J, Snow E C: T helper cell-dependent B cell activation. *FASEB J* 1991; **5:** 2770–6.

77. Kagan R J, Bratescu A, Jonasson O, *et al.* The relationship between the percentage of circulating B cells, corticosteroid levels, and other immunologic parameters in thermally injured patients. *J Trauma* 1989; **29:** 208–13.

78. Schluter B, Konig W, Koller M, *et al.* Differential regulation of T- and B-lymphocyte activation in severely burned patients. *J Trauma* 1991; **31:** 239–46.

79. Schluter B, Konig W, Koller M, *et al.* Studies on B-lymphocyte dysfunctions in severely burned patients. *J Trauma* 1990; **30:** 1380–9.

80. Miller-Graziano C L, Szabo G, Kodys K, Griffey K. Aberrations in post-trauma monocyte (MO) subpopulation: role in septic shock syndrome. *J Trauma* 1990; **30:** S86–96.

81. Solomkin J S. Neutrophil disorders in burn injury: complement, cytokines, and organ injury. *J Trauma* 1990; **30:** S80–5.

82. Jeyapaul J, Mehta L N, Arora S, Antia N H. Fc and complement receptor integrity of polymorphonuclear (PMN) cells following thermal injury. *Burns* 1984; **10:** 387–95.

83. Ogle C K, Alexander W, Nagy H, *et al.* A long-term study and correlation of lymphocyte and neutrophil function in the patient with burns. *J Burn Care Rehabil* 1990; **11:** 105–11.

84. Bjerknes R, Vindenes H, Pitkanen J, *et al.* Altered polymorphonuclear neutrophilic granulocyte functions in patients with large burns. *J Trauma* 1989; **29**(6): 847–55.

85. Bjerknes R, Vindenes H. Neutrophil dysfunction after thermal injury: alteration of phagolysosomal acidification in patients with large burns. *Burns* 1989; **15**(2): 77–81.

86. Bjornson A B, Knippenberg R W, Bjornson H S. Bactericidal defect of neutrophils in a guinea pig model of thermal injury is related to elevation of intracellular cyclic-3′,5′- adenosine monophosphate. *J Immunol* 1989; **143:** 2609–16.

87. Babcock G F, Alexander J W, Warden G D. Flow cytometric analysis of neutrophil subsets in thermally injured patients developing infection. *Clin Exp Immunol* 1990; **54**(1): 117–25.

88. Deitch E A. The relationship between thermal injury and neutrophil membrane functions as measured by chemotaxis, adherence and spreading. *Burns* 1984; **10:** 264–70.

89. Tchervenkov J I, Latter D A, Psychogios J, Christou N V. Altered leukocyte delivery to specific and nonspecific inflammatory skin lesions following burn injury. *J Trauma* 1988; **25:** 582–8.

90. Hasslen S R, Ahrenholz D H, Solem L D, Nelson R D. Actin polymerization contributes to neutrophil chemotactic dysfunction following thermal injury. *J Leukoc Biol* 1992; **52:** 495–500.

91. Killer M, Konig W, Brom J, *et al.* Studies on the mechanisms of granulocyte dysfunctions in severely burned patients – evidence for altered leukotriene generation. *J Trauma* 1989; **29:** 435–45.

92. Bergmann U, Konig W, Gross-Weege W, *et al.* Basophil releasability in severely burned patients. *J Trauma* 1990; **30**(11): 1372–9.

93. Cioffi W G Jr, Burleson D G, Jordan B S, Mason A D Jr, Pruitt B A Jr. Granulocyte oxidate activity after thermal injury. *Surgery* 1992; **112**(5): 860–5.

94. Mullen P, Windsor A, Walsh C, *et al.* Tumor necrosis factor (TNF-α) and interleukin-6 (IL-6) regulate neutrophil (PMN) function selectively. Presented at the meeting of the Association for Academic Surgeons, Montreal Nov. 18–21, 1992.

95. Carr D J. The role of endogenous opioids and their receptors in the immune system. *Proc Soc Exp Biol Med* 1991; **198:** 710–20.

96. Weber R J. Neutral and peripheral mechanisms involved in opioid regulation of immune function. Presented at the meeting for Research Perspectives in Psychoneuroimmunology IV, Boulder, Colorado 1993.

97. Elliot D, Everitt A S, Gault D, *et al.* The role of endorphins in septicaemic shock: a pilot study in burned patients. *Burns* 1985; **11:** 387–92.

98. Deitch E A, Xu D, Bridges R M. Opioids modulate human neutrophil and lymphocyte function: thermal injury alters plasma B-endorphin levels. *Surgery* 1988; **104:** 41–8.

99. Carter E A, Tompkins R G, Schiffrin E, Burke J F. Cutaneous thermal injury alters macromolecular permeability of rat small intestine. *Surgery* 1990; **107:** 335–41.

100. LeeVoyer T, Cioffi W G, Pratt L, *et al.* Alterations in intestinal permeability after thermal injury. *Arch Surg* 1992; **127:** 26–30.

101. Deitch E A. Intestinal permeability is increased in burn patients shortly after injury. *Surgery* 1990; **107:** 411–16.

102. O'Dwyer S T, Michie H R, Ziegler T R, *et al.* A single dose of endotoxin increases intestinal permeability in healthy humans. *Arch Surg* 1988; **123:** 1459–64.

103. Winchurch R A, Thupari J N, Munster A M. Endotoxemia in burn patients: levels of circulating endotoxins are related to burn size. *Surgery* 1987; **102:** 808–12.

104. Endo S, Inada K, Kikuchi M, *et al.* Are plasma endotoxin levels related to burn size and prognosis? *Burns* 1992; **18:** 486–9.

105. Zhong W, Hand T, Burke P, Forse R A. Human macrophage cytokine gene regulation to endotoxin is both dose and time dependent. *Surg Inf Soc Prog* 1992; **12:** 38.

106. Nichols F C, Garrison S W, Davis H W. Prostaglandin E_2 and thromboxane B_2 release from human monocytes treated with bacterial lipopolysaccharide. *J Leukoc Biol* 1988; **44:** 376–84.

107. Ulich T R, del Castillo J, Ni R X, Bikhazi N. Hematologic interactions of endotoxin, tumor necrosis factor alpha (TNF-α), interleukin 1, and adrenal hormones and the hematologic effects of TNF-α in *Corynebacterium parvum*-primed rats. *J Leukoc Biol* 1989; **45:** 546–57.

108. Megyeri P, Issekutz T B, Issekutz A C. An endotoxin-induced factor distinct from interleukin-1 and tumor necrosis factor α produced by the THP-1 human macrophage line stimulates polymorphonuclear leukocyte infiltration in vivo. *J Leukoc Biol* 1990; **47:** 70–8.

109. Bergmann U, Scheffer J, Koller M, *et al.* Induction of inflammatory mediators (histamine and leukotrienes) from rat peritoneal mast cells and human granulocytes by *Pseudomonas aeruginosa* strains from burn patients. *Infect Immun* 1989; **57**(7): 2187–95.

110. Blanchard D K, Djeu J Y, Klein T W *et al.* Interferon-γ induction by lipopolysaccharide: dependence on interleukin-2 and macrophages. *J Immunol* 1986; **136:** 963–70.

111. de Groote M A, Martin M A, Denesen P, *et al.* Plasma tumor necrosis factor alone does not explain the lethal effect of lipopolysaccharide. *Arch Surg* 1991; **126:** 231–5.

112. Sanchez–Cantu L, Rode H N, Yun T J, Christou N V. Tumor necrosis factor alone does not explain the lethal effect of lipopolysaccharide. *Arch Surg* 1991; **126:** 231–5.

113. Tobias P S, Mathison J C, Ulevitch R J. A family of lipopolysaccharide binding proteins involved in responses to gram-negative sepsis. *J Biol Chem* 1988; **263**(27): 13479–81.

114. Taylor F B Jr. Presented at the Seminar on Advances in Prevention and Treatment of Endotoxemia & Sepsis, Philadelphia June 22–23, 1992.

115. Birkenmaier C, Hong Y, Horn J. Modulation of the endotoxin receptor CD14 in septic patients. *J Trauma* 1992; **32:** 473–9.

116. Kruger C, Schutt C, Obertacke U, *et al.* Serum CD14 levels in polytraumatized and severely burned patients. *Clin Exp Immunol* 1991; **85**(2): 297–301.

117. Weingarten R, Sklar L A, Mathison J C, *et al.* Interactions of lipopolysaccharide with neutrophils in blood via CD14. *J Leukoc Biol* 1993; **53:** 518–24.

118. Richardson R P, Rhyne C D, Fong Y, *et al.* Peripheral blood leukocyte kinetics following in vivo lipopolysaccharide (LPS) administration to normal human subjects. *Ann Surg* 1989; **210:** 239–45.

119. Ogle C K, Arita H, Nagy H, *et al.* The immunosuppressive effects of the in vivo administration of endotoxin as influenced by macrophages. *J Trauma* 1989; **29:** 1015–20.

120. Tokyay R, Zeigler S T, Heggers J P, *et al.* Effects of anesthesia, surgery fluid resuscitation, and endotoxin administration on postburn bacterial translocation. *J Trauma* 1991; **31:** 1376–9.

121. Suffredini A F, Fromm R E, Parker M M, *et al.* The cardiovascular response of normal humans to the administration of endotoxin. *N Engl J Med* 1989; **321:** 280–7.

122. Callery M P, Mangino M J, Kamei T, Flye M W. Organ interactions in sepsis: host defense and the hepatic-pulmonary macrophage axis. *Arch Surg* 1991; **126**(1): 28–32.

123. Li J J, Sanders R L, McAdam K P W J, *et al.* Endotoxin suppresses surfactant synthesis in cultured rat lung cells. *J Trauma* 1989; **29:** 180–8.

124. Maier R V, Hannel G B, Pohlman T H. Endotoxin requirements for alveolar macrophage stimulation. *J Trauma* 1990; **30:** S49–S57.

125. Dean P, Yagi K, Naunheim K, Baudendistal L. Chronic endotoxin induced lung injury. Presented at the meeting of the Association for Academic Surgeons, Louisville, November 15–18, 1989.

126. Demling R H, LaLonde C. Effect of a body burn on endotoxin-induced lipid peroxidation: comparison with physiologic and histologic changes. *Surgery* 1990; **107:** 669–76.

127. Yirmiya R, Ovadia H, Rosen H, *et al.* Behavioral effects of LPS: involvement of endogenous opioids. Presented at the meeting for Research Perspectives in Psychoneuroimmunology IV, Boulder, Colorado 1993.

128. Jackson J J, Kropp H. β-Lactam antibiotic-induced release of free endotoxin: in vitro comparison of penicillin-binding protein (PBP) 2-specific imipenem and PBP 3-specific ceftazidime. *J Infect Dis* 1992; **165:** 1033–41.

129. Gelfand J A, Donelan M, Burke J F. Preferential activation and depletion of the alternative complement pathway by burn injury. *Ann Surg* 1983; **198:** 58–62.

130. Ferrara J J, Dyess D L, Luterman A, *et al.* In vitro effects of complement inactivation upon burn-associated cell-mediated immunosuppression. *Am Surgeon* 1990; **56**(9): 571–4.

131. Teodorczyk-Injeyan J A, Sparkes B G, Girotti M J. Induced immunologlobulin secretion by T-cell replacing products from blunt trauma patients. *J Trauma* 1982; **33:** 171–8.

132. Ertel W, Faist E, Nestle C, *et al.* Dynamics of immunologlobulin synthesis after major trauma. *Arch Surg* 1989; **124:** 1437–42.

133. Shorr R M, Ershler W B, Gamelli R L. Immunoglobulin production in burned patients. *J Trauma* 1984; **24:** 319–22.

134. Kawakami M, de Serres S, Meyer A A. Immunoglobulin synthesis by cultured lymphocytes from spleen and mesenteric lymph nodes after thermal injury. *J Burn Care Rehabil* 1991; **12:** 474–81.

135. Teodorczyk-Injeyan J A, Sparkes B G, Peters W J. Regulation of IgM production in thermally injured patients. *Burns* 1989; **15:** 241–7.

136. Faist E, Ertel W, Baker C C, Heberer G. Terminal B-cell maturation and immunoglobulin (Ig) synthesis in vitro in patients with major injury. *J Trauma* 1989; **29:** 2–9.

137. Peterson V, Hansbrough J, Buerk C, *et al.* Regulation of granulopoiesis following severe thermal injury. *J Trauma* 1983; **23:** 1923.

138. Parry-Billings M, Evans J, Calder P C, Newsholme E A. Does glutamine contribute to immunosuppression after major burns? *Lancet* 1990; 336: 523–5.

139. Ozkan A N, Hoyt D B, Tompkins S, *et al.* Immunosuppressive effects of a trauma-induced suppressor active peptide. *J Trauma* 1988; **28:** 589–92.

140. Ninnemann J L, Ozkan A N. Definition of a burn injury-induced immunosuppressive serum component. *J Trauma* 1985; **25:** 113–17.

141. Dyess D L, Ferrara J J, Luterman A, Curreri P W. Subeschar tissue fluid: a source of cell-mediated immune suppression in victims of severe thermal injury. *J Burn Care Rehabil* 1991; **12**(2): 101–5.

142. Bjornson A B, Somers S D, Knippenberg R W, Bjornson H S. Circulating factors contribute to elevation of intracellular cyclic-3′, 5′-adenosine monophosphate and depression of superoxide anion production in polymorphonuclear leukocytes following thermal injury. *J Leukoc Biol* 1992; **52:** 407–14.

143. Bautista A P, Meszaros K, Bojta J, Spitzer J J. Superoxide anion generation in the liver during the early stage of endotoxemia in rats. *J Leukoc Biol* 1990; **48:** 123–8.

144. Ablin R J, Holder I A. Immunologic sequelae of thermal injury: I. Frequency and relationship of epithelial antibodies to extent of burn. *Immunol Immunopathol* 1976; **5:** 195–207.

145. Leguit P Jr, Feltkamp T E W, van Rossum A L, *et al.* Immunological studies in burn patients: III. Autoimmune phenomena. *Int Arch Allergy* 1973; **45:** 392–404.

146. Moran K T, Anholt G T, O'Reilly T J, Thupari J N. Autoantibody formation in burn patients after inhibition of suppressor T cell activity with polymyxin B. *J Burn Care Rehabil* 1989; **10:** 213–15.

147. Katz D R. Immunosuppression as a physiological homeostatic mechanism. *Immunol Today* 1984; **5**(4): 96–7.

148. Polk H C Jr. The enhancement of host defenses against infection: search for the holy grail? *Surgery* 1986; **99:** 1–6.

149. Munster A M. Control of infection following major burns: the immunological approach. In: Imbach P, ed. *Immunotherapy with Intravenous Immunoglobulins*. London: Academic Press, 1991.

150. Faist T E, Ninneman J, Green D, Eds. *Symposium: Immune consequences of Trauma, Shock and Sepsis*. Berlin: Springer Verlag 1989.

151. Meakins J L. Surgeons, surgery, and immunomodulation. *Arch Surg* 1991; **126:** 494–8.

152. Hansbrough J F, Zapata-Sirvent R L, Peterson V M. Immunomodulation following burn injury. *Surg Clin North Am* 1987; **67:** 69–92.

153. Demling R H, LaLonde C. Early burn excision attenuates the postburn lung and systemic response to endotoxin. *Surgery* 1990; **108:** 28–35.

154. Stratta R H, Warden G D, Ninneman J L, *et al.* Immunologic parameters in burned patients: effect of therapeutic interventions. *J Trauma* 1986; **26:** 7–17.

155. Warden G D, Stratta R J, Saffle J R, *et al.* Plasma exchange therapy in patients failing to resuscitate from burn shock. *J Trauma* 1983; **23:** 945–51.

156. Benhaim P, Hunt T K. Natural resistance to infection: leukocyte functions. *J Burn Care Rehabil* 1992; **13:** 287–92.

157. Alexander J W, Gottschlich M M. Nutritional immunomodulation in burn patients. *Crit Care Med* 1990; **18:** S149–53.

158. Germenis A E, Achilleos O A, Stavropoulos-Giokas C, *et al.* The effect of very early enteral tube feeding on the humoral immunity of burned children. *Ann Medit Burns Club* 1992; **5:** 69–72.

159. Herndon D N, Stein M D, Rutan T C, *et al.* Failure of TPN supplement to improve liver function immunity and mortality in thermally injured patients. *J Trauma* 1987; **27:** 195–204.

160. Bone R C. A critical evaluation of new agents for the treatment of sepsis. *JAMA* 1991; **266:** 1686–91.

161. Meek M, Munster A M, Winchurch R A, Dickerson C. The Baltimore Sepsis Scale: measurement of sepsis in burn patients using a new scoring system. *J Burn Care Rehabil* 1991; **12:** 564–8.

162. Munster A M. Infections in burns. In: Morell A, Nydegger V E, eds. *Clinical Use of Intravenous Immunoglobulins*. London: Academic Press, 1986.

163. Frame J D, Everitt A S. Pilot study into the IgG_1 and IgG_2 subclass response to polyvalent pseudomonas vaccine in burned adults. *Burns* 1989; **15**(3): 167–70.

164. Waymack J P, Jenkins M E, Alexander J W, *et al.* A prospective trial of prophylactic intravenous immune globulin for the prevention of infections in severely burned patients. *Burns* 1989; **5:** 71–6.

165. Frame J D, Everitt A S, Gordon P W N, Hackett M E. IgG subclass response to gamma globulin administration in burned children. *Burns* 1990; **16:** 437–40.

166. Burleson D G, Mason A D, McManus A T, Pruitt B A Jr. Lymphocyte phenotype and function changes in burn patients after intravenous IgG therapy. *Arch Surg* 1988; **123:** 1379–82.

167. Munster A M, Moran K T, Thupari J, Allo M, Winchurch R A. Prophylactic intravenous immunoglobulin replacement in high-risk burn patients. *J Burn Care Rehabil* 1987; **8:** 376–80.

168. Cross A S. Use of hyperimmune immunoglobulin. Presented at the Seminar on Advances in Prevention and Treatment of Endotoxemia & Sepsis, Philadelphia June 17–18, 1993.

169. Dobke M K, Pearson G, Roberts C, *et al.* Effect of circulating fibronectin on stimulation of leukocyte oxygen consumption and serum opsonizing function in burned patients. *J Trauma* 1983; **23:** 882–9.

170. Mansberger A R, Doran J E, Treat R, *et al.* The influence of fibronectin administration on the incidence of sepsis and septic mortality in severely injured patients. *Ann Surg* 1989, **210:** 297–307.

171. Audibert F M, Lise L D. Adjuvants: current status, clinical perspectives and future prospects. *Immunol Today* 1993; **14:** 281–4.

172. Hadden J W. Immunostimulants. *Immunol Today* 1993; **14:** 275–80.

173. Hamilton G, *et al.* Thymopentin (TP5) in the treatment of the postburn and postoperative immunodeficiency syndrome. *Prog Clin Biol Res* 1989; **308:** 995–9.

174. Waymack J P, Miskell P, Gonce S J, Alexander J W. Effect of two new immunomodulators on normal and burn injury neutrophils and macrophages. *J Burn Care Rehabel* 1987; **8:** 9–14.

175. Visenti P. Extensive burn patients: Immunological problems. *Ann Medit Burns Club* 1989; **2:** 185.

176. Faist E, Ertel W, Salmen B, *et al.* The immune-enhancing effect of perioperative thymopentin administration in elderly patients undergoing major surgery. *Arch Surg* 1988; **123:** 1449–53.

177. Donati L, Lazzarin A, Signorini M, *et al.* Preliminary clinical experiences with the use of immunomodulators in burns. *J Trauma* 1983; **23:** 816–31.

178. Stinnett J D, Loose L D, Miskell P, *et al.* Synthetic immunomodulators for prevention of fatal infections in a burned guinea pig model. *Ann Surg* 1983; **198:** 53–7.

179. Sartorelli K H, Silver G M, Gamelli R L. The effect of granulocyte colony-stimulating factor (G-CSF) upon burn-induced defective neutrophil chemotaxis. *J Trauma* 1991; **31:** 523–30.

180. Mooney D P, Gamelli R L, O'Reilly M, *et al.* Recombinant human granulocyte colony-stimulating factor and pseudomonas burn wound sepsis. *Arch Surg* 1988; **123:** 1353–7.

181. Rusche J R. Preclinical studies with anti-integrin monoclonal antibodies for treatment of septic shock. Presented at the Seminar on Advances in Prevention and Treatment of Endotoxemia & Sepsis, Philadelphia June 22–23, 1992.

182. Evans D A, Jacobs D O, Revhaug A, Wilmore D W. The effects of tumor necrosis factor and their selective inhibition by ibuprofen. *Ann Surg* 1989; **209:** 312–20.

183. Demling R H, LaLonde C, Pequet Goad M D. Effect of ibuprofen on the pulmonary and systemic response to repeated doses of endotoxin. *Surgery* 1989; **105:** 421–9.

184. Byrne K, Carey D, Sielaff T D, *et al.* Ibuprofen prevents deterioration in static transpulmonary compliance and transalveolar protein flux in septic porcine acute lung injury. *J Trauma* 1991; **31:** 155–66.

185. Fukushima R, Giamotti L, Alexander W, Pyles T. The degree of bacterial translocation is a determinant factor for mortality after burn injury and is improved by prostaglandin analogs. *Ann Surg* 1992, **216:** 438–45.

186. Gadd M A, Hansbrough J F. Postburn suppression of murine lymphocyte and neutrophil functions is not reversed by prostaglandin blockade. *J Surg Res* 1990; **48:** 84–90.

187. Waymack J P, Guzman R F, Mason A D Jr, Pruitt B A Jr. Effect of prostaglandin E in multiple experimental models. VII: Effect on resistance to sepsis. *Burns* 1990; **16:** 9–12.

188. Bernard G R. Sepsis syndrome: current practice and new therapy. Presented at the Seminar on Advances in Prevention and Treatment of Endotoxemia & Sepsis, Philadelphia June 17–18, 1993.

189. Sheppard B C, Fraker D L, Norton J A. Prevention and treatment of endotoxin and sepsis lethality with recombinant human tumor necrosis factor. *Surgr* 1989; **106:** 156–62.

190. Alexander H R, Langstein H N, Doherty G M, *et al.* Human recombinant tumor necrosis factor (hrTNF) protection against endotoxin-induced shock and lethality in the rat. *Surg Forum* 1990; **41:** 103–5.

191. Fong Y, Tracey K J, Moldawer L L, *et al.* Antibodies to cachectin/tumor necrosis factor reduce interleukin 1B and interleukin 6 appearance during lethal bacteremia. *J Exp Med* 1989; **170:** 1627–33.

192. Doherty G M, Jensen J C, Alexander H A, *et al.* Pentoxifylline (PTX) suppression of tumor necrosis factor gene transcription. *Surgery* 1991; **110**(2): 192–8.

193. Ertel W, Morrison M H, Ayala A, *et al.* Passive immunization against cachectin (TNF-α) prevents hemorrhage-induced suppression of Kupffer cell functions. *Surg Forum* 1990; **41:** 91–30.

194. Ashkenazi A. Results with TNF receptor immunoadhesins for the treatment of sepsis. Presented at the Seminar on Advances in Prevention and Treatment of Endotoxemia & Sepsis, Philadelphia June 22–23, 1992.

195. Mohler D S, Torrance R V, Widmer M B. Therapeutic potential of soluble cytokine receptors in septic shock. Presented at the seminar on Advances in Prevention and Treatment of Endotoxemia & Sepsis, Philadelphia June 22–23, 1992.

196. Bodmer M. Pre-clinical evaluation of CDP571, a humanized anti-TNFα antibody. Presented at the Seminar on Advances in Prevention and Treatment of Endotoxemia & Sepsis, Philadelphia June 22–23, 1992.

197. Opal S M. Experience with interleukin-1 receptor antagonist in the treatment of sepsis. Presented at the Seminar on Advances in Prevention and Treatment of Endotoxemia & Sepsis, Philadelphia June 17–18, 1993.

198. Pribble J. Interleukin-1 receptor antagonist for the treatment of sepsis syndrome. Presented at the Seminar on Advances in Prevention and Treatment of Endotoxemia & Sepsis, Philadelphia June 22–23, 1992.

199. Silver G M, Gamelli R L, O'Reilly M, Herbert J C. The effect of interleukin 1 on survival in a murine model of burn wound sepsis. *Arch Surg* 1990; **125:** 922–5.

200. Polk H C Jr, Cheadle W G, Livingston D H, *et al* A randomized prospective clinical trial to determine the efficacy of interferon-gamma in severely injured patients. *Am J Surg* 1992; **163:** 191–6.

201. Redmond H P, Chavin K D, Bromberg J S, Daly J M. Inhibition of macrophage-activating cytokines is beneficial in the acute septic response. *Ann Surg* 1991; **214:** 502–9.

202. Lee J D, Swisher S G, Minehart E H, *et al.* Interleukin-4: a potent inhibitor of IL-6, TNF-α, IFN-γ, and IL-1β production. *Surg Forum* 1990; **41:** 441–4.

203. Yim J H, Tewari A, Pearce M K, *et al.* Monoclonal antibody against murine interleukin-6 prevents lethal effects of *Escherichia coli* sepsis and tumor necrosis factor challenge in mice. *Surg Forum* 1990; **41:** 114–17.

204. Barton B E. The anti-inflammatory effect of interleukin 6. Presented at the Seminar on Advances in Prevention and Treatment of Endotoxemia & Sepsis, Philadelphia June 17–18, 1993.

205. Etemadi A, Tempel G E, Farah B A, *et al.* Beneficial effects of a leukotriene antagonist on endotoxin-induced acute hemodynamic alterations. *Circ Shock* 1987; **22**(1): 55–63.

206. Teodorczyk–Injeyan J A, Sparkes B G, Mills G B, *et al.* Impaired expression of interleukin 2 receptor (IL-2R) in the immunosuppressed burned patient: reversal by exogenous IL2. *J Trauma* 1987; **27:** 180–6.

207. Howard M, Muchameul T, Andrade S, Menon S. Interleukin 10 protects mice from lethal endotoxemia. *J Exp Med* 1993; **177:** 1205–8.

208. Miller A S, Meredith J W, Meredith J H, *et al.* Immunoenhancement in the thermally injured guinea pig. *J Burn Care Rehabil* 1985; **6:** 358–62.

209. Munster A M, Leary A G. Treatment of pseudomonas sepsis in the rat with lymphocyte culture products. *Surg Forum* 1974; **25:** 33-4.

210. Fletcher J R, DiSimone A G, Earnest M A. Platelet activating factor receptor antagonist improves survival and attenuates eicosanoid release in severe endotoxemia. *Ann Surg* 1990; **211:** 312–16.

211. Hinshaw L B, Archer L T, Beller B K, *et al.* Evaluation of naloxone therapy for *E. coli* sepsis in the baboon. *Arch Surg* 1988; **123:** 700–4.

212. Hendrickson M, Shelby J, Sullivan J J, Saffle J R. Naloxone inhibits in the in vivo immunosuppressive effects of morphine and thermal injury in mice. *J Burn Care Rehabil* 1989; **10:** 494–8.

213. Lynn W A, Golenbock D T. Lipopolysaccharide antagonists. *Immunol Today* 1992; **13:** 271–6.

214. Magee G D, Hoper M, Halliday M I, *et al.* An in vitro study of the effect of centoxin on the production of tumor necrosis factor and interleukin-6 by normal human mononuclear cells. Presented at the meeting of the Surgical Infection Society, 1992.

215. Wedel N I. Update on the use of E5, an anti-endotoxin monoclonal antibody, in the treatment of gram-negative sepsis. Presented at the Seminar on Advances in Prevention and Treatment of Endotoxemia & Sepsis, Philadelphia June 22–23, 1992.

216. Quezado Z M N, Natanson C, Alling D W, *et al.* A controlled trial of HA-1A in a canine model of gram-negative septic shock. *JAMA* 1993; **269:** 2221–7.

217. Ziegler E F, Fisher C J Jr, Sprung C L, *et al.* Treatment of gram-negative bacteremia and septic shock with HA-1A human monoclonal antibody against endotoxin. *N Engl J Med* 1991; **324:** 429–36.

218. Warren H S, Danner R L, Munford R S. Sounding Board: anti-endotoxin monoclonal antibodies. *N Engl J Med* 1992; **326:** 1153–8.

219. Battafarano R J, Burd R S, Cody C S, Kellogg T A. Anti-lipopolysaccaharide monoclonal antibodies inhibit macrophage TNF messenger RNA synthesis in vitro. *J Surg Res* 1993; **54**(4): 342–8.

220. Burd R S, Cody C S, Raymond C S, Dunn D L. Anti-endotoxin monoclonal antibodies protect by enhancing bacterial and endotoxin clearance. *Arch Surg* 1993; **128:** 145–51.

221. Cody C S, Burd R S, Mayoral J L, Dunn D L. Protective anti-lipopolysaccharide monoclonal antibodies inhibit tumor necrosis factor production. *J Surg Res* 1992; **52**(4): 314–19.

222. Rubin R M, Noland J, Rosenbaum J T. Monoclonal antibodies directed against endotoxin reduce endotoxin-induced vascular permeability. *Clin Res* 1988; **36:** 147A.

223. Baumgartner J D, Glauser M P, McCutchan J A, *et al.* Prevention of gramnegative shock and death in surgical patients by antibody to endotoxin core glycolipid. *Lancet* 1985; **2:** 59–63.

224. Cometta A, Baumgartner J-D, Lee M L, *et al.* Prophylactic intravenous administration of standard immune globulin as compared with core-lipopolysaccharide immune globulin in patients at high risk of postsurgical infection. *N Engl J Med* 1992; **327:** 234–40.

225. Nys M, Damas P, Joassin L, Lamy M. Sequential anti-core glycolipid immunoglobulin antibody activities in patients with and without septic shock and their relation to outcome. *Ann Surg* 1993; **217:** 300–6.

226. Staubach K H, Kooistra A, Kujath P, *et al.* Extracorporeal absorption of endotoxin by a new polymyxin B detoxification column in pigs with endotoxin shock. Presented at the meeting of the Surgical Infection Society, 1992.

227. Hanasawa K, Tani T, Kodama M. New approach to endotoxic and septic shock by means of polymyxin B immobilized fiber. *Surg Gynecol Obstet* 1989; **168:** 323–31.

228. Crowley B M, O'Riodain G, Ellwanger K, Collins K H. Anti-endotoxin therapy improves survival in a model of thermal injury and sepsis. *Surg Forum* 1990; **41:** 72–4.

229. Cheadle W G, Hanasawa K, Gallinaro R N, *et al.* Endotoxin filtration and immune stimulation improve survival from gram-negative sepsis. *Surgery* 1991; **110:** 785–92.

230. Munster A M, Winchurch R A, Thupari J N, Ernst C B. Reversal of postburn immunosuppression with low-dose polymyxin B. *J Trauma* 1986; **26:** 995–8.

231. Munster A M, Meek M, Dickerson C, Winchurch R A. Translocation: true pathology of phenomenology. *Ann Surg* 1993; **218:** 321–7.

232. Nedeliaeva A V, Levin G Y. The influence of enterosorption on endotoxemia in burn illness. *Ann Medit Burns Club* 1992; **5:** 236–9.

233. Corradin S B, Mauel J, Gallay P, *et al.* Enhancement of murine macrophage binding of and response to bacterial lipopolysaccharide (LPS) by LPS-binding protein. *J Leukoc Biol* 1992; **52:** 363–8.

234. Gottardis M, Benzer A, Koller W, Luger T J. Improvement of septic syndrome after administration of recombinant human growth hormone (rhGH). *J Trauma* 1991; **31:** 81–6.

235. Noronha-Blob L. Leumedins and bradykinin receptor antagonists. Presented at the Seminar on Advances in Prevention and Treatment of Endotoxemia & Sepsis, Philadelphia June 17–18, 1993.

236. Pogrebniak H W, Merino M J, Hahn S M, *et al.* Spin trap salvage from endotoxemia: the role of cytokine down-regulation. *Surgery* 1992; **112:** 130–9.

237. Reilly P M, Schiller H J, Bulkley G B. Pharmacologic approach to tissue injury mediated by free radicals and other reactive oxygen metabolites. *Am J Surg* 1991; **161:** 488–503.

238. Aida Y, Pabst M J, Rademacher J M, *et al.* Effects of polymyxin B on superoxide anion release and priming in human polymorphonuclear leukocytes. *J Leukoc Biol* 1990; **47:** 283.

239. Lefer A M. Endothelial preserving agents in endotoxin shock. Presented at the Seminar on Advances in Prevention and Treatment of Endotoxemia & Sepsis, Philadelphia June 17–18, 1993.

240. Ertel W, Meldrum D R, Morrison M H, Ayala A. Immonoprotective effect of a calcium channel blocker on macrophage antigen presentation function, major histocompatibility class II antigen expression, and interleukin-1 synthesis after hemorrhage. *Surgery* 1990; **108:** 154–60.

241. French J F, Thomas C E, Downs T R, *et al.* Protective effects of a cyclic nitrone antioxidant in endotoxic shock. Presented at the Seminar on Advances in Prevention and Treatment of Endotoxemia & Sepsis, Philadelphia June 17–18, 1993.

242. Demling R H, Lalonde C. Identification and modifications of the pulmonary and biochemical changes caused by a skin burn. *J Trauma* 1990; **30:** S57–S62.

243. Demling R H, Lalonde C, Knox J, *et al.* Fluid resuscitation with deferoxamine prevents systemic burn-induced oxidant injury. *J Trauma* 1990; **30:** 918.

244. Thomson P D, Till G O, Prasad J K, Smith D J Jr. Enhancement of humoral immunity by heterologous lipid peroxidation products resulting from burn injury. *J Burn Care Rehabil* 1991; **12:** 38–40.

245. Mackensen A, Galanos C, Andreesen R, Engelhardt R. Cytokines in cancer patients treated with endotoxin in combination with ibuprofen. *J Leukoc Biol* 1989; **46:** 326.

246. Faist E, Markewitz A, Fuchs D, *et al.* Immunomodulatory therapy with thymopentin and indomethacin: successful restoration of interleukin-2 synthesis in patients undergoing major surgery. *Ann Surg* 1991; **214:** 264–75.

247. Malangoni M A, Lingston D H, Sonnenfeld G, Polk H C. Interferon gamma and tumor necrosis factor alpha. *Arch Surg* 1990; **125:** 444–6.

248. O'Riordain M G, Collins K H, Pitlz M, *et al.* Modulation of macrophage hyperactivity improves survival in a burn-sepsis model. *Arch Surg* 1992; **127:** 152–8.

249. Mendez M V, Molloy R G, O'Riordain D S, *et al.* Lymphokine activated killer cells enhance IL-2 prevention of sepsis-related death in a murine model of thermal injury. *J Surg Res* 1993; **54**(6): 565–70.

250. Silver G M, *et al.* The beneficial effect of granulocyte colony stimulating factor (G-CSF) in combination with gentamicin on survival after *Pseudomonas* infection. *Surgery* 1989; **106:** 452–6.

251. Oliva R G, Sica I. Intravenous immunoglobulin in severely burned patients five years of successful experience. *Ann Medit Burns Club* 1993; **6:** 20–4.

252. Missavage A E, Vaughan G M, McManus A T, *et al.* Alteration of host resistance in burned soldiers: therapy with IgG and T4 in burn patients. *Annual Research Progress Report for Fiscal Year 1987,* US Army Institute of Surgical Research, pp 188–99.

253. Munster A M, Winchurch R A. Unpublished data, 1987.

254. Ayala A, Lehmans D L, Herdar C D, Chaudry I H. Mechanism of enhanced susceptibility to sepsis following hemorrhage: interleukin 10 suppression of T-cell responses is mediated by eicosanoid-induced IL4 release. Presented to the 14th Annual Meeting of the Surgical Infection Society, Toronto, April 28–30, 1994.

CHAPTER TWENTY-EIGHT

Hematologic and Acute Phase Response

Richard H. C. Harries and Linda G. Phillips

Introduction

Over the last few decades, mortality from major burns has been reduced. This has been largely due to improved monitoring, broader spectrum antimicrobials, and, more recently, the practice of early total burn wound excision. These clinical advances would not have been possible without the information gleaned from ongoing burn research. The rapid progress of molecular biology and more specifically, DNA recombinant technology, has allowed investigation into the pathophysiology of thermal injuries to advance at a rapid rate. Clinicians now have a better understanding of the mechanisms of inflammation and burn wound sepsis, allowing more rational therapeutic interventions to be applied. In addition, various cytokines are now available in quantities large enough to allow a new chapter in burns management to be explored. Despite this progress, burn care continues to represent a significant challenge to modern medicine. Depending on their etiology and severity, burn injuries can disrupt the homeostasis of every system in the body. This chapter restricts its discussion to the hemopoietic system and the acute phase response to burns. Each cellular component of blood is discussed and humoral factors are covered with emphasis placed on clotting factors, cytokines, and acute phase response proteins. The pathophysiological disturbances caused by burns on each of these areas are addressed and following this, possible treatment strategies are elaborated. The reader should note that the hemopoietic system, as it pertains to immunity, is covered elsewhere in this text.

Red Blood Cells

Anemia is a frequent sequela of thermal injury and can be expected in full-thickness burns which involve greater than 10% of the total body surface area. The causes of reduced circulating red cell mass are multifactorial[1–11] (**Table 28.1**). The effects of direct heat on tissues can lead to red blood cell destruction within the burned area. It is possible that up to 10% of the circulating red blood cells could be lost as a direct and immediate sequela of thermal injury.[12,13] The extent of erythrocyte loss is related to burn severity. It has been reported that patients suffering 15–40% full-thickness burns have an average red cell loss of 12% with the first 6 hours of injury and 18% after 24 hours.[12] Direct heat alone does not account for all of these losses.

Table 28.1 The causes of anemia in the thermally injured patient

Increased red cell losses
- Direct effect of heat on tissues
- Surgical procedures
- Laboratory investigations
- Increased RBC clearance by the reticuloendothelial system
- Intravascular hemolysis
- Disseminated intravascular coagulation
- Gastrointestinal hemorrhage
- Heparin excesses

Reduced production of red cells
- Bone marrow suppression may be secondary to:
  - Infection
  - Burn toxin
  - Therapeutic drugs
  - Impaired iron metabolism
- Inadequate response to erythropoietin levels related to:
  - Bone marrow suppression
  - Erythropoietin inhibitory substance
  - Reduced erythroid stem cell sensitivity to erythropoietin
- Nutritional deficiencies
- Hepatorenal dysfunction

There is an interrelationship between the degree of burn and the extent of thrombosis in burned tissue. Vascular injury activates clotting mechanisms; red cells which are not initially present in the thermally injured area are consumed. Thrombi are readily seen in the venules of second degree burns while third degree burns have more extensive thrombosis involving both venules and arterioles.[14] Similarly, direct heat cannot account for ongoing erythrocyte losses in the days following the burn. There is little doubt that many circulating erythrocytes are partially damaged as a direct result of the burn, and these cells are quickly cleaned from the circulation by the spleen and other components of the reticuloendothelial system.[15] Apart from this intrinsic clearing system, red blood cells are also damaged as a result of factors extrinsic to the cell. Erythrocytes from normal donors, when transfused into burned patients, have significantly reduced half-lives, while red cells from burned patients, when transfused into normal individuals, exhibit normal survival.[13] In the thermally injured patient, normal red cells are thought to be damaged by oxygen free radicals which are released from complement-activated neutrophils.[16] The exact mechanisms whereby normal erythrocytes in thermally injured patients are rendered more susceptible to accelerated destruction is yet to be fully understood but is related to change in the properties of the erythrocyte membrane. These membrane changes cause an increase in the cells' osmotic fragility and a reduction in membrane deformability.[6,17] This results in morphologic changes in the red cells. Spherocytosis, fragmentation, and vesiculation of red blood cells can occur within hours of any major burn.[7] Such cells, if not cleared by the reticuloendothelial system, can undergo intravascular hemolysis, leading to acute hemoglobinuria. Hemoglobinemia of up to 300 mg/dl can occur but, in the presence of normal renal function, is a short-lived phenomenon because the high renal threshold for hemoglobin excretion is 130–140 mg/ml.[6,18]

Despite the loss of erythrocyte mass immediately following burns, the hematocrit of thermally injured patients actually rises during the acute phase of burns. This is due to well established plasma volume losses. The extent of hemoconcentration seen following burns depends on both the severity of the thermal injury and the adequacy of fluid resuscitation. Each of these factors is also related to the severity of anemia observed in patients once the resuscitative phase of burn management is over. Patients with extensive burns will continue to lose red blood cells at a rate of 1–2% per day until the burn is healed.[19,20] This is the result of ongoing blood loss secondary to surgery, laboratory tests, and usually intervening infection of variable degrees.

The body's usual response to anemia is to stimulate the bone marrow to produce more red cells. This is achieved via erythropoietin, a glycoprotein produced primarily by the kidney in response to hypoxia (**Table 28.2**). The structure, chemistry, and function of erythropoietin have recently been reviewed.[21] The erythropoietin response to thermal injury is currently controversial. Studies published in the last two decades have had conflicting results with both elevations and reductions in erythropoietin levels being reported.[13,22,23] These studies used varying techniques including bioassay or radioimmunoassay, and suffered from small sample sizes, widely varying burn sizes, or did not control for disordered iron metabolism and the need for serial blood transfusions. This may explain why results between studies varied. Recent investigations indicate that erythropoietin levels are in fact elevated following burns and that the bone marrow is able to produce reticulocytes.[9,10] Despite this, anemia persists. This paradox has several possible explanations. First, the reticulocytic anemia along with the decreased erythroid cellularity of the bone marrow seen in burns indicates that the marrow's response to anemia is submaximal.[1,20,24] The erythropoietic response may not equate to the degree of anemia due to an erythropoietic inhibitory substance. This serum factor is yet to be fully characterized, but may act by blocking the action of erythropoietin on erythroid progenitor cells.[1,4,10,25]

Disordered iron metabolism in thermally injured patients may significantly contribute to the submaximal erythropoietic responsiveness. Circulating iron levels are depressed in burned patients.[1,10] It is known that adequate iron availability is essential for effective erythropoietin responses.[26] If iron is not freely available, then new hemoglobin synthesis is not possible even in the presence of elevated erythropoietin levels. This fact underscores the rationale of iron supplementation during the postburn period.

Finally, it may be that under certain conditions as yet undefined, erythroid progenitor cells are insensitive to erythropoietin.[10] Cytokines, such as interleukin-1 and tumor necrosis factor (TNF), are known to interfere with the normal inverse relationship between hemoglobin levels and erythropoietin levels.[27] Elevated erythropoietin titers seen in burns may not be sufficient to overcome the dampening effect of these and other cytokines. In AIDS patients who are anemic, endogenous erythropoietin levels can be very high (500 U/ml).[28] Despite this, erythropoiesis can be stimulated by elevating erythropoietin titers further with exogenous recombinant human erythropoietin. Erythropoietin levels in thermally injured patients rarely exceed 500 U/ml.[9,10,23] If, for whatever reason, erythroid progenitor cells in a burn environment are insensitive to these endogenous erythropoietin levels, then anemia would not be reversed. Anemia may be reversed with exogenous erythropoietin; and early work in the thermally injured population is already occurring.[23]

White Blood Cells

It is important to discuss the role of granulocytes and their colony stimulating factors (CSFs). (Discussion involving macrophage and lymphocyte cell lines is covered in another chapter.) The phagocytic cell represents a two-edged sword for the burned patient. These cells are of great importance in providing resistance against opportunistic infection. When activated inappropriately, they can also be detrimental to the burned patient, as the tissue damage they cause can contribute to adult respiratory distress syndrome or even multiorgan failure.[28–32]

Burn-related changes in granulocyte numbers depend on the severity of the thermal injury, the presence or absence of infection, and individual patient characteristics. In the first 24 hours following injury, burned patients uniformly manifest a granulocytosis. This is not due to an increased production of phagocytic cells but rather a combination of intravascular demargination and mobilization of preexisting mature bone marrow reserves.[7,33–35] Serum factors such as complement products, interleukin-1 and interleukin-6 are responsible for the elevated peripheral leukocyte concentrations.[36,37]

Granulocytosis peaks during the first postburn day and then the white blood cell count starts to fall. This is related to dilutional effects during the resuscitative phase and margination of leukocytes, both within the burned area and at sites distant to damaged tissue.[38] This margination process can potentially deplete bone marrow stores within 24–48 hours. The burned patient is then dependent on the bone marrow to respond with increased granulocyte production.

Following this initial fall in white blood cell levels, the remaining postburn period can exhibit a leukocytosis or a leukopenia.[35,39,40] Postburn leukocytosis has been related to increasing burn size[28] and more recently, to a patient's capacity to produce hemopoietic colony stimulating factors in response to stress. Colony stimulating factors can be divided into two groups. Granulocyte-monocyte colony stimulating factor, interleukin-3 and interleukin-6 (GM-CSF, IL-3, IL-6) stimulate the proliferation and differentiation of pleuripotent stem and progenitor cells. Erythropoietin, monocyte colony stimulating factor and granulocyte colony stimulating factors (EPO, M–CSF, G–CSF) restrict their actions to the development of mature progenitor cells into specific cell lineages[41–43] (**Table 28.2**). No matter whether the patient manifests a leukocytosis or leukopenia postburn, in both situations a defect in granulocyte function exists. Such defects have been well reviewed.[44–48] These studies all report disorders in migration, phagocytosis and degranulation.

The last decade has seen the development of *in vitro* culture systems which can measure granulocyte regulatory factors. This, along with advances in recombinant DNA technology, has allowed further investigation of disorders of leukocyte function and kinetics. It has been proposed that the host's bacterial or antigenic load is the major stimulus for granulopoiesis.[49–51] Infection is thought to stimulate colony stimulating factor synthesis by circulating monocytes; rising colony stimulating factor levels trigger an increase in production and maturation of granulocyte precursors in the bone marrow. The resultant leukocytosis enables clearance of bacteria,

Table 28.2 Hemopoietic colony stimulating factors (CSF)

Name	Molecular unit	Synonyms	Chromosomal location	Cell sortes	Target cells	Biological effects
Granulocyte-monocyte CSF (GM-CSF)	118–22 kDa glycoprotein; 127 amino acids; monomer	CSF-2; neutrophil inhibitory factor; pluripoietin-α	5q21–5q21	Fibroblasts Monocytes Macrophages Endothelial cells Mesangial cells T lymphocytes Smooth muscle cells Epithelial cells Fibroblasts Mast cells	Mature progenitor granulocytes and macrophages eosinophils and neutrophils	Maturation of granulocytes and macrophage progenitors Promotes growth and differentiator of multipotential progenitor cells Proliferation of mature granulocyte macrophages and eosinophils
Granulocyte CSF (G-CSF)	18–32 kDa glycoprotein; 174 amino acids	DF, MG1–2, GSF-β, pleuripoietin	17	Fibroblasts Keratinocytes T cells Macrophages Neutrophils Endothelial cells Fibroblasts	Granulocyte progenitors	Maturation of granulocyte progenitors Enhances the differentiation activation of neutrophils Stimulates the production of neutrophils and macrophages *in vitro*
Macrophage CSF (M-CSF)	70–90 kDa glycosylated dimer; 223 amino acids or 158 homodimer. Also biologically, active membrane bound form	CSF-1	5	Fibroblasts Epithelial cells Macrophages Embryonic yolk sac Monocytes T cells Neutrophils Fibroblasts Endothelial cells	Macrophage progenitors	Maturation of macrophage progenitors Stimulates various functions of monocytes and macrophages
Erythropoietin (EPO)	34 kDa glycoprotein; 165 amino acids; monomer		7q11–7q22	Renal cells Hepatocytes Macrophages	Erythroid progenitors	Stimulates growth and differentiation of erythroid progenitors
Interleukin-3 (IL-3)	20 kDa glycoprotein; 133 amino acids; monomer	Mast cell growth factor T-cell stimulating factor Burst promoting activity Multicolony stimulating factor WEH1–3 growth factor CSF2α	5	T cells Thymic epithelial cells Keratinocytes Neutral cells Mast cells	Granulocytes Macrophages Erythrocyte progenitors Megakaryocytes Mast cells T cells B cells	Synergizes with lineage restricted factors to stimulate the production and differentiation of macrophages, neutrophils, eosinophils, basophils erythroid cells and megakeryocytes Supports the proliferation of multipotential progenitor cells
Interleukin-6 (IL-6)	23–30 kDa glycoprotein; 184 amino acids; monomer	1FN-β2 26 kDa protein BSF-2 MG 1–2A Cytotoxic T-cell and/or B-cell differentiating factor Hepatocyte stimulating factor	7q21	T cells/B cells Monocytes Macrophages Fibroblasts Hepatocytes Endothelial cells Neuronal cells Epithelial cells Mesangial cells	T cells B cells Myeloma cells Thymocytes Hemopoietic stem cells Hepatocytes Macrophages	Activates hemopoietic progenitor cells and shortens their G_0 phase Induces maturation of megakaryocytes and an increase in platelet number Induces growth and/or differentiation of T_2, B cells, hepatocytes, keratinocytes, nerve cells, cytotoxic T cells Stimulates the production of acute phase protein by hepatocytes

and this, in turn, provides a negative feedback, reducing colony stimulating factor production. Patients who are able to mount such a response to sepsis are better equipped to survive the trauma of burns. Nonsurvivors of burns have been observed to have delayed rises in colony stimulating factor levels and a monocytopenia. Such patients die of sepsis, presumably as a result of an aberration in their granulocyte regulatory function. It is difficult to dissect out whether sepsis itself directly causes bone marrow failure or whether the deficient colony stimulating factor response to infection leads to bone marrow quiescence, despite the presence of sepsis.[28,52,53] Generally when sepsis occurs, stem cell proliferation is compromised;[54] however, myeloid stem cell proliferative defects, as well as significant falls in colony stimulating factor levels, have both been described in patients well *before* the development of sepsis.[55,56] These reports indicate that in thermal injury, bone marrow failure is not a product of sepsis but is, instead, due to low colony stimulating factor levels. Leukopenia and sepsis are the sequelae.

The causes for colony stimulating factor deficiency states in some patients are not well understood. Serum factors, such as lactoferrin, are elevated following burns and these substances may inhibit colony stimulating factor production.[57] Whatever the cause, there is little doubt that the immunosuppression seen in major thermal injuries is related to a disorder in the colony stimulating factor–myeloid stem cell axis.

Early work with colony stimulating factor revealed that under physiologic conditions, colony stimulating factor could enhance phagocytic cell functions. Proliferation, chemotaxis, phagocytosis, and bacterial killing are all increased by colony stimulating factors.[41,43] As a result of this work, several groups have shown that the detrimental effects of suboptimal colony stimulating factor levels can now be ameliorated by treating patients with exogenous colony stimulating factor.[52,57–59] Similarly, immunomodulators may be helpful in preventing colony stimulating factor deficiency states in thermally injured patients.[28] Such studies all report increases in both granulocyte number and function. It is too early to say whether these effects will be beneficial to the burned patient as inappropriate activation of phagocytic cells can be detrimental. For example, activated macrophages are involved in the regulation of acute phase response proteins. Prolonged activation with exogenous colony stimulating factors may contribute to inappropriate hypercatabolism with rapid and harmful loss of protein.[60,61] Similarly, the use of colony stimulating factors in patients with inhalation injury could potentially increase inappropriate inflammatory responses in the lung, producing edema and progressive pulmonary failure.

PLATELETS

During the acute resuscitative phase of burns, platelet numbers usually fall. This is due to both dilutional and consumptive effects.[62] The large fluid volumes used during the shock phase of burns dilutes both platelets and clotting factors. The mechanisms underlying platelet consumption are less well understood. Like red blood cells, some platelets will be destroyed within the burn area as a direct result of heat. Large numbers of platelets may be consumed to support the integrity of the microvasculature within the burned area.[63] Additionally, the release of thromboplastins from damaged tissue can cause microthrombi to form in distant sites such as lung and renal vasculature.[64,65] The reticuloendothelial system also contributes to reductions in platelet numbers by removing these microthrombi from the circulation.[61,65] A serum effect has also been implicated in falls in platelet numbers, as chromium-51 labeled platelets from normal, unburned individuals have a reduced half-life if infused into a thermally injured patient in the first postburn week.[63] The bone marrow has no significant platelet reserves and there is a proportional relationship between the size of burn injury and the subsequent fall in platelet numbers during the first 3 days postburn.

Following this initial fall, platelet numbers return to more normal levels, although, from about 2 weeks postburn, a thrombocytosis is commonly observed. Thrombocytosis can persist for weeks after burn injury. The mechanisms for postburn thrombocytosis are yet to be fully characterized. The production of megakaryocytes by the bone marrow is stimulated by several colony stimulating factors. GM-CSF, IL-3, and IL-6 are all involved in platelet production. The interactions which occur between these colony stimulating factors are poorly understood. The derangements in colony stimulating factor levels caused by thermal injuries could contribute to thrombocytosis. Again, the level of thrombocytosis has been positively correlated with increasing burn severity.

Thrombocytosis does not always occur following thermal injury, however. Thrombocytopenia can occur and may be considered a bad prognostic sign. Thrombocytopenia has been correlated with poor outcome in extensive burns and may be considered an early and sensitive indicator of sepsis.[67] It is not currently known whether the low platelet counts are a product of increased megakaryocyte destruction or failed production. The role of colony stimulating factors in this scenario is also not documented.

Finally, a thrombocytosis, rather than a reduction in platelet numbers, has been reported during the first 3 postburn days.[7] Patients with greater than 70% burns who succumbed to their injuries within 57 hours all had intravascular hemolysis and an apparent thrombocytosis. On further investigation, this was actually a pseudothrombocytosis, due to incorrect recording of platelets by automated cell counters. Red cell microvesicles from fragmented and lysed red blood cells were incorrectly recorded as platelets. Clinicians should be alert to the fact that thrombocytosis occurring acutely in severe burns may be spurious and may actually be obscuring a thrombocytopenia which can occur in patients with disseminated intravascular coagulation.

CLOTTING FACTORS

The homeostasis of clotting is complex. It involves interactions between multiple clotting factors, the fibrinolytic system, and several cellular elements. A delicate balance between amplification and inhibition is required in order to avoid hemorrhagic or hypercoagulable disorders.

Homeostasis in 60 thermally injured patients has recently been reviewed.[8] This study determined that following burns, thrombotic and fibrinolytic mechanisms are activated, and that the extent of activation increased with the severity of thermal injury. Most homeostatic markers of coagulation fell during the early shock phase of burns and dilutional effects, along with loss of plasma proteins into interstitial tissues, are thought to contribute. The return of clotting factors to more normal levels after the resuscitative period of thermal injury supports dilution as a cause of their initial fall rather than a progressive consumption of clotting factors.[62] Later in the postburn course, thrombogenicity is increased due to a decrease in antithrombin III, protein C, and protein S levels, while fibrinolysis activation occurs via increases in tissue plasminogen activator levels. The loss of the natural anticoagulants antithrombin III, protein C, and protein S, along with the rise in fibrinolytic products, places the patient at an increased risk of thrombosis.[8] Components of the coagulation cascade are not the only elements contributing to the hypercoagulable state following burns. Hypoxia, tissue factors, shock, sepsis, and even the phospholipids from fragmented red blood cells all play a role.

This hypercoagulable state in the post burn period puts many burned patients at risk for disseminated intravascular coagulation (DIC). Postmortem studies in the past have indicated that 30% of severely burned patients have evidence of DIC. All major organs of the body can manifest microvascular thromboses, which in severe cases can lead to parenchymal damage.[64] These microvascular thrombi, along with the plasma losses and red blood cells' morphologic changes seen in burns, contribute to elevations in blood viscosity.[17] In the absence of adequate resuscitation, this causes a reduced tissue perfusion and results in the progression of both local and systemic effects of burn injury.

Disseminated intravascular coagulation should be suspected in thermally injured patients if shock is out of proportion with blood loss and extensive hemorrhagic oozing is noted around intravascular cannula and venipuncture sites. Prothrombin times, partial thromboplastin times, and fibrin degradation products should also be increased while fibrinogen levels and platelet numbers should be decreased.

Acute Phase Response

The acute phase response to injury is part of the body's natural defense mechanism whereby cells and tissues are protected from further damage and homeostasis is restored. The pathophysiologic changes which occur during the acute phase response have been elaborated.[68–73] The acute phase proteins and their response to thermal injury are shown in **Table 28.3**. The acute phase response commences as a local reaction to injury.[74] This encompasses activation of the clotting cascade, platelets, and phagocytic cells. Inherent to this is dilation and leakage of plasma fluid and proteins from blood vessels. Activated phagocytic cells, fibroblasts, and endothelial cells release cytokines (including IL-6, IL-1, and TNF) which lead to the systemic phase of the acute phase response. The systemic reaction affects the hypothalamus which leads to fever, the pituitary–adrenal axis so as to release steroid hormones, the liver which causes the synthesis and secretion of acute phase proteins, the bone marrow which promulgates further hemopoietic responses, and finally, the immune system, which allows the activation of the reticuloendothelial system and the proliferation of lymphocytes. If all these elements coalesce in a balanced fashion, then the burn insult is counteracted, and healing with eventual recovery ensues.[37] While the acute phase response is protective, it must also be self-limiting. Its effects, when prolonged, lead to a hypercatabolic state and an extended inflammatory response to injury which is ultimately harmful to the host.[61] Previously, patients with extensive thermal injuries died because the resulting inflammation and sepsis exceeded the reparative capacity of the acute phase response. Today, patients with major burns have ever-extending survival times; clinicians are now having to combat not only the initial effects of burn injury, but also the harmful effects of a prolonged acute phase response. Recent advances with exogenous cytokines and other immunomodulators have allowed this paradox to be addressed.

Table 28.3 The acute phase response proteins and their levels following thermal injury

Increased	Normal	Decreased
C-reactive proteins	α_2-Macroglobin	Inter-α-antitrypsin
Serum amyloid A	Hemopexin	Transferrin
α_1-Proteinase inhibitor	Serum amyloid P	α_1-Lipoprotein
α_2-Acid glycoprotein	Prothrombin	Prealbumin
α_1-Antichymotrypsin		Albumin
Fibrinogen		
Haptoglobin		
Ceruloplasmin		
C_3 (complement)		
α_2-Antiplasmin		
C_1-Inactivator		

The proteins involved in the acute phase response have now been largely identified (**Table 25.3**), although the exact role played by each is yet to be fully understood.[68–73] The major site of acute phase protein synthesis is the liver. These proteins can be produced after minor burn injury, and the intensity of the acute phase response increases as the severity of burn increases. The modulators of the acute phase response are yet to be characterized, but the elevations or reduction in levels of acute phase proteins is related at the molecular level to either an upregulation or downregulation of messenger RNA (mRNA). It should be realized that changes in mRNA levels within the cells do not always translate to corresponding changes in serum protein levels. For example, it has been shown by one group that burns produce an upregulation of albumin mRNA levels.[72] Albumin levels characteristically fall in the postburn period. It would appear that albumin clearance exceeds that of a synthesis. This is probably due to the massive expansion of the extravascular space available to albumin due to its loss into the burn wound and into intestinal tissues and the increased catabolic state seen in thermal injury.[17,19]

Several serum protein inhibitors have been found to be elevated during the acute phase response. α_1-Antitrypsin is one such inhibitor and is important in activating proteolytic enzymes released both from damaged tissue in the early postburn phase and dead bacteria during the infection stage of thermal injury. Following a burn injury the mRNA levels for α_1-antitrypsin are increased, suggesting an upregulation of this protein. Interestingly, animal studies have shown that rat species which have an inherent resistance to burn injury also have comparatively higher levels of α_1-antitrypsin mRNA. It may be that a capacity to increase the titer of such protective serum protein inhibitors could prove beneficial in burn injury.[72]

Many researchers are now turning their endeavors to the cytokines which initiate the acute phase response. It now appears that while IL-1 and TNF play a role, it is IL-6 which is the major regulator of the acute phase response in humans. IL-6, IL-1, and TNF are all elevated in the serum of thermally injured patients.[37,72,74] These three cytokines, of which IL-6 is the most important, represent an amplification system for the synthesis of acute phase proteins by the liver. IL-6 directly stimulates the production of C-reactive protein, haptoglobin, ceruloplasmin, fibrinogen, C_1 inhibitor, α_1-antitrypsin and α_1-acid glycoprotein, while inhibiting production of fibronectin, albumin, and transferrin.[37,75] IL-6 also acts on hemopoiesis, being synergistic with IL-3 and GM-CSF in the maturation of megakaryocytes and other myeloid stem cells. IL-6 contributes to the prolonged fever seen in the thermally injured and may be the source of the reactive thrombocytosis seen in burn patients.[75] The elevations in IL-1 and TNF following a burn are probably related to their role in stimulating IL-6 elevations, rather than any direct effect they may have on the acute phase response.[75] How IL-1 and TNF interact with IL-6 is not understood. IL-6 may also be a marker of survival outcome. Its levels are directly related to burn size. Survivors of burns have significant elevations in IL-6 with a proportional increase in the synthesis of acute phase proteins. Nonsurvivors, on the other hand, have been reported to have even greater IL-6 elevations, but fail to produce increased levels of acute phase reactants. In these studies, death may have occurred before IL-6 produced its effects, or this observation may provide a clue for the mechanism of death in these patients.[76,77] For example, C-reactive protein, whose levels are normally significantly increased following thermal injury, is involved in the activation of phagocytes and the reticuloendothelial system, activation of complement, and activation of nonspecific host defense systems.[78] A submaximal response of this and other acute phase reactants could mean that the patient is ill prepared to cope with the insult of a major thermal injury.

It is apparent that the efficacy of the acute phase response to tissue injury and infection is determined by the serum levels of acute phase proteins achieved. Failure of the acute phase response to respond appropriately to stress is detrimental to the host. As our understanding of cytokines improves, modulation of the acute phase response may become possible. Early work in this area suggests that cytokines, such as colony stimulating factors or interleukins, may be useful in either activating a suppressed bone marrow or acute phase response or conversely, in downregulating inappropriate acute phase reactions and, thereby, protect the host from further harm.[28,52,61,79,80] The unraveling of this series of very complex interrelationships will ultimately lead to further advances in burn care.

TREATMENT STRATEGIES

A suggested management scheme for the hemopoietic and acute phase response to burns is shown in **Figure 28.1**. Following admission to a burn unit, thermal injuries of greater than 15% total body surface area (TBSA) generally require some form of fluid resuscitation. Intravenous fluids are the most efficient, but depending on the circumstances, oral fluid resuscitation may also be acceptable. Numerous formulae exist to calculate resuscitative fluid needs, and many different fluids can be selected for use. A reasonable strategy is to use crystalloids in the acute resuscitative phase followed by blood and/or colloid solutions in the remaining postburn phase. From a hematologic standpoint, adequate resuscitation is important; for it has been shown in animal models that apart from improving perfusion, resuscitation also improves blood flow. This occurs due to a reduction in red cell osmotic fragility and an improvement in erythrocyte membrane deformability, leading to reduced blood viscosity. Additionally, renal function is maintained, allowing efficient clearance of free plasma hemoglobin.[17] This improved blood rheology maximizes blood flow to tissue injured by burns. This may minimize the production of serum factors which cause ongoing damage to red blood cells in the postburn period.[6]

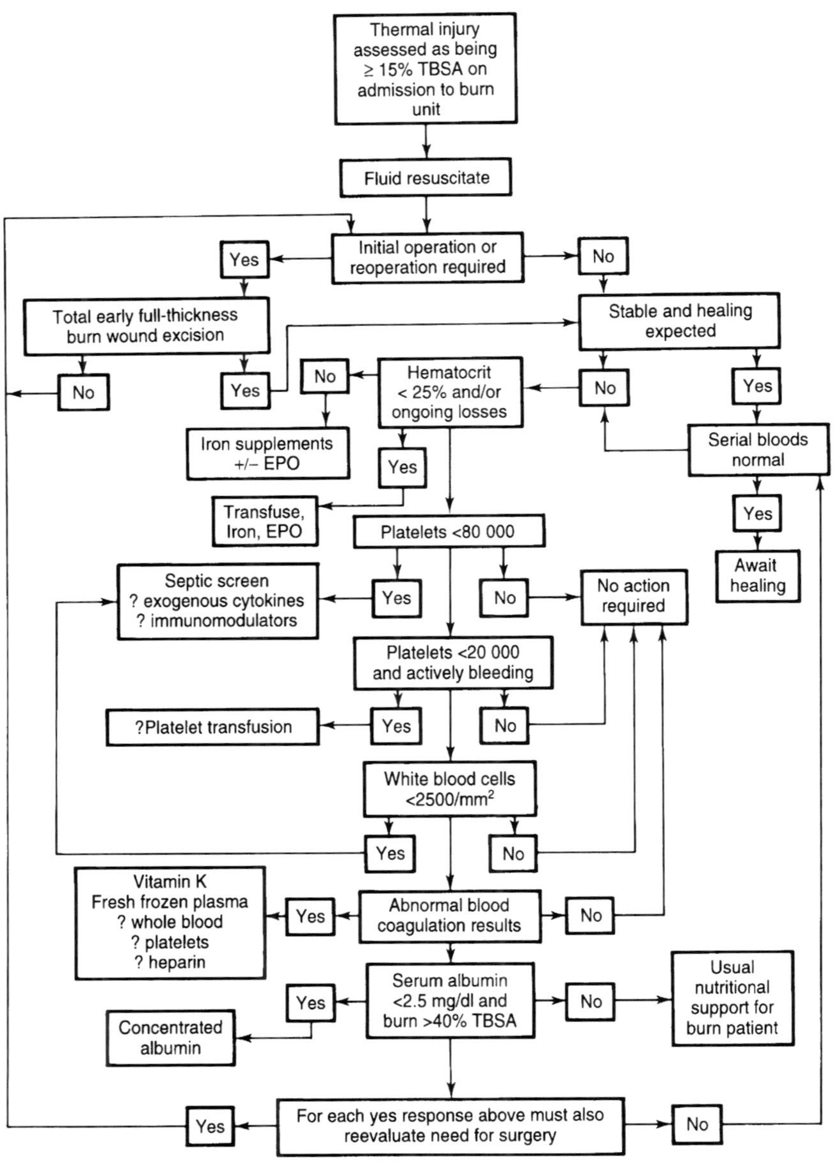

Fig. 28.1 Suggested management schedule for the hemopoietic and acute phase responses to burns.

If the thermal injury is partial thickness in nature, then surgery may be deferred on the assumption that healing will occur spontaneously. If such patients do not have a hospital stay complicated by sepsis or gastrointestinal hemorrhage, then their management is often trouble free. It is the patients with extensive full-thickness and partial-thickness burns who require multiple surgeries in order to cover their burn wounds who really represent a challenge to the burn unit. These patients can have a protracted hospital stay with their status oscillating between being stable and unstable depending on the outcomes of the inevitable septic episodes. Patients with severe partial-thickness burns are difficult to manage, as these partial-thickness areas can convert into full thickness burns; and this tissue can be the source of ongoing hematologic instability and acute phase responses.

On routine blood screens, this can manifest as falling hematocrits, platelets, and/or white cell counts, as persistently depressed serum albumin levels, and as abnormal coagulation parameters. In these cases, multiple interventions are possible, some accepted and some experimental.

Following initial burn wound excision or reoperation, patients who cannot be considered stable but whose hematocrit remains above 25% may reasonably have their anemia treated by iron supplementation alone. Patients with significant burns are known to be iron deficient; this not only promotes anemia but is thought by some to be directly related to the immunocompromised state of burned patients.[23] The latter is contested by some groups who believe hypoferremia is protective against infection[81] and so supplemental iron should not be provided.[10] Iron should certainly be given if erythropoietin treatment is instituted in these patients.[23] The use of erythropoietin when the hematocrit is over 25% should be considered unnecessary as the use of erythropoietin would not be cost-effective, especially as burned patients are comparatively sedentary and can readily tolerate hemoglobins of 7 g/dl. Hematocrits of less than 25% are not well tolerated, however, and this sort of patient probably benefits from both iron supplementation and erythropoietin therapy. While current literature remains largely undecided about the benefits of erythropoietin in the burn setting, there are certainly no contraindications to its use. Indeed, compared to the potential complications of transfusion, the erythropoietin alternative can be quite attractive. Currently, patients with hematocrits of less than 25% still warrant serial transfusions, but the inherent risks should not be ignored. Prior to 1985, the risk of HIV following transfusion within a burn unit had been reported as 2%.[82] With improved screening by blood banks, this risk should now be negligible. Hepatitis C, however, remains a real problem. Hepatitis C infection following multiple transfusions has been reported as high as 18% in some burn units.[83] This is especially alarming considering that up to 83% of hepatitis C infections can result in chronic hepatitis.[84] It should be remembered that chronic hepatitis is thought to be one of the antecedants for hepatocellular carcinoma, and this association is of concern when considering long-term outcomes in burn survivors. Finally, blood transfusion itself may have an immunosuppressive effect.[85–88]

In an attempt to avoid blood transfusion, clinicians should attempt to minimize postburn anemia. This may be possible by early total excision of full-thickness burns, thus, removing one of the major stimuli of prolonged postburn anemia. Once the patient is adequately resuscitated with crystalloid, early surgery is performed and operative blood losses are replaced on a strict volume for volume basis. A formula exists whereby operative blood losses can be calculated allowing accurate volume replacements.[89] Reductions of blood losses via early total excision may reduce the need for further transfusions in the postburn period. Indeed, the use of whole blood within the first 24 hours of burn injury has been reported to improve anemia and hypoproteinemia, among other things.[90]

Hypoalbuminemia is an early and consistent finding in burns. It is also considered to be a useful predictor of morbidity and mortality related to infection. Despite this, clinical studies to assess the potential benefits of its correction have yielded contradictory results. Albumin supplementation has been reported to reduce rates of both pneumonia and bacteremia.[91] It has also been shown to reverse intolerance to enteral feeding in burned children with hypoalbuminemia.[92] Other studies have reported no benefit with respect to either mortality or major morbidity.[93] Failure of serum albumin levels to increase with nutritional support identifies a group of patients at increased risk of dying following traumatic injury.[94] Therefore, despite the contradictory studies, it seems reasonable to give concentrated albumin in an attempt to elevate serum albumin levels in patients who are already severely injured. Patients with greater than 40% TBSA burns fall into this category.

In patients suffering leukopenia, overwhelming sepsis is a very real concern. Leukopenia in the thermally injured is related to bone marrow hyporesponsiveness in the presence of low CSF levels. A septic screen is mandatory and appropriate antimicrobials should be commenced. Other sources for the low white cell count should also be sought. Drug charts should be reviewed and the ongoing need for topical antimicrobials reviewed. Topical silver sulfadiazine and even plasma infusions have been reported to cause neutropenia in burned patients.[95,96] The ongoing presence of incompletely excised full-thickness burn tissue may also play a role, and the need for further surgery should be constantly reevaluated in the neutropenic patient. In the burns field, the support of leukopenic patients with exogenous cytokines and/or immunomodulators is still essentially experimental in nature.

Following the resuscitative phase of burns, patients are usually hypercoagulable. With the exception of DIC, hemorrhagic disorders of the clotting mechanism are unusual. Overwhelming sepsis can precipitate hemorrhage, but usually thrombosis and thromboembolism are more frequent problems.[62,63] Despite this, the use of prophylactic heparin in thermal injuries is controversial. Antithrombin III levels are reduced in burns,[8] and this natural anticoagulant is a co-factor for heparin activity. The use of antithrombin III and heparin have been shown to increase survival in uncontrolled studies.[97,98] Other investigators have indicated routine prophylactic heparin to be of little benefit.[99] The complications of heparin overdose and heparin-induced thrombocytopenia are well recognized. The use of heparin in frank DIC is more accepted. Patients who do develop hemorrhagic coagulopathies need clotting factors, and these are readily supplied in fresh frozen plasma. Fresh whole blood also supplies active clotting factors and platelets but is rarely available in the quantities required. Platelets can be used in cases of severe thrombocytopenia (<20 000 platelets/mm^3), particularly if the patient is actively bleeding, but should be used sparingly as they can generate platelet antibodies. Platelet transfusions, when platelet units fall to less than 12 000, have been advocated to prevent cerebrovascular accidents; few data exist to support the validity of this. The frequency of postburn coagulopathy can be reduced by aggressive fluid resuscitation and early total excision of the burn wound. This helps eliminate antecedants to any possible coagulation disorders by reducing the intravascular sludging due to increased blood viscosity or the ongoing release of thromboplastins, phospholipids, and other serum factors. If a coagulopathy does develop, underlying causes such as ongoing sepsis should be eliminated, the patient should be supported with supplemental clotting factors, and the need for further surgery should be reevaluated.

Conclusion

The systemic upheaval precipitated by thermal injuries is extraordinarily complex. With increased survival rates have come additional problems of prolonged inflammation and acute phase responses. Ongoing burn research is increasing our understanding of these processes and the advances in recombinant DNA technology will enable clinicians in the future to modulate the hemopoietic and acute phase response to burns.

REFERENCES

1. Andes W A, Rogers P W, Beason J W, Pruitt B A Jr. The erythropoietin response to the anemia of thermal injury. *J Lab Clin Med* 1976; **88:** 584–92.

2. Birdsell D C, Birch J R. Anemia following thermal burns: a survey of 109 children. *Can J Surg* 1971; **14:** 345–50.

3. Robinson H, Monato W W, Saver S M, Gallagher N I. The role of erythropoietin in the anemia of thermal injury. *Ann Surg* 1973; **178:** 565–72.

4. Wallner S F, Vautrin R M, Buerk C, Robinson W A, Peterson V M. The anemia of thermal injury: studies of erythropoiesis *in vitro*. *J Trauma* 1982; **22:** 774–80.

5. Boar S. Anemia of burns. *Burns* 1979; **6:** 1–8.

6. Endoh Y, Kawakami M, Orringer E P, Peterson H D, Meyer A A. Causes and time course of acute hemolysis after burn injury in the rat. *J Burn Care* 1992; **13:** 203–9.

7. Lawrence C, Bulent A. Hematological changes in massive burn injury. *Crit Care Med* 1992; **20:** 1284–8.

8. Kowal-Vern A, Gamelli R L, Walenga J, Hoppensteadt D, Sharp-Pucci M, Schumacher H R. The effect of burn wound size on hemostasis: a correlation of the hemostatic changes to the clinical state. *J Trauma* 1992; **33:** 50–7.

9. Vasko S D, Burdge J J, Ruberg R L, Verghese A S. Evaluation of erythropoietin levels in the anemia of thermal injury. *J Burn Care Rehabil* 1991; **12:** 437–41.

10. Deitch E A, Sittig K M. A serial study of the erythropoietic response to thermal injury. *Ann Surg* 1993; **217:** 293–9.

11. Wallner S F, Vautrin R M. The anemia of thermal injury: mechanism of inhibition of erythropoiesis. *Proc Soc Exp Biol Med* 1986; **181:** 144–50.

12. Topley E, Jackson D M, Cason J S, Davies J W L. Assessment of red cell loss in the first two days after severe burns. *Ann Surg* 1962; **155:** 581–90.

13. Loebl E C, Marvin J A, Curreri W, Baxter C R. The mechanism of erythrocyte destruction in the early postburn period. *Ann Surg* 1973; **178:** 681–6.

14. Robb H. Dynamics of the microcirculation during burn. *Arch Surg* 1967; **94:** 776.

15. Kimber R J, Lander H. The effect of heat on human red cell morphology, fragility and subsequent survival in vivo. *J Lab Clin Med* 1964; **64:** 922–33.

16. Heatherill J R, Till G O, Burner L H, Ward P A. Thermal injury, intravascular: hemolysis, and toxic oxygen products. *J Clin Invest* 1986; **78:** 629–36.

17. Kawakami M, Endoh Y, Orringer E P, Meyer A M. Improvements in rheologic properties of blood by fluid resuscitation after burn injury in rats. *J Burn Care Rehabil* 1992; **13:** 316–22.

18. Dacie J V, Lewis S M. Laboratory methods used in the investigation of hemolytic anaemia II. Hereditary haemolytic anaemias. In: *Practical Haematology*. 5th ed. Edinburgh: Churchill-Livingstone, 1975: 202–35.

19. Davies J W L. Anemia and red cell disorders. In: *Physiological Response to Burning Injury*. New York: Academic Press, 1982: 393–423.

20. Wallner S F, Warren G H. The haemopoietic response to burning: an autopsy study. *Burns* 1986; **12:** 22–77.

21. Krantz S B. Erythropoietin. *Blood* 1991; **77:** 419–34.

22. Sheldon G, Sanders S R, Fuchs R, Garcia J, Schooley J. Metabolism, oxygen transport and erythropoietin synthesis in the anemia of thermal injury. *Am J Surg* 1978; **35:** 406–11.

23. Fleming R Y, Herndon D N, Vaidya S I, *et al.* The effect of erythropoietin in normal healthy volunteers and pediatric patients with burn injuries. *Surgery* 1992; **112:** 424–32.

24. Erslev A J. Erythrokinetics. In: Williams W S, Beutley E, Erslev A J, Lichtman M D, eds. *Hematology*. New York McGraw–Hill Inc, 1990: 424–22.

25. Wallner S, Vautrin R, Katz J, Murphy J. The anemia of thermal injury: partial characterization of an erythroid inhibitory substance. *J Trauma* 1987; **27:** 639–45.

26. Van Wyck D B, Stivelman J C, Ruiz J *et al.* Iron status in patients receiving erythropoietin for dialysis associated anemia. *Kidney Int* 1989; **35:** 712–16.

27. Jelkman W, Wolff M, Fandrey J. Modulation of the production of erythropoietin by cytokines: in vitro studies and their clinical implications. *Contrib Nephrol* 1990; **87:** 68–77.

28. Peterson V M, Rundus M T, Reinoehl P J, Schroeter S R, McCall C A, Bartle E J. The myelopoietic effects of *Serratia marcescens*-derived biological response modifier in a mouse model of thermal injury. *Surgery* 1992; **11:** 447–54.

29. Henson P, Johnston R B. Tissue injury in inflammation: oxidants, proteinases and cationic proteins. *J Clin Invest* 1987; **79:** 669–74.

30. Weiss S J. Tissue destruction by neutrophils. *N Engl J Med* 1989; **320:** 365–76.

31. Callery M P, Kamei R, Mangino M J, Flye M W. Organ interactions in sepsis: host defense and the hepatic–pulmonary macrophage axis. *Arch Surg* 1991; **126:** 28–32.

32. Border J R. Hypothermia, sepsis, multiple systems organ failure and the macrophage. *Arch Surg* 1988; **123:** 285–6.

33. Eurenius K. Brouse R O. Granulocyte kinetics after thermal injury. *Am J Clin Pathol* 1973; **60:** 337–42.

34. Alexander J W, Wixon D. Neutrophil dysfunction and sepsis in burn injury. *Surg Gynecol Obstet* 1970; **130:** 431–8.

35. Emerson W A, Zieve P D, Krevans J R. Hematological changes in septicaemia. *John Hopkins Med J* 1970: **126:** 69–76.

36. Cannon J G, Friedberg J S, Gelfand J A, Tompkins R G, Burke J F, Dinarello C A. Circulating interleukin-1β and tumor necrosis factors – concentrations after burn injury in humans. *Crit Care Med* 1992; **20:** 1414–19.

37. Heinrich P C, Castell J V, Andus T. Interleukin-6 and the acute phase response. *Biochem J* 1990; **265:** 621–36.

38. Eriksson E, Straube R C, Robson M C. White blood cell consumption in the microcirculation after a major burn. *J Trauma* 1979; **19:** 94–7.

39. Wolach B, Coates T D, Hugli T E, *et al.* Plasma lactoferrin reflects granulocyte activation via complement in burn patients. *J Lab Clin Med* 1984; **103:** 284–93.

40. Peterson V, Hansbrough J, Buerk C, *et al.* Regulation of granulopoiesis following severe thermal injury. *J Trauma* 1983; **23:** 19–24.

41. Ruef C, Coleman D L. Granulocyte-macrophage colony stimulating factor: plieotropic cytokine with potential clinical usefulness. *Rev Infect Dis* 1990; **12:** 41–62.

42. Broxmeyer H E, Williams D E. Actions of hemopoietic colony stimulating factors in vivo and in vitro. *Pathol Immunopath Res* 1987; 207–220.

43. Bonnen E M, Morstyn C. Granulocyte macrophage colony stimulating factor (GM–CSF): current status and future development. *Semin Oncol* 1988; **15:** 46–51.

44. Falaky M H, Abdel Hafez A, Houta A H. Phagocytic activity of polymorphonuclear leucocytes in burns. *Burns* 1985; **11:** 185–91.

45. Nelson R D, Hasslen S R, Ahrenholz D H, *et al.* Mechanisms of loss of human neutrophil chemotaxis following thermal injury. *J Burn Care Rehabil* 1987; **8:** 496–502.

46. Marino J A, Gerding R L, Fratianne R B, *et al.* Neutrophil adhesive dysfunction in thermal injury. The role of fibronection. *J Infect Dis* 1988; **157:** 674–81.

47. Dobke M K, Deitch E A, Harner T J, *et al.* Oxidative activity of polymorphonuclear leukocytes after thermal injury. *Arch Surg* 1989; **124:** 856–9.

48. Solomkin J S. Neutrophil disorders in burn injury: complement, cytokines and organ injury. *J Trauma* 1990; **30(suppl):** 580–5.

49. Bolin R W, Robinson W A. Bacterial serum and cellular modulation of granulopoietic activity. *J Cell Physiol* 1977; **92:** 145–53.

50. Hertmann D, Entringer M, Vasil M, *et al.* The effect of bacterial infection on granulopoiesis. *Proc Soc Exp Biol Med* 1981; **167:** 6–11.

51. Robinson W A, Entringer M A, Bolin R W, *et al.* Bacterial stimulation and granulocytic inhibition of granulopoietic factor production. *N Engl J Med* 1977; **297:** 1129–34.

52. Cioffi W G, Burleson D G, Jordan B S, *et al.* Effects of granulocyte-macrophage colony stimulating factor in burn patients. *Arch Surg* 1991; **126:** 74–9.

53. Peterson V M, Robinson W A, Wallner S F, *et al.* Granulocyte stem cells are decreased in humans with fatal burns. *J Trauma* 1985; **25:** 413–18.

54. McEuen D D, Ogawa M, Eureniusk K. Myelopoiesis in the infected burn. *J Lab Clin Med* 1977; **89:** 540–3.

55. Peterson V M, Robinson W A, Rundus C A, Hansbrough J F. Granulocyte stem cells are decreased in humans with fatal burns. *J Trauma* 1985; **25:** 413–18.

56. Peterson V M, Renick M, Rundus C, Schroeter S, Hartford C, Ketch L. The granulocyte-colony stimulating factor (G-CSP) response to sepsis in badly burned patients (Abstract). *Blood* 1989; **74**(Suppl): 1017.

57. Peterson V M, Ambruso D R, Emmett M, Bartle E J. Inhibition of colony stimulating factor (CSF) production by post-burn serum. Negative feedback inhibition mediated by lactoferrin. *J Trauma* 1988; **28:** 1533–40.

58. Silver G M, Gamelli R L, O'Reilly M. The beneficial effect of granulocyte-colony stimulating factor (C-CSF) in combination with gentamicin on survival affect *Pseudomonas* burn wound infection. *Surgery* 1989; **106:** 452–6.

59. Sartorelli K H, Silver G M, Gamelli R L. The effect of granulocyte-colony stimulating factor (G-CSF) upon burn-induced defective neutrophil chemotaxis. *J Trauma* 1991; **31:** 523–30.

60. West M A, Billiar T R, Mazuski J E, Curran R J, Cerra F B, Simmons R L. Endotoxin modulation of hepatocyte secretory and cellular protein synthesis is mediated by kupfer cells. *Arch Surg* 1988; **123:** 1400–5.

61. O'Riordain M G, Collins K H, Pilz M, Saporoschetz I B, Mannick J A, Rodrick M L. Modulation of macrophage hyperactivity improves survival in a burn sepsis model. *Arch Surg* 1992; **127:** 152–8.

62. Bartlett R H, Fong S W, Marrujo G, Hardeman T, Anderson W. Coagulation and platelet changes after thermal injury in man. *Burns* 1981; **7:** 370–7.

63. Eurenius K, Mortensen P F, Meserol P M, Curreri P W. Platelet and megakaryocyte kinetics following thermal injury. *J Lab Clin Med* 1971; **79:** 147–257.

64. Wells D, Sissons M, Hasleton P S. Quantitation of pulmonary megakaryocytes and fibrin thrombi in patients dying from burns. *Histopathology* 1984; **8:** 517.

65. Goodwin M N. Selected anatomic burn pathology for the clinician and the pathologist. *Aviat Space Environ Med* 1989; **60:** 339.

66. Heideman M. The effect of thermal injury on hemodynamic, respiratory and hematological variables in relation to compliment activators. *J Trauma* 1979; **19:** 239–43.

67. Housinger T A, Brinkerhoff C, Warden G D. The relationship between platelet count, sepsis and survival in pediatric burn patients. *Arch Surg* 1993; **128:** 65–7.

68. Kushner I. The phenomenon of the acute phase response. *Ann NY Acad Sci* 1982; **389:** 39–49.

69. Weisman C. Metabolic response to stress: an overview and update. *Anesthesiology* 1990; **73:** 308.

70. Dinarello C A. Interleukin-1 pathogenesis of the acute phase response. *N Engl J Med* 1984; **311:** 1413–18.

71. Fey G H, Fuller T M. Regulation of acute phase gene expression by inflammatory mediators. *Mol Biol Med* 1987; **4:** 323–38.

72. Xia Z F, Coolbaugh M I, Feng H E, Herndon D N, Papaconstantinou J. The effects of burn injury on the acute phase response. *J Trauma* 1992; **32:** 245–51.

73. Hiyama, von Allmen, Rosenblum, Ogle C K, Hasselgren P O, Fisher J E. Synthesis of albumin and acute phase proteins in perfused liver after burn injury in rats. *J Burn Care Rehabil* 1991; 1–6.

74. Rodriguez J L, Miller C G, Garner W L, *et al.* Correlation of the local and systemic cytokine response with clinical outcome following thermal injury. *J Trauma* 1993; **34:** 684–94.

75. Nijsten M W N, Hack C E, Helle M, Ten Duis H J, Klasen H J, Aarden L A. Interleukin 6 and its relation to the humoral immune response and clinical parameters in burn patients. *Surgery* 1990; **109:** 761–7.

76. Guo Y, Dickerson C, Chrest F J, Adler W H, Munster A M, Winchurch R A. Increased levels of circulating interleukin 6 in burn patients. *Clin Immunol Immunopathal* 1990; **54:** 361–71.

77. Ueyama M, Maruyama I, Osame M, Sawada Y. Marked increase in plasma interleukin 6 in burn patients. *J Lab Clin Med* 1992; **120:** 693–8.

78. Li J J, Sanders R L, McAdam K P W J, *et al.* Impact of C-reactive protein (CRP) on surfactant function. *J Trauma* 1989; **29:** 690–7.

79. Silver G M, Gamelli R D, O'Reilly M, Hebert J C. The effect of interleukin 1 alpha on survival in a murine model of burn wounds sepsis. *Arch Surg* 1990; **125:** 922–5.

80. Alexander H R, Langstein H N, Doherty G M, Jensen J C, Norton J A. Human recombinant tumor necrosis factor (hrTNF) protection against endotoxin-induced shock and lethality in the rat. *Surg Forum* 1990; **41:** 103–5.

81. Letendre E D. Iron metabolism during infection and neoplasia. *Cancer Metastasis Rev* 1987; **6:** 41–53.

82. Rutan R L, Bjarnason D L, Desai M H, Herndon D N. Incidence of HIV seroconversion in pediatric burn patients. *Burns* 1992; **18:** 216–19.

83. Coursaget J P, Lesage G, Simpson B, Mayelo V, Le Cann P. Incidence of hepatitis C virus infection in burn patients: detection of anti-C100. anti-C33c and anti-core antibodies. *Biomed Pharmacother* 1991; **45:** 445–9.

84. Van derPool C L, Cuypers, HTM, Reesink H W, *et al.* Confirmation of hepatitis C virus infection by new four-antigen recombinant immunoblot assay. *Lancet* 1991; **337:** 317.

85. Tartter P L. Blood transfusion and post operative infections. *Transfusion* 1989; **29:** 456–9.

86. Graves T A, Cioffi W G, Mason A D Jr, McManus W F, Pruitt B A Jr. Relationship of transfusion and infection in a burn population. *J Trauma* 1989; **29:** 948–54.

87. Waymack J P, Robb E, Alexander R E. Effect of transfusion on immune function in a traumatized animal model. II. Effect on mortality rate following septic challenges. *Arch Surg* 1987; **122:** 935–9.

88. Waymack J P, Miskell P, Gonce S. Effect of blood transfusion on the immune function. VII. Identification of blood transfusion induced suppressive cell. *Surg Res Commun* 1990; **9:** 79–86.

89. Desai M H, Herndon D N, Broemeling L, Barrow R E, Nichols R J, Rutan R L. Early burn wound excision significantly reduces blood loss. *Ann Surg* 1990; **211:** 753–62.

90. Guo Z, Sheng Z, Wang D, *et al.* The use of blood in burn shock, clinical and experimental study. *J Burn Care Rehabil* 1989; **10:** 226–40.

91. Brown R O, Bradley J E, Bekemeyer W B, Luther R W. Effect of albumin supplementation during parenteral nutrition on hospital mortality. *Crit Care Med* 1988; **16:** 1177–83.

92. Ford E G, Jennings M, Andrassy R I. Serum albumin (oncotic pressure) correlates with enteric feeding tolerance in the pediatric surgical patient. *J Pediatr Surg* 1987; **22:** 597–600.

93. Foley E F, Borlase B C, Dzik W H, Bistrian B R, Benotti B N. Albumin supplementation in the critically ill. A prospective randomized trial. *Arch Surg* 1990; **125:** 739–45.

94. Ching N, Grossi C E, Angers J, *et al.* The outcome of surgical treatment as related to the response of serum albumin level to nutritional support. *Surg Gynecol Obstet* 1980; **151:** 199–206.

95. Jarrett F, Ellerbe S, Demling R. Acute leukopenia during topical burn therapy with silver sulfadiazine. *Am J Surg* 1978; **135:** 818–19.

96. Onyiah I D. Leukopenia in two burned patients treated with plasma infusion. *Burns* 1983; **9:** 118–20.

97. Rabinovitch M, Turner–Gomes S O. Platelet-endothelial factors. *Adv Pediatr* 1989; **36:** 91–6.

98. Seitz, R, Wolfe M, Egbring R, *et al.* The disturbance of hemostasis in septic shock: role of neutrophil elastase and thrombin, effects of antithrombin III in plasma substitution. *Eur J Hematol* 1989; **43:** 22–8.

99. Purdue G F, Hunt J L. Pulmonary emboli in burned patients. *J Trauma* 1988; **28:** 218–20.

CHAPTER TWENTY-NINE

Etiology and Prevention of Multisystem Organ Failure

ROBERT L. SHERIDAN AND RONALD G. TOMPKINS

Despite its common occurrence in critically ill burned patients, our understanding of the multisystem organ failure syndrome is fragmented and incomplete. The cascade of organ dysfunctions which typify the multisystem organ failure syndrome is driven by an unregulated inflammatory state, often, but not always, associated with uncontrolled infection.[1] Other potential 'engines' driving this cascade of organ dysfunctions are an impaired gastrointestinal barrier,[2,3] the open burn wound,[4] and inadequate delivery of oxygen to peripheral tissues.[5] The line between organ dysfunction and failure is admittedly unclear, but a set of organ-specific definitions of failure (**Table 29.1**) is helpful and has been developed.[6] Approximately 15% of patients admitted to surgical intensive care units have multisystem organ failure,[7] and perhaps 8% of burned patients ultimately develop the syndrome.[8]

The sequence of failures often follows a predictable course, although the cascade can be modified by various treatments, such as the prophylactic use of H_2 receptor blockers. In burned patients, two cascades have been described:[8] an early cascade characterized by resuscitation failure, adult respiratory distress syndrome, hemodynamic failure, renal failure, liver failure, gut failure, and infection; and a late cascade typified by pulmonary failure, hemodynamic instability, renal failure, gut failure, and liver failure. Frequently, vasomotor failure and death are seen at the end of both cascades. Mortality increases with increasing numbers of failed organ systems. When three organs have failed, mortality has been reported as 100%.[9] An understanding of the progression of the syndrome aids in prognostication and facilitates decisions regarding termination of futile efforts.[10,11] The management of specific organ failures will be presented in another chapter. The purpose of this chapter is to discuss the etiology and prevention of the syndrome.

Table 29.1 Organ-specific definitions of failure

If the patient had one or more of the following during a 24-hour period (regardless of the values), OSF existed on that day

Cardiovascular failure (presence of *one or more* of the following):
- Heart rate ≤ 54/min
- Mean arterial blood pressure ≤ 49 mmHg
- Occurrence of ventricular tachycardia and/or ventricular fibrillation
- Serum pH ≤ 7.24 with a $Pa\text{CO}_2$ of ≤ 49 mmHg

Respiratory failure (presence of *one or more* of the following):
- Respiratory rate ≤ 5/min or ≥ 40/min
- $Pa\text{CO}_2 \geq 50$ mmHg
- $A\text{aDO}_2 \geq 350$ mmHg ($A\text{aDO}_2 = 713\ F\text{IO}_2 - Pa\text{CO}_2 - Pa\text{O}_2$)
- Dependent on ventilator on the fourth day of OSF, e.g. *not* applicable for the initial 72 hours of OSF

Renal failure (presence of *one or more* of the following):*
- Urine output ≤ 479 ml/24 h or ≤ 159 ml/8 h
- Serum BUN ≥ 100 mg/dl
- Serum creatinine ≥ 3.5 mg/dl

Hematologic failure (presence of *one or more* of the following):
- WBC ≤ 1000 mm^3
- Platelets ≤ 20 000 mm^3
- Hematocrit ≤ 20%

Neurological failure
- Glasgow Coma Score ≤ 6 (in absence of sedation at any one point in day)
- Glasgow Coma Score: sum of best eye opening, best verbal, and best motor responses. Scoring of responses as follows: (points)
  - Eye – Open: spontaneously (4), to verbal command (3), to pain (2), no response (1)
  - Motor – Obeys verbal command (6); response to painful stimuli: localizes pain (5), flexion-withdrawal (4), decorticate rigidity (3), decerebrate rigidity (2); no response (1); movement without any control (4)
  - Verbal – Oriented and converses (5), disoriented and converses (4), inappropriate words (3), incomprehensible sounds (2), no response (1). If intubated, use clinical judgment for verbal responses as follows: patient generally unresponsive (1), patient's ability to converse in question (3), patient appears able to converse (5)

* Excluding patients on chronic dialysis before hospital admission.
Reproduced from reference 6 with permission.

Etiology

The etiology of multisystem organ failure is not understood, but is an area of active and intense research. All patients seem to share characteristics associated with an uncontrolled inflammatory state; and there are several proposed 'engines' which drive this uncontrolled inflammation, including sepsis, the open burn wound, the gut, and hypoperfusion.

Sepsis is clearly the most common initiator of the syndrome, and was recognized early on as the primary cause.[1] One single overwhelming infection is not required, as small repetitive infections may initiate the cascade,[12] perhaps by priming immune cells, making them react more intensely to each subsequent stimulus.[12] It was later recognized that many patients with multisystem organ failure did not have infection,[13] and this led the search for other 'engines'. Endotoxin liberated from the walls of gram-negative bacteria is a major, but not the only, intermediary,[14] as gram-positive bacteria cause similar aberrations in oxygen transport and hemodynamics[15] via similar cascades of mediators.[16]

In burned patients, the wound may also be a source of the inflammatory mediators leading to multiple organ failure. Certainly, an infected wound will do this, but wound sepsis is decreasing in incidence with the advent of early burn wound excision;[17] and most infectious deaths in burned patients today are caused by pneumonia rather than wound sepsis.[18] Complete wound closure, without donor sites, decreases oxygen consumption[19] and presumably ameliorates the inflammatory response to the open wound. Incomplete wound closure does not have this effect.[20] Increased levels of circulating mediators such as interleukin-6, interleukin-8, and tumor necrosis factor have been shown to originate from the burn wound[21] and contribute to the hypermetabolic and inflammatory state seen in burned patients. Interleukin-8 has been demonstrated to be upregulated in the lung after burn injury;[21] the stimulus for this upregulation, which is associated with pulmonary dysfunction, may come from the wound.[21]

Intensive recent work has demonstrated the importance of gut barrier function and the relation of gut barrier failure to the development of multisystem organ failure.[22] Normal barrier function prevents the movement of bacteria and their products from the gut lumen into the portal and lymphatic circulation. Bacterial densities range from near 0 in the stomach, to 10^4–10^5 in the distal small bowel, to 10^{11}–10^{12} per gram of stool in the normal colon.[23] That the normal gut can carry this bacterial load, without the frequent occurrence of gram-negative infection, is a tribute to normal barrier function. Although not seen immediately after trauma,[24] several insults have been shown to result in increased translocation of bacteria and their products into the portal and lymphatic circulations. Hemorrhagic shock,[25] endotoxin administration,[26] burns,[27] and burn wound sepsis[28] have each been shown to result in increased translocation of bacteria from the gut. Gut permeability to macromolecules, such as endotoxin, has been shown to increase with increasing burn wound size, using polyethylene glycol 3350 as a tracer.[29] Smaller molecules, with lactulose as the tracer, have also been shown to pass more readily through the gastrointestinal membrane after injury.[30] The exact mechanism by which bacteria and their products pass through the gastrointestinal barrier is not clear. Both intra- and transcellular processes may be involved.[31,32] The consequences of loss of the gastrointestinal barrier are profound. Translocating whole bacteria can be a direct source of sepsis or can activate Kupffer cells[2,3] and promulgate an inflammatory response in conjunction with bacterial products such as endotoxin.

Cellular dysfunction, caused by inadequate oxidative metabolism secondary to hypoperfusion, is another potential 'engine' resulting in multisystem organ failure. In ischemia–reperfusion models, oxygen radicals are generated, and this results in peroxidation of cell membrane lipids and accumulation of activated neutrophils,[33] with progressive cellular and whole-organ dysfunction. It has been proposed that critically ill patients suffer from supply dependent oxygen consumption because of defects in cellular oxygen extraction and utilization.[34,35] This results in inadequate aerobic metabolism unless supranormal levels of oxygen are supplied.[36] The reality of this proposal is still actively debated.[37,38] Certainly, a grossly inadequate amount of oxygen available to cells dependent on aerobic metabolism can lead to cellular dysfunction, and this may be followed by organ failures.[5] Maintaining oxygen delivery at least at normal, and possibly at supranormal, levels should help maintain cellular homeostasis and minimize the risk of multiple organ failure.[39] The requirement for a supranormal level of tissue oxygenation in critical illness is controversial and our ability to predict organ-specific oxygen delivery and consumption from whole-body data is poor;[40] so careful attention to whole-body hemodynamics is an integral part of the management of any critically ill patient.

Common Ground: Mediators

Sepsis, open burn wounds, impaired gut barrier function, and hypoperfusion are all associated with multiorgan failure. The similarity in the response to these differing events implies that there is some common ground. These processes all probably impact on individual organs via a number of mediators, whose complex interactions are still very poorly understood,[41] but are being unraveled by investigators using blocking antibodies, soluble receptors, and receptor antagonists.[42] At this point, these mediators, including endotoxin, arachidonic acid metabolites, cytokines, platelet-activating factor, activated neutrophils and adherence molecules, nitric oxide, complement, and oxygen free radicals will be briefly reviewed.

Endotoxin, a lipopolysaccharide component of gram-negative bacterial cell walls, induces many of the symptoms associated with sepsis, such as fever, hypotension, the release of acute phase proteins, and the production of multiple cytokines, including tumor necrosis factor and interleukin-1.[43] Endotoxin also activates complement,[44] causes activation of the coagulation cascade,[45] and results in the release of platelet-activating factor.[46] Potential sources of endotoxin include both gram-negative bacteria in foci of infection, as well as gram-negative bacteria within the gut when the gut barrier fails.

Arachidonic acid makes up approximately 20% of cell membranes, is released from these membranes in response to a multitude of stimuli which activate phospholipases A_2 and C, and is then metabolized by one of two major enzyme systems (**Figure 29.1**). The cyclooxygenase pathway results in production of prostaglandins and thromboxanes, and the lipoxygenase pathway results in the production of leukotrienes.[47] The prostaglandins and leukotrienes interact with other mediators in a complex fashion, and are later degraded by enzyme systems which are dispersed throughout the body.[48]

Arachidonic acid which is metabolized via the cyclooxygenase pathway results in the formation of prostaglandins and thromboxanes. Prostacyclin inhibits platelet aggregation, thrombus formation, and gastric secretion.[49] Thromboxane A_2 causes platelet aggregation, has profound vasoconstricting effects on both the splanchnic and pulmonary microvasculature, causes bronchoconstriction and increased membrane permeability.[50] It is studied via its longer lived but inactive metabolite, thromboxane B_2. Aspirin has physiologic effects by inhibiting thromboxane synthetase.[51]

Arachidonic acid metabolized via the lipoxygenase pathway results in the formation of leukotrienes. There are two types based on their metabolism after the action of 5-lipooxygenase, leukotrienes C_4, D_4, and E_4 (the sulfidopeptide group) and leukotriene B_4.[52] Leukotrienes are generated in response to multiple stimuli by several cell types including neutrophils, macrophages, and monocytes.[53] Vessel walls are also capable of generating leukotrienes.[54] Leukotrienes C_4, D_4, and E_4 have variable actions on vascular tone depending on the presence or absence of other

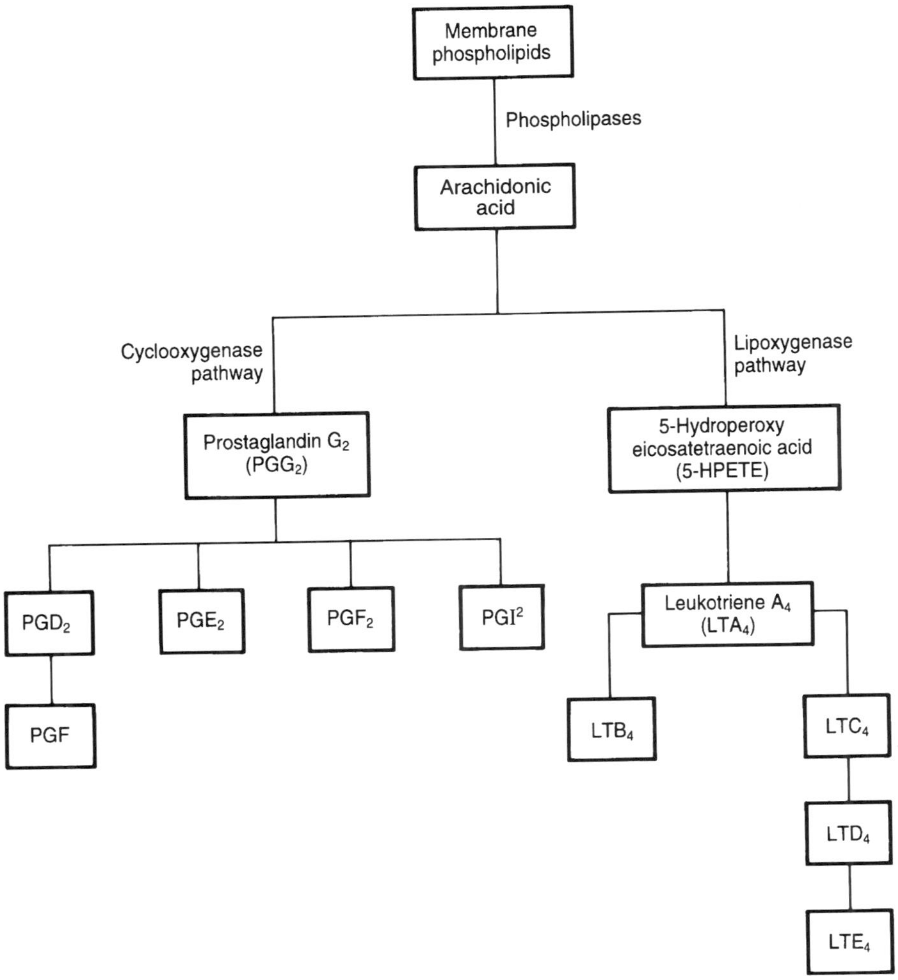

Fig. 29.1 The cyclooxygenase and lipoxygenase pathways of arachidonic acid metabolism.

mediators such as cyclooxygenase products.[55] In addition to their variable effects in redirecting blood flow, leukotrienes C_4, D_4, E_4 also increase vascular permeability[56] and have been observed to be elevated immediately prior to the development of pulmonary failure.[57] The major effect of leukotriene B_4 is an enhancement of neutrophil chemotaxis.[58] Thus, leukotrienes, as a group, may be involved in the edema formation and pulmonary and systemic vascular changes which are seen in the multisystem organ failure syndrome.

Cytokines are regulatory proteins which are secreted by immune cells and have multiple paracrine and endocrine effects. There are six major classes[59] including: interleukins, tumor necrosis factor, interferons, colony stimulating factors, chemotactic factors, and growth factors. Those which have been most extensively characterized are interleukin-1, interleukin-6, and tumor necrosis factor.

Interleukin-1 and interleukin-6 are elevated in septic states, and high levels are associated with a fatal outcome[60] and predict systemic infection.[61] Interleukin-1β causes hypotension and decreased systemic vascular resistance which may be synergistic with the effects of tumor necrosis factor.[62] Even better characterized is tumor necrosis factor, the administration of which causes hypotension, cardiac depression, and pulmonary dysfunction in animals.[63–65] When administered to humans, tumor necrosis factor causes fever, hypotension, decreased systemic vascular resistance, increased protein turnover, elevation of stress hormone levels,[66,67] and activation of coagulation cascade.[68]

Platelet-activating factor is a nonprotein phospholipid which is secreted by many cells including platelets, endothelial cells, and inflammatory cells[69] and is a major mediator of the pulmonary[70] and hemodynamic[71] effects of endotoxin. The major effects of platelet-activating factor are vasodilation, cardiac depression, and enhancement of capillary leak. Its complex interactions with other mediators are still poorly understood.

Although tissue injury can occur in the absence of neutrophils,[72] the inflammatory process results in local accumulation of activated inflammatory cells which release various local toxins such as oxygen radicals, proteases, eicosanoids, platelet-activating factor, and other substances. When unregulated, such accumulations of activated cells can cause tissue injury.[73] The initial attachment of neutrophils to the vascular endothelium at an inflammatory site is facilitated by the interaction of adherence molecules on the neutrophil and endothelial cell surfaces.[74]

These neutrophil adherence receptors are induced by numerous stimuli, but, interestingly, are reduced after major thermal and nonthermal injury,[75] perhaps explaining in part the increased incidence of infection in such patients. The importance of this adherence mechanism can be seen in patients who are deficient in one of the integrin class of neutrophil adherence receptors, CD18, and thereby suffer from frequent bacterial infections.[76] The biology of the transmembrane polypeptides which govern these complex cell-to-cell interactions is an active area of research[77] and holds promise for therapeutic interventions in the future.

Oxygen radicals, such as hydrogen peroxide and superoxide anion, are released by activated neutrophils in response to a variety of stimuli.[78] They are also released when xanthine oxidase is activated after reperfusion in ischemia–reperfusion models. These highly reactive products cause cell membrane dysfunction, increased vascular permeability, and release of eicosanoids.

Nitric oxide, released when citrulline is formed from arginine (**Figure 29.2**), was only recently identified as an endothelial product in the middle 1980s.[79] Its half-life is only a few seconds, as it is quickly oxidized, but it has profound local microvascular effects. Its synthesis is stimulated by various cytokines, endotoxin, thrombin, and by injury to the vascular endothelium. It is a potent vasodilator,[80] but its actions vary depending on the vascular bed and presence of other mediators.[81] It is one of the major mediators of the hypotensive response to sepsis.[82,83]

Antigen–antibody complexes activate the complement cascade; complement fragments, thus generated, can interact with other cytokines so as to promulgate the inflammatory response.[84] Diminished levels of a natural inhibitor of C5a have been demonstrated in patients with adult respiratory distress syndrome (ARDS),[85] and administration of anti-C5a antibody diminishes hypotension in an animal model endotoxemia.[86] Complement fragments may be involved in the development of burn wound edema.[87]

Obviously, our understanding of the incredibly complex cellular and subcellular biology, of which multisystem organ failure is but one manifestation, is poorly understood at the present time. This dim understanding highlights the important role which prevention plays in managing the syndrome.

Prevention of Multisystem Organ Failure

Once established, multisystem organ failure is very difficult to reverse, emphasizing the importance of prevention.[88] Prevention is based on our crude knowledge of the 'engines' which drive the process – sepsis, the gut, the wound, and inadequate perfusion (**Table 29.2**). Dealing with these issues is far more practical than dealing with an incompletely understood complex web of mediators. Also, this complex cascade has evolved in numerous species over thousands of years, and interference in the network may do more harm than good. The discussion which follows addresses prevention of sepsis via proper wound management and attention to unusual causes of sepsis, support of the gut, and prevention of inadequate oxygen delivery. Subsequently, the potential role of nutritional and specific immunomodulators are also addressed.

Table 29.2 Multiple organ failure etiology and established preventive measures

Etiology	*Prevention*
Sepsis	Early excision and biologic closure of deep wounds Anticipation and early treatment of occult septic foci
Gut barrier failure	Optimize whole-body hemodynamics +/– Early enteral feedings
Inadequate organ perfusion	Optimize whole-body hemodynamics +/– Enhanced oxygen delivery

Prevention of Sepsis

In the burned patient, prevention of multisystem organ failure is greatly facilitated by prevention of wound sepsis via an aggressive surgical approach to deep wounds. The increasing survival of burn patients has paralleled the evolution of this approach to burn wounds.[89–91] Not only is overt wound sepsis prevented by early removal of devitalized tissue, but multiple smaller septic insults are also prevented, as manipulation of heavily colonized burn wounds is a frequent source of transient bacteremia.[92,93] Such multiple occult bacteremias occurring during frequent manipulation of heavily colonized wounds could contribute to the development of multisystem organ failure by priming immune cells, making them react more intensively to each subsequent insult.[12] The role of perioperative antibiotics in minimizing bacteremias in the perioperative period has yet to be clearly defined; however, they are clearly beneficial in patients with injuries greater than 60% of total body surface area and in any other patient in whom the probability of bacteremia with wound manipulation is felt to be high.[94] Appropriate perioperative antibiotics are guided by surface cultures. Burned patients are prone to a large number of unusual and often occult infectious complications[95] which can result in sepsis and potentially contribute to

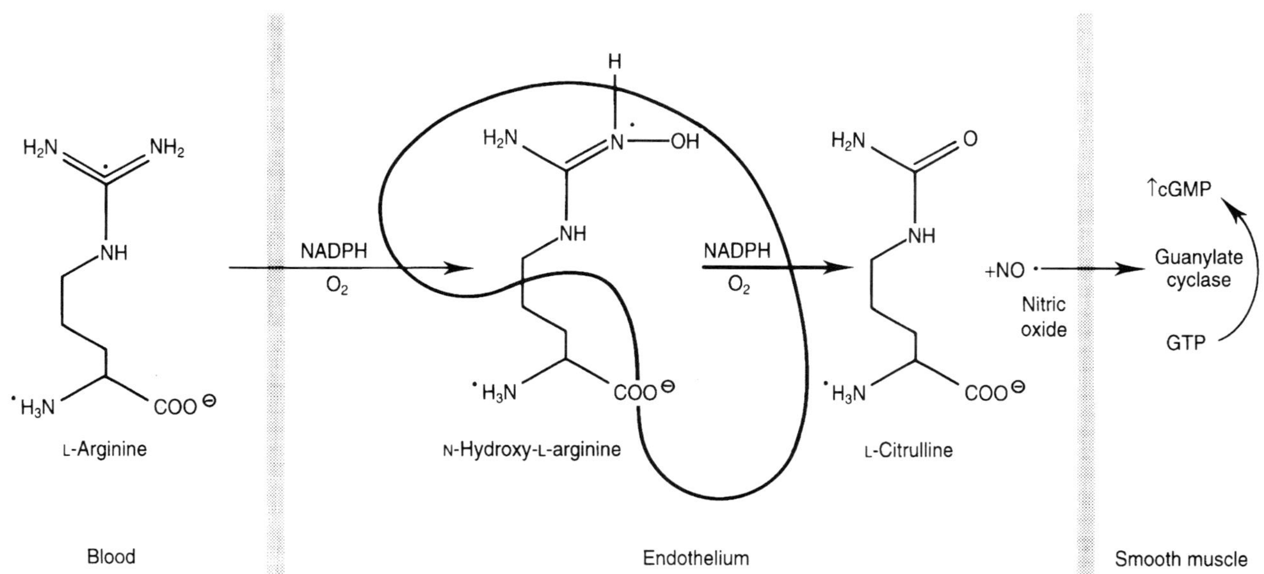

Fig. 29.2 Nitric oxide metabolism (reproduced from reference 189 with permission).

the development of multiorgan failure. Rapid diagnosis and treatment are facilitated by a high index of suspicion.

Intravascular infections, such as suppurative thrombophlebitis and endocarditis, typically present in burn patients with fever and bacteremia without localizing signs. Burned patients with endocarditis develop a new murmur in only 9% of cases,[96] and only 10% have been reported to present antemortem.[97] Of those with septic thrombophlebitis, 68% have no localizing signs and present with fever and positive blood cultures only.[98] The diagnosis is made in patients without localizing signs only by thorough examination of all sites of prior cannulation with surgical exposure of any suspicious sites and complete excision of any involved veins.[99] Vigilant care and scheduled replacement of intravascular devices will minimize the occurrence of catheter-related sepsis. Occult intracompartmental sepsis can also present with fever and bacteremia without localizing signs, and is diagnosed only by careful examination and exploration of suspicious compartments.[100]

Pneumonia, seen in approximately 35% of patients with inhalation injury, adds between 20 and 60% to the expected mortality of burned patients.[101] Although a difficult diagnosis to make in critically ill patients, pneumonia should be vigilantly anticipated and aggressively treated with appropriate endobronchial toilet and specific antibiotics. The incidence of nosocomial pneumonia increases with longer durations of intubation,[102] emphasizing the importance of judicious use of mechanical ventilation.

Suppurative sinusitis is being recognized with increasing frequency in the intensive care unit and may be more frequent in patients who are nasotracheally intubated.[103] Diagnosis may require examination and culture of material obtained by antral puncture, in addition to plain radiographs and computerized tomography. Although there is some controversy about the role of the nasotracheal tube in causing sinusitis,[104] treatment involves removing all nasotracheal devices, administering topical decongestants, and providing appropriate antibiotics. Surgical drainage is reserved for recalcitrant cases.

Acalculous cholecystitis often presents with generalized sepsis without localizing signs in the burned patient and, like intravascular infection, is a very difficult diagnosis to make.[105] Recently, bedside placement of percutaneous cholecystostomy tubes under ultrasonic guidance has become an option in the management of suspected cholecystitis in critically ill patients.[106] This technique allows an accurate diagnosis to be made and the condition to be temporarily treated in patients too unstable for immediate operation.

Sepsis accounts for at least half of cases of multisystem organ failure. In perhaps no other area can the vigilance of the burn team have a greater impact in multisystem organ failure prevention than in the early detection and aggressive treatment of occult septic foci.

Support of the Gut

Bacteria and their products which are released when the gut barrier fails, may fuel the multiorgan failure syndrome. Gut mucosal integrity suffers when mesenteric flow is inadequate and gut blood flow is decreased after burn injury, a response exacerbated by the release of thromboxane A_2.[107] Thus, support of splanchnic blood flow is an important aspect of multisystem organ failure prevention, and this is best done by careful attention to whole-body[108] hemodynamics. There is no substitute for a carefully monitored burn resuscitation.

The enterocyte may be better supported by intraluminal, rather than parenteral, feedings as a gut which is deprived of intraluminal feedings develops mucosal atrophy.[109] Early enteral feedings are tolerated in burned patients[110] and may reduce the magnitude of the hypermetabolic response to the injury.[111] Parenteral feedings do not prevent gut mucosal atrophy as well as isocaloric and isonitrogenous intraluminal feeds,[112] although convincing human data are not available to support the clinical significance of this point.

The value of specific nutrients to support the enterocycte is far less clear than the value of providing adequate mesenteric blood flow and perhaps intraluminal nutrition; however, this is an exciting and active area of research. Glutamine, a nonessential amino acid, is the preferred fuel of the small bowel enterocyte[113] as well as other rapidly dividing cells. Sepsis has been shown to decrease glutamine uptake by the small bowel enterocyte which may result in barrier failure,[114] and the addition of glutamine to the nutritional regimen has been theorized to improve barrier function. Glutamine is not a component of commercial parenteral nutritional formulae because of its short shelf life, although the dipeptide is well tolerated parenterally and has a longer shelf life.[115] While supplemental glutamine may improve protein balance in surgical patients[115] and may partially reverse gut atrophy,[116] it has not been shown to improve gut barrier function when given parenterally.[117] The role of specific nutrients in support of the large intestinal mucosa is less clear, but butyrate, a fatty acid liberated by fiber fermentation, is a favored fuel of the colonic mucosal cell.[118] Enteral pectin may help support the colonic mucosa;[119] the value of such support in the hypermetabolic burned patient is as yet unclear.

A decontaminated gut lumen might diminish the impact of gastrointestinal barrier failure. Attempts have been made to access the impact of selective decontamination of the gut[120] and coating enteric bacteria in order to inhibit their ability to attach to the intestinal mucosa and translocate.[121] Although there is a suggestion that the rate of pneumonia may be decreased by such maneuvers, there is no apparent impact on mortality.

Support of the gut, in an effort to prevent multisystem organ failure, is certain to have real value. Maintenance of adequate mesenteric perfusion via careful attention to whole-body hemodynamics is crucial. There are some data to support the contention that enteral feedings have beneficial effects on outcome in injured patients when compared with parenteral feedings, possibly via an enhancement of gastrointestinal barrier integrity.[122] These data require confirmation prior to general application. Data supporting the administration of specific mucosal substrates or gut decontamination are less convincing, but further research in these important areas may show such benefit.

Insuring Adequate Oxygen Delivery

The normal intracellular partial pressure of oxygen is 0.5 mmHg and this small amount of mitochrondial oxygen allows for the aerobic generation of most of the cell's adenosine triphosphate (ATP). When cells have to adapt to a lower oxygen tension, ATP generation continues at a lower rate by anaerobic channels,[123] possibly triggered by the build-up of adenosine diphosphate (ADP). As outlined by Gutierrez, the anaerobic reactions which generate ATP are glycolysis, the creatine kinase reaction, and the adenylate kinase reaction.[123] Glycolysis describes the conversion of glucose to lactate with the generation of two ATP molecules. The creatine kinase reaction is the breakdown of the high energy phosphate storage molecule, phosphocreatine, with the generation of ATP and creatine. The adenylate kinase reaction describes the combination of nucleotides to form ATP and AMP which, although generating ATP, depletes the cells of adenine nucleotides. In conjunction with this conversion to anaerobic ATP generation, the intracellular concentration of hydrogen ion increases, the amount of adenine nucleotides within the cell decreases, and intracellular calcium levels increase with decreased function of the ATP driven sodium–calcium pump.[124] There also may be an increase in the liberation of intracellular oxygen free radicals with the activation of xanthine oxidase.[125] If low oxygen tensions continue, membrane phospholipids may be degraded by the combined effects of elevated calcium, oxygen free radicals, and the decreased synthetic capabilities coincident with decreased levels of ATP.[126] These effects may be magnified if there is also systemic sepsis, as cellular oxygen extraction may be impaired. That such cellular hypoxic dysfunction occurs is implied by the fact that cocarboxylase, which enhances ATP generation by ischemic cells, ameliorates some of the metabolic and hemodynamic consequences of endotoxic shock in an animal model.[27]

An understanding of progressive cell destruction and dysfunction which is caused by low intracellular oxygen tensions, coupled with the perception of oxygen extraction abnormalities associated with sepsis, has led to an intense interest in the delivery of supranormal amounts of oxygen to prevent organ dysfunction, as clinical data suggest that inadequate oxygen delivery is associated with the development of multisystem organ failure.[128] Clinically, it is somewhat cumbersome to measure and follow oxygen delivery; other markers of the adequacy of tissue oxygenation have been tried, including the use of lactate and the lactate/pyruvate ratio, base deficit, mixed venous oxygen tension and pH, and gut tonometry. None of these secondary markers of oxygen delivery has proven to be as reliable as the direct determination of oxygen delivery and consumption by the reverse Fick technique.

Normal physiologic oxygen supply dependency is different from the pathologic supply dependency seen in septic states. In this circumstance, supranormal oxygen delivery is said to be required, as consumption is increased while extraction is decreased.[129] The exact reasons for this pathologic supply dependence are unclear but may involve microcirculatory shunting or aberrations of intracellular physiology. It has been proposed that the purposeful delivery of supranormal amounts of oxygen is associated with a decreased incidence of multiple organ failure and increased survival.[130] The reality of the proposal is still controversial, with data showing no increase in oxygen consumption with transfusion of blood in critically ill children[131] and the absence of a consumption plateau in patients with ARDS.[132] Also, regional blood flow is poorly predicted by whole-body oxygen delivery and consumption data,[133] implying that whole-body delivery and consumption data may be of no value even if pathologic supply dependency was real. Normally, oxygen consumption is approximately 25% of oxygen delivery, and delivery can be maximized by optimizing the hemoglobin, partial pressure of oxygen, and cardiac output, which are the major determinants of oxygen delivery, although total flow may be more important than the blood's oxygen carrying capacity.[134]

Inadequate oxygen delivery clearly leads to organ dysfunction. At a minimum, the clinician should insure that injured patients are resuscitated to the conventional clinical endpoints of appropriate urine output, skin perfusion, blood pressure, and sensorium. In selected critically ill patients, invasive monitoring is justified in order to document oxygen delivery and consumption, extraction ratio, and the possible presence of supply dependency in which case the provision of supranormal levels of oxygen delivery with plateau of oxygen consumption is an appropriate resuscitation endpoint.

The Potential Role of Nutritional and Specific Immunomodulators

The holy grail for those who study the complex biology of the multisystem organ failure syndrome is an ability to modulate the common pathways which lead to organ dysfunction and death. The three general approaches to this goal are nutritional, nonspecific, and specific immunomodulation.

Nutritional Immunomodulation

Three categories of substances show some promise as potential nutritional immunomodulators in burned patients: long-chain fatty acids; arginine, glutamine, and branched-chain amino acids; and nucleotides. Short- and medium-chain fatty acids are commonly utilized for energy, whereas long-chain fatty acids are important constituents of cell membranes and can profoundly influence cell function.[135] Omega-3 long-chain fatty acids play a particularly important role in the membranes of immunocompetent cells.[136] There are animal data suggesting that supplementation of the diet with long-chain fatty acids may improve immune function after burn injury;[137] however, there are no clear clinical data yet available to support the routine administration of long-chain fatty acids as a dietary supplement in injured patients.

The potential immunostimulating effects of specific amino acids, particularly arginine, glutamine, and the branched-chain amino acids leucine, isoleucine and valine, is an active area of research. Arginine is a nonessential amino acid with important functions in the urea cycle and in the generation of nitric oxide.[138] It also may have important effects in insuring immune cell competence.[139,140] Although there are some animal data suggesting improved immunocompetence and outcome after burn with supplementation of arginine,[141–143] human data are not yet adequate to support its routine administration to burned patients. Glutamine, the most common amino acid in the body and a preferred fuel of rapidly dividing cells, may be conditionally essential in hypermetabolic patients,[113–114] and its administration has been proposed as a method to support the gut barrier, thereby abrogating the consequences of barrier failure. Early human data suggest that administration of supplemental glutamine may improve amino acid protein economy in stressed surgical patients,[115] but there are inadequate data as yet to support the routine administration of glutamine as an immune stimulant.

The branched-chain amino acids leucine, isoleucine, and valine are important energy sources in stressed surgical patients. Although there was an early enthusiasm for the supplemental administration of these substrates, subsequent data have suggested that the supplemental administration of branched-chain amino acids does not benefit stressed surgical patients.[144]

Based on limited animal and human data, it has been suggested that the administration of adenine nucleotides may have beneficial effects on immune function in stressed patients.[145] Again, at the present time, there are inadequate human data to support the routine use of supplemental nucleotides.

The concept of nutritional immunomodulation via supplementation of specific substances is exciting; however, despite preliminary human studies suggesting a beneficial effect of supplemental arginine and long-chain fatty acids,[146] with additional nucleotides[145] and glutamine,[115] there do not yet exist adequate data to support nutritional immunomodulation as a routine maneuver in the management of burned patients.

Nonspecific and Specific Immunomodulation

It seems intuitively unlikely that there exists a magic immunomodulating bullet which will prevent the development of multisystem organ failure in critically ill surgical patients, particularly if sepsis is uncontrolled, the integrity of the gut barrier is compromised, burn wounds are unaddressed, or patients are inadequately supported hemodynamically. On the other hand, such efforts have tremendous potential to facilitate our understanding of cellular and subcellular biology and may, in time, provide a clinical dividend. Efforts at nonspecific immunomodulation have included the use of steroids,[147] immunoglobulin G,[148] and naloxone[149] with no significant impact on patient outcomes. With the exception of steroids for those with suspected adrenal insufficiency[150] and naloxone for those with opiate intoxication, there is no role for these substances in the critically ill burned patient.

Although there have been efforts to absorb lipopolysaccharide[151] and to prevent endotoxemia with prophylactic polymyxin B in burned patients,[152] the greatest efforts at specific immunomodulation have been applied to the development of anti-endotoxin antibodies. The earliest clinical efforts used human serum with anti-J5 activity; these studies demonstrated an enhanced survival in patients with gram-negative septic shock.[153] Later, two monoclonal IgMs were developed, and human trials were completed. The first development involved anti-E5, a murine monoclonal antibody. Clinical trials suggested a benefit in septic patients without refractory shock.[154] Large numbers of treated patients developed antibodies to the murine monoclonal; although these patients were not re-treated, attention turned more toward a human product. A subsequent effort with this murine monoclonal did not show statistically significant improvements in outcome.[155]

HA-1A, a human monoclonal IgM, was trialed in a large multicenter effort without statistically significant improvement in outcome, except in a subgroup of patients who had gram-negative bacteremia and shock.[156] Multiple confounding factors made these marginally beneficial results suspect and left the ultimate utility of HA-1A still unclear.

Anti-endotoxin monoclonal therapy, which may have a potential to be beneficial if significantly refined, has also been criticized for its expense. It is estimated that it would cost $24 100 per year of life saved should this technology be used widely.[157] Integrating such advanced and expensive technology into common practice poses tremendous practical problems and is therefore very unlikely to happen soon when one considers its lack of clear efficacy and high expense.

Significant efforts have also been made toward modifying the actions of arachidonic acid metabolites or eicosanoids, both cyclooxygenase and lipoxygenase products. Numerous animal models of sepsis and endotoxemia exist; cyclooxygenase pathway blockade with nonsteroidal anti-inflammatory agents has demonstrated improved survival,[158,159] improved pulmonary hemodynamics,[160] and improved mesenteric blood flow.[161] There has been little work documenting outcome improvement in human patients, but it has been suggested that nonsteroidal anti-inflammatory agents improve symptoms associated with endotoxin infusion in normal volunteers[162] and septic patients,[163] and may improve immune function after surgical trauma.[164] In an animal model, infusion of the vasodilating arachidonic acid metabolite, prostacyclin, ameliorates the pulmonary dysfunction associated with endotoxin infusion.[165] Less work has been done with lipoxygenase pathway inhibitors. Survival is enhanced in a murine model of endotoxin infusion with lipoxygenase pathway blockade.[166] Endotoxin-associated pulmonary dysfunction is diminished in sheep[167] and pigs[168] when this pathway is blocked. The ultimate role of lipoxygenase blockade in humans remains uninvestigated.

Cytokines are difficult to accurately measure and their complex interactions are poorly understood. The production of interleukin-1 receptor antagonist is increased in human endotoxemia;[169] in an animal model, its administration enhances survival.[170] Infusion of interleukin-1 may improve immune function in humans.[171] Clearly our understanding of the complex functions of this cytokine are inadequate to allow intelligent intervention.

Tumor necrosis factor is produced by macrophages and other inflammatory cells when stimulated by endotoxin.[172] In animal models, the physiologic effects of both endotoxin infusion and gram-negative sepsis[173,174] are attenuated by the TNF blockade with monoclonal antibodies. Circulating levels of TNF are high immediately after sepsis begins and then fall, implying that only anti-TNF pretreatment would be beneficial.[175] Even anti-TNF administration prior to experimental sepsis[176] and endotoxemia[177] has, at best, variable effects on survival. Again, our incomplete understanding precludes effective intervention.

Interference with the effects of platelet-activating factor (PAF) has been shown to decrease neutrophil priming by human burn serum,[178] to improve endotoxin-induced pulmonary dysfunction,[179] to decrease eicosanoid release,[180] and to attenuate thromboxane release and improve survival[181] in various animal models of endotoxemia. These exciting initial results, and the availability of several blockers and receptor antagonists, portend a future use for PAF modification.

Efforts to modulate both the adherence and function of inflammatory cells is an exciting area of research, as activated neutrophils clearly play an important role in the development of multiple organ failure. Blockade of neutrophil adhesion receptors with monoclonal antibodies enhances survival in animal models of endotoxic and hemorrhagic shock.[182,183] Again, our basic understanding is not yet adequate to intelligently modify such important processes.

Oxygen free radicals generated by activated neutrophils or xanthine oxidase may oxidize membrane lipids, forming lipid peroxides, resulting in membrane dysfunction.[184] Native antioxidant systems do exist, but can be overwhelmed. Circulating levels of vitamin E, a natural antioxidant, are low in patients with ARDS.[185] Efforts to modify oxidant activity have included blockade of free radical generation, addition of free radical scavengers, augmentation of host antioxidant defenses, and prevention of amplification of tissue damage by neutrophils.[184] Particularly exciting are free radical scavengers such as superoxide dismutase[186] and spin-trapping nitrones[187] which improve survival in animal models of endotoxic and hemorrhagic shock. Despite such encouraging initial animal work, such therapy is not yet appropriate in human patients.

The continuous synthesis of nitric oxide (see **Figure 29.2**) plays an important role in the regulation of pulmonary systemic vascular tone in sepsis;[188] and this presents potential opportunities for intervention.[189] Aerosolized nitric oxide has been shown to be useful in reversing the pulmonary hypertension associated with ARDS,[190] and nitric oxide synthesis blockade may improve the hypotension[191] and renal dysfunction[192] associated with sepsis. Its complex interactions with other cytokines and variable effects on different vascular beds render any nitric oxide based interventions investigational at the present time.

Most patients who die in the burn unit after surviving resuscitation, succumb to multiple organ failure.[193] Although modification of the cascade of events leading to multiorgan failure at the cellular and subcellular level is an enticing possibility, our fragmented understanding of these processes mitigates against such therapy in human patients at the present time. That tumor necrosis factor enhances the ability of neutrophils to kill invading bacteria[194] and of rats to survive gram-negative sepsis;[195] that cyclooxygenase inhibition increases TNF production after burn;[196] that prostaglandin E_2 is important in renal autoregulation;[197] and that cytokine levels do not predict survival as well as conventional variables[198] makes one loathe to interfere in such complex, and poorly understood processes. Vigilant clinical care in the intensive care unit, with the prevention of sepsis, proper management of burn wounds, support of the gut barrier, and careful attention to whole-body hemodynamics, is a much more fruitful area in which a vigilant clinician can make a difference.

REFERENCES

1. Fry D E, Pearlstein L, Fulton R L, Polk H C Jr. Multiple system organ failure. The role of uncontrolled infection. *Arch Surg* 1980; **115:** 136–40.

2. Marshall J C, Lee C, Meakins J L, Michel R P, Christou N V. Kupffer cell modulation of the systemic inflammatory response. *Arch Surg* 1987; **122:** 191–6.

3. Saadia R, Schein M, McFarlane C, Boffard K D. Gut barrier function and the surgeon. *Br J Surg* 1990; **77:** 487–92.

4. Echinard C E, Sajdel-Sulkowska E, Burke P A, Burke J F. The beneficial effect of early excision on clinical response and thymic activity after burn injury. *J Trauma* 1982; **22:** 560–5.

5. Schumacker P T, Samsel R W. Oxygen delivery and uptake by peripheral tissues: physiology and pathophysiology. *Crit Care Clin* 1989; **5:** 255–69.

6. Knaus W A, Droper E A, Wagner D P, Zimmerman J E. Prognosis in acute organ-system failure. *Ann Surg* 1985; **202:** 685–93.

7. Knaus W A, Draper E A, Wagner D P, Zimmerman J E. APACHE II: a severity of disease classification system. *Crit Care Med* 1985; **13:** 818–29.

8. Goodwin C W. Multiple organ failure: clinical overview of the syndrome. *J Trauma* 1990; **30:** S163–S165.

9. Carrico C J, Meakins J L, Marshall J C, Fry D, Maier R V. Multiple-organ-failure syndrome. *Arch Surg* 1986; **121:** 196–208.

10. Schneiderman L J, Jecker N S, Jonsen A R. Medical futility: its meaning and ethical implications. *Ann Intern Med* 1990; **112:** 949–54.

11. Meisel A. Legal myths about terminating life support. *Arch Intern Med* 1991; **151:** 1497–502.

12. Meakins J L. Etiology of multiple organ failure. *J Trauma* 1990; **30:** S165–S168.

13. Bone R C, Fisher C J Jr, Clemmer T P, Slotman G J, Metz C A, Balk R A. Sepsis syndrome: a valid clinical entity. *Crit Care Med* 1989; **17:** 389–93.

14. Suffredini A F, Fromm R E, Parker M M, *et al.* The cardiovascular response of normal humans to the administration of endotoxin. *N Engl J Med* 1989; **321:** 280–7.

15. Ahmed A J, Kruse J A, Haupt M T, Chandrasekar P H, Carlson R W. Hemodynamic responses to gram-positive versus gram-negative sepsis in critically ill patients with and without circulatory shock. *Crit Care Med* 1991; **19:** 1520–5.

16. Wakabayashi G, Gelfand J A, Jung W K, Connolly R J, Burke J F, Dinarello C A. *Staphylococcus epidermidis* induces complement activation, tumor necrosis factor and interleukin-1, a shock-like state and tissue injury in rabbits without endotoxemia. Comparison to *Escherichia coli*. *J Clin Invest* 1991; **87:** 1925–35.

17. Merrell S W, Saffle J R, Larson C M, Sullivan J J. The declining incidence of fatal sepsis following thermal injury. *J Trauma* 1989; **29:** 1362–6.

18. Peck M D, Heimbach D M. Does early excision of burn wounds change the pattern of mortality? *J Burn Care Rehabil* 1989; **10:** 7–10.

19. Lalonde C, Demling R H. The effect of complete burn wound excision and closure on postburn oxygen consumption. *Surgery* 1987; **102:** 862–8.

20. Demling R H, Lalonde C. Effect of partial burn excision and closure on postburn oxygen consumption. *Surgery* 1988; **104:** 846–52.

21. Rodriguez J L, Miller C G, Garner W L, *et al.* Correlation of the local and systemic cytokine response with clinical outcome following thermal injury. *J Trauma* 1993; **34:** 684–94.

22. Deitch E A. The role of intestinal barrier failure and bacterial translocation in the development of systemic infection and multiple organ failure. *Arch Surg* 1990; **125:** 403–4.

23. Schaedler R W, Goldstein F. Bacterial populations of the gut in health and disease; basic microbiologic aspects. In: Brochus H L, Beck J E, Haubrich W S, *et al.*, eds. *Gastroenterology*. Philadelphia: W B Saunders, 1976: 147–9.

24. Peitzman A B, Udekwu A O, Ochoa J, Smith S. Bacterial translocation in trauma patients. *J Trauma* 1991; **31:** 1083–6.

25. Baker J W, Deitch E A, Li M, Berg R D, Specian R D. Hemorrhagic shock induces bacterial translocation from the gut. *J Trauma* 1988; **28:** 896–906.

26. Deitch E A, Berg R, Specian R. Endotoxin promotes the translocation of bacteria from the gut. *Arch Surg* 1987; **122:** 185–90.

27. Deitch E A, Winterton J, Berg R. Thermal injury promotes bacterial translocation from the gastrointestinal tract in mice with impaired T-cell-mediated immunity. *Arch Surg* 1986; **121:** 97–101.

28. Jones W G, Minei J P, Barber A E, *et al.* Bacterial translocation and intestinal atrophy after thermal injury and burn wound sepsis. *Ann Surg* 1990; **211:** 399–405.

29. Ryan C M, Yarmush M L, Burke J F, Tompkins R G. Increased gut permeability early after burns correlates with the extent of burn injury. *Crit Care Med* 1992; **20:** 1508–12.

30. Deitch E A. Intestinal permeability is increased in burn patients shortly after injury. *Surgery* 1990; **107:** 411–16.

31. Fink M P. Gastrointestinal mucosal injury in experimental models of shock, trauma, and sepsis. *Crit Care Med* 1991; **19:** 627–41.

32. Alexander J W, Boyce S T, Babcock G F, *et al.* The process of microbial translocation. *Ann Surg* 1990; **212:** 496–510.

33. Schoenberg M H, Beger H G. Reperfusion injury after intestinal ischemia. *Crit Care Med* 1993; **21:** 1376–86.

34. Bihari D, Smithies M, Gimson A, Tinker J. The effects of vasodilation with prostacyclin on oxygen delivery and uptake in critically ill patients. *N Engl J Med* 1987; **317:** 397–403.

35. Kaufman B S, Rackow E C, Falk J L. The relationship between oxygen delivery and consumption during fluid resuscitation of hypovolemic and septic shock. *Chest* 1984; **85:** 336–40.

36. Cain S M, Curtis S E. Experimental models of pathologic oxygen supply dependency. *Crit Care Med* 1991; **19:** 603–12.

37. Barone J E, Lowenfels A B. Maximization of oxygen delivery: a plea for moderation. *J Trauma* 1992; **33:** 651–3.

38. Hotchkiss R S, Karl I E. Reevaluation of the role of cellular hypoxia and bioenergetic failure in sepsis. *JAMA* 1992; **267:** 1503–10.

39. Shoemaker W C, Kram H B, Appel P L, Fleming A W. The efficacy of central venous and pulmonary artery catheters and therapy based upon them in reducing mortality and morbidity. *Arch Surg* 1990; **125:** 1332–7.

40. Ruokonen E, Takala J, Kari A. Regional blood flow and oxygen transport in patients with low cardiac output syndrome after cardiac surgery. *Crit Care Med* 1993; **21:** 1304–13.

41. Cerra F B. The systemic septic response: concepts of pathogenesis. *J Trauma* 1990; **30:** S169–S174.

42. Dinarello C A. The proinflammatory cytokines interleukin-1 and tumor necrosis factor and treatment of the septic shock syndrome. *J Infect Dis* 1991; **163:** 1177–84.

43. Molvig J, Baek L, Christensen P, *et al.* Endotoxin-stimulated human monocyte secretion of interleukin-1, tumor necrosis factor alpha, and prostaglandin E_2 shows stable interindividual differences. *Scand J Immunol* 1988; **27:** 705–16.

44. Morrison D C, Kline L F. Activation of the classical and the properdin pathways of complement by bacterial lipopolysaccharides (LPS). *J Immunol* 1977; **118:** 362–8.

45. Morrison D C, Ulevitch R J. The effects of bacterial endotoxins on host mediation systems. A review. *Am J Pathol* 1978; **93:** 526–617.

46. Chang S W, Fedderson C O, Henson P M, Voelkel N F. Platelet-activating factor mediates hemodynamic changes and lung injury in endotoxin-treated rats. *J Clin Invest* 1987; **79:** 1498–509.

47. Ramwell P W, Leovey E M, Sintetos A L. Regulation of arachidonic acid cascade. *Biol Reprod* 1977; **16:** 70–87.

48. Henderson W R Jr. Eicosanoids and lung inflammation. *Am Rev Respir Dis* 1987; **135:** 1176–85.

49. Whittle B J, Moncada S. Pharmacological interactions between prostacyclin and thromboxanes. *Br Med Bull* 1983; **39:** 232–8.

50. Ogletree M L. Overview of physiological and pathophysiological effects of thromboxane A_2. *Fedn Proc* 1987; **46:** 133–8.

51. Fitzgerald G A, Reilly I A, Pedersen A K. The biochemical pharmacology of thromboxane synthase inhibition in man. *Circulation* 1985; **72:** 1194–201.

52. Sprague R S, Stephenson A H, Dahms T E, Lonigro A J. Proposed role for leukotrienes in the pathophysiology of multiple systems organ failure. *Crit Care Clin* 1989; **5:** 315–29.

53. Lewis R A, Austen K F. The biologically active leukotrienes. Biosynthesis, metabolism, receptors, functions, and pharmacology. *J Clin Invest* 1984; **73:** 889–97.

54. Feinmark S J. Cooperative synthesis of leukotrienes by leukocytes and vascular cells. *Ann N Y Acad Sci* 1988; **524:** 122–32.

55. Folco G C, Omini C, Vigano T, Brunelli G, Rossoni G, Berti F. Biological activity of leukotriene C_4 in guinea-pigs: in vitro and in vivo studies. *Adv Prostaglandin Thromboxane Leukotriene Res* 1982; **9:** 153–67.

56. Hedqvist P, Dahlen S E, Bjork J. Pulmonary and vascular actions of leukotrienes. *Adv Prostaglandin Thromboxane Leukotriene Res* 1982; **9:** 187–200.

57. Davis J M, Meyer J D, Barie P S, *et al.* Elevated production of neutrophil leukotriene B_4 precedes pulmonary failure in critically ill surgical patients. *Surg Gynecol Obstet* 1990; **170:** 495–500.

58. Goetzl E J, Pickett W C. The human PMN leukocyte chemotactic activity of complex hydroxy-eicosatetraenoic acids (HETEs). *J Immunol* 1980; **125:** 1789–91.

59. Arai K I, Lee F, Miyajima A, Miyatake S, Arai N, Yokota T. Cytokines: coordinators of immune and inflammatory responses. *Annu Rev Biochem* 1990; **59:** 783–836.

60. Waage A, Brandtzaeg P, Halstensen A, Kierulf P, Espevik T. The complex pattern of cytokines in serum from patients with meningococcal septic shock. Association between interleukin-6, interleukin-1, and fatal outcome. *J Exp Med* 1989; **169:** 333–8.

61. Fassbender K, Pargger H, Muller W, Zimmerli W. Interleukin-6 and acute-phase protein concentrations in surgical intensive care unit patients: diagnostic signs in nosocomial infection. *Crit Care Med* 1993; **21:** 1175–80.

62. Okusawa S, Gelfand J, Ikejima T, Connolly R J, Dinarello C A. Interleukin-1 induces a shock-like state in rabbits. Synergism with tumor necrosis factor and the effect of cyclooxygenase inhibition. *J Clin Invest* 1988; **81:** 1162–72.

63. Wheeler A P, Jesmok G, Brigham K L. Tumor necrosis factor's effects on lung mechanics, gas exchange, and airway reactivity in sheep. *J Appl Physiol* 1990; **68:** 2542–9.

64. Hollenberg S M, Cunnion R E, Parrillo J E. The effect of tumor necrosis factor on vascular smooth muscle. In vitro studies using rat aortic rings. *Chest* 1991; **100:** 1133–7.

65. Heard S O, Perkins M W, Fink M P. Tumor necrosis factor-α causes myocardial depression in guinea pigs. *Crit Care Med* 1992; **20:** 523–7.

66. Warren R S, Starnes H F Jr, Gabrilove J L, Oettgen H F, Brennan M F. The acute metabolic effects of tumor necrosis factor administration in humans. *Arch Surg* 1987; **122:** 1396–400.

67. Michie H R, Spriggs D R, Manogue K R, *et al.* Tumor necrosis factor and endotoxin induce similar metabolic responses in human beings. *Surgery* 1988; **104:** 280–6.

68. van der Poll T, Buller H R, ten Cate H, *et al.* Activation of coagulation after administration of tumor necrosis factor to normal subjects. *N Engl J Med* 1990; **322:** 1622–7.

69. Anderson B O, Bensard D D, Harken A H. The role of platelet activating factor and its antagonists in shock, sepsis and multiple organ failure. *Surg Gynecol Obstet* 1991; **172:** 415–24.

70. Rabinovici R, Esser K M, Lysko P G, *et al.* Priming by platelet-activating factor of endotoxin-induced lung injury and cardiovascular shock. *Circ Res* 1991; **69:** 12–25.

71. Qi M, Jones S B. Contribution of platelet activating factor to hemodynamic and sympathetic responses to bacterial endotoxin in conscious rats. *Circ Shock* 1990; **32:** 153–63.

72. Yonemaru M, Hatherill J R, Hoffmann H, Zheng H, Ishii K, Raffin T A. Pentoxifylline does not attenuate acute lung injury in the absence of granulocytes. *J Appl Physiol* 1991; **71:** 342–51.

73. Weiss S J. Tissue destruction by neutrophils. *N Engl J Med* 1989; **320:** 365–76.

74. Horgan M J, Ge M, Gu J, Rothlein R, Malik A B. Role of ICAM-1 in neutrophil-mediated lung vascular injury after occlusion and reperfusion. *Am J Physiol* 1991; **261:** H1578–H1584.

75. White-Owen C, Alexander J W, Babcock G F. Reduced expression of neutrophil CD11b and CD16 after severe traumatic injury. *J Surg Res* 1992; **52:** 22–6.

76. Anderson D C, Springer T A. Leukocyte adhesion deficiency: an inherited defect in the Mac-1, LFA-1, and p150,95 glycoproteins. *Annu Rev Med* 1987; **38:** 175–94.

77. Benton L D, Khan M, Greco R S. Integrins, adhesion molecules, and surgical research. *Surg Gynecol Obstet* 1993; **177:** 311–27.

78. Bautista A P, Shuler A, Spolarics Z, Spitzer J J. Tumor necrosis factor-α stimulates superoxide anion generation by perfused rat liver and Kupffer cells. *Am J Physiol* 1991; **261:** G891–G895.

79. Palmer R M, Ferrige A G, Moncada S. Nitric oxide release accounts for the biological activity of endothelium-derived relaxing factor. *Nature* 1987; **327:** 524–6.

80. Moncada S, Palmer R M, Higgs E A. Nitric oxide physiology, pathophysiology, and pharmacology. *Pharmacol Rev* 1991; **43:** 109–42.

81. Bernard C, Szekely B, Philip I, Wollman E, Payen D, Tedgui A. Activated macrophages depress the contractility of rabbit carotids via an L-arginine/nitric oxide-dependent effector mechanism. Connection with amplified cytokine release. *J Clin Invest* 1992; **89:** 851–60.

82. Nava E, Palmer R M, Moncada S. Inhibition of nitric oxide synthesis in septic shock: how much is beneficial? *Lancet* 1991; **338:** 1555–7.

83. Ochoa J B, Udekwu A O, Billiar T R, *et al.* Nitrogen oxide levels in patients after trauma and during sepsis. *Ann Surg* 1991; **214:** 621–6.

84. Hosea S, Brown E, Hammer C, Frank M. Role of complement activation in a model of adult respiratory distress syndrome. *J Clin Invest* 1980; **66:** 375–82.

85. Allen J N, Pacht E R, Gadek J E, Davis W B. Acute eosinophilic pneumonia as a reversible cause of noninfectious respiratory failure. *N Engl J Med* 1989; **321:** 569–74.

86. Smedegard G, Cui L X, Hugli T E. Endotoxin-induced shock in the rat. A role for C5a. *Am J Pathol* 1989; **135:** 489–97.

87. Friedl H P, Till G O, Trentz O, Ward P A. Roles of histamine, complement and xanthine oxidase in thermal injury of skin. *Am J Pathol* 1989; **135:** 203–17.

88. Livingston D H. Management of the surgical patient with multiple system organ failure. *Am J Surg* 1993; **165:** 8S–13S.

89. Tompkins R G, Burke J F, Schoenfeld D A, *et al.* Prompt eschar excision: a treatment system contributing to reduced burn mortality. A statistical evaluation of burn care at the Massachusetts General Hospital (1974–1984). *Ann Surg* 1986; **204:** 272–81.

90. Tompkins R G, Remensnyder J P, Burke J F, *et al.* Significant reductions in mortality for children with burn injuries through the use of prompt eschar excision. *Ann Surg* 1988; **208:** 577–85.

91. Herndon D N, Barrow R E, Rutan R L, Rutan T C, Desai M H, Abston S. A comparison of conservative versus early excision. Therapies in severely burned patients. *Ann Surg* 1989; **209:** 547–52.

92. Sasaki T M, Welch G W, Herndon D N, Kaplan J Z, Lindberg R B, Pruitt B A Jr. Burn wound manipulation-induced bacteremia. *J Trauma* 1979; **19:** 46–8.

93. Beard C H, Ribeiro C D, Jones D M. The bacteraemia associated with burns surgery. *Br J Surg* 1975; **62:** 638–41.

94. Piel P, Scarnati S, Goldfarb I W, Slater H. Antibiotic prophylaxis in patients undergoing burn wound excision. *J Burn Care Rehabil* 1985; **6:** 422–4.

95. Luterman A, Dacso C C, Curreri P W. Infections in burn patients. *Am J Med* 1986; **81** (1A): 45–52.

96. Baskin T W, Rosenthal A, Pruitt B A. Acute bacterial endocarditis: a silent source of sepsis in the burn patient. *Ann Surg* 1976; **184:** 618–21.

97. Srivastava R F, MacMillan B G. Cardiac infection in acute burned patients. *Burns* 1979; **6:** 48–54.

98. Pruitt B A Jr, Stein J M, Foley F D, Moncrief J A, O'Neil J A Jr. Intravenous therapy in burn patients. Suppurative thrombophlebitis and other life threatening complications. *Arch Surg* 1970; **100:** 399–404.

99. Pruitt B A Jr, McManus W F, Kim S H, Treat R C. Diagnosis and treatment of cannula-related intravenous sepsis in burn patients. *Ann Surg* 1980; **191:** 546–54.

100. Sheridan R L, Tompkins R G, McManus W F, Pruitt B A Jr. Intracompartmental sepsis in burn patients. *J Trauma* 1994; **36:** 301–305.

101. Shirani K Z, Pruitt B A Jr, Mason A D Jr. The influence of inhalation injury and pneumonia on burn mortality. *Ann Surg* 1987; **205:** 82–7.

102. Langer M, Mosconi P, Cigada M, Mandelli M. Long-term respiratory support and risk of pneumonia in critically ill patients. *Am Rev Respir Dis* 1989; **140:** 302–5.

103. Deutschman C S, Wilton P, Sinow J, Dibbell D Jr, Konstantinides F N, Cerra F B. Paranasal sinusitis associated with nasotracheal intubation: a frequently unrecognized and treatable source of sepsis. *Crit Care Med* 1986; **14:** 111–14.

104. Halzapfel L, Shervet S, Madinier G, *et al.* Influence of long-term oro- or nasotracheal intubation on nosocomial maxillary sinusitis and pneumonia: results of a prospective, randomized, clinical trial. *Crit Care Med* 1993; **21:** 1132–8.

105. Slater H, Goldfarb I W. Acute septic cholecystitis in patients with burn injuries. *J Burn Care Rehabil* 1989; **10:** 445–7.

106. Vauthey J N, Lerut J, Martini M, Becker C, Gertsch P, Blumgart L H. Indications and limitations of percutaneous cholecystostomy for acute cholecystitis. *Surg Gynecol Obstet* 1993; **176:** 49–54.

107. Herndon D N, Zeigler S T. Bacterial translocation after thermal injury. *Crit Care Med* 1993; **21:** S50–S54.

108. Wilmore D W, Smith R J, O'Dwyer S T, Jacobs D O, Ziegler T R, Wang X D. The gut: a central organ after surgical stress. *Surgery* 1988; **104:** 917–23.

109. Johnson L R, Copeland E M, Dudrick S J, Lichtenberger L M, Castro G A. Structural and hormonal alterations in the gastrointestinal tract of parenterally fed rats. *Gastroenterology* 1975; **68:** 1177–83.

110. McDonald W S, Sharp C W, Deitch E A. Immediate enteral feeding in burn patients is safe and effective. *Ann Surg* 1991; **213:** 177–83.

111. Saito H, Trocki O, Alexander J W, Kopcha R, Heyd T, Joffee S N. The effect of route of nutrient administration on the nutritional status, catabolic hormone secretion, and gut mucosal integrity after burn injury. *J Parenter Enteral Nutr* 1987; **11:** 1–7.

112. Levine G M, Deren J J, Steiger E, Zinno R. Role of oral intake in maintenance of gut mass and disaccharide activity. *Gastroenterology* 1974; **67:** 975–82.

113. Souba W W, Smith R J, Wilmore D W. Glutamine metabolism by the intestinal tract. *J Parenter Enteral Nutr* 1985; **9:** 608–17.

114. Souba W W, Herskowitz K, Klimberg V S, *et al.* The effects of sepsis and endotoxemia on gut glutamine metabolism. *Ann Surg* 1990; **211:** 543–9.

115. Stehle P, Zander J, Merts N, *et al.* Effect of parenteral glutamine peptide supplements on muscle glutamine loss and nitrogen balance after major surgery. *Lancet* 1989; **1:** 231–3.

116. Platell C, McCauley R, McCulloch R, Hall J. The influence of parenteral glutamine and branched-chain amino acids on total parenteral nutrition-induced atrophy on the gut. *J Parenter Enteral Nutr* 1993; **17:** 348–54.

117. Spaeth G, Gottwald T, Haas W, Holmes M. Glutamine peptide does not improve gut barrier function and mucosal integrity in total parenteral nutrition. *J Parenter Enteral Nutr* 1993; **17:** 317–23.

118. Roediger W E. Utilization of nutrients by isolated epithelial cells of the rat colon. *Gastroenterology* 1982; **83:** 424–9.

119. Koruda M J, Rollandelli R H, Settle R G, Saul S H, Rombeau J L. The effect of pectin-supplemented elemental diet on intestinal adaptation to massive small bowel resection. *J Parenter Enteral Nutr* 1986; **10:** 343–50.

120. Gastinne H, Wolff M, Delatour F, Faurisson F, Chevret S. A controlled trial in intensive care units of selective decontamination of the digestive tract with nonabsorbable antibiotics. The French Study Group on Selective Decontamination of the Digestive Tract. *N Engl J Med* 1992; **326:** 594–9.

121. Wang X, Andersson R, Soltesz V, Guo W, Bergmark S. Water-soluble ethylhydroxyethyl cellulose prevents bacterial translocation induced by major liver resection in the rat. *Ann Surg* 1993; **217:** 155–67.

122. Moore F A, Moore E E, Jones T N, McCroskey B L, Petersen V M. TEN versus TPN following major abdominal trauma – reduced septic morbidity. *J Trauma* 1989; **29:** 916–22.

123. Gutierrez G. Cellular energy metabolism during hypoxia. *Crit Care Med* 1991; **19:** 619–26.

124. Dixon I M, Elyolfson D A, Ohalla N S. Sarcolemmal Na^{+}-Ca^{2+} exchange activity in hearts subjected to hypoxia reoxygenation. *Am J Physiol* 1987; **253:** H1026–H1034.

125. Granger D N. Role of xanthine oxidase and granulocytes in ischemia-reperfusion injury. *Am J Physiol* 1988; **255:** H1269–H1275.

126. Das D K, Engelman R M, Rousou J A, Breyer R H, Otani H, Lemeshow S. Role of membrane phospholipids in myocardial injury induced by ischemia and reperfusion. *Am J Physiol* 1986; **251:** H71–H79.

127. Lindenbaum G A, Larrieu A J, Carroll S F, Kapusnick R A. Effect of cocarboxylase in dogs subjected to experimental septic shock. *Crit Care Med* 1989; **17:** 1036–40.

128. Shoemaker W C, Appel P L, Kram H B. Role of oxygen debt in the development of organ failure sepsis, and death in high risk surgical patients. *Chest* 1992; **102:** 208–15.

129. Cain S M. Supply dependency of oxygen uptake in ARDS; myth or reality? *Am J Med Sci* 1984; **288:** 119–24.

130. Shoemaker W C, Appel P L, Kram H B, Waxman K, Lee T S. Prospective trial of supranormal values of survivors as therapeutic goals in high risk surgical patients. *Chest* 1988; **94:** 1176–86.

131. Mink R B, Pollack M M. Effect of blood transfusion on oxygen consumption in pediatric septic shock. *Crit Care Med* 1990; **18:** 1087–91.

132. Clarke C, Edwards J D, Nightingale P, Mortimer A J, Morris J. Persistence of supply dependency of oxygen uptake at high levels of delivery in adult respiratory distress syndrome. *Crit Care Med* 1991; **19:** 497–502.

133. Ruokonen E, Takala J, Kori A, Saxen H, Mertsala J, Hansen E D. Regional blood flow and oxygen transport in septic shock. *Crit Care Med* 1993; **21:** 1296–303.

134. Lorente J A, Landin L, DePablo R, Renes E, Rodrigues-Diez R, Liste D. Effects of blood transfusion on oxygen transport variables in severe sepsis. *Crit Care Med* 1993; **21:** 1312–18.

135. Kinsella J E, Lokesh B, Broughton S, Whelan J. Dietary polyunsaturated fatty acids and eicosanoids: potential effects on the modulation of inflammatory and immune cells: an overview. *Nutrition* 1990; **6:** 24–44.

136. Barton R G, Wells C L, Carlson A, Singh R, Sullivan J J, Cerra F B. Dietary omega-3 fatty acids decrease mortality and Kupffer cell prostaglandin E_2 production in a rat model of chronic sepsis. *J Trauma* 1991; **31:** 768–73.

137. Alexander J W, Saito H, Trocki O, Ogle C K. The importance of lipid type in the diet after burn injury. *Ann Surg* 1986; **204:** 1–8.

138. Daly J M, Reynolds J, Thom A, *et al.* Immune and metabolic effects of arginine in the surgical patient. *Ann Surg* 1988; **208:** 512–23.

139. Reynolds J V, Daly J M, Zhang S, *et al.* Immunomodulatory mechanisms of arginine. *Surgery* 1988; **104:** 142–51.

140. Barbul A, Wasserkrug H L, Seifter E, Rettura G, Levenson S M, Efron G. Immunostimulatory effects of arginine in normal and injured rats. *J Surg Res* 1980; **29:** 228–35.

141. Madden H P, Breslin R J, Wasserkrug H L, Efron G, Barbul A. Stimulation of T cell immunity by arginine enhances survival in peritonitis. *J Surg Res* 1988; **44:** 658–63.

142. Barbul A, Wasserkrug H L, Yoshimura N, Tao R, Efron G. High arginine levels in intravenous hyperalimentation abrogate post-traumatic immune suppression. *J Surg Res* 1984; **36:** 620–4.

143. Saito H, Trocki O, Wang S L, Gonce S J, Jaffe S N, Alexander J W. Metabolic and immune effects of dietary arginine supplementation after burn. *Arch Surg* 1987; **122:** 784–9.

144. Yu Y M, Wagner D A, Walesreswski J C, Burke J F, Young V R. A kinetic study of leucine metabolism in severely burned patients. Comparison between a conventional and a branched-chain amino acid-enriched nutritional therapy. *Ann Surg* 1988; **207:** 421–9.

145. Daly J M, Lieberman M D, Goldfine J, *et al.* Enteral nutrition with supplemental arginine, RNA, and omega-3 fatty acids in patients after operation: immunologic, metabolic, and clinical outcome. *Surgery* 1992; **112:** 56–67.

146. Gottschlich M M, Jenkins M, Warden G D, *et al.* Differential effects of three enteral dietary regimens on selected outcome variables in burn patients. *J Parenter Enteral Nutr* 1990; **14:** 225–36.

147. Bone R C, Fisher C J Jr, Clemmer T P, Slotman G J, Metz C A, Balk R A. A controlled clinical trial of high-dose methylprednisolone in the treatment of severe sepsis and septic shock. *N Engl J Med* 1987; **317:** 653–8.

148. Dominioni L, Dionigi R, Zanello M, *et al.* Effects of high-dose IgG on survival of surgical patients with sepsis scores of 20 or greater. *Arch Surg* 1991; **126:** 236–40.

149. Hackshaw K V, Parker G A, Roberts J W. Naloxone in septic shock. *Crit Care Med* 1990; **18:** 47–51.

150. Sheridan R L, Ryan C M, Tompkins R G. Acute adrenal insufficiency in the burn intensive care unit. *Burns* 1993; **19:** 63–6.

151. McCune S, Short B L, Miller M K, Lotze A, Anderson K D. Extracorporeal membrane oxygenation therapy in neonates with septic shock. *J Pediatr Surg* 1990; **25:** 479–82.

152. Munster A M, Xiao G X, Guo Y, Wong L A. Control of endotoxemia in burn patients by use of polymyxin B. *J Burn Care Rehabil* 1989; **10:** 327–30.

153. Ziegler E J, McCutchan J A, Fierer J, *et al.* Treatment of gram-negative bacteremia and shock with human antiserum to a mutant *Escherichia coli*. *N Engl J Med* 1982; **307:** 1225–30.

154. Greenman R L, Schein R M, Martin M A, *et al.* A controlled clinical trial of E5 murine monoclonal IgM antibody to endotoxin in the treatment of gram-negative sepsis. *JAMA* 1991; **266:** 1097–102.

155. Wentzel R P. Anti-endotoxin monoclonal antibodies – a second look [editorial; comment]. *N Engl J Med* 1992; **326:** 1151–3.

156. Zeigler E J, Fisher C J Jr, Sprung C L, *et al.* Treatment of gram-negative bacteremia and septic shock with HA-1A human monoclonal antibody against endotoxin. A randomized, double blind, placebo-controlled trial. *N Engl J Med* 1991; **324:** 429–36.

157. Shulman K A, Glick H A, Ruben H, Eisenberg J M. Cost-effectiveness of HA-1A a monoclonal antibody for gram-negative sepsis. Economic assessment of a new therapeutic agent. *JAMA* 1991; **266:** 3466–71.

158. Wise W C, Cook J A, Eller T, Halushka P V. Ibuprofen improves survival from endotoxic shock in the rat. *J Pharmacol Exp Ther* 1980; **215:** 160–4.

159. Fletcher J R, Ramwell P W. Indomethacin treatment following baboon endotoxin shock improves survival. *Adv Shock Res* 1980; **4:** 103–11.

160. Adams T Jr, Traber D L. The effects of a prostaglandin synthetase inhibitor, ibuprofen, on the cardiopulmonary response to endotoxin in sheep. *Circ Shock* 1982; **9:** 481–9.

161. Temple G E, Cook J A, Wise W C, Halushka P V, Corral D. Improvement in organ blood flow by inhibition of thromboxane synthetase during experimental endotoxic shock in the rat. *J Cardiovasc Pharmacol* 1986; **8:** 514–19.

162. Revhaug A, Michie H R, Manson J M, *et al.* Inhibition of cyclo-oxygenase attenuates the metabolic response to endotoxin in humans. *Arch Surg* 1988; **123:** 162–70.

163. Bernard G R, Reines H D, Halushka P V, *et al.* Prostacyclin and thromboxane A_2 formation is increased in human sepsis syndrome. Effects of cyclooxygenase inhibition. *Am Rev Respir Dis* 1991; **144:** 1095–101.

164. Faist E, Ertel W, Cohnert T, Huber P, Inthorn D, Heberer G. Immunoprotective effects of cyclooxygenase inhibition in patients with major surgical trauma. *J Trauma* 1990; **30:** 8–17.

165. Demling R H, Smith M, Gunther R, Gee M, Flynn J. The effect of prostacyclin infusion on endotoxin-induced lung injury. *Surgery* 1981; **89:** 257–63.

166. Matera G, Cook J A, Hennigar R A, *et al.* Beneficial effects of a 5-lipoxygenase inhibitor in endotoxic shock in the rat. *J Pharmacol Exp Ther* 1988; **247:** 363–71.

167. Coggeshall J W, Christman B W, Lefferts P L, *et al.* Effect of inhibition of 5-lipoxygenase metabolism of arachidonic acid on response to endotoxemia in sheep. *J Appl Physiol* 1988; **65:** 1351–9.

168. Fink M P, Kruithoff K L, Antonsson J B, Wang H, Rothschild H R. Delayed treatment with an LTD_4/E_4 antagonist limits pulmonary edema in endotoxic pigs. *Am J Physiol* 1991; **260:** R1007–R1013.

169. Granowitz E V, Santos A A, Poutsiaka D D, *et al.* Production of interleukin-1 receptor antagonist during experimental endotoxaemia. *Lancet* 1991; **338:** 1423–4.

170. Ohlsson K, Bjork P, Bergenfeldt M, Hageman R, Thompson R C. Interleukin-1 receptor antagonist reduces mortality from endotoxin shock. *Nature* 1990; **348:** 550–2.

171. Watters J M, Bessey P Q, Dinarello C A, Wolff S M, Wilmore D W. The induction of interleukin-1 in humans and its metabolic effects. *Surgery* 1985; **98:** 298–305.

172. Beutler B A, Milsark I W, Cerami A. Cachectin/tumor necrosis factor: production, distribution, metabolic fate in vivo. *J Immunol* 1985; **135:** 3972–7.

173. Tracey K J, Fong Y, Hesse D G, *et al.* Anti-cachectin/TNF monoclonal antibodies prevent septic shock during lethal bacteremia. *Nature* 1987; **330:** 662–4.

174. Hinshaw L B, Tekamp-Olson P, Chang A C, *et al.* Survival of primates in LD_{100} septic shock following therapy with antibody to tumor necrosis factor. *Circ Shock* 1990; **30:** 279–92.

175. Marks J D, Marks C B, Luce J M, *et al.* Plasma tumor necrosis factor in patients with septic shock. Mortality rate, incidence of adult respiratory distress syndrome, and effects of methylprednisolone administration. *Am Rev Respir Dis* 1990; **141:** 94–7.

176. Franks A K, Kujawa K I, Yaffe L J. Experimental elimination of tumor necrosis factor in low-dose endotoxin models has variable effects on survival. *Infect Immun* 1991; **59:** 2609–14.

177. Eskandari M K, Bolgos G, Miller C, Nguyen D T, DeForge L E, Remick D G. Anti-tumor necrosis factor antibody therapy fails to prevent lethality after cecal ligation and puncture or endotoxemia. *J Immunol* 1992; **148:** 2724–30.

178. Pitman J M, 3d, Thurman G W, Anderson B O, *et al.* WEB2170, a specific platelet-activating factor antagonist, attenuates neutrophil priming by human serum after clinical burn injury: the 1991 Moyer Award. *J Burn Care Rehabil* 1991; **12:** 411–19.

179. Chang S-W, Fernyak S, Voelkel N F. Beneficial effect of a platelet-activating factor antagonist, WEB 2086, on endotoxin-induced lung injury. *Am J Physiol* 1990; **258:** H153–H158.

180. Fletcher J R, DiSimone A G, Earnest M A. Platelet activating factor receptor antagonist improves survival and attenuates eicosanoid release in severe endotoxemia. *Ann Surg* 1990; **211:** 312–16.

181. Moore J M, Earnest M A, DiSimone A G, Abumrad N N, Fletcher J R. A PAF receptor antagonist, BN 52021, attenuates thromboxane release and improves survival in lethal canine endotoxemia. *Circ Shock* 1991; **35:** 53–9.

182. Eichacker P Q, Farese A, Hoffman W D, *et al.* Leukocyte CD11b/18 antigen-directed monoclonal antibody improves early survival and decreases hypoxemia in dogs challenged with tumor necrosis factor. *Am Rev Respir Dis* 1992; **145:** 1023–9.

183. Vedder N B, Winn R K, Rice Cl, Chi E Y, Arfors K E, Harlan J M. A monoclonal antibody to the adherence-promoting leukocyte glycoprotein, CD18, reduces organ injury and improves survival from hemorrhagic shock and resuscitation in rabbits. *J Clin Invest* 1988; **81:** 939–44.

184. Schiller H J, Reilly P M, Bulkley G B. Tissue perfusion in critical illnesses. Antioxidant therapy. *Crit Care Med* 1993; **21:** S92–S102.

185. Richard C, Lemonnier F, Thibault M, Couturier M, Auzepy P. Vitamin E deficiency and lipoperoxidation during adult respiratory distress syndrome. *Crit Care Med* 1990; **18:** 4–9.

186. Rhee P, Waxman K, Clark L, Tominaga G, Soliman M H. Superoxide dismutase polyethylene glycol improves survival in hemorrhagic shock. *Am Surg* 1991; **57:** 747–50.

187. Novelli G P. Oxygen radicals in experimental shock: effects of spin-trapping nitrones in ameliorating shock pathophysiology. *Crit Care Med* 1992; **20:** 499–507.

188. Lorente J A, Landin L, DePablo R, Renes E, Liste D. L-arginine pathway in the sepsis syndrome. *Crit Care Med* 1993; **21:** 1287–95.

189. Cobb J P, Cunnian R E, Donner R L. Nitric oxide as a target for therapy in septic shock. *Crit Care Med* 1993; **21:** 1261–3.

190. Pepke-Zaba J, Higenbottam T W, Dinh-Xuan A T, Stone D, Wallwork J. Inhaled nitric oxide as a cause of selective pulmonary vasodilatation in pulmonary hypertension. *Lancet* 1991; **338:** 1173–4.

191. Nava E, Palmer R M, Moncada S. Inhibition of nitric oxide synthesis in septic shock: how much is beneficial. *Lancet* 1991; **338:** 1555–7.

192. Lieberthal W, McGarry A E, Sheils J, Valeri C R. Nitric oxide inhibition in rats improves blood pressure and renal function during hypovolemic shock. *Am J Physiol* 1991; **261:** F868–F872.

193. Saffle J R, Sullivan J J, Tuohig G M, Larson C M. Multiple organ failure in patients with thermal injury. *Crit Care Med* 1993; **21:** 1673–83.

194. Shalaby M R, Aggarwal B B, Rinderknecht E, Svedersky L P, Finkle B S, Palladino M A Jr. Activation of human polymorphonuclear neutrophil functions by interferon-gamma and tumor necrosis factors. *J Immunol* 1985; **135:** 2069–73.

195. Alexander H R, Sheppard B C, Jensen J C, *et al.* Treatment with recombinant human tumor necrosis factor-alpha protects rats against the lethality, hypotension, and hypothermia of gram-negative sepsis. *J Clin Invest* 1991; **88:** 34–9.

196. Dong Y L, Herndon D N, Yan T Z, Waymack J P. Blockade of prostaglandin products augments macrophage and neutrophil tumor necrosis factor synthesis in burn injury. *J Surg Res* 1993; **54:** 480–5.

197. Schael G L, Fink M P, Chernow B, Ahmed S, Parrillo J E. Renal hemodynamics and prostaglandin E_2 excretion in a nonhuman primate model of septic shock. *Crit Care Med* 1990; **18:** 52–9.

198. Calandra T, Baumgartner J D, Grau G E, *et al.* Prognostic values of tumor necrosis factor/cachectin, interleukin-1, interferon-α, and interferon-γ in the serum of patients with septic shock. *J Infect Dis* 1990; **161:** 982–7.

CHAPTER THIRTY

Renal Failure in Burned Patients

Yotaro Shinozawa and Naoki Aikawa

Acute renal failure is one of the major complications of burns and is accompanied by a high mortality rate. Most renal failure occurs either immediately after the injury or at a later period when sepsis develops. Owing to recent advances in cardiovascular management, acute renal failure has become a much less frequent complication than in the past; renal failure itself is no longer life threatening because hemodialysis is available. The renal failure occurring in extensively burned patients, however, is usually associated with failure or dysfunction of other organs in a form of multiple organ dysfunction syndrome, which has an adverse influence on the prognosis. Acute renal failure occurring immediately after burns is mostly due to reduced cardiac output, which is mainly caused by fluid loss. It is usually reversible.

Renal Failure in Burned Patients

In an experimental shock model[1] it was demonstrated that acute renal failure developing 2 hours after scalding is associated with a marked reduction in glomerular filtration rate (GFR) and almost complete reabsorption in the normally functioning distal tubule. Under such circumstances, the reduced GFR depends not only on decreased blood pressure but on the regulation of the filtration rate via tubuloglomerular feedback. Proximal tubular damage and organic and/or nonorganic glomerular damage develop when acute renal failure becomes irreversible.[2]

Acute renal failure occurring in the second week or later after injury is sometimes irreversible. This may be the result of renal damage in the early period. In most cases of acute renal failure developing in patients surviving beyond 48 hours after burns, the patients are polyuric.[3] A primary glomerular impairment,[4] osmolar regulatory disturbance[5] due to the lack of an osmolar gradient in the papilla of the renal medulla, and impairment of tubuloglomerular feedback mechanisms have been hypothesized. Proximal tubular dysfunction causes a modest 'downstream' solute diuresis in spite of intact distal exchange function. A reduction in GFR, low urinary sodium concentration and high urinary potassium concentration are present; and a consequent nonresorbable solutes load causes osmotic diuresis.[3] Polyuria in acute renal failure is also believed to reflect inadequate response to aldosterone in the distal tubule.[2]

Etiologic Factors in Renal Failure

The major etiologic factors in the development of early acute renal failure after burns are hypovolemia and a decrease in cardiac output. The resultant decrease in renal blood flow is primarily responsible for the oliguria seen immediately after burns. Two major mechanisms are involved in the pathophysiologic changes in the kidneys: filtration failure and tubular dysfunction caused by various factors and interacting with each other (**Figure 30.1**).[6]

Fluid Shifts and Hypovolemia

In burned patients, increased vascular permeability causes extensive fluid shifts manifested as both local and generalized edema. This results in hypovolemia and centralization of circulation, inducing oliguria early after burns. Sodium retention in collagen fibers and sodium–potassium pump impairment also participate in giving rise to generalized edema. Excess free water given in this period lowers the tonicity of plasma, which also results in renal edema, followed by acute renal failure.[7]

Myocardial Depression

Besides the decreased circulatory volume and plasma tonicity, myocardial depression, due to a presumed myocardial depressant factor and/or oxygen free radicals, serves to reduce renal flow and is followed by tubular necrosis.

Stress-related Hormones

Burn stress and the associated circulatory derangement induce elevated levels of catecholamines, angiotensin II, aldosterone, and

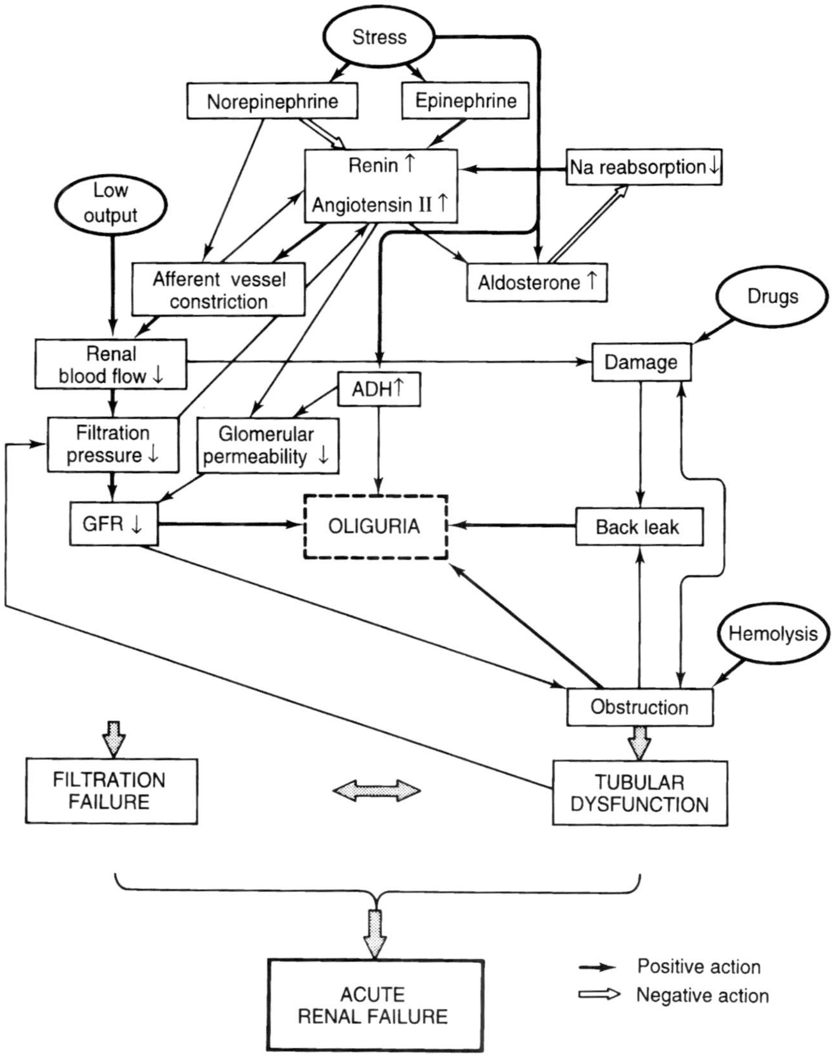

Fig. 30.1 Etiologic factors and mechanisms in the development of acute renal failure in the early postburn period.

vasopressin. These hormonal changes cause vasoconstriction and fluid retention as well as alteration of regional blood flow, especially in the kidney. On the other hand, plasma atrial natriuretic polypeptide (ANP) levels are elevated for sustained periods after burns. ANP counterbalances the actions of the stress-related hormones through vasodilatation and natriuresis.[6] Excessively high levels of stress-related hormones and/or impairment of ANP secretion may participate in reduced renal function.

Inflammatory Mediators

Besides the hormonal mediators mentioned above, many mediators including cytokines (TNF, IL-1, etc.), eicosanoids (prostaglandins [PGs], thromboxane, leukotrienes), and platelet-aggregating (activating) factor (PAF) are produced or released in the early postburn period. They act variably to increase vascular permeability and to induce tissue damage. These mediators are also involved in the development of disseminated intravascular coagulation (DIC), in which microthrombi are formed in the capillaries of the glomeruli and renal tubule. Vasodilator PGE_2 is a specific PG in the kidney and works to counteract the above vasoconstrictor substances, but its production is inhibited in the early phase of burns. Similar inflammatory changes occur when a burn patient develops sepsis in the late period.

Denatured Proteins (Pigmenturia)

Free hemoglobin released from degraded red blood cells by heat is conjugated by haptoglobin and transferred to the liver. When a large amount of free hemoglobin is produced in extensive third degree burns, unconjugated free hemoglobin passes through the glomeruli and is excreted in the urine. This could cause degenerative changes in the tubule cells, occlusion of the renal tubules by the formation of hemoglobin casts, and eventually renal failure, especially when combined with dehydration, acidosis, shock, or endotoxemia.[8,9] The free hemoglobin absorbed by tubular epithelium is degraded into globin and heme; the latter may induce tubular damage by generating oxygen free radicals via iron ions. Increased serum myoglobin has also been reported in patients with destroyed muscle in deep thermal injury, electrical injury, distal ischemia due to persistent hypotension or sustained compression, high fever, and drug-induced myolysis.[10] These proteins can be etiologic factors of acute renal failure in the first 1–2 days after injury.

Nephrotoxic Agents

Antibiotics, such as aminoglycosides and certain cephalosporins, are known to be nephrotoxic. Acute or chronic intoxication with alcohol, barbiturates, chlorpromazine, toluene, and paint thinner have been reported as possible associated agents inducing renal failure in burned patients. In some of these patients, early resuscitation therapy was delayed.[11]

Respiratory Dysfunction

Associated respiratory dysfunction adversely affects renal function because of reduced oxygen supply to the kidney. Reduced cardiac output caused by mechanical ventilation with continuous positive airway pressure modes decreases renal flow.

Incidence of Renal Failure

Ten to thirty percent of burned patients are reported to suffer renal failure, depending on the criteria used to define renal failure and on the patient population.[3] Generally, the more severely burned the patients are, the higher the incidence of renal failure is. In severely burned patients, the incidence of renal failure ranges from 1.3 to 38%.[2] In a report on 1785 children with 67 ± 5% TBSA burns, only four developed acute renal failure. All of the cases of renal failure occurring more than 1 week after burn were associated with sepsis.[12]

Prognosis

The prognosis of burned patients with acute renal failure is usually unfavorable. Mortality rates of 73–100% have been reported.[2] The survival rate of patients with renal failure (defined as serum creatinine levels above 2.5 mg/dl) was 30%; this was lower than the survival rate of 75% in patients having normal renal function, although the former patients were older and more severely burned than the latter.[13] In patients in whom serum creatinine increased to a level greater than 1.5 mg/dl above initial values in the absence of shock,[3] the mortality rate was 72.7%; this was much higher than among patients without renal dysfunction (16.6%). Moreover, in patients with multiple organ failure, the mortality rate was 88% among patients with acute renal failure, the criteria for which was C_{H_2O}>–0.5 ml/min, blood urea nitrogen level >50 mg/dl and serum creatinine level >2.0 mg/dl.[14]

Diagnosis of Acute Renal Failure

Urinary output is the key parameter in evaluating both renal function and the patient's circulatory state. Generally a urine volume of 0.8–1.0 ml/kg/h reflects adequate perfusion pressure. In an oliguric state, however, it must be determined whether the reduced urine volume is due to functional renal (or prerenal) failure or due to organic (or renal) failure (**Table 30.1**). Prolonged functional renal failure is often observed before organic failure develops. In nonoliguric renal failure, urine volume is of no value in the diagnosis. Urine and serum osmolality and electrolyte concentrations are useful in the differential diagnosis (**Table 30.2**).

Table 30.1 Differential diagnosis of acute renal failure

	Functional (prerenal)	Organic (renal)
U_{osm} (mosmol/l)	>500	<350
U_{osm}/P_{osm}	>2	<1.2
U_{Na} (mEq/l)	<20	>40
FE_{Na} (%)	<1	>3
C_{H_2O} (ml/min)	<–1.0	–0.5 ~ 0
U_{cr}/P_{cr}	>40	<20

U_{osm}, urine osmolality; P_{osm}, plasma osmolality; U_{Na}, urine sodium; FE_{Na}, fractional excretion of filtered sodium, $FE_{Na} = (U_{Na}/P_{Na})/(U_{cr}/P_{cr})$; C_{H_2O}, free water clearance, $C_{H_2O}=UV(1-U_{osm}/P_{osm})$; UV, urine volume; U_{cr}, urine creatinine; P_{cr}, plasma creatinine.

Table 30.2 Differential diagnosis of oliguric and nonoliguric renal failure

	Oliguric	Nonoliguric
Urine volume (ml/day)	<400~500	>500
Serum K (mEq/l)	Increased	Normal range
Serum creatinine (mg/dl)	Increased	Gradually increased
Furosemide test*	No response	Response
U_{Na} (mEq/l)	40–80	Various
C_{H_2O} (ml/min)	–0.25~0.25	–0.25~0.25
FE_{Na} (%)	>3	>3
C_{cr} (ml/min)	<5	5~30

* 'Response' to the furosemide test means doubled urine volume in 2 hours, compared with the urine volume (UV) during the 2 hours before administration 40–200 mg of furosemide or 40 ml/h urinary excretion by diuretics; U_{Na}, urine sodium; C_{H_2O}, free water clearance, C_{H_2O}=UV$(1-U_{osm}/P_{osm})$; FE_{Na}, fractional excretion of filtered sodium, $FE_{Na}=(U_{Na}/P_{Na})/(U_{cr}/P_{cr})$; C_{cr}, creatinine clearance, $C_{cr}=UV \times U_{cr}/P_{cr} \times 1.48/m^2$.

Prevention of Renal Failure

Circulatory Stabilization

Adequate fluid therapy is crucial in maintaining renal function. In extensively burned patients, fluid formulas, such as the Parkland formula, are just general guidelines; the argument as to what kind of fluid to use has not been settled. Thus, initial fluid resuscitation should be carried out according to an individualized fluid resuscitation program in order to maintain optimal ranges of the various hemodynamic parameters.[15] Monitoring by Swan–Ganz catheterization and thermodilution cardiac output determination is useful in the circulatory management of severely burned patients.[16] Particularly in extensive third degree burns or in patients with inhalation injury, more fluid than the calculated volume[17] is needed in order to maintain circulatory status. Dopamine, 3–5 μg/kg/min, for dilatation of renal blood vessels is useful in oliguric burn patients who have received adequate fluid therapy. When cardiac output is reduced in spite of full fluid resuscitation, higher doses of dopamine (5–12 μg/kg/min) and dobutamine (5–12 μg/kg/min) are used.

Monitoring Renal Functions

Early diagnosis of renal failure is very important. To evaluate renal failure, monitoring glomerular and tubular function, persistent proteinuria, and urinary tubule enzymes are recommended in addition to taking measurements of urine volume, blood urea nitrogen, and serum creatinine.

Creatinine clearance reflects the glomerulofiltration rate (GFR), and is useful in evaluating the prognosis in renal dysfunction. Increased serum concentrations of β_2-microglobulin reflect a decreased GFR. Free water clearance (C_{H_2O}) is a useful parameter for the early diagnosis of renal failure. C_{H_2O} falls to nearly zero before organic renal failure is established. Fractional excretion of filtered sodium (FE_{Na}) is another parameter reflecting tubular function, but it is not useful in evaluating renal function in burn patients. In spite of normal tubular function, FE_{Na} becomes abnormally high when a large amount of sodium is administered in the early postburn phase and also when the sequestered sodium is excreted in the urine in the late phase. Temporarily increased FE_{Na} immediately after a burn and on postburn days 2–4 has been reported in patients with burn >30% who did not develop renal failure.[18]

Glomerular dysfunction is associated with increased renal excretion of higher molecular weight proteins, and tubular dysfunction is associated with lower molecular weight proteins (<60 000 daltons) due to tubular impairment of reabsorption and/or degradation of these proteins. In some burned patients, a transient glomerular lesion may cause albuminuria immediately after the burn, followed by increased excretion of higher molecular weight proteins, such as α_1-acid glycoprotein, α_1-antichymotrypsin and γ-glutamyltransferase (GT), around 5 days after the burn.[19] There is no correlation, however, between proteinuria and the development of renal dysfunction.

Urinary α-glucosidase is specific for the epithelium of the proximal renal tubule. Its elevation above a level of 1.5 unit/l indicates proximal renal tubule injury. Urinary *N*-acetyl-β-D-glucosamidase (NAG) is not exclusive for lesions of the proximal renal tubule. Increased urinary β_2-microglobulin suggests proximal renal tubular damage. These enzymes were elevated even in burn patients who were not suffering from acute renal failure, but who finally died.[2] The excretion of β_2-microglobulin, coinciding with the maximal liberation of tissue breakdown products, increases 2–3 weeks postburn when sepsis develops, and it is correlated with the extent and depth of the burn.[20]

Haptoglobin Administration

Haptoglobin combines specifically with free hemoglobin, forming a conjugate which is metabolized in the liver. In extensive third degree burns, haptoglobin administration is useful in preventing or decreasing hemoglobinuria[8] (**Figure 30.2**). It was approved for clinical use in Japan in 1985, but not yet in the United States. Haptogloblin preparations must be administered immediately after

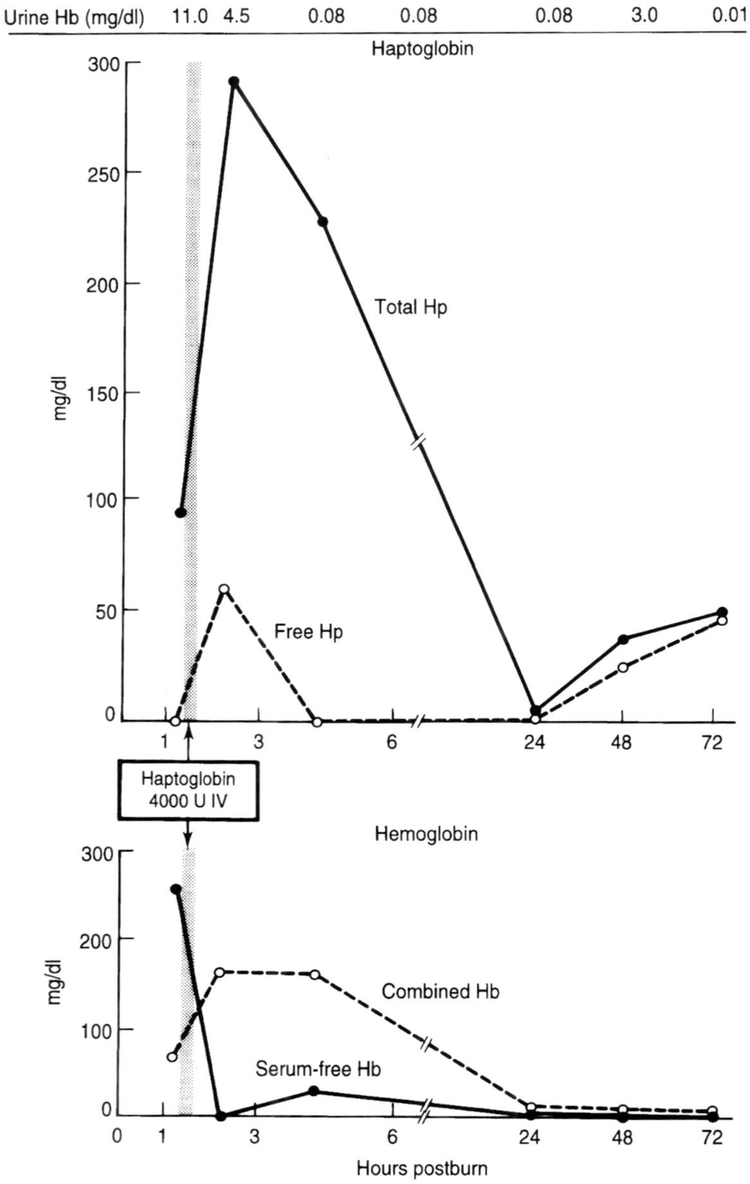

Fig. 30.2 Changes in serum haptoglobin (Hp) and hemoglobin (Hb) in a 60-year-old man with 58% full-thickness burn. Free Hp increased following Hp infusion.

burns when hemoglobulinemia is anticipated or trace hemoglobulinemia is detected. Alkalinizing urine by administering sodium bicarbonate and increasing urine output by massive fluid loading or diuretics prevents hemoglobin precipitation in the tubules, but may not prevent the possible toxic effects of hemoglobin on tubular cells.[6]

Other Measures to Prevent Renal Failure

Correction of hypoxia and acidosis are important measures in preventing the development of renal failure.[21] Anticoagulation therapy, such as antithrombin III and heparin, is indicated in the hypercoagulatory state, which is mostly associated with sepsis. More importantly, early excision of deep second degree and third degree burns, followed by immediate grafting, decreases the incidence of renal failure which develops in sepsis.

Management of Renal Failure

Fluid Balance

If a hemofiltration device, such as hemodialysis, is not indicated, then urine volume, insensible water loss, and gastrointestinal fluid loss must be determined. Fluid overload should be avoided in order to prevent pulmonary edema and heart failure. In burn patients with extensive raw surfaces, fluid loss through the wound is not accurately assessed. Central venous pressure and/or pulmonary capillary wedge monitoring is recommended.[16]

Diuretics

Diuretics are indicated in prerenal oliguria but not in established organic renal failure. Intravenous furosemide (20–80 mg/day) is given to maintain urine output when oliguria continues in spite of adequate fluid replacement. The required minimum urine volume (*UV*) necessary to prevent an increase in blood urea nitrogen or creatinine is calculated using the following formula:

$UV=P_{urea}/U_{urea}\times 10$ (l/day) to maintain urea clearance at 10 l/day

$UV=P_{cr}/U_{cr}\times 30$ (l/day) to maintain creatinine clearance at 30 l/day.

Management of Hyperkalemia

Serum potassium levels above 6.0 mEq/l and/or abnormal EKG (tenting of the T wave, flattening of the P wave, and widened QRS complex) are indications of the need for immediate treatment. Intravenous administration of 500 ml of 10% dextrose with 20 units of regular insulin will lower the serum potassium level by approximately 2 mEq/l. When metabolic acidosis is present, elevating pH by intravenous sodium bicarbonate also lowers the serum potassium concentration. Until the serum potassium levels are reduced, calcium chloride is given intravenously in order to counteract the cardiac abnormalities due to hyperkalemia. In less critical settings, ion-exchange resins (sodium polystyrene sulfonate: Kayexalate^{R}) are administered by mouth or by retention enema.

Hemodialysis (HD)

Early and frequent hemodialysis is recommended. The criteria for the introduction of HD to treat acute renal failure in burned patients are listed in **Table 30.3**. Although HD is most effective in the management of renal failure, it is sometimes difficult to insure stable circulation. Also, in extensive burns, bleeding through burns may be a problem due to the use of anticoagulants. In hypotensive patients, albumin or blood should be transfused prior to HD. To remove excess water and circulating toxic substances other than creatinine and urea, continuous hemofiltration may be combined with HD. In burned patients, the blood access site must be chosen as far away from the burn site as possible. Peritoneal dialysis has little value in the treatment of acute renal failure in burns.

Table 30.3 Criteria for hemodialysis

BUN >70 mg/dl
Creatinine >5 mg/dl
K >6 mEq/l
Base excess <–15 mEq/l
Pulmonary edema
Systemic signs of uremia

Nutritional Support

In burned patients, energy requirements are high, and adequate nutritional support is critical to the outcome. The renal failure itself does not increase the metabolic rate, but the stress causing the renal failure may induce a hypermetabolic state. Energy requirements can be assessed by indirect calorimetry (IC). When IC is not available, a daily energy supply of (23–26) kcal/kg × (1.5–2.0) should be given.[22] The major substrate is glucose, and 30% of the energy is provided as lipid products. As for the nitrogen administration, amino acids, 0.5–1.0 g/kg/day, balanced with essential amino acids and nonessential amino acids, is recommended. When urea nitrogen (calculated by increased nitrogen in the body, urinary nitrogen loss, and nitrogen loss into the dialysis water) is 10 g or more, then more than 1.0 g/kg/day of amino acids, rich in branched-chain amino acids, should be administered. Nutritional support requires much carrier water to be infused; if more than 1000 ml/day of water is administered into anuric patients, then continuous hemofiltration is applied in order to remove the excess water.

References

1. Loew D, Meng K. Acute renal failure in experimental shock due to scalding. *Kidney Int* 1976; **10:** S81–S85.
2. Schiavon M, DiLandro D, Baldo M, *et al.* A study of renal damage in seriously burned patients. *Burns* 1988; **14:** 107–14.
3. Planas M, Wachtel T, Frank G, *et al.* Characterization of acute renal failure in the burned patient. *Arch Intern Med* 1982; **142:** 2087–91.
4. Sevitt S. Renal function after burning. *J Clin Pathol* 1965; **18:** 572–8.
5. Eklund J. Studies on renal function in burns: II. Early signs of impaired renal function in lethal burns. *Acta Chir Scand* 1970; **136:** 735–40.
6. Aikawa N, Wakabayashi G, Ueda M, *et al.* Regulation of renal function in thermal injury. *J Trauma* 1990; **30:** S174–S178.
7. Hauben D J. Invited comment on acute renal failure in burned patients. *Burns* 1988; **14:** 113–14.
8. Aikawa N, Ishibiki K, Okusawa S, *et al.* Use of haptoglobin to prevent renal damage due to hemolysis in extensive third-degree burns. *J Burn Care Rehabil* 1984; **5:** 20–4.
9. Yoshioka T, Sugimoto T, Ukai T, *et al.* Haptoglobin therapy for possible prevention of renal failure following thermal injury: a clinical study. *J Trauma* 1985; **25:** 281–7.
10. Cynober L, Guechot J, Lioret N, *et al.* Rhabdomyolysis and acute renal failure in a patient with thermal injury. *Int Care Med* 1986; **12:** 159–60.
11. Sawada Y, Momma S, Takamizawa A, *et al.* Survival from acute renal failure after severe burns. *Burns* 1984; **11:** 143–7.

12. Tweddell J S, Waymack J P, Warden G D, *et al.* Hematuria in the burned child. *J Pediat Surg* 1987; **22:** 899–903.

13. Vanholder R, Bogaerde J V D, Vogelaers D, *et al.* Renal function in burns. *Acta Anaesth Belg* 1987; **38:** 367–71.

14. Aikawa N, Shinozawa Y, Ishibiki K, *et al.* Clinical analysis of multiple organ failure in burned patients. *Burns* 1987; **13:** 103–9.

15. Aikawa N, Ishibiki K, Naito C, *et al.* Individualized fluid resuscitation based on haemodynamic monitoring in the management of extensive burns. *Burns* 1982; **8:** 249–55.

16. Aikawa N, Martyn J A J, Burke J F. Pulmonary artery catheterization and thermodilution cardiac output determination in the management of critically burned patients. *Am J Surg* 1978; **135:** 811–17.

17. Herndon D N, Barrow R E, Traber D L, *et al.* Extravascular lung water changes following smoke inhalation and massive burn injury. *Surgery* 1987; **102:** 341–9.

18. Naito C, Aikawa N, Yamamoto S, *et al.* FENa test in burned patients. *Jap J Burn Injury* 1981; **6:** 187–92.

19. Shakespeare P G, Coombes E J, Hambleton J, *et al.* Proteinuria after burn injury. *Ann Clin Biochem* 1981; **18:** 353–60.

20. Barison A S, Graziani M G, Rigotti G, *et al.* B_2-Microglobulins and renal dysfunction in burned patients. *Burns* 1988; **14:** 369–72.

21. Walsh M B, Miller S L, Kagen L J. Myoglobinemia in severely burned patients; correlations with severity and survival. *J Trauma* 1982; **22:** 6–10.

22. Wesson D E, Mitch W E, Wilmore D W. Nutritional considerations in the treatment of acute renal failure. In: Brenner B M, Lazarus J M (eds). *Acute Renal Failure*, Philadelphia: WB Saunders, 1983: 618 pp.

CHAPTER THIRTY-ONE

31

Critical Care of Burn Complications

Werner W. Lingnau, Thuan T. Nguyen, Lee C. Woodson, David N. Herndon and Donald S. Prough

Introduction

Burn injuries in the United States result in approximately 30–50 acute admissions per year per 100 000 people.[1,2] About 65% are burned severely, defined as burns exceeding 41% of total body surface area (TBSA), and require the facilities of a designated Burn Intensive Care Unit (BICU) staffed by specially trained personnel. Many severely burned patients require invasive monitoring during hemodynamic stabilization; about 10% of burned patients require long-term cardiovascular or respiratory treatment because of inhalation injury, hypovolemic shock, burn shock, or nonthermal injuries. Some patients, after admission to a nonintensive burn unit, require transfer to a BICU for treatment of systemic infections or developing organ dysfunction.

Teamwork between multiple specialties is needed to support or replace vital organ function until recovery occurs. Vasoactive infusions, ventilatory management, and continuous hemofiltration are examples of treatments requiring intensive care facilities. Surgeons provide expert knowledge about wound management. Surgeons, anesthesiologists, and critical care specialists have experience in supporting various organ systems, including the heart and lungs. Experienced BICU nurses play an essential role in bedside care. Respiratory therapists provide pulmonary support.

This chapter describes the special requirements of critically ill, burned patients. BICU organization is outlined, as are requirements for personnel, equipment, and clinical expertise. Technological advances have made possible resuscitation of patients from burns that once were lethal; however, improving support has revealed a new spectrum of disease: multiple systems organ dysfunction and failure.

Organization of the Burn Intensive Care Unit

A BICU should be developed within a designated burn center or within a major trauma center, the latter providing the capability to treat both thermal and nonthermal injuries. The number of BICU beds required may be calculated from the incidence of severe burn injuries in the catchment area. The reported incidence of severe burn injuries is about 20 per 100 000 people.[1] American Burn Association (ABA) guidelines suggest an average census of at least four patients and at least 75 admissions annually to maintain both sufficient experience and acceptable access to specialized burn care.

Physical Plant

The capacity of a BICU can be estimated using figures for the surrounding population and the expected incidence of severe burns. In addition to 20 primary BICU admissions per 100 000 population, six readmissions per 100 000 are required for delayed complications. Most severely burned patients need intensive care at least on the day of admission. Inhalation injury, hypovolemic shock, burn shock, nonthermal injuries, and preexisting diseases mandate prolonged cardiopulmonary monitoring and support in approximately 10% of all burned in-patients. In this fraction, an average length of stay of 25 days, including readmission for delayed complications, results in a requirement of 170–200 BICU-patient-days per year per 100 000 population. The smallest, cost-effective BICU consists of four beds; because eight-bed units are more efficient, such a unit can serve a population of 1.5 million people.

An eight-bed BICU should be approximately 3000 ft^2. The minimum space required for each BICU bed, about 180 ft^2, is necessary to allow access for procedures, monitoring, and daily care. Support space is necessary for nursing and charting areas, office space, and storage. Additional capacity to permit isolation of severely infected patients is strongly recommended, but adds further space requirements.

Personnel

A BICU functions best with a team approach, including surgeons, intensivists, nurses, microbiologists, therapists, and psychologists. The ABA recommends a full-time BICU director to coordinate treatment protocols and education of personnel. A BICU also should have an alternate director and experienced medical staff. In teaching hospitals, two to three residents may be assigned to an eight-bed unit. To provide sufficient experience, the rotation should be at least 4 months in total duration. Both residents and faculty should be available around the clock to ensure continuous care by experienced medical personnel who are familiar with each patient.

Nursing personnel should be specially trained. One full-time registered nurse should be administratively responsible and should have an alternate. A nurse administrator should have 2 years of experience in intensive care and burn care, as well as appropriate training and experience in management.[1] Due to the high intensity of burn intensive care, at least three full-time equivalents are required per BICU bed to provide sufficient care around the clock.[3] Additional personnel are required for respiratory care, physical therapy, and clerical support. Students should be assigned for training rather than patient care.

Equipment

Each bed should be equipped to measure and record heart rate, EKG, noninvasive blood pressure, invasive pressures (at least two channels), and cardiac output. Continuous mixed venous saturation monitoring is optional. Weight and body temperature should be recorded. Ventilatory support must be available for all beds. Oxygen sources and central vacuum are required. A cardiac emergency cart with a battery-powered electrocardiograph, a defibrillator, and bag and mask resuscitators must be available. Infusion pumps for controlled fluid replacement, parenteral feeding, vasoactive drugs, and sedation are needed. A laboratory providing blood gas analysis and plasma electrolyte determinations should be readily accessible to the BICU.

At least one fiberoptic bronchoscope should be available for diagnosis and treatment; personnel should be experienced in bronchoscopy. To manage acute renal failure (ARF), occurring as an accompaniment of shock or sepsis, continuous hemofiltration,[4,5] continuous arteriovenous or venovenous hemodialysis, or conventional hemodialysis should be available. An eight-bed BICU should be capable of handling two patients with ARF.

Hospital Equipment and Consultants

Portable radiography must be available around the clock. Sonography, angiography, and computed tomography may be needed for diagnosis of accompanying nonthermal injuries and brain edema. To provide frequent, routine bacterial cultures, a microbiological laboratory must be available within the hospital. Consultants who should be available are listed in the guidelines of the ABA;[1] however, it is especially important to have access to internists, pediatricians, neurologists, infectious disease specialists, dermatologists, orthopedic surgeons, nephrologists, and radiologists.

Discharge from the BICU

A separate medical and nursing report should accompany the patient when transferred from the BICU to a burn unit or normal ward. Effective transfer of care requires communication about the initial injury, related injuries, coexisting diseases, diagnostic and therapeutic interventions, microbiological cultures, and recent treatments.

The nurse who has cared for the patient should personally transfer the patient to counteract anxiety about separation from the constant attention in the BICU. Most long-term patients regress to less mature behavior, may exhibit psychological disorders, and usually become psychologically dependent on the environment of the BICU. When faced with transfer, some patients report new symptoms and become so anxious that hypertension and tachycardia develop. In such cases, insensitivity and hasty reassurance are counterproductive. Patients must be carefully prepared for discharge, sometimes days in advance. It is important to review the hospital course, including early events that the patient may not recall. A frank and honest explanation of potential disabilities and rehabilitation needs is important.[6] Only with a realistic understanding of the extent of injuries can patients accept responsibility and make the efforts needed during recovery and rehabilitation to adjust to a new life.

Among the controversies in critical care is the dilemma of withdrawing care.[7,8] The central questions are when to stop and who makes the decision. Decisions ranging from 'Do not resuscitate' orders to reduction of organ support or to discontinuation of all life-supporting treatments should be individualized.[9] Though this decision rests ultimately with the responsible physician, structured conferences are recommended to address these issues and to develop consensus regarding a decision to continue interventions or to allow a patient to 'die with dignity'.[10] Inviting nonphysician members of the staff to participate in the decision builds their personal and professional self-esteem and binds the team members into a more cohesive group. A decision to forego additional therapy is then discussed with the patient and the patient's family. If the patient's wishes about continuing therapy are not known, the role of the family in decision making has been limited by the US Supreme Court.[11]

Organ System-Specific Management

Overview

Shock due to hemorrhage, trauma, sepsis, or burns produces cellular injury and death through similar common pathways. Preserving tissue perfusion or, theoretically, blocking mediator pathways may prevent or ameliorate life-threatening complications.[12] During shock, bacteria and endotoxin enter the systemic circulation from the large pool of bacteria in the gut. During circulatory failure, the splanchnic region experiences reduced blood flow due to the vasoconstricting properties of a variety of mediators, including thromboxane A_2. Reduced flow leads to ischemic mucosal injury[13] and may result in infection and sepsis, complications associated with mortality rates that may exceed 60%.[14,15] Once shock injures the microvasculature, resuscitation and restoration of tissue perfusion may be associated with reperfusion injury, in part due to production of oxygen free radicals. Infections, sepsis, and the systemic inflammatory response syndrome (SIRS) may lead to organ dysfunction, finally progressing to multiple systems organ failure (MSOF) and death.

MSOF, recognized only for the past 30 years, is defined as a combination of cardiovascular, respiratory, renal, hepatic, gastrointestinal, and neurological failure. Usually associated with a hyperdynamic hemodynamic and metabolic state, MSOF results from a generalized inflammatory reaction involving a cascade of mediating factors (i.e. tumor necrosis factor and interleukins) produced by macrophages, lymphocytes, and vascular endothelium.

The prevention as well as the treatment of MSOF depend on early correction of tissue hypoperfusion. Support and temporary replacement of the function of impaired organ systems and, perhaps, in the future, antagonism of mediators or immunotherapy may allow more specific treatment. Currently, only cardiopulmonary support, supplementation of impaired renal function, nutritional support, and antibiotics provide support.

After thermal injury, pathophysiological changes fall into three general phases: an initial critical phase, an intermediate phase, and a second critical phase. The *initial phase* is determined by the magnitude of the burn wound, the presence of inhalation injury, and the extent of associated injuries. The principal physiological derangement is loss of intravascular volume, mediated in part by locally increased microvascular permeability in the wound area. Fluid shifts to the interstitial space, causing wound edema, reducing venous return, and finally compressing arterial inflow. A decrease in the reflection coefficient (σ) produces massive losses of plasma into the interstitium. In burns affecting more than 40% TBSA, the release of inflammatory mediators from damaged tissues may cause systemic permeability changes. During the initial phase, the primary therapeutic goal is aggressive fluid resuscitation to rapidly achieve hemodynamic stability. If resuscitation is delayed or inadequate, the incidence of later, shock-induced complications increases.

The initial or acute phase after the burn injury lasts for about 24–48 hours. An *intermediate phase* is characterized by markedly increased metabolic rates. Core temperature is increased because the thermostatic control center in the hypothalamus is reset. During this catabolic phase, associated with rapid consumption of energy reserves, adequate calories must be provided. The mediators of the inflammatory response have been implicated in causing this hypermetabolic stress period as have catecholamines, corticosteroids, and glucagon. Heart rate is frequently increased to about 50% above normal.[16,17] Modulating the hypermetabolic response with β-blocking agents decreases caloric requirements and protein catabolism but permits an adequate cardiovascular response.[18] During this hypermetabolic state, human recombinant growth factor may restore positive nitrogen balance, an effect that appears to be most dramatic in burned children.[19–23] Insulin-like growth factor-1, a second messenger of growth factor, appears to produce similar effects in adult burned patients.[24,25] Due to insulin deficiency and peripheral insulin resistance, glucose intolerance may develop; hyperglycemia may cause an osmotic diuresis which can be misinterpreted as volume repletion. During the intermediate phase, the therapeutic goals are optimal tissue perfusion, nutritional support, and early wound closure to prevent sepsis and MSOF.

Pneumonia, sepsis, and organ failure are the most common complications during the *second critical phase*, characterized by generalized increased microvascular permeability. Mortality rates increase to more than 60% once these complications have occurred.[14] Although thermal injury leads to depressed immunity, the mechanism remains controversial.[26] This stage, which begins with SIRS, reflects activation of the immune system in response to bacteria and their toxins or to the secretion of various mediators by injured tissues. During this phase, the primary therapeutic goal is preservation of oxygen delivery.

Cardiovascular System

Physiological principles and monitoring

Treatment of the cardiovascular responses to acute burns requires an understanding of both cardiac and vascular responses and the effects of treatment on each component. The effects of interventions should be monitored carefully and reevaluated frequently.

The four main determinants of cardiac function are: (1) ventricular preload or end-diastolic resting fiber length, (2) myocardial contractility, (3) ventricular afterload, and (4) heart rate and rhythm (**Table 31.1**). Ventricular preload, best measured clinically as end-diastolic volume (EDV), is not routinely assessable, although transthoracic echocardiography or transesophageal echocardiography (TEE)[27] noninvasive techniques provide data about the functional state of the ventricle, the cardiac valves, flow characteristics, and ventricular dimensions. Instead, we measure end-diastolic *pressures*: central venous pressure (CVP), right atrial pressure (RAP), or pulmonary artery occlusion pressure (PAOP). These estimates of preload do not accurately reflect changes in fiber length; in addition, the cardiac pressure–volume relationship can be altered in burned or septic patients.

Table 31.1 Determinants of cardiac function

Physiological variable	Clinical estimation
Preload	PAOP; CVP; end-diastolic volume (by radionuclide scan or echocardiography)
Contractility	LVSWI; RVSWI; ejection fraction (radionuclide scan, echocardiography, or RVEF pulmonary artery catheter)
Afterload	SVRI; PVRI
Heart rate and rhythm	Electrocardiography

PAOP, pulmonary artery occlusion pressure; CVP, central venous pressure; LVSWI, left ventricular stroke work index; RVSWI, right ventricular stroke work index; RVEF, right ventricular ejection fraction; SVRI, systemic vascular resistance index; PVRI, pulmonary vascular resistance index.

Although many factors, including intrathoracic and transmural pressures, influence PAOP, this pressure provides the best estimate of left atrial pressure and therefore left ventricular preload. Pulmonary vasoconstriction, associated with burns or sepsis,[28,29] can result in striking differences between left and right heart pressure.[30,31] High central venous or right atrial pressures, elevated pulmonary arterial pressures and normal or low PAOPs may result from increased right ventricular outflow resistance. Using a canine sepsis model, Parrillo *et al.* demonstrated that reversible ventricular dilatation (also evident in septic humans) was necessary to allow the increased cardiac output seen in hyperdynamic sepsis.[32] Therefore, because of changes in myocardial compliance, neither CVP nor PAOP may give adequate information about volume status.

Myocardial contractility cannot be assessed clinically; calculating left ventricular stroke work index (LVSWI) as a function of PAOP provides an alternative estimate of contractility which may be monitored in response to interventions. LVSWI is calculated from the formula:

$$\text{LVSWI} = \text{SVI}\ (\text{MAP} - \text{PAOP}) \times 0.0136$$

where SVI is the stroke volume index (cardiac index ÷ heart rate). Left ventricular afterload can be estimated clinically by calculating systemic vascular resistance index (SVRI), by the formula:

$$\text{SVRI} = \frac{\text{MAP} - \text{CVP}}{\text{CI}} \times 80$$

where MAP is the mean arterial pressure and CI is the cardiac index.

Heart rate and rhythm are monitored by continuous electrocardiography. In addition to cardiac function, the adequacy of peripheral circulation must be assessed indirectly, e.g. by using urinary output to assess renal perfusion or mixed venous oxygen saturation ($S\bar{v}O_2$) to assess total systemic perfusion.

Cardiovascular monitoring should be appropriate to the severity of illness. Without invasive procedures, clinicians can assess blood pressure, heart rate and rhythm, oxygen saturation, temperature, urinary output, respiratory pattern, mental status, and capillary refill. In critically ill patients, more invasive measurements may provide important information which justifies the risk of morbidity.

In hemodynamically unstable patients, direct measurement of blood pressure using an arterial catheter provides beat-to-beat monitoring and allows repeated blood sampling. In addition, in patients in whom the extremities are edematous or injured, blood pressure cuffs may be impractical. Inspection of the arterial waveform provides subjective information regarding volume status and myocardial contractility, especially during rapid resuscitation. In hypovolemic patients, positive-pressure ventilation causes an exaggerated fall in blood pressure and greater changes in the amplitude of the arterial waveform. The upslope of the arterial wave is less steep in the presence of reduced myocardial contractility.

CVP measurements can be helpful when large fluid shifts are expected or infusion of large volumes is necessary. CVP catheters also permit repeated blood sampling and provide secure intravenous access in patients who have limited peripheral access. Although blood gas samples from a CVP catheter are not truly mixed venous blood, such samples may show trends in venous oxygenation that reflect systemic oxygen extraction and peripheral perfusion. Pulmonary artery catheters, inserted through the antecubital, jugular, subclavian or femoral veins, are useful to measure cardiac output, pulmonary arterial pressure and PAOP, and to provide access for intermittent measurement of $S\bar{v}O_2$. More expensive pulmonary artery catheters allow continuous oximetric measurement of $S\bar{v}O_2$ or calculation of right ventricular ejection fraction.

Although pulmonary artery catheters provide important information for the management of critically ill patients, the mechanical and infectious risks of catheterization must be weighed against the therapeutic goals of preventing subclinical tissue hypoperfusion and late MSOF. Autopsy studies of nonburned patients have shown a high incidence (from 33 to 91%) of endocardial damage in patients with pulmonary artery catheters in place at the time of death; the incidence of endocardial lesions is 20 times greater in patients dying with than without pulmonary artery catheters.[33] These endocardial lesions may serve as sites for infection, especially in burned patients. Although invasive monitoring can be terminated after the patient has been stabilized, it is far more difficult to reverse multiple organ failure and septic complications.

Hemodynamic therapy: preload augmentation

During the initial phase, intravascular volume must be restored. Associated injuries or hemorrhage may increase fluid requirements. Various formulas have been used to guide acute repletion of intravascular volume and avoid under-resuscitation. Due to fluid and protein losses, most patients require fluid in addition to the quantities proposed by the Parkland/Baxter formula (i.e. 4 ml lactated Ringer's solution/kg/% TBSA burned during the first 24 hours, one-half within the first 8 hours. Burned children require 5000 ml/m^2 TBSA for burned areas plus an additional 2000 ml/m^2 TBSA for unburned areas (one-half within the first 8 hours).

Inhalation injury requires fluid administration of approximately 2 ml/kg/% area burned in addition to the calculated resuscitation volume. This additional volume may actually decrease the development of pulmonary edema by reducing polymorphonuclear leukocyte deposition in the pulmonary microcirculation. In sheep with burns plus inhalation injury, under-resuscitation produced more pulmonary dysfunction than over-resuscitation (**Table 31.2**).[34]

Fluid resuscitation should be assessed at least hourly, basing on monitored criteria. The single best monitor of initial fluid replacement, urinary output, should exceed 0.5 ml/kg/h in an adult and 1 ml/kg/h in a child. In patients with high-voltage electrical burns and crush injuries, which increase the risk for renal tubular obstruction from myoglobinuria and hemoglobinuria, urinary output should be maintained at 1–2 ml/kg/h.

In shocked, vasoconstricted patients, heart rate and pulse pressure are more sensitive indicators of hemodynamic status than blood pressure; arterial hypotension occurs later. Clear mental status and brisk capillary refill are additional clinical indicators of adequate perfusion. With adequate resuscitation, cardiac output begins to rise and usually returns to normal by 18–24 hours postinjury; however, plasma volume and blood volume continue to fall for another 12–24 hours and return to normal only after 48 hours postburn.[35] By this time, cardiac output has increased to supranormal levels, reflecting the onset of postburn hypermetabolism. This sequence emphasizes the value of cardiac output measurements as a guide to resuscitation.[36]

In the *second* critical phase, in which secondary infectious complications develop, hypovolemia, a major factor contributing to circulatory instability and failure in septic patients,[37–39] must be treated adequately. Venous pooling, increased microvascular permeability, and fluid losses due to vomiting, diarrhea, and inappropriate polyuria reduce intravascular volume and ventricular preload. Besides splanchnic and hepatic venous pooling, a generalized increase in systemic venous capacitance, including skeletal muscle, lung and other vascular beds causes effective hypovolemia. Fluid shifts from the plasma volume to the interstitial space occur systemically in sepsis, causing tissue edema. The decreased σ produces losses of water and protein.

Resuscitation with crystalloid solutions further decreases colloid osmotic pressure, resulting in additional fluid shifting from the intravascular to the interstitial space. Reduced colloid osmotic pressure may negatively influence the matrix of the endothelial

Table 31.2 Response of sheep 12 hours after smoke inhalation combined with two levels of fluid resuscitation (maintenance vs. resuscitation)

Group	*n*	Cardiac index (l/min/m^2)	PaO_2 (mmHg)	LQ (ml/h)	PAP (mmHg)	L/P Ratio
Smoke, maintenance (SM)	6	3.5 ± 0.3*	66 ± 3*	40 ± 9*	24 ± 4	0.81 ± 0.05†
Smoke, resuscitation (SR)	6	4.1 ± 0.4	89 ± 7	17 ± 3‡	21 ± 2	0.73 ± 0.03
Control, maintenance (CM)	6	4.7 ± 0.5	96 ± 8	7 ± 1.9	20 ± 1	0.66 ± 0.05

LQ, lymph flow; LP, lymph-to-plasma protein concentration ratio; PAP, pulmonary arterial pressure.
* $p < 0.05$, SM versus CM + SR; † $p < 0.05$, SM versus CM; ‡ $p < 0.05$, SR versus CM + SM by three-way analysis of variance and Duncan's multiple-range test.
Animals in the smoke maintenance group (inhalation injury; *n*=6) were given 70 ml/m^2/24 h (maintenance) 5% dextrose in lactated Ringer's solution; animals in the smoke resuscitation group (inhalation injury; *n*=6) received 140 ml/m^2/24 h of 5% dextrose in lactated Ringer's solution; the control group (smoke-free air inhalation; *n*=6) received maintenance fluids.
Reprinted with permission from Herndon *et al.*[34]

membrane.[40,41] Clinical experience suggests that colloid osmotic pressure should be maintained > 16 mmHg during this phase.

Another therapeutic goal in sepsis is to maintain an appropriate hematocrit.[42–44] In critically ill patients, systemic oxygen delivery ($\dot{D}O_2$) and oxygen consumption ($\dot{V}O_2$) are maximal with a hematocrit ranging between 27 and 33%.[45,46] Data inadequately clarify whether higher or lower hematocrits improve $\dot{V}O_2$ and prevent lactic acidemia; continued controversy underscores the balance between arterial oxygen content (CaO_2) and blood rheology, i.e. increased hematocrit increases blood viscosity which reduces capillary blood flow.

Preload can be excessively augmented, exceeding the optimal point on the ventricular function curve, as a consequence of over-resuscitation, fluid mobilization from the interstitial space, or myocardial depression. The risk of fluid overload should be weighed carefully against the consequences of under-resuscitation. Peripheral edema is often a consequence of increased microvascular permeability or decreased colloid osmotic pressure rather than excessive fluid administration. If preload must be reduced, furosemide is especially appropriate for patients with normal cardiac and renal function. Hemodialysis or hemofiltration are appropriate for patients with normal cardiac function and renal failure. Vasodilators, i.e. nitroglycerin or angiotensin-converting enzyme inhibitors, are appropriate for patients with reduced cardiac function.

Hemodynamic therapy: inotropic support

Although inotropic support may be necessary during any phase after burn injury, it is most likely to be required during the second critical phase. Two stages of sepsis, a hyperdynamic (early) and a hypodynamic (late), can be distinguished. The hyperdynamic response with low systemic vascular resistance (SVR) and increased cardiac output[47] appears in part to be a response to increased metabolic needs in peripheral tissues. Maldistribution of flow and arteriovenous shunting necessitate even higher cardiac output. Antagonism of vasodilation, though arithmetically reasonable, is relatively ineffective. Despite increased cardiac output, myocardial depression is evident in experimental and human sepsis (**Figure 31.1**).[48–50] Various mediators, including nitric oxide, have

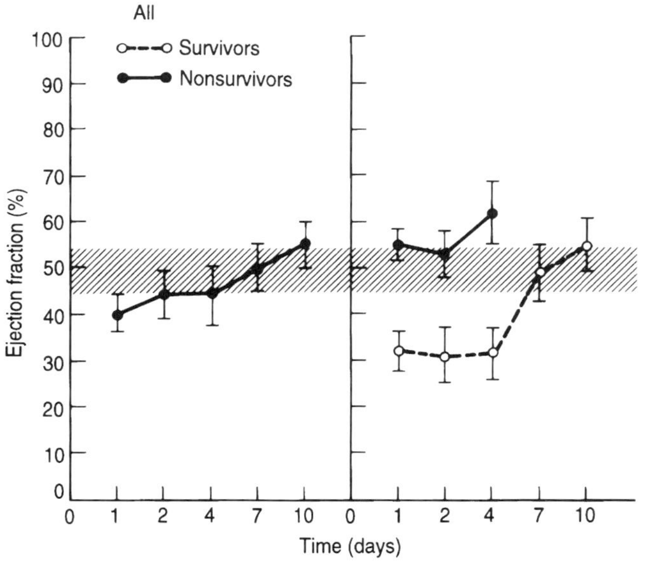

Fig. 31.1 Ejection fraction (EF) in patients surviving and not surviving severe sepsis. During days 1–10 of severe sepsis, EF was profoundly, but reversibly depressed, with the depression actually more evident in those who survived (open circles) than in nonsurvivors (closed circles). The hatched area shows the normal range of EF. Reprinted with permission from Parker et al.[50]

been implicated in septic peripheral vasodilation.[51,52] The magnitude and severity of myocardial depression have been directly related to the severity of the septic process, the extent of the systemic inflammatory response, and outcome.[32] The apparent paradox of increased cardiac output and decreased contractility is explained by physiological afterload reduction (vasodilation) and tachycardia. The later, hypodynamic stage of sepsis, in which cardiac output is low and SVR is normal or high, often is characterized by failing responsiveness to cardiovascular support. The cardiovascular treatment of sepsis is based on early detection and correction of physiologic abnormalities.

If intravascular volume is restored and $\dot{D}O_2$ remains inadequate, positive inotropic drugs should be considered. In general, hemodynamic monitoring is required to guide acute inotropic or vasodilator interventions in critically ill patients. Noninvasive assessment of preload is notoriously inaccurate. Complex hemodynamic interventions can be quantified and refined using the measurements and calculations available from pulmonary artery catheterization. Myocardial performance can be enhanced pharmacologically to increase systemic blood flow, improve $\dot{D}O_2$, and reverse anaerobic metabolism.

To individualize therapy, pharmacological effects on both the myocardium and the vascular smooth vessel must be considered. Myocardial contractility can be increased either by activation of β_1-receptors, activating adenylate cyclase and increasing cyclic AMP (cAMP), or α_1-receptors, causing cAMP-independent inotropy. Adenylate cyclase transforms AMP to its cyclic form cAMP, a second messenger that promotes calcium influx into cells. Experimentally, direct activators of adenylate cyclase and calcium channels also have been investigated.[53,56] The enzyme phosphodiesterase (PDE) metabolizes cAMP to ADP. Blocking PDE increases intracellular cAMP concentrations.

In vascular smooth vessel cells, α_1-receptor agonists produce vasoconstriction, whereas β_2-agonists, PDE inhibitors, and calcium channel blockers cause vasodilation by changing intracellular calcium concentrations and elevating intracellular cAMP and cyclic GMP (cGMP). Endothelial-derived relaxing factors (EDRF), one of which is nitric oxide (NO), play a role in regulating vascular smooth vessel tone.[57] In normal individuals, NO is metabolized from L-arginine by a constitutive, calcium-dependent form of the enzyme nitric oxide synthase. A calcium-independent, inducible form of this enzyme, demonstrated in experimental sepsis, may be partially responsible for septic vasodilation (**Figure 31.2**).[58] Elevated levels of nitrite and nitrate, the stable end products of NO, have been found in the plasma after trauma[59] and in adults[59–61] and newborn infants with sepsis.[62] In addition, NO mediates the endothelial-dependent relaxation caused by α_2-receptor agonists.[63,64]

Positive inotropic therapy increases stroke volume and improves $\dot{D}O_2$. Norepinephrine, epinephrine, and dopamine, which combine inotropic and vasoconstricting properties, can be termed 'inoconstrictors'. Dobutamine, dopexamine, and PDE inhibitors amrinone, milrinone, and enoximone combine positive inotropic and vasodilatory effects, hence the term 'inodilators'. The PDE inhibitors possess a positive lusitropic effect, i.e. they promote myocardial relaxation by increasing intracellular concentrations of cAMP and cGMP. NO may exert similar effects. In sepsis, PDE inhibitors, which do not act through β-receptor stimulation, may improve inotropic effects or cause vasodilation even though adrenergic receptors are downregulated as a consequence of continuous adrenergic stimulation. Dopamine in low concentrations (<4 μg/kg per min) and dopexamine are dopaminergic agonists in the splanchnic and renal vasculature, resulting in increased regional blood flow.[65] Renal vasodilation produced by dopamine may protect against renal ischemia by antagonizing norepinephrine-induced

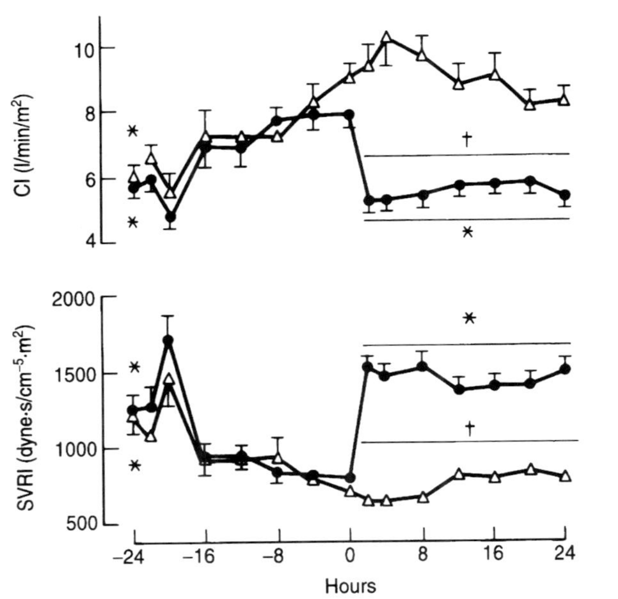

*Fig. 31.2 Cardiac index (CI) and systemic resistance index (SVRI) as a function of time during continuous infusion of low-dose endotoxin in awake, chronically instrumented sheep. The endotoxin infusion continued from –24 hours to +24 hours. At 0 hours, 12 sheep (closed circles, treatment group) received 25 mg/kg of the nitric oxide synthase inhibitor N^{ω}-nitro-L-arginine methyl ester (L-NAME); eight sheep (open triangles, control group) received the carrier. The hyperdynamic state persisted in the control group, whereas it was immediately reversed by L-NAME. Data are presented as mean ± SEM. If the error bars are not seen, they are within the symbol. *p < 0.05 vs. 0 hour; †p < 0.05 treatment vs. control. Reprinted with permission from Meyer* et al.[58]

vasoconstriction.[66] Myocardial oxygen consumption is increased by norepinephrine, epinephrine, isoproterenol, and dopamine, whereas dobutamine has only minor effects and PDE inhibitors actually reduce myocardial oxygen uptake.[67]

Hemodynamic therapy: afterload manipulation

In sepsis, right and left ventricular afterload are strikingly different. Increases in right ventricular afterload, caused in part by thromboxane-induced vasoconstriction, contrast with systemic vasodilation, which reduces left ventricular afterload.[68,69] Intravenously administered drugs affect both the pulmonary and systemic circulations.

Some vasodilators selectively dilate the pulmonary circulation; others dilate both the pulmonary and systemic circulations. Prostaglandin E_2 demonstrates nearly specific pulmonary vasodilation in pulmonary hypertension induced by U-46619, a thromboxane A_2 agonist.[70] In contrast, nitroglycerin, sodium nitroprusside, and hydralazine, which are nonspecific vasodilators, cause systemic vasodilation and may precipitate hypotension, especially in septic patients.

In some septic patients, pathologic vasodilation is so severe that regional perfusion pressure to the brain, heart, and kidneys may be inadequate. Arterial constrictors may then be needed to increase cerebral, coronary, and renal perfusion (**Table 31.3**).[71] Increased perfusion pressure must be balanced against excessive vasoconstriction.

During the acute phase of hypovolemic shock, increased afterload may be desirable as a temporizing treatment until intravascular volume has been restored. To achieve this goal, α-receptor agonists, such as norepinephrine or high-dose dopamine, may be used. Vasoconstrictors can normalize blood pressure and improve myocardial and cerebral perfusion until sufficient volume is infused to increase $\dot{D}O_2$. Prolonged use of vasoconstriction may improve regional perfusion at the expense of the splanchnic circulation, resulting in ischemic damage to the gut.

Vasodilators are of greatest value in patients in whom blood pressure is acceptable, left ventricular function is compromised, and $\dot{D}O_2$ is inadequate. Systemic vascular resistance is a dynamic variable, reflecting both pharmacological effects and secondary physiological influences. Thus, it is common to observe a dramatic decrease in endogenous vasoconstriction as resuscitation progresses.

Table 31.3 Hemodynamic values during the control period and 20 min after beginning a 0.5 μg/kg·min NE infusion (mean ± SD)

Variable	Control	NE 0.5 μg/kg·min	*p* Value
HR (beat/min)	142 ± 22	136 ± 19	<0.02
MPAP (mmHg)	16 ± 4	15 ± 4	NS
PAOP (mmHg)	8 ± 3	7 ± 3	NS
SAP (mmHg)	77 ± 10	99 ± 15	<0.01
DAP (mmHg)	32 ± 12	44 ± 12	<0.001
MAP (mmHg)	48 ± 11	62 ± 10	<0.001
CI (L/min·m^2)	5.2 ± 2.4	5.4 ± 2.4	NS
SVI (ml/beat·m^2)	37 ± 15	39 ± 14	NS
SVRI (dyne·s/cm^5·m^2)	700 ± 290	899 ± 277	<0.001
UF (ml/h)	22 ± 21	51 ± 37	<0.01

NE, norepinephrine; HR, heart rate; MPAP, mean pulmonary artery pressure; PAOP, pulmonary artery occlusion pressure; SAP, systolic arterial pressure; DAP, diastolic arterial pressure; MAP, mean arterial pressure; CI, cardiac index; SVI, stroke volume index; SVRI, systemic vascular resistance index; UF, urinary flow; NS, nonsignificant.
Reprinted with permission from Desjars *et al.*[71]

Goals of hemodynamic therapy

The conventional approach to circulatory failure is to restore hemodynamic variables to normal values and to titrate hemodynamic support by using urinary output as an indicator of peripheral perfusion. The renal circulation is one of the first regional circulations compromised during hypovolemia and after thermal injury.[72,73] In addition, prevention of renal failure greatly simplifies care of the critically ill and improves mortality.

In septic, critically burned, or otherwise traumatized patients, restoration of normal blood pressure and hemoglobin and maintenance of urinary output may not insure adequate tissue perfusion. In prospective clinical studies, Bland and Shoemaker[74] demonstrated that mean blood pressure is not different in survivors and nonsurvivors of critical illness. Despite a normal blood pressure and cardiac output, microvascular blood flow may be unevenly distributed and tissue hypoxia may occur; subclinical tissue hypoperfusion, a cause of delayed MSOF, may not be detected by routine hemodynamic monitoring.[75] Calculation of $\dot{D}O_2$ and $\dot{V}O_2$ provides the best hemodynamic means of predicting which patients will survive and may provide the most appropriate goals for resuscitation. $\dot{D}O_2$ is calculated from the equation:

$$\dot{D}O_2 = CI \times CaO_2$$

where CI is the cardiac index and $CaO_2 = PaO_2 \times 0.0031 + Hb \times SaO_2 \times 1.36$. To maintain adequate $\dot{D}O_2$, a Hb concentration of 10–11.5

g/dl or a hematocrit of 30–35% appears desirable. If Hb is less, CI must be proportionally increased to maintain $\dot{D}O_2$.

To prevent the progression from subclinical hypoperfusion to MSOF, invasive monitoring and aggressive therapy should be introduced early. The common approach of continuing noninvasive, basic monitoring until therapeutic interventions have failed may waste important time. If empirical volume expansion is ineffective or hazardous, invasive monitoring is essential. CVP or pulmonary artery catheters should be positioned percutaneously through a nonburned area to reduce the risk of catheter-related bacteremia, and tip placement should be confirmed radiographically. Placement of a pulmonary artery catheter through an indwelling introducer permits volume replacement through the additional lumen.

Pulmonary System

Pathophysiology of ARDS

Burn injury is one of the systemic insults which may initiate the Adult Respiratory Distress Syndrome (ARDS), the clinical manifestation of acute lung injury characterized by dyspnea, severe hypoxemia, and decreased lung compliance with radiographic evidence of diffuse bilateral pulmonary infiltrates.[76] In burned patients, lung damage is more commonly the result of a systemic process initiated by products of burned tissue, infection, or inflammation, but ARDS also can be the result of a direct lung injury from smoke inhalation. Characteristically, alveolar consolidation with fluid, protein, and inflammatory cells accompanies a normal PAOP (i.e. pulmonary edema is noncardiogenic). Increased pulmonary capillary permeability results in increased movement of fluid from the intravascular to the interstitial space.

Respiratory insufficiency after major thermal injury generally occurs at two intervals after injury. During the *early* period, smoke inhalation injury or chemical burns to the airways result in increased capillary permeability, mucosal irritation with bronchorrhea, and cough. Ciliary dysfunction increases the risk of bronchopulmonary infection. Three to four days after smoke inhalation, the damaged mucosa becomes necrotic and begins to slough. Increasingly viscous secretions may lead to distal airway obstruction and atelectasis. As airway inflammation and bronchial blood flow increase, diffuse interstitial edema may develop. During the early interval, the occurrence of secondary pulmonary infection and the subsequent development of ARDS depends on the integrity of host defenses and the aggressiveness of pulmonary support.

In the *late* interval after burn injury, bacteria and bacterial products, derived from burn wound tissue or gut contents, initiate the systemic inflammatory response. Cytokines are secreted by resident tissue macrophages. Furthermore, endotoxin and bacteria promote a proinflammatory, procoagulant endothelial cell phenotype, stimulate production of neutrophil proteases and oxidants, and activate multiple humoral protein cascades, including complement and coagulation systems.[77] Products of these activated leukocytes and protein cascades may, in turn, further impair microcirculatory flow. Increased endothelial permeability and impaired lymphatic function result in noncardiogenic pulmonary edema, producing a mild-to-moderate decrease in lung compliance and functional residual lung capacity (FRC). The pulmonary shunt fraction (Q_S/Q_T) increases as does ventilation/perfusion (V/Q) inhomogeneity; initially hypoxemia improves if inspired oxygen is increased.

Pulmonary venous and capillary congestion, accompanied by endothelial cell swelling and necrosis, is a characteristic feature of early ARDS. Most patients develop pulmonary arterial hypertension within a few days. Vasoconstriction (in part mediated by thromboxane A_2) and increased pulmonary interstitial pressure increase pulmonary vascular resistance. Increasing interstitial and alveolar edema contributes to collapse of distal airways. Atelectasis further increases Q_S/Q_T. Using the multiple inert gas elimination technique, Dantzker *et al.*[78] demonstrated that most of the hypoxemia in ARDS was explained by distribution of blood flow to unventilated lung regions. Ralph *et al.*[79] also found pure shunt in half of their ARDS patients; in the remainder perfusion to low V_A/Q regions always contributed less than Q_S/Q_T to hypoxemia.

When increasing inspired oxygen no longer adequately improves hypoxemia, positive end-expiratory pressure (PEEP) may reduce Q_S/Q_T, in part by recruiting closed airway units, as evidenced by an increased FRC.[80] For patients with ARDS, the magnitude of Q_S/S_T versus V/Q inhomogeneity determines the response of PaO_2 to an increase in FiO_2. If Q_S/S_T is high and 'fixed', only PEEP may improve oxygenation;[81] however, PEEP does not change the severity and extent of lung damage, i.e. extravascular lung water is not decreased.[82] In patients with ARDS, lung density measured by computerized tomographic scanning (CT) correlated with gas exchange, as the quantity of radiodense, and presumably nonventilated, lung regions increased in concert with both V_D/V_T and Q_S/Q_T, while PaO_2 decreased.[83]

In contrast to cardiogenic pulmonary edema, the efflux of protein-rich fluid occurs at a considerably lower hydrostatic pressure in patients with ARDS.[84] Because microvascular permeability is increased, pulmonary capillary pressure (P_c)[85,86] is the major driving force for fluid from the pulmonary microvasculature, exceeding capillary oncotic pressure (π_c) as a key factor in Starling's equation:

$$Q = kA\,[(P_c - P_i) + \sigma\,(\pi_i - \pi_c)]$$

where Q is the fluid filtration, k the capillary filtration coefficient (conductivity of water), A the area of the capillary membrane, P_c the capillary hydrostatic pressure, P_i the interstitial hydrostatic pressure, σ the reflection coefficient for albumin, π_i the interstitial colloid osmotic pressure, and π_c the capillary colloid oncotic pressure. As plasma enters the interstitial space, the transvascular colloid osmotic pressure gradient ($\pi_i - \pi_c$) disappears; P_c and the rate of lymphatic drainage become the major determinants of extravascular fluid accumulation. There is no evidence that changing π_c alters pulmonary edema formation in ARDS.

As the alveolar lining deteriorates and fluid moves into the alveoli, proteins, particularly fibrinogen, accumulate in alveolar fluid and may inactivate surfactant, further increasing the tendency to atelectasis. Type I alveolar cells, which cover 90% of the gas exchange surface, are rapidly destroyed as they are highly vulnerable and incapable of reproduction, leaving a denuded alveolar basement except where the cuboidal type II epithelial cells are present. Protein and other debris in the alveoli begin to precipitate as hyaline-like membranes that progressively organize to line the alveoli. The alveolar septum thickens as it is infiltrated by increasing numbers of fibroblasts, plasma cells, leukocytes, and histiocytes. Capillary injury along with severe diffuse microatelectasis becomes increasingly apparent at this stage.[87]

As gas exchange deteriorates, hypoxic vasoconstriction plays an important role in diverting blood flow from low V/Q units towards better ventilated units, reducing Q_S/Q_T and improving PaO_2, but potentially increasing pulmonary vascular resistance (PVR) and pulmonary artery pressure (PAP). Vasodilator therapy, using an agent such as nitroprusside to reduce PVR, thus decreasing right ventricular afterload, may increase cardiac output, antagonize hypoxic pulmonary vasoconstriction,[88] increase Q_S/Q_T, and decrease PaO_2.[89–91] Cardiac output-mediated changes in Q_S/Q_T are less prominent at high levels of PEEP.[90,91]

The four clinical phases of ARDS

The pulmonary pathophysiological abnormalities produced by this inflammatory process can be divided into four clinical phases:[92–94]

- Phase I. The injury and resuscitation phase of ARDS is characterized by altered tissue perfusion and metabolism. Arterial PaO_2 is normal and $PaCO_2$ is normal or slightly decreased. Q_S/Q_T is < 15%. Auscultation of the lungs reveals only scattered rales. Chest radiography is unremarkable.
- Phase II. The subclinical respiratory distress phase is characterized by hypocapnia and an increased alveolar-arterial oxygen difference. Mild, diffuse infiltrates appear on chest x-ray, suggesting patchy atelectasis and perihilar pulmonary congestion.
- Phase III. Established respiratory distress includes continued hypocapnia, now often more severe ($PaCO_2$ ~ 20 mmHg), and hypoxemia (PaO_2<60 mmHg on room air). Q_S/Q_T is > 20%. Increasing pulmonary edema and progressive confluence of the diffuse infiltrates are apparent on chest radiography.
- Phase IV. Severe respiratory distress is characterized by increasingly severe hypoxemia (Q_S/Q_T>30%). The dead space ventilation ratio (V_D/V_T, normally 0.3) may exceed 0.6. Metabolic acidosis may develop. Chest x-rays often show nearly complete opacification ('white-out').

Clinical management of ARDS

Management of ARDS combines supportive measures along with treatment of the initial disorder, i.e. excision of infected burn wounds, volume replacement, and antimicrobial and/or antifungal agents. Unfortunately, at present, no specific therapeutic modality exists which will halt or reverse either the capillary leak or the later pulmonary fibrosis.

Physiotherapy, including chest percussion, vibration therapy, and dependent drainage, is a method to prevent or treat secretion retention and atelectasis. Position changes ('side–side–back') help to mobilize secretions, and, by changing *V/Q* relationships, may improve gas exchange. Elevation of the head and chest decreases the pressure put on the diaphragm by the abdominal viscera and improves FRC. Nasogastric drainage, to decrease abdominal distension, also improves thoracic compliance.

Airway Support. In patients with ARDS, a secure airway is essential. Oxygen administration and continuous positive airway pressure (CPAP) by mask are noninvasive, but usually serve only as short-term or temporizing measures. Severe hypoxemia accompanied by labored breathing, tachypnea, and difficulty clearing secretions usually must be treated with an artificial airway as part of therapy.

Tracheostomy vs. Endotracheal Intubation. Endotracheal intubation is the technique of choice to secure the airway in acutely burned patients. Early tracheostomy is associated with multiple complications, including higher infection rates, tracheomalacia, and tracheal stenosis.[95] Oral intubation often is preferable to nasotracheal intubation because the latter carries the risk of infections of the maxillary sinus and subsequent sepsis. The advantages of the nasotracheal route include placement without direct laryngoscopy, and greater ease in caring for neck or mouth burns.[96] Only nasotracheal routes are used at some children's burn units. Orotracheal tubes may be somewhat less comfortable, but long-term mechanical ventilation in sedated patients can be performed with few complications, when using high-volume, low-pressure cuffed tubes.

It is mandatory to properly secure the endotracheal tube, but this can be difficult in the presence of facial burns. Continuous movements of the tube cause increased requirements for sedation and may damage the tracheal epithelium. Unplanned self-extubation, usually resulting in the need for prompt reintubation, is not entirely avoidable; however, careful use of sedation, passive restraint, and vigilant bedside personnel reduce the incidence.

Mechanical Ventilatory Support. **Table 31.4** summarizes an approach to the management of ARDS. Three key respiratory functions, oxygenation, CO_2 elimination, and clearance of secretions, may fail in concert or separately. Failure of a single component may require an artificial airway and respiratory support. Continued subjective and objective assessment of these functions determines the timing of intubation and extubation. Clinical observation of respiratory rate, respiratory pattern, nasal flaring, and use of accessory muscles provides important information. Quantitative measurements of peak negative pressure and forced vital capacity provide objective data. Trends in blood gases and in oxygen saturation by pulse oximetry are more important than isolated values. A patient should be provided with ventilatory support if these observations suggest a high probability of further deterioration.

Table 31.4 Strategy for managing ARDS

Humidified gas for spontaneous or artificial ventilation
Artificial airway for bronchial toilet if secretions unmanageable
Increase FRC (using PEEP) to reduce toxic FiO_2 (ideally ≤ 0.5)
Add mechanical ventilation if WOB excessive
Adjust tidal volumes and PEEP according to PaO_2, FiO_2, and PIP
Avoid neuromuscular blockers if possible
Consider specialized measures (ECMO, permissive hypercapnia) to improve gas exchange and oxygen delivery while reducing pulmonary trauma

ARDS, adult respiratory distress syndrome; FRC, functional residual capacity; PEEP, positive end-expiratory pressure; WOB, work of breathing; PIP, peak inspiratory pressure; ECMO, extracorporeal membrane oxygenation

In clinical practice, a variety of ventilatory techniques are used in the management of acute lung injury. All ventilatory techniques have in common several key control functions (**Figure 31.3**): those that initiate the mechanical ventilatory cycle, those that limit the cycle, and those that terminate the cycle. Clinical and investigational modes will be briefly described below.

Continuous positive airway pressure (CPAP), in spontaneously breathing patients, is a simple technique to improve FRC. CPAP may be applied either by tight face mask or through an artificial airway. Exhalation should occur through a threshold resistor rather than a flow-restricting device. Mask CPAP requires an awake, unrestrained patient with adequate gastric decompression to avoid passive or active regurgitation and aspiration.

Positive end-expiratory pressure (PEEP). As CPAP improves FRC in spontaneously breathing patients, PEEP improves FRC when added to mechanical ventilation. PEEP often allows reduction of FiO_2 to nontoxic levels; however, the 'optimal' level of PEEP is controversial.[97,98] PEEP is adjusted to provide at least adequate oxygenation (PaO_2> mmHg) on a nontoxic oxygen concentration (FiO_2 < 0.6) without adversely affecting cardiac output or $\dot{D}O_2$. In severe ARDS, these conflicting goals may be unobtainable. Hemodynamic monitoring and augmentation of cardiac output by increasing preload or adding inotropic agents is usually necessary at high levels (<15 cmH_2O) of PEEP.

PEEP may be adjusted by determining the level at which

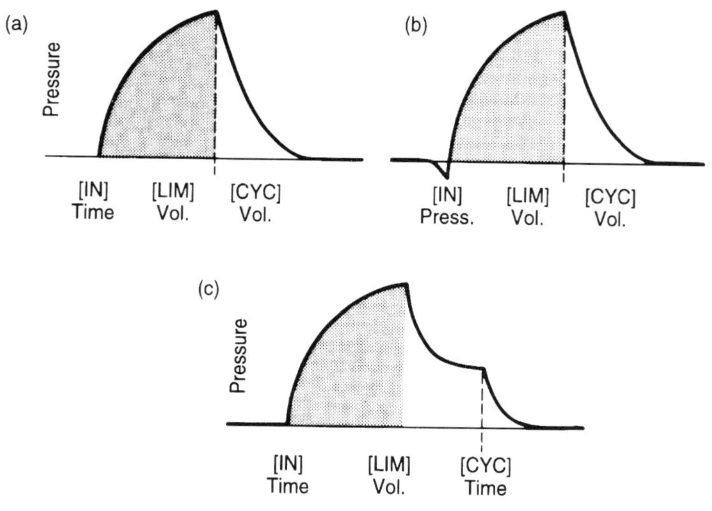

Fig. 31.3 Airway pressure curves illustrating the three mechanical functions: IN, initiation of the cycle; LIM, the preset limit (i.e. pressure or volume) imposed on the positive pressure cycle; CYC, the function (i.e. time or volume) ending the cycle. Each mechanical function is preset to be governed by one of four physical factors: volume, pressure, flow, time. (A) A time-initiated, volume-limited, volume-cycled mode. (B) A pressure-initiated (sub-baseline pressure produced by the patient's effort to breathe), volume-limited, volume-cycled mode. (c) A time-initiated, volume-limited, time-cycled mode that extends inspiration beyond the time the volume is delivered. A plateau is evident after flow has stopped but before the ventilator cycles into exhalation. Reprinted with permission from Shapiro et al.[329]

dynamic lung compliance is maximal;[97] this technique is variably effective. Another common objective is the reduction of intrapulmonary shunt to 15%, an approach termed 'optimal PEEP'.[98] Simple techniques have been described to adjust tidal volume and PEEP level in poorly compliant lungs at the bedside, using automated incremental and decremental PEEP levels in ventilated patients with computerized calculation of quasi-static lung compliance. **Table 31.5** summarizes the calculations of dynamic and static lung compliance.

Table 31.5 Calculation of static and dynamic compliance and airway resistance

1. Estimated static lung compliance (C_{es})

$$C_{es} = \frac{V_{et}}{P_{plat} - \mathrm{PEEP}_{appl} - \mathrm{PEEP}_{i}}$$

2. Dynamic lung compliance (C_{dyn})

$$C_{dyn} = \frac{V_{et}}{\mathrm{PIP} - \mathrm{PEEP}_{appl} - \mathrm{PEEP}_{i}}$$

3. Airway resistance (R_{aw})

$$R_{aw} = \frac{\mathrm{PIP} - P_{plat}}{\mathrm{flow}}$$

V_{et}, expiratory tidal volume; P_{plat}, inspiratory plateau pressure; PEEP_{appl}, applied positive end-expiratory pressure; PEEP_{i}, inadvertent positive end-expiratory pressure; PIP, peak inspiratory pressure; flow, inspiratory gas flow.

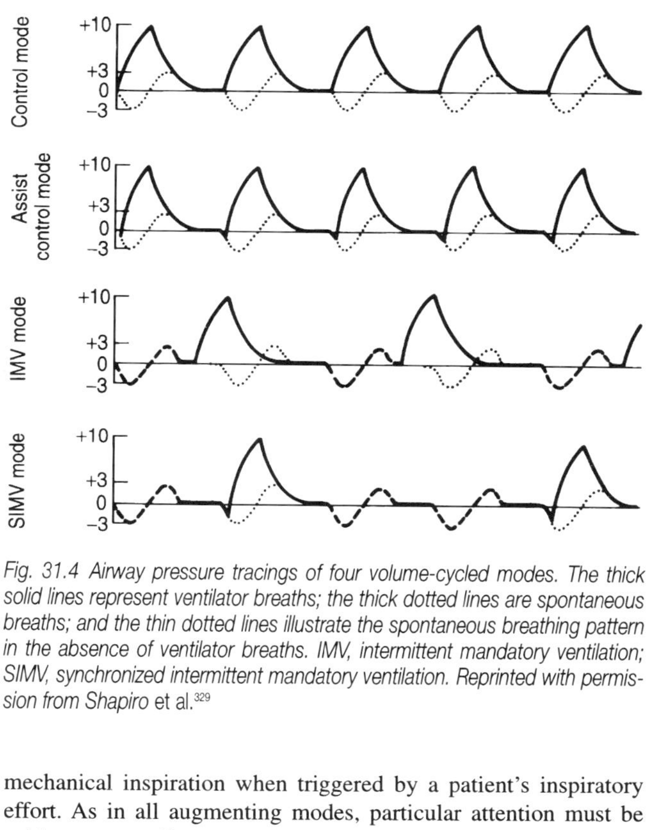

Fig. 31.4 Airway pressure tracings of four volume-cycled modes. The thick solid lines represent ventilator breaths; the thick dotted lines are spontaneous breaths; and the thin dotted lines illustrate the spontaneous breathing pattern in the absence of ventilator breaths. IMV, intermittent mandatory ventilation; SIMV, synchronized intermittent mandatory ventilation. Reprinted with permission from Shapiro et al.[329]

Controlled mechanical ventilation (CMV) (**Figure 31.4**), the simplest form of mechanical ventilatory support, initiates all mechanical breaths at preset intervals and permits no spontaneous ventilation. Most patients require sedation, narcotics, or muscle relaxants with this form of ventilation. Continuous positive pressure ventilation (CPPV) describes CMV with PEEP. CPPV is performed nearly exclusively in a time-cycled mode, being either volume-controlled or pressure-controlled.

Evidence from animal studies suggests that mechanical ventilation using conventional tidal volumes of 12–15 ml/kg can produce iatrogenic lung damage, probably by overdistension of more compliant lung regions. Techniques of ventilation have been modified to reduce this risk. With few exceptions, however, the efficacy and safety of newer techniques remain clinically unproven.

Assist/control mechanical ventilation (A/CMV) (**Figure 31.4**), in addition to providing a fixed default rate of CMV, initiates a full mechanical inspiration when triggered by a patient's inspiratory effort. As in all augmenting modes, particular attention must be paid to proper adjustment of the sensitivity of the triggering mechanism to avoid extremely high rates or increased work of breathing. Respiratory alkalosis and air trapping are potential complications of this mode of ventilation.

Intermittent mandatory ventilation (IMV) (**Figure 31.4**) is a time-cycled, volume-controlled mode. A patient breathes spontaneously on a preset CPAP, intermittently assisted by a mechanical cycle at the desired rate. Synchronized IMV (SIMV) (**Figure 31.4**) initiates a preset number of breaths when triggered by an inspiratory effort or the time-cycled default. SIMV is often chosen for weaning patients from mechanical support, and may produce less hemodynamic compromise than CMV or A/CMV.[99] In a crossover protocol comparing SIMV and ACMV in 40 patients who required mechanical ventilation for acute respiratory failure, SIMV was associated with significantly greater systemic blood pressure and cardiac output, lower mean airway pressure, peak airway pressure, ventilator rate, and arterial pH and higher $Pa\mathrm{CO}_2$.[100] Despite differences in minute ventilation, resting energy expenditure, and $\dot{D}O_2$ in specific subgroups of patients, the authors found no evidence to support any clear-cut advantage of SIMV or A/CMV in the acute management of respiratory failure.

Clinicians continue to debate the advantages of weaning patients with various forms of mechanical ventilation. Some clinicians prefer to use pressure support ventilation (PSV) or SIMV because of the ease with which the level of support can gradually be reduced. Some investigators propose that intermittent trials of abrupt discontinuation of mechanical ventilation will result in more rapid weaning[101] (**Figure 31.5**). It must be noted, however, that the rate of weaning for mechanical ventilation is critically dependent upon the rate at which the patient recovers from respiratory failure and also upon the aggressiveness with which the clinician pursues weaning.

Pressure support ventilation (PSV) (**Figure 31.6**), another form of partial ventilatory support, is a pressure-preset, flow-cycled mode intended to aid each spontaneous breathing cycle. By augmenting spontaneous inspiratory efforts, PSV helps to overcome the resistances of both the endotracheal tube and respirator valves in patients breathing spontaneously during mechanical ventilation. By varying pleural pressure, the patient determines both the duration of mechanical support and the flow profile of the tidal volume. Pressure support ventilation reduces the inspiratory work of breathing,[102] decreases energy expenditure by 10–18% in ARDS,[103] and can lower airway pressures compared with controlled positive pressure ventilation.[104] By enhancing spontaneous tidal volume, PSV reduces respiratory frequency.

Inverse ratio ventilation (IRV) has been developed to reduce peak end-inspiratory pressures in poorly compliant lungs by prolonging inspiratory time to allow lower inspiratory flow rates to produce the same tidal volume. Applied for the treatment of ARDS in 1980 by Baum and Benzer[105] IRV, a time-cycled, volume-controlled mode, improved oxygenation. By providing more homogeneous distribution of PEEP-induced increases in lung volume, this technique may help to diminish iatrogenic lung damage due to hyperinflation. Subsequently, pressure-controlled ventilation (PCV), a pressure-limited, time-cycled mode, was added to IRV in deeply sedated, paralyzed subjects.[106,107] PC-IRV limits the risk of alveolar overdistension and may reduce the risk of barotrauma but reduces control of mechanical tidal volume.

Airway pressure-release ventilation (APRV)[108,109] *and biphasic positive airway pressure (BiPAP)*[110] are time-cycled, pressure-

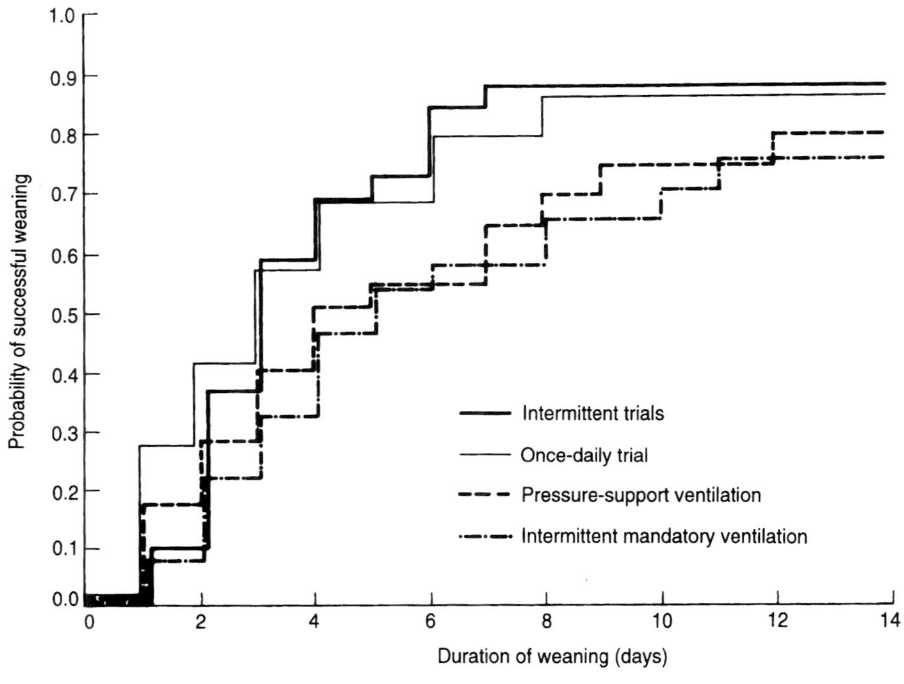

Fig. 31.5 The probability of successful weaning with intermittent mandatory ventilation, pressure-support ventilation, intermittent trials of spontaneous breathing, and a once-daily trial of spontaneous breathing (Kaplan–Meier curves). After adjustments for baseline characteristics (using a Cox proportional-hazards model), the rate of successful weaning with a once-daily trial of spontaneous breathing was 2.83 times higher than that with intermittent mandatory ventilation (p < 0.006) and 2.05 times higher than that with pressure-support ventilation (p < 0.04). Reprinted with permission from Esteban et al.[101]

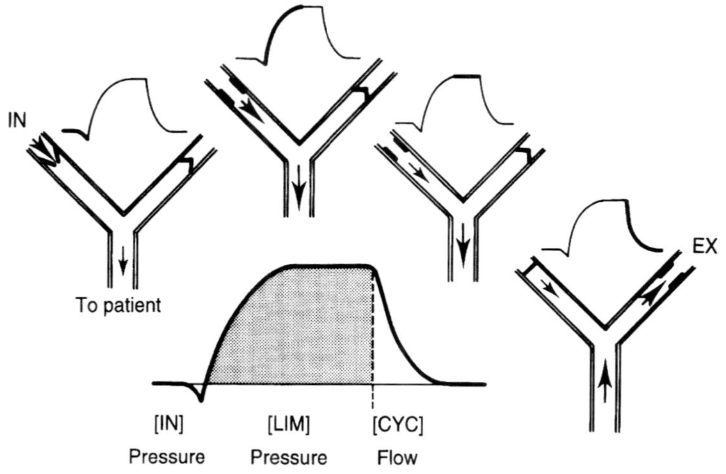

Fig. 31.6 Schematic illustration of pressure support ventilation. IN, initiation (by spontaneous breathing); LIM, limit (pressure); CYC, cycle (derived from decreasing inspiratory flow); EX, exhalation. Reprinted with permission from Shapiro et al.[329]

controlled modes of ventilation that depend on a high flow of fresh gas. Switching alternately between two preset CPAP levels allows spontaneous breathing at any time. Pressure differences between these CPAP levels determine the mechanical tidal volume, augmenting spontaneous breathing efforts. The principal goal of APRV was to reduce the danger of high CPAP levels by intermittently reducing pressure to zero. BiPAP, developed contemporaneously with APRV, was intended to augment ventilation in patients breathing spontaneously on CPAP. It supports CO_2 elimination by switching between a low and a high CPAP level at preset time intervals. The major theoretical advantage of APRV or BiPAP is provision of ventilatory support at lower airway pressures than conventional positive pressure ventilation.

High-frequency ventilation (HFV) may recruit and stabilize collapsed, diseased lung segments[111,112] and may improve clearance of secretions. Cioffi *et al.* showed improvement in survival rate and a decrease in the incidence of pneumonia in patients treated prophylactically with HFV, as compared with a historical control group of patients treated in the 7 years before the trial.[113] In 113 patients at risk for the development of ARDS, Hurst *et al.* randomized prophylactic therapy to ventilatory support with either HFV or conventional modes.[114] The incidence of ARDS was similar in the two groups; however, in those patients who developed ARDS, HFV achieved therapeutic endpoints at lower peak airway pressures and lower levels of PEEP.

Permissive hypercapnia. A management technique usually feasible only in well sedated patients, reduces inflation pressure and may decrease the risk of barotrauma and iatrogenic lung injury. If conventional respiratory modes, adjusted to limit peak inspiratory pressure to a maximum of 35 cmH_2O, are used in patients with ARDS, $Paco_2$ increases.[115] Even profound hypercapnia ($Paco_2$ ≥ 100 mmHg), if it develops gradually, is well tolerated.[115] To maintain oxygenation despite reduced airway pressures, PEEP or IRV is often used with permissive hypercapnia. In experimental animals, permissive hypercapnia appears to exert few adverse effects on hemodynamics or regional blood flow.[116,117] Gradually developing respiratory acidosis is limited by renal compensatory mechanisms; $NaHCO_3$ can be given acutely to maintain pH > 7.25.

Intratracheal pulmonary ventilation. For many years, investigators have been interested in bypassing the anatomical deadspace of the upper airway in order to improve ventilatory efficiency. The validity of this concept has been successfully demonstrated in two neonates with congenital diaphragmatic hernia.[118] Although some technical details remain to be solved, intratracheal ventilation may provide an adjunctive technique to a volume-targeted pressure-targeted strategy of mechanical ventilation

Extracorporeal membrane oxygenation (ECMO). ECMO describes prolonged, partial cardiopulmonary bypass achieved with a membrane oxygenator and extrathoracic vascular cannulation. In patients with severe ARDS, ECMO reduces the need to administer a toxic Fio_2 to provide oxygenation and high positive airway pressures to achieve CO_2 elimination. Thus, ECMO may provide life-sustaining gas exchange and may promote recovery by minimizing the harmful effects of continuing high-pressure mechanical ventilation. Using now outdated techniques and equipment, a multicenter prospective randomized study of ECMO in adults with severe ARDS reported no significant difference in survival (9.5% in the ECMO group; 8.3% in those receiving conventional treatment). Improved ventilators, better inclusion criteria, earlier intervention, a lower Fio_2, and less traumatic ventilator settings could further improve survival rates with ECMO. Gattinoni *et al.* used a modified technique, combining low-frequency positive pressure ventilation with extracorporeal CO_2 removal, and achieved 49% survival in a group of adults with ARDS.[120]

Although modified venovenous ECMO supports gas exchange, it may exacerbate lung injury.[121] In addition, ECMO is extremely labor intensive and requires expensive equipment and maintenance. Venoarterial ECMO requires ligation of the carotid artery, potentially resulting in cerebrovascular insufficiency or strokes. An alternate device (IVOX®, CardioPulmonics; Salt Lake City, UT) is positioned within the inferior vena cava.[122] IVOX® consists of multiple long, crimped, hollow fibers which provide CO_2 removal and partial blood oxygenation. Based upon studies in normal animals,[123] animals with acute lung injury,[124] and patients with severe ARDS,[125,126] in which IVOX® only partially supported (25–30%) gas exchange, this device seems to be of limited value.

Nonventilatory Therapy of ARDS. Bronchodilators are indicated if there is evidence of bronchospasm. To gauge efficacy, one can estimate changes in airway resistance before and after bronchodilators. Calculation of the relative contributions to peak inspiratory pressure due to airway resistance and lung compliance can be derived from the difference between the peak inspiratory pressure and the inspiratory plateau pressure, if an inspiratory hold is applied for more than 20% of the total inspiratory time. Calculations of airway resistance, dynamic compliance, and static compliance can be performed using readily available data (see **Table 31.5**).

Although corticosteroids appear to have little value in ARDS, some data suggest circumstances under which they might be beneficial. In established ARDS, high-dose corticosteroids may increase mortality and morbidity, although successful use has been reported.[127]

Hooper and Kear noted that in studies not demonstrating benefits of high-dose corticosteroid therapy, the duration of ARDS before treatment had been brief and the initial cause of ARDS was not mentioned. They reported 10 apparently uninfected patients with established ARDS which was treated with prolonged courses (> 21 days in eight of ten patients) of methylprednisolone, exceeding 40 mg/day for 12 days. Because all of these patients survived, corticosteroids may be beneficial in selected, uninfected ARDS patients in the late proliferative phase of the disease.

Pulmonary vasodilators have been used to reduce PAP and PVR in moderate and severe ARDS. In some ARDS patients, pulmonary vascular filling defects, possibly due to multiple embolism or thrombosis, may increase right ventricular afterload.[129] In several prospective studies, prostaglandin E_1 (PGE_1), in doses up to 30 ng/kg/min, lowered PAP and PVR while Pao_2 tended to increase, suggesting that PGE_1 acted as a pulmonary vasodilator without increasing Q_S/Q_T.[130,131] Although PGE_1 may block inflammation by inhibiting platelet aggregation and neutrophil activation, a multicenter study did not show significant benefits.[132]

Recently, the administration of low concentrations of nitric oxide (NO) has been proposed for the treatment of ARDS patients by the groups of Falke and Zapol.[133] Theoretically, inhaled NO would act as a microvascular vasodilator only in ventilated lung regions. By avoiding vasodilatation of nonventilated parts of the lung, Q_S/Q_T is not increased, and overall V/Q matching and oxygenation improve.

Gastrointestinal System

The gastrointestinal tract is a vitally important system in burned patients. First, as the preferred route for nutritional support, the gut assumes a central role in limiting protein loss during the catabolic response to acute illness. Second, the stomach and duodenum, as targets for mucosal injury, ulceration, and hemorrhage, are major sites of complications. Third, increasing evidence suggests that bacterial translocation, occurring through damaged gut mucosa, may play a key role in generating SIRS and MSOF in burned patients. This section will emphasize stress-related gastrointestinal bleeding and bacterial translocation.

The intestinal mucosa is impaired even by short intervals of starvation. Enteral feeding is one of the most important means of preventing mucosal breakdown and increased permeability. Early enteral feeding has been associated with reduced mortality rates and sepsis in burned children.[134] Reduced motility and ileus are common in burned patients. If gut function is severely compromised, parenteral nutrition is necessary to meet hypermetabolic energy demands. While both intraluminal and circulating substrates are necessary to supply energy to the gut mucosa, glutamine from skeletal muscles is utilized by the gut as a major substrate. Glutamine is metabolized to citrulline and, through the urea cycle, to pyruvate and tricarboxylic acids for gluconeogenesis, and to ammonia. Alanine is produced in the gut from pyruvate by transamination from L-glutamate. During starvation, stress, and catabolism, alanine and ketone bodies are transported in high concentrations to the liver as substrates for gluconeogenesis. Hepatic consumption of glutamine was elevated in endotoxemia.[135,136] To overcome intestinal mucosal damage and to prevent subsequent bacterial translocation, a glutamine-enriched diet, investigated in rats after abdominal radiation injury,[137] resulted in decreased bacterial colonization of mesenteric lymph nodes and conserved mucosal mass.

Prophylaxis of stress ulceration

Before the mid 1970s, stress-induced gastroduodenal ulceration (called Curling's ulcers in burned patients) caused substantial morbidity and mortality from hemorrhage and perforation. Gastric ulcers occur primarily in the watershed zones between capillary beds, areas particularly sensitive to ischemia. Mucosal injury is promoted by gastric acid. The mechanism of injury is in part dependent on the imbalance between injurious and protective factors. Most critically ill patients show reduced acid secretion, reduced gastric mucosal blood flow, decreased mucus production and decreased bicarbonate secretion. Tissue protective factors, including prostaglandins, modify injurious factors such as gastric acid.

Prophylactic antacid therapy to increase gastric pH has reduced the incidence of stress ulceration.[138] The increased pH, however, allowed gram-negative bacteria and fungi to colonize the stomach, esophagus, and oropharynx and to gain access to the trachea.[139] In mechanically ventilated patients with impaired reflexes, aspiration of these organisms contributes to nosocomial pneumonia.[140,141] Histamine type 2 (H_2) blockers such as cimetidine[142] and ranitidine also reduced the incidence of stress ulcers, but with comparable side effects.[143] Side effects other than an increased risk of nosocomial pneumonia also limit the utility of H_2 blockers. H_2 receptor blockers inhibit oxidative processes that require cytochrome P-450. This group of drugs also may cause central nervous side effects, especially in elderly patients; some neurological side effects are mediated by interaction with other drugs.[143]

Problems with antacids and H_2 blockers has led to the introduction of other mucosal protective agents that do not influence gastric pH. Pirenzepine provides stress ulcer protection equivalent to ranitidine, but is associated with a lower incidence of pneumonia.[144] Sucralfate, a nonabsorbable complex of sulfated glucose and aluminum hydroxide, was at least as effective in children as antacids and H_2 blockers,[145] but with a reduced risk of pneumonia. Sucralfate enhances mucosal defensive mechanisms.[146,147] Because sucralfate has only a minor influence on gastric pH yet exerts proven bactericidal effects,[148] gastric and gut bacterial overgrowth is less prominent. These effects may explain the reduced incidence of pneumonia in contrast to alkalinizing drugs.[149]

Intestinal permeability and bacterial translocation

In healthy persons, normal intestinal motility and absorption maintain an intact mucosal barrier. Short periods of starvation and stress, in concert with total parenteral nutrition, interrupt luminal nutrient flow and cause rapid mucosal atrophy and increased permeability to macromolecules.[150] Impaired function of the reticuloendothelial system and liver may interfere with clearance of bacteria and bacterial products. Moreover, during a prolonged critical illness accompanied by administration of antimicrobial agents,[151] selection of resistant microorganisms within the intestinal flora occurs; subsequent infections caused by translocated organisms are more difficult to treat. Prolonged infections and a septic state increase the risk of multiple organ failure and death. The gut has been therefore called the 'motor of organ failure' with liver failure as an essential prerequisite.[152]

Even in the absence of frank circulatory shock, decreases in systemic perfusion redistribute blood flow within the layers of the gut. In shock, the splanchnic circulation acts as a reservoir for 'autotransfusion.' Although reduction of venous capacitance increases venous return and preserves cardiac preload, excessive vasoconstriction of the precapillary arterial resistance vessels by activation of local and systemic mediators may cause splanchnic ischemia.[153]

Although gut mucosal flow may be limited in sepsis, mucosal oxygen consumption actually may increase. In septic trauma patients, splanchnic oxygen demands were increased and a discrepancy developed between oxygen supply and demand.[154] In addition to increased sympathetic tone, other mediators also influence splanchnic resistance. In hemorrhagic shock, vasopressin produces disproportionately greater vasoconstriction in the splanchnic arterioles than in the remainder of the systemic circulation.[155,156] Angiotensin II, generated by renin released from the kidney in response to hypotension, appears to mediate nonocclusive mesenteric ischemia.[157] This potent vasoconstrictor exhibits important mesenteric selectivity thought to be caused by an increased affinity of the angiotensin II receptors for splanchnic vascular smooth muscle receptors.[158] Other humoral agents, such as glucagon[159] and some arachidonate metabolites, are potent modulators of splanchnic vascular tone.[160–162]

Bacterial translocation occurs when live bacteria or their toxins cross the intestinal mucosal barrier into the portal and systemic circulation or into the mesenteric lymph nodes. In healthy individuals, bacteria are then cleared by the liver and the lymph nodes. In mesenteric ischemia after major burn injury,[163] hypovolemic or septic shock, portal bacteremia exceeds the clearing capacity of the liver and lymphatic system and live organisms pass into the systemic circulation. **Figure 31.7** illustrates a theoretical relationship between thermal injury, mesenteric vasoconstriction, and bacterial products (endotoxin) in the genesis of bacterial translocation.

In response to burn injury and sepsis, the intestinal membrane becomes more permeable.[163–170] In minipigs subjected to 40% flame burn and fluid resuscitation, superior mesenteric blood flow was dramatically reduced immediately after the burn, then recovered (**Figure 31.8a**); in association with the reduction splanchnic blood flow, bacteria were translocated, resulting in increased culture of bacteria from lymph nodes, organs, and blood (**Figure 31.8b**). Using the ratio of absorption of two nonmetabolizable sugars, lactulose and mannitol, as markers of intestinal permeability, Deitch *et al.* demonstrated that patients following major burn injuries had substantial increases in intestinal permeability (**Figure 31.9**). Early endotoxemia, occurring less than 24 hours after burn injury, is proportional to the burn size[171,172] and may represent increased permeability. Endotoxin itself increases intestinal permeability[173] and promotes bacterial translocation as well as mesenteric

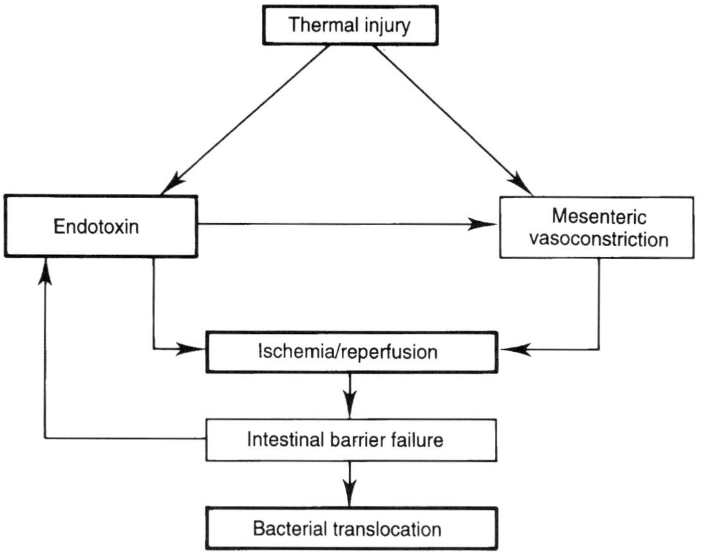

Fig. 31.7 Schematic diagram of the relationship between thermal injury and bacterial translocation. In response to thermal injury, mesenteric vasoconstriction occurs. With resuscitation, an ischemia/reperfusion sequence results in failure of the intestinal barrier, leading to bacterial translocation and to release of endotoxin into the circulation, precipitating further mesenteric vasoconstriction and perpetuation of the ischemia/reperfusion sequence.

hypoperfusion,[174] Alexander *et al.* demonstrated that organisms in the lamina propria were commonly phagocytized by macrophages but were also found free in lymphatics and blood vessels.[175] Translocation of *E. coli* and endotoxin also occurred directly through enterocytes as well as between myocytes.[175]

Normal intestinal microflora consists predominantly of anaerobic organisms, which are thought to play an important role as a protection from changes in intestinal colonization with nosocomial bacteria.[176] As anerobes are highly susceptible to several antibiotics used against aerobic bacteria, they are reduced in number, freeing an ecological niche to be filled subsequently by overgrowth of aerobic gram-negative and gram-positive organisms. Other barriers to colonization of the gut are secretions, such as gastric acid, bile and mucosal IgA, and intestinal motility; together, these prevent bacteria from ascending to the oropharynx and colonizing and infecting the respiratory tract.[177] Consequently, Stoutenbeek *et al.*[178,179] suggested a method of selective decontamination of the digestive tract by administering, via nasogastric tube, nonabsorbable antibiotics that are effective against aerobic gram-negative strains. This strikingly reduced the infection rate from 81% in a historic control group to 15% in a treated group of patients; however, there is insufficient evidence that this prophylactic regimen improves outcome in critically ill patients,[180] perhaps because reducing the pool of intestinal bacteria and endotoxin pool does not influence the cytokine cascade induced by the underlying injury.[181]

One possible approach to reducing bacterial translocation is to pharmacologically enhance gut regeneration, thereby reducing the postburn problems with permeability. Huang *et al.* studied insulin-like growth factor-1 in rats subjected to 50% full-thickness burns that demonstrated improved gut atrophy and reduced bacterial translocation.[25] They demonstrated that the administration of insulin-like growth factor-1 slightly increased the combined weight of proximal and distal small bowel in sham animals, but caused a dramatic effect in burned animals (**Figure 31.10**). In conjunction with the improved gut mass, there was a reduction in the rate of bacterial translocation to mesenteric lymph nodes on the second postburn day (**Figure 31.11**).

In summary, prevention of gastrointestinal failure is a cornerstone in the prevention of multiple organ failure after major injury. The means to achieving this goal include maintenance of adequate mesenteric perfusion, control of bacteria in the gastrointestinal tract, stress ulcer prophylaxis without alkalinization, parenteral nutrition, and early enteral nutrition.

Renal System

Acute renal failure

Acute renal failure (ARF) represents a potentially lethal complication of burns, multiple trauma, and other critical illness. Despite substantial technical developments in hemodialysis and other renal replacement therapy, mortality exceeds 50% in virtually all series. If ventilatory support is required, the mortality approaches 100%.[182] Military casualty experience provides valuable insights into prevention of ARF. In World War II, the incidence of ARF was 42% and mortality exceeded 90%. During the Korean War, improved evacuation and more liberal resuscitation with blood and plasma reduced the incidence of ARF to 35%; mortality remained above 50% despite the intercurrent introduction of dialysis. During the Vietnam War, evacuation and field resuscitation further improved, reducing the incidence of ARF to 0.17%,[183] perhaps because of increased use of isotonic crystalloid and the use of urinary output as a monitor; however, mortality was still 77%. The introduction of dialytic therapy accounted for the modest decrease in mortality, an improvement of far less quantitative importance than the dramatic reduction in incidence.

The clinical presentation of ARF has changed from an early to a late finding. In the early posttraumatic period, hypovolemia or delayed or inadequate resuscitation causes circulatory impairment and subsequent reduction of renal blood flow; this type of ARF should occur rarely with modern resuscitation techniques. Later, approximately 2 weeks after burn injury, infection and sepsis cause ARF as one expression of MSOF. Renal insufficiency may be manifest as a wide variety of deficits, ranging from nonoliguric ARF to oliguria to anuria.

Pathogenesis. ARF, alternatively termed acute tubular necrosis, may be produced by a variety of factors that interfere with glomerular filtration and tubular reabsorption. The pathogenesis of ARF conventionally is divided into an initiation period, a maintenance period (**Table 31.6**), and a recovery period.[184] Renal hypoperfusion, nephrotoxic insults, or both, may initiate ARF. In surgical patients, hypoperfusion, produced either by external or internal fluid loss or sepsis, constitutes a frequent cause. Experimental renal hypoperfusion, whether induced by hemorrhagic shock or intrarenal norepinephrine infusion at supraphysiologic doses, impairs renal function in proportion to the depletion of high-energy phosphates.[185,186] One promising hypothesis states that

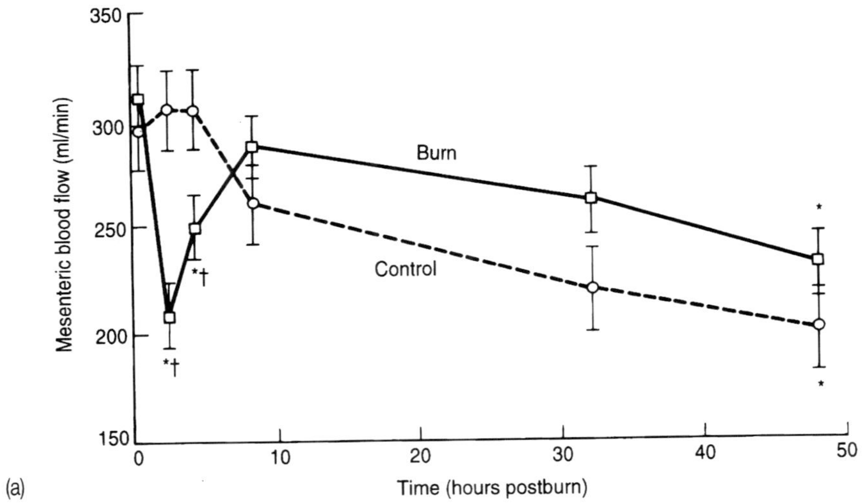

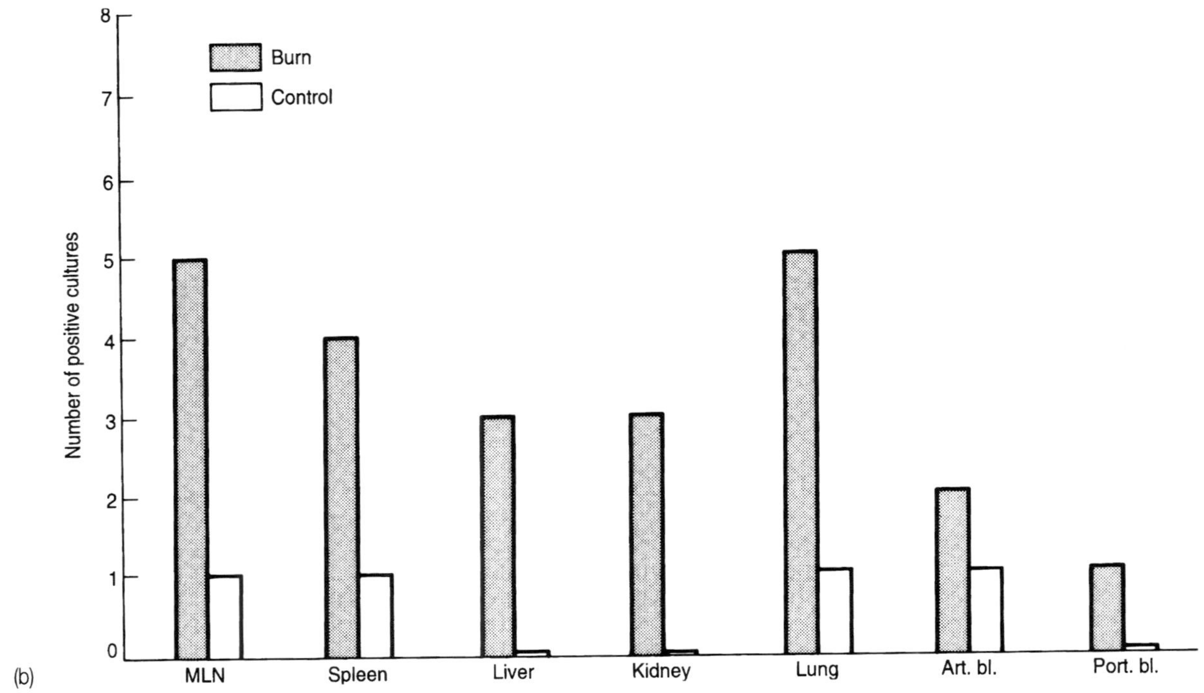

*Fig. 31.8 (a) After flame-burn injury in minipigs, superior mesenteric blood flow (solid line) decreased abruptly, then recovered with resuscitation. *p ≤ 0.05 vs. baseline; †p ≤ 0.05, burn vs. the unburned control group (dotted line). (b) Bacterial tissue culture results from mesenteric lymph nodes (MLN), spleen, liver, kidney, lung, arterial blood (Art.bl.) and portal blood (Port.bl.) after sham injury (open bars) and thermal injury (solid bars) in flame-burned minipigs. Reprinted with permission from Tokyay et al.*[170]

Table 31.6 Pathogenesis of acute renal failure (ARF)

Initiation	Maintenance
Renal hypoperfusion	Tubular dysfunction
Hemodynamic factors	Tubular obstruction
Nephrotoxins	Descreased glomerular filtration
	Decreased renal blood flow

the renal medulla, because of its disproportionately low baseline flow, is particularly at risk for damage if total renal blood flow is reduced.[187,188]

The initiating insult ultimately culminates in the development of one or more of the maintenance factors (e.g. decreased tubular function, tubular obstruction, decreased glomerular filtration, and decreased renal blood flow) that reduce urinary flow and osmolar excretion. In hypovolemia, renal blood flow is reduced by afferent arterial vasoconstriction. Activation of the renin–angiotensin system and endothelial cell swelling also may contribute to reduced renal blood flow. Prostaglandin E_2, an endogenous vasodilator, counteracts vasoconstriction and plays a major role in renal blood flow regulation. Atrial natriuretic peptide, elevated after burn injury,[72] may protect the kidneys by increasing blood flow and urinary output. At the level of the renal tubules, inappropriate secretion of antidiuretic hormone,[189] washout of the medullary osmotic gradient,[190] tubular epithelial damage, or reduced blood flow in the vasa recta may create ARF. Other tubular causes of ARF include obstruction by cellular debris, hemoglobin, or myoglobin in patients with crush injuries or rhabdomyolysis.[191]

In sepsis, the hyperdynamic septic circulation may be associated with inappropriate polyuria even while creatinine clearance is

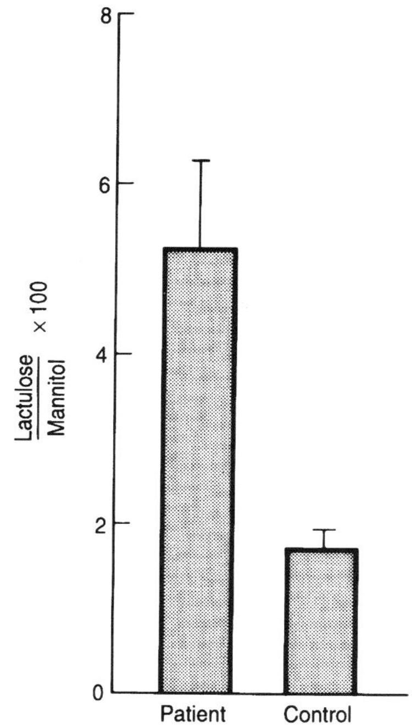

Fig. 31.9 The lactulose/mannitol ratio (a marker of intestinal permeability) was higher in burn patients than in unburned controls ($p < 0.05$). The ratio demonstrates that increased urinary lactulose excretion was not simply secondary to alterations in intestinal motility or renal excretion. Reprinted with permission from Deitch,[330] with permission from Mosby Yearbook Inc., St Louis.

depressed.[190] In managing this inappropriate polyuria, it is mandatory to obtain data about kidney function such as serum creatinine, urinary osmolality, and urinary and blood urea and electrolytes to calculate clearances. In response to this spontaneous diuresis, falsely interpreted as fluid repletion, inappropriate fluid restriction may result in hypovolemia and further renal compromise.

Although decreased renal blood flow characterizes both the initiation and the maintenance phases, once the maintenance phase begins, pharmacological improvement in renal blood flow will not reverse ARF. In contrast, the hemodynamic factors that initiate perioperative ARF often prove amenable to acute therapeutic intervention during the period when the anesthesiologist or intensivist is directly responsible for the patient's welfare.

In general, improved management of acute prerenal oliguria has resulted in both a decreasing incidence of ARF and an increase in the proportion of patients with ARF who remain nonoliguric.[192] Myers and Moran[192] recently proposed a practical, clinical classification of hemodynamically mediated ARF, dividing it into abbreviated, overt, and protracted ARF, on the basis of the pattern of reduction in creatinine clearance, and the increase in serum creatinine (**Figure 31.12**). The categories emphasize the frequency of nonoliguric ARF and provide a useful framework for grouping patients with similar prognoses. This classification is clinically pertinent because it emphasizes the role of secondary insults, such as sepsis, in protracted ARF. Sepsis often complicates the course of patients with protracted critical illness.[192,193] Prognostically, one can anticipate low mortality in abbreviated ARF and high mortality in protracted ARF.[192]

Nonoliguric ARF, once uncommon, now occurs frequently. In contrast to oliguric ARF, nonoliguric ARF is somewhat easier to manage clinically, since it requires less scrupulous control of fluid and electrolyte intake. The first extensive clinical description of nonoliguric ARF stressed its lower mortality rate.[194] In that study, a larger percentage of patients with nonoliguric ARF had a nephrotoxic injury, whereas oliguric patients developed ARF in association with surgery, with prolonged volume depletion, or with impaired cardiac output. Therefore, it appears that nonoliguric ARF, occurring spontaneously in a hospitalized population, is associated with a lower mortality. Nonoliguric ARF occurring as a complication of trauma may also carry a better prognosis than oliguric ARF. Shin *et al.*[195] reported on two consecutive groups (groups 1 and 2) of trauma patients. In group 2, more liberal fluid administration and less frequent diuretic administration increased the incidence of nonoliguric ARF and decreased the incidence of oliguric ARF in comparison with group 1, which received fluid in lower volumes and was more frequently chemically diuresed. Mortality and morbidity in group 2 were substantially less than in group 1.[195]

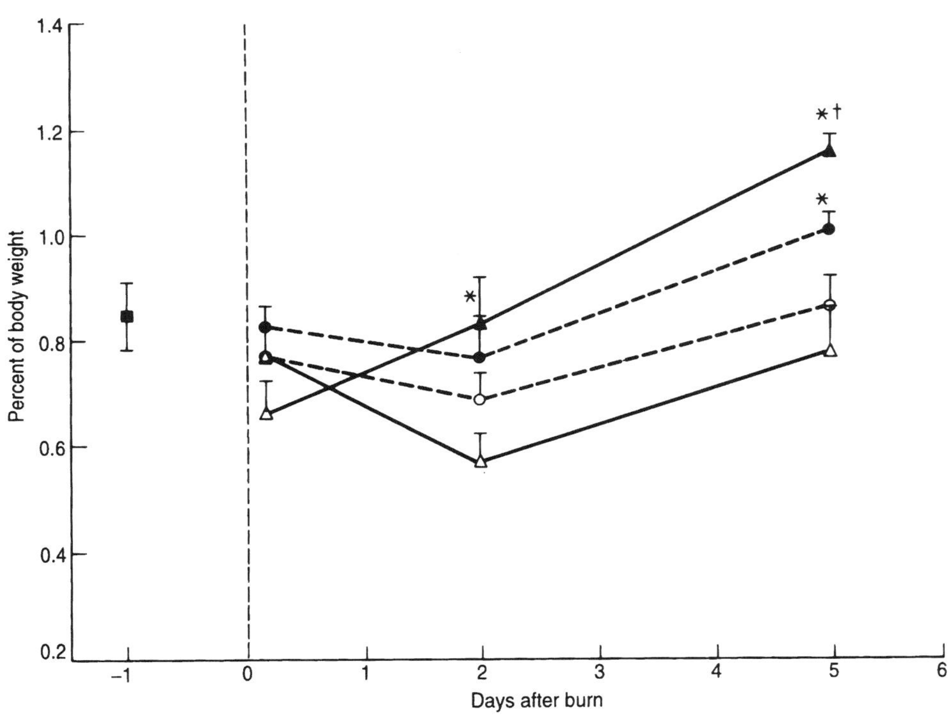

*Fig. 31.10 The total mucosal wet weight (as a percent of body weight) of the combined proximal and distal small bowel in sham animals (circles) and burned animals (triangles). Treatment with insulin-like growth factor-1 increased mucosal wet weight slightly in the sham animals (closed symbols = treated group), but caused a much more dramatic improvement in wet weight in burned animals treated with insulin-like growth factor-1 (closed triangles). *$p < 0.05$ vs placebo control animals (unpaired t test); †$p < 0.05$ vs sham groups (Bonferronis multiple comparison). Reprinted from Huang* et al.,[25] *with permission from the American Medical Association.*

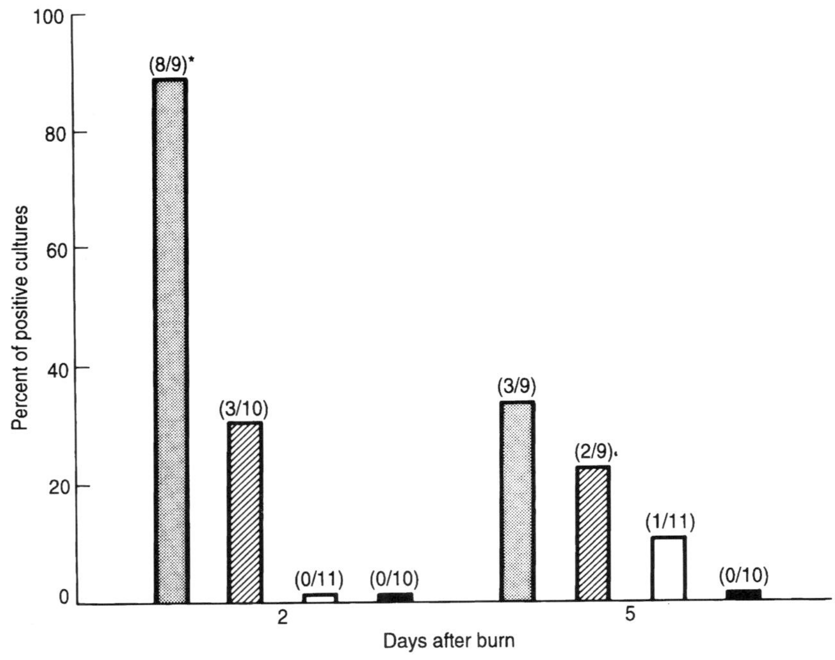

*Fig. 31.11 Insulin-like growth factor-1 decreased the rate of bacterial translocation to mesenteric lymph nodes after burn injury on postburn day 2. (*p < 0.01, Fisher's exact test.) The first solid bar represents burned, placebo-treated animals; the hatched bar represents burned animals treated with insulin-like growth factor-1; and the open and shaded bars represent sham animals with and without treatment. Reprinted from Huang et al.,[25] with permission from the American Medical Association.*

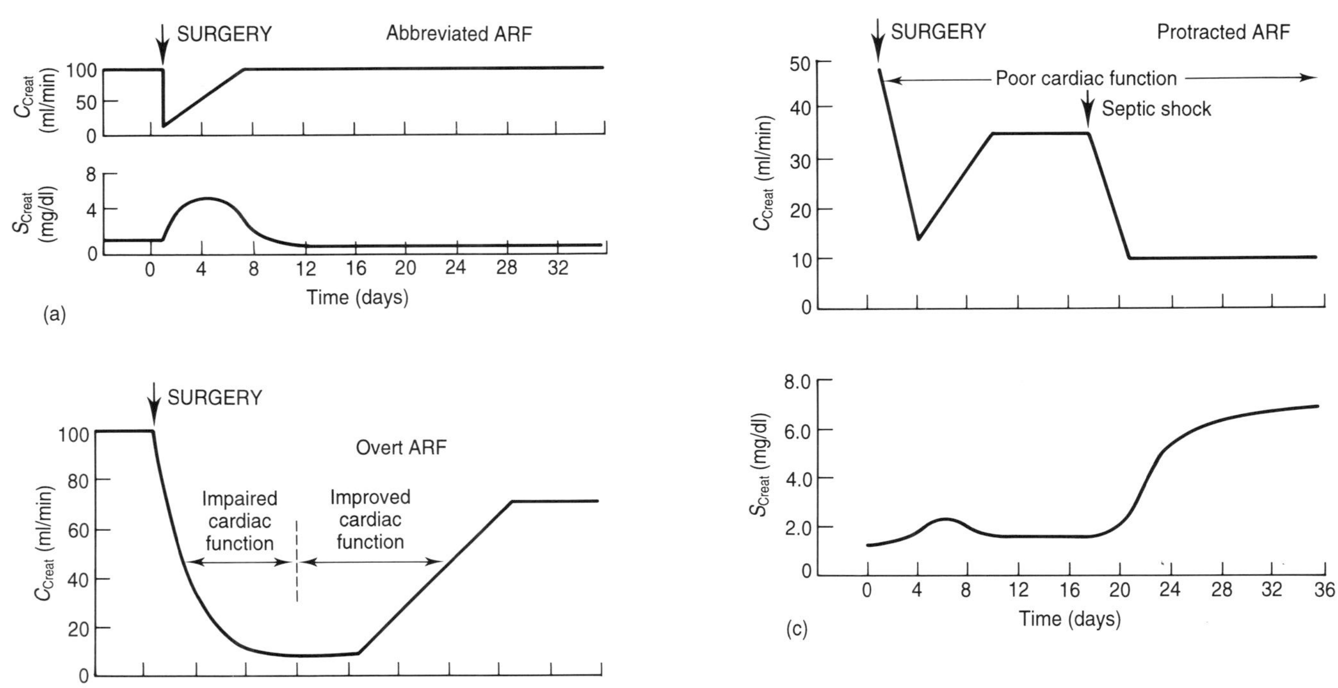

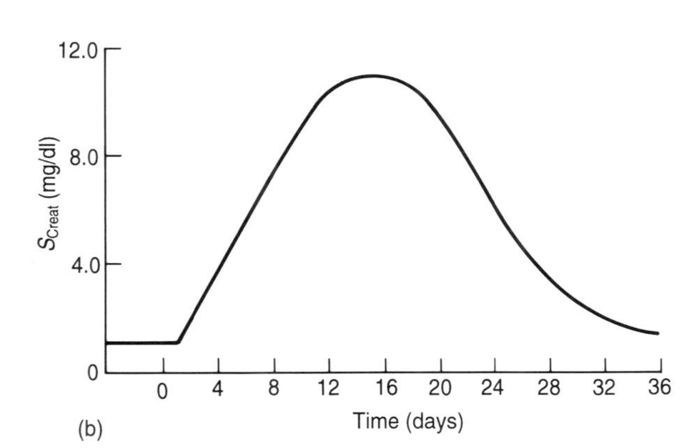

Fig. 31.12 Three patterns of hemodynamically mediated acute renal failure (ARF) occur after major trauma or surgery. (A) Abbreviated ARF consists of an acute reduction in creatinine clearance (C_{creat}) with prompt recovery. Serum creatinine (S_{Creat}) may be increasing even as C_{Creat} recovers. (B) Overt ARF consists of concurrent, mirror-image decreases in C_{Creat} and increases in S_{Creat}, usually in association with compromised cardiac function followed by recovery. (C) Protracted ARF develops as a consequence of prolonged hemodynamic compromise, often complicated by systemic sepsis. Reproduced with permission from Myers and Moran.[192]

Because of the reported improved mortality and morbidity in patients with nonoliguric ARF, several investigators have attempted to convert established oliguric ARF to nonoliguric ARF using diuretic drugs with or without dopamine. Uncontrolled series emphasized the efficacy of induced diuresis,[196,197] however, controlled randomized trials have failed to demonstrate that conversion of oliguric ARF to nonoliguric ARF improves mortality, morbidity, the duration of renal failure, or the number of necessary dialyses.[198,199] In addition, direct intrarenal administration of furosemide (275 mg over 30 minutes) failed to improve renal function or renal blood flow in patients with ARF.[200] The aforementioned data support the conclusion that early, aggressive hemodynamic support of the patient with prerenal oliguria may produce a better outcome, even if nonoliguric ARF develops. Conversely, the chemical conversion of oliguric to nonoliguric ARF does not improve outcome.

Assessment of renal function

Table 31.7 summarizes typical laboratory findings in patients with prerenal oliguria, secondary to hypoperfusion, and renal oliguría. Prerenal oliguria is associated with physiologic mechanisms that conserve salt and water, resulting in excretion of waste products in a minimal volume of urine; therefore, patients with prerenal oliguria classically produce urine with high osmolality and low sodium. In patients with a chronic reduction in concentrating ability owing to preexisting renal disease, urinary sodium and osmolality may not achieve 'prerenal' values during acute prerenal insults. In addition, diuretics increase urinary sodium and decrease urinary osmolality.

Table 31.7 Diagnostic tests in acute oliguria

Test	Prerenal	Renal
Urinary osmolality (mosmol/kg)	>400	<400
Urine/plasma osmolality	>1.3	<1.1
Urinary sodium (mEq/l)	<20	>40
Urine/plasma creatinine	>40	<20
FE_{Na} (%)*	<1	>2

*FE_{Na}, fractional excretion of sodium, calculated as: $\frac{U/P_{Na}}{U/P_{Cr}} \times 100$ where *U* is urinary concentration, *P* is plasma concentration, Na is sodium and Cr is creatinine.

In an effort to clarify ambiguous laboratory findings, several investigators have proposed the fractional excretion of sodium (FE_{Na}) as a laboratory guide that can more accurately differentiate patients according to those with prerenal oliguria and those with renal oliguria. The (FE_{Na}) is calculated as follows:

$$FE_{Na} = \frac{U_{Na}/P_{Na}}{U_{Cr}/P_{Cr}} \times 100$$

where *U* is urine; Na is sodium; *P* is plasma; and Cr is creatinine. Values less than 1% suggest prerenal azotemia. Despite early enthusiasm for this derived index, it is now apparent that it has limited diagnostic and prognostic use in the acute situation.[201,202] The most critical limitation is that the FE_{Na} may suggest established parenchymal ARF at a time when hemodynamically mediated prerenal factors are still reversible. Moreover, these tests are unreliable in sodium-avid patients (those with liver failure, nephrotic syndrome, and cirrhosis) in whom urinary sodium may be low despite inexorably progressive renal failure.[203]

Oliguria *per se*, the diagnostic test that responds most quickly to changes in renal perfusion, should be considered neither a specific nor sensitive marker of acute renal insufficiency (ARI).[204,205] Patients can have normal urinary outputs with clinically significant renal insufficiency. An equally important consideration for the clinician caring for postoperative, critically ill patients at risk for ARI is whether the glomerular filtration role (GFR) is abnormal, and whether it is improving or deteriorating. Clinically this can best be evaluated using serial evaluations of creatinine clearances (C_{Cr}). This has been determined clinically using collection periods as short as 1 and 2 hours.[206,207] Short-term C_{Cr} may overestimate GFR when compared to measurements using inulin.[208] In several studies in critically ill patients, C_{Cr} seems to be superior to other diagnostic tests, i.e. serum creatinine, blood urea nitrogen (BUN), free water clearance, FE_{Na}, urinary flow rate, or (for monitoring purposes) 24-hour C_{Cr}. Specifically, serum creatinine may not change significantly during the first 24 postoperative hours in the setting of ARI because of the diluting effects of aggressive fluid administration. By actually measuring serial 2-hour C_{Cr}, renal function monitoring probably can be improved.

The indications for pulmonary artery catheterization in patients with ARF resemble those in other critically ill patients. Hemodynamic monitoring proves especially useful for those patients in whom a conflict exists regarding the need for aggressive dialytic removal of sodium and water. The estimation of PAOP before and during dialysis may assist the dialysis personnel in managing fluid removal during dialysis and in determining appropriate therapy if hypotension develops.

One of the greatest limitations of current monitoring techniques is the lack of an effective means for determining the rate of recovery of renal function in patients with ARF. The inability to accurately estimate renal blood flow and GFR means that dialysis will frequently continue for an unnecessarily long period of time. Myers and Moran[192] suggest that limiting the number of dialyses, and their attendant risk of hypotension, would hasten recovery from renal failure in some patients.

In the acute situation, most therapeutic decisions should not rely on urinary sediment, electrolytes, osmolality, or complex formulas derived from urinary and plasma sodium and creatinine measurements. The discriminatory value of those measurements is too limited for application in the perioperative setting. Unfortunately, the readily available tests are insufficiently sensitive and specific, require excessive time for completion, and provide little information that can guide therapy. All acutely oliguric patients at risk for ARF should receive fluids and should undergo monitoring and hemodynamic support in the same fashion, using the same endpoints, regardless of the results of those tests.

Prevention of acute renal failure

The key to preventing early ARF is providing adequate renal blood flow by administering adequate fluid. Maintenance of urinary output > 60 ml/h suggests adequate resuscitation. In infected or septic patients, the septic focus should be eliminated, if possible, and appropriate antibiotic treatment instituted. To prevent sepsis-associated ARF, the highest priority is maintaining renal perfusion. Both cardiac output and perfusion pressure must be monitored. In hemoglobinuric or myoglobinuric patients, hydration to maintain urinary flow is essential. If necessary, mannitol may be added; however, increasing urinary production by osmotic or loop diuretics will not increase creatinine clearance.

Systemic $\dot{D}O_2$ should be addressed with aggressive volume expansion, and if cardiac index is not improved to a normal or 'supranormal level', inotropic agents should be added. Commonly in severe sepsis and septic shock, renal perfusion pressure (mean arterial pressure – central venous pressure) remains low (i.e. below the renal autoregulatory threshold of 50 mmHg) despite a markedly increased cardiac index. In this situation, in which cardiac index is adequate but systemic vascular resistance and perfusion pressure are severely reduced, several studies in animals and humans have shown norepinephrine to have beneficial effects[71,209–211] (see **Table 31.3**). Some of these studies have shown improvement in perfusion pressure and urinary flow in patients even when used as a 'last resort' for patients who were refractory to high doses of dopamine (≥80 μg/kg/min). Norepinephrine used in this manner improves urinary output without decreasing renal blood flow. When used in combination with low-dose (i.e. 'renal dose') dopamine, norepinephrine significantly increases renal blood flow, relative to baseline values, by increasing the fraction of cardiac output perfusing the kidneys and even lowering renal vascular resistance.[211]

In an attempt to improve outcome in high-risk surgical patients, Shoemaker *et al.* adjusted hemodynamic therapy to achieve the higher values for cardiac output and systemic oxygen delivery previously associated with improved survival.[212] In the first of two studies they compared conventional management of a control surgical group to a protocol which utilized hemodynamic values of previous survivors as goals for therapy. In the protocol group, in which cardiac output and oxygen delivery were elevated above baseline values as guided by pulmonary artery catheterization, survival was improved, complications were reduced, and, importantly, the incidence of ARF was less.[212] The control group received conventional monitors, including a central venous pressure catheter. In a second study, combined with the first study for publication, an additional control group received conventional monitoring, supplemented by pulmonary artery catheterization without specific management guidelines. As in the first series, the protocol group demonstrated improved mortality and reduced total complications, including ARF. The control group that underwent pulmonary artery catheterization and treatment without specific hemodynamic goals had a mortality and complication rate equal to the group managed without a pulmonary artery catheter.[212] These data suggest that aggressive, so-called 'supranormal', goal-directed hemodynamic support avoids clinically inapparent hypoperfusion and as a consequence limits the incidence of mortality and morbidity, such as ARF, secondary to that process. It is worth noting that the target for oxygen delivery (600 ml/min/m^2) used by Shoemaker *et al.*[212] is equivalent to a 'normal' cardiac index (3.0 l/min/m^2) multiplied by a 'normal' oxygen content (20 ml/min/m^2). The benefit of 'supranormal' oxygen transport is still controversial. While some clinical investigations show support for the association of 'supranormal' oxygen transport with improved outcome in high-risk critically ill patients[213] and in septic patients,[214] a more recent study could not demonstrate positive effects on outcome of these patients when boosting cardiac index with positive inotropic agents.[332] (See **Figure 31.13**.)

Many pharmacologic approaches to reducing the incidence and severity of perioperative ARF and ARI are based upon inferences from animal models of acute, norepinephrine-induced renal ischemia.[215] Mannitol, dopamine, and furosemide promote urinary flow and reduce the renal damage produced by experimental renal ischemia.[196,198,199,216–223] Mannitol improves renal cortical blood flow and may exert a renal cellular protective effect.[217–219] By maintaining high tubular flow, it may decrease the incidence and severity of ARF secondary to contrast media or pigmenturia. Mannitol is ineffective in reversing profound reductions in GFR and renal blood flow induced by suprarenal aortic cross-clamping for 60 minutes in dogs.[220] Dopamine, like mannitol, is ineffective in reversing the renal injury produced by thoracic aortic cross-clamping.[220] Dopamine, used in doses of 1–3 μg/kg/min to achieve selective renal vasodilation, increases renal cortical blood flow with minimal systemic effects.[221] Dopamine induces natriuresis, increases GFR, improves urinary flow,[221,222] and is a useful adjunct to the treatment of oliguria. One of the mechanisms for increased urinary output with dopamine in critically ill patients who have oliguria may be inhibition of aldosterone secretion by dopamine.[224] Fenoldopam, a novel dopamine-1 receptor agonist, substantially enhances urinary flow, sodium excretion, and creatinine clearance, while reducing systemic vascular resistance.[225–228] Although fenoldopam will likely become a valuable perioperative adjunct, its precise role remains to be demonstrated.

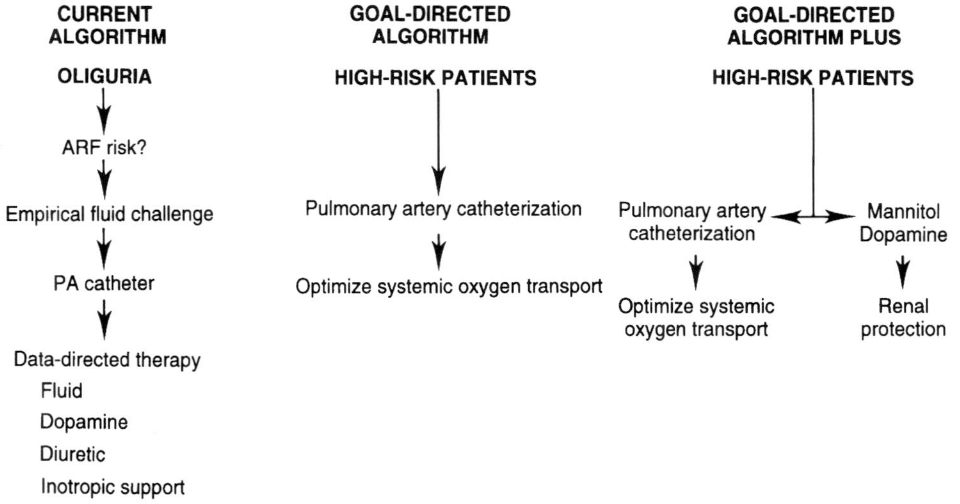

Fig. 31.13 Three possible approaches to prevention of acute renal failure (ARF). The left-hand algorithm is derived from the approach used by many clinicians. Once oliguria is recognized, the diagnostic and therapeutic approach consists of empirical volume expansion, supplemented if necessary by pulmonary artery (PA) catheterization with subsequent data-directed therapy consisting of fluid, dopamine, inotropic support, mannitol, or furosemide. In contrast, the goal-directed algorithm is based upon identification of high-risk patients. Such patients would undergo pulmonary artery catheterization with subsequent support of systemic oxygen transport (cardiac output × arterial oxygen content) at levels associated with improved survival in high-risk surgical patients. The right-hand figure combines goal-oriented therapy with early pharmacologic support, based on the assumption that early pharmacologic intervention is most likely to be effective, but that induced diuresis may perpetuate hypovolemia and interfere with monitoring of urinary output. Reproduced with permission from Prough and Foreman.[331]

Furosemide is effective in experimental models of complete renal ischemia,[218,219] though generally less effective than mannitol. In an effort to combine the potentially beneficial effects of both dopamine and furosemide, Lindner and colleagues infused both dopamine and furosemide in a canine model of nephrotoxic canine ARF and demonstrated a synergistic renal protective effect.[223] Subsequently, in an uncontrolled trial in a small group of patients who had oliguric ARF, the combination of low-dose dopamine (1–3 μg/kg/min) and furosemide resulted in production of a brisk diuresis and stabilization of renal function.[196] This has not been duplicated in a controlled, randomized trial.

In addition to the commonly discussed renal protective effects of volume expansion, mannitol, dopamine, and furosemide, a variety of agents demonstrate efficacy in experimental models of ARF.[229–264] Numerous recent reviews address potential mechanisms that may produce therapeutic progress.[215,265–270]

Renal replacement therapy

Treatment of ARF is less satisfactory than prevention. If creatinine clearance is severely decreased, the plasma concentrations of metabolic products excreted by the kidney will increase. To avoid inadvertent overdosage, it is crucial to know about the pharmacokinetic and pharmacodynamic profiles of any drug used in renal insufficiency. Ideally, drugs that are excreted through the liver and bile should be selected. If available, drug levels should be monitored closely.

In critically ill patients, intermittent hemodialysis can effectively remove fluid but is associated with hemodynamic instability and mandates a specially trained team. To permit care by bedside personnel, continuous arteriovenous hemofiltration (CAVH) was introduced in clinical practice in Europe in 1977 by Kramer *et al.*[271,272] and approved by the United States Food and Drug Administration in 1982. CAVH, and later, continuous venovenous hemofiltration (CVVH), replicates the clearance profile of glomerular filtration.[273] More recently, continuous venovenous hemodiafiltration (CVVHD), which markedly enhances solute clearance, has been widely used. Simple to monitor by the critical care nurse,[274] CAVHD, using continuous low-dose heparin administration[275] into the afferent loop, provides 24 hours of dialysis per membrane without systemic complications; however, fluid balances must be carefully calculated as ultrafiltrate volumes may range from 20 to 50 liters per day. Venous access is available through the subclavian, internal jugular, or the femoral vein by double lumen catheters. Despite the successful removal of metabolic products, maintenance of plasma levels of metabolites within the normal range, and cardiocirculatory and respiratory improvement, the mortality of ARF remains prohibitively high, with the persistent systemic inflammatory response and MSOF leading to mortality.

Pharmacological Interventions

Burns, trauma, and sepsis are associated with a variety of mediators, many of which appear to be critical in the pathogenesis of cardiorespiratory, gastrointestinal, and renal dysfunction and in the development of SIRS and MSOF. Consequently, a variety of interventions, designed to block the effects of mediators, have been tested in animals and humans. Thus far, those efforts have not altered the outcome of organ system injury, although research continues.

Endotoxin (lipopolysaccharide, LPS), a component of the cell wall of Gram-negative bacteria, is present in the gut in considerable amounts. Burns, trauma, hypovolemia, hypoxemia, and intestinal ischemia as well as LPS itself may lead to increased mucosal permeability,[164,173] allowing endotoxins to enter the systemic circulation.[170] Immunotherapy, using *murine*[276,277] and human[278] anti-lipopolysaccharide IgG (E5, HA-1A), inactivates LPS, helps to destroy gram-negative bacteria, and was expected to become a major component of therapy, although blockade of LPS theoretically would be effective only in gram-negative sepsis. Immunotherapy directed against LPS has not been effective[279,280] and is unacceptably expensive.[281] Consequently, HA-1A has not been approved by the Food and Drug Administration.

Pseudomonas immunoglobulin has been given prophylactically to major burn-trauma patients with and without inhalation injury. Burned patients with inhalation injury who received 250 mg/kg of *Pseudomonas* immunoglobulin intravenously shortly after injury showed an earlier return of immunoglobulin serum levels to normal, a significantly reduced number of positive blood cultures, improved pulmonary function, and lower mortality.[282,283] However, prophylaxis with *Pseudomonas* immunoglobulin did not benefit other categories of burn-trauma patients.[282]

Host-derived factors, not bacterial products, are ultimately responsible for the development of septic shock. The cytokine, tumor necrosis factor (TNF), is produced by cells derived from the monocyte/macrophage line in response to gram-positive and gram-negative bacteria,[284] endotoxin and enterotoxins, antibodies to the CD14 receptor, products of complement activation, toxic shock syndrome toxin, mycobacterial cell wall products, viruses, parasites, and tumors.[285–291] Quantities of TNF undetectable by commercially available assays may cause lethal shock and tissue injury.[284] LPS binds to the liver-derived carrier protein (LPBP),[292,293] which is necessary for LPS to bind to the CD14 receptor on macrophages.[294,295] When LPBP is blocked, LPS no longer stimulates release of TNF.

After LPS binds to CD14, transcription and translation of TNF is upregulated within macrophages and other immunocompetent cells, and large amounts of TNF are released within minutes,[296] after which macrophages become refractory to LPS for 12–24 hours.[297] Regulation of TNF secretion is influenced by interferon-γ and prostaglandin E_2. Both interleukin-1 (IL-1) and interferon-γ synergistically influence the toxicity of TNF. Downregulation of TNF is promoted by corticosteroids and by pentoxifylline.

The development of the septic shock syndrome is dependent in part on the phasic release of TNF. Once induced, TNF produces both beneficial and deleterious effects, depending upon the quantity in which it is produced and the time period over which production is sustained. Circulating TNF binds to both cell-bound and soluble binding proteins, which are then cleared by the liver and kidneys. After administration of interferon-γ, LPS, or other cytokines, increased quantities of soluble receptors are present in serum and urine. Increased 'detoxifying' proteins may protect against excessive amounts of TNF, whereas 'appropriate' amounts of TNF are protective in listeriosis, malaria, and infections with *Legionella pneumophila*.

Two ways to reduce the toxicity are to neutralize TNF or to reduce the host's responsiveness. Neutralization, accomplished using anti-TNF monoclonal antibodies, also prevented the later increase of IL-1 and IL-6.[298,299] Another approach is to enhance elimination by administering soluble TNF receptors[300] or the extracellular portion of the type 1 TNF receptor,[301] one of two TNF receptors that have been characterized. Tolerance against TNF may be induced by repetitive administration of small quantities of TNF.[302] Moreover, granulocyte colony stimulating factor,[303] IL-10, and leukemia inhibitory factor[304] reduce responsiveness to TNF.

Another important mediator of the septic syndrome, IL-1, acts synergistically with TNF but increases 90–120 minutes after a TNF peak.[305,306] More prolonged circulation of this cytokine may provide a therapeutic window in which to administer antagonists.

An IL-1 receptor antagonist, a naturally occurring monocyte product that acts as a competitive inhibitor, reduced the mortality of experimental septic shock even when administered after the onset.[307]

Multiple interventions have been designed to inhibit or block other mediators. Thromboxane A_2 antagonists or thromboxane synthetase inhibitors reduce experimental pulmonary vasoconstriction and mesenteric ischemia. Prostaglandin E_2 and prostacyclin, which counteract thromboxane A_2 and participate in the regulation of organ blood flow, are, like thromboxane A_2, dependent on metabolism of arachidonate by cyclooxygenase. Leukotrienes, synthesized by lipoxygenase, may increase microvascular permeability. Blocking cyclooxygenase alone will increase the substrate for lipoxygenase activity, while inhibiting both vasoconstricting and vasodilating eicosanoids.[308] This illustrates the general principle that interventions designed to reduce mediator-related injury have multiple consequences.

Pulmonary injury in sepsis is mediated at least in part by generation of free radicals. Inflammatory cells, especially neutrophils, are one source of these toxic oxygen species, but generation of free radicals within lung cells may also contribute to pulmonary injury. The observations that free radicals inactivate antiproteinases and that antiproteinases act as free radical scavengers suggest a complex relationship among the mediators of injury.

The vasodilator NO may contribute to the decreased SVR and increased CI which is characteristic of hyperdynamic sepsis.[309–311] Two important forms of NO synthase have been identified.[312–314] A constitutive form participates in the regulation of microvascular blood flow.[309] A second, inducible NO synthase is increased by various mediators, including endotoxin, TNF, and IL-1.[315–318] Once induced, this enzyme generates NO rapidly in an autonomous and nonreceptor-mediated fashion.[312–314] NO synthase inhibitors restore normal responsiveness to catecholamines in septic rats,[319] an observation of some potential importance because septic patients tend to develop tachyphylaxis to pressors. When patients with vasopressor-treated hypotension were given NO synthase inhibitors,[60] blood pressure increased and cardiac output decreased, either because of restored responsiveness to catecholamines or attenuated vasodilation. Perhaps part of the toxicity of TNF is mediated by NO as a second messenger.[316] Prospective clinical trials of NO synthase inhibition are necessary because of the risk that reversal of septic vasodilation could actually worsen tissue perfusion.

On the other hand, NO has been administered by inhalation to ventilated patients with ARDS.[133] By vasodilating ventilated lung regions only, NO reduces Q_s/Q_T and improves ventilation/perfusion matching. Since one side effect of systemic NO synthase inhibition is pulmonary vasoconstriction, the combination of NO inhalation and systemic inhibition of NO production may be a promising treatment in the future.

Another future approach to septic complications and multiple organ failure in burn patients may be the elimination of inflammatory mediators.[320] Hemofiltration improves pulmonary function in septic ARDS in pigs[321] and children,[322] even if no net fluid is removed.[321] Hemofiltration also improved hemodynamic function[323] and right ventricular ejection fraction,[324] suggesting the removal of vasoactive and myocardial depressant factors. In septic patients with renal failure, hemofiltration was able to reduce significantly circulating levels of TNF and IL-2.[325]

After hemodiafiltration using acetate dialysate, release of IL-1, PGE_2, and leukotriene B_4 (LTB_4) was greater than with bicarbonate,[326] whereas after bicarbonate dialysis, TNF production was significantly higher.[326] Acetate-free filtration did not increase production of cytokines.[326] Acetate dialysis may directly activate circulating monocytes to produce IL-1, PGE_2, and LTB_4, whereas bicarbonate-induced TNF production is mediated by endotoxin.[326]

Hemofiltration and hemodialysis membranes show distinct clearance characteristics.[327] Polymethacrylate and polyacrylonitrile but not polysulfone membranes reduced TNF and IL-1 blood levels.[327] Detectable amounts of TNF and IL-1 were spontaneously produced by peripheral-blood monocytes 6 hours after the end of hemodialysis, but not after hemodiafiltration.[327] Continuous or intermittent blood-membrane contact alters endothelial responses.[328]

Summary

Treatment of complications in burned patients is a challenge for critical care physicians. The main goal of therapy is to monitor and preserve or support organ function. To preserve cardiopulmonary homeostasis, therapeutic efforts should be goal-directed. The gastrointestinal tract appears to be a critical link in the pathogenesis of sepsis. Although physiologic support is currently the hallmark of therapy, future interventions may specifically antagonize inflammatory mediators.

References

1. American Burn Association. Hospital and prehospital resources for optimal care of patients with burn injury: guidelines for development and operation of burn centers. *J Burn Care Rehabil* 1990; **11:** 98–104.

2. Herndon D N, Rutan R L, Rutan T C. Management of the pediatric patient with burns. *J Burn Care Rehabil* 1993; **14:** 3–8.

3. Snelling C F. The comprehensive burn unit. *Can J Surg* 1985; **28:** 478–81.

4. Paradiso C. Hemofiltration: an alternative to dialysis. *Heart Lung* 1989; **18:** 282–90.

5. Zobel G, Ring E, Kuttnig M, Grubbauer H M. Five years experience with continuous extracorporeal renal support in paediatric intensive care. *Intensive Care Med* 1991; **17:** 315–19.

6. Imbus S H, Zawacki B E. Encouraging dialogue and autonomy in the burn intensive care unit. *Crit Care Clin* 1986; **2:** 53–60.

7. Petro J A, Salzberg C A. Ethical issues of burn management. *Clin Plast Surg* 1992; **19:** 615–21.

8. Fratianne R B, Brandt C, Yurko L, Coffee T. When is enough enough? Ethical dilemmas on the burn unit. *J Burn Care Rehabil* 1992; **13:** 600–4.

9. Slater A L, Fassnacht Hanrahan K, Slater H, Goldfarb I W. From hopeful to hopeless. When do we write 'do not resuscitate'? *Focus Crit Care* 1991; **18:** 476–9.

10. Konigova R. Ethical problems in burn injury in the past decade. *Acta Chir Plast* 1992; **34:** 178–81.

11. McDermott J F, Waldron J A, Ponce D E. The right to die as an ethical dilemma for new physicians in Hawaii. *Hawaii Med J* 1992; **51:** 44–5.

12. Rush B F Jr. The bacterial factor in hemorrhagic shock. *Surg Gynecol Obstet* 1992; **175:** 285–92.

13. Rush B F, Sori A J, Murphy T F, Smith S, Flanagan J J, Machiedo G W. Endotoxemia and bacteremia during hemorrhagic shock. The link between trauma and sepsis? *Ann Surg* 1988; **207:** 549–54.

14. Crowley K, Phelan D. Septicaemia and the prevention of multiorgan failure – the intensive care perspective. *Ir Med J* 1990; **83:** 121–4.

15. Messahel F M, Seraj M A. Mortality in the surgical intensive care unit – the role of sepsis and organ failure. *Middle East J Anesthesiol* 1989; **10:** 299–305.

16. Gore D C, Honeycutt D, Jahoor F, Barrow R E, Wolfe R R, Herndon D N. Propranolol diminishes extremity blood flow in burned patients. *Ann Surg* 1991; **213:** 568–73.

17. Herndon D N, Barrow R E, Rutan T C, Minifee P, Jahoor F, Wolfe R R. Effect of propranolol administration on hemodynamic and metabolic responses of burned pediatric patients. *Ann Surg* 1988; **208:** 484–92.

18. Honeycutt D, Barrow R, Herndon D. Cold stress response in patients with severe burns after beta-blockade. *J Burn Care Rehabil* 1992; **13:** 181–6.

19. Fleming R Y, Rutan R L, Jahoor F, Barrow R E, Wolfe R R, Herndon D N. Effect of recombinant human growth hormone on catabolic hormones and free fatty acids following thermal injury. *J Trauma* 1992; **32:** 698–702.

20. Herndon D N, Hayward P G, Rutan R L, Barrow R E. Growth hormones and factors in surgical patients. *Adv Surg* 1992; **25:** 65–97.

21. Gore D C, Honeycutt D, Jahoor F, Rutan T, Wolfe R R, Herndon D N. Effect of exogenous growth hormone on glucose utilization in burn patients. *J Surg Res* 1991; **51:** 518–23.

22. Ziegler T R, Young L S, Ferrari Baliviera E, Demling R H, Wilmore D W. Use of human growth hormone combined with nutritional support in a critical care unit. *J Parenter Enteral Nutr* 1990; **14:** 574–81.

23. Herndon D N, Barrow R E, Kunkel K R, Broemeling L, Rutan R L. Effects of recombinant human growth hormone on donor-site healing in severely burned children. *Ann Surg* 1990; **212:** 424–9.

24. Dong Y L, Fleming R Y, Huang K F, Herndon D N, Yan T Z, Waymack J P. Effect of insulin-like growth factor 1 on host response to tumor. *J Surg Oncol* 1993; **53:** 121–7.

25. Huang K F, Chung D H, Herndon D N. Insulin like growth factor 1 (IGF-1) reduces gut atrophy and bacterial translocation after severe burn injury. *Arch Surg* 1993; **128:** 47–53.

26. Deitch E A. Infection in the compromised host. *Surg Clin North Am* 1988; **68:** 181–97.

27. Parker M M, Cunnion R E, Parrillo J E. Echocardiography and nuclear cardiac imaging in the critical care unit. *JAMA* 1985; **254:** 2935–9.

28. Knobel E, Fernandes C J, Akamine N, *et al.* Right ventricular influence on left ventricular performance in septic patients. *Crit Care Med* 1987; **15:** 1158–9.

29. Theissen J L, Loick H M, Traber L D, Herndon D N, Traber D L. Carbon monoxide and pulmonary circulation in an ovine model. *J Burn Care Rehabil* 1992; **13:** 623–7.

30. Sibbald W J, Driedger A A, Cunningham D G, Cheung H. Right and left ventricular performance in acute hypoxemic respiratory failure. *Crit Care Med* 1986; **14:** 852–7.

31. Redl G, Abdi S, Traber L D, *et al.* Inhibition of thromboxane synthesis reduces endotoxin-induced right ventricular failure in sheep. *Crit Care Med* 1991; **19:** 1294–302.

32. Parrillo J E, Parker M M, Natanson C, *et al.* Septic shock in humans. Advances in the understanding of pathogenesis, cardiovascular dysfunction, and therapy. *Ann Intern Med* 1990; **113:** 227–42.

33. Johnston W E. Complications from the use of pulmonary artery catheters. In: Lumb P D, Bryan-Brown C W, eds. *Complications in Critical Care Medicine*. Chicago, IL: Year Book Medical Publishers, Inc, 1988.

34. Herndon D N, Traber D L, Traber L D. The effect of resuscitation on inhalation injury. *Surgery* 1986; **100:** 248–51.

35. Pruitt B A Jr, Mason A D Jr, Moncrief J A. Hemodynamic changes in the early postburn patient: the influence of fluid administration and a vasodilator (hydralazine). *J Trauma* 1971; **11:** 36–40.

36. Goodwin C W, Finkelstein J L, Madden M R, Marano M A. Resuscitation of the burned patient. In: Barie P S, Shires G T, eds. *Surgical Intensive Care*. Boston/Toronto/London: Little, Brown and Company (Inc), 1993: 1123–36.

37. Carroll G C, Snyder J V. Effect of bacteremia and fluid resuscitation on cardiac output. *Circ Shock* 1983; **11:** 217–22.

38. Carroll G C, Snyder J V. Hyperdynamic severe intravascular sepsis depends on fluid administration in cynomolgus monkey. *Am J Physiol* 1982; **243:** R131–R141.

39. Rackow E C, Kaufman B, Falk J. Hemodynamic response to fluid repletion in patients with septic shock. *Circ Shock* 1987; **22:** 11–22.

40. Savin V J, Sharma R, Lovell H B, Welling D J. Measurement of albumin reflection coefficient with isolated rat glomeruli. *J Am Soc Nephrol* 1992; **3:** 1260–9.

41. Lucas C E, Ledgerwood A M, Rachwal W J, Grabow D, Saxe J M. Colloid oncotic pressure and body water dynamics in septic and injured patients. *J Trauma* 1991; **31:** 927–31.

42. Steffes C P, Bender J S, Levison M A. Blood transfusion and oxygen consumption in surgical sepsis. *Crit Care Med* 1991; **19:** 512–17.

43. McCormick M, Feustel P J, Newell J C, Stratton H H, Fortune J B. Effect of cardiac index and hematocrit changes on oxygen consumption in resuscitated patients. *J Surg Res* 1988; **44:** 499–505.

44. Conrad S A, Dietrich K A, Hebert C A, Romero M D. Effect of red cell transfusion on oxygen consumption following fluid resuscitation in septic shock. *Circ Shock* 1990; **31:** 419–29.

45. Fortune J B, Feustel P J, Saifi J, Stratton H H, Newell J C, Shah D M. Influence of hematocrit on cardiopulmonary function after acute hemorrhage. *J Trauma* 1987; **27:** 243–9.

46. Czer L S, Shoemaker W C. Optimal hematocrit value in critically ill postoperative patients. *Surg Gynecol Obstet* 1978; **147:** 363–8.

47. Astiz M E, Tilly E, Rackow E D, Weil M H. Peripheral vascular tone in sepsis. *Chest* 1991; **99:** 1072–5.

48. Ognibene F P, Parker M M, Natanson C, Shelhamer J H, Parrillo J E. Depressed left ventricular performance. Response to volume infusion in patients with sepsis and septic shock. *Chest* 1988; **93:** 903–10.

49. Parrillo J E, Burch C, Shelhamer J H, Parker M M, Natanson C, Schuette W. A circulating myocardial depressant substance in humans with septic shock. *J Clin Invest* 1985; **76:** 1539–53.

50. Parker M M, Shelhamer J H, Bacharach S L, *et al.* Profound but reversible myocardial depression in patients with septic shock. *Ann Intern Med* 1984; **100:** 483–90.

51. Hollenberg S M, Cunnion R E, Zimmerberg J. Nitric oxide synthase inhibition reverses arteriolar hyporesponsiveness to catecholamines in septic rats. *Am J Physiol* 1993; **264:** H660–H663.

52. Vicaut E, Hou X, Payen D, Bousseau A, Tedgui A. Acute effects of tumor necrosis factor on the microcirculation in rat cremaster muscle. *J Clin Invest* 1991; **87:** 1537–40.

53. Preiser J C, Moulart D, Cosyns B, Vincent J L. Administration of the calcium agonist BAY K 8644 in endotoxic shock. *Circ Shock* 1991; **35:** 199–206.

54. Rump A F, Ratke R, Fricke U, Klaus W. Influence of (–)-S-Bay K 8644, (+/–)-Bay W 5035 and (+/–)-Bay T 5006 on hemodynamics and FITC-dextran 3 elution kinetics in isolated rat hearts. *Gen Pharmacol* 1993; **24:** 631–6.

55. Rupp H, Berger H J, Pfeifer A, Werdan K. Effect of positive inotropic agents on myosin isozyme population and mechanical activity of cultured rat heart myocytes. *Circ Res* 1991; **68:** 1164–73.

56. Furukawa Y, Ogiwara Y, Akahane K, Chiba S. Different antagonism of the positive chronotropic and inotropic responses of the isolated, blood-perfused dog atrium to Bay K 8644 by nicardipine and verapamil. *Eur J Pharmacol* 1988; **156:** 231–7.

57. Furchgott R F, Jothianandan D. Endothelium-dependent and -independent vasodilation involving cyclic GMP: relaxation induced by nitric oxide, carbon monoxide and light. *Blood Vessels* 1991; **28:** 52–61.

58. Meyer J, Lentz C W, Stothert J C Jr, Traber L D, Herndon D N, Traber D L. Effects of nitric oxide synthesis inhibition in hyperdynamic endotoxemia. *Crit Care Med* 1994; **22:** 306–12.

59. Ochoa J B, Udekwu A O, Billiar T R, *et al.* Nitrogen oxide levels in patients after trauma and during sepsis. *Ann Surg* 1991; **214:** 621–6.

60. Lorente J A, Landin L, De Pablo R, Renes E, Liste D. L-Arginine pathway in the sepsis syndrome. *Crit Care Med* 1993; **21:** 1287–95.

61. Evans T, Carpenter A, Kinderman H, Cohen J. Evidence of increased nitric oxide production in patients with the sepsis syndrome. *Circ Shock* 1993; **41:** 77–81.

62. Shi Y, Li H-Q, Shen C-K, *et al.* Plasma nitric oxide levels in newborn infants with sepsis. *J Pediatr* 1993; **123:** 435–8.

63. Pepke Zaba J, Higenbottam T W, Dinh Xuan A T, Ridden C, Kealey T. Alpha-adrenoceptor stimulation of porcine pulmonary arteries. *Eur J Pharmacol* 1993; **235:** 169–75.

64. Tschudi M, Richard V, Buhler F R, Luscher T F. Importance of endothelium-derived nitric oxide in porcine coronary resistance arteries. *Am J Physiol* 1991; **260:** H13–H20.

65. Vincent J L. Do we need a dopaminergic agent in the management of the critically ill? *J Auton Pharmacol* 1990; **10** (Suppl 1): S123–S127.

66. Schaer G L, Fink M P, Parrillo J E. Norepinephrine alone versus norepinephrine plus low-dose dopamine: enhanced renal blood flow with combination pressor therapy. *Crit Care Med* 1985; **13:** 492–6.

67. Baim D S. Effect of phosphodiesterase inhibition on myocardial oxygen consumption and coronary blood flow. *Am J Cardiol* 1989; **63:** 23A–26A.

68. Thijs L G, Schneider A J, Groeneveld A B. The haemodynamics of septic shock. *Intensive Care Med* 1990; **16** (Suppl 3): S182–S186.

69. Schneider A J, Groeneveld A B, Teule G J, Nauta J, Heidendal G A, Thijs L G. Volume expansion, dobutamine and noradrenaline for treatment of right ventricular dysfunction in porcine septic shock: a combined invasive and radionuclide study. *Circ Shock* 1987; **23:** 93–106.

70. Prielipp R C, Rosenthal M H, Pearl R G. Vasodilator therapy in vasoconstrictor-induced pulmonary hypertension in sheep. *Anesthesiology* 1988; **68:** 552–8.

71. Desjars P, Pinaud M, Potel G, Tasseau F, Touze M. A reappraisal of norepinephrine therapy in human septic shock. *Crit Care Med* 1987; **15:** 134–7.

72. Aikawa N, Wakabayashi G, Ueda M, Shinozawa Y. Regulation of renal function in thermal injury. *J Trauma* 1990; **30:** S174–S178.

73. Asch M J, Feldman R J, Walker H L, *et al.* Systemic and pulmonary hemodynamic changes accompanying thermal injury. *Ann Surg* 1982; **178:** 218–21.

74. Bland R D, Shoemaker W C. Probability of survival as a prognostic and severity of illness score in critically ill surgical patients. *Crit Care Med* 1985; **13:** 91–5.

75. Dries D J, Waxman K. Adequate resuscitation of burn patients may not be measured by urine output and vital signs. *Crit Care Med* 1991; **19:** 327–9.

76. Ashbaugh D G, Bigelow D B, Petty T L, Levine B E. Acute respiratory distress in adults. *Lancet* 1967; **2:** 319–23.

77. Drost A C, Burleson D G, Cioffi W G, Mason A D, Pruitt B A. Plasma cytokines after thermal injury and their relationship to infection. *Ann Surg* 1993; **218:** 74–8.

78. Dantzker D R, Brook C J, Dehart P, Lynch J P, Weg J G. Ventilation-perfusion distributions in the adult respiratory distress syndrome. *Am Rev Respir Dis* 1979; **120:** 1039–52.

79. Ralph D D, Robertson H T, Weaver L J, Hlastala M P, Carrico C J, Hudson L D. Distribution of ventilation and perfusion during positive end-expiratory pressure in the adult respiratory distress syndrome. *Am Rev Respir Dis* 1985; **131:** 54–60.

80. Falke K J, Pontoppidan H, Kumar A, Leith D E, Geffin B, Laver M B. Ventilation with end-expiratory pressure in acute lung disease. *J Clin Invest* 1972; **51:** 2315–23.

81. Lamy M, Fallat R J, Koeniger E, *et al.* Pathologic features and mechanisms of hypoxemia in adult respiratory distress syndrome. *Am Rev Respir Dis* 1976; **114:** 267–84.

82. Hopewell P C, Murray J F. Effects of continuous positive-pressure ventilation in experimental pulmonary edema. *J Appl Physiol* 1976; **40:** 568–74.

83. Gattinoni L, Pesenti A, Bombino M, *et al.* Relationships between lung computed tomographic density, gas exchange, and PEEP in acute respiratory failure. *Anesthesiology* 1988; **69:** 824–32.

84. Boyd J E, Bewman J H, Brigham K L. Permeability pulmonary edema. Diagnosis and management. *Arch Intern Med* 1984; **144:** 143–7.

85. Holloway H, Perry M, Downey J, Parker J, Taylor A. Estimation of effective pulmonary capillary pressure in intact lungs. *J Appl Physiol* 1983; **54:** 846–51.

86. Collee G G, Lynch K E, Hill R D, Zapol W M. Bedside measurement of pulmonary capillary pressure in patients with acute respiratory failure. *Anesthesiology* 1987; **66:** 614–20.

87. Anderson R R, Holliday R L, Driedger A A, Lefcoe M, Reid B, Sibbald W J. Documentation of pulmonary capillary permeability in the adult respiratory distress syndrome accompanying human sepsis. *Am Rev Respir Dis* 1979; **119:** 869–77.

88. Benumof J L. Hypoxic pulmonary vasoconstriction and infusion of sodium nitroprusside. *Anesthesiology* 1979; **50:** 481–3.

89. Radermacher P, Santak B, Wust H J, Tarnow J, Falke K J. Prostacyclin for the treatment of pulmonary hypertension in the adult respiratory distress syndrome: effects on pulmonary capillary pressure and ventilation-perfusion distributions. *Anesthesiology* 1990; **72:** 238–44.

90. Hemmer M, Suter P M. Treatment of cardiac and renal effects of PEEP with dopamine in patients with acute respiratory failure. *Anesthesiology* 1979; **50:** 399–403.

91. Lemaire F, Regnier B, Simoneau G, Harf A. Positive end-expiratory pressure (PEEP) ventilation suppresses the increase of shunting caused by dopamine infusion. *Anesthesiology* 1980; **52:** 376–7.

92. Andreadis N, Petty T L. Adult respiratory distress syndrome: problems and progress. *Am Rev Respir Dis* 1985; **132:** 1344–6.

93. Jacobs E R, Bone R C. Clinical indicators in sepsis and septic adult respiratory distress syndrome. *Med Clin North Am* 1986; **70:** 921–32.

94. Murray J F, Matthay M A, Luce J M, Flick M R. An expanded definition of the adult respiratory distress syndrome. *Am Rev Respir Dis* 1988; **138:** 720–3.

95. Moylan J A, West J T, Nash G, Bowen J A, Pruitt B A. Tracheostomy in thermally injured patients: a review of five years' experience. *Am Surg* 1972; **38:** 119–23.

96. Herndon D N, Curreri P W, Abston S, Rutan T C, Barrow R E. Treatment of burns. *Curr Probl Surg* 1987; **24:** 341–97.

97. Suter P M, Fairley B, Isenberg M D. Optimum end-expiratory airway pressure in patients with acute pulmonary failure. *N Engl J Med* 1975; **292:** 284–9.

98. Gallagher T J, Civetta J M, Kirby R R. Terminology update: optimal PEEP. *Crit Care Med* 1978; **6:** 323–6.

99. Mathru M, Rao T L, Venus B. Ventilator-induced barotrauma in controlled mechanical ventilation versus intermittent mandatory ventilation. *Crit Care Med* 1983; **11:** 359–61.

100. Groeger J S, Levinson M R, Carlon G C. Assist control versus synchronized intermittent mandatory ventilation during acute respiratory failure. *Crit Care Med* 1989; **17:** 607–12.

101. Esteban A, Frutos F, Tobin M J, *et al.* A comparison of four methods of weaning patients from mechanical ventilation. *N Engl J Med* 1995; **332:** 345–50.

102. Brochard L, Harf A, Lorino H, Lemaire F. Inspiratory pressure support prevents diaphragmatic fatigue during weaning from mechanical ventilation. *Am Rev Respir Dis* 1989; **139:** 513–21.

103. Fassoulaki A, Eforakopoulou M. Cardiovascular, respiratory, and metabolic changes produced by pressure-supported ventilation in intensive care unit patients. *Crit Care Med* 1989; **17:** 527–9.

104. Wong D H, Stemmer E A, Gordon I. Acute massive airleak and pressure support ventilation. *Crit Care Med* 1990; **18:** 114–15.

105. Baum M, Benzer H, Mutz N, Pauser G, Tonczar L. Inverse ratio ventilation (IRV). Role of the respiratory time ratio in artificial respiration in ARDS. *Anaesthesist* 1980; **29:** 592–6.

106. Cole A G, Weller S F, Sykes M K. Inverse ratio ventilation compared with PEEP in adult respiratory failure. *Intensive Care Med* 1984; **10:** 227–32.

107. Mercat A, Graini L, Teboul J L, Lenique F, Richard C. Cardiorespiratory effects of pressure-controlled ventilation with and without inverse ratio in the adult respiratory distress syndrome. *Chest* 1993; **104:** 871–5.

108. Stock M C, Downs J B, Frolicher D A. Airway pressure release ventilation. *Crit Care Med* 1987; **15:** 462–6.

109. Garner W, Downs J B, Stock M C, Rasanen J. Airway pressure release ventilation (APRV). A human trial. *Chest* 1988; **94:** 779–81.

110. Baum M, Benzer H, Putensen C, Koller W, Putz G. Biphasic positive airway pressure (BIPAP) – a new form of augmented ventilation. *Anaesthesist* 1989; **38:** 452–8.

111. Brichant J F, Rouby J J, Viars P. Intermittent positive pressure ventilation with either positive end-expiratory pressure or high frequency jet ventilation (HFJV), or HFJV alone in human acute respiratory failure. *Anesth Analg* 1986; **65:** 1135–42.

112. El Baz N, Faber L P, Doolas A. Combined high-frequency ventilation for management of terminal respiratory failure: a new technique. *Anesth Analg* 1983; **62:** 39–49.

113. Cioffi W G, Rue L III, Graves T A, McManus W F, Mason A D, Pruitt B A. Prophylactic use of high-frequency percussive ventilation in patients with inhalation injury. *Ann Surg* 1991; **213:** 575–80.

114. Hurst J M, Branson R D, Davis K, Barrette R R, Adams K S. Comparison of conventional mechanical ventilation and high-frequency ventilation. A prospective, randomized trial in patients with respiratory failure. *Ann Surg* 1990; **211:** 486–91.

115. Hickling K G, Henderson S J, Jackson R. Low mortality associated with low volume pressure limited ventilation with permissive hypercapnia in severe adult respiratory distress syndrome. *Intensive Care Med* 1990; **16:** 372–7.

116. Nguyen T T, Cox C S, Tzounakis A, *et al.* Carotid blood flow during permissive hypercapnia in an ovine model. *Crit Care Med* 1993; **21:** S190 (Abstract).

117. Tzounakis A, Nguyen T T, Tao W, *et al.* Effect of permissive hypercapnia on renal and mesenteric blood flow in an ovine model. *Am Rev Respir Dis* 1993; **147:** A891–A890 (Abstract).

118. Wilson J M, Thompson J R, Schnitzer J J, *et al.* Intratracheal pulmonary ventilation and congenital diaphragmatic hernia: a report of two cases. *J Pediatr Surg* 1993; **28:** 484–7.

119. Zapol W M, Snider M T, Hill J D, *et al.* Extracorporeal membrane oxygenation in severe acute respiratory failure. A randomized prospective study. *JAMA* 1979; **242:** 2193–6.

120. Gattinoni L, Pesenti A, Mascheroni D, *et al.* Low-frequency positive-pressure ventilation with extracorporeal CO_2 removal in severe acute respiratory failure. *JAMA* 1986; **256:** 881–6.

121. Zwischenberger J B, Cox C S, Minifee P K, *et al.* Pathophysiology of ovine smoke inhalation injury treated with extracorporeal membrane oxygenation. *Chest* 1993; **103:** 1582–6.

122. Mortensen J D, Berry G. Conceptual and design features of a practical, clinically effective intravenous mechanical blood oxygen/carbon dioxide exchange device (IVOX). *Int J Artif Organs* 1989; **12:** 384–9.

123. Tao W, Zwischenberger J B, Nguyen T T, *et al.* Performance of an intravenous gas exchanger (IVOX) in a venovenous bypass circuit. *Ann Thorac Surg* 1994; **57:** 1484–90.

124. Cox C S, Zwischenberger J B, Traber L D, Traber D L, Herndon D N. Use of an intravascular oxygenator/carbon dioxide removal device in an ovine smoke inhalation injury model. *ASAIO Trans* 1991; **37:** M411–M413.

125. Gentilello L M, Jurkovich G J, Gubler K D, Anardi D M, Heiskell R. The intravascular oxygenator (IVOX): preliminary results of a new means of performing extra-pulmonary gas exchange. *J Trauma* 1993; **35:** 399–404.

126. High K M, Snider M T, Richard R, *et al.* Clinical trials of an intravenous oxygenator in patients with adult respiratory distress syndrome. *Anesthesiology* 1992; **77:** 856–63.

127. Ashbaugh D G, Maier R V. Idiopathic pulmonary fibrosis in adult respiratory distress syndrome. Diagnosis and treatment. *Arch Surg* 1985; **120:** 530–5.

128. Hooper R G, Kearl R A. Established ARDS treated with a sustained course of adrenocortical steroids. *Chest* 1990; **97:** 138–43.

129. Greene R, Lind S, Jantsch H, *et al.* Pulmonary vascular obstruction in severe ARDS: angiographic alterations after i.v. fibrinolytic therapy. *Am J Roentgenol* 1987; **148:** 501–8.

130. Holcroft J W, Vassar M J, Weber C J. Prostaglandin E1 and survival in patients with the adult respiratory distress syndrome. A prospective trial. *Ann Surg* 1986; **203:** 371–8.

131. Shoemaker W C, Appel P L. Effects of prostaglandin E1 in adult respiratory distress syndrome. *Surgery* 1986; **99:** 275–83.

132. Silverman H J, Slotman G, Bone R C, *et al.* Effects of prostaglandin E1 on oxygen delivery and consumption in patients with the adult respiratory distress syndrome. Results from the prostaglandin E1 multicenter trial. *Chest* 1990; **98:** 405–10.

133. Rossaint R, Falke K J, Lopez F, Slama K, Pison U, Zapol W M. Inhaled nitric oxide for the adult respiratory distress syndrome. *N Engl J Med* 1993; **328:** 399–405.

134. Alexander J W, MacMillan B G, Stinnett J D, *et al.* Beneficial effects of aggressive protein feeding in severely burned children. *Ann Surg* 1980; **192:** 505–17.

135. Austgen T R, Chen M K, Flynn T C, Souba W W. The effects of endotoxin on the splanchnic metabolism of glutamine and related substrates. *J Trauma* 1991; **31:** 742–51.

136. Pacitti A J, Austgen T R, Souba W W. Mechanisms of increased hepatic glutamine uptake in the endotoxin-treated rat. *J Surg Res* 1992; **53:** 298–305.

137. Souba W W, Klimberg V S, Hautamaki R D, *et al.* Oral glutamine reduces bacterial translocation, following abdominal radiation. *J Surg Res* 1990; **48:** 1–5.

138. Hastings P R, Skillman J J, Bushnell L S, Silen W. Antacid titration in the prevention of acute gastrointestinal bleeding. A controlled, randomized trial of 100 critically ill patients. *N Engl J Med* 1978; **298:** 1041–5.

139. Driks M R, Craven D E, Celli B R, *et al.* Nosocomial pneumonia in intubated patients given sucralfate as compared with antacids or histamine type 2 blockers. The role of gastric colonization. *N Engl J Med* 1987; **317:** 1376–82.

140. Craven D E, Driks M R. Nosocomial pneumonia in the intubated patient. *Semin Respir Infect* 1987; **2:** 20–33.

141. Tryba M. The gastropulmonary route of infection – fact or fiction? *Am J Med* 1991; **91:** 135S–146S.

142. Priebe H J, Skillman J J, Bushnell L S, Long P C, Silen W. Antacid versus cimetidine in preventing acute gastrointestinal bleeding. A randomized trial in 75 critically ill patients. *N Engl J Med* 1980; **302:** 426–30.

143. Tryba M. Side effects of stress bleeding prophylaxis. *Am J Med* 1989; **86:** 85–93.

144. Tryba M. Prevention of stress bleeding with ranitidine or pirenzepine and the risk of pneumonia. *J Clin Anesth* 1988; **1:** 12–20.

145. Lopez Herce J, Dorao P, Elola P, Delgado M A, Ruza F, Madero R. Frequency and prophylaxis of upper gastrointestinal hemorrhage in critically ill children: a prospective study comparing the efficacy of almagate, ranitidine, and sucralfate. *Crit Care Med* 1992; **20:** 1082.

146. Tryba M. Risk of acute stress bleeding and nosocomial pneumonia in ventilated intensive care unit patients: sucralfate versus antacids. *Am J Med* 1987; **83:** 117–24.

147. Borrero E, Ciervo J, Chang J B. Antacid vs sucralfate in preventing acute gastrointestinal tract bleeding in abdominal aortic surgery. A randomized trial in 50 patients. *Arch Surg* 1986; **121:** 810–12.

148. Tryba M, Mantey Stiers F. Antibacterial activity of sucralfate in human gastric juice. *Am J Med* 1987; **83:** 125–7.

149. Tryba M. Sucralfate versus antacids or H_2-antagonists for stress ulcer prophylaxis: a meta-analysis on efficacy and pneumonia rate. *Crit Care Med* 1991; **19:** 942–9.

150. Ryan C M, Schmidt J, Lewandrowski K, *et al.* Gut macromolecular permeability in pancreatitis correlates with severity of disease in rats. *Gastroenterology* 1993; **104:** 890–5.

151. Deitch E A, Maejima K, Berg R. Effect of oral antibiotics and bacterial overgrowth on the translocation of the GI tract microflora in burned rats. *J Trauma* 1985; **25:** 385–92.

152. Meakins J L, Marshall W. The gastrointestinal tract: the 'motor' of MOF. *Arch Surg* 1986; **121:** 197–201.

153. Carter E A, Tompkins R G, Burke J F. Hepatic and intestinal blood flow following thermal injury. *J Burn Care Rehabil* 1988; **9:** 347–50.

154. Dahn M S, Lange P, Lobdell K, Hans B, Jacobs L A, Mitchell R A. Splanchnic and total body oxygen consumption differences in septic and injured patients. *Surgery* 1987; **101:** 69–80.

155. McNeill J R. Role of vasopressin and angiotensin in response of splanchnic resistance vessels to hemorrhage. In: Hinshaw L B, Cox J B, eds. *The Fundamental Mechanisms of Shock*. New York: Plenum, 1983: 127–44.

156. Kerr J C, Jain K M, Swan K G, Rocko J M. Effects of vasopressin on cardiac output and its distribution in the subhuman primate. *J Vasc Surg* 1985; **2:** 443–9.

157. Banks R O, Gallavan R H, Zinner M H, *et al.* Vasoactive agents in control of the mesenteric circulation. *Fed Proc* 1985; **44:** 2743–9.

158. Gunther S, Gimbrone M A Jr, Alexander R W. Identification and characterization of the high affinity vascular angiotensin II receptor in rat mesenteric artery. *Circ Res* 1980; **47:** 278.

159. Oshima A, Kitajima M, Sakai N, Ando N. Does glucagon improve the viability of ischemic intestine? *J Surg Res* 1990; **49:** 524–33.

160. Tokyay R, Traber D L, Herndon D N. Thromboxane synthetase inhibition prevents the increased mesenteric vascular resistance seen after major burn in a chronic porcine model. *Surg Forum* 1990; **41:** 47–9.

161. Aoki N, Siegfried M, Tsao P, Lento P, Lefer A M. Beneficial mechanisms of action of a prostacyclin enhancing agent in splanchnic artery occlusion shock. *Res Commun Chem Pathol Pharmacol* 1988; **60:** 275–89.

162. Aoki N, Lefer A M. Protective effects of thromboxane receptor blockade in splanchnic artery occlusion shock. *Methods Find Exp Clin Pharmacol* 1988; **10:** 413–18.

163. Jones W, Minei J P, Barber A E, Fahey T III, Shires G III, Shires G T. Splanchnic vasoconstriction and bacterial translocation after thermal injury. *Am J Physiol* 1991; **261:** H1190–H1196.

164. Ziegler T R, Smith R J, O'Dwyer S T, Demling R H, Wilmore D W. Increased intestinal permeability associated with infection in burn patients. *Arch Surg* 1988; **123:** 1313–319.

165. Tokyay R, Zeigler S T, Heggers J P, Loick H M, Traber D L, Herndon D N. Effects of anesthesia, surgery, fluid, resuscitation, and endotoxin administration on postburn bacterial translocation. *J Trauma* 1991; **31:** 1376–9.

166. Tokyay R, Zeigler S T, Loick H M, *et al.* Mesenteric lymphadenectomy prevents postburn systemic spread of translocated bacteria. *Arch Surg* 1992; **127:** 384–8.

167. Jones W, Barber A E, Minei J P, Fahey T J, Shires G III, Shires G T. Antibiotic prophylaxis diminishes bacterial translocation but not mortality in experimental burn wound sepsis. *J Trauma* 1990; **30:** 737–40.

168. Deitch E A, Berg R. Bacterial translocation from the gut: a mechanism of infection. *J Burn Care Rehabil* 1987; **8:** 475–82.

169. Deitch E A. Bacterial translocation of the gut flora. *J Trauma* 1990; **30:** S184–S189.

170. Tokyay R, Zeigler S T, Traber D L, *et al.* Postburn gastrointestinal vasoconstriction increases bacterial and endotoxin translocation. *J Appl Physiol* 1993; **74:** 1521–7.

171. Ryan C M, Yarmush M L, Burke J F, Tompkins R G. Increased gut permeability early after burns correlates with the extent of burn injury. *Crit Care Med* 1992; **20:** 1508–12.

172. Winchurch R A, Thupari J N, Munster A M. Endotoxemia in burn patients: levels of circulating endotoxins are related to burn size. *Surgery* 1987; **102:** 808–12.

173. O'Dwyer S T, Michie H R, Ziegler T R, Revhaug A, Smith R J, Wilmore D W. A single dose of endotoxin increases intestinal permeability in healthy humans. *Arch Surg* 1988; **123:** 1459–64.

174. Fink M P, Antonsson J B, Wang H L, Rothschild H R. Increased intestinal permeability in endotoxic pigs. Mesenteric hypoperfusion as an etiologic factor. *Arch Surg* 1991; **126:** 211–18.

175. Alexander J W, Boyce S T, Babcock G F, *et al.* The process of microbial translocation. *Ann Surg* 1990; **212:** 496–510.

176. van der Waaij D, Berghuis-de Vries J M, Lekkerkerk-van der Wees J E C. Colonization resistance in conventional and antibiotic-treated mice. *J Hyg Camb* 1971; **69:** 405–11.

177. Lingnau W. Selektive Florasuppression bei traumatisierten Intensivpatienten. *Intensivbehandlung* 1990; **15:** 89–91.

178. Stoutenbeek C P, van Saene H K F, Miranda D R, Zandstra D F. The effect of selective decontamination of the digestive tract on colonization and infection rate in multiple trauma patients. *Intensive Care Med* 1984; **10:** 185–92.

179. Stoutenbeek C P, van Saene H K F, Miranda D R, Zandstra D F. The effect of oropharyngeal decontamination using topical nonabsorbable antibiotics on the incidence of nosocomial respiratory tract infections in multiple trauma patients. *J Trauma* 1987; **27:** 357–64.

180. Vandenbroucke Grauls C M, Vandenbroucke J P. Effect of selective decontamination of the digestive tract on respiratory tract infections and mortality in the intensive care unit. *Lancet* 1991; **338:** 859–62.

181. Munster A M, Smith–Meek M, Dickerson C, Winchurch R A. Translocation: incidental phenomenon or true pathology? *Ann Surg* 1993; **218:** 321–7.

182. Spiegel D M, Ullian M E, Zerbe G O, Berl T. Determinants of survival and recovery in acute renal failure patients dialyzed in intensive-care units. *Am J Nephrol* 1991; **11:** 44–7.

183. Tilney N L, Lazarus J M. Acute renal failure in surgical patients. Causes, clinical patterns, and care. *Surg Clin North Am* 1983; **63:** 357–77.

184. Wilkes B M, Mailloux L U. Acute renal failure. Pathogenesis and prevention. *Am J Med* 1986; **80:** 1129–36.

185. Sinsteden T D, O'Neil T J, Hill S, Lifschitz M D, Stein J H. The role of high-energy phosphate in norepinephrine-induced acute renal failure in the dog. *Circ Res* 1986; **49:** 93–104.

186. Ratcliffe P J, Moonen C T W, Holloway P A H, Ledingham J G G, Radda G K. Acute renal failure in hemorrhagic hypotension: cellular energetics and renal function. *Kidney Int* 1986; **30:** 355–60.

187. Brezis M, Rosen S, Silva P, Epstein F H. Renal ischemia: a new perspective. *Kidney Int* 1984; **26:** 375–83.

188. Brezis M, Rosen S, Hypoxia of the renal medulla – its implications for disease. *N Engl J Med* 1995; **332:** 647–55.

189. Hermreck A S. Renal response in sepsis. *Arch Surg* 1973; **107:** 169–75.

190. Lucas C E. The renal response to acute injury and sepsis. *Surg Clin North Am* 1976; **56:** 953–75.

191. Hackl J M, Neumann M, Weirather E, Stroschneider E. Myoglobin release and renal function in polytraumatized patients in intensive care. *Anaesthesist* 1990; **39:** 319–22.

192. Myers B D, Moran S M. Hemodynamically mediated acute renal failure. *N Engl J Med* 1986; **314:** 97–105.

193. Wardle N. Acute renal failure in the 1980s: the importance of septic shock and of endotoxaemia. *Nephron* 1995; **66:** 380–5.

194. Anderson R J, Linas S L, Berns A S, *et al.* Non-oliguric acute renal failure. *N Engl J Med* 1977; **296:** 1134–8.

195. Shin B, Mackenzie C F, McAslan T C, Helrich M, Cowley R A. Postoperative renal failure in trauma patients. *Anesthesiology* 1979; **51:** 218–21.

196. Lindner A. Synergism of dopamine and furosemide in diuretic-resistant, oliguric acute renal failure. *Nephron* 1983; **33:** 121–6.

197. Myers B D, Miller D C, Mehigan J T, *et al.* Nature of the renal injury following total renal ischemia in man. *J Clin Invest* 1984; **73:** 329–41.

198. Kleinknecht D, Ganeval D, Gonzales–Duque L A, Fermanian J. Furosemide in acute oliguric renal failure. A controlled trial. *Nephron* 1976; **17:** 51–8.

199. Brown C B, Ogg C S, Cameron J S. High dose frusemide in acute renal failure: a controlled trial. *Clin Nephrol* 1981; **15:** 90–6.

200. Krasna M J, Scott G E, Scholz P M, Spotnitz A J, Mackenzie J W, Penn F. Postoperative enhancement of urinary output in patients with acute renal failure using continuous furosemide therapy. *Chest* 1986; **89:** 294–5.

201. Oken D E. On the differential diagnosis of acute renal failure. *Am J Med* 1981; **71:** 916–20.

202. Pru C, Kjellstrand C M. The FE_{Na} test is of no prognostic value in acute renal failure. *Nephron* 1984; **36:** 20–3.

203. Diamond J R, Yoburn D C. Nonoliguric acute renal failure associated with a low fractional excretion of sodium. *Ann Intern Med* 1982; **96:** 597–600.

204. Prough D S, Zaloga G P. Monitoring renal function. *Crit Care Clin* 1988; **4:** 573–89.

205. Kellen M, Aronson S, Roizen M F, Barnard J, Thisted R A. Predictive and diagnostic tests of renal failure: a review. *Anesth Analg* 1994; **78:** 134–42.

206. Shin B, Mackenzie C F, Helrich M. Creatinine clearance for early detection of posttraumatic renal dysfunction. *Anesthesiology* 1986; **64:** 605–9.

207. Sladen R N, Endo E, Harrison T. Two-hour versus 22-hour creatinine clearance in critically ill patients. *Anesthesiology* 1987; **67:** 1013–16.

208. Kim K, Onesti G, Ramirez O. Creatinine clearance in renal disease: a reappraisal. *BMJ* 1969; **4:** 11.

209. Meadows D, Edwards J D, Wilkins R G, Nightingale P. Reversal of intractable septic shock with norepinephrine therapy. *Crit Care Med* 1988; **16:** 663–6.

210. Martin C, Papazian L, Perrin G, Saux P, Gouin F. Norepinephrine or dopamine for the treatment of hyperdynamic septic shock? *Chest* 1993; **103:** 1826–31.

211. Schaer G L, Fink M P, Parrillo J E. Norepinephrine alone versus norepinephrine plus low-dose dopamine: enhanced renal blood flow with combination pressor therapy. *Crit Care Med* 1985; **13:** 492–6.

212. Shoemaker W C, Appel P L, Kram H B, Waxman K, Lee T S. Prospective trial of supranormal values of survivors as therapeutic goals in high-risk surgical patients. *Chest* 1988; **94:** 1176–86.

213. Yu M, Levy M M, Smith P, Takiguchi S A, Miyasaki A, Myers S A. Effect of maximizing oxygen delivery on morbidity and mortality rates in critically ill patients: a prospective, randomized, controlled study. *Crit Care Med* 1993; **21:** 830–8.

214. Tuchschmidt J, Fried J, Astiz M, Rackow E. Elevation of cardiac output and oxygen delivery improves outcome in septic shock. *Chest* 1992; **102:** 216–20.

215. Finn W F. Diagnosis and management of acute tubular necrosis. *Med Clin North Am* 1990; **74:** 873–91.

216. Cronin R E, de Torrente A, Miller P D, Bulger R E, Burke T J, Schrier R W. Pathogenic mechanisms in early norephinephrine-induced acute renal failure: functional and histological correlates of protection. *Kidney Int* 1978; **14:** 115–25.

217. Burke T J, Cronin R E, Duchin K L, Peterson L N, Schrier R W. Ischemia and tubule obstruction during acute renal failure in dogs: mannitol in protection. *Am J Physiol* 1980; **238:** F305–F314.

218. Patak R V, Fadem S Z, Lifschitz M D, Stein J H. Study of factors which modify the development of norepinephrine-induced acute renal failure in the dog. *Kidney Int* 1979; **15:** 227–37.

219. Hanley M J, Davidson K. Prior mannitol and furosemide infusion in a model of ischemial acute renal failure. *Am J Physiol* 1981; **241:** F556–F564.

220. Pass L J, Eberhart R C, Brown J C, Rohn G N, Estrera A S. The effect of mannitol and dopamine on the renal response to thoracic aortic cross-clamping. *J Thorac Cardiovasc Surg* 1988; **95:** 608–12.

221. Henderson I S, Beattie T J, Kennedy A C. Dopamine hydrochloride in oliguric states. *Lancet* 1980; **2:** 827–8.

222. Schwartz L B, Gewertz B L. The renal response to low dose dopamine. *J Surg Res* 1988; **45:** 574–88.

223. Lindner A, Cutler R E, Goodman W G. Synergism of dopamine plus furosemide in preventing acute renal failure in the dog. *Kidney Int* 1979; **16:** 158–66.

224. Dick M, Dasta J, Choban P, Sinha R, Flancbaum L. Urine output (UO) and serum aldosterone (ALDO) concentrations in oliguric ICU patients (PTS) receiving low dose dopamine. *Crit Care Med* 1993; **21:** S177 (Abstract).

225. Elliott W J, Weber R R, Nelson K S, Oliner C M, Fumo M T. Renal and hemodynamic effects of intravenous fenoldopam versus nitroprusside in severe hypertension. *Circulation* 1990; **81:** 970–7.

226. Allison N L, Dubbs J W, Ziemniak J A, Alexander F, Stote R M. The effect of fenoldopam, a dopaminergic agonist, on renal hemodynamics. *Clin Pharmacol Ther* 1987; **41:** 282–8.

227. Murphy M B, McCoy C E, Weber R R, Frederickson E D, Douglas F L, Goldberg L I. Augmentation of renal blood flow and sodium excretion in hypertensive patients during blood pressure reduction by intravenous administration of the dopamine$_1$ agonist fenoldopam. *Circulation* 1987; **76:** 1312–18.

228. Hughes J M, Ragsdale N V, Felder R A, Chevalier R L, King B, Carey R M. Diuresis and natriuresis during continuous dopamine-1 receptor stimulation. *Hypertension* 1988; **11:** I69–I74.

229. Nouwen E J, Verstrepen W A, De Broe M E. Epidermal growth factor in acute renal failure. *Ren Fail* 1994; **16:** 49–60.

230. Pollock D M, Opgenorth T J. Atrial natriuretic peptides in the treatment of acute renal failure. *Ren Fail* 1993; **15:** 439–49.

231. Badr K F. Novel mediators of sepsis-associated renal failure. *Semin Nephrol* 1994; **14:** 3–7.

232. Lake E W, Humes H D. Acute renal failure: directed therapy to enhanced renal tubular regeneration. *Semin Nephrol* 1994; **14:** 83–97.

233. Epstein M. Calcium antagonists and the kidney: future therapeutic perspectives. *Am J Kidney Dis* 1993; **21:** 16–25.

234. Eliahou H E, Ben-David A, Blau A. Recovery can be enhanced in acute renal failure of multisystem organ failure. *Contrib Nephrol* 1994; **106:** 59–62.

235. Agmon Y, Brezis M. Acute renal failure: a multifactorial syndrome. *Contrib Nephrol* 1993; **102:** 23–6.

236. Safirstein R. Gene expression in nephrotoxic and ischemic acute renal failure. *J Am Soc Nephrol* 1994; **4:** 1387–95.

237. Humes H D. Potential molecular therapy for acute renal failure. *Cleve Clin J Med* 1993; **60:** 166–8.

238. Brezis M, Epstein F H. Cellular mechanisms of acute ischemic injury in the kidney. *Annu Rev Med* 1993; **44:** 27–37.

239. Goligorsky M S, Lieberthal W, Racusen L, Simon E E. Integrin receptors in renal tubular epithelium: new insights into pathophysiology of acute renal failure. *Am J Physiol* 1993; **264:** F1–F8.

240. Vetterlein F, Petho A, Schmidt G. Distribution of capillary blood flow in rat kidney during postischemic renal failure. *Am J Physiol* 1986; **251:** H510–H519.

241. Ratcliffe P J, Endre Z H, Tange J D, Ledingham J G G. Ischaemic acute renal failure: why does it occur? *Nephron* 1989; **52:** 1–5.

242. Mason J, Torhorst J, Welsch J. Role of medullary perfusion defect in the pathogenesis of ischemic renal failure. *Kidney Int* 1984; **26:** 283–93.

243. Hirasawa H, Odaka M, Soeda K, *et al.* Experimental and clinical study on ATP-$MgCl_2$ administration for postischemic acute renal failure. *Clin Exp Dial Apheresis* 1983; **7:** 37–47.

244. Siegel N J, Glazier W B, Chaudrey I H, *et al.* Enhanced recovery from acute renal failure by the postischemic infusion of adenine nucleotides and magnesium chloride in rats. *Kidney Int* 1980; **17:** 338–49.

245. Zager R A, Gmur D J, Bredl C R, Eng M J. Degree and time sequence of hypothermic protection against experimental ischemic acute renal failure. *Circ Res* 1989; **65:** 1263–9.

246. Wait R B, White G, Davis J H. Beneficial effects of verapamil on postischemic renal failure. *Surgery* 1983; **94:** 276–82.

247. Goldfarb D, Iaina A, Serban I, Gavendo S, Kapuler S, Eliahou H E. Beneficial effect of verapamil in ischemic acute renal failure in the rat. *Proc Soc Exp Biol Med* 1983; **172:** 398–92.

248. Silverman M, Rose H, Puschett J B. Modification in proximal tubular function induced by nitrendipine in a rat model of acute ischemic renal failure. *J Cardiovasc Pharmacol* 1989; **14:** 799–802.

249. Russell J D, Churchill D N. Calcium antagonists and acute renal failure. *Am J Med* 1989; **87:** 306–15.

250. Leahy A L, Galla J, Fitzpatrick J M, Wait R B. The canine kidney in haemorrhagic shock: effect of verapamil. *Eur Urol* 1987; **13:** 401–6.

251. Loutzenhiser R D, Epstein M. Renal hemodynamic effects of calcium antagonists. *Am J Med* 1987; **82:** 23–8.

252. Diamond J R, Cheung J Y, Fang L S T. Nifedipine-induced renal dysfunction. Alterations in renal hemodynamics. *Am J Med* 1984; **77:** 905–9.

253. Canavese C, Stratta P, Vercellone A. The case for oxygen free radicals in the pathogenesis of ischemic acute renal failure. *Nephron* 1988; **49:** 9–15.

254. Ratych R E, Bulkley G B. Free-radical-mediated postischemic reperfusion injury in the kidney. *J Free Radic Biol Med* 1986; **2:** 311–19.

255. Mauk R H, Patak R V, Fadem S Z, Lifschitz M D, Stein J H. Effect of prostaglandin E administration in a nephrotoxic and a vasoconstrictor model of acute renal failure. *Kidney Int* 1977; **12:** 122–30.

256. Mandal A K, Miller J. Protection against ischemic acute renal failure by prostaglandin infusion. *Prostaglandins Leukot Med* 1982; **8:** 361–73.

257. Tobimatsu M, Konomi K, Saito S, Tsumagari T. Protective effect of prostaglandin E_1 on ischemia-induced acute renal failure in dogs. *Surgery* 1985; **98:** 45–52.

258. Torsello G, Schror K, Szabo Z, *et al.* Effects of prostaglandin E1 (PGE1) on experimental renal ischemia. *Eur J Vasc Surg* 1989; **3:** 5–13.

259. Lifschitz M D, Barnes J L. Prostaglandin I_2 attenuates ischemic acute renal failure in the rat. *Am J Physiol* 1984; **247:** F714–F717.

260. Klausner J M, Paterson I S, Goldman G, *et al.* Postischemic renal injury is mediated by neutrophils and leukotrienes. *Am J Physiol* 1989; **256:** F794-F802.

261. Lelcuk S, Alexander F, Kobzik L, Valeri C R, Shepro D, Hechtman H B. Prostacyclin and thromboxane A_2 moderate postischemic renal failure. *Surgery* 1985; **98:** 207–12.

262. Kaufman R P Jr, Klausner J M, Anner H, *et al.* Inhibition of thromboxane (Tx) synthesis by free radical scavengers. *J Trauma* 1988; **28:** 458–64.

263. Andrews P M, Bates S B. Dietary protein prior to renal ischemia dramatically affects postischemic kidney function. *Kidney Int* 1986; **30:** 299–303.

264. Seguro A C, Shimizu M H M, Monteiro J L, Rocha A S. Effect of potassium depletion on ischemic renal failure. *Nephron* 1989; **51:** 350–4.

265. Bonventre J V. Mediators of ischemic renal injury. *Annu Rev Med* 1988; **39:** 531–44.

266. Corwin H L, Bonventre J V. Acute renal failure. *Med Clin North Am* 1986; **70:** 1037–54.

267. Cronin R E. Drug therapy in the management of acute renal failure. *Am J Med Sci* 1986; **292:** 112–19.

268. Corwin H L, Bonventre J V. Acute renal failure in the intensive care unit. Part 2. *Intensive Care Med* 1988; **14:** 86–96.

269. Epstein F H, Brown R S. Acute renal failure: a collection of paradoxes. *Hosp Pract* 1988; **23:** 171–94.

270. Madal A K, Lightfoot B O, Treat R C. Mechanisms of protection in acute renal failure. *Circ Shock* 1983; **11:** 245–53.

271. Kramer P, Wigger W, Rieger J, Matthaei D, Scheler F. Arteriovenous haemofiltration: a new and simple method for treatment of over-hydrated patients resistant to diuretics. *Klin Wochenschr* 1977; **55:** 1121–2.

272. Kramer P, Matthaei D, Rieger J, Scheler F. A new automatic haemofiltration machine with continuously monitored fluid balance. *Proc Eur Dial Transplant Assoc* 1977; **14:** 613–17.

273. Henderson L W, Besarab A, Michaels A, Bluemle L W Jr. Blood purification by ultrafiltration and fluid replacement (diafiltration). *Trans Am Soc Artif Intern Organs* 1967; **12:** 216–22.

274. Kramer E, Wohl M. Nursing participation in hemofiltration. *J Am Assoc Nephrol Nurses Tech* 1981; **8:** 27–30.

275. Kramer P, Kaufhold G, Grone H J, *et al.* Management of anuric intensive-care patients with arteriovenous hemofiltration. *Int J Artif Organs* 1980; **3:** 225–30.

276. Ziegler E J, McCutchan J A, Fierer J, *et al.* Treatment of gram-negative bacteremia and shock with human antiserum to a mutant *Escherichia coli. N Engl J Med* 1982; **307:** 1225–30.

277. Baumgartner J D, Glauser M P, McCutchan J A, *et al.* Prevention of gram-negative shock and death in surgical patients by antibody to endotoxin core glycolipid. *Lancet* 1985; **2:** 59–63.

278. Ziegler E J, Fisher C J, Sprung C L, *et al.* Treatment of gram-negative bacteremia and septic shock with HA-1A human monoclonal antibody against endotoxin. A randomized, double-blind, placebo-controlled trial. *N Engl J Med* 1991; **324:** 429–36.

279. Fujihara Y, Lei M G, Morrison D C. Characterization of specific binding of a human immunoglobulin M monoclonal antibody to lipopolysaccharide and its lipid A domain. *Infect Immun* 1993; **61:** 910–18.

280. Luce M. Introduction of new technology into critical care practice: a history of HA-1A human monoclonal antibody against endotoxin. *Crit Care Med* 1993; **21:** 1233–41.

281. Chalfin D B, Holbein M E, Fein A M, Carlon G C. Cost-effectiveness of monoclonal antibodies to gram-negative endotoxin in the treatment of gram-negative sepsis in ICU patients. *JAMA* 1993; **269:** 249–54.

282. Stuttmann R, Hebebrand D, Hartert M, Spilker G, Doehn M. Prevention with pseudomonas immune globulin in burn injury patients with inhalation trauma: does it have an effect on lung function and outcome? *Klin Wochenschr* 1991; **69**(Suppl 26): 168–77.

283. Stuttmann R, Hartert M, Jahn M, Spilker G, Doehn M. [Serum IgG concentrations and antibody titer of burn patients after preventive intravenous IgG substitution with a Pseudomonas immunoglobulin]. *Infusionsther Transfusionsmed* 1993; **20**(Suppl 1): 48–55.

284. Hesse D G, Tracey K J, Fong Y, *et al.* Cytokine appearance in human endotoxemia and primate bacteremia. *Surg Gynecol Obstet* 1988; **166:** 147–53.

285. Beutler B, Mahoney J, Le Trang N, Pekala P, Cerami A. Purification of cachectin, a lipoprotein lipase-suppressing hormone secreted by endotoxin-induced RAW 264.7 cells. *J Exp Med* 1985; **161:** 984–95.

286. Tracey K J, Lowry S F, Fahey T III, *et al.* Cachectin/tumor necrosis factor induces lethal shock and stress hormone responses in the dog. *Surg Gynecol Obstet* 1987; **164:** 415–22.

287. Beutler B, Milsark I W, Cerami A C. Passive immunization against cachectin/tumor necrosis factor protects mice from lethal effect of endotoxin. *Science* 1985; **229:** 869–71.

288. Hinshaw L B, Emerson T E Jr, Taylor F B Jr, *et al.* Lethal *Staphylococcus aureus*-induced shock in primates: prevention of death with anti-TNF antibody. *J Trauma* 1992; **33:** 568–73.

289. Wayte J, Silva A T, Krausz T, Cohen J. Observations on the role of tumor necrosis factor-alpha in a murine model of shock due to *Streptococcus pyogenes*. *Crit Care Med* 1993; **21:** 1207–12.

290. Nordmann P, Ronco E, Guenounou M. Involvement of interferon-gamma and tumor necrosis factor-alpha in host defense against *Rhodococcus equi*. *J Infect Dis* 1993; **167:** 1456–9.

291. Miethke T, Duschek K, Wahl C, Heeg K, Wagner H. Pathogenesis of the toxic shock syndrome: T cell mediated lethal shock caused by the superantigen TSST-1. *Eur J Immunol* 1993; **23:** 1494–500.

292. Schumann R R, Leong S R, Flaggs G W, *et al.* Structure and function of lipopolysaccharide binding protein. *Science* 1990; **249:** 1429–31.

293. Tobias P S, Mathison J C, Ulevitch R J. A family of lipopolysaccharide binding proteins involved in responses to gram-negative sepsis. *J Biol Chem* 1988; **263:** 13479–81.

294. Ulevitch R J, Mathison J C, Schumann R R, Tobias P S. A new model of macrophage stimulation by bacterial lipopolysaccharide. *J Trauma* 1990; **30:** S189–S192.

295. Pugin J, Schurer Maly C C, Leturcq D, Moriarty A, Ulevitch R J, Tobias P S. Lipopolysaccharide activation of human endothelial and epithelial cells is mediated by lipopolysaccharide-binding protein and soluble CD14. *Proc Natl Acad Sci USA* 1993; **90:** 2744–8.

296. Han J, Beutler B, Huez G. Complex regulation of TNF mRNA turnover in lipopolysaccharide-activated macrophages. *Biochim Biophys Acta* 1991; **1090:** 22–8.

297. Zuckerman S H, Evans G F. Endotoxin tolerance: *In vivo* regulation of tumor necrosis factor and interleukin-1 synthesis at the transcriptional level. *Cell Immunol* 1992; **140:** 513–19.

298. Fong Y, Tracey K J, Moldawer L L, *et al.* Antibodies to cachectin/tumor necrosis factor reduce interleukin 1 beta and interleukin 6 appearance during lethal bacteremia. *J Exp Med* 1989; **170:** 1627–33.

299. Fisher C J, Opal S M, Dhainaut J F, *et al.* Influence of an anti-tumor necrosis factor monoclonal antibody on cytokine levels in patients with sepsis. The CB0006 Sepsis Syndrome Study Group. *Crit Care Med* 1993; **21:** 318–27.

300. Mathison J, Tobias P, Wolfson E, Ulevitch R. Regulatory mechanisms of host responsiveness to endotoxin (lipopolysaccharide) 1. *Pathobiology* 1991; **59:** 185–8.

301. Haak-Frendscho M, Marsters S A, Mordenti J, *et al.* Inhibition of TNF by a TNF receptor immunoadhesin. Comparison to an anti-TNF monoclonal antibody. *J Immunol* 1994; **152:** 1347–53.

302. Sheppard B C, Norton J A. Tumor necrosis factor and interleukin-1 protection against the lethal effects of tumor necrosis factor. *Surgery* 1991; **109:** 698–705.

303. Gorgen I, Hartung T, Leist M, *et al.* Granulocyte colony-stimulating factor treatment protects rodents against lipopolysaccharide-induced toxicity via suppression of systemic tumor necrosis factor α. *J Immunol* 1992; **149:** 918–24.

304. Alexander H R, Wong G H, Doherty G M, *et al.* Differentiation factor/leukemia inhibitory factor protection against lethal endotoxemia in mice: Synergistic effect with interleukin 1 and tumor necrosis factor. *J Exp Med* 1992; **175:** 1139–42.

305. Dinarello C A. Interleukin-1 and the pathogenesis of the acute-phase response. *N Engl J Med* 1984; **311:** 1413–18.

306. Michie H R, Manogue K R, Spriggs D R, *et al.* Detection of circulating tumor necrosis factor after endotoxin administration. *N Engl J Med* 1988; **318:** 1481–6.

307. Ohlsson K, Bjork P, Bergenfeldt M, *et al.* Interleukin-1 receptor antagonist reduces mortality from endotoxic shock. *Nature* 1990; **348:** 550–2.

308. Brigham K L, Meyrick B. Endotoxin and lung injury. *Am Rev Respir Dis* 1986; **133:** 913–27.

309. Moncada S, Palmer R M, Higgs E A. The discovery of nitric oxide as the endogenous nitrovasodilator. *Hypertension* 1988; **12:** 365–72.

310. Siegel J H, Giovannini I, Coleman B. Ventilation: perfusion maldistribution secondary to the hyperdynamic cardiovascular state as the major cause of increased pulmonary shunting in human sepsis. *J Trauma* 1979; **19:** 432–60.

311. Suffredini A F, Fromm R E, Parker M M, *et al.* The cardiovascular response of normal humans to the administration of endotoxin. *N Engl J Med* 1989; **321:** 280–7.

312. Palmer R M, Rees D D, Ashton D S, Moncada S. L-Arginine is the physiological precursor for the formation of nitric oxide in endothelium-dependent relaxation. *Biochem Biophys Res Commun* 1988; **153:** 1251–6.

313. Salvemini D, Masini E, Anggard E, Mannaioni P F, Vane J. Synthesis of a nitric oxide-like factor from L-arginine by rat serosal mast cells: stimulation of guanylate cyclase and inhibition of platelet aggregation. *Biochem Biophys Res Commun* 1990; **169:** 596–601.

314. Rees D D, Cellek S, Palmer R M, Moncada S. Dexamethasone prevents the induction by endotoxin of a nitric oxide synthase and the associated effects on vascular tone: an insight into endotoxin shock. *Biochem Biophys Res Commun* 1990; **173:** 541–7.

315. Busse R, Mulsch A. Induction of nitric oxide synthase by cytokines in vascular smooth muscle cells. *FEBS Lett* 1990; **275:** 87–90.

316. Kilbourn R G, Gross S S, Jubran A, *et al.* N^G-methyl-L-arginine inhibits tumor necrosis factor-induced hypotension: implications for the involvement of nitric oxide. *Proc Natl Acad Sci USA* 1990; **87:** 3629–32.

317. Gross S S, Stuehr D J, Aisaka K, Jaffe E A, Levi R, Griffith O W. Macrophage and endothelial cell nitric oxide synthesis: cell-type selective inhibition by N^G-aminoarginine, N^G-nitroarginine and N^G-methylarginine. *Biochem Biophys Res Commun* 1990; **170:** 96–103.

318. Hibbs J B Jr, Taintor R R, Vavrin Z. Macrophage cytotoxicity: role of L-arginine deiminase and imino nitrogen oxidation to nitrite. *Science* 1987; **235:** 473–6.

319. Gray G A, Schott C, Julou-Schaeffer G, Fleming I, Parratt J R, Stoclet J C. The effect of inhibitors of the L-arginine/nitric oxide pathway on endotoxin-induced loss of vascular responsiveness in anaesthetized rats. *Br J Pharmacol* 1991; **103:** 1218–24.

320. Grootendorst A F, van Bommel E F. The role of hemofiltration in the critically-ill intensive care unit patient: present and future. *Blood Purif* 1993; **11:** 209–23.

321. Stein B, Pfenninger E, Grunert A, Schmitz J E, Deller A, Kocher F. The consequences of continuous haemofiltration on lung mechanics and extravascular lung water in a porcine endotoxic shock model. *Intensive Care Med* 1991; **17:** 293–8.

322. DiCarlo J V, Dudley T E, Sherbotie J R, Kaplan B S, Costarino A T. Continuous arteriovenous hemofiltration/dialysis improves pulmonary gas exchange in children with multiple organ system failure. *Crit Care Med* 1990; **18:** 822–6.

323. Stein B, Pfenninger E, Grunert A, Schmitz J E, Hudde M. Influence of continuous haemofiltration on haemodynamics and central blood volume in experimental endotoxic shock. *Intensive Care Med* 1990; **16:** 494–9.

324. Grootendorst A F, van Bommel E F, van der Hoven B, van Leengoed L A, van Osta A L. High volume hemofiltration improves right ventricular function in endotoxin-induced shock in the pig. *Intensive Care Med* 1992; **18:** 235–40.

325. Bellomo R, Tipping P, Boyce N. Continuous veno-venous hemofiltration with dialysis removes cytokines from the circulation of septic patients. *Crit Care Med* 1993; **21:** 522–6.

326. Carozzi S, Nasini M G, Caviglia P M, Schelotto C, Santoni O, Atti M. Acetate free biofiltration. Effects on peripheral blood monocyte activation and cytokine release. *ASAIO J* 1992; **38:** 52–4.

327. Tetta C, Camussi G, Turello E, *et al.* Production of cytokines in hemodialysis. *Blood Purif* 1990; **8:** 337–46.

328. von Appen K, Ivanovich P, Mujais S, Klinkmann H. Endothelium: the next frontier in biocompatibility. *Artif Organs* 1993; **17:** 985–95.

329. Shapiro B A, Kacmarek R M, Cane R D, *et al. Clinical Application of Respiratory Care*. St Louis: Mosby Year Book Publishers, 1991.

330. Deitch E A. Intestinal permeability is increased in burn patients shortly after injury. *Surgery* 1990; **107:** 411–16.

331. Prough D S, Foreman A S. Anesthesia and the renal system. In: Barash P G, Cullen B F, Stoelting R K, eds *Clinical Anesthesia*. Philadelphia: JB Lippincott Company, 1992: 1125–85.

332. Hayes M A, Timmins A C, Yau E H, Palazzo M, Hinds C J, Watson D. Elevation of systemic oxygen delivery in the treatment of critically ill patients. *N Engl J Med* 1994; **330:** 1717–22.

CHAPTER THIRTY-TWO

Burn Nursing

Denise M. Tompkins

Acute Burn Nursing Care

The burn injury requires a dedicated team of health care professionals to produce the most satisfactory outcome for each patient. As the emphasis in treatment changes, so does the role of each team member. At various times, one or another team member will have a central role; so open communication and cooperation among the burn care team are key factors in all successful outcomes. Nursing care of the burn victim is both an art and a science, and experienced burn nurses play a critical role in long-term outcomes. The professional nurse is a key member of the burn team throughout the hospital course.

In an emergency room, the team's first concern is to stop the burning process, assess the patient's overall condition, and deal at once with any life-threatening issues. These include acute airway obstruction, continued burning from smoldering clothes or chemical action, cardiovascular collapse, and massive bleeding. The nurse should watch and listen for signs and symptoms of airway impairment: stridor, dyspnea, grunting sounds in expiration, cyanosis, restlessness and agitation due to anoxia. All of these signs of respiratory distress must be evaluated and treated immediately. In a struggle for oxygen, a patient may kick or flail about. In a burn injury, this extreme agitation may be mistaken for pain. Oxygen, a functioning laryngoscope, a set of endotracheal tubes, and suction equipment should be immediately available to remedy breathing difficulties.[1] To check for cardiovascular collapse, a nurse should take the blood pressure, feel the pulse (noting both quality and rate), and look for external bleeding.

Since many burn accidents also involve falls or violent impacts in automobile collisions or explosions, there may be related internal injuries such as a ruptured spleen or skull fracture. Information about a burn accident is of great value in evaluating the injury. As soon as possible a careful history should be taken in order to learn the cause and the circumstances (flame, steam, chemicals, electric current) of the burn. If the patient is unable to speak, the staff should question those who brought the patient to the hospital. If the patient was in an enclosed space when the injury occurred, the chances of respiratory involvement are greater. Careful examination of the clothing is necessary because some fabrics continue to burn for a long time. The remains of the patient's clothing may still be smoldering when the patient arrives in the emergency room, and the continuing heat can cause a deeper injury. Rinsing with cool water or saline will stop the burn and loosen fabric from the flesh. Continual monitoring of the patient while rinsing is important in order to maintain body temperature and hemodynamics. In the case of acid or alkali chemical burns, the damaging action will continue until all remaining chemical has been washed away with large volumes of water or has been neutralized with the appropriate agent.[2]

Once the team has dealt with any immediate life-threatening issues, an IV line is established and fluid, usually lactated Ringer's solution, is given. The IV line should be a large enough bore catheter to deliver large volumes of fluid at a high flow rate. In the case of a moderate to large injury, a CVP line is often required. As soon as possible, the exact fluid requirement for a patient is calculated and fluid resuscitation continues on the schedule.

At the time the IV line is inserted, blood samples are taken and sent to the laboratory for baseline studies and to the blood bank for typing and cross-matching. If the burns cover a large area, the choice of sites for IV insertion may be limited. The ideal location is an unburned site where maximum security and stability can be assured. This is not always possible; sometimes the IV must be inserted through burn tissue. Often surgical cutdowns may also be required. The nurse must assure adequate preparation of all sites and observe all requirements for sterile technique.[3]

The Burn Unit

As soon as possible, a burn victim should be transferred to a burn unit for ongoing evaluation and care by an experienced team. Once the patient is on the burn unit, a thorough history is taken and the complete assessment, intervention, and plan of nursing care is implemented and evaluated on a continuous basis. For the acute burn patient, major nursing issues which need to be continually assessed include: impaired gas exchange, fluid volume deficit, impairment of skin integrity, potential for infection, nutrition, pain management, and impaired physical mobility. For a moderate to large burn, skin grafting, perioperative care, and long-term rehabilitation must also be considered.[4]

Impaired Gas Exchange

Inhalation injury of facial edema from wounds may quickly lead to airway problems. Early on, frequent assessment, often hourly, of respiratory status is essential. Trends and changes must be documented and shared with the team. These should be correlated with ongoing monitoring of laboratory results, although, the key role of physical assessment cannot be overstated. Suctioning with aseptic technique must be done as needed in order to maintain a patent airway. It is most prudent to keep resuscitative equipment at the bedside at all times when inhalation injury is suspected and/or when facial and neck wounds are present. Aggressive respiratory toilet, including coughing, deep breathing, turning the patient, and PRN suctioning are key nursing interventions and must be performed at regular intervals and adapted to the patient's changing condition.[5] The frequency will often vary from every 1 or 2 hours to twice daily. Constant nursing assessment and physician communication will determine the exact frequency.

In the event that impaired gas exchange or a large inhalation injury leads to ineffective gas exchange, an artificial airway and mechanical ventilation may be required. The nursing care associated with the respiratory care of the intubated ventilated patient is similar to other critical care patients with a few burn injury related adaptations. As in all intubated patients, the desired outcomes for the intubated burned patient include: adequate tissue perfusion, clear and equal breath sounds with full expansion, stable artificial airway in proper position, and ultimately, successful weaning and extubation. Of particular complexity with a burn patient is stabilizing an artificial airway, particularly in the presence of facial wounds. Often nurses need to be creative in order to stabilize the endotracheal tube over facial dressings. Whenever possible, an assistant to be in charge of the endotracheal tube during facial dressing changes is an excellent safety measure. When nasal tubes are used, integrity of the columnella and nares must be watched for long-term tissue breakdown. Additional padding fashioned from gauze bandage material may be applied between the endotracheal tube and the nares/columnella intersection in order to preserve cosmetic integrity. Respiratory care for the intubated burned patient should follow hospital standards of care and routine nursing policy and procedure. These important care routines must be integrated with the total care of the burned patient and must not be overlooked because of extensive wound care. They are equally important.

Burn Wound Care: Impairment of Skin Integrity

There are many modes of burn wound care, and many theories concerning which is the most effective. In all cases, the primary goal for burn wound care remains focused on closure of the burn wound as soon as possible. With the surgical intervention of prompt eschar excision and grafting for wound closure, wound healing is achieved in a more timely fashion, and mortality rates have been reduced.[6–8] Often a nurse will be working with multiple wounds in various stages of healing. These can include: eschar, newly excised and grafted areas, donor sites, and healing partial-thickness wounds. The ongoing assessment of effectiveness for each treatment modality and the routine application of these modalities are within the domain of a professional nurse. At each dressing change, the nurse assesses the wound and documents the appearance of each wound, including the character and amount of drainage and the progress toward healing. Any deterioration should promptly be brought to the physician's attention. Removal of necrotic tissue and mechanical cleaning of any purulent drainage is done with each dressing change. A wound care flow sheet or a total body diagram may be used to document care and healing and to promote consistency in care. In addition, it is important to provide skin care to all unburned and healed areas so as to diminish the likelihood of secondary skin breakdown and increased open wound areas.

Skin Integrity: Potential for Infection

The primary goal of all wound care is to promote optimal healing and prevent introduction of additional bacteria to the wound. In addition to a patient's own burn wound flora, sources for bacteria include the environment, as well as the patient's own respiratory, gastrointestinal, or skin flora. Barriers maintained between different wound sites prevent transfer of organisms from one wound site to another. The nurse should be alert in assessing signs and symptoms of infection such as malodorous wound drainage, elevated leukocyte count, and elevated body temperature.

In addition to burn wound infections, a nurse needs to be alert for signs and symptoms of bloodstream infections. They are more apt to occur in patients with 30% TBSA injury or greater, or in patients with an inhalation injury. Pathogens usually originate in the burn wound; however, they also have been associated with invasive intravascular devices such as arterial, central venous, and pulmonary artery catheters, as well as altered host defenses and immune system function. Strategies for preventing blood stream infections include: careful wound management and strict adherence to clean/sterile technique protocols when performing wound care; appropriate handling of intravascular devices; monitoring blood cultures when a patient has temperature elevations; and administration of appropriate antibiotic therapy as indicated. Success in prevention and control of infections in burn patients depends upon a consistent and coordinated team effort.[9]

Potential for Fluid Volume Deficit

There are many hemodynamic changes in burn injuries, and strategies for maintaining a patient in a hemodynamically stable state are a constant challenge to a burn care team. Fluid resuscitation formulas are used as guidelines to monitor a patient and prevent burn shock. The Parkland formula is a common guideline for many burn units.[10] In the first 48 hours, capillary integrity is lost as a result of burn trauma. Fluid shifts from intravascular spaces into the interstitial spaces; thus edema forms and dehydration may occur. A patient should be weighed as soon as possible after admission. Vital signs should be monitored every hour until stable. The nurse must be alert for trends and must report fluctuations immediately. Accurate records of fluid intake and output are critical to titrating fluid replacement. All burned extremities should be elevated in order to promote venous return. Pulse must be continuously monitored, using Doppler if necessary, particularly in areas of circumferential burns. In the second 48 hours, as the capillaries heal, the interstitial fluid is gradually reabsorbed into intravascular spaces and excreted by the kidneys. Laboratory results must be monitored, and all abnormalities reported. Again, the importance of noting trends for each patient must be continually emphasized.

Pain Management: Alteration in Comfort

The importance of pain management cannot be overemphasized in providing optimal comfort for a patient (see Chapter 54). Pain should be assessed using both objective and subjective criteria.[11] Vital sign changes such as increased blood pressure and heart rate as well as restlessness, irritability, facial grimacing, body rigidity, or other nonverbal behaviors may indicate discomfort. Patients subjectively report their experiences of pain; this task is often helped by the use of a visual analog scale. Nursing interventions to promote patient comfort are key to pain management in a burned patient. A careful pain history including the patient's past experiences with pain and ways of handling those events may provide clues to guide management of the current situation. Family members of the patient may relate past coping strengths which will help the patient through this crisis. Family involvement is especially important with the very young and the very old where reporting skills or memory may not be totally present and accurate. Most importantly, the patient must be medicated as ordered. The nurse should continuously assess the patient's response to pain medication and report the results to the physician so that appropriate pain medication orders can be made available. The IV and PO routes are amenable to most patients; injections should be avoided when possible, especially in children.[12] Background pain may be dealt with by regular routine administration of an analgesic agent. This keeps the blood level constant and does not subject the patient to the peaks and troughs of intermittent medication administration. Anti-anxiety medications are also frequently titrated with analgesics in order to handle background pain. Additional medication should be given as needed for specific procedures and for the occurrence of breakthrough pain. Many units now also utilize patient controlled analgesia (PCA) protocols to assist in pain relief. Knowing that they have control over their next analgesic dose seems to decrease the anxiety associated with pain for many patients.[13]

In addition to medication, the nurse can also use nonpharmacological techniques such as deep breathing and progressive relaxation to help ease a patient's pain. For some patients, imagery and diversional activities assist in pain relief. For others, active participation in painful procedures (such as assisting in removing bandages) provides some pain relief, presumably by allowing the patient control.[14] Frequent position changes will also aid in the patient's comfort. Advance warning of uncomfortable procedures and age-appropriate explanations of the rationale for actions of the caregivers seem to enhance comfort by reducing anxiety.

Nutrition

A patient must maintain adequate calorie requirements in order to meet the unique metabolic demands for healing from burn trauma (see Chapter 22). Nutritional support beyond voluntary intake is required for most burns greater than 30% TBSA. Whenever possible, enteral nutritional support is provided. When this is not feasible, total parenteral nutrition (TPN) may be indicated. The goals for calorie and protein requirements are usually based on ideal body weight.[15] The nurse is continually involved in assessing, delivering and evaluating nutritional needs for patients. An accurate record of intake, output, and daily calorie count is essential. The nurse should work with the dietitian in order to insure that a prescribed diet along with appetizing supplemental snacks are delivered to the patient. The patient often requires physical assistance in eating because of the location of burn wounds and splinting or positioning requirements. In moderate to large burns, the nurse should also monitor the pH of gastric aspirate and be aware of the potential for an occurrence of a stress ulcer and administer antacid as ordered. The nurse also needs to routinely ausculate bowel sounds and administer stool softeners, laxatives, or bulking agents as ordered so as to promote and maintain routine bowel and elimination patterns.

Impaired Physical Mobility

The goal throughout the burn wound healing process is for the patient to achieve maximum function of all involved body parts and return to regular activities of daily living to the extent possible. Nurses must insure proper positioning and immobilization of burn wound and graft sites, routinely assessing the appearance of the wound bed or graft site. Splints should be applied by nurses as ordered in conjunction with physical and occupational therapy services. Skin integrity under and around splints must be monitored so as to avoid pressure areas and subsequent skin breakdown. Active and passive range of motion exercises must also be done as soon as possible. Ambulation should proceed in conjunction with the patient's overall condition. Until the time of ambulation, frequent repositioning will be necessary and the patient should be turned every 2 hours.[16]

Discharge Planning

As in most areas of burn care, discharge planning is a team process. It requires a multidisciplinary approach with tremendous amounts of communication, cooperation, and flexibility. There are three general criteria which must be considered in comprehensive discharge planning: status of wound; status of mobility; and readiness of family/home environment. As these criteria are being met, discharge teaching is ongoing. Specific written discharge instructions are valuable. Many units use generic discharge booklets with blank spaces to customize instructions, while others personalize boiler plate discharge instructions from a master computer program. Generally, four main areas need to be covered:

- wound care and dressing;
- skin care;
- physical therapy and occupational therapy; and
- return to previous life style, including information about expected psychological and social issues.

Wound care/dressings

Generally clean technique is taught for any residual wound dressings required after discharge. Sterile technique is not practical, cost-effective, or usually medically necessary for home care. Clearly written instructions with a step-by-step procedure are most effective (see **Table 32.1**). The nurse should demonstrate the entire wound dressing for the responsible person and then evaluate a return demonstration at a later date. The patient's insurance and other resources should be reviewed in order to insure the patient's capability to buy the needed dressing materials. For some insurance plans, prescriptions for dressing materials as well as appropriate ointments or creams are needed. If money is an issue, other resources and adaptation of procedures are best explored while the patient is still in the hospital.

Skin care

Skin care to all healed wounds, donor sites, and grafted areas needs to be reviewed with each patient. Bathing and recommended applications of emollient creams need to be emphasized. Since a deep burn may have destroyed oil-producing glands, cream may need to be applied at least twice a day. The nurse must remind the patient to check for dryness and flaking, because these signs would indicate that more lubricating cream is required. Medication, such as

Table 32.1 Sample silver sulfadiazine dressing instructions for home care

1. Wash hands.
2. Set up equipment, paper bag, gauze pad, gauze bandage, tongue blade, bowl with soap and water.
3. Remove soiled dressing from area. Discard in paper bag. Be careful to hold only on edge.
4. If there is a lot of drainage on dressing, wash hands again.
5. Gently wash around with gauze pad dipped in bowl with soap and water. Try and remove any leftover silver sulfadiazine cream.
6. Note any drainage or smell from wound. Call *(burn unit/clinic)* if there is any change from previous day.
7. Dip tongue blade in jar of silver sulfadiazine cream and smooth thin layer on gauze pad to cover open wound.
8. Secure gauze pad in place by strapping with gauze bandage. Use figure 8 wrap if possible.
9. Return to follow-up appointment date. Please call us if you have any questions.

Benadryl and Atarax, may be necessary to reduce itchiness, one of the biggest complaints with burn scars and healing. Blisters may also form on and around scars and healed areas. If they break, the patient should be instructed to apply mercurochrome or a recommended cream or ointment to any superficial breakdown areas. Healed burns, skin grafts, and donor sites are also more prone to sun sensitivity. Patients need to be cautious in their sun exposure, using sun block and barrier clothing as recommended.

Physical therapy/occupational therapy

Burn unit rehabilitation therapists will also spend time with discharge teaching. They will review, in depth, instructions on exercise, splints, and pressure garments needed by each patient. It is prudent for the nurse also to review these areas with the patient and emphasize areas where future compliance or learning needs are in doubt. The occupational therapist will also insure the patient's capability of performing regular activities of daily life. Adaptive devices may be required, and these should all be available for use in the hospital prior to discharge.

Return to previous life style

Healing the physical wounds is not enough. Physical, emotional, and psychological preparation of the patient and family is a necessary team effort for a truly successful discharge (see Chapter 57). The team must work just as hard to prevent social death as it has done to prevent physical death. The nurse plays an active role in the psychological adaptation of the patient and family. At discharge, the nurse continues this role by encouraging questions and verbalization of anxieties regarding post-hospital life. All members of the burn team need to encourage return to normality, including preburn autonomy and socialization.[17]

Out-Patient Management

As in all areas of medicine, there is trend toward increased out-patient management of burns. Generally only small, partial-thickness burns should be treated in the ambulatory setting. The following criteria are considered in distinguishing minor from major burns:

- depth of the wound;
- percentage of the body affected;
- indication of respiratory burn;
- presence of high tension wire in electrical injury; and
- child abuse/neglect.

Generally, burn injuries to the very young or very old as well as burns affecting the face, hands, or genitalia are best managed as in-patients. Nursing assessment in the out-patient area is key to evaluating patient/family potential for ability to perform wound care and to comply with an optimal care plan, including returning for follow-up appointments.

Once the decision has been made to treat a patient in an ambulatory setting, the nurse will initiate the out-patient care plan and begin teaching the home care instructions to the patients and family. Referrals to community agencies should also be utilized as necessary to assist the family. With each subsequent ambulatory visit, the nurse will continue to evaluate compliance with the care plan and progress of healing. Admission to in-patient care should be considered whenever routine progress does not continue.

References

1. Surveyor J A. Smoke inhalation injuries. *Heart Lung* 1980; **9:** 825–32.

2. Nebraska Burn Institute. *Advance Burn Life Support Provider's Manual.* Lincoln, NE: Nebraska Burn Institute, 1987.

3. Faldmo L, Kravitz M. Management of acute burns and burn shock resuscitation. *AACN Clin Issues Crit Care Nurs* 1993; **4:** 351–66.

4. Walter P H. Burn wound management. *AACN Clin Issues Crit Care Nurs* 1993; **4:** 378–87.

5. Carrougher G J. Inhalation injury. *AACN Clin Issues Crit Care Nurs* 1993; **4:** 367–77.

6. Tompkins R G, Burke J F, Schoenfeld O A, *et al.* Prompt eschar excision: a treatment system contributing to reduced burn mortality. *Ann Surg* 1986; **204:** 272–81.

7. Herndon D N, Gore D, Cole M, *et al.* Determinants of mortality in pediatric patients with greater than 70% full thickness total body surface area thermal injury treated by early total excision and grafting. *J Trauma* 1987; **27:** 208–12.

8. Tompkins R G, Remensnyder J P, Burke J F, *et al.* Significant reductions in mortality for children with burn injuries through the use of prompt eschar excision. *Ann Surg* 1988; **208:** 577–85.

9. Weber J M, Tompkins D M. Improving survival: Infection control and burns. *AACN Clin Issues Crit Care Nurs* 1993; **4:** 414–23.

10. Baxter C R, Marvin J, Curreri P W. Fluid and electrolyte therapy of burn shock. *Heart Surg* 1973; **2:** 707–13.

11. McCaffery M. *Nursing Management of the Patient with Pain.* Philadelphia: JB Lippincott Co, 1979.

12. Osgood P F, Szyfelbein S K. Management of burn pain in children. *Pediatr Clin North Am* 1989; **36:** 1001–13.

13. Gureno M A, Reisinger C L. Patient controlled analgesia for the young pediatric patient. *Pediatr Nurs* 1991; **17:** 251–4.

14. Kavanagh C. A new approach to dressing change in the severely burned child and its effect on burn-related psychopathology. *Heart Surg* 1983; **12:** 612–19.

15. Tompkins R G, Burke J F. Care of burns. In: Tinker J, Zapol W M, eds. *Care of the Critically Ill Patient.* 2nd ed. London: Springer-Verlag, 1993: 893–908.

16. Surveyer J A, Clougherty D M. Burn scars: fighting the effects. *Am J Nursing* 1983; **83:** 746–51.

17. Molter N G. When is the burn injury healed? *Psychosoc Impl Care* 1993; **4:** 424–32.

CHAPTER THIRTY-THREE

Special Considerations of Age: The Pediatric Burned Patient

Randi L. Rutan and Deb Benjamin

Each year more than 1000 children under the age of 15 die in house fires in the US and about two-thirds of these fire-related deaths involve children younger than 4 years of age.[1] Approximately 440 000 children receive medical treatment each year or have at least one day of restricted activity due to burn injuries,[2] and more than 20 000 of these require hospital admission. Two-thirds of burns in children are scalds due to household accidents or deliberate abuse. The burn injury produces overwhelming physiological and psychological challenges to a pediatric victim. The unique anatomical and physiological attributes of the child require the attention of physicians and nurses who are trained not only in burn care, but also in the specifics of pediatric care. The provision of medical care can induce an additional trauma if developmental needs are not addressed.

Great strides have been made in the reduction of mortality related to thermal injuries over the past few decades. Although fires and burn injuries are the second leading cause of death in children, current approaches to care have altered the mortality curves such that a child with an uncomplicated burn injury of 95% total body surface area (TBSA) has a 50% chance of survival.[3] The unprecedented survival of these severely injured children can be attributed to the advances in surgical techniques, infection control, and nutritional support.

The most obvious differences between adults and children are in size and body proportion. Shorter lengths, tighter angles, and smaller diameters of various anatomic structures and spaces make certain manipulations more difficult. These differences also require the provision of special equipment and supplies which reflect the configurations of pediatric anatomy. There are also physiological differences between children and adults which must be considered when treating the pediatric patient.

Alterations in Resuscitation

Due to their small body sizes, fluid losses are proportionally greater in children. Normal blood volume in children is approximately 80 ml/kg body weight, compared to the adult whose normal volume is 60 ml/kg. A 20% TBSA burn in a 10 kg child causes the evaporative loss of 475 ml or 60% of the circulating volume, while the same size burn in a 70 kg adult causes the loss of 1100 ml or only 25% of the blood volume.

Infants possess a larger cranial surface area with less area in the extremities than do adults; therefore the standard relationships between surface area and weight in adults do not hold true in growing children. Surface area is a function of weight. Although fluid losses following a burn injury are directly proportional to the burned surface area, the commonly used 'rule of nines', useful in adults, does not accurately reflect the surface area of children under 15 years of age (**Figure 33.1**). Most routinely used resuscitation formulae were developed using adult patients and are almost exclusively weight-based. Since the linear relationship between weight and surface area does not exist in children, use of these formulas in children results in gross under- or over-resuscitation (**Table 33.1**).

Pediatric burned patients should be resuscitated using formulas based on body surface area, which can be calculated from height and weight using standard nomograms (**Figure 33.2**) and which also consider maintenance fluid needs. The most commonly used resuscitation formula used in pediatric patients calls for the administration of 5000 ml/m^2 body surface area (BSA) burn plus 2000 ml/m^2 BSA given over the first 24 hours after burn, with half the volume administered during the first 8 hours. The subsequent 24 hours call for 3750 ml/m^2 BSA burn plus 1500 ml/m^2 BSA.[4] As in the adult patient, resuscitation formulas offer *guides* to the amounts necessary for replacing lost volume.

Fluid administration should be titrated to achieve a urine output of 0.5–2 ml/kg/h. An indwelling urinary catheter is essential during the early phase of resuscitation as urine output should be assessed as frequently as every 15 minutes during early titration. Fluid boluses should be administered in amounts appropriate for the size of the child and should represent no more than 25% of the total circulating volume (10 ml/kg).

Intravenous resuscitation fluid should be isotonic and replace lost electrolytes. Lactated Ringer's is the most suitable solution for the first 24 hours postburn and should be replaced by 5% dextrose during subsequent days. Rarely, infants can become hypoglycemic, and for them a small part of the resuscitation fluid should contain glucose during the first 24 hours postburn.

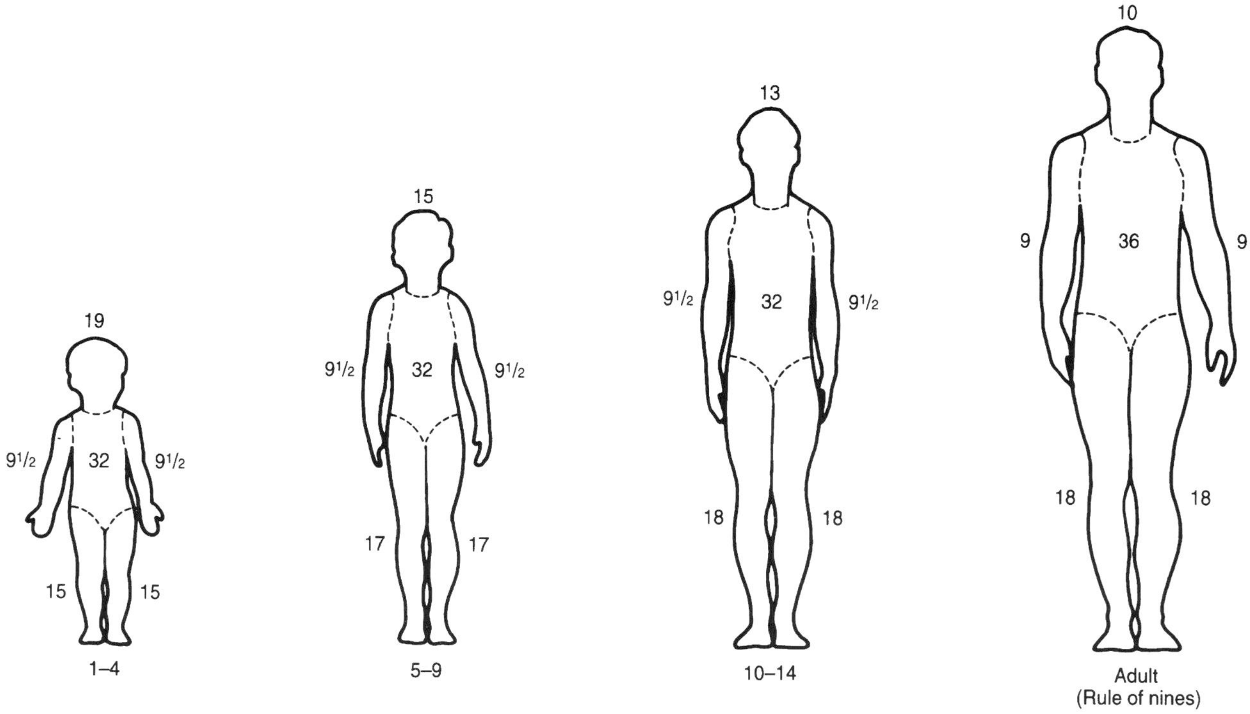

Fig. 33.1 The 'rule of nines' altered for the anthropomorphic differences of infancy and childhood. Reprinted with permission from Eichelberger MR, ed. Pediatric Trauma Prevention, Acute Care and Rehabilitation. *St Louis: Mosby Year Book, 1993: p 570.*

Table 33.1 Resuscitation and maintenance fluid requirement

		Calculated needs		Replacement burn loss	
Example	% Burn	Resuscitation*	Maintenance†	ml	ml/kg/%
1 year old	15	600	800	–200	–1.33
10 kg	30	1200	800	400	1.33
0.48 m² BSA	60	2400	800	1600	2.67
	90	3600	800	2800	3.11
4 years old	15	990	1200	–210	–0.85
16.5 kg	30	1980	1200	780	1.58
0.68 m² BSA	60	3900	1200	2760	2.79
	90	5940	1200	4940	3.33
12 years old	15	2400	2250	1150	1.92
40 kg	30	4800	2550	2550	2.12
1.13 m² BSA	60	9600	2250	7350	3.06
	90	14 400	2250	12 150	3.38

* 4 ml/kg/% burn.
† 2000 ml/m² BSA.

Route of administration

It is crucial that venous access be obtained early postburn, even though such access may be extremely difficult to obtain. Due to the small circulating volume, delays in resuscitation for periods as short as 30 minutes can result in profound shock. Small bore catheters limit the rates at which fluid can be administered; therefore, children with large burn injuries may require two large vessels to be cannulated so that sufficient fluid can be given. Intravenous cannulation of the major central vessels is arduous in children. The short thick necks of children makes jugular access difficult. The subclavian vein lies within a protective triangle of shoulder, jaw, and neck; attempted cannulation of this vein often results in pneumo- and hemothoraces. The femoral or the saphenous veins offer the best temporary alternative for large vein access via surgical cut-down when percutaneous cannulation is unsuccessful.

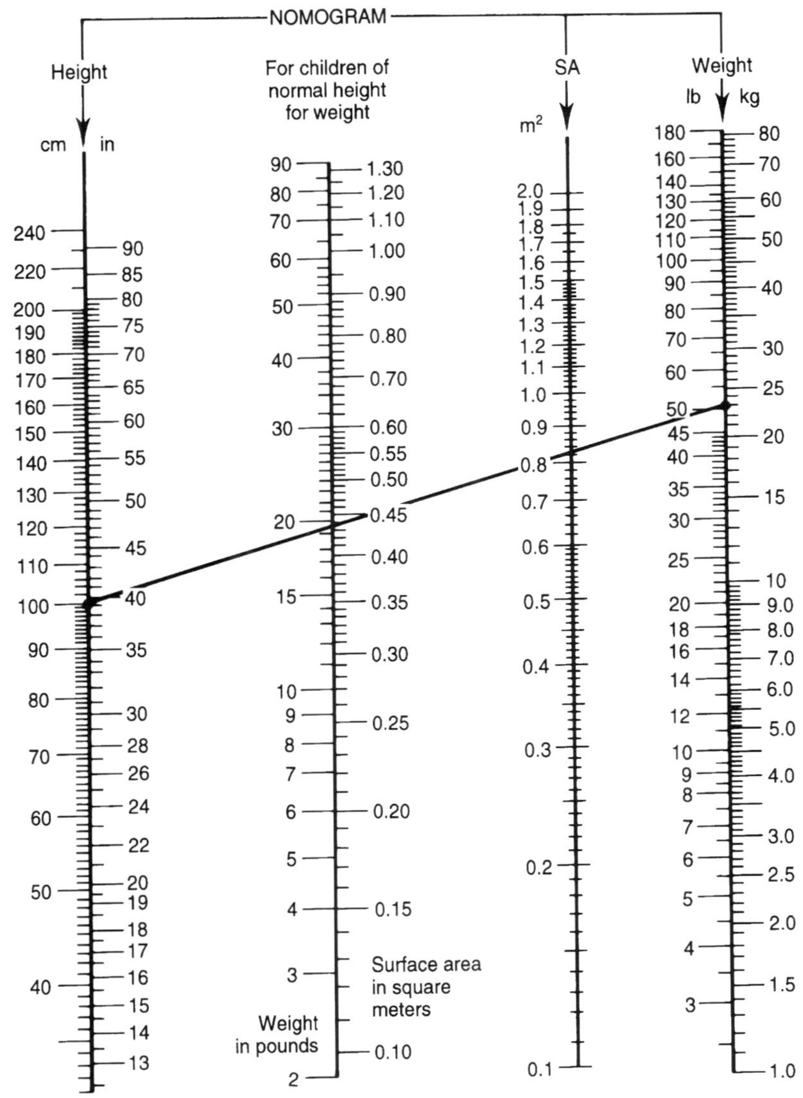

Fig. 33.2 Standard nomogram for the determination of body surface area based on height and weight. The example depicted is for a child of 100 cm in height (closed circle) and 23 kg in weight (closed triangle). Reprinted with permission from Eichelberger MR, ed. Pediatric Trauma: Prevention, Acute Care and Rehabilitation. *St Louis: Mosby Year Book, 1993: p 572.*

When venous cannulation cannot be accomplished with dispatch, children can be administered fluid volumes in excess of 100 ml/h directly into the bone marrow.[5] The low fat content of the marrow in children may account for the rare incidence of embolic complications with this procedure. A 16–18 gauge bone marrow aspiration needle can be used to cannulate the bone marrow compartment, although spinal needles and even butterfly needles can be pushed through the porous bone of a child. Although previously advocated only for children younger than 3 years of age, intraosseous fluid administration can be safely performed in children under 8 years of age, if the bone is sufficiently soft to allow needle penetration.[6] The anterior tibial plateau, medial maleolus, anterior iliac crest, and the distal femur are preferred sites for intraosseous infusion. The needle should be introduced into the bone, taking care to avoid the epiphysis, either perpendicular to the bone or at a 60° angle with the bevel facing the greater length of bone (**Figure 33.3**). The needle has been properly inserted when bone marrow can be freely aspirated.

Assessment of Resuscitation

Evaluation of the efficacy of resuscitation is difficult. The routine clinical signs of hypovolemia for the adult burn victim, such as tachycardia, low blood pressure, and decreased urine output, are late manifestations in the pediatric patient. Children have remarkable cardiopulmonary reserve, often not exhibiting clinical signs of hypovolemia until more than 25% of the circulating volume has been lost and complete cardiovascular decompensation is imminent. They frequently develop a reflex tachycardia after even the most trivial injury due to an overexuberant catecholamine response to the emotional trauma or anxiety. Due to smaller body sizes, lower vascular pressures are needed to circulate the blood (**Table 33.2**). Systolic blood pressures of less than 100 mmHg are common in children younger than 5 years of age. Additionally, young children with immature kidneys have less tubular concentrating ability than adults, and urine production may continue in spite of hypovolemia. Mental clarity, pulse pressures, arterial blood gases, distal extremity color, capillary refill, and body temperature reflect volume status. The Glasgow Coma Scale has been modified to reflect the immature cognition and verbal skills of the infant and young child (**Table 33.3**). A child with normal blood pressure and acceptable heart rate, but with cool clammy extremities, mental obtundation, and a delayed capillary refill, is a child in dire danger.

Volume overload must be avoided. Although children possess a large cardiopulmonary reserve, the young heart is less compliant, and stroke volumes plateau at relatively low filling pressures, shifting the Starling curve to the left. Cardiac output is almost

Table 33.2 Normal pediatric vital signs

Age	Minimum heart rate (beats/min)	Systolic BP (mmHg)	Respirations (breaths/min)	Minimal hemoglobin (g/dl)	Minimal hematocrit (%)
< 2 years of age	100–160	60	30–40	11.0	33.0
2–5 years of age	80–140	70	20–30	11.0	33.0
6–12 years of age	70–120	80	18–25	11.5	34.5
< 12 years of age	60–110	90	16–20	12.0	36.0

Table 33.3 Modification of the Glasgow Coma Scale for the altered cognition and verbalization skills of the young child

Glasgow Coma Scale		'Pediatric' modifications	
Eye opening			
Spontaneous	4	Spontaneous	4
To speech	3	To speech	3
To pain	2	To pain	2
None	1	None	1
Best verbal response			
Oriented	5	Coos, babbles	5
Confused	4	Irritable cries	4
Inappropriate words	3	Cries to pain	3
Incomprehensible sounds	2	Moans to pain	2
None	1	None	1
Best motor response			
Obeys commands	6	Spontaneous movement	6
Localizes pain	5	Withdraws to touch	5
Withdraws	4	Withdraws to pain	4
Flexion posturing	3	Abnormal flexion	3
Extensor posturing	2	Abnormal extension	2
None	1	None	1

completely dependent upon heart rate, and the immature heart is more sensitive to volume and pressure overload.

Children are particularly prone to the development of edema from both vasogenic and hydrostatic sources. Vasogenic edema occurs within the early postburn period when vascular integrity is impaired. Of particular concern is the development of cerebral edema. Care should be taken in order to maintain cerebral elevation, particularly during the initial 24–48 hours postburn. The maintenance of intravascular osmotic pressures decrease the likelihood of edema development. Salt-poor albumin can be expected to remain in the intravascular space if administered after 6 hours postburn in amounts necessary to maintain serum albumin levels at more than 2.5 g/dl. Albumin deficit can be calculated using the formula of:

$$[2.5 \text{ g/dl} - \text{current serum albumin (g/dl)}] \times [\text{wt (kg)} \times 3]$$

The deficit can be administered as 25% albumin and given in three divided doses.

Pulmonary edema is more frequently caused by hydrostatic pressures. If identified during the early postburn period without the presence of an inhalation injury, it is diagnostic of overhydration. Management of volume overload should include restriction of fluid intake and pharmacologic diuresis.

Following the first 24 hours postburn, evaporative water loss of 1500 ml/m^2 for maintenance and 3750 ml/m^2 burn area can be expected. Loss of renal medullary concentrating capacity is usual secondary to washout of the medulla during resuscitation. Delivery of volume to achieve sufficient calories to support the hypermetabolic response usually exceeds fluid requirements. Hyponatremia is the most frequently observed complication in pediatric patients after the first 48 hours post-injury. Frequent monitoring of serum sodium is necessary to guide appropriate salt or water supplementation. Children of less than 1 year of age may require more sodium supplementation due to higher urinary sodium losses. Further, potassium losses should usually be replaced with potassium phosphate rather than potassium chloride as hypophosphatemia is frequently observed in this population.[7]

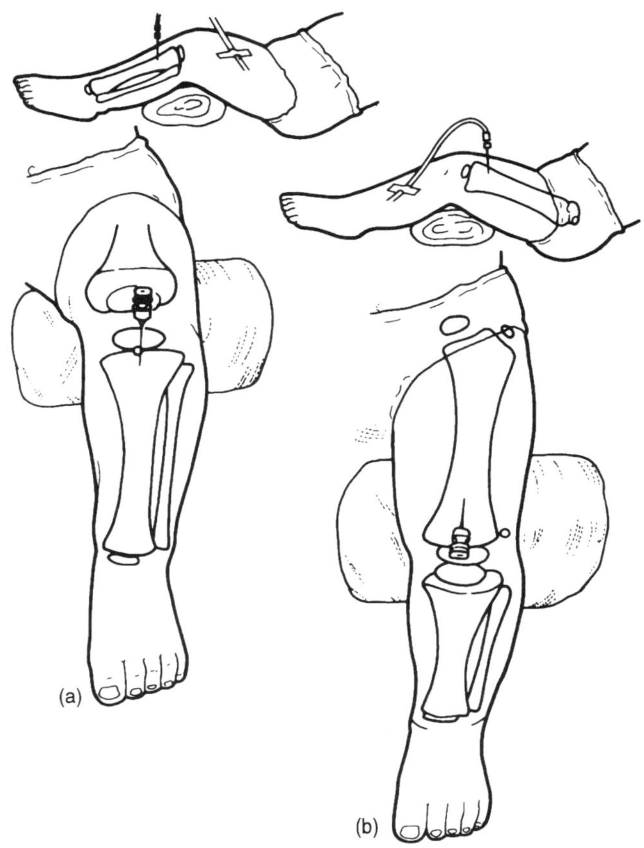

Fig. 33.3 Intraosseous line placement in the proximal tibia (a) and distal femur (b). Reprinted with permission from Fleisher G, Ludwig S, eds. Textbook of Pediatric Emergency Medicine. *2nd ed. Baltimore: Williams & Wilkins, 1988: p 268.*

EVALUATION OF AIRWAYS

Inhalation injury, and its sequelae of infection and pulmonary failure, are major determinants of mortality after thermal injury. Often children are discovered within the burned shells of their homes, huddled deep within closets where the flames did not touch them, but they are nevertheless dead. Carbon monoxide poisoning coupled with hypoxia are the causes of deaths due to 'smoke inhalation'. Any flame-related injury, particularly if it is incurred indoors, should be evaluated for an inhalation component. Children may be spared some of the overt signs of inhalation injury due to their short stature and proximity to the floor-level cool air. Yet, as with adults, the only definitive method to diagnose an inhalation injury is through direct visualization of the airway.

The smaller aperture of the pediatric trachea predisposes it to obstruction. Equal amounts of airway edema in pediatric and adult airways results in significantly disproportionate increases in amounts of resistance and decreases in cross-sectional area. A 1 mm increase in tissue thickness of a 4 mm diameter pediatric trachea results in a 16-fold increase in resistance with a 75% decrease in cross-sectional area, while the same edema in an adult airway would increase the airway resistance but threefold and reduce airway area by only 44%.[8] As edema develops promptly following injury, airway evaluation and management must be given priority in pediatric patients. During emergent conditions when edema is present, inability to secure the airway with an endotracheal tube is a clear indication of the need for surgical airway control.

Hyperextension of the neck is contraindicated in the pediatric patient. Due to the tight angle between the mouth, pharynx, and trachea, hyperextension will obstruct the airway. Additionally, due to the relatively large tongue and hypertrophied tonsils in young children, hyperextension encourages epiglottal obstruction in the unconscious. The head should be positioned with a slight tilt so that the chin and tip of the nose are level. This should provide optimal alignment of the oropharynx and trachea. Direct laryngoscopy is necessary to inspect the larynx and cords for accumulation of soot or the development of erythema or edema. In children under 6 years of age, a straight blade should be inserted below the epiglottis and gently lifted to allow clear visualization of the vocal cords. Care should be taken to avoid the highly vascular adenoidal tissue.

Potential hemorrhage and prompt edema formation make emergency intubation difficult. Concurrent placement of an endotracheal tube during bronchoscopy should be considered. A readily available estimate of airway diameter is the width of the patient's little finger. Those practitioners accustomed to intubating adults will likely intubate the right mainstem bronchus in children, because of the shorter distance between the mouth and the bronchial carina. In children under 8 years of age, the developing cricoid cartilage creates the narrowest part of the airway just below the glottis, so cuffed endotracheal tubes are rarely needed. The cricoid cartilage is the only circumferential support for the trachea. Open cricothyroidotomy is discouraged in children under the age of 12.[9]

Metabolic Considerations

Hypermetabolism, fed by protein and lipid catabolism, is a characteristic response to major trauma and infection. No other disease state produces as dramatic an effect on the metabolic rate as burn injury. In the pediatric patient, there are limited glycogen stores to meet the augmented energy demands; therefore, the initiation of protein and lipid catabolism for gluconeogenesis is accelerated. Available stores to support prolonged starvation are critically absent in children.

Body Composition

Weight gain is extremely rapid during the first 3 years of life, particularly during the first year. Gains in height are not as rapid, rendering the infant chubby. As height growth rates increase, toddlers take a more 'child like' body silhouette and are said to be '... losing their baby fat'. During the remainder of childhood, children 'leapfrog' their growth by first gaining weight and then height. Fat is, therefore, the most variable body tissue component.

Fat and subcutaneous tissue provide some protection from injury. During the last trimester of pregnancy, the fetus rapidly gains fat; this accumulation continues after birth, reaching maximal thickness at about 9 months of age. The thickness of this tissue then begins to slowly decrease until about age 6 years, but it accumulates again during preadolescence, allowing the postpubertal sex-specific fat deposition. In girls, the percentage of body fat increases gradually up to about 25% in adult women. In contrast, pubescent boys gradually lose fat, eventually reaching about 12% total body fat in adult men. Lean muscle comprises about 25% of birth weight and gradually increases to about 40% in both sexes at puberty; shortly after this time, boys gain an additional 10% in muscle mass.

Growth

Metabolic rates of growing children are significantly higher than those predicted by the Harris–Benedict equation. This elevation is necessary to meet the metabolic demands of growth. Major catastrophic illnesses and traumas have been demonstrated to produce both transient and permanent changes in growth patterns,[10] which may be an adaptive mechanism designed to promote reparative processes. In severely burned patients, nail and hair growth are attenuated during the acute postburn period, and bone growth is slowed.[11–13] Dampened height and weight gain velocities have been documented in children during the first 3 years postburn without a subsequent period of catch-up growth, thereby rendering these burned children slighter and shorter than their age-matched peers.[14]

Thermoregulation

Core body temperature is consistently elevated after a major trauma. A hypothalamic reset induced by various inflammatory cytokines causes this elevation even in the absence of infection. The temperature reset is thought to be an adaptive mechanism to bolster host defense against potential pathogens. Burned patients strive for temperatures of about 38°C. Depressed or 'normal' temperatures are more likely indicative of overwhelming sepsis or exhausted physiological capabilities and should be viewed as an ominous sign. After major thermal injuries, routine methods of heat conservation are inadequate due to the extensive heat loss through convection and evaporation. Infants and toddlers, with their increased surface area/volume ratios, less insulating fat, and lower muscle mass for shivering are particularly susceptible to hypothermia.

Hypothermia produces numerous consequences. The heart is particularly sensitive to temperature, and ventricular arrhythmias are not uncommon. Hypothermia also increases the susceptibility of the myocardium to changes in electrolyte concentrations. The oxyhemoglobin dissociation curve is shifted to the left by lowered body temperature, impairing peripheral oxygenation. In extreme cases, hypothermia produces central nervous system and respiratory depression, coagulopathies, and loss of peripheral vasomotor tone.

Every effort should be made to reduce the heat loss experienced by pediatric patients. Ambient temperatures and humidity should be maintained at 28–33°C and 80%, respectively, in order to decrease energy demands and evaporative water losses. Wet dressings should be avoided or at least wrapped, and wet bedding promptly changed so as to decrease evaporative or conductive cooling. The patient should be positioned so that drafts are avoided, including the inlets and outlets for air-conditioning and heating ducts. Bathing or showering should be expeditiously completed, avoiding undue environmental exposure.

Nutritional Support

In addition to the increased metabolic demands made by the burn injury itself, essentially all the routine events associated with burn care increase the catecholamine release and metabolic rate through increasing pain and anxiety. Adults rarely are able to voluntarily consume adequate calories needed to meet metabolic demands, despite mature cognitive function. Children will simply refuse, and rational conversation will not sway their adamant refusals.

Those children with small injuries (i.e. less than 30% TBSA) can usually be coaxed to take sufficient calories to support their metabolic response; sometimes their wounds are closed sufficiently quickly so that their endogenous calorie stores are not depleted during their acute postburn period. On the other hand, those children with injuries of greater than 30% TBSA burn will require some form of caloric supplementation.

Calories should be provided through the enteral route. Most children will tolerate enteral feedings as early as 3–6 hours postburn, if not immediately. Several studies have demonstrated the efficacy of early alimentation and the additional salutary effects.[15–16] Enteral feedings can be given through a flexible silastic duodenal feeding tube, bypassing the stomach, which may be experiencing decreased peristaltic action.

Enteral milk has been demonstrated to be one of the least expensive and best tolerated of all enteral formulas. Additionally, it is palatable and easily recognized by children when they are able to take oral feedings. Because of the low sodium content of milk, sodium supplementation may be needed. Hyperosmolar feedings, commercially available, should be avoided because of the high incidence of subsequent diarrhea. Diarrhea is particularly troublesome in children because of their increased sensitivity to volume deficits.

Since caloric demands are related to burn size, caloric support should be given in amounts calculated on body surface area. A series of different formulae have been developed at Shriners Burns Institute – Galveston to meet the differing requirements of the various age groups.[17–19] The Curreri formula has likewise been amended to reflect the differing demands of the pediatric group (**Table 33.4**). Pediatric patients lack the endogenous calorie stores which permit lengthy fasts in adults. Preoperative NPO orders should consider this unique physiologic aspect of the pediatric patient.

Neurocognitive development

Delivery of care must be tailored to the specific needs of each patient. The maturing cognitive abilities of the growing child dictate the need for a variety of interactive models for primary care providers. Additionally, knowledge of the neurocognitive stage of the child may indicate the probable method of injury. With recognition of the particular needs of the child within a particular developmental stage, medical care can be safely and effectively delivered with the cooperative participation of the pediatric burned patient.

An infant under 1 year of age is completely dependent; consequently, burn injuries in children of this age are most frequently a result of abuse or neglect. Infants are relatively immobile and unable to verbalize needs, so their requirements must be anticipated and met by the health care team. During this period, the infant is developing a trusting relationship with his care providers. This relationship is essential as it forms the basis for all subsequent social development. A hospitalization during this period is a terrifying experience for which the infant possesses no coping skills. Parental or primary caretaker involvement in care is requisite and should be initiated as soon as possible.

During toddler years, children attempt to separate self from others and the environment and this results in two relevant consequences. Burn injuries to children between 1 and 2 years of age are frequently the result of exploratory behaviors, whereby toddlers differentiate themselves from objects in their environments, including electrical cords and boiling pots. Also, toddlers are frightened by strangers and unfamiliar environments; this may create difficulties for caregivers. Although verbal skills remain immature, cognitive skills have developed sufficiently that children of this age are receptive to simple verbal explanations and assurances given by the burn care team or parents. These verbalizations must be given in friendly tones and with simple language. Parental or primary caretaker involvement remains critical, for they provide necessary security to the toddler. Comfort may also be sought from special toys, blankets, or other objects brought from home.

Preschool children, aged 2–5 years, can be characterized by their imitative behaviors, which occasionally result in burn injuries due to their immature judgment skills. The propensity of these children for this type of behavior, however, can be used to facilitate their care. Children of this age can assist with their dressing changes and other wound care activities. Additionally, exercise routines can be facilitated with imitative games such as 'Simon says'. Preschool children, although possessing a limited vocabulary, can directly express their fears and anxieties. Regression to toddler-like behavior is to be expected, and parents should be prepared for this occurrence.

Most often, burn injuries to the school-aged child are the results of true accidents or inappropriate judgment. Cognitively, these children can understand basic explanations of the procedures to be performed, and such explanation usually elicits the cooperation of a child with the health care provider. The child of 6–10 years is attempting to gain competence in basic interpersonal and social skills and has a well developed gender identification. Modesty should be scrupulously observed; intimate procedures, such as catheterization or bedpan assistance, should be performed by a same-sexed individual.

Table 33.4 Nutritional requirements for children

	Galveston	Modified Curreri
Infant	2100 kcal/m^2 + 1000 kcal/m^2 burn	BMR + 15 kcal/% burn
Toddler		BMR + 25 kcal/% burn
Child	1800 kcal/m^2 + 1300 kcal/m^2 burn	BMR + 40 kcal/% burn
Adolescent	1500 kcal/m^2 + 1500 kcal/m^2 burn	

Preadolescent children draw their personal identities from their peer group. They prefer to be grouped with other similarly aged and sexed children or in a private room. Most commonly, injuries in this group are the result of true accidents. Health care providers should interact with these children with the same consideration they would give to adults, observing their rights to privacy and confidentiality. The preadolescent often reacts to hospitalization with withdrawal, particularly if isolated from the peer group. If similarly aged children are unavailable, social stimulation can be provided by facilitating their interaction with younger children in an 'older sibling' role.

Adolescents are preparing to assume adult roles. Their judgment is limited by their experience, however, and their emotional responses are dramatized. Burn trauma in this group may be the result of homicidal or suicidal attempts in addition to accidents. All interactions with these young people should be conducted as with other adults, and they must feel respected. They will refuse to cooperate with procedures which they perceive to be forced on them autocratically.

With injury, illness, and hospitalization, children can be expected to exhibit regressive behavior, reverting to behaviors which brought comfort at an earlier developmental age. Parents and caretakers should understand these behaviors as the child attempts to cope with a very difficult situation. Adult responses to the child should promote comfort and security and should not punish the child. As the child recovers, the behaviors also can be expected to return to preburn maturity.

Family Support

Parents and other family members can provide necessary support, comfort, and guidance for their children. Health care providers can promote family involvement in patient care by encouraging a parent to sleep in the room with a frightened child or by showing the adult how to safely hold the child for cuddling and rocking. Family members can also be invited to feed the patient, participate in dressing changes, or simply to sit and talk or play games. On the other hand, parents and other family members may themselves require psychological support, encouragement, and specific guidance from the health care team in order to interact optimally with the child. Such care of the family is an inseparable aspect of good care of the pediatric patient.

References

1. Center for Disease Control. *1986 Mortality Data*. Atlanta, GA: CDC, 1987.

2. Division of Injury Control, Centers for Disease Control. Childhood injuries in the United States. *Am J Dis Child* 1990; **133:** 627–52.

3. Herndon D N, Rutan R L, Alison W E, Cox C S. Management of burn injuries. In: Eichelberger M R, ed. *Pediatric Trauma: Prevention, Acute Care and Rehabilitation*. St Louis: Mosby Year Book, 1993, 568–90.

4. Carvajal H F. A physiologic approach to fluid therapy in severely burned children. *Surg Gynecol Obstet* 1980; **150:** 379–84.

5. Tocantins L M, O'Neill J F. Infusions of blood and other fluids into the general circulation via the bone marrow. *Surg Gynecol Obstet* 1941; **73:** 281–7.

6. Fiser H D. Intraosseous infusion. *N Engl J Med* 1990; **322:** 1579–81.

7. Kruesser W, Ritz E. The phosphate depletion syndrome. *Contrib Nephrol* 1978; **14:** 162–6.

8. Ryan J F, Todres I D, Cotes C J, *et al.*, eds. *A Practice of Anesthesia for Infants and Children*. New York: Grune & Stratton, 1986: 39.

9. Magnason D K, Maier R V. Pathophysiology of injury. In: Eichelberger MR, ed. *Pediatric Trauma: Prevention, Acute Care and Rehabilitation*. St Louis: Mosby Year Book, 1993: 61.

10. Prader A. Catchup growth. *Postgrad Med J* 1978; **54**(S): 133–46.

11. Artz C P, Moncrief JA. *Treatment of Burns*. 3rd ed. Philadelphia PA: WB Saunders Co, 1974.

12. Artz L P, Stern P J, Wurick J D. Skeletal changes after burn injuries in an animal model. *J Burn Care Rehabil* 1988; **9:** 148–51.

13. Klein G L, Herndon D N, Rutan T C, *et al.* Bone disease in burn patients. *J Bone Miner Res* 1993; **8**(3): 337–45.

14. Rutan R L, Herndon D N. Growth delay in postburn pediatric patients. *Arch Surg* 1990; **125:** 392–5.

15. Enzi G, Casadei A, Sergi G, *et al.* Metabolic and hormonal effects of early nutritional supplementation after surgery in burn patients. *Crit Care Med* 1990; **18:** 719–21.

16. McDonald W S, Sharp C W, Deitch E A. Immediate enteral feeding in burn patients is safe and effective. *Ann Surg* 1991; **213:** 177–83.

17. Hildreth M A, Herndon D N, Desai M H, Broemeling D L. Caloric requirements of patients with burns under 1 year of age. *J Burn Care Rehabil* 1993; **14**(1): 108–12.

18. Hildreth M A, Herndon D N, Desai M H, Duke M A. Caloric needs of adolescent patients with burns. *J Burn Care Rehabil* 1989; **10**(6): 523–6.

19. Hildreth M A, Herndon D N, Desai M H, Broemeling L D. Current treatment reduces calories required to maintain weight in pediatric patients with burns. *J Burn Care Rehabil* 1990; **11**(5): 405–9.

CHAPTER THIRTY-FOUR

Care of Geriatric Patients

Manuhbai H. Desai

Burn injuries rank fourth among causes of injury-related deaths in the geriatric age group.[1] Age and concomitant chronic disease processes contribute to a high mortality rate in this group of patients so that they require specialized care.[2,3] Diminished manual dexterity, reaction time, vision, hearing and judgment render the elderly vulnerable to burn injuries.[4] Many older people live alone and are often physically or mentally unable to respond appropriately in an emergency. Smoking materials and stoves/ovens are reported as frequent sources of injury in older persons, suggesting that they are most frequently burned during the course of routine daily tasks associated with self-care or homemaking (**Figure 34.1**).[5] The seriousness of burn injuries in this group is enhanced by a characteristic delay in seeking medical attention for the treatment of these injuries. The relatively superficial appearance and small surface area of the majority of these injuries are deceptive and do not cause immediate concern. Lack of definitive care predisposes the injury to develop cellulitis and subsequent infection. As many as 35% of elderly individuals who are burned delay seeking medical attention for at least 1 day following their injuries.[5,6]

Care of the elderly patient involves treatment of many medical conditions. The major causes of mortality and morbidity in the elderly following thermal injury are not the burn, but rather the alterations imposed by concomitant chronic disease processes. Linn[7] compared complications of burn injury by age groups and determined a statistically higher rate of burn shock (15%), inhalation injury (12%), pulmonary pathology (22%), septicemia (8%), and renal failure (11%) in the elderly age group than in younger patients. Preexisting cardiovascular or pulmonary pathology contributes to difficulties in providing adequate and appropriate fluid resuscitation as well as to high mortality.[8] Although it is not routine practice to administer fluid resuscitation to patients with less than a 10–15% body surface area (TBSA) burn, there is evidence to suggest that the elderly, like children, are particularly volume sensitive and may be at risk for hypotensive renal damage.[9] Herd[10] has advocated the administration of resuscitation fluid to elderly patients with injuries of more than 5% TBSA. A relatively high rate of mortality during the early postburn period has been cited in this population due to over- or under-resuscitation, despite careful fluid management.[11] Adequacy of resuscitation can be surmised by 30–50 ml/h urine output, clear mentation, and appropriate blood pressure. Mental confusion is a particularly sensitive indicator of cerebral perfusion and, thus of adequacy of resuscitation, but it may be difficult to determine in a patient whose mental faculties were impaired pre-injury, especially if there are no informants accompanying the patient who can report cognitive changes.

Resuscitation with crystalloid or crystalloid/colloid solutions should be initiated at a rate of 3–4 ml/kg/% burn and titrated to specific outcome parameters while carefully evaluating evidence of systemic overload or underhydration. Hypertonic saline/dextran solutions have been used[12] and may be of benefit in those select patients in whom fluid overload would be particularly troublesome. There is some evidence to suggest that the sodium load with these solutions may enhance cardiovascular recovery more than the colloid content.[13]

Due to diminished reaction time in geriatric individuals, the severity of burn injury and the incidence of inhalation injury is increased in this segment of the population.[7] Manktelow[3] reported a

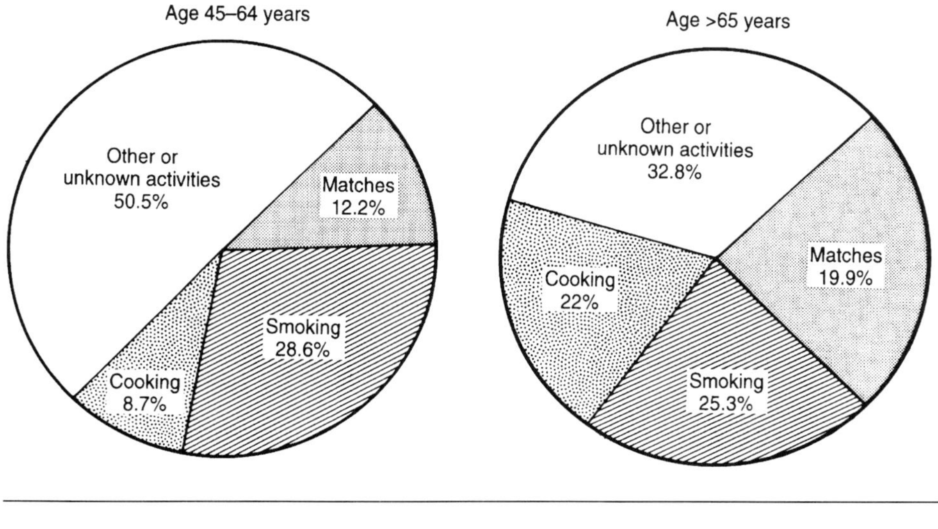

Fig. 34.1 Most frequent activities associated with fabric ignition accidents among middle age and older persons. Adapted from Beverley (1976)[4] with permission from Advanstar Communications, Inc.

39% incidence of inhalation injury in the elderly and a concomitant reduction in the size of survivable burn injuries. Older patients more frequently require mechanical ventilatory support following an inhalation injury and are more prone to iatrogenic complications; additionally, elderly patients with inhalation injury have more frequent episodes of pneumonia and sepsis.[14]

Pneumonias developed post-injury may be due to inhalation injury, nosocomial infection, or a combination of both. Prolonged immobilization and ongoing physiologic stress contribute to the significant morbidity related to inhalation injury. In this patient group, it is imperative that every effort be made to prevent endotracheal intubation and, if intubation occurs, that aggressive therapy be implemented to permit early extubation. Mobilization of pulmonary secretions should be encouraged through the use of humidified oxygen, nebulization of mucolytic agents and the judicious use of bronchodilators. Adjunctively, frequent position changes, chest physiotherapy and early ambulation discourage the development of pneumonias or attenuate their clinical course.

Wound Care

Wound healing is of great concern in older patients. Skin changes associated with the aging process predispose this group to poor or delayed wound healing of not only partial-thickness wounds, but also skin graft recipient beds and split-thickness skin graft donor sites.[15,16] Because of this, conservative wound care has historically been advocated for this group of burned patients. Application of antimicrobial agents, frequent dressing changes, and daily hydrotherapy accompanied by blunt debridement to encourage eschar separation and subsequent split-thickness skin grafting have been the treatment plan of choice for older individuals.[17] Responses of the elderly to other types of major surgery indicate that geriatric patients can tolerate the stress of surgery provided that no complications occur. At least one study suggests that improved survival and reduced hospital stays can be achieved with early excision and grafting of burn wounds in older patients, and that elderly patients may tolerate the stress of early excision better than they tolerate the ravages of chronic burn wound sepsis.[18–20] Investigators have reported that early excision of burn wounds less than 20% total body surface area (TBSA) has a salutary effect on mortality and length of hospital stay in the geriatric age group.[14,20] Deitch[20] reported a significantly larger burn size at 50% mortality (LA_{50}) than previous studies when geriatric patients were treated with early excision and grafting (see **Table 34.1**). The general consensus from the literature is that early excision of small wounds (i.e. less than 20%) is probably beneficial to elderly patients, and decreases the mortality and morbidity of their injuries. Large wounds, however, should be conservatively managed with staged excisions of areas of less than 20% TBSA.

Infectious Complications

Infection is a constant danger with a geriatric patient. Older patients frequently have a diminished capacity to respond to the bacterial challenge which follows a burn injury. Additionally, there is an increased likelihood that the elderly have preexisting malnutrition, which further impairs their immunocompetence. Even identifying the presence of an infection in this group of patients is somewhat challenging because they frequently are unable to mount a febrile response to bacterial or viral invasion and may manifest such phenomena with vague, ill-defined symptoms. The use of systemic antibiotics should be reserved for documented infection. Systemic levels of drugs excreted by the kidneys should be carefully monitored in elderly patients as renal function frequently has been impaired preburn injury and may have been further denigrated by subsequent hypovolemia or the elimination of toxic burn products.

Table 34.1 Burn size (%) to cause a 50% mortality (LA_{50})

	50–59 years	60–74 years	> 75 years
Feller	45.9	30.6	18.0
Bowser *et al.*	51.7	40.7	18.4
Deitch	65.5	41.7	34.0

* From Deitch (1985).[20]

Recovery

It has been reported that the long-term prognosis of geriatric trauma victims is poor. Fewer than one out of ten trauma survivors return to an independent life style within 1 year of discharge. More than 70% of such survivors require continuing nursing home care for more than 1 year post-injury.[21] In sharp contrast to these data are reports of the recovery of burned geriatric patients.[19,22,23] Keys *et al.*[24] reported 94 of 99 patients over 55 years of age were discharged home following the closure of their burn wounds. Because the overall social environment was not assessed, it is impossible to determine how many of these patients returned to spouses and/or families and how many returned to solitary living. Manktelow *et al.*[3] reported that 47% of geriatric patients surviving a burn injury were reduced to a less independent level of living when discharged from the hospital. They also reported that although 21% required nursing home care upon discharge, only 11% required this type of care at 1 year postburn. Similarly, Larson[23] reported 27 of 31 patients over the age of 61 returned home following recovery, almost all to spouses or other family members. In general, the reports in the literature appear to indicate that geriatric victims of thermal injury have a more satisfactory functional outcome than do elderly victims of other traumas which involve broken bones or damaged organs. Functional outcome depends greatly on the nursing and other medical care received during hospitalization. With this group, it is particularly important to keep them oriented and cognitively stimulated to the degree possible. It is also critical to institute a regimen of passive and active exercise in order to maintain functional mobility.

As with children, providing support and guidance for family or caretakers is an integral part of the care of the elderly who will depend on these individuals for their well-being upon discharge. Discharge planning for elderly patients should be initiated upon admission to a hospital.[25] The elderly are not a homogeneous group and will require varying levels of both social and medical support upon discharge. Special attention must be paid to the limitations imposed by aging, such as communication deficits; limitations of mobility; decreased muscle tone, strength, and function; and slowed cognitive abilities.

References

1. *Accident Facts.* Chicago IL: National Safety Council, 1982.

2. Anous M M, Heimbach D M. Causes of death and predictors in burned patients more than 60 years of age. *J Trauma* 1986; **26:** 135–9.

3. Manktelow A, Meyer A A, Herzog S R, Peterson H D. Analysis of life expectancy and living status of elderly patients surviving a burn injury. *J Trauma* 1989; **29:** 203–7.

4. Beverley E V. Reducing fire and burn hazards among the elderly. *Geriatrics* 1976; **31**(5): 106–10.

5. Rossignol A M, Locke J A, Boyle C M, Burke J F. Consumer products and hospitalized burn injuries among elderly Massachusetts residents. *J Am Geriatr Soc* 1985; **33:** 768–72.

6. MacKay A M, Chang A, Branch L D, *et al.* Delay of treatment of elderly burned patients. *APHA 108th Meeting*, Detroit MI, 1980.

7. Linn B S. Age differences in the severity and outcome of burns. *J Am Geriatr Soc* 1980; **28**(3): 118–23.

8. Le H Q, Zamboni W, Eriksson E, Baldwin J. Burns in patients under 2 and over 70 years of age. *Ann Plast Surg* 1986; **17**(1): 39–44.

9. Housinger T, Saffle J, Ward S, *et al.* Conservative approach to the elderly patient with burns. *Am J Surg* 1984; **148:** 817–19.

10. Herd B M, Herd A N, Tanner N S B. Burns to the elderly: a reappraisal. *Br J Plast Surg* 1987; **40:** 278–91.

11. Pruitt B A Jr, Mason A D Jr, Hunt J L. Burn injury in the aged or high risk patient. In: Seige J H, Chadoff P D, eds. *The Aged and High Risk Surgical Patient.* New York: Grune and Stratton, 1976: 523–46.

12. Bowser-Wallace B H, Cone J B, Caldwell F T. Hypertonic lactated saline resuscitation of severely burned patients over 60 years of age. *J Trauma* 1985; **25**(1): 22–6.

13. Munster A M. *Burn Care for the House Officer.* Baltimore: Williams & Wilkins Co, 1980: 9–21.

14. Kara M, Peters W J, Douglas L G, Morris S F. An early surgical approach to burns in the elderly. *J Trauma* 1990; **30**(4): 430–2.

15. Goldstein S. The biology of aging. *N Engl J Med* 1977; **285:** 1120–9.

16. Cameron I L. Cell proliferation and renewal in aging mice. *J Gerontol* 1972; **27:** 162–9.

17. Long J M III. Burns in geriatric patients. In: Artz C P, Moncrief J A, Pruitt B A Jr, eds *Burns: A Team Approach.* Philadelphia: WB Saunders, 1979: 334–40.

18. Heimbach D M. Early burn excision and grafting. *Surg Clin North Am* 1987; **67:** 93–107.

19. Burdge J J, Katz B, Edwards R, Ruberg R. Surgical treatment of burns in elderly patients. *J Trauma* 1988; **28:** 214–17.

20. Deitch E A. A policy of early excision and grafting in elderly burn patients shortens the hospital stay and improves survival. *Burns* 1985; **12:** 109–14.

21. Oreskovich M R, Howard J S, Copass M K, Carrico C J. Geriatric trauma: injury patterns and outcome. *J Trauma* 1984; **24:** 565–72.

22. Kravitz M, Elliott S, Weissman M, Saffle J R, Warden G D. Thermal injury in the elderly: incidence and cause. *J Burn Care Rehabil* 1985; **6:** 487–9.

23. Larson C M, Saffle J R, Sullivan J. Lifestyle adjustments in elderly patients after burn injury. *J Burn Care Rehabil* 1992; **13**(1): 48–52.

24. Keys T C, Moresi J M, Deitch E A. Thermal injury in the elderly. The limited need for nursing home care. *J Burn Care Rehabil* 1989; **10**(5): 429–31.

25. Suter-Gut D, Metcalf A M, Donnelly M A, Smith I A. Post-discharge care planning and rehabilitation of the elderly surgical patient. *Clin Geriatr Med* 1990; **6**(3): 69–83.

CHAPTER THIRTY-FIVE

SURGICAL MANAGEMENT OF COMPLICATIONS OF BURN INJURY

DANIEL K. ROBIE AND DAVID N. HERNDON

INTRODUCTION

General surgical problems which are secondary to both a burn injury and a body's physiological response to burn injury can occur in burned patients. These problems can occur immediately coincident with a burn injury, or during a postburn course. One immediate problem involves traumatic injuries sustained from associated blunt or penetrating trauma. Additional problems include gastrointestinal ulceration, suppurative thrombophlebitis, acalculous cholecystitis, superior mesenteric artery (SMA) syndrome, enterocolitis, as well as infections and complications related to enteral feeding and surgical incisions. Upon initial examination, a concerted effort is needed on the part of an attending physician in order to insure that nonthermal injuries are not overlooked while the burns are treated. Other injuries could, in fact, be more immediately life threatening. Hypoperfusion, or burn shock, which results from excessive loss of fluid, also needs immediate attention in patients with large burn wounds. After initial treatment, many burned patients develop additional complications which are overlooked because symptoms are attributed directly to burn wounds. Ulcers can be prevented or treated if an attending physician is aware of their likelihood and presenting symptoms. Catheter-related infections frequently occur and must be diagnosed early if treatment is to be successful. Acaculous cholecystitis is a more rare complication, but its effects are often deadly. SMA syndrome is also rare and can be successfully managed if it is diagnosed; however, the presenting symptoms for this condition can be easily mistaken for other burn injury complications. Cutaneous burns can obscure the diagnosis of enterocolitis which frequently occurs in burned patients and often is fatal. Further complications can result from enteral feeding and surgical incisions which can lead to additional infections and trauma to an already injured body. Early detection of these conditions and complications is essential if treatment is to be effective. Thus, a surgeon must remain constantly vigilant in order to recognize causes other than burn wound sepsis and 'burn shock' for the clinical deterioration of a burned patient.

Three previously published reports show the significance of general surgical problems in burned patients[1–3] (**Table 35.1**). Counce and associates identify the cause of occult sepsis in ten patients to be from intra-abdominal sources (ischemic bowel, acute cholecystitis, abscess formation, and gastric perforation).[1] Marzek and associates report ten deaths among 45 burned patients resulting from general surgical problems.[2] Kirksey reports a large series of burned patients with general surgical problems of whom 210 (65%) suffered gastroduodenal ulceration or gastritis.[3] All three reports demonstrate that problems occur in older and more severely burned patients. Delay in diagnosis of surgical complications leads to a poor prognosis.

Recently, SBI–Galveston reported 15 general surgical problems occurring in 14 patients (**Table 35.1**). These patients required a total of 31 operations and exhibited a mortality rate of 50%. Specific problems encountered included: enterocolitis, gastrointestinal ulceration, septic thrombophlebitis, mesenteric ischemia, and small bowel obstruction. In addition, 18 patients underwent tracheostomy. There were six deaths with three attributable to sud-

Table 35.1 Reported series of nonthermal complications in burned patients

	No.	%*	Age(avg)	TBSAB(avg)	Comp(*n*)	Mort(%)
Kirksey (1968)[3]	322	45	–	–	322	18(–)
Counce (1988)[1]	26	0.02	35	43	32	15(58)†
Marzek (1991)[2]	23	7	52	36	45	10(44)†
SBI–Galveston (1994)	14	0.01	7	61	15	7(50)†

* Percent of total burned patients.
† Significant difference vs. all burns.

den decannulation at home. Clearly, these secondary and sometimes fatal complications in burn-injured patients deserve attention. This chapter reviews the often encountered general surgical problems in burned patients with respect to diagnosis, management, and prevention.

Blunt and Penetrating Trauma

Proper management of a multiply injured patient who has sustained burns follows well established guidelines. Knowing the mechanism of injury helps to predict the type of traumatic injury. Diagnostic procedures such as abdominal computed tomography scans and diagnostic peritoneal lavage are used as they would be with the nonburned patient. Unique to the burned patient are adjustments which are necessary to manage associated inhalation injury, 'burn shock', and electrical injuries.

The incidence of associated injuries in burned patients is approximately 5%;[4] however, some mechanisms of injury result in a very high incidence of associated injury. For example, 88% of burned patients injured in motorcycle accidents and 36% of burned patients in motor vehicle accidents have additional injuries other than burns[5] (**Table 35.2**). Musculoskeletal injuries are the most common (59%) and include vertebral fractures/dislocations and pelvic fractures.[5] Other organ systems injured include: cardiothoracic (26%), head (24%), abdomen (12%), and genitourinary (9%). Abdominal injuries often involve spleen, liver/pancreas, and kidney, with 58% of these requiring operative intervention. Fractures account for 82% of nonthermal injuries in burned patients according to another series.[6] Admitting physicians may be distracted by the overwhelming impression of a major burn and thus be far diverted from recognizing associated injuries. Delay in diagnosis of associated injuries occurs frequently and leads to an increase in morbidity and mortality.

Controversy exists concerning the optimal management of combined orthopedic and burn injuries. Ideally, fractures and dislocations are stabilized early while providing maximal access for burn wound care and allowing patient mobilization for postburn rehabilitation. This stabilization is best achieved by either internal or external fixation with the former being optimal. The role of both internal and external fixation is controversial due to the presumed risk of infection from adjacent or overlying burns. Also, fixation of orthopedic injuries must be performed early (within 24–48 hours) prior to burn wound colonization and, therefore, during the resuscitative phase of a postburn period and during relative patient instability.

Dislocations are managed with closed reduction when possible.[7] When open reduction is required through burned skin, the wound is closed to fascia only and drainage avoided. In an unstable patient, splinting or use of external fixators may be necessary. Fracture management follows standard techniques of closed reduction and casting. Access for wound care to overlying burns is provided by cast bivalving or traction/suspension systems. Open fractures underlying burned skin should be cleansed and reduction maintained preferably with skeletal suspension (with pins placed distant to the burn when possible). The traditional approach calls for internal fixation to be avoided due to the theoretical but unproven risk of infection, and fracture stabilization should be performed early (<24 hours postburn) with minimal hardware when necessary.[7]

More recently, an aggressive approach to orthopedic injuries in burned patients has been shown to be very successful.[4,8] Thirty-four fractures in 28 patients were managed with internal fixation. In follow-up, no clinically significant infections occurred, and only two fractures healed poorly. No metallic hardware subsequently required removal. Wound management was made noticeably easier and orthopedic morbidity was reduced. Other authors report similar success with early operative fixation of orthopedic injuries in burned patients.[6,9,10] No increased incidence of infection, poor fracture healing, or amputation has been noted. Notably, it is essential that internal fixation be performed early and a patient be stable enough to undergo anesthesia. The burn wound itself is best managed with early excision and grafting, including operative incisions through the burn. This process removes potential sources of bacterial contamination and infection at the surgical site.

Table 35.2 Association between number of organ systems injured and mortality

Systems injured	Patients	Age (years)	TBSA burned	Mortality %
One	29	28.3	35.7	17.2
Two	23	31.7	29.0	21.7
Three or more	13	26.8	28.1	36.4
Totals	65	29.2	31.8	23.1

Reproduced with permission from Purdue and Hunt.[4]

Pathophysiology

A burned patient is host to a vast array of pathophysiological alterations initiated by a burn injury. Burn wounds of sufficient size (>30% in the average size adult) initiate a generalized physiologic response which is not limited to burned areas alone. These pathophysiologic alterations include hypoperfusion (burn shock) which is due to massive fluid loss and vasoactive hormones, hypermetabolism which leads to profound catabolic state and malnutrition, and immunosuppression with a breakdown of normal barriers to bacterial invasion. These derangements alone and in combination lead to organ dysfunction and nonthermal complications of burn injury.

The effect of hypoperfusion in a massively burned patient is ischemic injury to vital organs. Gallbladder ischemia alone or along with bile stasis and systemic sepsis can lead to acalculous cholecystitis.[11] Gastrointestinal ischemia can result in mucosal ulceration (Curling's ulcer) and enterocolitis severe enough to cause intestinal perforation.[12] Poor renal and hepatic perfusion results in organ dysfunction and failure which leads to high mortality. Finally, decreased wound perfusion results in poor wound healing and increased incidence of wound infection. The effect of thermal injury on splanchnic blood flow has been extensively studied experimentally.[13–21] Splanchnic blood flow includes that to the stomach, intestine, spleen, pancreas, and liver. Massive burn injury results in diffuse capillary leak, hypovolemia, and release of vasoconstrictive hormones which cause a selective decrease in splanchnic blood flow (**Figure 35.1**).[22,23]

Redistribution of blood flow with decreased regional splanchnic perfusion has been shown to occur in the early postburn period.[13,16,18] The duration of splanchnic ischemia and the adequacy of fluid resuscitation may be critical in determining the extent of gastrointestinal injury. Cardiac output is maintained while blood flow to the gut is decreased by one-third. A selective reduction in blood flow to specific abdominal organs (liver, small intestine, kidney) and preservation of blood flow to others (stomach, duodenum, large intestine, spleen, pancreas) has been demonstrated.[13] A 40% flame-burned pig model, receiving adequate fluid resuscitation, showed an early reduction in superior mesenteric blood flow associated with intestinal mucosal hypoxia and acidosis and increased

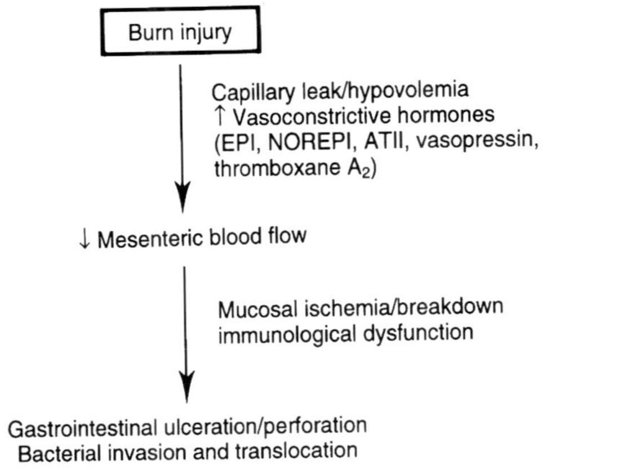

Fig. 35.1 Massive burn injury initiates events which can cause mesenteric ischemia. The diffuse capillary leak reduces intravascular volume with resultant hypoperfusion. A massive outpouring of vasoconstrictive hormones contributes to hypoperfusion and selective organ ischemia. The reduction in splanchnic circulation can cause mucosal ischemia, intestinal perforation, breakdown of immunological barriers, and bacterial translocation.

bacterial translocation.[14] Decreased small bowel blood flow in a nonresuscitated rat burn model could be reversed by administration of enalapril.[16] Sepsis and burn injury have additive effects on intestinal integrity despite intestinal blood flow.[17] There is evidence that intestinal blood flow may be improved by enteral feeding.[18] Further, in burned patients, large increases in thromboxane levels with no change in prostacyclin levels have been noted both in the acute stage (<3 days postburn) and in association with sepsis.[24] The unmatched increase in thromboxane levels could, in part, be responsible for diminished splanchnic perfusion in burned patients.

The hypermetabolic response to burn injury and alterations in immunological function can also cause nonthermal complications in burn-injured patients. The hypermetabolic response causes a profound catabolic state which can inhibit wound healing and immunological function. The increase in metabolic rate approaches twice the normal; this can result in excessive weight loss in the absence of adequate caloric intake.[25] This pathophysiological response includes activation of the hypothalmic–pituitary axis, sympathetic outflow, and the acute phase response.[26] The result includes fat and protein breakdown, and increased gluconeogenesis. Defective fibroblast function occurs with possible delayed wound healing. Leukocyte dysfunction and reduced cellular immunity cause immunological compromise. Various attempts at blunting the hypermetabolic response have been studied.[27–31] Maintaining a higher ambient temperature, administering systemic steroids, and adrenalectomy have failed in clinical and experimental trials.[25] Intravenous propranolol leads to increased protein catabolism despite decreasing myocardial workload.[27] Excess administration of glucose and insulin improves protein synthesis but increases metabolic rate.[25] Early enteral feeding blunts the response period.[28–30] Growth hormone, monoamine oxidase inhibitors, adrenalectomy, and prostaglandin synthetase inhibitors have all resulted in a decreased hypermetabolic response.[25,31]

The combined effects of splanchnic hypoperfusion and the hypermetabolic response to burn injury can lead to a breakdown of immunological barriers and, specifically, translocation of bacteria from the gut. Numerous studies have shown the association of burn injury and bacterial translocation.[32–36] Intervention aimed at preventing splanchnic perfusion and the hypermetabolic response to burn injury may prevent immunological dysfunction and the occurrence of many nonthermal complications of burn injury.

Curling's Ulcer

The changing incidence of gastroduodenal stress ulceration in burned patients reflects both improvement in the treatment of acutely burned patients and success of specific prophylactic measures. The incidence of gastroduodenal disease was previously reported as high as 86%, depending on the method of diagnosis (postmortem, gastrointestinal bleeding, routine endoscopic evaluation).[37,38] Since the introduction of early aggressive fluid resuscitation, antacid therapy, and early enteral feeding, the incidence of clinically significant gastroduodenal disease has fallen below 2%.[37,39] An extensive review of stress ulcers in burned patients shows that they occur more frequently in those with larger burns and in the presence of sepsis.[37] While gastric ulcers are usually multifocal, and duodenal ulcers are usually solitary, 15% of these patients have both gastric and duodenal ulcerations. Patients present predominantly with hemorrhage which is often massive. Ulcer perforation occurs in 12% of the patients, but only one-third of these will experience pain.

The natural history of acute gastroduodenal disease in burned patients has been reported in a classic series.[38] Admitted patients were serially examined with an endoscope during their early postburn course. Most patients with large burns had mucosal changes within 72 hours of a burn injury. Frank ulceration developed in the stomach in 22% of the cases and in the duodenum in 28% of the patients. Progression of the disease occurred in half of those afflicted, predominantly in association with subsequent septic episodes and hypoxemia. Multiple factors are implicated as potentially causative of stress ulcers in burned patients.[37] These include: mucosal ischemia, increased acid production, increased acid backdiffusion, energy depletion, duodenogastric reflux of bile, and direct mucosal injury due to the presence of intraluminal tubes. The state of mucosal perfusion is controversial and is dependent on a complex interplay of local and systemic factors; however, even in the absence of any measurable decrease in gastric blood flow, perfusion may be inadequate to meet the energy demands for maintaining the mucosal acid barrier.

Preventing stress ulcers requires eliminating or minimizing factors which are important in mucosal injury. Aggressive fluid resuscitation aids in minimizing the reduction in mucosal blood flow. Also important is the administration of agents to minimize gastric acid production. Excellent prospective studies have shown the efficacy of either H_2 blockers or antacids in decreasing the incidence of stress ulceration.[40,41] The ease of administering cimetidine and the low incidence of side effects favors the selection of this agent except in selected patients (with hepatic or renal failure, concomitant anticoagulant use, or neutropenia).[37] Notably, the most important step after resuscitation may be early administration of enteral feedings. This provides both acid buffering and nutrition. In 4107 patients treated at the SBI–Galveston burn center since 1964, only four patients have undergone ulcer surgery. This relatively low incidence is considered supportive of a policy of aggressive early enteral feeding in all burned patients.

Proper treatment of established stress ulcers includes those measures currently in use for prevention. More aggressive medical therapy may include combined treatments involving: intravenous or intra-arterial vasopressin, intravenous somatostatin, and/or interventional endoscopy. The surgical option should be utilized early in order to prevent the profound effects of bleeding and hypotension on a maximally stressed burned patient. Specific surgical indications include ongoing uncontrolled blood loss, massive bleeding (>2.5 liters in adult, >60% blood volume in child), and gastroduodenal perforation. Pruitt recommends definitive surgery with vagotomy and antrectomy as the operation of choice.[37] Death occurs in approximately half of patients who undergo surgical correction for ulcers due to the severity of their burn injuries.

Although Curling's ulcers are far less frequent today, they remain a potential hazard to all burned patients. The low incidence of stress ulceration is due to successful aggressive burn injury management and the use of specific prevention measures. Surgical therapy is required in a small number of patients with resective procedures favored.

SUPPURATIVE THROMBOPHLEBITIS

The significance of suppurative thrombophlebitis in burned patients was first reported by Pruitt and associates.[42] In 1980, their updated report included 193 patients treated over an 18-year period. This sample represented 4% of all burns seen at the United States Army Institute for Surgical Research (USAISR).[43] Other centers have, since then, also reported experience with suppurative thrombophlebitis in burned patients.[2] Cases have predominantly been catheter-related and involved peripheral veins for which the management is well described. More recently, experience with catheter-related septic central venous thrombosis has been reported along with recommendations for its management.[44,45] The incidence of catheter-related infections is best measured in patient-days of catheter use (no. of infective episodes/1000 patient-days of catheter use).[46] Peripheral catheter infections occur at an average rate of 3.35. Central venous catheter infections occur at an average rate of 1.37. Not all of these infections occur in association with venous thrombosis. Specific risk factors for developing suppurative thrombophlebitis include both burn injury and prolonged intravenous catheterization (**Table 35.3**).[47]

The presentation of suppurative thrombophlebitis is often occult with approximately 20% of patients showing no local clinical signs (**Table 35.4**).[47] In burned patients, occult suppurative thrombophlebitis is most frequent; only 36% of patients reported by Pruitt exhibited local signs.[43] Burned patients most frequently display a positive culture and clinical sepsis having no obvious source. Clinical sepsis is accompanied by hyperpyrexia, hypothermia, change in mental status, hyperglycemia, and hypotension. Diagnosis in these cases requires sequential exploration of all previous catheter sites. The absence of pus at the site or within the vein does not rule out suppurative thrombophlebitis.[43,47] Proper exploration of a vein requires surgical cut-down and expression of vein contents. If pus or clot is found, the vein is excised to a normal appearing vein (usually at the first uninvolved tributary). Complete

Table 35.3 Factors that increase risk of septic thrombophlebitis

Prolonged catheterization (greater than 72 hours)
Concentrated intravenous solutions (K^+, antibiotics)
Venous cut-downs
Plastic catheters
Lower extremity access
Poor sterile technique
Emergency catheterization
Frequent intravenous line manipulation
Burns

Reproduced with permission from Golueke and Zinner.[47]

Table 35.4 Local clinical signs of septic phlebitis

Clinical sign	Percentage of patients
Erythema	50.9
Edema	49.0
Local tenderness	45.1
Palpable cord	35.3
Purulent drainage	16.6
Asymptomatic	20.4

Reproduced with permission from Golueke and Zinner.[47]

excision is critical as demonstrated in 12 patients inadequately excised in the series by Pruitt.[43] A wound may be closed to the site of percutaneous entry with no reported increased incidence of wound infection.[47] If exploration is negative at one site, then sequential exploration of other sites is absolutely necessary until the source of infection is identified. Besides surgical excision, treatment for suppurative thrombophlebitis includes systemic antibiotics. The most commonly found organisms recovered from infected veins in burned patients reflect those cultured from a burn wound.[43] In nonburned patients, *Staphlococcus*, *Klebsiella*, and *Candida* are cultured in descending order of frequency.[47] Antibiotics are chosen based on sensitivities; the duration of treatment ranges from 3 to 5 days for common bacterial pathogens or up to weeks for *Candida* sepsis.

Catheter-related septic central venous thrombosis has increasingly been recognized in the burn population as paralleling the increased use of central venous catheters (**Figure 35.2**).[43] Two recent reports emphasize the success of nonoperative therapy.[44,45] Kaufman and associates reported five patients diagnosed with septic evidence

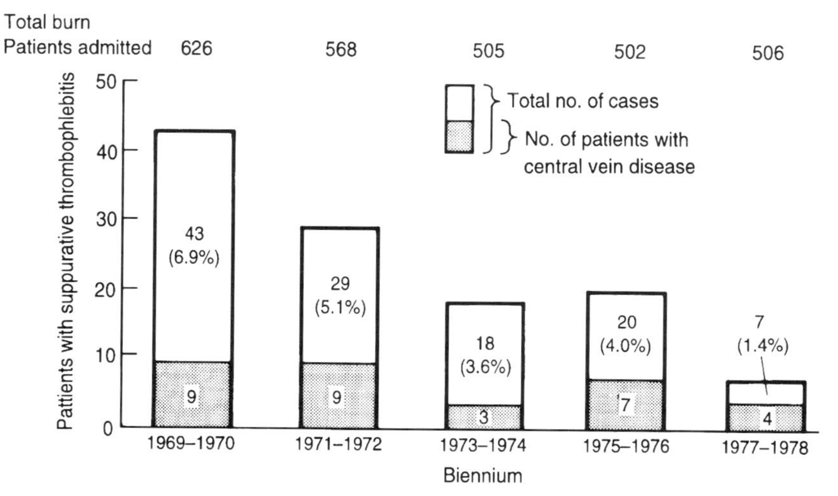

Fig. 35.2 Occurrence of suppurative thrombophlebitis in toto and in central veins by binnium. Reproduced with permission from Pruitt et al.[41]

of thrombosis, catheter infection diagnosed by positive tip and blood culture, and ongoing bacteremia after catheter removal. All of these patients had local evidence of disease manifested by ipsilateral swelling. Treatment encompassed systemic antibiotics and full heparinization (partial thromboplastin time twice normal). No surgical intervention was required in these cases; however, surgical therapy may be warranted if medical therapy fails. In the presence of a mediastinal phlegmon as evidenced on computed tomography, drainage is necessary with only a rare need for central venous excision. Three burned patients with septic central venous thrombosis, reported by Pruitt, survived with nonoperative therapy.[43] The prevention of catheter-related suppurative thrombophlebitis requires avoidance of specific risk factors (see **Table 35.3**). When infection occurs without an identifiable source, a sequential exploration of all catheter sites should be performed early in order to avoid the potential catastrophe of death from suppurative thrombophlebitis.

Acalculous Cholecystitis

Acalculous cholecystitis is a rare complication of burn injury. Multiple etiologies have been proposed for the condition, including bile stasis, ischemia, and sepsis. Diagnosis depends on recognizing a combination of signs and symptoms which are often attributed to other problems in a burned patient. Mortality is high in such cases, and the treatment method chosen depends on a patient's overall stability.

Forty cases of acute acalculous cholecystitis have been reported since 1960.[11,48–52] Its occurrence is estimated at 0.4–0.5% in burned patients.[52] The acalculous form of cholecystitis predominates in postburned cases as it does in post-traumatic and postoperative patients. Patient data from 17 cases have been reported since 1981 (**Table 35.5**).[11,48–52] The mean TBSAB was 51%. The male to female ratio was 5:1. Ages ranged from 3 to 65 with an average of 30 years. Disease onset occurred between 17 and 30 days postburn. Interestingly, two cases immediately followed the initiation of enteral feeds after long-term parenteral nutrition. Two other cases occurred in patients exclusively fed enterally. Clinical sepsis and positive blood cultures were common.

Proposed etiologies for acalculous cholecystitis include bile stasis, acute decrease in perfusion, and systemic sepsis.[48–50] All these conditions are common in a severely burned patient. The effect is local ischemia of the gallbladder wall leading to inflammation, gangrene, and perforation in unrecognized cases. The common histological finding consists of intense injury to blood vesels within the muscularis and serosa. Lack of enteral feeding and resultant decreased secretion of cholecystokinin, along with narcotic use, leads to bile stasis within the gallbladder. The composition of the bile changes locally, and, concurrently, the load of bile may increase due to multiple blood transfusions. The effect is increased intraluminal pressure within the gallbladder and wall ischemia. The state of hypoperfusion present in acutely burned patients due to third space fluid loss and circulating vasoactive substances can lead to gallbladder ischemia and injury. Finally, sepsis and endotoxemia can cause decreased perfusion and bacterial invasion of the gallbladder wall.

Acute acalculous cholecystitis commonly presents with fever, right upper quadrant pain and tenderness, leukocytosis, and elevated liver function tests. These findings are also common in any severely burned patient, especially when the overlying abdominal wall is burned. Therefore, a high degree of suspicion is necessary in order to avoid a delay in diagnosis. The percentage of gangrenous changes (33–100%) and rate of gallbladder perforation (12%) noted in recent burn cases of acalculous cholecystitis underlies the continuing difficulty of diagnosis. Ultrasound findings include thickened gallbladder wall, pericholecystic fluid, and intraluminal sludge. A positive HIDA scan confirms the diagnosis but is often unavailable for severely ill patients. Once diagnosed, the best choice of treatment for acalculous cholecystitis is cholecystectomy in an otherwise stable patient.

Superior Mesenteric Artery Syndrome

An acute form of superior mesenteric artery syndrome may be precipitated by rapid and substantial weight loss and is a rare complication of major trauma and burns. Symptoms include: bilious emesis, abdominal distension and pain, and intolerance to tube or oral feeds. The diagnosis is established by findings on upper gastrointestinal series of x-rays. Symptoms include a dilated duodenum and extrinsic compression of the third part of the duodenum. The management is primarily medical via improved nutrition and weight gain. Surgical procedures previously performed on patients with superior mesenteric artery syndrome include: gastrojejunostomy, duodenoduodenostomy, duodenojejunostomy, and takedown of the ligament of Treitz.[53–55]

Lescher reported a series of 37 patients treated for SMA syndrome at the United States Army Institute of Surgical Research.[56] Eighteen patients were successfully medically managed, mainly with intravenous nutrition and nasogastric decompression. Operative intervention was necessary in 30%, either for failed medical therapy or perforated ulcer. The operation of choice was a side-to-side duodenojejunostomy. There were three postoperative deaths and eight deaths following medical therapy alone for an overall 27% mortality rate. They recommended intravenous nutri-

Table 35.5 Published series of acute acalculous cholecystits in burn patients

	No.	Sex (m:f)	Age (avg)	Sepsis	G/P*	Rx(E/O/PM)†	Outcome (S/D)‡
Glenn (1981)[49]	3	2:1	42	3	0/0	1/0/2	0/3
Gately (1983)[52]	1	1:0	19	–	–	1/0/0	1/0
McDermott (1985)[48]	4	4:0	29	2	2/1	2/3/0	4/0
Ross (1987)[50]	3	2:1	39	2	2/0	2/0/1	3/0
Slater (1989)[11]	5	–	26	4	5/0	4/1/0	4/1
Polacek (1991)[51]	1	1:0	3	–	0/1	0/0/1	0/1
Total	17	10:2	30	11	9/2	10/3/4	12/5

* G, gangrenous; P, perforation; † E, cholecystectomy; O, cholecystostomy; PM, postmortem diagnosis; ‡ S, survival; D, death.

tion and nasogastric decompression as the treatment of choice for superior mesenteric artery syndrome in burned patients. Today, placement of a jejunal tube beyond the point of obstruction is the preferred treatment.

The experience with superior mesenteric artery syndrome in children at both SBI–Cincinnati and SBI–Galveston has shown uniform success with medical management alone and no mortality. MacMillan reported a series of 11 patients treated over a 15-year period.[57] The average burn size for these patients was 64% and their weight loss ranged from 10 to 30%. Only one case occurred during the second 5 years of their review. This was attributed to more aggressive enteral nutritional support limiting weight loss to under 5% of preburn weight. They recommended bowel rest with nasogastric decompression and intravenous nutrition for a period of 3–4 weeks in order to relieve the obstruction. At SBI–Galveston, only one patient received intravenous nutrition while the other six were managed with nasojejunal feeds and positioning. Nasojejunal tubes were easily placed under fluoroscopic guidance. Positional therapy required placement in either a left-side down or prone position for feeding. The overall incidence of superior mesenteric syndrome was low (0.03%), attributed to a policy of aggressive early enteral feeding of all burned children.

Comparing the experience at three institutions, the severity of the burns and amounts of weight loss were similar (**Figure 35.3**). Operative intervention was not necessary in any patients in the two Shriner series and no mortality occurred. The difference is likely not fully explained by the varied populations treated. In addition to a lower incidence of superior mesenteric artery syndrome, 86% of the patients in the SBI–Galveston series avoided potential complications of central intravenous nutrition.

Superior mesenteric artery syndrome occurs due to extrinsic compression of the duodenum by the superior mesenteric vascular pedicle. Loss of retroperitoneal fat through malnutrition and weight loss, laxity of abdominal wall muscles, and a recombinant position occurs in burned patients and contributes to the severity of this compression. A policy of aggressive early enteral feeding as well as ongoing physical rehabilitation results in a very low incidence of superior mesenteric artery syndrome. Almost all patients can be managed medically through positioning and nasojejunal feeding. The potential complications of central venous hyperalimentation or surgical intervention are thereby avoided, and the benefits of enteral feeding are realized.

Enterocolitis

A burned patient experiences many pathophysiological alterations caused by a burn injury. Splanchnic hypoperfusion may occur as a result of hypovolemia and circulating vasoactive mediators. The degree and extent of resultant intestinal injury is related to the severity and duration of ischemia. Complications of intestinal

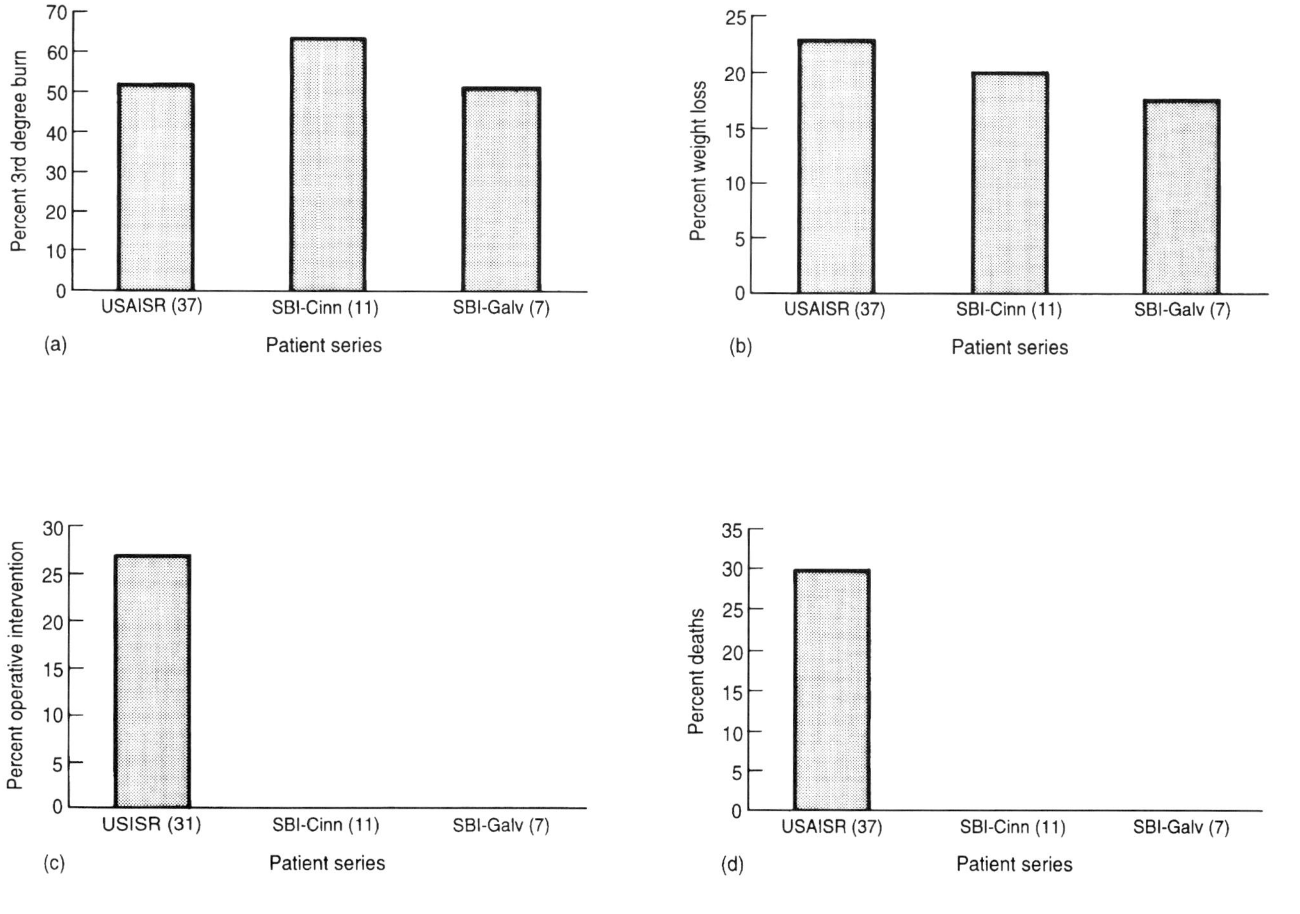

Fig. 35.3 Comparison of experience with superior mesenteric artery (SMA) syndrome at three burn centers: (a) average percent burn; (b) average percent weight loss; (c) percent undergoing operation for SMA syndrome; (d) percent mortality.

injury may include both intestinal necrosis with perforation as well as bacterial invasion and translocation. An intra-abdominal catastrophe may go unrecognized due to the presence of a cutaneous burn. Also, systemic sepsis may be attributed to complications of a burn wound and not bacterial translocation originating from a compromised bowel. A high index of suspicion and an aggressive surgical approach must be maintained in order to successfully treat this complication.

Enterocolitis can occur due to causes other than ischemia (infectious, etc.); so a more descriptive term for changes related to decreased mesenteric perfusion might be ischemic intestinal complications. Desai and associates reported a series of both clinically recognized ischemic intestinal complications in burned patients (incidence 1%) and those identified at autopsy (incidence 55%).[12] Seven children and nine adults underwent initial laparotomy for suspected necrotic intestine. Fourteen additional laparotomies were performed in the children with three survivors. One patient underwent seven laparotomies after initial presentation with enterocolitis and survived. Another patient, exhibiting symptoms of sepsis and abdominal distension, underwent five laparotomies for continued clinical deterioration and subsequently died. The nine adult patients underwent 11 additional laparotomies with two survivors. Additional resection of necrotic bowels was required at each reoperation. All the children and 89% of the adults were septic and had positive blood cultures during their postburn courses. Sixty-one percent of autopsies performed on children who had succumbed to burn injury showed ischemic intestinal changes. Of these, 66% had been septic at the time of death. At autopsy, 53% of adults had ischemic intestinal findings and 86% had been septic at the time of death. These results show both the high mortality associated with intestinal ischemic complications in burned patients as well as the high incidence of sepsis in patients with compromised intestines. Other series report additional experience with ischemic intestinal complications in burned patients.[2,3]

The clinical approach to necrotizing enterocolitis in premature infants may provide insight into the optimal approaches for enterocolitis in burned patients.[58] Mesenteric hypoperfusion is considered the underlying mechanism of injury initiated by stressors (enteral feeding, sepsis, hypovolemia). Infants who exhibit abdominal distension, tenderness, and signs of sepsis may be suspected. Diagnosis follows examination and recognition of pneumatosis intestinalis on an abdominal radiograph. Treatment includes broad spectrum antibiotics, bowel rest, and operative intervention for perforation or clinical deterioration despite maximal medical therapy. A similar approach, but with earlier surgical intervention, may be most appropriate in a burned patient.

Although the incidence of clinically recognized intestinal ischemic complications is low (1–3%), early recognition and intervention requires a high level of suspicion. Signs and symptoms may be falsely attributed to a burn wound and delay abdominal exploration. An aggressive approach to reexploration, either at a predetermined second look or when clinically indicated, is also essential, given the high likelihood of finding additional compromised bowel.

Sepsis, electrolyte imbalance, narcotic use, and renal failure are common conditions in a burned patient and are associated with complications such as pseudo-obstruction of the colon (Ogilvie's syndrome).[59] Diagnosis is established by a plain abdominal radiograph which shows massive colonic distension. Signs and symptoms are usually minimal or attributable to the burns. A proposed treatment algorithm emphasizes the amount of cecal distension in deciding optimal therapy. Distension which is less than 10 cm is treated conservatively. Colonoscopy is performed for persistent distension lasting more than 3 days or having a size greater than 10 cm. Only rarely is operative intervention necessary with the creation of a cecostomy or occasionally with resection accompanied by diversion.

Finally, acute pancreatitis may affect a burned patient.[3] The etiology is usually idiopathic but may be attributable to ischemia, sepsis, and medication use. The diagnosis may be difficult and masked by burn injuries. Treatment is supportive and includes NPO, fluid resuscitation, and intravenous nutrition. Close surveillance is necessary in order to identify early complications such as pseudocyst formation, pancreatic necrosis, and pancreatic abscess. Operative intervention is rarely indicated unless complications occur.

Enteral Feeding

The excessive caloric intake required in a burned patient, coupled with associated appetite suppression, necessitates alternative means of delivering calories. The superiority of enteral nutrition over the intravenous route has been well established to specifically avoid complications of central venous lines and concomitant intestinal atrophy and bacterial overgrowth. The optimal method and type of enteral formula, however, remains controversial. Nasogastric, nasojejunal, gastrostomy, and jejunostomy tubes all deliver enteral nutrition but have unique advantages and disadvantages. Selecting the incorrect enteral formula can cause diarrhea and malabsorption which complicate wound healing and local wound care. The optimal choice would include a method of delivery which impacts least on patient care and a formula which rapidly achieves a positive nitrogen balance without associated diarrhea.

A clear advantage of nasogastric tubes is the avoidance of an abdominal operation and associated complications. Nasogastric tubes are soft, thin, and pliable; they avoid the gastric, pulmonary, and nasal complications of large decompression nasogastric tubes. These tubes are difficult to maintain, however, and can inadvertently be placed or migrate into the pulmonary tree. Gastrostomy tubes are maintained for long periods and require minimal experience to manage (**Table 35.6**).[60] Alternate methods of placement are now available which avoid large abdominal incisions. The percutaneous endoscopic technique has proven to be safe and feasible in large series.[61] When compared with traditional Stamm gastrostomies, it has significantly fewer major and overall complications (3% and 9%, n=1758 vs. 7% and 15%, n=1293).[62] Importantly, Hollands and associates significantly reduced the occurrence of peristomal (exit-site) wound infections with single-dose systemic antibiotic prophylaxis.[63] It is presently recommended also to coat the tube with antibiotic ointment prior to transesophageal placement. Jejunostomy tubes offer the theoretical advantage of avoiding gastroesophageal reflux often associated with gastric feeds.[60,64] This may be especially important in a burned patient because of gastric atony during the early postburn course (49–72 hours). Nasojejunal feeding tubes have proven useful in burned patients and can accurately be placed with the aid of fluoroscopy. Jejunal feeding tubes can also be placed either via a gastrostomy (open or percutaneous) or by open creation of a jejunostomy. This, again, requires the disadvantage of an operative incision. Laparoscopic placement of gastrostomy and jejunostomy tubes has proven technically feasible. The advantage over the percutaneous technique is not yet apparent and experience in burned patients is lacking. Although the ideal enteral feeding method is controversial, certain recommendations are appropriate. Nasojejunal tubes have proven efficacy, minimize reflux, and are best for the short-term requirements often present in a burned patient. When chronic delivery of feeds is necessary (neurologically impaired patients), percutaneous insertion techniques offer a great advantage over open techniques.

Table 35.6 Gastrostomy and nasogastric tubes

Category	Advantages	Disadvantages
Nasogastric tubes		
Feeding	Readily available Insertion – minimal skill Inexpensive	Unintentional removal Reinsertion may be difficult Social stigma – visibility Requires fixation Caliber may restrict diets Migration
Decompression	Readily available Insertion – minimal skill Inexpensive	Requires large stiff tubes Uncomfortable Nasal, pharyngeal, esophageal, gastric irritation Occlude frequently Increase pulmonary complications
Gastrostomy		
Decompression	Comfort Less fluid and electrolyte loss Fewer respiratory complications	Require surgery or PEG Increased cost Potential complications Decompression may be inadequate May leave permanent fistula

Reproduced with permission from Gauderer and Stellano.[60]

The occurrence of diarrhea in enterally fed patients has been extensively reviewed by Gottschlich and associates.[65] They prospectively followed the course of 50 patients enterally fed postburn. Enteral formulas were chosen at the discretion of an attending physician or nutritional specialist. One formula available was a modular tube feeding recipe specifically prepared for burned patients. It was composed of 85% carbohydrate (nonlactose), 15% fat (50% fish oil, 50% safflower oil), provided 1 kcal/ml, and had a osmolality of 549 mosmol/kg H_2O. Of the patients studied, 50% received this formula. The incidence of diarrhea (defined by >4 bowel movements per day, or large (>200 gms) liquid stools) was 32%. All stool cultures were negative, including those for *Clostridium difficile* toxin. Significant variables for the increased occurrence of diarrhea were age (older patients), percent of third degree burn (average 40%), treatment with antibiotics, high fat intake (>25 g), inadequate vitamin A intake (<10 000 IU), late initiation of tube feedings (>48 hours postburn), and use of a formula other than the modular tube feeding recipe. Neither osmolality of the formula nor low serum albumin correlated with the occurrence of diarrhea. Given these findings, Gottschlich and associates recommend early initiation of enteral feeding, specifically formulated to avoid diarrhea. The common practice of diluting feeds should be avoided to maximize caloric value.

The Surgical Incision

Bacterial contamination of a burn wound, stress response to injury, altered host defenses with immunosuppression, malnutrition, and local factors delay and complicate healing of surgical incisions in burned patients. Wound complications are frequent and include infection, dehiscence, and fistula formation. The type of incision, technique of fascial closure, and management of an overlying burn may have an impact on the incidence of wound complications.

Goodwin reported a series of 149 intra-abdominal operations in 103 burned patients.[66] The mean TBSA burned was 43% and the overall mortality was 63%. The most common operative indications were for complications of Curling's ulcer and placement of feeding tubes. Wound dehiscence occurred in 32% of these patients, most commonly on the sixth postburn day. The rate of dehiscence was not attributable to the presence of burned abdominal skin, the number of prior abdominal operations, or the presence of perforated viscus. Paramedian incisions dehisced more frequently than midline or transverse incisions. Properly placed retention sutures resulted in fewer dehiscences when compared with wounds closed with no retention sutures (**Table 35.7**). Many incisions were closed by mass closure with retention sutures only. They conclude that the ideal wound is midline or transverse and is closed with mass retention sutures alone (wire recommended) placed 1.5–4 cm from the wound edge and spaced 1–1.5 cm apart, and remaining in place for a minimum of 4 weeks.

The experience at SBI–Galveston with 29 abdominal operations in 13 burned children has been reviewed. Initial operative indications were for enterocolitis, gastrointestinal ulcer/perforation, and one each for obstruction, possible appendicitis, pneumoperitoneum, and open gastrostomy. There were three wound dehiscences and one enterocutaneous fistula of the initial 13 operations (31%). Four patients died following the first operation (31%). The overall mortality was 54% and the average TBSA burned was 58%. Wound complications occurred despite the type of incision or technique of wound closure (wire mass closure, continuous prolene, Vicryl mesh) with or without primary skin closure.

Although an optimal technique for wound closure has not been defined, retention sutures or mass closure techniques should be utilized as described above. The skin may be closed if unburned, but it should be excised and covered with allograft or autograft if burned.

Table 35.7 Effect of retention sutures on incidence of dehiscence

Closure	No. of closures	No. of dehiscences	(%)
With retention sutures	91	18	(20)
Without retention sutures	35	15	(43)

Reproduced with permission from Goodwin *et al.*[66]

SUMMARY

Surgical problems which are secondary to burn injury can cause devastating physiological responses while remaining unidentified. Attending physicians must be on the alert for nonburn injuries when presented with a burned patient. Fractures and dislocations should be handled within 24–48 hours of injury. Further, infections which result from burns as well as other sources must be checked. Ulcers and other complications must be prevented when possible and detected and treated when present. Finally, medical professionals must be constantly on the alert for problems related to intravenous catheters and tube feedings, as related infections and complications can be fatal.

REFERENCES

1. Counce J S, Cone J B, McAlister L, Wallace B, Caldwell F T. Surgical complications of thermal injury. *Am J Surg* 1988; **156:** 556–7.

2. Marzek P A, Miller F B, Cryer H M, Polk H C. Nonthermal surgical complications in burn patients. *South Med J* 1991; **84:** 689–91.

3. Kirksey T D, Moncrief J A, Pruitt B A, O'Neill J A. Gastrointestinal complications in burns. *Am J Surg* 1968; **116:** 627–33.

4. Purdue G F, Hunt J L. Multiple trauma and the burn patient. *Am J Surg* 1989; **158:** 536–9.

5. Purdue G F, Hunt J L, Layton T R, Copeland C E, delMundo A G, Baxter C R. Burns in motor vehicle accidents. *J Trauma* 1985; **25:** 217–19.

6. Wong L. Grande C M, Munster A M. Burns and associated nonthermal trauma: an analysis of management, outcome, and relation to the injury severity score. *J Burn Care Rehabil* 1989; **10:** 512–16.

7. Kaplan J Z, Pruitt B A. Burns and fractures. In: Hupperstad, R B, ed. *Fracture Treatment and Healing*. Philadelphia: W B Saunders, 1979.

8. Dossett A B, Hunt J L, Purdue G F, Schlegel J D. Early orthopedic intervention in burn patients with major fractures. *J Trauma* 1991; **31:** 888–93.

9. Saffle J R, Achnelby A, Hofmann O, Warden G D. The management of fractures in thermally injured patients. *J Trauma* 1983; **23:** 902–10.

10. Curtis M J, Clarke J A. Skeletal injury in thermal trauma: a review of management. *Br J Accid Surg* 1989; **20:** 333–6.

11. Slater H, Goldfarb I W. Acute septic cholecystitis in patients with burn injuries. *J Burn Care Rehabil* 1989; **10:** 445–7.

12. Desai M H, Herndon D N, Rutan R L. Abston S, Linares H A. Ischemic intestinal complications in patients with burns. *Surg. Gynecol Obstet* 1991; **172:** 257–61.

13. Asch M J, Meseral P M, Mason A D, Pruitt B A. Regional blood flow in the burned unanesthetized dog. *Surg Forum* 1971; **22:** 55–6.

14. Tokyay R, Ziegler S T, Traber D L, *et al.* Postburn gastrointestinal vasoconstriction increases bacterial and endotoxin translocation. *J Appl Physiol* 1993; **74:** 1521–7.

15. Kiviluoto T, Gronbech J E, Kivilaakso E, *et al.* Acute gastric mucosal lesions, haemodynamic and microcirculatory changes in the thermally injured rat. *Burns* 1989; **15:** 365–70.

16. Jones W G, Minei J P, Barber A E, Fahey T J, Shires G T III, Shires G T. Splanchnic vasoconstiction and bacterial translocation after thermal injury. *Am J Physiol* 1991; **261:** H1190–H1196.

17. Jones W G, Minei J P, Barber A E, *et al.* Additive effects of thermal injury and infection on the small bowel. *Surgery* 1990; **108:** 63–70.

18. Inoue S, Lukes S, Alexander J W, Trocki O, Silberstein E B. Increased gut blood flow with early enteral feeding in burned guinea pigs. *J Burn Care Rehabil* 1989; **10:** 300–8.

19. Cartger E A, Tompkins R G, Burke J F. Hepatic and intestinal blood flow following thermal injury. *J Burn Care Rehabil* 1988; **9:** 347–50.

20. Carter E A, Udall J N, Kirkham S E, Walker W A. Thermal injury and gastrointestinal function I. Small intestinal nutrient absorption and DNA synthesis. *J Burn Care Rehabil* 1986; **7:** 469–74.

21. Bohlen H G. Tissue Oxygenation and Splanchnic Blood Flow. In: Shepard A P & Granger D N (eds). *Physiology of the Intestinal Circulation* 1948; pp 143–51.

22. Banks R O, Gallavan R H, Zinner M J, *et al.* Vasoactive agents in control of the mesenteric circulation. *Fedn Proc* 1985; **44:** 2743–9.

23. Hilton J G, Marullo D S. Trauma induced increases in plasma vasopressin and angiotensin II. *Life Sci* 1987; **41:** 2195–200.

24. Herndon D N, Abston S, Stein M D. Increased Thromboxane B2 Levels in the Plasma of Burned and Septic Burned Patients. *Surg. Gynecol & Obstet* 1984; **159:** 210–13.

25. Herndon D N, Curreri P W, Abston S, Rutan T C, Barrow R E. Treatment of burns. *Curr Prob Surg* 1987; **6:** 349–57.

26. Kupper T S, Deitch E A, Baker C C, Wong W. The human burn wound as a primary source of interleukin-1 activity. *Surgery* 1986; **100:** 409–41.

27. Herndon D N, Barrow R E, Rutan T C, *et al.* Effect of propranolol administration on haemodynamic and metabolic responses of burned pediatric patients. *Ann Surg* 1988; **208:** 484–92.

28. McArdle A H, Palmason C, Brown R A, Brown H C, Williams H B. Early enteral feeding of patients with major burns: prevention of catabolism. *Ann Plastic Surg* 1984; **13**.

29. Mochizuki H, Trocki O, Dominioni L, Brackett K A, Joffe S N, Alexander J W. Mechanism of prevention of postburn hypermetabolism and catabolism by early enteral feeding. *Ann Surg* 1984; **200:** 297–310.

30. Sologub V K, Zeats T L, Tarasov A V, Mordkovitch M R, Yashin A Y. Enteral hyperalimentation of burned patients: the possibility of correcting metabolic disorders by the early administration of prolonged high calorie evenly distributed tube feeds. *Burns* 1992; **18:** 245–9.

31. Fleming Y D, Rutan R L, Jahoor F, Barrow R E, Wolfe R R, Herndon D N. Effect of recombinant human growth hormone on catabolic hormones and free fatty acids following thermal injury. *J Trauma* 1992; **32:** 698–703.

32. Jones W G, Minei J P, Barber A E, *et al.* Bacterial translocation and intestinal atrophy after thermal injury and burn wound sepsis. *Ann Surg* 1990; **211:** 399–405.

33. Carter E A, Tompkins R G, Schiffrin E, Burke J F. Cutaneous thermal injury alters macromolecular permeability of rat small intestine. *Surgery* 1990; **107:** 335–41.

34. Levoyer T, Cioffi W G, Pratt L, *et al.* Alterations in intestinal permeability after thermal injury. *Arch Surg* 1992; **127:** 26–30.

35. Deitch E A, Winterton J, Berg R. Thermal injury promotes bacterial translocation from the gastrointestinal tract in mice with impaired T-cell mediated immunity. *Arch Surg* 1986; **121:** 97–101.

36. Alexander J W, Gianotti L, Pyles T, Carey M A, Babcock G F. Distribution and survival of *Escherichia coli* translocation from the intestine after thermal injury. *Ann Surg* 1990: 558.

37. Pruitt B A, Goodwin C W. Stress ulcer disease in the burned patient. *World J Surg* 1981; **5:** 209–22.

38. Czaja A J, McAlhany J C, Pruitt B A. Acute gastroduodenal disease after thermal injury. *N Engl J Med* 1974; **18:** 925–9.

39. Yao-Liang L, Ke-Jian Y. Clinical characteristics and operative treatment of postburn stress ulcers. *Burns* 1983; **10:** 30–3.

40. McAlhany J C, Czaja A J, Pruitt B A. Antacid control of complications from acute gastroduodenal disease after burns. *J Trauma* 1976; **16:** 645–

41. McElwee H P, Sirinek K R, Levine B A. Cimetidine affords protection equal to antacids in prevention of stress ulceration following thermal injury. *Surgery* 1979; **86:** 620.

42. Pruitt B A, Stein J M, Foley F D, Moncrief J A, O'Neill J A. Intravenous therapy in burn patients. *Arch Surg* 1970; **100:** 399–404.

43. Pruitt B A, McManus W F, Kin S H, Treat R C. Diagnosis and treatment of cannula-related intravenous sepsis in burn patients. *Ann Surg* 1980; **191:** 546–54.

44. Kaufman J, Demas C, Stark K, Flancbaum L. Catheter-related septic central venous thrombosis – current therapeutic options. *West J Med* 1986; **145:** 200–3.

45. Topiel M S, Bryan R T, Kessler C G, Simon G L. Case report: treatment of silastic catheter-induced central vein septic thrombophlebitis. *Am J Med Sci* 1986; **291:** 425–8.

46. Clarke D E, Raffin T A. Infectious Complications of Indwelling Long-Term Central Venous Catheters. *Chest* 1990; **97:** 966–72.

47. Golueke P J, Zinner M J. Management of septic thrombophlebitis. In: Ernst C B, Stanley J C, eds. *Current Therapy in Vascular Surgery*. Philadelphia: B C Decker, Inc, 1991: 1014–19.

48. McDermott M W, Scudamore C H, Boileau L O, Snelling C F T,

Kramer T A. Acalculous-cholecystitis: its role as a complication of major burn injury. *Can J Surg* 1985; **28:** 529–33.

49. Glenn F, Becker C G. Acute acalculous cholecystitis. *Ann Surg* 1981; **195:** 131–6.

50. Ross D C, Lee K C, Peters W J, Douglas L G. Acalculous cholecystitis in association with major burns. *Burns* 1987; **13:** 488–91.

51. Polacik V, Broz L, Kripner J, Bouska I, Liska E. Unexpected gastrointestinal complications in severely burned children. *Acta Clir Plast* 1991; **33:** 98–109.

52. Gately J F, Thomas E J. Acute cholecystitis occurring as a complication of other diseases. *Arch Surg* 1983; **118:** 1137–41.

53. Ortiz C, Cleveland R H, Blickman J G, Jaramillo D, Kim S H, Familial superior mesenteric artery syndrome. *Radiology* 1990; 588–9.

54. Lundell L, Thulin A. Wilkie's syndrome – a rarity? *Br J Surg* 1980; **67:** 604–6.

55. Jones P A, Wastell C. Superior mesenteric artery syndrome. *Postgrad Med J* 1983; **59:** 376–9.

56. Lescher T J, Sirinek K R, Pruitt B A. Superior mesenteric artery syndrome in thermally injured patients. *J Trauma* 1979; **19:** 567–71.

57. Ogbuokiri C G, Law E J, MacMillan B G. Superior mesenteric artery syndrome in burned children. *Am J Surg* 1972; **124:** 75–9.

58. Amoury R A. Necrotizing enterocolitis. In: Ashcraft K W, Holder T M, eds. *Pediatric Surgery*. Philadelphia: W B Saunders, 1993: 341–57.

59. Talamani M A. Ogilvie's syndrome. In: Cameron J L, ed. *Current Surgical Therapy*. 4th ed. St Louis: Mosby-Year Book, Inc, 1992: 168–70.

60. Gauderer M W, Stellano T A. Gastrostomy tubes. *Curr Prob Surg* 1986; **9:** 658–717.

61. Grant J P. Percutaneous endoscopic gastrostomy: initial placement by single endoscopic technique and long term follow up. *Ann Surg* 1993; **217:** 168–74.

62. Grant J P. Comparison of percutaneous endoscopic gastrostomy with Stamm gastrostomy. *Ann Surg* 1988; **207:** 598–603.

63. Hollands M J, Fletcher J P, Young J. Percutaneous feeding gastrostomy. *Med J Aust* 1989; **151:** 328–31.

64. MacFayden B V Jr, Ghobria R, Catalano M, Raijman I. Concomitant placement of percutaneous endoscopic gastrostomy and jejunostomy. *Surg Endosc* 1992; **6:** 289–93.

65. Gottschlich M M, Warden G D, Michel M, *et al.* Diarrhea in tube-fed burn patients: incidence, etiology, nutritional impact, and prevention. *J Parenter Enteral Nutr* 1988; **12:** 338–45.

66. Goodwin C W, McManus W F, Mason A D, Pruitt B A. Management of abdominal wounds in thermally injured patients. *J Trauma* 1982; **22:** 92–7.

CHAPTER THIRTY-SIX

The Burn Problem: A Pathologist's Perspective

Hugo A. Linares

Introduction

As Long stated in 1840,[1] 'burns are not a simple injury, but a very complicated disease, of which the numerous and various degrees constitute so many affections, which present marked characters, variable results, particular complications, and which may require various kinds of treatment, and that in them we find combined all the internal complications which severally attend upon irritation of the cutaneous surface, whether produced by erysipelas, measles, scarlatina, small-pox, etc'. Indeed, the morphologic observations during the past two centuries, specially after the report on five burn autopsies by Cumin[2] and the works by Dupuytren,[3] have confirmed that a vast ensemble of morphologic multisystem lesions evolves from the severe physiologic derangement occurring in a burned patient. Although inflammatory processes, hemodynamic and metabolic disorders, fluid imbalance and other alterations are also seen within the general pathologic frame of some clinicosurgical diseases, the magnitude and the pattern of changes in burned patients are unique. The contribution of the pathomorphologic approach to the advancement of the understanding of the burn problem continues to be very significant. Pathology combines anatomy, physiology, and theories of disease, and it is a point of convergence for medicine and the biological disciplines.

Sedillot, in 1781, suggested that the study of the anatomical changes occurring in tissues could lead to a more rational therapy.[4] It logically followed that morphologic descriptions of loss of fluid into tissues[5–7] and subsequent production of shock resulted in procedures aimed at restoring fluid homeostasis after burn injury.[8,9] The concept of a burn as an inflammatory process, seen today in some publications as a novelty, evolved through centuries of clinical observations. It was the anatomical description of the internal inflammatory reactions after burn reported by Oliveira and Cumin in 1823, which gave confirmation and meaning to clinical observations.[2,10] A better understanding of postburn gastrointestinal hemorrhages began to evolve after the description of gastroduodenal ulcerations seen in autopsies by Swan[11] and later on by Dupuytren,[3] Cooper,[12] Long,[1] and Curling.[13]

The first anatomical description of smoke inhalation occurred in 1822. A patient who died 4 days after a moderate burn involving face and thorax showed, at autopsy, a black pigmented tracheobronchial mucosa.[14] It is well acknowledged that awareness about the effects of smoke inhalation were learned after the pathomorphologic examination of the victims of the Coconut Grove fire in Boston, 1942.[15] The treatment of burned skin with tannic acid proposed by Nikolsky[16] and reintroduced by Davidson in 1925 was a popular treatment until a striking degeneration of the liver was described in autopsies of tannic acid treated burned patients and later confirmed experimentally.[17] Through the evaluation of the morphologic lesions and their clinical correlation, these and many other examples reflect the major contribution of the pathologic approach to advance the understanding of the burn problem.

The complex physiopathologic responses elicited by a severe burn injury affect different tissues and organs which may react by promoting a variety of changes leading to multiorgan dysfunction. Thus, a cumulative sequence of organ failures may involve vital areas such as the cardiorespiratory system, kidneys, liver, the gastrointestinal tract, or the central nervous system. Burn tissue may also release tissue thromboplastin and other cellular enzymes into the systemic circulation, triggering a disseminated intravascular coagulation-like process which is almost always present to some degree at the early period of critical burns. The initiation of coagulation may also be triggered by bacterial, fungal, or viral procoagulant activators. In fact, disseminated intravascular coagulation and sepsis are a frequently described cause–effect mechanism. Similarly, sepsis and the development of multiorgan failure has been described as a frequent concurrence. Therefore, it would not be uncommon to find severe burn injuries associated with a series of complications including sepsis, disseminated intravascular coagulation, and multisystem organ failure.

Many significant changes are set in motion by the burn itself, starting with acute severe hypovolemia which requires prompt and efficient management. Plasma loss as the result of local injury and increased permeability of the microvasculature, a clearly inflammatory type of response, leads to the hemodynamic changes of burn shock. Several pathomorphologic complications may arise during this period, such as structural red cell damage, hemorrhages, pulmonary edema, or intravascular microthrombosis.

Pathologic Problems

The systemic inflammatory response syndrome (SIRS) is a complex response to burn injury. A thermal burn is essentially an inflammatory reaction as already described in the early 1800s. If severe enough, it may elicite a wide spectrum of systemic manifestations.[2,10] These are expressed by an ample variety of complex biochemical actions, reactions, and interactions, which share the commonalities of the newly defined systemic inflammatory response syndrome (SIRS).[18] In a burned patient, the basic event seems to be the nonspecific activation of a generalized inflammatory response with the active participation of leading elements such as leukocytes, macrophages and endothelial cells. The histamine released from mast cells during the first hours of thermal injury lead to vasodilation and edema.[19,20] Furthermore, intracellular proteases released as a result of the thermally induced cell damage seems to activate the kallikrein–kinin system, leading to the synthesis of prostaglandins, vasodilation, and leukocyte migration.[21] A delayed phase can be reproduced by a number of mediators, especially those related to arachidonic acid. This phase is characterized by a marked increase in microvascular permeability and changes in vasomotor control together with the margination of leukocytes and platelets and the release of prostaglandins, prostacyclins, thromboxanes, leukotrienes, and lipoxins. Postburn inflammatory response involves activation of the coagulation and fibrinolytic systems which together with the kallikrein–kinin system may be activated by the Hageman factor. As a result, the fibrin polymerization in burned tissue and platelet aggregation induce the formation of intravascular microthrombi which lead to ischemia and necrosis through perfusion blockage.[22]

A number of mediators have been implicated in neutrophil chemotaxis such as the components of the complement cascade, metabolites derived from arachidonic acid, lymphokines, or components associated with the coagulation system (fibrinogen, kallikrein, platelet-derived growth factor, platelet-activating factor, etc.). The activation of the complement system, and particularly fragment C5a, not only results in widespread leukostasis but may constitute a source of potential pathogenic mediators of the hemodynamic disturbances related to sepsis and organ failure.[23] The chemotaxis agents produce aggregation, adherence, diapedesis, and degranulation of the polymorphonuclear leukocytes. This leukocyte activation generates metabolites of arachidonic acid (prostanoids, thromboxane, leukotrienes), releases proteolytic enzymes, and forms products of oxidative metabolism (superoxide, hydrogen peroxide, oxygen free radicals, singlet oxygen).[24–26] These mediators produce severe endothelial damage with increased capillary permeability, tissue damage, and further organ dysfunction.

Endothelial integrity is of paramount importance due to the complex and multifunctional activity of endothelial cells. Biological processes such as the production of vasoactive substances and procoagulants, immunoreactions, lipid metabolism, and endocrinological interactions are among the variety of endothelial cell actions.[27] The integrity or failure of the reticuloendothelial system may also contribute to these complex mechanisms which evolve from severe burns. Hypovolemia may significantly depress the activity of the hepatic reticuloendothelial system, promoting not only an impaired clearance of microorganisms of intestinal origin and toxic substances from the gut but also the nonremoval of circulating procoagulants and the activation of pulmonary macrophages so as to establish another link among burns, sepsis, DIC and multiorgan failure (MOF).[28–30]

Sepsis can readily develop in burned patients. When the inflammatory response supervenes as the result of a documented infection (bacterial, fungal, viral or its toxic products) with not merely the presence of microorganisms in the bloodstream but also the invasion of normally sterile tissues, then sepsis has developed. Sepsis is a complex clinical entity recently defined as sepsis syndrome when the systemic response to infection is expressed by tachycardia, hyperthermia or hypothermia, tachypnea, and evidence of organ dysfunction; it is defined as septic shock if the sepsis syndrome is accompanied by hypotension.[18] Sepsis remains one of the most dangerous complications of burn injury and a primary contributory cause of death in the burn population around the world.[31,32] In our series of 100 consecutive autopsies,[33] documented sepsis (positive blood cultures and invasion of viable tissues) was present in 73 cases. The most frequent source of infection was the burn wound (80.8%) followed by air-borne infections (6.4%). The predominant infecting microorganisms were (in order of importance) *Pseudomonas aeruginosa* (43%), *Staphylococcus aureus* (20%), *Klebsiella pneumoniae* (19%) *Escherichia coli* (15%), *Enterobacter* sp. (13%) and *Candida* sp. (13%).

The risk of infection is proportional to the severity of burn, the time before the initiation of fluid therapy, the presence of metabolic alterations, the development of immunological deficiency, the concurrence of trauma, the local evolution of wounds, and the age of a patient. Also, the risk of infection increases parallel to the increase in virulence and resistance of microorganisms. An infection may begin in a burn wound, the respiratory system, the gastrointestinal tract (whence it may be spread by translocation), the urinary tract, the blood vessels (where it is caused by catheters), and also from localized infections in any area of the body or by nosocomial contamination.

Burn wound sepsis is suspected when a burn wound is the site of proliferating microorganisms exceeding 10^5/g of tissue, and there is active invasion of subjacent unburned tissue.[34] The presence of microorganisms on or within the necrotic eschar cannot be considered sufficient evidence of burn wound sepsis; but as a site of primary colonization, it has a potential capability for bacterial overgrowth and invasion of surrounding viable tissue.

At autopsy, it is necessary to take an adequate number of sections from burned and unburned skin as well as sections from venous cut-down areas. Multiple, deep, parallel incisions of a burn wound should be made, looking for discoloration of subcutaneous tissue, hemorrhages, or other suspicious zones. If no suspicious areas are seen, random sections should be taken for histologic studies and bacterial or fungal cultures. Cardiac blood cultures, if properly obtained, can also be very valuable in assessing sepsis. Cultures from different organs (especially from lungs and spleen), may be taken as well.[35]

Disseminated intravascular coagulation (DIC, microcirculatory thrombosis) is another serious complication in burned patients.[36–39] The extensive tissue necrosis occurring in severe burns along with the inflammatory response, damage to erythrocytes, platelets, and endothelial cells, or the exposure to subendothelial collagen can promote disseminated intravascular coagulation by the release of procoagulants or thromboplastin-like substances (extrinsic pathway). The systemic circulation of thrombin promotes the cleavage of fibrinopeptides from fibrinogen. The resultant fibrin monomers polymerize into fibrin aggregates; this leads to intravascular thrombosis, tissue ischemia, and in some cases to a microangiopathic hemolytic anemia (red cell fragmentation). Thrombocytopenia may result from the entrapment of platelets within a fibrin clot; the systemic circulation of plasmin may promote the formation of fibrinogen degradation products (FDP). FDP interference with fibrin monomer polymerization, as well as the consumption of blood coagulation factors, the depletion of platelets and fibrinogen, and the activation of plasminogen may lead to hemorrhages. The activation of the kallikrein pathway leads to an increased vascular permeability, hypotension, and shock.[40]

Burned patients have supranormal *in vitro* clotting activity and may develop the syndrome of DIC coincidentally with septicemia or hypotension.[39] Bleeding tendency in the early phase and hypercoagulability in the late phase of acute burn care are common clinical observations. During the period of high coagulation (3–10 days after injury) in which acute burned patients may exhibit hyperfibrinogenemia and elevated fibrin–fibrinogen split products, DIC might be precipitated by shock or sepsis.[38,41]

DIC can occur without depression of all the intrinsic clotting factors below the accepted normal values because of the common elevation in burns of factor VIII, fibrinogen or platelets. Therefore, the laboratory diagnosis of DIC may be masked. The diagnosis may be confirmed by the histologic presence of fibrin thrombi, hyaline thrombi, platelet thrombi, and/or hemorrhages, although these morphological features are not always present because microthrombi may be lysed by *in vivo* or postmortem fibrinolysis.[37,42,43] In our series of 100 autopsies,[33] there were 69 cases of verified DIC. In 64 of them, fibrin microthrombi were present at autopsy. The thrombi were observed most frequently in the lung (81%), followed by the skin (21.7%), kidneys (11.5%), gastrointestinal tract (11.5%), spleen (8.6%), heart (4.3%) and, in lesser percentage, in other organs such as thymus, pancreas, liver, adrenals, ovaries, muscle, airways, and gallbladder.

Multiorgan dysfunction and failure has a very high mortality rate and is the main cause of death in surgical and trauma patients in intensive care units.[44] Ironically, it has evolved under the shadow of improvements which occurred in intensive care units. The increased survival achieved by artificial support and monitoring of vital systems (i.e. cardiorespiratory, renal, gastrointestinal) has permitted the recognition of frequently fatal complications which are usually only indirectly related to the original illness.

The incidence of multisystem organ failure (MOF) in burned patients is still unclear. In a 4-year review of 117 severe burns averaging 48.4% total body surface area, Mohan[45] showed 67.5% of patients developing one or more organ system failures with a mortality rate of 72% for those with three or more organ system failures. The organ system most frequently affected was the respiratory system, followed by the immunological, cardiovascular, hematologic, renal, hepatic, and gastrointestinal systems. Aikawa[46] reported an incidence of 16.5% MOF of 158 burned patients or 48.1% of the severe burns (more than 30% body surface area burned and/or inhalation injury). The mortality rate was 76.9% in MOF and 1.5% in non MOF patients. The most frequently affected organ was the lung, followed by the heart, kidney, liver, and the blood clotting system. In our series of autopsies,[33] the incidence of MOF was very high (94%) and the organ system which most commonly failed was the respiratory system, followed by heart, kidney, GI, and liver.

Respiratory System

Pulmonary complications are frequent in patients with severe thermal injuries and, along with sepsis, constitute the most important factors influencing morbidity and mortality in burned patients (**Figure 36.1**). As can be shown from our series,[33] the lung is the main target organ, with respiratory failure being the most conspicuous contributory cause of morbidity and death.[47,48] All the patients in this series had severe lung lesions, ranging from the classical bacterial pneumonia to a distinctive acute respiratory distress syndrome. Sepsis, burn shock, and inhalation injury were the most common determinants of respiratory system failure. Respiratory insufficiency is manifested by an increased respiratory effort followed by a progressive decrease in compliance, increased resistance, decreased arterial oxygen tension, and pulmonary arteriovenous shunting.[49] This clinical syndrome and its variants have been described under a variety of terms such as post-traumatic pulmonary insufficiency, congestive atelectasis, traumatic wet lung, Da Nang lung, and others.[49,50] The lung has a limited reactional pattern, and different types of injuries usually elicit a similar anatomical pathologic response. Thus, this type of 'pulmonary distress' (ARDS) may also result as a nonspecific pulmonary response to body tissue injury, inhalation injuries, or sepsis.[51] In our series,[33] 60% of the patients died with 'pulmonary distress', 23% with bacterial pneumonia, and the remaining 17% with a variety of other lesions such as aspiration pneumonia, pulmonary embolism, fluid and electrolyte imbalance, etc.

The more common morphologic features seen in patients dying with progressive respiratory insufficiency were interstitial and intra-alveolar edema and hemorrhages, atelectasis, intra-alveolar proteinaceous and cellular debris, hyaline membranes, leukocytosis, and fibrin microthrombi (**Figure 36.2**). Although numerous factors have been implicated in the genesis of this type of lung damage, its pathogenetic mechanisms remain unclear.[52] Clinical and experimental evidence accumulated through the past several years seems to implicate the sequestration of polymorphonuclear leukocytes in the pulmonary microvasculature with the subsequent fragmentation and release of lysosomal enzymes.[53,54] Nevertheless, some reports also indicate a developing of ARDS without pulmonary leukostasis.[55,56] A common histologic feature in our series[33] was the existence of leukostasis even in the presence of peripheral leukopenia. The acute leukostasis observed in the lung seems to be caused by the activation of humoral systems, particularly of the complement system.[57] The activation of the sequestered leukocytes in the pulmonary circulation may originate multiple mediators which in turn may contribute to a variety of pathophysiologic changes. Although the neutrophil is a sufficient promoter of the acute lung injury, the presence of activated neutrophils in the pulmonary vascular bed and interstitium may not signify tissue damage or make the neutrophil a necessary mediator of the tissue injury.[56]

The diagnosis of inhalation injury at autopsy is not always possible. The classical coagulation necrosis of the tissues and the deposition of carbonaceous material may no longer be present if a patient had a prolonged survival or if there are laryngotracheal lesions secondary to intubation. In many cases, carbonaceous material may be detected in the pulmonary parenchyma. Direct thermal injury to the lower airways is extremely rare except in those patients subjected to the effect of hot gases or high-pressure steam from sudden explosions or similar accidents. The extent of damage usually depends on the time of exposure, intensity, and type of inhalant. Hot, dry air almost never reaches the lower respiratory tract with a damaging temperature. This is because of rapid dissipation of heat through air passages. In contrast, steam can produce serious damage even to the pulmonary parenchyma because of its high thermal conductivity.

The most common occurrence of inhalation injury takes place when a fire occurs in a closed area, thus exposing a patient to the inhalation of smoke. Smoke contains a variety of toxic products of combustion, which may cause a severe inflammatory reaction in the entire tracheobronchial tree, including lung parenchyma. The resulting respiratory injury is associated with a high mortality rate. The predominant morphologic features of inhalation injury include acute tracheobronchitis which varies in severity from marked congestion, edema, and leukocytosis, to a severe necrotizing process accompanied by sloughing of the mucosa. The progressive separation of the necrotic epithelium with the formation of pseudomembranous casts may cause a complete or partial obstruction of the airways and result in atelectasis and pneumonia. The pseudomembranous exudate is mainly composed of cellular debris, mucus, fibrin, and polymorphonuclear leukocytes. Usually there are no pseudomembranes in bronchioles; but this nonpathological state changes, progressing to a peribronchial pneumonia. The pulmonary parenchyma shows lesions similar to that described in 'pulmonary distress' including: congestion, interstitial and alveolar edema, neutrophilic infiltration, occasional hyaline membranes and microthrombi, septal edema, atelectasis, hyperplasia of pneumono-

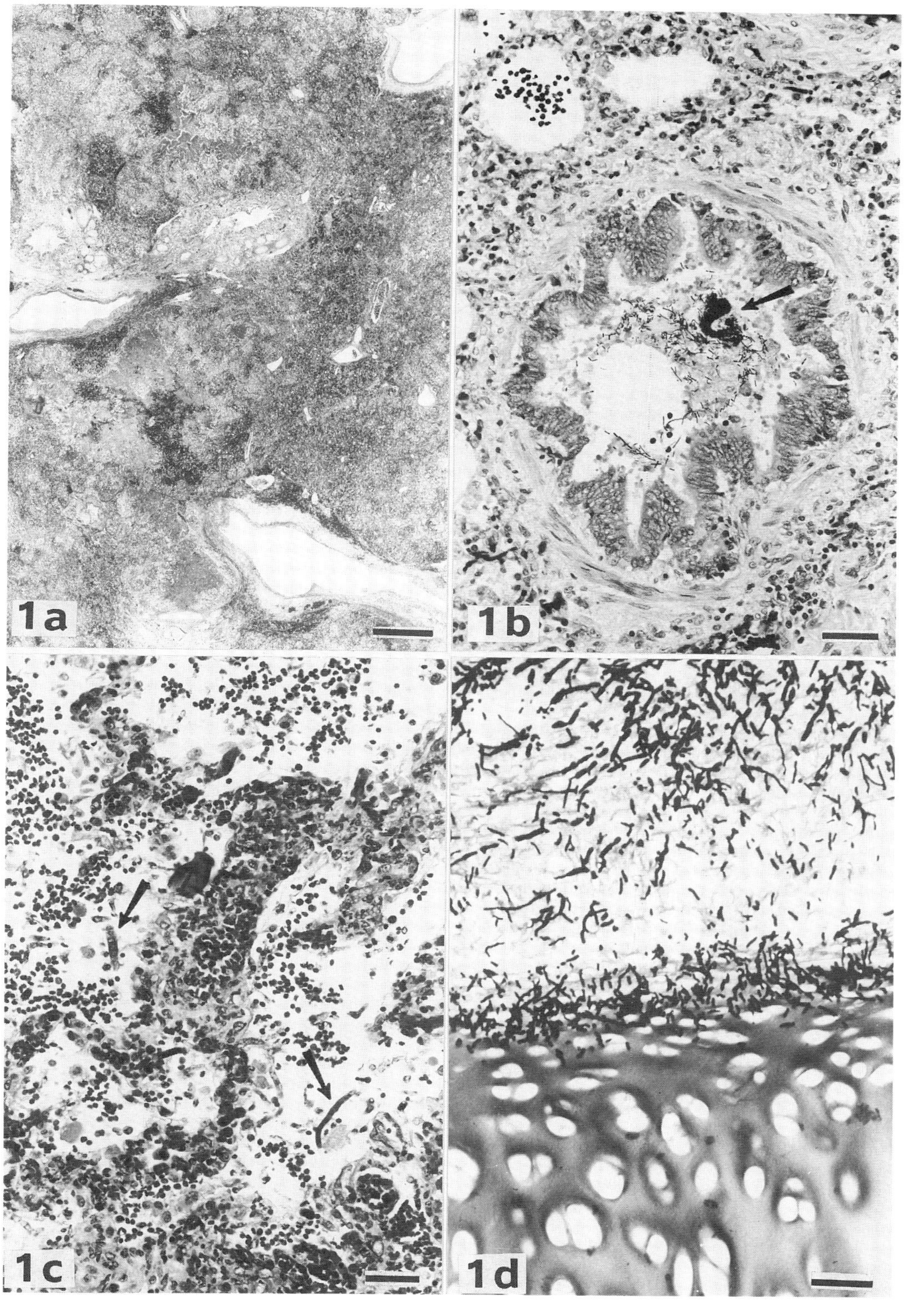

Fig. 36.1 Lung infection. (a) Pseudomonas aeruginosa *pneumonia. HE stain. Bar=250 µm. (b) Bronchus filled with aspirated material (aspiration pneumonia) and superimposed bacterial infection. Gram stain. Bar=100 µm. (c) Alveoli invaded by fungal filaments. Groccott stain. Bar=100 µm. (d)* Candida *sp. tracheitis. PAS stain. Bar=50 µm.*

cytes (type II), macrophage activity, and edema of subpleural septa and peribronchiovascular spaces.[58]

Cardiovascular System

Postburn hypovolemia due to the early loss of plasma volume (microvascular and cellular alterations) leads to a noticeable cardiovascular instability. It is still controversial as to whether a postburn depression of cardiac output is due to hypovolemia secondary to inadequate volume resuscitation or to a circulating myocardial depressant factor.[59,60] Most of the physiopathologic cardiovascular complications found in severely burned patients are secondary to sepsis or burn shock, usually related to inotropic disturbances (i.e. ischemia). In our series,[33] the heart disclosed anatomical lesions in

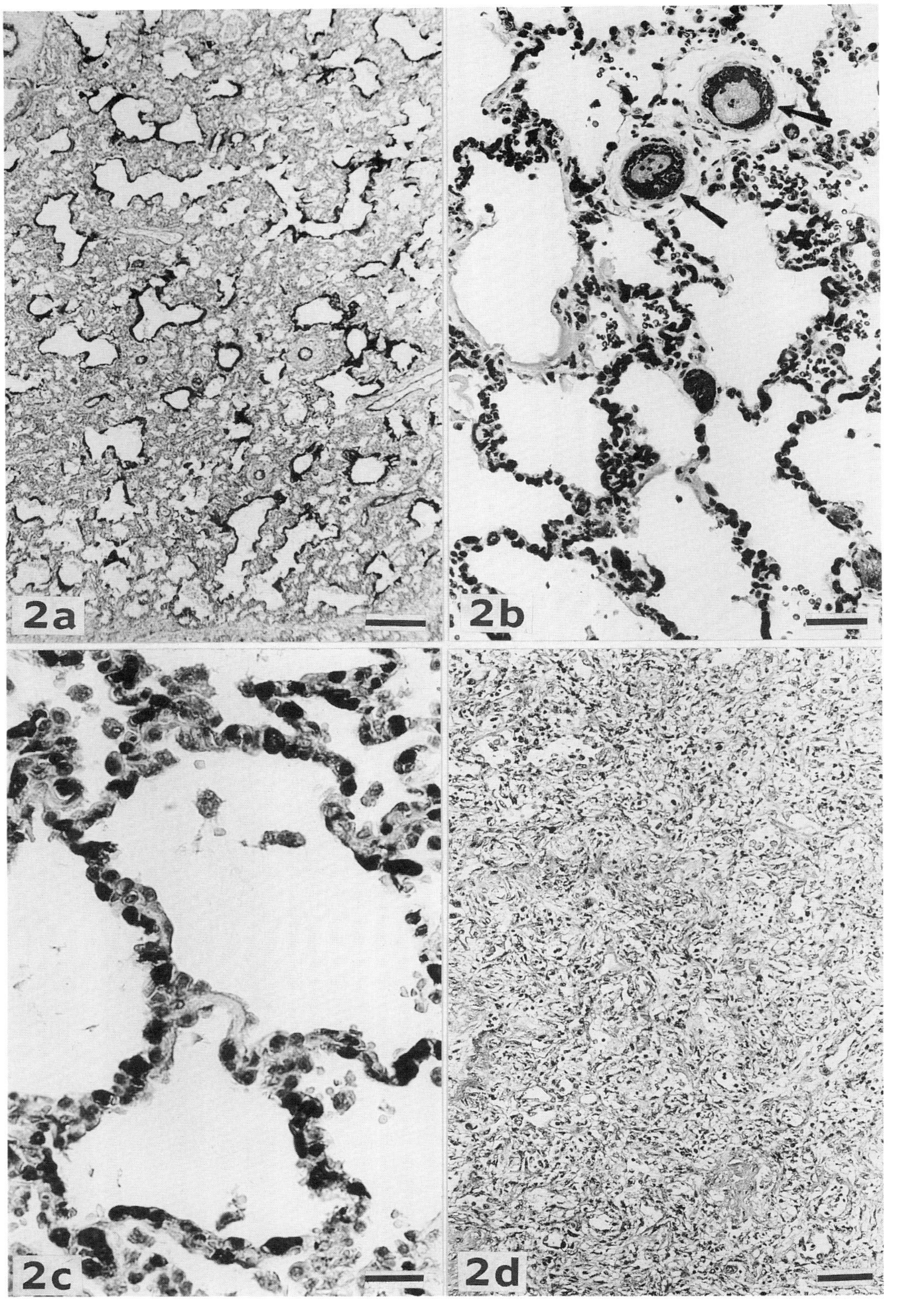

Fig. 36.2 ARDS. (a) Hyaline membrane formation. PAS stain. Bar= 200 μm. (b) Fibrin microthrombi (arrows) HE stain. Bar=50 μm. (c) Leukocytosis (black dots). Leder stain. Bar=40 μm. (d) Lung fibrosis. Masson stain. Bar=200 μm.

57% of the cases. Most of them consisted of subendocardial ischemia, and to a very lesser degree, focal myocardial necrosis, hemorrhages or septic processes (**Figure 36.3a**). Adding anatomical lesions to significant clinical symptoms within 48 hours of demise, the number of cardiovascular failures in this series reached 79%, with most associated with concomitant sepsis.

Kidneys

Advances in fluid resuscitation therapy have greatly diminished or altogether prevented renal complications following a severe burn injury. The kidneys are able to function properly even with only 20% of their normal capacity; however, this enormous reserve can

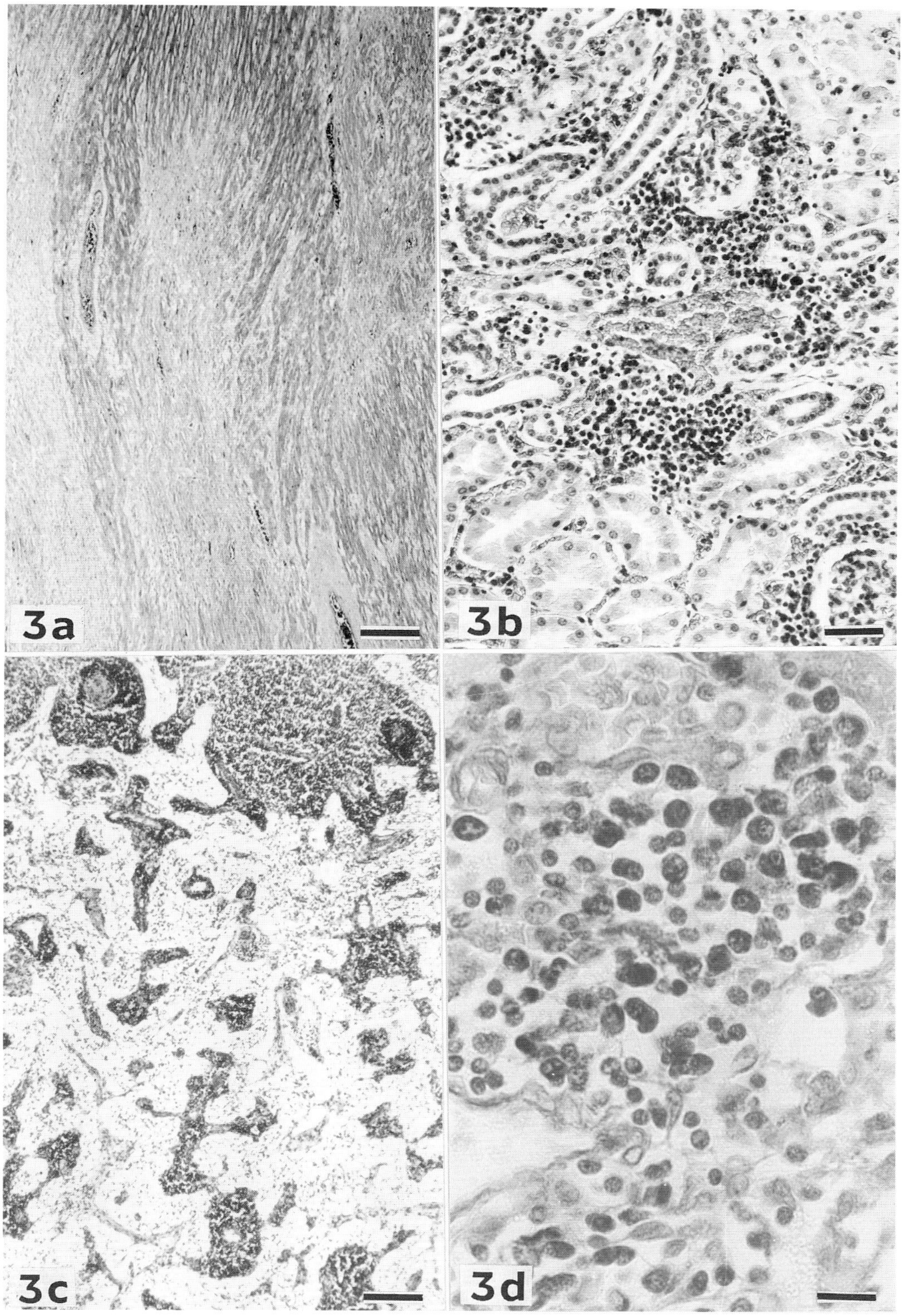

Fig. 36.3 (a) Myocardial ischemia. HE stain. Bar=200 μm. (b) Interstitial nephritis. HE stain. Bar=50 μm. (c) Lymph node with lymphocyte depletion. HE stain. Bar=100 μm. (d) Medullary cord of a lymph node with a marked pyroninophilic cell response. Methyl-green-pyronine stain. Bar=50 μm.

be jeopardized because of the severe hemodynamic changes which occur during the shock phase. Thus, a state of kidney dysfunction is frequently present in extensive burns during the immediate postburn period and in sepsis and shock from other causes.

Morphologic lesions observed in the kidney do not always coincide with the degree of the functional impairment, but an association between acute renal failure and the so-called 'acute tubular necrosis' can usually be demonstrated. Martineau and Hartman reviewed the renal pathological changes reported in extensive burns since 1823.[61] The most frequent lesions observed in the early and late postburn period were congestion; interstitial and submucosal hemorrhages; hyaline thrombi in the glomerular loops and granular thrombi in the large vessels; hemorrhagic and anemic infarctions; glomerular endothelial hyperplasia; interstitial edema;

hyaline, granular, and hemoglobin casts; and a variety of degenerative changes in the tubules (albuminous and vacuolar degeneration, degenerative fatty infiltration, and tubular necrosis, particularly involving the proximal convoluted tubule and Henle's loop). Tubular hemoglobin casts and bilateral necrosis were found only in the first 72 hours, while acute interstitial nephritis and metastatic abscesses were late findings (after 72 hours) (**Figure 36.3b**). In their own study of 84 experimentally burned dogs and 20 human cases, Martineau and Hartman found degenerative tubular changes, capillary congestion, tubular casts from the products of intravascular hemolysis, and lesions due to infection.[61]

The most common lesion in our series of autopsies[33] was acute tubular necrosis (68%). All cases of acute tubular necrosis were associated with clinical renal failure; however, in 12 cases of clinical renal failure, no morphologic changes were seen at autopsy. Acute tubular necrosis and renal failure, developing later in the course of the illness, were always associated with pulmonary lesions and/or septicemia.

Digestive System

Esophagus

Thermal burns of the esophagus are rare. Injuries to the esophagus are usually self-limited and superficial due to the immediate reflex ejection elicited by the heat. In contrast, chemical burns constitute a significant problem, not only because of the difficulties in the immediate management, but also because of the frequent complications and unavoidable sequelae which frequently develop. The severity of the lesion is related to the nature, amount, contact time, and concentration of the agent ingested. The severity of the injury varies depending on the consistency of the corrosive agent, esophageal peristalsis, and/or spasm. As a result, the irregular topography of an ulceration will also lead to irregular scarring and stenosis. In most cases, the damage is progressive because of the sequential chemical reactions produced within cells or tissues which persist even after the death of a patient.

The rapid transit time of concentrated acids (usually thin liquids) and the resistance of the esophageal squamous epithelium lead to major corrosive effects in the stomach rather than in the esophagus. The latter is only rarely affected; however, injury to the esophagus can also occur after vomiting of a corrosive substance. This can also produce further injury to the lips, skin around the mouth, and even the larynx. In addition, strong acids cause almost immediate coagulative necrosis of the tissue, probably due to protein precipitation. This will impede further penetration, and, therefore, will produce more superficial lesions than alkalis.

Strong alkalis are at least partially neutralized by the acid gastric environment but produce maximum effects in the esophagus where the transit time is decreased due to the thickness of the liquids involved. The cardial spasm is most likely to succeed in making the passage of the substance to the stomach more difficult. Alkalis remove water from cells and tissues and have a saponifying effect on lipids and precipitate proteins forming alkali–albuminate linkages. The precipitates redissolve in an excess of water and produce the so-called colliquation necrosis, as opposed to the coagulation necrosis caused by acids. Thus, the lesions produced by alkalis are highly destructive, leading in some cases to the perforation of the organ. The corroded areas are soft, gelatinous, and friable, showing a brownish discoloration.

In a broad sense, the healing process of esophageal lesions follows the characteristics of burns elsewhere in the body. The necrotic tissue is sloughed and replaced by a granulating bed. The elicited inflammatory process, fibroblastic activity, contraction, and scar formation will eventually result in fibrosis and stricture formation. The severity of the lesion and the length of healing time will depend on the depth of necrosis and extent of injury. The esophagus, like other organs, can occasionally be affected by the systemic effects of burn sepsis. Hyperemia, edema, petechiae, and superficial ulcerations or erosions may be present. In addition, bacteria, fungi, or viruses can seed the organ via the bloodstream or from the oral cavity (**Figure 36.4a**). These types of lesions are not very common, seldom cause severe problems *per se* in the course of the disease, and, at most, constitute a final event in a critically burned patient.

Stomach and duodenum

Acute digestive tract bleeding constitutes a common gastrointestinal complication of severe burn injury. The initial postburn congestion and hyperemia of the mucosa frequently evolves into a diffuse bleeding. This can also originate not only in a nonspecific, superficial, and inflammatory process, but also in erosions and/or ulcerations, with a subsequent possibility of hemorrhage and perforation, a life-threatening complication[13] (**Figure 36.4b**). These lesions are compatible with the so-called 'stress ulcer syndrome' and have been associated not only with burns but also with several other conditions such as trauma, major surgery, sepsis, central nervous system lesions, respiratory disturbances, acute myocardial infarction, hepatic cirrhosis, and anti-inflammatory drugs. Erosions and ulcers can be seen through the entire gastrointestinal tract from esophagus to rectum, but the stomach and the duodenum have been the sites of greatest predilection for these types of lesions. This may be due to the fact that gastroduodenal mucosa (especially stomach) is likely to be affected by any stressing stimulus.[13] Through the years, confusion has arisen concerning the definition of the lesions according to the depth of penetration. Thus, ulcerations which do not penetrate the muscularis mucosa have been reported by some authors as erosions, while others use the term ulcers for any lesion ranging from superficial loss of the mucosa to transmural penetration.

Within the first hours after a severe burn, gastroduodenal congestion and edema are likely to occur; by the end of the first day, a focal or diffuse hemorrhagic gastroduodenitis may be established. In this case, confluent pinpoint mucosal hemorrhages, sometimes alternating with focal areas of ischemia, can be seen mainly over the fundus and great curvature of the stomach and in the first pars of the duodenum. The mucosa appears pink-red in color. It is soft and friable and bleeds easily. Also, it shows scattered dark-red or black blood clots which, when wiped off, reveal minute, shallow, round to oval erosive lesions. These lesions lie between the rugal crests and involve only the mucosa. The rugal pattern of the stomach does not show significant alterations. At any given time, a varying age and severity of the lesions may be present. These vary from simple focal hyperemia or small yellowish edematous areas with hyperemic margins to petechial hemorrhages and mucosal erosions. The bleeding is usually diffuse, originating from the multiple erosive areas.

By the end of the first week, the superficial erosive lesions have a tendency to heal; in a certain number of cases, the loss of substance can involve the muscularis mucosae and penetrate deeply, constituting a frank ulceration. The superficial or deep lesions are generally unique or double in the duodenum where they are mainly located over the posterior wall of the first pars. They usually exist in multiples in the stomach and are found predominantly in the fundus and the anterior wall of the great curvature. The lesions show minimal to moderate inflammatory edema and induration of the margins (especially in the duodenum) and have a circumscribed, punched-out appearance. The sizes vary from 1 or 2 mm in diame-

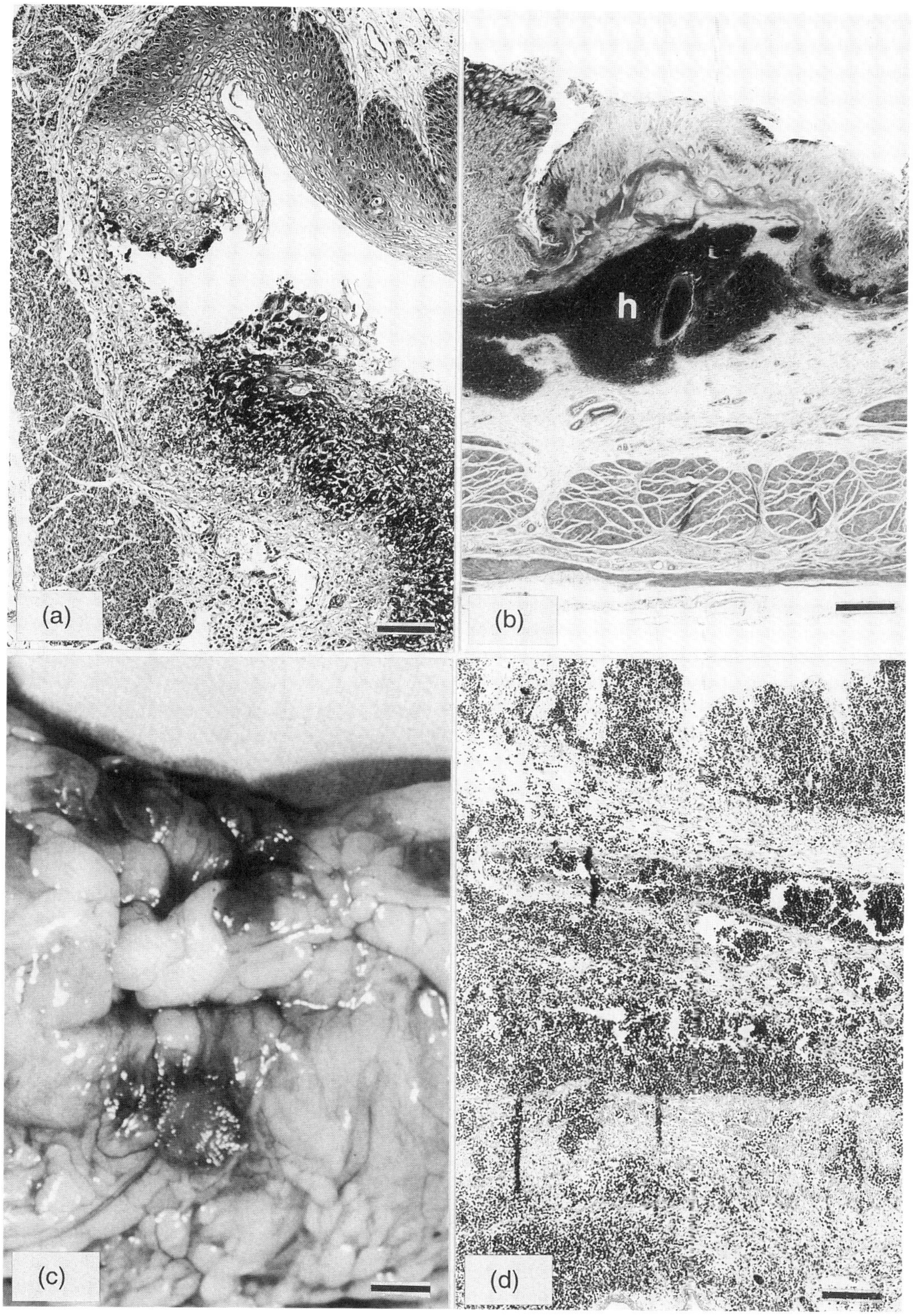

Fig. 36.4 (a) Herpes virus esophagitis. HE stain. Bar= 200 μm. (b) Stomach ulcer showing full-thickness mucosal necrosis with submucosal hemorrhage (h). HE stain. Bar=200 μm. (c) Gross anatomy of a section of large intestine showing hemorrhagic spots with abscess formation (arrow) protruding to the peritoneal layer. Bar=500 μm. (d) Intestinal transmural hemorrhagic necrosis. HE stain. Bar=250 μm.

ter to 3 or 4 cm in diameter. The larger lesions are predominantly located in the duodenum. The shape also has a wide geometrical variety from an irregular, dentate, stellate, or serpentine appearance to a linear, oval, or circular configuration. The ulcer base is generally clear and gray-yellow; occasionally a bleeding vessel can be seen. A dark-brown staining of the floor of a lesion may be seen as the result of acid digestion of blood originating from exposed tiny vessels of the floor. Hemorrhages (with hematemesis, 'coffee-ground' vomitus, melena) and, sometimes, perforation are the most frightening complications. Acute ulcers have a tendency to heal in a relatively short time and no scars will form if the process has not reached the muscular coat of the organ.

Occasionally, a focal necrosis has a linear appearance which may be due to a mechanical action of a nasogastric tube, although in these cases no severe complications are likely to occur. The incidence of acute focal gastroduodenal necrosis in burns is very difficult to determine due to the multiple variables involved. In many cases, the gastrointestinal complaints are minimal and are not even reported. Also, the results of the studies based on clinical cases or autopsy reports will differ considerably. Often the gastroduodenal lesions of burned patients who have died are not detected because an autopsy is only partially realized or is not performed at all. Significant variations can be observed if a pathologist differentiates between erosions and ulcerations or reports only lesions invading the muscularis mucosae. Some of the patients die in the first days after burn, before an erosion or ulceration can develop. On the other hand, there are also a number of ulcerations following burn injury which go on to heal without significant clinical symptoms.[32]

Intestine

The most frequent lesion associated with burn shock and sepsis is ischemic enterocolitis. These lesions range from a metaplasia of mucous cells to a complete transmural necrosis and may be focal or involve large areas of the organ (**Figure 36.4c, d**). This type of ischemia is of the so called 'nonocclusive' type, usually related to hypotension and/or disseminated intravascular coagulation. Both of these are frequent complications of severe burns. During the past decade, an increasing number of reports show evidence, mostly based on animal experimentation, which implicates the gastrointestinal tract as a possible source of infection. Our series was unable to show evidence of the gut as a source of sepsis.[33] In 57% of the cases of sepsis there were digestive tract lesions, but they appeared to be more the consequence rather than the source of infection. Also, in 25% of the cases without sepsis, there were anatomical lesions in the digestive tract. Furthermore, in 80% of the cases of sepsis, documented burn wound sepsis was the source of the infection.

As far back as the end of the last century, the presence of viable bacteria in the internal organs of humans and animals has been reported.[62] Furthermore, it has been suggested that under certain conditions bacteria may pass through the intestinal wall and colonize in internal organs.[63] This phenomenon is currently known as bacterial translocation and implies the passage of viable bacteria from the gastrointestinal tract through the epithelial mucosa to mesenteric lymph nodes and other organs.[64] Translocation is promoted by disruption of the ecology of the indigenous gastrointestinal microflora which results in bacterial overgrowth, impaired host defenses, or physical disruption of the gut mucosal barrier.[65]

The mechanisms involved in this translocation process remain obscure; and numerous hypotheses have been proposed, such as the presence of a functional defect in the macrophages of the intestinal submucosa interfering in the intracellular bacterial killing;[66] the passage through the brush border or through the intercellular functional complex as has been described in the case of the *Salmonella typhimurium*;[67] through capture and transport of bacteria within host macrophages from the intestinal epithelium to the lamina propria;[68] by disruption of the mucosal barrier due to increased local protease activity;[69] the activity of the oxygen free radicals generated during the period of intestinal reperfusion;[70] intestinal ischemia;[71] hemorrhagic shock;[72] endotoxin and xanthine oxydase activity;[73] or immunosuppression and intestinal bacterial overgrowth.[74] It is not clear if the term bacterial translocation means that viable indigenous bacteria pass through an intact intestinal mucosa,[64,75–77] through an epithelium with alteration of its permeability,[78] or through necrotic mucosa.[79] Obviously, if there is a necrosis of the mucosa, bacterial colonization with invasion of viable tissue is likely to occur. This mechanism is similar to the bacterial infection in any tissue of the body.

Liver

A variable degree of liver dysfunction is often present in a burned patient, and it is usually related to the severity of an injury. Fatty changes, a common finding, are *per se* reversible and their significance depends on the cause and severity of accumulation[32] (**Figure 36.5a**). The 12% incidence of liver necrosis in our series[33] did not differ significantly from other reports.[80,81] It was generally focal or zonal (central or paracentral), sometimes microfocal, and related to burn shock and sepsis (**Figure 36.5c**). Intrahepatic cholestasis, which is one of the prime manifestations of hepatocellular injury, was present in 26% of these cases; all of these were concurrent with sepsis (**Figure 36.5b**). The cellular damage observed in sepsis is most likely the result of decreased effective hepatic blood flow rather than direct cellular injury.[82]

Cholestasis appears to be an important finding, and occurs without demonstrable extrahepatic obstruction. It has been described in association with a number of processes such as sepsis, hypoxia, drug toxicity, or total parenteral nutrition.[83,84] The mechanisms of intracholestasis remain uncertain, and a variety of hypotheses have been proposed in the past several years. Because of the liver's innumerable functions, hepatic failure has many dimensions, although the clinical features of hepatic failure are much the same, and the histologic changes may not be conspicuous.

Lymphoid Tissue

Considerable interest has focused on the immune system and the immunological defects in patients with severe thermal injury. In one of our series of autopsies, lymphocyte depletion was the common denominator in all the lymphoid tissues examined (nodes, spleen, thymus, gastrointestinal tract).[32] A marked depletion of lymphocytes from the thymic-dependent areas was a common finding early in the postburn period and for as long as 114 days postburn (the longest survival time in our series of autopsies). This change was associated with a progressive increase of pyroninophilic cells resembling plasmablasts and plasma cells in the bursal-dependent areas of the nodes[85] (**Figure 36.3c, d**).

Brain

Cerebral symptoms in burned patients are increasingly being reported in recent years, and although it is not usually fatal, burn encephalopathy may be a relatively common process. More than 90% of the cases in a series of autopsies showed generalized edema and a focal or diffuse loss of neurons as well as perivascular transudates, diapedesis hemorrhages, and other lesions associated with toxic–hypoxic alterations.[86].

Other Lesions

Miscellaneous complications which affect different organs may occur. True adrenal insufficiency is rare in burned patients. The most common findings are lipid depletion and focal hemorrhages; they are usually terminal and associated with sepsis or irreversible burn shock (**Figure 36.6a, b**). Pancreatic lesions are rare and also usually related to sepsis or severe uremia such as acinar

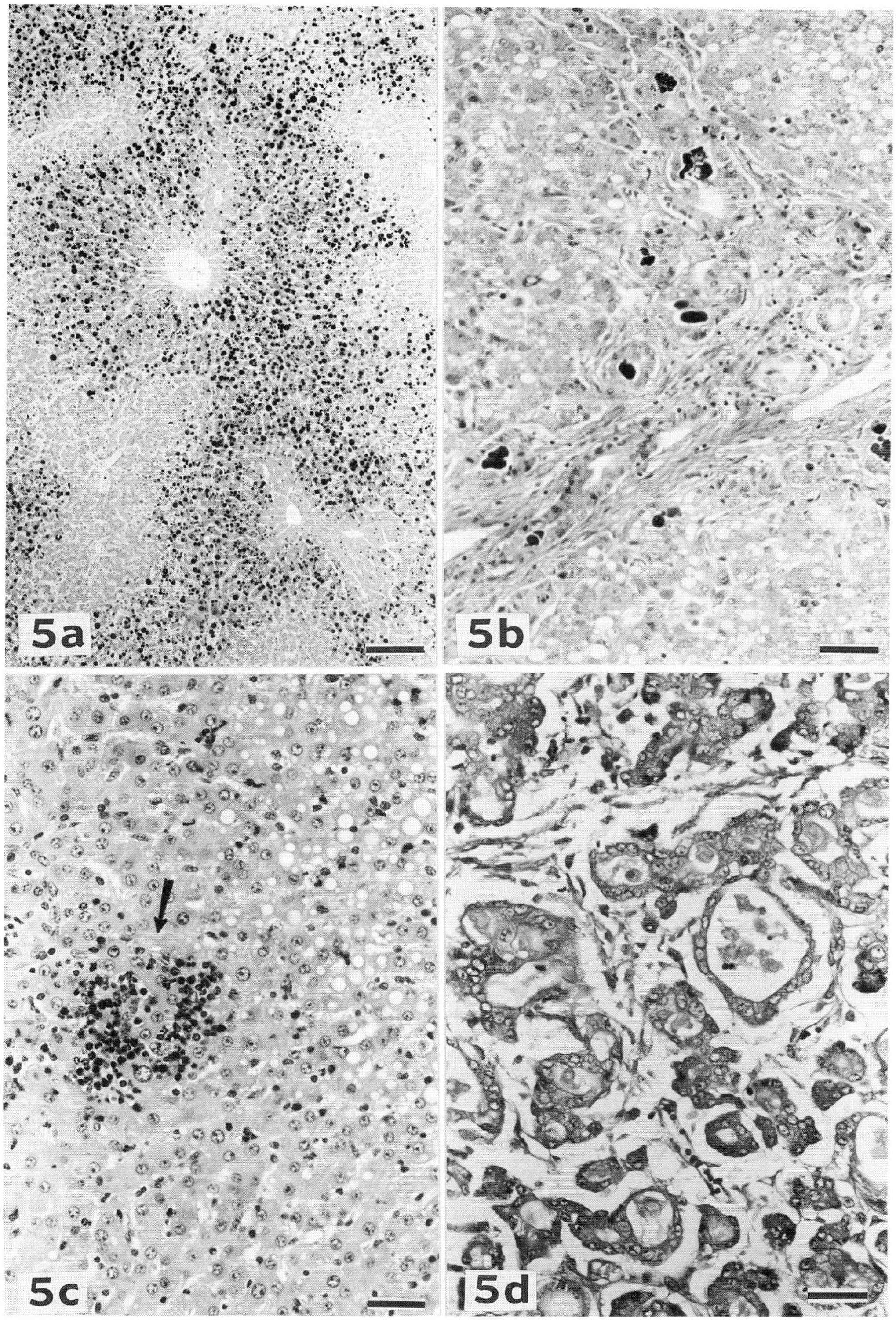

Fig. 36.5 (a) Liver with fatty metamorphosis (black dots). Osmic acid stain. Bar=250 µm. (b) Intrahepatic cholestasis (black spots). HE stain. Bar=100 µm. (c) focal micronecrosis in liver (arrow). Leder stain. Bar=100 µm. (d) Baggentoss changes in pancreas. HE stain. Bar=50 µm.

ectasia with dilatation of the pancreatic ducts and inspissation of pancreatic secretion[87] (**Figure 36.5d**). Thromboembolism is not as frequent as it used to be, probably due to improved prophylactic measures, although the use of invasive monitoring may be a source of high potential risk of complications. Aspiration pneumonia and airway lesions post-intubation are also some of the many complications which may arise during the course of a severe burn (**Figure 36.6c**). Fine filaments of inert material (parenteral therapy) may be introduced into pulmonary circulation where they tend to lodge in arteries between 150 and 500 µm in diameter. Eventually they become incorporated in the intima, and gradually the whole lesion is forced through the media and into perivascular tissues as far as the surrounding alveoli (**Figure 36.6d**).

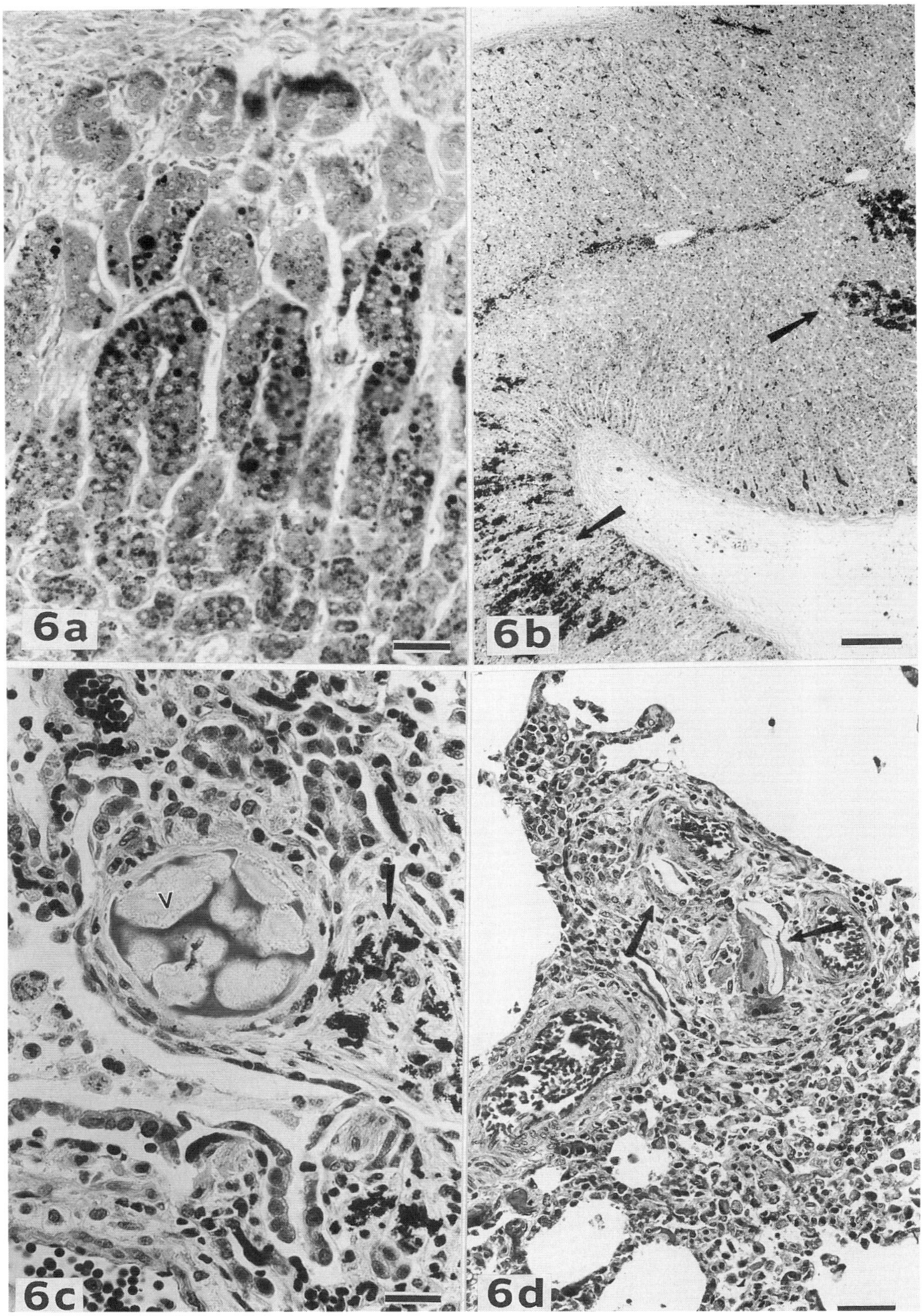

Fig. 36.6 (a) Adrenal with a moderate lipid depletion. Osmic acid stain. Bar=50 μm. (b) Focal hemorrhage in adrenal (arrows). HE stain. Bar=200 μm. (c) Section of lung showing an aspirated vegetal material (v) and carbonaceous pigment (arrow) indicating a concomitant inhalation injury. HE stain. Bar=50 μm. (d) Section of lung showing several periarterial foreign body granuloma (arrow) constituted of gauze filaments. HE stain. Bar=50 μm.

The Burn Autopsy

Five centuries ago, Bernard Tornius, asking permission of a parent to perform an autopsy of a child, said: 'To lose one's offspring is hard, harder to lose a son, and hardest by a disease not yet fully understood by doctors. But for the sake of the other children, I think that to have seen his organs will be of the greatest utility'.[88] Indeed, even in these modern times with so many sophisticated procedures and technological advances in diagnostic accuracy, the autopsy remains the best way to correlate anatomical morphology with physiopathologic processes, to evaluate known diseases and to describe new entities, to enlighten clinical judgments, to learn, and to teach. The availability of human tissue, so significant as a tool for learning and research in the past, remains of significant value in the study of many areas of vital interest such as cell biology, genetics, virology, immunology and endocrinology. Progress in diagnosis and treatment, which signifies medical progress, is definitively linked to postmortem examination of human tissues or animal research.

The contribution of autopsies to the better understanding of the perplexities of burn illness cannot be underestimated. Despite the simplicity of burn etiology, there is no disease with more complex clinical and physiopathologic derangements than an extensive burn. A careful morphologic evaluation of the anatomohistologic lesions and their clinical correlation can provide an invaluable critical analysis and give relevant information about important complications, unsuspected lesions, therapeutic effects, or previous diseases. The burn autopsy can provide not only an appropriate morphologic analysis but a dynamic interpretation of sequential pathogenesis. The autopsy should be oriented to an adequate investigation and retrospective evaluation of the entire clinical course of a burned patient. The history and magnitude of the injury and the clinical course and complications of therapy should be reconstituted so as to achieve a dynamic sequence of events. Thus, a properly conducted autopsy has as much practical value as it represents a learning experience.

REFERENCES

1. Long J. Post-mortem appearances found after burns. *Lond Med Gaz* 1840; **25:** 743–50.

2. Cumin W. Cases of severe burn with dissections, and remarks. *Edinb Med Surg J* 1823; **19:** 337–44.

3. Dupuytren G. Leçons orales de clinique chirurgicale: XII. Des brulures. Paris: G. Gailliere, 1839, vol. 4.

4. Sedillot J. Theses de ambustione. Dissertation. Paris, 1781.

5. Baraduc H. *Des Causes de la Mort à la Suite des Brulures Superficielles.* Paris: Bailliere, 1862.

6. Harkins H N. Experimental burns. I. The rate of fluid shift and its relation to the onset of shock in severe burns. *Arch Surg* 1935; **31:** 71–85.

7. Underhill F P, Kapsinow R, Fisk M E. Studies on the mechanism of water exchange in the animal organism. *Am J Physiol* 1930; **95:** 302–14.

8. Cope O, Moore F D. The redistribution of body water and the fluid therapy of the burned patient. *Ann Surg* 1947; **126:** 1010–45.

9. Evans E I, Purnell O J, Robinett P W, Batchelor A, Martin M. Fluid and electrolyte requirements in severe burns. *Ann Surg* 1952; **135:** 804–17.

10. Oliveira A. De ambustione. Dissertation. Leyden, 1823.

11. Swan J. Case of a severe burn. *Edinb Med Surg J* 1823; **19:** 344–5.

12. Cooper S. Pathology of burn and scalds. *Lond Med Gazette* 1839; **23:** 837–8.

13. Curling T B. On acute ulceration of duodenum in cases of burn. *Trans R Med Chir Soc Lond* 1842; **25:** 260–81.

14. Coates B H. On burns and scalds. *Phil J M Phys Sc* 1822; **4:** 113–25.

15. Aub J C, Beecher H K, Cannon B, *et al. Management of the Coconut Grove Burns at the Massachusetts General Hospital.* Philadelphia: JB Lippincott Co, 1943.

16. Nikolsky P W. Pinselungen von Verbrennungen mit Gerbsauretinctur. *Deutsch Med Wochenschr* 1888; **14:** 648.

17. McClure R D, Lam C R, Romence H. Tannic acid and the treatment of burns: an obsequy. *Ann Surg* 1944; **120:** 387–98.

18. Bone R C, Sibbald W J, Sprung C L. The ACCP-SCCM consensus conference on sepsis and organ failure. *Chest* 1992; **101:** 1481–2.

19. Fredholm B, Hagermark O. Studies on histamine release from skin and from peritoneal mast cells of the rat induced by heat. *Acta Derm Venereol* 1970; **50:** 273–7.

20. Horakova Z, Beaven M A. Time course of histamine release and edema formation in the rat paw after thermal injury. *Eur J Pharmacol* 1974; **27:** 305–12.

21. Olsson P. Clinical views on the kinin system. *Scand J Clin Lab Invest* 1969; **24:** 123–4.

22. Zimmerman T J, Krizek T J. Thermally induced dermal injury: a review of pathophysiologic events and therapeutic intervention. *J Burn Care Rehabil* 1984; **5:** 193–201.

23. Schirmer W J, Schirmer J M, Naff G B, Fry D E. Systemic complement activation produces hemodynamic changes characteristic of sepsis. *Arch Surg* 1988; **123:** 316–21.

24. Berringer R, Harwood-Nuss A L. Septic shock. *J Emerg Med* 1985; **3:** 475–83.

25. Carmona R, Catalano R, Trunkey D D. Septic shock. In: Shires GT, ed. *Shock and Related Problems.* Edinburgh: Churchill Livingstone, 1984; 156.

26. Sprague R S, Stephenson A H, Dahns T E, Lonigro A J. Proposed role for leukotrienes in the pathophysiology of multiple systems organ failure. *Crit Care Clin* 1989; **5**: 315–29.

27. Wagner B M. A new look at the endothelial cell. *Mod Pathol* 1989; **2:** 186.

28. Border J R. Hypothesis: sepsis, multiple systems organ failure and the macrophage. *Arch Surg* 1988; **123:** 285–6.

29. Pardy B J, Dudley H A F. Post-traumatic pulmonary insufficiency. *Surg Gynecol Obstet* 1977; **144:** 259–69.

30. Effeney D J, Blaisdell F W, McIntyre K E, Graziano C J. The relationship between sepsis and disseminated intravascular coagulation. *J Trauma* 1978; **18:** 689–95.

31. Karyoute S M, Badran D H. Analysis of 100 patients with thermal injury treated in a new burn unit in Amman, Jordan. *Burns* 1989; **15:** 23–6.

32. Linares H A. Autopsy findings in burned children. In: Carvajal H F, Parks D H, eds, *Burns in Children* Chicago: Year Book Medical Publishers, 1988.

33. Linares H A Sepsis, disseminated intravascular coagulation and multi-organ failure: catastrophic events in severe burns. In: Schlag G, Redl H, Siegel J H, Traber D L, eds. *Shock, Sepsis, and Organ Failure.* Berlin: Springer-Verlag, 1991; 370–98.

34. Teplitz C, Davis D, Mason A D, Moncrief J A. Pseudomonas burn wound sepsis. 1. Pathogenesis of experimental pseudomonas burn wound sepsis. *J Surg Res* 1964; **4:** 200–22.

35. Smith R F, Linares H A, Jorgensen J H. Bacteremia and postmortem bacteriology in burned children. *Am J Clin Pathol* 1975; **63:** 502–8.

36. Alkjaersig N, Fletcher A P, Peden J C, Monafo W W. Fibrinogen catabolism in burned patients. *J Trauma* 1980; **20:** 154–9.

37. Curreri P W, Kak A F, Dotin L N, Pruitt B A. Coagulation abnormalities in the thermally injured patient. In: Skinner D B, Ebert P A, eds. *Current Topics in Surgical Research.* New York London: Academic Press, 1970: 401.

38. Eurenius K, Rossi T D, McEuen D, Arnold J, McManus W F. Blood coagulation in burn injury. Proc Soc Exp Biol Med 1974; **147:** 878–82.

39. McManus W F, Eurenius K, Pruitt B A. Disseminated intravascular coagulation in burned patients. *J Trauma* 1973; **13:** 416–22.

40. Bick R L. Disseminated intravascular coagulation and related syndromes: a clinical review. *Semin Thromb Hemost* 1988; **14:** 299–337.

41. Bartlett R H, Fong S W, Marrujo G, Hardeman J, Anderson W. Coagulation and platelet changes after thermal injury in man. *Burns* 1980; **7:** 370–7.

42. Neame P B, Lechago J, Ling E T, Koval A. Thrombotic thrombocytopenic purpura: report of a case with disseminated intravascular platelet aggregation. *Blood* 1973; **42:** 807–14.

43. Watanabe T, Imamura T, Nakagaki K, Tanaka K. Disseminated intravascular coagulation in autopsy cases: its incidence and clinico-pathologic significance. *Pathol Res Pract* 1979; **165:** 311–22.

44. Goris R J A, Boekhorst T P A, Nuytinck J K S, Gimbrere J S F. Multiple-organ failure: generalized autodestructive inflammation? *Arch Surg* 1985; **120:** 1109–15.

45. Mohan N, Leslie K, Sandor G, Douglas L G, Peters W J. Multisystem organ failure in burn patients. *Canadian Trauma Association Meeting, 1988.* Ottawa, September 23–24.

46. Aikawa N, Shinozawa Y, Ishibiki K, Abe O. Clinical analysis of multiple organ failure in burned patients. *Burns* 1987; **13:** 103–9.

47. Demling R H, Wong C, Jin L J, Hechtman H, Lalonde C, West K. Early lung dysfunction after major burns: role of edema and vasoactive mediators. *J Trauma* 1985; **25:** 959–66.

48. Petroff P, Pruitt B A. Pulmonary disease in the burn patient. In: Artz C, Moncrief W, Pruitt B, eds. *Burns, A Team Approach*. Philadelphia: W B Saunders, 1979: 95.

49. Blaisdell F W. Respiratory insufficiency syndrome: clinical and pathological definition. *J Trauma* 1973; **13:** 195–9.

50. Fishman A P. Shock lung: a distinctive nomentity. *Circulation* 1973; **47:** 921–9.

51. Clowes G H A, Zuschneid W, Dragacevic S, Turner M. The nonspecific pulmonary inflammatory reactions leading to respiratory failure after shock, gangrene and sepsis. *J Trauma* 1968; **8:** 899–914.

52. Demling R H. Wound inflammatory mediators and multisystem organ failure. *Progr Clin Biol Res* 1987; **236A:** 523–37.

53. Craddock P R, Hammerschmidt D E, Moldow C F, Yamada O, Jacob H S. Granulocyte aggregation as a manifestation of membrane interactions with complement: possible role in leukocyte margination, microvascular occlusion, and endothelial damage. *Semin Hematol* 1979; **16:** 140–7.

54. Henson P M, McCarthy K, Larsen G L, *et al.* Complement fragments, alveolar macrophages, and alveolitis. *Am J Pathol* 1981; **97:** 93–110.

55. Ognibene F P, Martin S E, Parker M M, *et al.* Adult respiratory distress syndrome in patients with severe neutropenia. *N Engl J Med* 1986; **315:** 547–51.

56. Swank D W, Moore S B. Roles of the neutrophil and other mediators in adult respiratory distress syndrome. *Mayo Clin Proc* 1989; **64:** 1118–32.

57. Craddock P R, Fehr J, Dalmasso A P, Brigham K L, Jacob H S. Pulmonary leukostasis resulting from complement activation of dialyzer cellophane membranes. *J Clin Invest* 1977; **59:** 879–88.

58. Linares H A, Herndon D N, Traber D L. Sequence of morphologic events in experimental smoke inhalation. *J Burn Care Rehabil* 1989; **10:** 27–37.

59. Demling R H. Fluid replacement in burned patients. *Surg Clin North Am* 1987; **67:** 15–30.

60. Redl H, Hallstrom S, Lieners C, Furst W, Schag G. Proteoglysis and lipid peroxidation – two aspects of cell injury in experimental hypovolemic traumatic shock. In: Horl W H, Heidland A, eds, *Proteases II – Potential Role in Health and Disease*. New York: Plenum, 1988: 449–55.

61. Martineau P P, Hartman F W. The renal lesions in extensive cutaneous burns. *JAMA* 1947; **134:** 429–36.

62. Ford W W. On the bacteriology of normal organs. *J Hyg* 1901; **1:** 277–84.

63. Arnold L. Alterations in the endogenous enteric bacterial flora and microbic permeability of the intestinal wall in relation to the nutritional and meterological changes. *J Hypertens* 1929; **29:** 82–116.

64. Berg R D, Garlington A W. Translocation of certain indigenous bacteria from the gastrointestinal tract to the mesenteric lymph nodes and other organs in a gnotobiotic mouse model. *Infect Immun* 1979; **23:** 403–11.

65. Deitch E A, Berg R. Bacterial translocation from the gut: a mechanism of infection. *J Burn Care Rehabil* 1987; **8:** 475–82.

66. Wells C L, Maddaus M A, Simmons R L. Proposed mechanisms for the translocation of intestinal bacteria. *Rev Infect Dis* 1988; **10:** 958–79.

67. Takeuchi A. Electron microscope studies of experimental salmonella infection. *Am J Pathol* 1967; **50:** 109–36.

68. Popiel I, Turnbull P C B. Passage of *Salmonella enteritidis* and *Salmonella thompson* through chick ileocecal mucosa. *Infect Immun* 1985; **47:** 786–92.

69. Bounous G, Menard D, DeMedicis E. Role of pancreatic proteases in the pathogenesis of ischemic enteropathy. *Gastroenterology* 1977, **73:** 102–8.

70. Parks D A, Bulkley G B, Granger D N, Hamilton S R, McCord J M. Ischemic injury in the cat small intestine: role of superoxide radicals. *Gastroenterology* 1982; **82:** 9–15.

71. Ahren C, Haglund V. Mucosal lesions in the small intestine of the cat during low flow. *Acta Physiol Scand* 1973; **88:** 541–50.

72. Baker J W, Deitch E A, Berg R D, Specian R D. Hemorrhagic shock induces bacterial translocation from the gut. *J Trauma* 1988; **28:** 896–906.

73. Deitch E A, Taylor M, Grisham M, Ma L, Bridges W, Berg R. Endotoxin induces bacterial translocation and increases xanthine oxidase activity. *J Trauma* 1989; **29:** 1679–83.

74. Berg R D, Wommack E, Deitch E A. Immunosuppression and intestinal bacterial overgrowth synergistically promote bacterial translocation. *Arch Surg* 1988; **123:** 1359–64.

75. Deitch E A, Maejima K, Berg R. Effect of oral antibiotics and bacterial overgrowth on the translocation of the GI tract microflora in burned rats. *J Trauma* 1985; **25:** 385–92.

76. Inoue S, Wirman J A, Alexander J W, Trocki O, Cardell R R. *Candida albicans* translocation across the gut mucosa following burn injury. *J Surg Res* 1988; **44:** 479–92.

77. Maejima K, Deitch E A, Berg R D. Bacterial translocation from the gastrointestinal tracts of rats receiving thermal injury. *Infect Immun* 1984; **43:** 6–10.

78. Berg R D. Translocation of indigenous bacteria from the intestinal tract. In: Hentges D J, ed. *Human Intestinal Microflora in Health and Diseases*. Orlando: Academic Press Inc, 1983: 333.

79. Ma L, Ma J, Deitch E A, Specian R D, Berg R D. Genetic susceptibility to mucosal damage leads to bacterial translocation in a murine burn model. *J Trauma* 1989; **29:** 1245–51.

80. Teplitz C. The pathology of burns and the fundamental of burn wound sepsis. In: Artz C L, Moncrief J A, Pruitt B A, eds. *Burns: A Team Approach*. Philadelphia: WB Saunders, 1979: 45.

81. Yi-sheng C, Ngao L, Jing-quan S, Yuan-ping L, Davies J W L. Histopathological and ultrastructural changes in liver tissue from burned patients. *Burns* 1985; **11:** 408–18.

82. Hurd T, Lysz T, Dikdan G, McGee J, Rush B F, Machiedo G W. Hepatic cellular dysfunction in sepsis: an ischemic phenomenon? *Curr Surg* 1988; **45:** 114–19.

83. Cano N, Gerolami A. Intrahepatic cholestasis during total parenteral nutrition. *Lancet* 1983; **1:** 985.

84. Phillips M J, Poucell S. Cholestasis: surgical pathology, mechanism, and new concepts. In: Farber E, Phillips M J, Kaufman N, eds. *Pathogenesis of Liver Diseases*. Baltimore: Williams & Wilkins, 1987: 65–94.

85. Linares H A, Beathard G A, Larson D L. Morphological changes of lymph nodes of children following acute thermal burns. *Burns* 1978; **4:** 165–70.

86. Unterharnscheidt F J, Linares H A. Morphological findings in the CNS after thermal burn: a preliminary report. *Proceedings of the Sixth American Burn Association Meeting*. Cincinnatti, 1974: 52.

87. Baggenstoss A H. The pancreas in uremia: a histopathologic study. *Am J Pathol* 1948; **24:** 1003–17.

88. Thorndike L. *A Fifteenth Century Autopsy in Science and Thought in the Fifteenth Century*. Reprint edition. New York: Hafner Publ Co, 1967: 123–32, 290–4.

CHAPTER THIRTY-SEVEN

Pathophysiology of the Burn Scar

Hugo A. Linares

Introduction

Cutaneous wound repair is a complex, multi-step physiologic, biochemical, cellular, and molecular process of restoring the anatomical and biological integrity of damaged skin. Skin, the largest organ of the body, is multistructural and multifunctional and exhibits substantial regional variations. It is composed of two distinct layers of different embryonic origins, the ectodermal vascular epidermis and the vascularized mesodermal dermis, lying over a fibroadipose connective tissue which, in turn, attaches the skin to the underlying musculoskeletal system. Separating, but at the same time binding, the epidermis and dermis is a zone of attachment called the basement membrane or epidermal–dermal junction. This biological complex zone (basal membrane zone) is composed of both ectodermal and mesodermal elements. It forms a specialized bridge which integrates epidermis and dermis, and it contains at least three major matrix molecules (laminin, type IV collagen, and bullous pemphigoid antigen) and provides a functional supporting structure for cellular and extracellular activities.[1]

Restoration of skin continuity requires ectodermal and mesodermal repair with epithelial resurfacing, synthesis of connective tissue, and active centripetal movements aimed at diminishing a defect. The ability to replace destroyed tissue with identical anatomical and functional structures has been lost during the evolutionary process for most mammalian tissues. Only certain tissues with expanding cell population (i.e. liver) or with cell renewal systems (i.e. epithelium) are capable of a certain degree of regeneration. In general, mesodermal injuries will be repaired through a fibroplastic mechanism (scar formation). Clearly, acceptable wound repair will depend not only on the ability of cells to proliferate, but also on the degree of preservation and reconstruction of the stromal architecture.

Wounds and Loss of Tissue

Vertical cutaneous injuries, such as surgical incisions which have a minimal loss of tissue, will essentially heal through the formation of a blood clot (fibronectin, plasma glycoprotein), rapid epithelialization, and fibroblast proliferation. Progressive collagenization and increased strength, which reach normal levels within weeks, will complete the healing process and leave imperceptible scarring, in most cases. On the other hand, cutaneous wounds with a predominant horizontal loss of tissue (ulcerations, lacerations, burns) exhibit a healing which proceeds through a variety of mechanisms according to the extent and level of the involved structures. Superficial epidermal damage, with intact basal membrane, requires only the replacement of epithelial cells. Stimulation of physiologic epimorphic mechanisms of epithelial renewal leads to rapid repair. Lesions involving epidermis and superficial dermis (i.e. deep donor site, superficial partial-thickness burns) which leave intact hair follicles or sweat glands, heal by migration of epithelial cells from the edge of the wound and from epithelial appendages together with a prompt and fairly uncomplicated mesenchymal activity. Burn injuries delay epithelial migration, proliferation, and intercellular adhesions (integrins) by 1–2 weeks; and infection further retards this process. Burn injury may also interfere with the normal sequence of growth factors involved in this form of repair.[2] The combined epidermal and dermal healing may leave minimal or no scarring especially in areas where skin appendages are numerous (i.e. scalp). In full-thickness skin loss where all epithelial sources are destroyed, the reepithelialization occurs only from the edges.

There is a critical level of damage (deep partial-thickness burns) in which mesodermal healing takes between 2 and 6 weeks, and frequently results in abnormal scarring. Most mesenchymal wounds, which are caused by horizontal damage, heal through the formation of granulation tissue. Granulation tissue is a specialized young connective tissue, so called because of its bright red granular surface created by multiple, raised capillary loops which form a structural axis surrounded by cells and extracellular matrix. It is basically a highly cellular, vascular, and fairly organized anatomical, physiologic, and functional structure directed primarily 'to clean' damaged areas (via macrophages), 'to fill' existent gaps (via collagen) and 'to feed' growing active new mesenchymal tissue (via neovessels). It is a very dynamic cellular and extracellular matrix which, in time, will progressively be replaced by a permanent, distinct, mature connective tissue called a scar.[3]

The Burn Wound

Cutaneous repair after burning is accomplished through a series of complex, biological mechanisms. Burns are very peculiar injuries because they force an organism into a tremendous biological task of equilibrating its deranged internal homeostasis and, at the same time, reconstituting its destroyed protective barrier against the external environment. Paradoxically, the same systemic and potentially damaging inflammatory response triggered by extensive thermal destruction of the cutaneous envelope will provide the basic stimulus for the reconstitution of the skin barrier. A burn wound becomes ischemic, hypoxic, and highly edematous; so healing follows a slow course in comparison with other types of wounds.

The immediate first response is to control the damage produced to the vascular system. A hemorrhage is always sensed by the body as a threat. The first reaction is prompt vasoconstriction, platelet aggregation, and activation of the coagulation system. The ensuing response starts a wide spectrum of structural physiologic actions and reactions guided by molecular signals within the frame of a nonspecific inflammatory response. The initial neurohormonal and immune response is followed by release of mediators (cytokines), by macrophages, and by lymphocytes within a wound. With this active intervention of the host environment, cellular and extracellular elements will converge in order to achieve epidermal and mesenchymal closure of the defect followed by a lengthy period of remodeling (maturation) which may last several months or years. Permanent scarring will result.

The Mesenchymal Response

Platelets, in contact with thrombin and subendothelial collagen surrounding a vascular gap, not only contribute to hemostasis but trigger the healing process by releasing a variety of local and circulating growth factors, fibrinopeptides, Willebrand factor VIII, glycoproteins, vasoactive substances, adenosine diphosphate, chemoattractants and other inflammatory mediators.[4,5] A classic inflammatory response involving intravascular and extravascular processes is then evoked. Proteases not only attack the damaged tissue but, as a product of their activity, promote the formation of important peptides which locally and systemically elicit the activity of different systems of defense. Liberated peptides provide the signals for chemotactic attraction of leukocytes, monocytes, and mast cells; they also provide the amino acid essentials for the protein synthesis which is required for the reparative process.

Polymorphonuclear leukocytes, in a rapid response to the messages sent by platelets and also through factors produced by the activation of the complement system, form the first line of defense against local bacterial contamination. Usually within 24–72 hours, the polymorphonuclear cells will gradually be superseded by monocytes which acquire the characteristics of tissue macrophages and become a central mediator of the process. The macrophages not only help to clean a wounded area of undesirable debris and bacteria (including effete neutrophils) but, through the release of biologically active mediators (growth factors, enzymes, reactive oxygen intermediates, prostaglandins, etc.), they stimulate the attraction of the fibroblasts to the area.[6]

It has been demonstrated that activated T lymphocytes, following the influx of neutrophils and macrophages, enter a wound area by day 4 or 5 and become an important part of the modulation of the healing process.[7,8] The polymorphonuclear leukocyte has been claimed to be nonessential to the wound healing process in the absence of bacterial contamination. On the contrary, activated macrophages and T lymphocytes are a consistent part of the repair mechanisms. Macrophages are essential for fibroblast function; the presence of an intact T-cell immune system is essential, at least indirectly, for a normal healing outcome.[9] An adequate balance of monokines and cytokines, which have both stimulatory and inhibitory activity, will lead to a regulated normal repair.[7]

Granulation Tissue

Granulation tissue is the framework for the repair processes and provides provisional support for the resurfacing epithelium.[4–6,10] Fibroblasts, macrophages and new blood vessels form a structural trinity embedded in a loose, gel-like, extracellular matrix of collagen, hyaluronic acid, fibronectin, and other glycosaminoglycans which move into a wound space as a unit under the direction and regulation of orchestrated biomolecular messages.[10] Fibronectin, a glycoprotein found in serum, precedes the appearance of collagen which later is deposited in a fibronectin-bearing matrix. Fibronectin gives direction to migrating processes and disappears as soon as mature collagen bundles are formed.[11] Through a variety of still not well understood mechanisms, an ambivalent activity will promote the growth of this reparative tissue. The same cellular and molecular structures aimed at destroying and eliminating wounded tissue will now change functions and will proceed to a very opposite task, which is the build up of a new connective tissue (cells and extracellular matrix), first as a provisory assurance of tissue continuity and later as a permanent fibrous bridge between the edges of the wound (scarring).

There is increasing evidence that the complex processes involving the formation and activity of granulation tissue, as well as other aspects of wound healing, are highly influenced by a group of multifunctional polypeptides (growth factors, cytokines). These substances may influence *angiogenesis* by transforming growth factor alfa and beta (TGFα, TGFβ), fibroblast growth factor (FGF), tumor necrosis factor alfa (TNFα), or platelet-derived endothelial cell growth factor (PDECGF). They also affect *collagenogenesis* by transforming growth factor beta (TGFβ), platelet-derived growth factor (PDGF), or insulin-like growth factor (IGF). Further, they influence *fibroblast proliferation and activation* via platelet-derived growth factor (PDGF) and macrophage-derived proliferation factor (MDPF). *Epithelial cell proliferation* is altered via epidermal growth factor (EGF), transforming growth factor-alfa (TGFα) and basic fibroblast growth factor (bFGF). These polypeptides can also regulate *chemotaxis* by influencing Interleukin-1 (I1–1) and Interleukin-6 (I1–6) or *contraction* via endothelin-1.[12–14] TGFβ seems to be essential in attracting the right cells to a wound area and promoting the stimulation of angiogenesis as well as a variety of cells involved in wound healing, including epithelial cells and fibroblasts.[15] The TGFβ family of five different peptides seems to have a unique and specific intervention in the building regulation of the extracellular matrix and in control over cell-to-matrix and cell-to-cell interaction mediated by integrin receptors.[16] Multifunctional activities of most of these polypeptides are unclear. At different times or concentrations, they may be stimulators or inhibitors to one another and to other wound healing processes.[17–19]

The 'Feeding' Network

One of the main developing features of granulation tissue is the formation of a capillary network. Capillaries originating as sprouts of proliferating endothelial cells from the vascular net of viable connective tissue, which surrounds the hyperlactated, acidotic, and hypoxic wounded area, form the axis of each of the 'red granules' of the wound bed. The anoxic environment of the wound not only stimulates fibroblasts but induces macrophages to secrete angiogenic factors.[20] The newly formed vessels run predominantly parallel to each other and perpendicular to the open surface of the wound; to some extent, they send off lateral sprouts to their neighbors' capillaries, thereby producing an arced plexus. The development of new capillaries follows a sequence of structural and biochemical steps, beginning with the vasodilation of a preexisting vessel (usually another capillary or a venule). This facilitates the arrival of messages sent through angiogenic factors to stimulate the migration of endothelial cells from the donor vessel. The stimulated endothelial cell produces plasminogen activator and collagenase, which degrade the basement membrane of the vessel wall. The endothelial cells then migrate, proliferate, and mature. In as little as 24–36 hours, it is possible histologically to detect the formation of capillary sprouts and the progressive formation of a capillary tube which includes a new basement membrane and pericytes.[21] The leakiness of the new interendothelial junctions frequently results in edema.[22]

Fibroblasts

Fibroblasts are of the juvenile type, with a large and hyperchromatic nucleus, one or more prominent nucleoli, intense cytoplasmic basophilia and a plump fusiform or stellate appearance. They demonstrate an increased amount of ribonucleoproteins and an active synthesis of proteoglycans and collagen. In the beginning, the fibroblasts are loosely and irregularly arranged and lay down collagen fibers which first run in a predominantly parallel orientation with respect to the neovessels. As the granulation tissue matures and gets older, the new formed collagen fibers tend to be oriented parallel to the surface, at right angles to the direction of the growing neovessels and usually parallel also to the lines of tension. This pattern of orientation is lost on hypertrophic scars as will be described later[23] (**Figure 37.1**). Because of the sequenced growing of the granulation tissue, it is possible to distinguish in the same histological section the younger, superficial, unorganized layer from the progressively dense fibroplastic organized, older and deeper layer. Fibroblasts synthetize many of the components of the extracellular matrix, including glycosaminoglycans (proteoglycans), fibronectin, laminin, and elastic fibers.

Collagen

Collagen, the most common mammalian protein and an essential product of fibroblasts, will undergo structural modifications so as to provide adequate tensile strength. At least 17 types of collagen have been already described. Of those, the most known in skin are the types I, III, IV, V, VI and VII. The fibrillar type I, III, and V, and the beaded filaments type VI, are normal components of dermal collagen. The sheet forming collagen IV, fibrillar type V, anchoring forming collagen VII, and collagen XVII are found at the dermo-epidermal interface.[24,25] Fibrillar collagens I and III are the primary fibroplastic molecules associated with granulation tissue and the development of scars. Type III is already forming within 24 hours after injury, while type I and its precursor molecules can be seen between 4 and 7 days.[26,27] Type III fibrillar collagen is produced first and is the most abundant.[28] The high lactate and low oxygen concentration in the wound alters the normal skin I:III collagen ratio and regulates collagen synthesis and deposition.[29] This is gradually reversed, and as healing progresses, type I collagen becomes predominant. Mature dermal tissue has a normal I:III collagen ratio of 4:1;[30] however, this normal proportion is never achieved by scar tissue.

Proteoglycans

Fibroblasts produce and secrete several complex carbohydrates, and many of them are associated with proteins (glycosaminoglycans/proteoglycans). Proteoglycans are very versatile and striking molecules with essential functions. They interact with other substances and cells, and they bind to several extracellular matrix molecules, cell-to-cell adhesion molecules, and growth factors.[31] Proteoglycans have one or more attached glycosaminoglycan chains covalently bound to a core protein. The core protein molecular structure has been recommended as the base for the classification of proteoglycans.[32] It is possible to differentiate at least five groups according to their molecular sizes and site of activity:[33]

- large extracellular proteoglycans with multiple glycosaminoglycan chains (aggrecan, versican, perlecan);
- small connective tissue proteoglycans with no more than two chains (decorin, biblycan, fibromodulin);
- basement membrane heparan sulfate proteoglycans;
- cell surface proteoglycans (syndecan, betaglycan, thrombomodulin); and
- intracellular proteoglycans (serglycin).

The role of proteoglycans in the wound healing process (i.e. regulation of collagen fibrillogenesis) is currently a subject of great interest.[34,35] Early in granulation tissue, fibroblasts deposit a matrix of fibronectin and hyaluronic acid which promotes cell migration and proliferation. Later, fibroblasts produce collagen and proteoglycan matrix which increase tissue tensile strength and resilience.[6,36] It has been suggested that fibronectin may be essential in the organization of the granulation tissue matrix and may form the scaffold in which collagen is organized, in addition to sending chemotactic signals for neutrophils and macrophages.[37]

Hyaluronic acid is the most abundant glycosaminoglycan present during the first week of healing and has its highest concentration at about 5 days after injury. It is required for fibroblast mitosis.[38] Gradually, the concentration of hyaluronic acid diminishes in favor of dermatan sulfate and chondroitin sulfate (decorin, versican, aggrecan) which peak at about 2 weeks after wounding so as to progressively decline in the following weeks.[39] These macromolecules are an integral part of the healing process and are the proteoglycans which actively participate in the differentiation and stabilization of the connective tissue extracellular matrix.

Contraction

About 1 week post-injury, when fibrillar collagen type I starts to build up the strength of the fibrous tissue, another mechanism commences. Along with efforts to epithelialize a denuded area, an

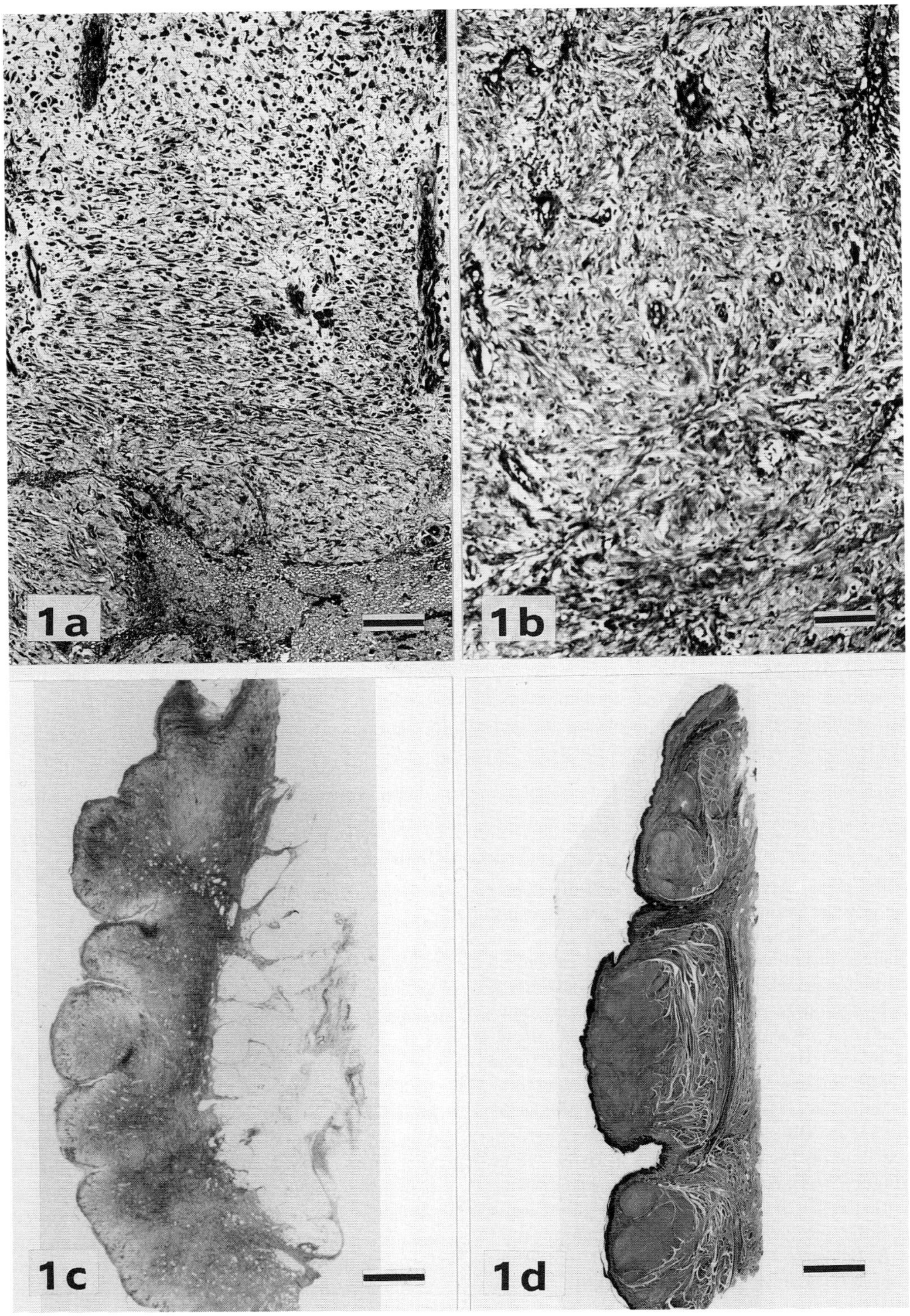

Fig. 37.1 Granulation tissue. (a) Normal healing with a predominant parallel orientation of collagen fibers. Masson stain. Bar=100 μm. (b) Granulation tissue leading to a hypertrophic healing showing the collagen fibers in a predominant whorl-like pattern. Masson stain. Bar=100 μm. (c) and (d) Hypertrophic granulation tissue matching the developed hypertrophic scar depicted in (d). Masson stain c: Bar=1 mm; (d) Bar=2.5 mm.

organism tries also to achieve a spatial reduction of a wounded area by means of centripetal movements of the surrounding skin and shrinkage of the wound contents. This active process of contraction is in contrast to the deforming contracture which is a late end result. The contractile forces, it is suggested, are produced by fibroblasts and their functional and structural phenotypic modulated versions, the myofibroblast.[40,41] A specialized interconnection of intracellular actin-like microfilaments and extracellular fibronectin across the cellular membrane of the myofibroblast form a cohesive complex of cell-to-cell and cell-to-matrix links, called a 'fibronexus'.[42] Contraction should cease when its force is exceeded by the opposite force of the surrounding skin[43] (**Figure 37.2**).

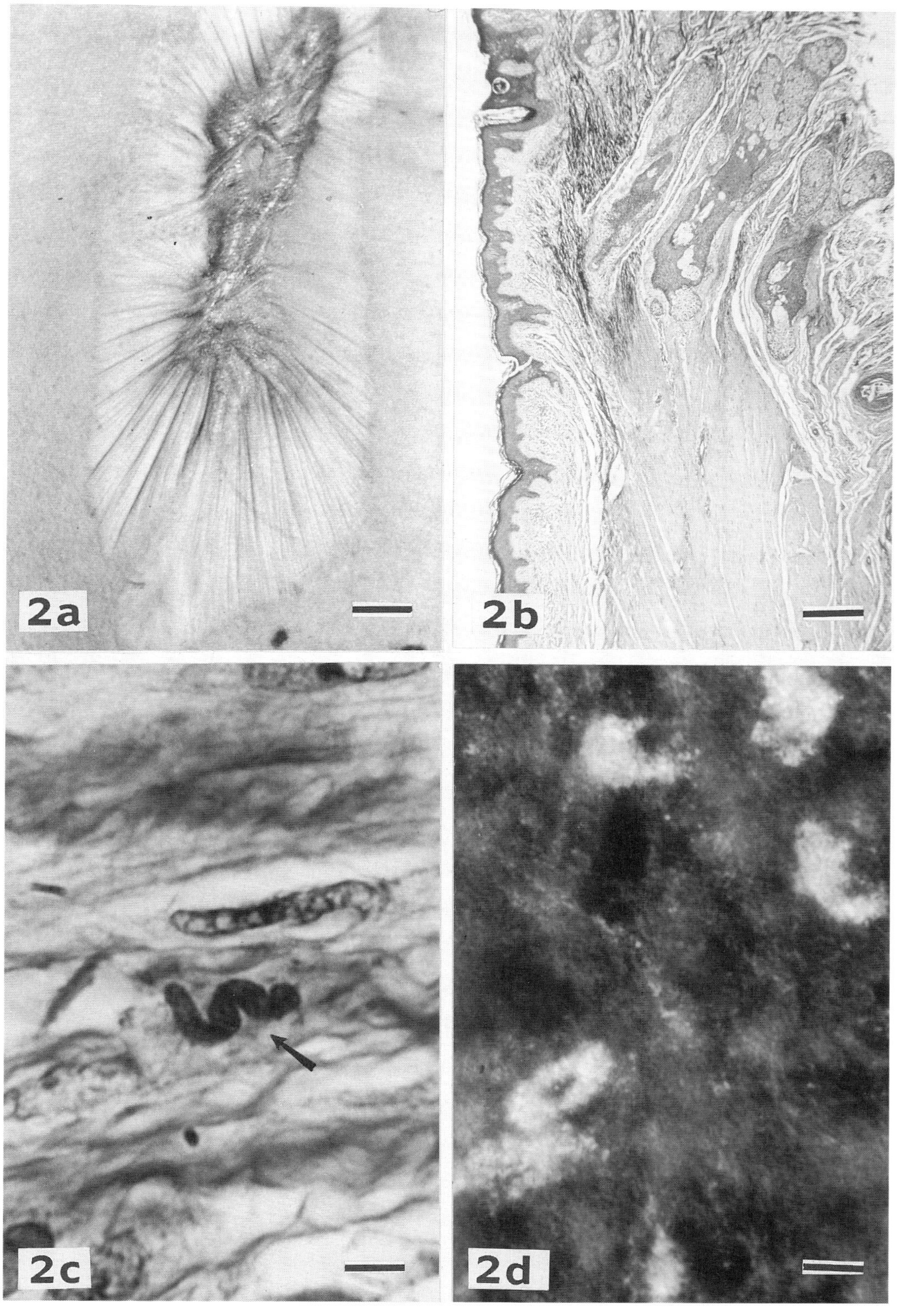

Fig. 37.2 Contraction. (a) Clinical appearance of a scar with clear contraction marks. Bar=1 cm. (b) Histological appearance showing the stretched morphology of the dermal tissue due to contraction. Movat stain. Bar=100 μm. (c) Contracted myofibroblast (arrow) Masson stain. Bar=10 μm. (d) Immunocytoplasmic labeling of myofibroblasts with human antismooth muscle serum followed by antihuman IgG. Immunofluorescence. Bar=10 μm.

The Process of Reepithelialization

Within hours after injury, epithelial cells from wound margins or adnexal structures, if a wound is superficial, will initiate a series of specific mechanisms, directed to cover a new surface. In burns, this epithelial response may be delayed up to several days. The early phases of the reepithelialization process are marked by the centripetal and epibolic migration of epithelial cells from the margins of the wound. This is followed within 24–48 hours by the proliferation of new cells behind the migrating front to provide an additional population of cells to cover the gap.[44] The rate of movement varies from 0.1 mm to 1 mm per day according to local conditions.

The initial stimulus is largely unknown, but several possible mechanisms have been suggested. The migration may be induced by loss of attachment to neighboring damaged cells ('free edge effect'), active contact guidance, or the presence of soluble mediators such as fibronectin, chalones, epibolin, or platelet-derived growth factors. Cellular proliferation may be assisted by epidermal growth factors.[45,46] Through phenotype modulation (cellular metamorphosis), the epidermal basal cells lose their desmosomes and hemidesmosomes; and the intracellular tonofilaments are retracted, form peripheral actin filaments (pseudopodia), and express fibronectin receptors.[46] This change in phenotype, similar to the one observed in cultured epidermal cells, has been called regenerative maturation.[47,48] The cells, without hemidesmosomal links, start their lamellipodial crawling over a provisional matrix of fibrin, fibrinogen, fibronectin, and tenascin while secreting plasminogen activators and collagenases in order to open a way through desiccated tissues. The cells migrate on fibronectin using integrin receptors.[49] Fibronectin and thrombospondin promote keratinocyte mobility while laminin, an adhesion factor in intact epidermis, is lost after wounding.[1] The mechanisms involved in the epithelial movement are controversial and include the 'leapfrog model' (pulling and sliding), whereby cells above and behind the leading cell stream over the latter to attach to the wound bed,[50] or the model of the formation of a chain of cells which advances while individual cells maintain their original position in the chain.[46] It seems that in the skin the epithelial cells migrate in clusters or sheets of cells rather than in a single dissociated cell migration as seen in the monolayer epithelia of the cornea.[44] These cellular activities need a new supporting structure to replace the damaged original basement membrane and facilitate movement. Epithelial cells traverse the surface of granulation tissue by gliding over a new provisional matrix synthesized by themselves.[51] It seems that a fibronectin substrate, a critical component, appears first and is gradually supplemented by collagen IV, heparin sulfate, and, finally, laminin.[52]

Epithelial reparation and granulation tissue formation take place simultaneously. Both of these processes advance through devitalized tissue to cover a wound. This is accomplished by the release from the advancing epithelium of several proteases, including collagenase to denature collagen and plasminogen to dissolve blood clots. Epithelial cells advance more rapidly if the wound bed has adequate humidity.[53,54] For this reason, if enough devitalized tissue still covers the area, the leading cellular front seeks a more favorable environment by gliding underneath the eschar, crust, or scab. The epithelial migration ceases when the advancing epithelium meets its counterpart growing from the opposite direction. The microvillous processes of the encountering cells contact one another and form attachments which could result in contact inhibitions. The cells which were migrating in a lateral motion across the wound surface then regain the normal vertical direction of differentiation toward the surface so as to become cornified cells. Probably laminin is the 'stop signal' to cease the horizontal motion and start ascending vertically.[55] The same migrating epidermal cells, from the wound margins inwards, will reconstitute the basal membrane which is discernible by day 5 and exhibits complete development 2 weeks post-injury.[26]

The Beginning of a Permanent Scar

When the migrating epithelium has completed resurfacing the new connective tissue matrix, the building up of granulation tissue stops. The mechanisms involved in the termination of the healing processes are largely unknown, although the intervention of angiogenic inhibitor factors may be an important feature. The former granulation tissue becomes true scar tissue, and is inelastic and somewhat brittle. The tensile strength, which initially is very low, increases in subsequent weeks as the scar matures, although it never regains the strength of the original tissue.[56]

The remodeling of the collagen meshwork includes increased cross-linking, breakdown activity of collagenases, decrease in glycosaminoglycans, regression of the capillary neovascularity, maintenance of an adequate I:III collagen ratio, and reorientation of collagen fibers in response to mechanical stress. The latter is a very characteristic feature of normal scarring in which collagen bundles of the dermis run in a distinct parallel orientation with respect to the surface of the skin. Clinically, the original redness, elevation, and firm consistency of the new scar tissue gradually evolves into a pale, flat, soft scar tissue which is level with the adjacent skin surface. This phase of 'maturation' includes a gradual replacement of the original scar tissue over a period of at least 6 months.

Wound Healing Interferences

It is obvious that any factor capable of disturbing the complex mechanisms of tissue repair will interfere with adequate wound healing. The more common problems are associated with:

- local factors (impaired circulation, denervation, infection, mechanical stress, foreign bodies, dehiscence, trauma);
- systemic factors (age, nutritional deficits, illness, metabolic disturbances); or
- iatrogenia (surgical technique and material, medications, physicochemical treatments).

These adverse wound conditions will increase the possibility of abnormal healing, either hypotrophic or hypertrophic.

Abnormal Healing

The healing of a wound is a very complex nonspecific process which requires a delicate equilibrium of opposing actions. Cell proliferation must be balanced by cell necrosis, and collagenosis must be paired with collagenolysis, and angiogenesis with capillary obliteration. A resulting scar may be depressed with respect to the surrounding normal skin level, show hypotrophic or even atrophic tissue features, be darker or lighter than the surrounding skin, or become hypertrophic.

The Distinction Between Keloids and Hypertrophic Scars

The differentiation between true, genuine, spontaneous, or idiopathic keloid, and false, spurious, traumatic, or cicatricial keloid was introduced by Alibert almost 200 years ago, leading to a controversy which still continues.[57]

According to Alibert, true keloids have a lancinating, pungent, and burning pruritus with a painful sensation, while false keloids result only from inflammation of a scar after burns or ulcerations. Although this division was generally accepted in the beginning, the false keloid started to be designated as a cicatrix, warty tumor of the cicatrix, or vegetations of the cicatrix. By the end of the 19th century, 'hypertrophic scar' became a differentiating term. It is in Kaposi's chapter on keloids, in 1874,[58] that the differentiation among 'true keloid, cicatricial keloid, and hypertrophied scar' was first made. He stated that scars 'which remain within the limits of the loss of substance of the skin represent so-called hypertroid scars, looking, however, exactly like keloids. Does this kind of scar belong also to the class of false, or cicatricial keloids? Where does keloid cease; and where does hypertrophied scar commence? Or is it probable that the so-called spontaneous keloid is only hypertrophied scar?' Since then, repeated efforts have been made to solve such a controversial issue. Perhaps two of the most currently used criteria of differentiation are that keloids exceed the limits of the initial injury as defined by Kaposi in 1874[58] and that keloids have conspicuous thick, glassy, faintly retractile collagen bundles, as described by Blackburn and Cosman in 1966.[59] Histologic studies show that the growing of scars over the limits of a wound is related not only to the activity of the scar itself but also to the structure and opposing forces of the surrounding normal tissue. This 'trespass' of boundaries may be seen in clinically diagnosed hypertrophic scars as well as in scars clinically classified as keloids. Also, thick, glassy, faintly retractile collagen bundles may be seen in the same histologic section of a scar sharing large areas with collagen bundles of opposite characteristics[60] (**Figure 37.3**). Several biochemical profiles of skin and scar samples have shown that hypertrophic scar and keloid are not distinct pathologic entities, but are similar aberrations with quantitative differences, and keloids show greater deviation from normal healing.[61–63] We support the concept that the differences are essentially quantitative and that keloids are extreme variants of hypertrophic scars. Therefore, no distinction will be made, and thus hypertrophic scars as well as keloids will be termed either as hypertrophic healing or as hypertrophic scars, unless the term keloid is used to maintain a specific reference.

Toward a Hypertrophic Healing

The development of a new mesenchymal matrix in granulation tissue follows a fairly predictable pattern, as was previously described for normal wound healing. At the surface of normal granulation tissue, fibroblasts and collagen fibers have a predominant parallel orientation with respect to the vertical proliferating neovessels. In the lower layer, however, collagen fibers and fibroblasts adopt a transverse orientation with respect to the neovessels and a parallel orientation with respect to the surface of the skin (see **Figure 37.1a**). By the time a wound is completely reepithelialized and the granulation phase is complete, all the collagen fibers of the dermis will present the predominant parallel orientation which is characteristic of normotrophic scars (see **Figure 37.4b**).

In previous works, we have shown that the events differentiating normal healing from hypertrophic healing actually start during the development of granulation tissue and become fairly evident 3–5 weeks after injury.[64,65] One of the most notable differences is the orientation of collagen fibers. If the healing process will result in hypertrophic healing, it is possible to see, in the granulation tissue, a tendency for collagen fibers to run in a haphazard direction with a tendency toward a whorl-like pattern which is characteristic of hypertrophic scars (see **Figure 37.1b**).

Although the cell population of granulation tissue, as seen with light microscopy, does not show qualitative differences between normal and hypertrophic development, they show a marked difference in their cyclic evolution. The structural characteristic of immature connective tissue, which normally disappears within several weeks, will persist for several months if hypertrophic healing develops. In many cases, a chronic inflammatory reaction of variable degree may persist. The collagen pattern, persistent cellularity, abundance and composition of proteoglycans, and the prolonged chronic inflammatory reaction are the most common morphologic features which distinguish hypertrophic healing from normal healing.[66–68]

Clinical Appearance and Histiotypic Organization

Hypertrophic scars are depicted as tumor-like lesions raised above the level of the skin with a wide spectrum of variations in shape, size, color, and consistency. These characteristics usually correspond to the site and extent of an injury, time of evolution, and individual susceptibility. In certain areas (chest, shoulders, lobules of the ears) the hypertrophic healing tends to be prominent, nodular, pedunculated or semipedunculated, round or oval, smooth and shiny, hard, and somewhat elastic. In other areas, it usually has an irregular surface and is rarely elevated more than 15–20 mm above the level of the surrounding skin. The edges are usually prominent and end abruptly, sometimes with fingerlike or chain-like prolongations. Initially, a scar is red or pink (so-called immature); but after a period of time, months or even years, the scar flattens, softens, and blanches (maturation). In immature scars, redness and turgidity are due to increased active vascularity. Immature scars sometimes display a minute pinkish, bluish, or purplish superficial net of small blood vessels. The scar does not adhere to the subcutaneous tissue and appears to grossly exceed the limits of the original injury[60] (see **Figure 37.3b**).

Histologically, the appearance of a scar depends on the evolutionary state during which a sample is taken. Also, scars from different anatomical sites display histologic differences. Those located on ears or shoulders show very broad, thick collagen fibers more frequently than scars from other sites. It is also possible to observe that there is no 'invasion' of surrounding normal tissues but that the overgrown healing really pushes apart the surrounding normal tissue without invading it. The gross anatomy appearance of lesions which exceed the limits of the original injury appears to be produced by tumor-like growth pushing the epithelium upward. This suggests that the clinical appearance will depend, in part, on the forces generated by the opposing superficial layers of the skin in the area and on the skin's resistance to deformation.

The histologic appearance of the epidermis is also variable. It many appear hyperplastic, with visible rete ridges, or thin and smooth. The typical histologic features of the hypertrophic healing reside in the reticularis layer of the dermis. In early stages, there is hypercellularity (fibroblasts, myofibroblasts) and hypervascularity. The collagen fibers run in curvilinear, whorl-like arrangements which, in most cases, progress to distinct nodular forms. Whorls and nodules may be seen in the same histologic section[66] (**Figure 37.4**). These structures never involve the subcutaneous tissue, from which they are often separated by somewhat compact parallel bands of connective tissue with nearly normal characteristics. The increased cellular population is composed of young, active fibroblasts and myofibroblasts. Mast cells appear increased over the number observed in normal skin. Plasma cells and lymphocytes are usually present at the beginning of the formation of a scar and form a perivascular cuff, which may persist for a long time as scattered foci or chronic inflammation. The vascular structure is prominent and the capillary network appears to follow the arrangement of the collagen fibers. Skin appendages are atrophic, destroyed, or displaced by the scar. At times they do not slough, but elicit a foreign-body reaction. Usually, no elastic tissue can be found except in the papillary areas of the dermis and in the normal dermal areas surrounding the scar. The interstitium shows a significant amount of ground substance (glycosaminoglycans), which has been shown to contain an elevated amount of chondroitin-4-sulfate.[68]

With time, the thickened hyaline fibers of nodules and whorls become elongated and elastic fibers reappear. This is indicative of a regression pattern, which proceeds toward 'mature' scar. The reorientation of the collagen fibers in a parallel arrangement, as

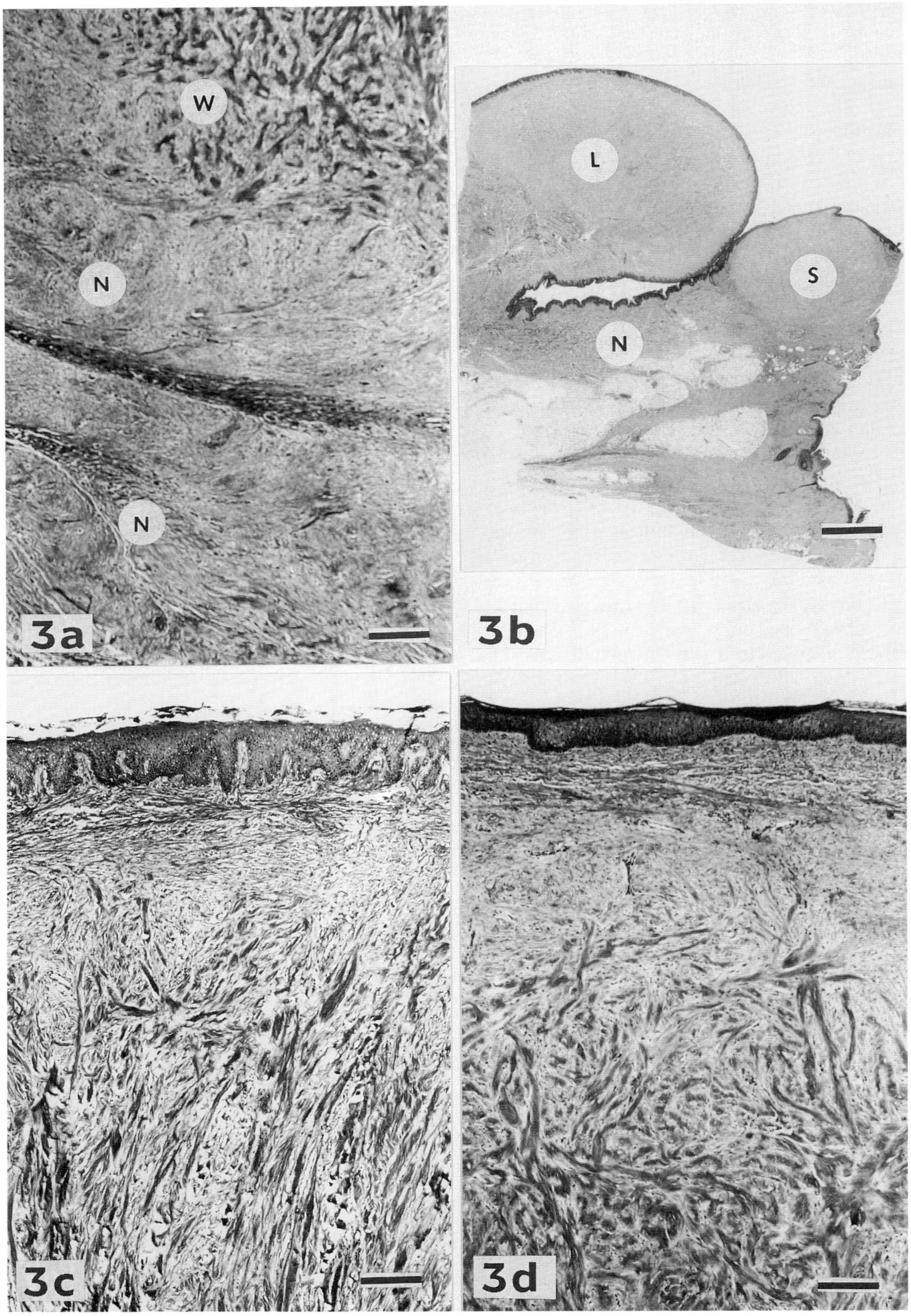

Fig. 37.3 Scars differentiation. (a) Hypertrophic healing showing two different collagen patterns in the same section: whorls (W) and nodules (N). Masson stain. Bar=100 µm. b. Two hypertrophic scars (S and L) bridged by a section of normal skin (N). The hypertrophic scar (S) shows a moderate expansion above the level of the normal skin (N) while the hypertrophic scar (L) shows the excessive tumor-like growth producing the 'trespass' of the original limits of the wound. H E stain. Bar=3 mm. (c) and (d) Hypertrophic healing with rete ridges (c) compared to a hypertrophic healing without rete ridges as depicted in (d) Masson stain. Bar=100 µm.

found with nonhypertrophic healing, is accompanied by a progressively reduced number of fibroblasts and myofibroblasts, and a pronounced decrease in vascularization, which corresponds to the flattening, blanching, and softening of a mature scar described above. Tissue structure never recovers its original appearance.

Scanning Electron Microscopy

Under a scanning electron microscope (SEM), nodules appear as fused masses of tissue in stark contrast to the adjacent collagen filaments and fibers. The individual collagen filaments present in normal skin are rarely seen. The dermal matrix appears as an adhesive

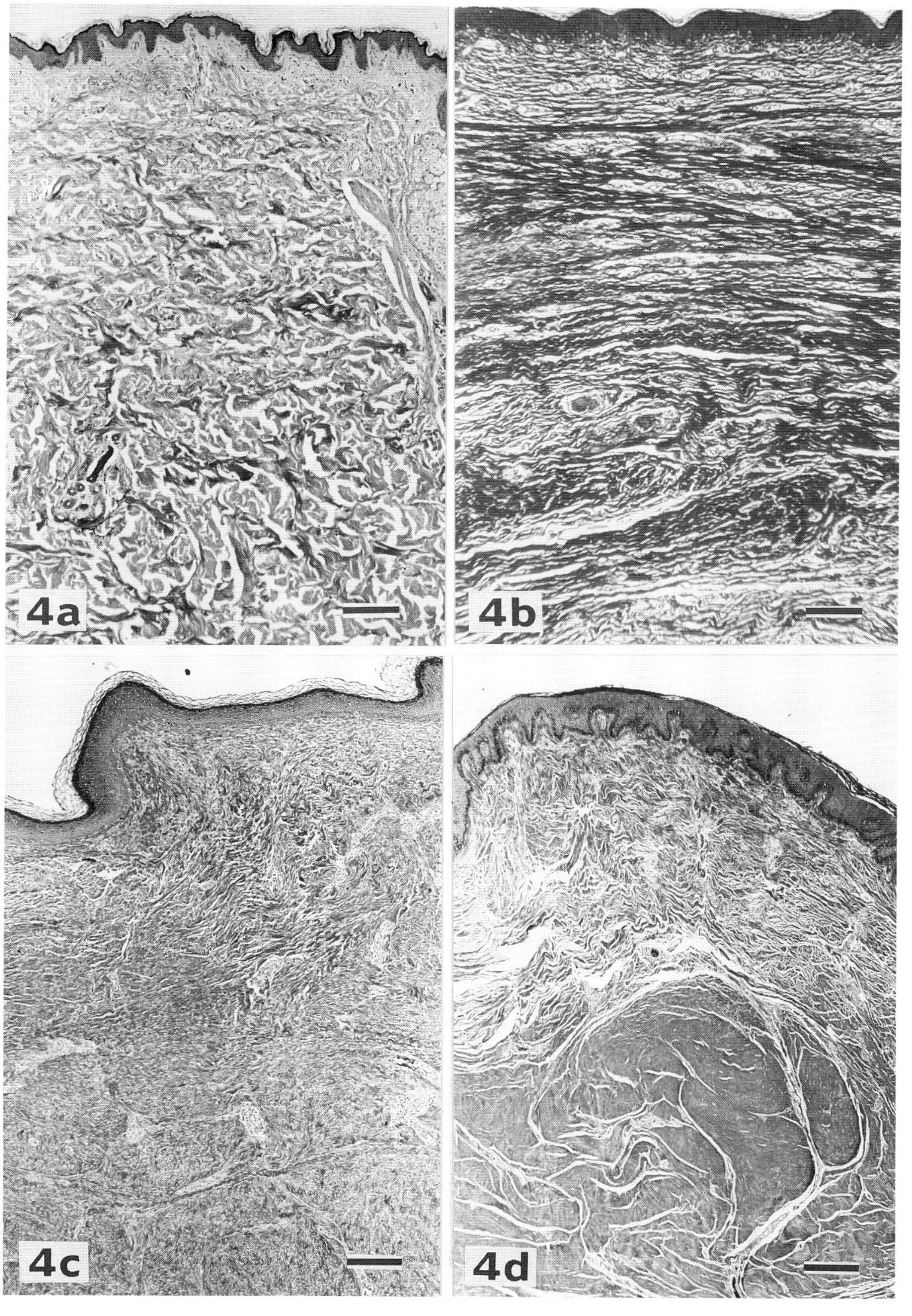

Fig. 37.4 Histomorphology. (a) Normal skin. Dermal collagen in a tridimensional regular pattern. Masson stain. Bar=200 μm. (b) Normotrophic healing. Dermal collagen in a parallel orientation. Masson stain. Bar=100 μm. (c) Hypertrophic healing. Dermal collagen in a predominant whorl-like pattern. Masson stain. Bar=100 μm. (d) Hypertrophic healing. Dermal collagen in a predominant nodular pattern. Masson stain. Bar=100 μm.

mass of material, as though the filaments were 'glued' together. Fiber diameter is about one-half to three-quarters that of normal skin, and cross-stranding is frequent. The large bands of collagen appear also to be oriented in every direction except directly across the wound.[69,70]

Transmission Electron Microscopy

The nodules of active hypertrophic scars consist of tightly packed collagen with a reduced amount of total interstitial space. The collagen filaments have a predominant diameter of 600 Å (60 nm).

The lumen of the vessels is often partially or completely occluded, and the basal lamina in most of the vessels is greatly thickened. In early stages, the number of fibroblasts and myofibroblasts is significant. Fibroblasts have an active appearance, with vast arrays of rough endoplasmic reticulum and Golgi membranes. Myofibroblasts appear with folded or grooved nuclei containing fine contractile filaments, and with a variable number of free ribosomes, mitochondria, glycogen, vacuoles, and pinocytotic vesicles. The structural appearance of hypertrophic scars under electron microscopy parallels that under light microscopy at any stage of hypertrophic healing.[70]

In Search of Etiopathogenic Explanations

The biological mechanisms responsible for the deviation of the normal healing process toward an excessive reparative response are still elusive. The lack of a reproducible laboratory animal models adds a very frustrating circumstance. On the other hand, increasing technology and firm interest from many researchers are providing, piece by piece, the elements which hopefully will solve the hypertrophic healing puzzle.

The Collagen/Fibroblast Factor

Evidently, the most visible feature of a hypertrophic scar is the excess of collagen deposition, suggesting that the essential balance between collagen synthesis and degradation is missing. An increased proline hydroxylase activity and an increased collagenase activity insufficient to counteract the exuberant collagen synthesis have been described by many authors.[71–73] Despite equal or increased levels of activity of lysyl oxidase, it seems that hypertrophic scars have a decreased content of highly cross-linked collagen and also an increased amount of soluble collagen.[63,74,75] A proper degradation of collagen may be inhibited by the action of α_1-antitrypsin and α_2-macroglobulin which were found in the extracellular matrix of hypertrophic scars.[71,76] Some researchers report a significant increase in the I:III collagen ratio,[77] while others describe just the opposite.[78,79] Since the report from Conway *et al.*[80] which describes the characteristics of cultured fibroblasts in keloids and hypertrophic scars, an increased number of workers have followed this line of research. Diegelmann[81] shows that cultured keloid fibroblasts synthesize two to three times more collagen than normal skin fibroblasts, without significant differences in collagen degradation rate.

An intriguing observation was made by Abergel *et al.*[77] that the increase in collagen synthesis was not a constant characteristic of keloids. It was speculated that the heterogeneous population of normal skin fibroblasts which can strongly differ in the amount of collagen synthesized among them may be also reflected in keloid fibroblast cultures. Thus, it may be that keloids have a normal or a very high production of collagen.[82,83] Although the growth of keloid fibroblasts is normal, the cells seem to be modulated to some specific function, such as the production of more collagen.[81] Cultures with an excessive production of collagen may also have high levels of type 1 collagen-specific mRNA which suggest a loss of regulatory control at the transcriptional level.[77,82]

Two conflicting reports of similar studies raise some speculation about the possibility of racial factors and also reflect the concept that production of collagen is not the sole problem in hypertrophic healing. Procollagen synthesis was found to be increased in five of nine keloid fibroblast cultures from black patients,[77] while, despite increased levels of intracellular prolyl-4-hydroxylase and glucosyltransferase, a normal synthesis was found in eight of nine keloid fibroblast cultures from white patients.[83] The initial rate of collagen synthesis in hypertrophic scars is about twice that in normotrophic scars and fell to the same level as in normal scars about 2–3 years after injury.[84]

The Glycosaminoglycan/Proteoglycan Factor

Proteoglycans affect the ultimate physical characteristic of the mature collagen within a scar because of their intervention in the extracellular formation of collagen fibrils. They influence the aggregation of collagen monomers.[85] There is evidence from a variety of studies that the composition of glycosaminoglycans and proteoglycans in wound healing and in hypertrophic healing differs from normal skin. While, in normal skin, human dermis shows a much greater amount of decorin than chondroitin sulfate proteoglycans, the reverse occurs in granulation tissues and scars.[86] Particularly, chondroitin-4-sulfate has been identified as the main contributor to the striking increase of proteoglycan levels in hypertrophic scars.[68,87] It has also been demonstrated that the strong association between collagen and proteoglycans in hypertrophic scars may prevent collagenase from breaking down collagen. The excessive presence of chondroitin-4-sulfate may contribute to the overabundance of collagen deposition which is characteristic of hypertrophic scars.[67,88] Furthermore, it has been observed that, in hypertrophic scars, there is a persistent presence of a perivascular cuff of variable density, mainly composed of lymphocytes[60,66] and that the proteoglycan associated with this perivascular T-cell infiltration is mainly chondroitin-4-sulfate.[89] Fibroblasts derived from hypertrophic scars incorporated proportionally more radiolabeled precursors into chondroitin sulfate and hyaluronic acid *in vitro* than did normal skin fibroblasts.[90]

Other Factors

The immunological explanation has been explored by several researchers. Chytilova *et al.* were able to produce hypertrophic healing in rabbits, during the course of autoimmune disease, by the repeated injection of lyophilized autologous skin.[91] People who carry HLA-B14 or HLA-Bw16 antigens have been shown to have a greater risk of developing hypertrophic healing;[92,93] but it was also found that there were no significant differences in the incidence of HLA-A and B antigens in keloid and nonkeloid formers.[94] Abdalla-Osman *et al.* developed a sebum autoimmune theory.[95] Other researchers found antinuclear antibodies directed against fibroblasts in those who form keloids and increased levels of IgA, IgG, and IgM.[96] Immunoperoxidase techniques performed on hypertrophic scar sections showed an anomalous expression of HLA class II molecules on keratinocytes and fibroblasts and dense infiltrates of IL-2R positive cells and Langerhans (CD1+) cells.[97,98] Fibroblasts from hypertrophic healing were shown as having an increased fibronectin production, suggesting the presence of specific mechanisms controlling fibronectin expression.[99] A heavy fibronectin deposition was found to be predominantly located in the nodular structures of hypertrophic healing sections.[100] A recent study showed an increased production of IL-6, TNFα and IFN in hypertrophic healing, suggesting that the altered levels of immunoregulatory cytokines may play a significant role in the overproduction of collagen.[101] It has been also suggested that the excessive and inappropriate action of TGFβ may promote abnormal healing.[102–105]

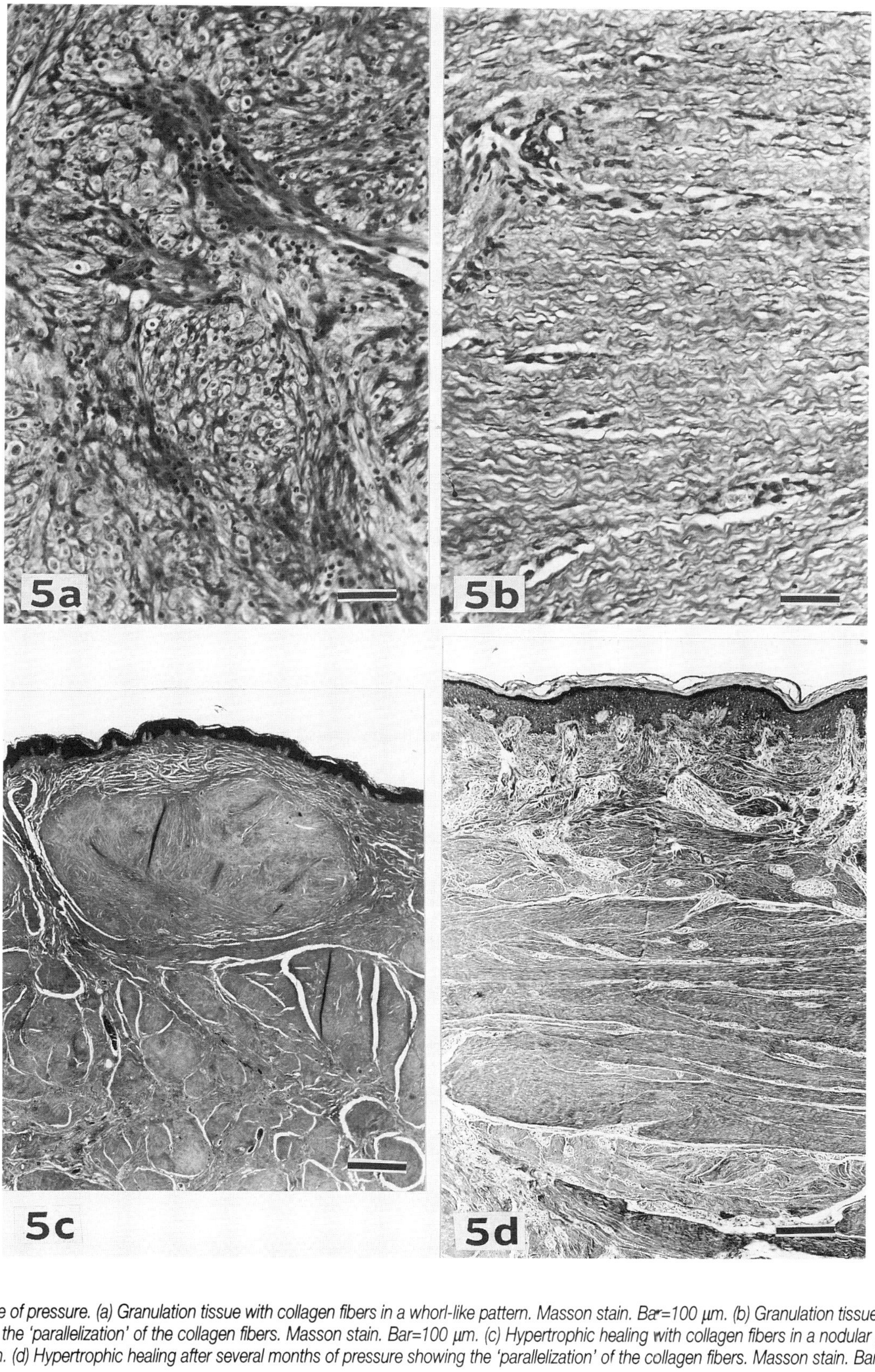

Fig. 37.5 Influence of pressure. (a) Granulation tissue with collagen fibers in a whorl-like pattern. Masson stain. Bar=100 μm. (b) Granulation tissue after 25 days of pressure showing the 'parallelization' of the collagen fibers. Masson stain. Bar=100 μm. (c) Hypertrophic healing with collagen fibers in a nodular pattern. Masson stain. Bar=250 μm. (d) Hypertrophic healing after several months of pressure showing the 'parallelization' of the collagen fibers. Masson stain. Bar=150 μm.

The Search for Solutions

Therapeutic solutions to hypertrophic scars have been met with the same degree of confusion and controversy as their morphologic and etiopathogenic descriptions. Proposed solutions have been innumerable, but in most instances frustration has been the net result. Unfortunately, the present state of knowledge of the etiopathogenic mechanisms responsible for hypertrophic healing is still inadequate to formulate a sound biological basis for a routinely effective treatment. It is possible to achieve, if not ideal, at least satisfactory results with several different approaches using surgical, pharmacologic, and physical methods. Surgery, corticoids, and

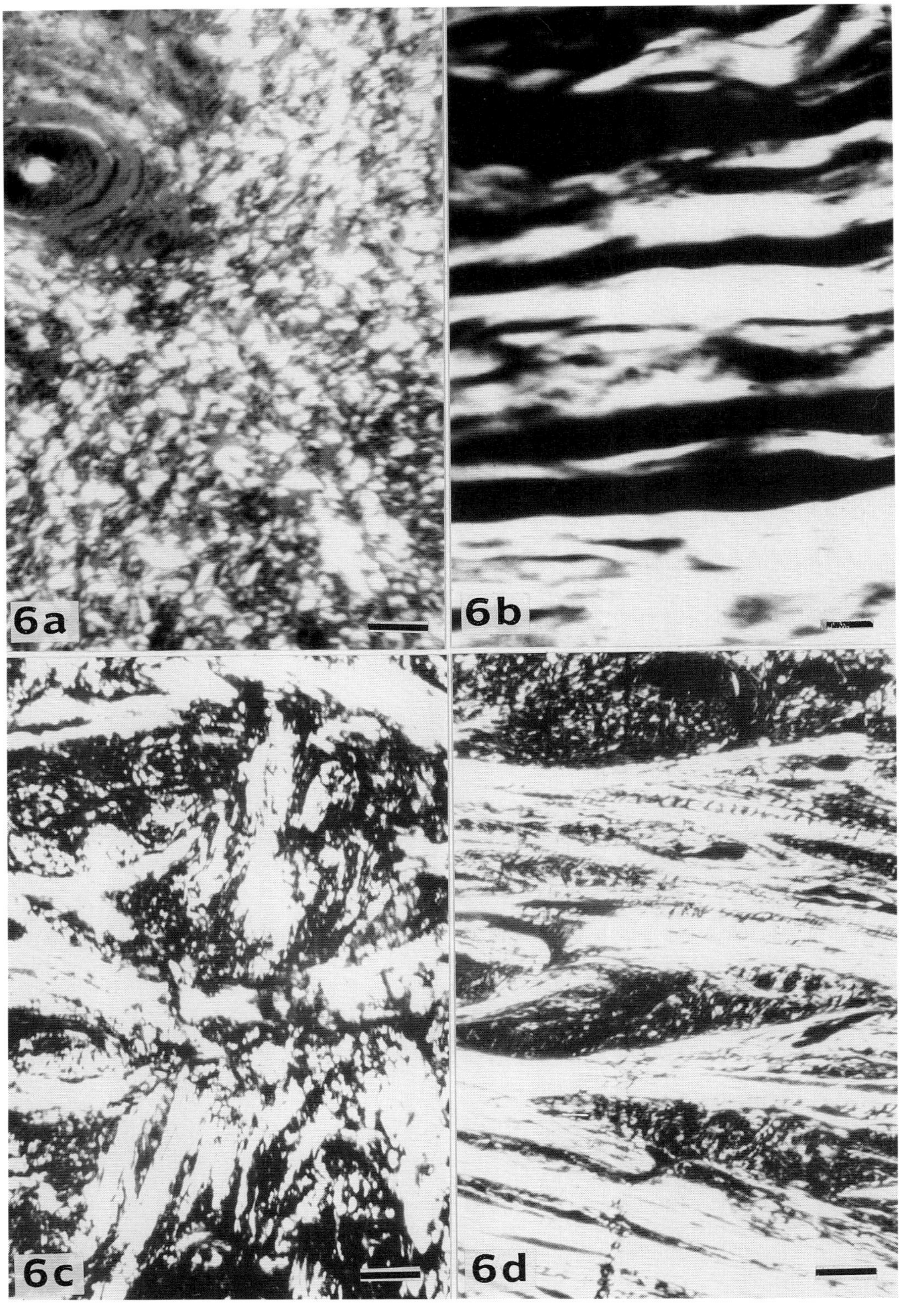

Fig. 37.6 Polarized light pictures of collagen fibers depicting (a) the tridimensional pattern of collagen in normal skin, (b) the parallel orientation in normotrophic scars, (c) the whorl-like arrangement in hypertrophic scars, and (d) the 'parallelization' of collagen fibers after pressure. (a)–(d) Bar=200 μm.

pressure, alone or in combination, are currently the most universally used methods of treatment.

Because of the altered disposition of collagen fibers in dermal hypertrophic healing and the possibility of modifying it by mechanical methods, a special consideration concerning the use of pressure may be worthwhile (**Figure 37.5**). The influence of mechanical forces on the clinical course of hypertrophic scarring has been known for centuries, although it was not until recent years that its use was particularly stressed. As early as in the sixteenth century, Ambroise Paré advised: 'if the scar be too big, or high, it shall be plained by making convenient ligation and straight binding to the part a Plate of Lead rubbed over with Quick Silver'.[106] It was not until the early 1970s that the use of pressure for the treatment of hypertrophic scars and contractures after burns became a standard

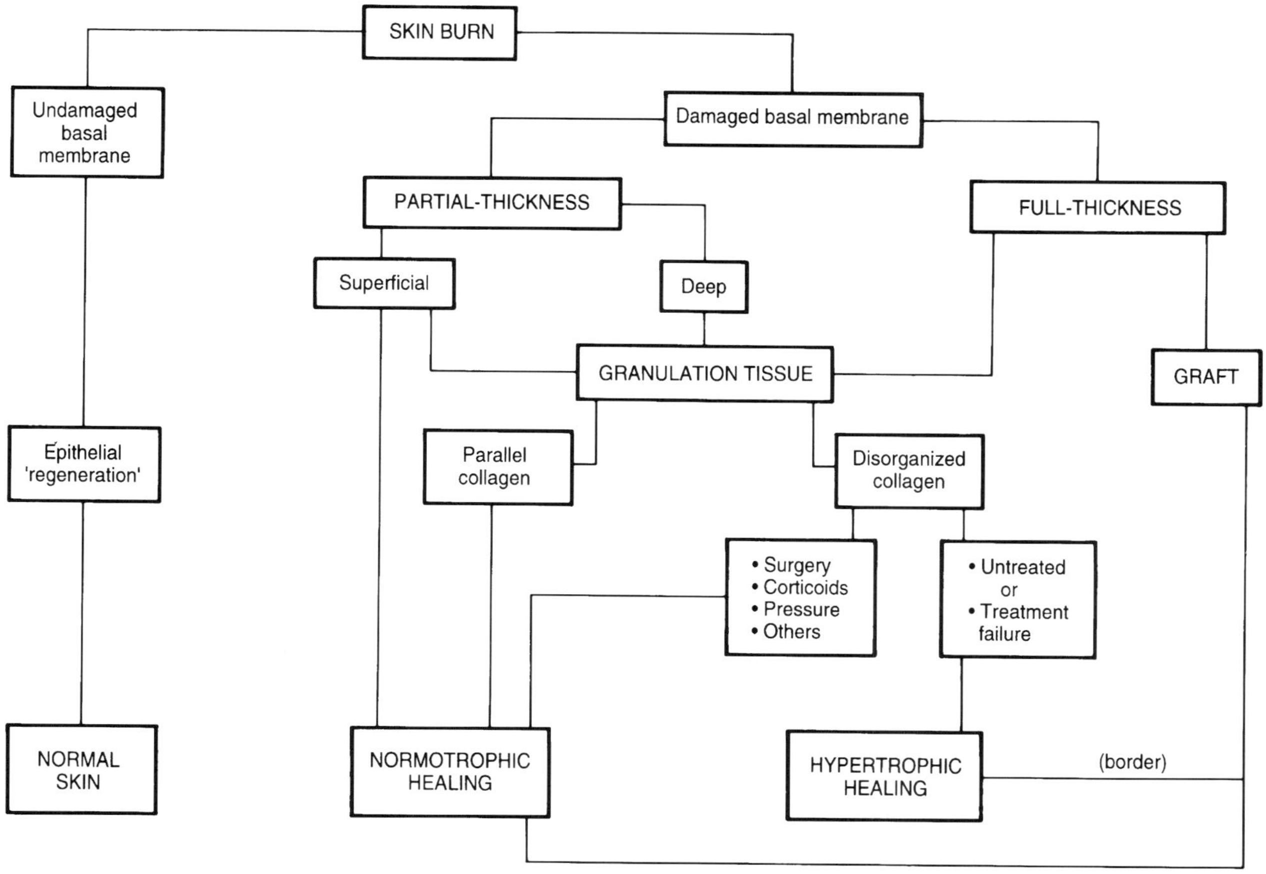

Fig. 37.7 The healing of skin after a burn injury.

treatment in every burn facility. This universal use of pressure originated and was promoted by the Shriners Burns Institute at Galveston.[106] As was described in the preceding pages, a granulation tissue showing collagen fibers in a disorganized, whorl-like arrangement will develop into hypertrophic scarring. If pressure is applied for a variable period of time, however, the collagen fibers will modify their disorganized orientation and will adopt a definite parallel arrangement which is characteristic of the pattern of the granulation tissue which leads to normotrophic healing. Likewise, under constant pressure, the whorl-like arrangement of collagen fibers and nodular formation seen in immature hypertrophic scars assumes a progressive predominantly parallel arrangement similar to that found in normotrophic scars (**Figure 37.6**). Constant pressure will decrease the vascularity, decrease the tissue partial pressure of oxygen, decrease the amount of proteoglycans, and decrease the cellular response as well as the collagen deposition, **Figure 37.7**.[107–110]

Toward the Future

Recent progress in molecular biology has shown that many cell functions are brought about by an interaction among macromolecules. The binding between macromolecules, therefore, has far-reaching physiologic implications. The study of proteoglycans in hypertrophic scars can be of great interest because the organization of collagen fibrils in tissues may be related to amounts and kinds of proteoglycans, and because the binding of proteoglycans to collagen can influence fibril formation.

Research should include the study of factors which influence the structure, migration, function, and modulation of the cells which control the synthesis and degradation of the intercellular matrix. The immunologic and genetic interference should be thoroughly explored. Biochemical analysis and structural events could be important in determining the role of the sulfate glycosaminoglycans in the development and aggregation of collagen fibers. Several possible mechanisms might be involved in producing the excessive amount of collagen deposition which is characteristic of these scars including: an actual increase in the rate of collagen synthesis; the presence of inhibitors for the enzymatic breakdown of collagen and/or glycosaminoglycans; the absence or defective production of the specific enzymes; the presence of physical barriers opposing a proper enzymatic attack; growth activity promoted by sulfated proteoglycans; or other causes, yet unknown.

References

1. Gamelli R L. Wound healing. In: Gamelli R L, Dries D J, eds. *Trauma 2000*. Austin: R G Landes Company, 1992: 139–45.

2. Dover R & Wright N A. The cell proliferation kinetics of the epidermis. In: Goldsmith L A, ed. *Physiology, Biochemistry, and Molecular Biology of the Skin*. New York: Oxford University Press, 1991: 239–65.

3. Larson D L, Abston S, Dobrkovsky M, *et al. The Prevention and Correction of Burn Scar Contracture and Hypertrophy.* Galveston: Shriners Burns Institute, 1973: 1–21.

4. Kloth L C, Miller K H. The inflammatory response to wounding. In: Kloth L C, McCulloch J M, Feedar J A, eds. *Wound Healing: Alternatives in Management*. Philadelphia: F A Davis Company, 1990: 3–13.

5. Knighton D R, Fiegel V D. Regulation of cutaneous wound healing by growth factors and the microenvironment. *Invest Radiol* 1991; **26:** 604–11.

6. Clark R A F. Cutaneous wound repair. In: Goldsmith L A, ed. *Physiology, Biochemistry, and Molecular Biology of the Skin*. New York: Oxford University Press, 1991: 576–601.

7. Barbul A. Immune aspects of wound repair. *Clin Plast Surg* 1990; **17:** 433–42.

8. Efron J E, Frankel H L, Lazarou S A, Wasserkrug H L, Barbul A. Wound healing and T-lymphocytes. *J Surg Res* 1990; **48:** 460–63.

9. Regan M C, Barbul A. Immune control of wound healing. In: Gamelli R L, Dries D J, eds. *Trauma 2000*. Austin: R G Landes Company, 1992: 146–50.

10. Hunt T K. Physiology of wound healing. In: Clowes G H A, ed. *Trauma, Sepsis and Shock*. New York: Marcel Dekker. Inc, 1988: 443–71.

11. Lambert W C, Cohen P J, Klein K M, Lambert M W. Cellular and molecular mechanisms in wound healing: selected concepts. *Clin Dermatol* 1984; **2:** 7–23.

12. Appleton I, Tomlinson A, Chander C L, Willoughby D A. Effects of endothelin-1 on croton oil-induced granulation tissue in rat: a pharmacological and immunohistochemical study. *Lab Invest* 1992; **67:** 703–10.

13. Kingsnorth A N, Slavin J. Peptide growth factors and wound healing. *Br J Surg* 1991; **78:** 1286–90.

14. Dijke P T, Iwata K K. Growth factors for wound healing. *Biotechnology* 1989; **7:** 793–8.

15. Schultz G, Bennett N, Rotatori S, Macaully S, Moser M. EGF and TGF-β in wound healing: analysis of wound fluids and effects of exogenous factors on wound healing. *J Cell Biol* 1993; **S17E:** 109.

16. Roberts A B, Flanders K C, Heine U I. Transforming growth factor-β multifunctional regulator of differentiation and development. *Phil Trans R Soc Lond B* 1990; **327:** 145–54.

17. Sporn M B, Roberts A B. Peptide growth factors are multifunctional. *Nature* 1988; **332:** 217–18.

18. Hunt T K, La Van F B. Enhancement of wound healing by growth factors. *N Engl J Med* 1989; **321:** 111–12.

19. Hunt T K. Wound fluid: the growth environment. In: Barbul A, Caldwell M D, Eaglstein W H, *et al.*, eds. *Clinical and Experimental Approaches to Dermal and Epidermal Repair: Normal and Chronic Wounds*. New York: Wiley-Liss, Inc, 1991: 223–30.

20. Anderson G R, Stoler D L. Anoxia, wound healing, VL30 elements, and the molecular basis of malignant conversion. *Bioessays* 1993; **15:** 265–72.

21. Folkman J, Brem H. Angiogenesis and inflammation. In: Gallin J I, Goldstein I M, Snyderman R, eds. *Inflammation: Basic Principles and Clinical Correlates*. New York: Raven Press, 1992: 821–39.

22. Schoefl G I. Studies of inflammation. III. Growing capillaries: their structure and permeability. *Virchows Arch Pathol Anat* 1963; **337:** 97–104.

23. Linares H A, Kischer C W, Dobrkovsky M, Larson D L. The histiotypic organization of the hypertrophic scar in humans. *J Invest Dermatol* 1972; **59:** 323–31.

24. Claudy A L. Les Collagenes. *Ann Dermatol Venereol* 1988; **115:** 767–71.

25. Uitto J, Christiano A M, Chung-Honet L C, Greenspan D S, Li K, Tamai K. Molecular complexity of the cutaneous basement membrane zone: perspectives on wound healing. *J Cell Biol* 1993; **S17E:** 109.

26. Eisenmenger W, Nerlich A, Gluck G. Die Bedeutung des Kollagens bei der Wundaltersbestimmung. *Z Rechtsmed* 1988; **100:** 79–100.

27. Hopkinson I. The extracellular matrix in wound healing: collagen in wound healing. *Wounds* 1992; **4:** 124–32.

28. Gay S, Viljanto J, Raekallio J, Penttinen R. Collagen types in early phases of wound healing in children. *Acta Chir Scand* 1978; **144:** 205–11.

29. Hunt T K. The physiology of wound healing. *Ann Emerg Med* 1988; **17:** 1265–73.

30. Peakcock E E, Cohen I K. Wound healing. In: McCarthy L, ed. *Plastic Surgery*. Philadelphia: W B Saunders, 1990: 161–85.

31. Ruoslahti E. Proteoglycans in cell regulation. *J Biol Chem* 1989; **264:** 13369–72.

32. Kjellen L, Lindahl U. Proteoglycans: structures and interactions. *Annu Rev Biochem* 1991; **60:** 443–75.

33. Templeton D M Proteoglycans in cell regulation. *Crit Rev Clin Lab Sci* 1992; **29:** 141–84.

34. McPherson J M, Piez K A. Collagen in dermal wound repair. In: Clark RAF, Henson P M, eds. *The Molecular and Cellular Biology of Wound Repair*. New York: Plenum Press, 1988: 471–96.

35. Sugumaran G, Baldwin C T. The diversity of proteoglycans. *Wounds* 1992; **4:** 248–55.

36. Hascall V C, Hascall G K. Proteoglycans. In: Hay E D, ed. *Cell Biology of Extracellular Matrix*. New York: Plenum Press, 1981: 39–63.

37. Grinnell F. Fibronectin and wound healing. *J Cell Biochem* 1984; **26:** 107–16.

38. Turley E A, Torrance J. Localization of hyaluronate-binding protein on motile and non-motile fibroblasts. *Exp Cell Res* 1984; **16:** 17–28.

39. Bently J P. Rate of chondroitin sulfate formation in wound healing. *Ann Surg* 1967; **165:** 186–91.

40. Gabbiani G, Ryan G D, Majno G. Presence of modified fibroblasts in granulation tissue and their possible role in wound contraction. *Experientia* 1971; **27:** 549–53.

41. Ehrlich H P. Wound closure: evidence of cooperation between fibroblasts and collagen matrix. *Eye* 1988; **2:** 149–57.

42. Singer II. The fibronexus: a transmembrane association of fibronectin-containing fibers and bundles of 5 nm filaments in hamster and human fibroblasts. *Cell* 1979; **16:** 675–85.

43. Pollack S V. The wound healing process. *Clin Dermatol* 1984; **2:** 8–16.

44. Stenn K S, Malhotra R. Epithelialization. In: Cohen I K, Diegelmann R F, Lindblad W J, eds. *Wound Healing*. Philadelphia: W B Saunders, 1992: 115–27.

45. Goslen J B. Wound healing for the dermatologic surgeon. *J Dermatol Surg Oncol* 1988; **14:** 959–72.

46. Daly T J. The repair phase of wound healing – re-epithelialization and contraction. In: Kloth L C, McCulloch J M, Feedar J A, eds. *Wound Healing: Alternatives in Management*. Philadelphia: F A Davis Company, 1990: 14–30.

47. Hennings H, Michael D, Cheng D, Steinert P, Holbrook K, Yuspa S A. Calcium regulation of growth and differentiation of mouse epidermal cells in culture. *Cell* 1980; **19:** 245–54.

48. Mansbridge J N, Knapp A M. Changes in keratinocyte maturation during wound healing. *J Invest Dermatol* 1987; **89:** 253–63.

49. Grinnell F. Fibronectin and wound healing. *Am J Dermatopathol* 1982; **4:** 185–8.

50. Krawczyk W S. The pattern of epidermal cell migration during wound healing. *J Cell Biol* 1971; **49:** 247–63.

51. Stenn K S, Madri J A, Roll F J. Migrating epidermis produces AB2 collagen and requires continued collagen synthesis for movement. *Nature* 1979; **277:** 229–32.

52. Davidson J M. Wound repair. In: Gallin J I, Goldstein I M, Snyderman R, eds. *Inflammation: Basic Principles and Clinical Correlates*. New York: Raven Press, 1992: 809–19.

53. Winter G D. Formation of the scar and the rate of epithelialization of superficial wounds in the skin of the young domestic pig. *Nature* 1962; **193:** 293–4.

54. Hinman C D, Maibach H. Effect of air exposure and occlusion on experimental human skin wounds. *Nature* 1963; **200:** 377–8.

55. Woodley D T, Bachmann P M, O'Keefe E D. The role of matrix components in human keratinocyte re-epithelialization. In: Barbul A, Caldwell M D, Eaglstein W H, *et al.*, eds. *Clinical and Experimental Approaches to Dermal and Epidermal Repair*. New York: Wiley–Liss, 1991: 129–40.

56. Forrest L. Current concepts in soft connective tissue wound healing. *Br J Surg* 1983; **70:** 133–40.

57. Alibert J L M. *Description des Maladies de la Peau Observées à l'Hôpital Saint-Louis et Exposition des Meilleurs Methodes Suivés pour leur Traitement*. Paris: Barrois l'Ainé et Fils, 1806: 113 pp.

58. Hebra F, Kaposi M. *On Diseases of the Skin Including the Exanthemata*. London: The New Sydenham Society, 1874: 272 pp.

59. Blackburn W R, Cosman B. Histologic basis of keloid and hypertrophic scar differentiation. *Arch Pathol* 1966; **82:** 65–71.

60. Linares H A. Hypertrophic healing: controversies and ethiopathogenic review. In: Carvajal H F, Parks D H, eds. *Burns in Children*. Chicago: Year Book Medical Publishers, 1988: 305–19.

61. Murray J C, Pinnell S R. Keloids and excessive dermal scarring. In: Cohen I K, Diegelmann R F, Lindblad W J, eds. *Wound Healing, Biochemical and Clinical Aspects*. Philadelphia: W B Saunders Co, 1992: 500–22.

62. Craig P. Collagenase activity in cutaneous scars. *Hand* 1973; **5:** 239–43.

63. Knapp T R, Daniels J R, Kaplan E N. Pathologic scar formation. *Am J Pathol* 1977; **86:** 47–67.

64. Linares H A, Kischer C W, Dobrkovsky M, *et al.* On the origin of the hypertrophic scar. *J Trauma* 1973; **13:** 70–5.

65. Linares H A, Larson D L. Early differential diagnosis between hypertrophic and nonhypertrophic healing. *J Invest Dermatol* 1974; **62:** 514–16.

66. Linares H A, Kischer C W, Dobrkovsky M, *et al.* The histiotypic organization of the hypertrophic scar in humans. *J Invest Dermatol* 1972; **59:** 323–31.

67. Linares H A, Larson D L. Proteoglycans and collagenase in hypertrophic scar formation. *J Plast Reconstr Surg* 1978; **62:** 589–93.

68. Shetlar M R, Shetlar C L, Linares H A. The hypertrophic scar: location of glycosaminoglycans within scars. *Burns* 1977; **4:** 14–19.

69. Hunter J A A, Finlay J B. Scanning electron microscopy of normal human scar tissues and keloids. *Br J Surg* 1976; **63:** 826–30.

70. Kischer C W, Linares H A, Dobrkovsky M, Larson D L. Electron microscopy of the hypertrophic scar. In: Arceneaux C J ed. *29th Ann Proc. Electron Microscopy Soc Amer.* Boston, MA 1971: 302–3.

71. Cohen I K, Keiser H R, Sjoerdsma A. Collagen synthesis in human keloid and hypertrophic scar. *Surg Forum* 1971; **22:** 488–9.

72. Craig R D P, Schofield J D, Jackson S S. Collagen biosynthesis in normal human skin, normal and hypertrophic scar and keloid. *Eur J Clin Invest* 1975; **5:** 69–74.

73. McCoy B J, Cohen I K. Collagenase in keloid biopsies and fibroblasts. *Connect Tissue Res* 1982; **9:** 181–92.

74. Harris E D Jr, Sjoerdsma A. Collagen profile in various clinical conditions. *Lancet* 1966; **2:** 707–19.

75. Di Cesare P E, Cheung D T, Perelman N, Libaw E, Peng L, Nimni M E. Alteration of collagen composition and cross-linking in keloid tissues. *Matrix* 1990; **10:** 172–8.

76. Cohen I K, Beaven M A, Horakova Z, Keiser H R. Histamine and collagen synthesis in keloid and hypertrophic scar. *Surg Forum* 1972; **23:** 509.

77. Abergel R P, Pizzurro D, Meeker C A, *et al.* Biochemical composition of the connective tissue in keloids and analysis of collagen metabolism in keloid fibroblast cultures. *J Invest Dermatol* 1985; **84:** 384–90.

78. Bailey A J, Bazin S, Sims T J, LeLous M, Nicoletis C, Delaunay A. Characterization of the collagen of human hypertrophic and normal scars. *Biochim Biophys Acta* 1975; **405:** 412–21.

79. Weber L, Meigel W N, Spier W. Collagen polymorphism in pathologic human scars. *Arch Dermatol Res* 1978; **261:** 63–71.

80. Conway H, Gillette R, Smith J W, Findley A. Differential diagnosis of keloids and hypertrophic scars by tissue culture technique with notes on therapy of keloids by surgical excision and decadron. *Plast Reconstr Surg* 1960; **25:** 117–32.

81. Diegelmann R F, Cohen I K, McCoy B J. Growth kinetics and collagen synthesis of normal skin, normal scar and keloid fibroblasts in vitro. *J Cell Physiol* 1979; **98:** 341–6.

82. Abergel R P, Chu M L, Bauer E A, Uitto J. Regulation of collagen gene expression in cutaneous diseases with dermal fibrosis: evidence for pretranslational control. *J Invest Dermatol* 1987; **88:** 727–31.

83. Ala-Kokko L, Rintala A, Savolainen E R. Collagen gene expression in keloids: analysis of collagen metabolism and type I, III, IV, and V procollagen mRNAs in keloid tissue and keloid fibroblast cultures. *J Invest Dermatol* 1987; **89:** 238–44.

84. Craig R D P, Schofield J D, Jackson D S. Collagen biosynthesis in normal and hypertrophic scars and keloid as a function of the duration of the scar. *Br J Surg* 1975; **62:** 741–4.

85. Hardingham T E, Fosang A J. Proteoglycans: many forms and many functions. *FASEB J* 1992; **6:** 861–70.

86. Yeo T K, Brown L, Dvorak H F. Alterations in proteoglycan synthesis common to healing wounds and tumors. *Am J Pathol* 1991; **138:** 1437–50.

87. Shetlar M R, Larson D L, Sheltar C L, *et al.* The hypertrophic scar, glycoprotein and collagen components of burn scars. *Proc Soc Exp Biol Med* 1971; **138:** 298–300.

88. Linares H A. Measurement of collagen–proteoglycans interaction in hypertrophic scars. *Plast Reconstr Surg* 1983; **71:** 818–19.

89. Linares H A. Proteoglycan–lymphocyte association in the development of hypertrophic scars. *Burns* 1990; **16:** 21–4.

90. Savage K, Swann D A. A comparison of glycosaminoglycan synthesis by human fibroblasts from normal skin, normal scar, and hypertrophic scar. *J Invest Dermatol* 1985; **84:** 521–6.

91. Chytilova M, Kulhankek V, Horn V. Experimental production of keloids after immunization with autologous skin. *Acta Chir Plast* 1959; **1:** 72–9.

92. Laurentaci G, Dioguardi D. HLA antigens in keloids and H S. *Arch Dermatol* 1977; **113:** 1726.

93. Castagnoli C, Peruccio D, Stella M, *et al.* The HLA-DR 16 allogenotype constitutes a risk factor for hypertrophic scarring. *Human Immunol* 1990; **29:** 229–32.

94. Cohen I K, McCoy B J, Mohanakumar T, Diegelmann R F. Immunoglobulin, complement, and histocompatibility antigen studies in keloid patients. *Plast Reconstr Surg* 1979; **63:** 689–92.

95. Abdalla-Osman A A, Gumma K A, Satir A A. Highlights on the etiology of keloid. *Int Surg* 1978; **63:** 33–7.

96. Kischer C W, Shetlar M R, Sheltar C L, Chavapil M. Immunoglobulins in hypertrophic scars and keloids. *Plast Reconstr Surg* 1983; **71:** 821–5.

97. Castagnoli C, Stella M, Magliacani G, Alasia S T, Richiard P. Anomalous expression of HLA class II molecules on keratinocytes and fibroblasts in hypertrophic scar consequence to thermal injury. *Clin Exp Immunol* 1990; **82:** 350–4.

98. Cracco C, Stella M, Alasia S T, Filogamo G. Comparative study of Langerhans cells in normal and pathological human scars. II. Hypertrophic scars. *Eur J Histochem* 1992; **36:** 53–65.

99. Babu M, Diegelmann R, Oliver N. Fibronectin is overproduced by keloid fibroblasts during abnormal wound healing. *Mol Cell Biol* 1989; **9:** 1642–50.

100. Kischer C W, Hendrix M J C. Fibronectin (FN) in hypertrophic scars and keloids. *Cell Tissue Res* 1983; **231:** 29–37.

101. McCauley R L, Chopra V, Li Y Y, Herndon D N, Robson M C. Altered cytokine production in black patients with keloids. *J Clin Immunol* 1992; **12:** 300–8.

102. Davidson J M, Broadley K N, Benn S I. Cytokine influences on ECM metabolism during wound healing. *J Cell Biol* 1993; **S17E:** 109.

103. Sporn M B, Roberts A B. Introduction: what is TGF -β. In: *Clinical Applications of TGF-Beta. Ciba Foundation Symposium 157.* Wiley, Chichester, 1991: 1–6.

104. Babu M, Diegelmann R, Oliver N. Keloid fibroblasts exhibit an altered response to TGF-β. *J Invest Dermatol* 1992; **99:** 650–5.

105. Martin P, Hopkinson-Woolley J, McCluskey J. Growth factors and cutaneous wound repair. *Prog Growth Factor Res* 1992; **4:** 25–44.

106. Linares H A, Larson D L, Willis-Galstaun B A. Historical notes on the use of pressure in the treatment of hypertrophic scars or keloids. *Burns* 1993; **19:** 17–21.

107. Larson D L, Evans E B, Abston S, Dobrkovsky M, Linares H A. Techniques for decreasing scar formation and scar contractures in the burn patient. *J Trauma* 1971; **11:** 807–23.

108. Linares H A, Larson D L, Baur P S. Influence of mechanical forces on burn scar contracture and hypertrophic. In: Krizek Th J, Hoopes J E, eds. *Symposium on Basic Science in Plastic Surgery.* St Louis: C V Mosby, 1976: 101–27.

109. Larson D L, Willis B, Linares H A, Shetlar M R, Kischer C W. Burn scar changes associated with pressure. In: Longacre J J, ed. *The Ultrastructure of Collagen.* Springfield: C C Thomas, 1976: 269–74.

110. Larson D L, Huang T T, Linares H A, Dobrkovsky M, Baur P S, Parks D H. Prevention and treatment of scar contractures. In: Artz C P, Moncrief J A, Pruitt B, eds. *Burns, A Team Approach.* Philadelphia: W B Saunders, 1979: 466–91.

NON THERMAL INJURIES

CHAPTER THIRTY-EIGHT

Electrical Injuries

JAMES M. SHAW AND MARTIN C. ROBSON

Introduction

An electrical injury is a unique form of trauma. The clinical pictures following cellular damage due to electrical current comprise more of a syndrome than a specific injury.[1] Clinicians arbitrarily divide electrical injuries into high- and low-tension injuries as determined by the voltage which is responsible for the damage. The dividing line is 1000 volts. All current in the United States is 60 Hz, or cycles per second. Low-voltage injuries mimic thermal burns and have zones of injury from the surface extending into the tissue.[2] The syndrome from high-voltage injury consists of varying degrees of cutaneous burn combined with 'hidden' destruction of deep tissue.[1,3] The electrical insult results in progressive tissue necrosis in excess of the originally apparent trauma, and somewhat resembles the injury of crush trauma.[4,5] Controversy exists as to whether this is a slow manifestation of irreversible muscle damage secondary to the original current of passage,[6–8] or if it is actively progressive ischemic necrosis secondary to ongoing macrovascular or microvascular compromise.[3,9–11]

Pathophysiology

The cause of the controversy over electrical injury damage is a poor understanding of the relevant pathophysiology. Because electrical injuries comprise a syndrome, the inciting cellular mechanism(s) for the resulting pathologic course may be multiple.[1] Historically, the mechanism was thought to be heat. Passage of electric current through a solid conductor results in conversion of electrical energy into heat, the joule effect. The amount of heat can be determined by Ohm's law and the joule effect. Ohm's law states that the current traveling through tissue is determined by the voltage (V) divided by the resistance (R). Heat production in joules is proportional to the power dissipated multiplied by the duration of contact and is expressed by the equation $J = I^2RT$ where J is the heat production, I is the current, R is the tissue resistance, and T is the time of contact.[3] The extent of injury depends on the type of current, the pathway of flow, the local tissue resistance, and the duration of contact.[7,12–16]

Two theories attributing the pathologic changes seen following electrical injury to generated heat have been postulated.[1] The first emphasizes the differences in tissue resistance to current flow in order to explain the observed changes following electrical injury.[9] Tissue resistance progressively increases from nerve to blood vessels, muscle, skin, tendon, fat, and bone. Bone, having the greatest resistance, generates the most heat according to the joule effect. This would cause greater necrosis in the deep periosseous tissues, a situation frequently observed in this syndrome. The majority of current would preferentially travel along the lines of lesser resistance, particularly the blood vessels.[17,18] These vessels are injured, but not immediately thrombosed.[19] According to this theory, the progressive muscular necrosis is attributed to these vascular lesions leading to delayed arterial occlusion and progressive ischemic necrosis.[9–11]

Another theory questions the existence of progressive muscle necrosis.[1] Hunt *et al.* found that the internal milieu of an experimental animal's body acts like a volume conductor of a single resistance and not as if it were composed of tissues of varying resistances.[7] With the onset of current flow, amperage and temperature rise in parallel throughout the limb. By the time of current arcing, both muscle and bone temperatures are equal. They also observed that it takes bone longer to dissipate the heat and suggested that it was this prolonged elevation in temperature which accounted for the periosseous 'core' of necrotic muscle seen clinically. They also thought that involved muscle and vessels sustained irreversible damage at the time of current passage with immediate microscopic muscular coagulation necrosis and small nutrient artery thrombosis. To support this concept are reports that progressive occlusion of major-sized vessels have not been documented arteriographically in the experimental situation or clinically.[6,8,20]

Progressive microvascular deterioration beyond the resolution of radiographic evaluation is not ruled out by a failure to delineate progressive changes arteriographically.[1] Quinby *et al.* and Luce *et al.* in describing the microscopic changes of questionably viable muscle emphasized the mixed 'patchy' nature of the electrical injury.[21,22] Normal muscle cells can be seen immediately adjacent to necrotic cells with pyknotic nuclei, and normal patent vessels can exist adjacent to thrombosed vessels, reminiscent of the 'zone of stasis' in a thermal burn.[14] Progressive small vessel thrombosis and deterioration of the microvasculature could convert these areas of patchy necrosis into complete tissue loss.

The entire pathophysiology responsible for the syndrome of electrical injury cannot be attributed to heat. Lee and Kolodney have demonstrated, through electrical and mathematical modeling, that joule heating is often not sufficient to explain the tissue necrosis seen.[23] When a current passes transversely across a limb, the tissue with lower conductivity and higher resistance would generate the greatest amount of heat. This situation would mimic the theory suggested by Baxter.[9] Lee and Kolodney suggest, however, that most clinical situations probably place the tissues electrically in parallel.[23] When current enters an upper extremity and transverses the entire body to another contact point on a lower extremity, this is the case. They have also shown that the tissue with the greatest conductivity generates the most heat.[1] They suggested that muscle would generate the greatest intensity of joule heating and the adjacent bone would be heated secondarily. This would corroborate the theory proposed by Hunt *et al.*[7] The bone heated secondarily would dissipate heat quite slowly. Lee and Kolodney showed this dissipation to be prolonged in a state of poor perfusion.[23] Although the mathematical modeling appeared to explain the different theories for joule heating as a cause for cellular damage in electrical injuries, it also showed that often the amount of heat is not sufficient to explain tissue damage at sites distant from current contact.[23] Lee and Kolodney have demonstrated that an electric field can be of sufficient magnitude to cause electrical breakdown of cells and cell lysis.[23] They point out that rupture of cells by strong electric fields is well documented.[24] Electrical fields, which are stronger than a threshold magnitude and turned on faster than the mechanical response of a membrane, can rupture bilaminate lipid membranes.[25]

The various observations are all correct in select situations following electrical trauma. That is the reason for describing the clinical response as a syndrome.[1] Perhaps a way of unifying these theories is to look at the cellular response to the initial electrical insult. To do this, one needs to look at the immediate and delayed cellular damage following contact with an electrical field. This unifying concept is the same as for other causes of soft tissue trauma such as thermal burning, frostbite, or other injuries in which patients present to an emergency department with what appears to be relatively minor injuries and, after a period of days, lose large amounts of tissue.[26] The immediate damage is similar and fairly well delineated for all of these injuries, including electrical trauma.[1] The traumatic insult results in a degree of cell shock. The intracellular energy system changes stored adenosine triphosphate (ATP) to cyclic adenosine monophosphate (AMP), and the sodium pump becomes ineffective as the cell membrane becomes permeable to sodium and calcium ions.[27,28] As part of the immediate cellular injury, proteases are released and these can trigger both the coagulation cascade and complement degradation. Degradation products such as chemotactic factor (C5a) begin the immunological cascade, and the soft tissue responds by increased vascular permeability and chemotaxis.[26] The mast cell, stimulated by these tissue proteases coming out of the injured cell, produces more cyclic AMP. Penneys has shown that injury also actives phospholipase A, which cleaves the phospholipids that are bound to cholesterol and triglycerides in the cell membrane.[29] This results in the metabolism of arachidonic acid which, when released, helps to activate the platelet plug. The other activity from the proteases is the initiation of chemotaxis. The respiratory burst of the leukocyte occurs and produces more arachidonic acid metabolites. This also produces free oxygen radicals which are necessary for the initial control of bacteria at the site of injury.

All traumatic soft tissue injury results in these immediate effects; but, except in the most severe cases, these immediate effects do not result in tissue necrosis. This is the case in clinical electrical injuries in which tissue proximal to the site of contact often appears uninjured.[1] The major causes of tissue loss in the various clinical presentations of the electrical syndrome are due to delayed effects. Robson *et al.* suggested an etiology and a method to control these delayed effects in an experimental electrical injury.[3] Their laboratory had previously shown that progressive tissue loss in burns and frostbite was due to progressive dermal ischemia mediated by various metabolites of arachidonic acid.[30–33] Heggers and Robson have postulated that cellular integrity depends on a homeostatic relationship between PGE_2 and $PGF_{2\alpha}$.[34] Injury to the cells disrupts this balance and causes a shunt in arachidonic acid metabolism in favor of thromboxane production. Production of this vasoactive prostanoid in large amounts leads to vasoconstriction, thrombosis, progressive ischemic necrosis, and further thromboxane production.

Because Arturson[35] suggested that various forms of trauma could activate phospholipase A to cleave the phospholipids from the cell membrane and thereby begin the arachidonic cascades and because heat and electrical disruption of the cell membrane were forms of trauma, the definitive experiment linking arachidonic acid metabolites to the pathophysiology of electrical trauma was reported in 1984.[3] A rat model, modified from that described by Buchanan *et al.*, was used to provide a reproducible electrical injury to a limb.[20] This model appeared to mimic the progressive tissue damage of a high-voltage injury in the human since the limb progressed from normal to autoamputation over a 72-hour period. Using this rat model, Robson *et al.* showed increasing levels of arachidonic acid metabolites, chiefly thromboxane, in the deep periosseous tissue beneath what appeared to be uninjured skin.[3] With time, the thromboxane increased progressively toward the limb surface until that apparently uninjured skin necrosed, just as in clinical situations. In this electrical injury, the elevated thromboxane production by the injured cells appeared to provide the impetus for converting areas of 'patchy' necrosis into areas of complete tissue loss, resulting in amputation.

Treatment with agents capable of blocking thromboxane production produced a 30–40% decrease in the incidence of autoamputation. More striking than the modest decrease in amputation rate, however, was the change in the marginally injured tissue when thromboxane production was blocked. This change was manifested as an increase in the eventual surviving length of electrically burned hind limbs. All treatment groups exhibited a significant tissue salvage, with mean lengths of electrically burned limbs up to twice that in control animals.[1,3] Surviving limb length was the measure of success. All attempts were successful compared to the untreated controls, with the best results due to the combination of systemic and topical antithromboxane agents. In this group, surviving limb length was 79.8% compared to 37.2% in the control animals.[3] Total salvage of the limb occurred in some animals.

The demonstration of arachidonic acid metabolites in increasing amounts in tissue following electrical trauma allows a unifying concept for the various theories regarding the pathophysiology of these injuries. Both joule heating and cell membrane disruption can activate the arachidonic acid cascade. Once initiated, the various immediate effects of trauma produce more of these mediators.[26] This concept allows other clinical observations to be clarified. Many of the inflammatory mediators can cause marked vasoconstriction of the microcirculation. This would decrease perfusion of an anatomical part and markedly decrease the rate of cooling. Another concept difficult to explain by previous theories is that of 'patchy necrosis'. This has been reported in most clinical and experimental electrical injuries.[3,22,23] Since tissue perfusion can be both macroscopic and microscopic, local production of ischemia-causing mediators due to cell rupture in an electrical field could result in 'patchy necrosis'. Certainly, in the experiment reported by Robson *et al.*, tissue was stained specifically for TXA_2 and a patchy distribution was seen.[3] They postulated that the elevated thromboxane production by the injured cells could easily provide the impetus for converting areas of 'patchy' necrosis into areas of complete tissue loss.

The observed and reported increase in tissue necrosis in periosseous tissue becomes quite clear when one combines all of the theories. In Baxter's scenario, the bone provides the greatest amount of joule heating.[9] In the theories by Hunt *et al.* and Lee and Kolodney, the muscle produces the highest immediate heat, but the bone prolongs the time of heating.[7,23] If mediators are produced by the two mechanisms discussed above, perfusion next to the bone will be less because of vasoconstriction of the microvasculature, temperatures will rise, and more injurious mediators will be produced. Therefore, the increased death of tissue needs no further explanation. It now seems quite straightforward to explain the presence of deep necrosis beneath unaffected skin. Skin temperature distant from the point of contact may never rise to the lethal range in an electrical injury.[23] The fact that this apparently uninjured skin may develop signs of necrosis could be due to progressive ischemia caused by inflammatory mediators and not the electrical event itself. This would be similar to other forms of trauma which activate the arachidonic acid cascade and would allow a unifying concept regarding progressive tissue loss.[1]

Diagnostic Measures

Often the integumentary wounds of a victim of electrical trauma are impressive. Clinically, three types of skin damage may result from electric injury: (1) contact burns at points of current entry and exit from the body; (2) arc burns caused by current exiting and reentering adjacent parts or body parts in close proximity; and (3) thermal burns from ignition of clothing because of the degree of heat generated by the current passing through the body.[36] These injuries, no matter how dramatic, cannot take precedence over a systematic history and physical examination.

The history of an electrical contact event is very useful. Determining the site where the injury occurred helps to approximate the voltage. Injuries in the home probably equal 110–220 volts, whereas industrial injuries or powerline injuries are typically high tension. This information is usually readily available from coworkers or superintendents. It must be determined whether, as frequently occurs, the patient suffered a cardiac arrest at the injury scene. Because coworkers or bystanders perform cardiopulmonary resuscitation, the patient can arrive in the emergency department in a resuscitated state, and the arrest event may not be communicated to the staff. Similarly, it should be determined whether the patient was thrown a distance or fell from a height after contacting the electric source, and if loss of consciousness occurred.[36]

The physical examination is similar to that following all major trauma. Airway patency should be established, and chest expansion should be assessed as well as uniformity of breath sounds bilaterally. Pneumothorax is not uncommon in high-tension injuries.[36] Health care providers should examine cardiac rate and rhythm, and consider electrocardiographic monitoring. The peripheral circulation is assessed to determine the need for escharotomy or fasciotomy. Muscle compartmental pressures may be an adjunct in making this determination.[36] The mental and neurological status needs to be assessed, noting the level of consciousness and orientation as to person, place, and time. A rapid neurological examination is performed to check for focal motor and sensory deficits.

Following the initial history and cursory physical examination, a more detailed evaluation is required. In severe electrical injuries, death of large volumes of muscle will occur, and this results in extremely large fluid loss.[37] Significant blood loss may occur as a consequence of vascular injury or from associated fractures or chest or abdominal trauma. Shock should not be attributed to an uncomplicated electrical injury. The possibility of associated hemorrhage or perforation of an intra-abdominal viscus should always be considered.[36] A detailed examination of the nervous system will be necessary. Respiratory paralysis and extremity paralysis are not uncommon.[36] Although these disturbances may subside spontaneously, Silversides has reported permanent residual disability as well as hemiplegia, aphasia, cerebellar dysfunction, and epilepsy after electrical injuries.[38] In one reported series, physiologic spinal cord transection developed in 25% of patients with high-voltage electrical injury.[9] Nausea, vomiting, and prolonged paralytic ileus are common after electrical injuries. It must be determined that these problems are not a result of a perforated viscus or transmural injury of the colon. If signs of peritoneal irritation exist, an exploratory laparotomy should be considered.[36]

Health care providers should make a recording of the burn degree, realizing that determination is difficult because much of the injured tissue is 'hidden' beneath apparently uninjured skin.[36] Contact area wounds should be located if possible. This examination requires a careful look at the scalp, as well as the soles of the feet. The amount of thermal burn should be illustrated on a Lund and Browder chart. Areas of potential vascular or nerve compression should be noted.[36]

Laboratory tests are useful in evaluating a victim of an electrical injury. Significant hemoglobinemia may appear after electrical accidents as a result of lysis of red blood cells. Similarly, the result of myoglobin from destroyed muscle may further increase the levels of circulating chromoproteins. Both hemoglobin and myoglobin may be present in the urine, and this needs to be determined. If not detected and cleared from the renal tubules, these pigments will precipitate and cause renal failure.[36] Blood chemistry abnormalities can occur as a result of massive tissue destruction, especially of muscle. Creatinine and creatine phosphokinase levels may be elevated. Damage to cardiac muscle will be reflected by a rise in the cardiac enzyme levels, such as those for aspartate aminotransferase (AST), SGOT, and lactate dehydrogenase. A standard 12-lead electrocardiogram (ECG) should be obtained. If the ECG findings are normal, the patient has no history of cardiac arrest or cardiopulmonary resuscitation, and no abnormality in the cardiac rate or rhythm exists, then Purdue and Hunt suggest that cardiac problems are unlikely to occur.[39] If the ECG findings or any other study findings are abnormal, then they recommend continuous cardiac monitoring.[36] Other laboratory tests may be useful. A chest radiograph should be obtained if any sign of electrical burn exists on the thorax or the patient has fallen to rule out a pneumothorax–hemothorax of transected aortic root. Similarly, cervical, thoracic, and lumbar spine radiographs are usually indicated in high-voltage injury or if a patient has fallen.[36] Falls can result from electrical contact, and Baxter has reported bony fractures in 10% of electrical injuries.[9] In addition, the violent tetanic muscular contraction which results from contact (particularly with alternating current sources) may cause a variety of fractures and dislocations.[40] Direct damage and extensive destruction of bone is common in electrical injuries from very high voltages. Grossly, the bone is avascular and may be exposed. Even nonexposed bone may be damaged. After injuries from very high voltage, about 15% of patients develop bone sequestration.[9] The gradual sequestration and discharge of devitalized areas of bone result in a prolonged delay in healing. Extremity or skull radiographs are obtained if indicated by examination. Finally, barium or Gastrografin contrast studies may be indicated for a suspected perforated viscus.

Treatment

Immediate first aid at the scene of an injury may have required cardiopulmonary resuscitation; thus, if the initial ECG findings are abnormal, continued cardiac monitoring is necessary along with pharmacologic treatment for any dysrhythmia.[36] Prolonged respiratory support may be required because coma occasionally occurs after electrical injury. Continuous nasogastric suction is usually required for 24–48 hours more than in thermal burns. Associated injuries detected on initial evaluation require treatment and may require the services of other specialists such as orthopedic surgeons or neurosurgeons.

Maintenance of adequate fluid to support the intravascular volume is difficult in patients with major electrical injuries. Because of the 'hidden' underlying deep muscle damage, fluid requirements exceed anything predicted by formulas which are based on surface wounds.[36] As a starting point, a balanced salt solution is begun at about 4 ml/kg/% TBSA burn. Because of the possibility of renal failure from precipitation of myoglobin and hemoglobin, a brisk urine flow must be encouraged. To help obtain this, an osmotic diuretic such as mannitol is useful. After obtaining urine, a sample is tested for pigment. The presence of chromogens indicates a need to maintain the urine output at 70–100 ml/h in order to clear the pigments.[36] Alkalinizing the blood will help increase the solubility of these pigments in the urine. Therefore, additional bicarbonate is added to the balanced salt solution for resuscitation. After the pigment has cleared, the urine flow is titrated to 0.5–1 ml/kg.

The key to managing a patient with electrical injuries lies in the treatment of the wound. This is where the most recent thoughts on the pathophysiology have suggested changes. There has been resistance to accepting this unifying concept for the pathophysiology of tissue injury following electrical trauma. Part of this has been due to semantics. Historically, many held the idea that there was delayed muscle necrosis and, therefore, early debridement and wound closure was contraindicated. This led to weeks of serial debridement, desiccation of the open wound, and infection. This vicious cycle indeed led to further tissue necrosis. Kuzon *et al.* and Zelt *et al.* designed a model in a primate which showed that this delayed muscle necrosis did not occur and suggested that debridement and definitive wound closure could occur much earlier.[41,42] Similarly, Silverberg *et al.* have advocated early debridement and closure.[43]

The arachidonic acid metabolites are activated immediately after injury. Their effects begin at that time, and most of the ischemia produced by them would be expected to be complete by 72–96 hours. Any attempt to pharmacologically block their effects must be done in the immediate post-traumatic period. Therefore, Zelt's and Daniel's recommendation to decompress and adequately explore the injury immediately and to provide definitive debridement and wound closure between the third and the fifth day is totally compatible with the concept of a progressive mediator-induced injury over a limited time span.[8] To delay beyond that time has no physiologic basis; to allow the wound to remain open invites further loss of tissue. Dessication alone actually stimulates the production of thromboxane.

Nonoperative wound care involves consideration for topical antithromboxane treatment and topic antibacterials.[36] The most frequent cause of death after electrical injury is systemic infection. In one series, 7% of deaths were a result of sepsis.[9] In another series, sepsis developed in approximately one-third of the patients during their hospitalization.[44] Sepsis can arise from necrotic muscle mass, bacterial invasion from associated thermal burn, or perforations of the gastrointestinal tract. Because of the vascularity changes noted in the pathophysiology, topical therapy is indicated. Mafenide acetate is particularly well suited for these wounds. It can penetrate to the deep levels of injury, and the operative management can be divided into those procedures which must be performed early and those which can be postponed until the injury has completely evolved. Life-threatening and limb-threatening problems should be operatively managed acutely, and definitive wound closure should be delayed until the progressive injury is complete or has been pharmacologically aborted.

Because the injured cells are most heavily concentrated in the periosseous core in a high-voltage injury, edema will occur beneath what appears clinically to be uninjured skin. Therefore, escharotomy and fasciotomy may be necessary soon after injury. Physical examination can usually determine the need for these measures and compartmental pressure measurements can be used as an adjunct.[45] Because major nerves are susceptible to increased pressure in closed compartments, escharotomy or fasciotomy alone (or in combination) may not be sufficient to decompress nerves in an arm. Therefore, decompression of the median and ulnar nerves as an emergency procedure in high-voltage injury to the hands is recommended[36] (**Figure 38.1**).

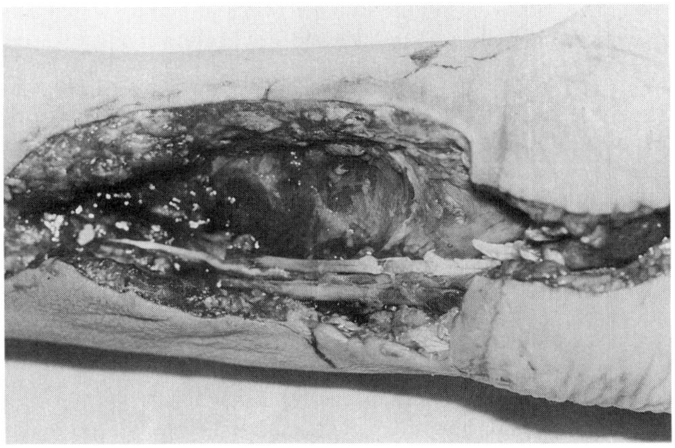

Fig. 38.1 Carpal tunnel and Guyon's canal releases must be performed early to decompress the median and ulnar nerves.

We believe that debridement of obviously necrotic tissue should be performed as early as possible, preferably soon after the patient's admission, while performing escharotomies, fasciotomies, and nerve decompressions.[36] If the wound is truly progressive, definitive wound close at the time of initial debridement should be avoided. Most clinicians who advocate early wound closure in electrical injuries suggest the definitive debridement and closure not be done in the first 48–72 hours.[1] This makes sense as it allows the progressive or 'nonimmediate' cellular effects to manifest. If, as Lee and Kolodney suggest, those cells not coagulated by joule heating die because of membrane disruption, this will not be recognized grossly at the time of initial decompression and exploration.[23] It will be recognized several days later when the arachidonic acid metabolites have caused microvascular ischemic cell death. It is at that time that the necrotic tissue can be excised and the wound closed.

Debridement in high-voltage injury, when indicated, remains difficult. Obvious necrotic tissue may extend beneath what appears to be normal uninjured skin and subcutaneous tissue.[36] Ponten *et al.* reported that this coagulation necrosis may exist in the contiguous deeper tissues as far as 25 cm from the point of current entry and exit.[10] It is useful to observe the muscles at the time of initial fasciotomy in order to determine whether they are viable. Among the different tests suggested to make that determination, the most reliable are those that assess the ability of the muscle to bleed and contract.[36] Technetium-99m pyrophosphate muscle scans may be useful in assessing nonperfused muscle. 'Cold' areas on the skin may suggest irreversibly necrosed nonsalvageable tissue, and 'hot' areas correspond to 20–80% necrotic muscle fiber.[46] Clayton *et al.* showed that muscle blood flow can be directly measured with xenon-133 washout to determine muscle viability. Another adjunct is the use of frozen microscopic sections at the time of debridement so as to insure completeness of debridement while minimizing tissue loss.[22]

After completing the definitive debridement of nonviable tissue, one can proceed with wound closure. Exposed normal tissue or minimally injured (yet still viable) tissue should be covered so as to prevent further damage by desiccation (**Figure 38.2**). A final exploration and debridement should be performed immediately before closure in order to prevent coverage of nonviable tissue. Whereas skin grafts will almost always suffice as closure for thermal burn wounds, flaps may frequently be required for closure of electrical burn wounds. Recently, Robson *et al.* reported that an increasing number of early wound closures are being done with the use of free-tissue transfers[48] (**Figure 38.3**). Also, as part of wound debridement, amputations may be required.[36] These are best delayed until the limb is threatening to cause overwhelming sepsis. Even exposed, charred, and superficially infected bone can be salvaged with coverage by a vascularized flap.[36] If amputations are necessary, they should be performed in an open circular method, maintaining maximum length, and closed at a later date.

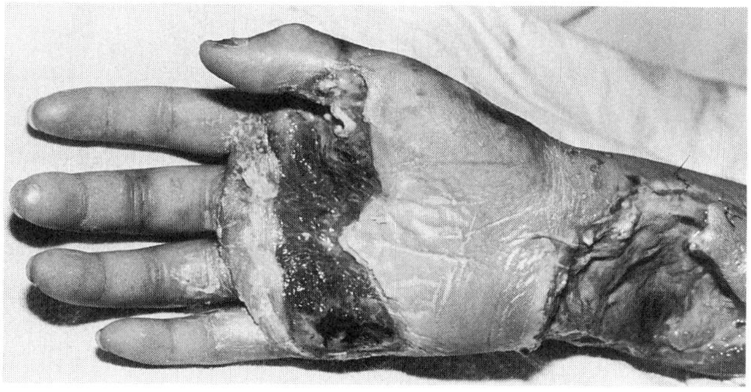

Fig. 38.2 Exposed tendons and nerves covered with allograft.

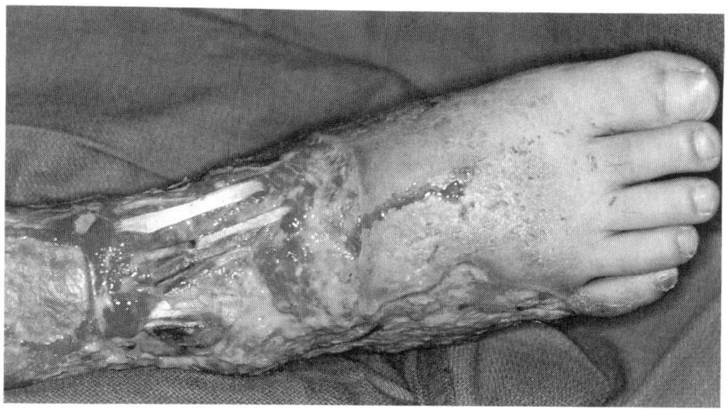

(a)

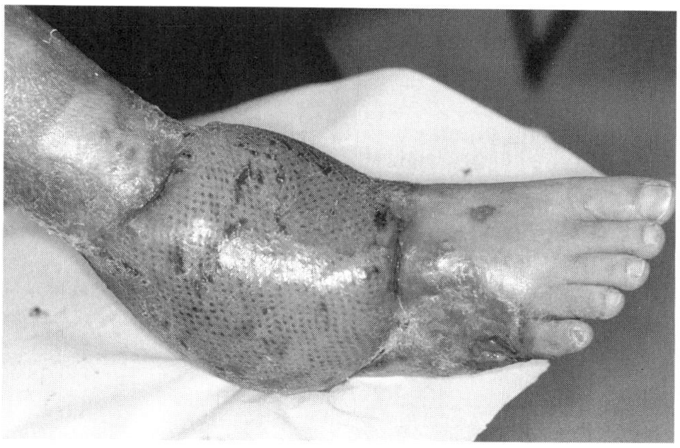

(b)

Fig. 38.3 Exposed tendons and open joint covered early with free flap shown (a) before and after (b).

Patients with electrical injuries may require other operations in addition to those for the visible wounds. Intraperitoneal injuries are common. Suspicion of these injuries requires a laparotomy and exteriorization or resection of compromised bowel. A second procedure may be considered, depending on the appearance of the visceral organs at initial laparotomy. Long bones or vertebrae may have been fractured as a result of tetanic contracture or an accompanying fall or injury. These fractures should be operatively managed after removing necrotic tissue.

Long-term Management and Sequelae

A patient surviving high-voltage electrical injury may need more extensive rehabilitation because he or she may be a single or multiple amputee. Proper choice and fitting of prostheses may be challenging in those patients with less than optimal stumps. Frequently, the patient needs occupational retraining because returning to the work that he or she performed before being injured may no longer be a possibility.[36] Also, the patient requires long-term follow-up because complications often result for some time after injury.

Some of these complications are caused by the complex pathophysiology of the injury, which is not yet completely understood. Early complications include myocardial damage, arterial mural necrosis and rupture, and occult injuries to the abdominal viscera. The complications which can be most perplexing are those with delayed onset, such as complications involving the cardiac system, central and peripheral nervous systems, and the eyes. Cardiac dysrhythmias or ECG changes exist initially in 10–30% of cases[13] Right bundle branch block, supraventricular tachycardia, and focal ectopic dysrhythmias, however, may occur later and persist.[36]

Christensen *et al.* reported cortical encephalopathy, hemiplegia with or without aphasia, striatal syndrome, and brain stem dysfunction.[49] Temporally, these complications may be delayed for 6–9 months after injury. Convulsive disorders also can appear late. Spinal cord symptoms similar to progressive muscular atrophy, amyotrophic lateral sclerosis, or transverse myelitis may occur, with a latent period of days to months.[50] Peripheral nerve lesions can appear up to 3 years after injury. Histopathologic changes have shown perivascular hemorrhage, demyelination with vacuolization, reactive gliosis, and neuronal death.[51] Another devastating complication of electrical injury is the slow progressive onset of cataracts. Cataracts can often be delayed for several years, although the onset of blurred vision usually begins about 6 months after injury.[51] Because this complication can occur in as many as 30% of persons receiving an electrical burn with contact above the clavicles, physicians must check for this complication in all patients and make patients aware of its possibility.[36]

The flowchart shown in **Figure 38.4** may be used to organize the initial management of the patient who has sustained electrical

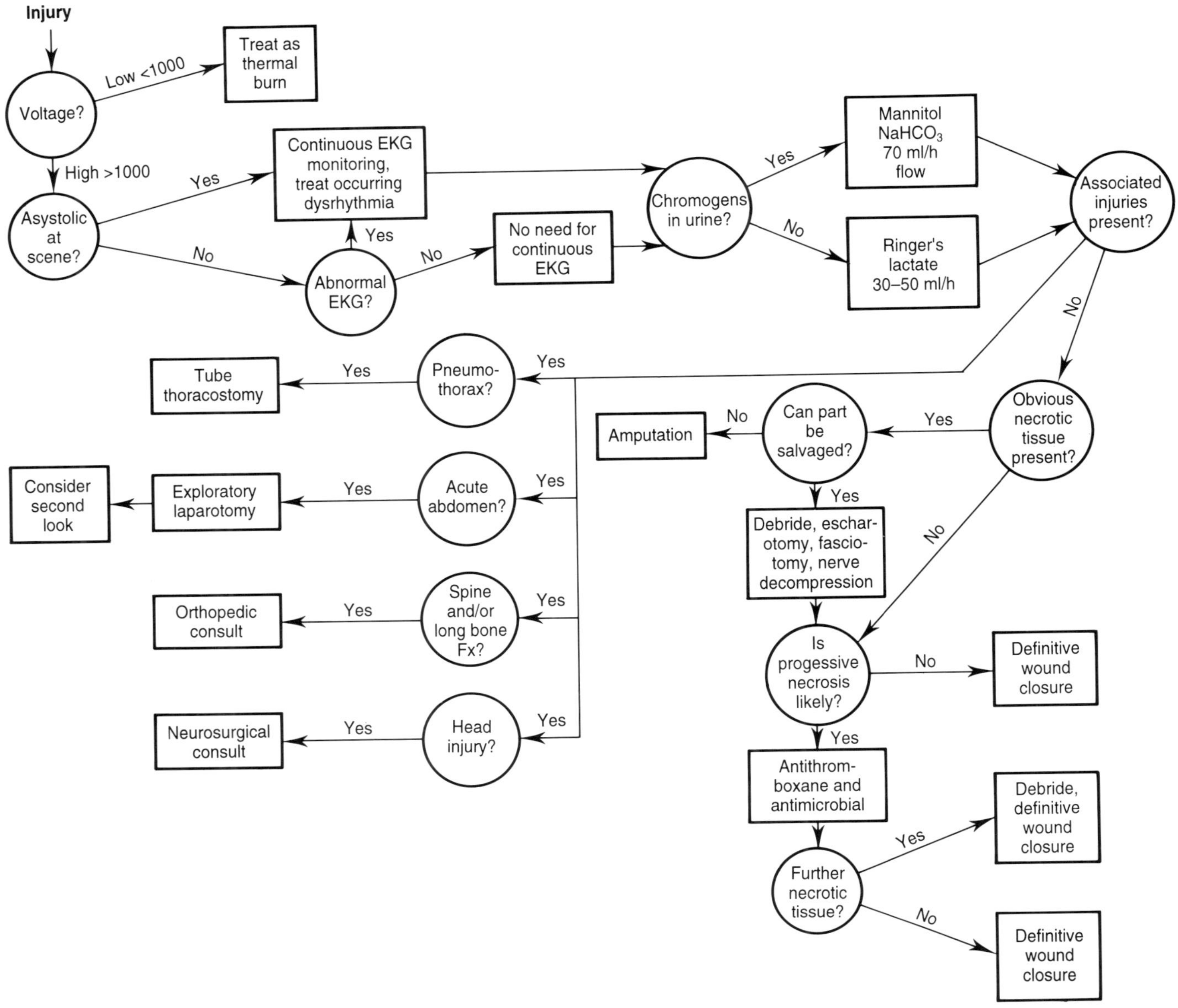

Fig. 38.4 Flow chart showing the proper management of a patient with electrical injuries.

trauma. The management of such patients is undergoing many changes based on newer studies elucidating the cellular mechanisms underlying the pathophysiologic changes seen in the syndrome. If electroporation of the cell membrane can be stabilized and the mediators responsible for progressive tissue destruction blocked, this injury may become much less severe than in the past. With better reconstructive techniques being applied earlier in the time course, hopefully the outcome from electrical trauma will be greatly improved.

Summary

Recent evidence has unified what appeared to be conflicting theories regarding the pathophysiology of electrical injuries. A single concept of cellular injury either due to heat or electroporation causing membrane disruption propagates production of inflammatory mediators which can account for the various pathologic changes seen in the injury syndrome following electrical trauma. Based on the unifying concept of tissue injury, clinical treatment of patients with high-voltage electrical injuries has changed. After admission and stabilization, the muscular compartments are immediately released, the nerves decompressed, and a topical antithromboxane agent applied. It is believed that the progressive injury is thereby limited. This appears to allow earlier definitive reconstruction than was seen historically with delayed necrosis due to desiccation and infection which frequently would have resulted in an amputation.

References

1. Robson M C, Hayward P G, Heggers J P. The role of arachidonic acid metabolism in electrical injury. In: Lee R C, Carvalhol E G, Burke J F, eds. *Electrical Trauma: Pathophysiology and Clinical Management.* Cambridge: Cambridge University Press, 1992: 179–88.

2. Laberge L C, Ballard P A, Daniel R K. Experimental electrical burns low voltage. *Ann Plast Surg* 1984; **13:** 185–90.

3. Robson M C, Murphy R C, Heggers J P. A new explanation for the progressive tissue loss in electrical injuries. *Plast Reconstr Surg* 1984; **73:** 431–7.

4. Rouse R G, Dimick A R. Treatment of electrical injury compared to burn injury. *J Trauma* 1978; **18:** 43–7.

5. Artz C P. Electrical injury simulates crush injury. *Surg Gynecol Obstet* 1967; **125:** 1316–17.

6. Hunt J L, McManus W F, Haney W P, Pruitt B A. Vascular lesions in acute electrical injuries. *J Trauma* 1974; **14:** 461–73.

7. Hunt J L, Mason A D, Masterson T S, Pruitt B A. Pathophysiology of acute electrical injuries. *J Trauma* 1976; **16:** 335–40.

8. Zelt R C, Daniel R K. Electrical injury. In: Marsh J, ed. *Current Therapy in Plastic and Reconstructive Surgery*. Toronto: B C Decker Inc, 1989: 29–33.

9. Baxter C R. Present concepts in the management of major electrical injuries. *Surg Clin North Am* 1970; **50:** 1401–18.

10. Ponten B, Erikson U, Johansson S H, *et al.* New observation on tissue changes along the pathway of the current in an electrical injury. *Scand J Plast Reconstr Surg* 1970; **4:** 75–80.

11. Skoog T. Electrical injuries. *J Trauma* 1970; **10:** 816–30.

12. Sances A, Larson S J, Myklebust J, Cusick J F. Electrical injuries. *Surg Gynecol Obstet* 1979; **149:** 97–108.

13. Esses S I, Peters W J. Electrical burns: pathophysiology and complications. *Can J Surg* 1981; **24:** 11–14.

14. Mann R J, Wallquist J M. Early decompression fasciotomy in the treatment of high voltage electrical injury of the extremities. *Scand Med J* 1985; **68:** 1103–8.

15. Jaffe R H. Electropathology: a review of the pathologic changes produced by electric currents. *Arch Pathol* 1928; **5:** 837–42.

16. Sances A, Mydlebust J B, Larson S J, *et al.* Experimental electrical injury studies. *J Trauma* 1981; **21:** 589–97.

17. Solem L, Fischer R P, Strate R G. Natural history of electrical injury. *J Trauma* 1977; **17:** 487–92.

18. Sturim H S. The treatment of electrical injuries. *J Trauma* 1971; **11:** 959–65.

19. Jaffe R H, Willis D, Bachem A. The effect of electrical current on arteries. *Arch Pathol* 1929; **7:** 244–9.

20. Buchanan D L, Erk Y, Spira M. Electrical current arterial injury: a laboratory model. *Plast Reconstr Surg* 1983; **72:** 199–205.

21. Quinby W C, Burke J F, Trelstad R L, Caulfield J. The use of microscopy as a guide to primary excision of electrical burns. *J Trauma* 1978; **18:** 423–31.

22. Luce E A, Dowden W L, Su C T, Hoopes J E. High tension electrical injury of the upper extremity. *Surg Gynecol Obstet* 1978; **147:** 38–42.

23. Lee R C, Kolodney M S. Electrical injury mechanisms: dynamics of the thermal response. *Plast Reconstr Surg* 1987; **80:** 663–71.

24. Teissie J, Dnutson V P, Tsang T Y, Lane M C. Electric pulse-induced fusion of 3T3 cells in monolayer culture. *Science* 1982; **216:** 537–8.

25. Benz R, Beckers F, Zimmerman U. Reversible electrical breakdown of lipid bilayer membranes: a charge-pulse relaxation study. *J Membr Biol* 1979; **48:** 181–204.

26. Robson M C. The immediate and delayed cellular damage following soft tissue. In: Zarins C K, ed. *Essays in Surgery*. New York: Churchill Livingstone, 1989: 153–8.

27. Teissie J, Tsang T Y. Evidence of voltage-induces channel opening in Na/K ATPase of human erythrocyte membrane. *J Membr Biol* 1980; **55:** 133–40.

28. Lee R C, Gaylor D C, Bhatt D, Isreal D. Role of cell membrane rupture in the pathogenesis of electrical trauma. *J Surg Res* 1988; **44:** 709–19.

29. Penneys N S. Prostaglandins and the skin. *Current Concepts*. Kalamazoo, Michigan: The Upjohn Co, 1980: 34–9.

30. Robson M C, DelBeccaro E J, Heggers J P. The effect of prostaglandins on the dermal microcirculation after burning and the inhibition of the effect by specific pharmacological agents. *Plast Reconstr Surg* 1979; **63:** 781–7.

31. DelBeccaro E J, Robson M C, Heggers J P, Swaminathan R. The use of specific thromboxane inhibitors to preserve the dermal microcirculation after burning. *Surgery* 1980; **87:** 137–41.

32. Robson M C, DelBeccaro E J, Heggers J P, Loy G L. Increasing dermal perfusion after burning by decreasing thromboxane production. *J Trauma* 1980; **20:** 722–5.

33. Raine T J, London M D, Goluch L, Heggers J P, Robson M C. Antiprostaglandins and antithromboxanes for treatment of frostbite. *Surg Forum* 1980; **31:** 557–9.

34. Heggers J P, Robson M C. Prostaglandins and thromboxanes. In: Ninneman J, ed. *Traumatic Injury – Infection and Other Immunologic Sequelae*. Baltimore: University Park Press, 1983: 79–102.

35. Arturson G. How are prostaglandins and leukotrienes involved in immunological alterations? A discussion. *J Trauma* 1984; **24:** S128–37.

36. Robson M C, Smith D J. Care of the thermally injured victim. In: Jurkiewicz M J, Krizek T J, Mathes S J, Ariyan S, eds. *Plastic Surgery: Principles and Practice*. St Louis: CV Mosby Company, 1990: 1355–410.

37. Sachatello C R, Stephenson S E. High voltage burns. *Am Surg* 1965; **31:** 807–13.

38. Silversides J. The neurological sequelae of electrical injury. *Can Med Assoc J* 1964; **91:** 195–204.

39. Purdue G, Hunt J L, Gillespie R W, *et al.* Biosynthetic skin substitute versus frozen human cadaver allograft for temporary coverage of excised burn wounds. *J Trauma* 1987; **27:** 155–7.

40. Robson M C, Krizek T J, Wray R C Jr. Care of the thermally injured patient. In: Zuidema G D, Rutherford R B, Ballinger W F II eds. *The Management of Trauma*. Philadelphia: W B Saunders Co, 1979: 666–730.

41. Kuzon W M, Zelt R G, Green H J, *et al.* Skeletal muscle energy metabolism following high voltage electrical injury. *Surg Forum* 1986; **37:** 621–3.

42. Zelt R G, Ballard P A, Common A A, Heroux P, Daniel R K. Experimental high voltage electrical burns: role of progressive necrosis. *Surg Forum* 1986; **37:** 624–6.

43. Silverberg B, Banis J C, Verdi G D, *et al.* Microsurgical reconstruction for the electrical and deep thermal injury. *Proc Am Burn Assoc* 1985; **17:** 129.

44. Moncreif J A, Pruitt B A. Electric injury. *Postgrad Med* 1970; **48:** 189–94.

45. Saffle J R, Zeluff G R, Warden G D. Intramuscular pressure in the burned arm: measurement and response to escharotomy. *Am J Surg* 1980; **140:** 825–31.

46. Lewis B K. Chemical burns. *Am J Surg* 1959; **98:** 928–33.

47. Clayton J M, Hayes A C, Hammel J, Boyd W C, Hartford C E, Barnes R W. Xenon-133 determination of muscle blood flow in electrical injury. *J Trauma* 1977; **17:** 293–8.

48. Robson M C, Smith D J Jr, Heggers J P. Innovations in burn wound management. In: Habal M B, Morain W D, Lewin M L, Parsons R W, Woods J E, eds. *Advances in Plastic Surgery*. Chicago: Yearbook Medical Publishers, 1987: 149–76.

49. Christensen J A, Sherman R T, Balis G A, Waumett J D. Delayed neurologic injury secondary to high-voltage currents with recovery. *J Trauma* 1980; **20:** 166–8.

50. Farrell D F, Staff A. Delayed neurological sequelae of electrical injuries. *Neurology* 1968; **18:** 601–6.

51. Monafo W W, Freedman B M. Electrical and lightning injury. In: Boswick J A, ed. *The Art and Science of Burn Care*. Rockville: Aspen Publishers Inc, 1987: 241–54.

CHAPTER THIRTY-NINE

39

COLD-INDUCED INJURY: FROSTBITE

JOHN P. HEGGERS, ROBERT L. MCCAULEY, LINDA G. PHILLIPS AND MARTIN C. ROBSON

Progressive tissue necrosis commences with a traumatic insult to the integrity of a host's outer covering, 'the skin', triggering a variety of mediators which are either beneficial or detrimental. Thermal injuries encompass both ambient and tissue temperatures below 32°F (0°C; hypothermia/frostbite) and above 110°F (43.3°C burns). An important clinical and scientific question is whether the mechanism of tissue necrosis could be similar in frostbite and burns. Cold-induced injuries are almost exclusively a result of man's inability to properly protect himself from his environment. Cold injuries may be either systemic or localized, depending upon the temperature and the length of exposure. Systemic injury is hypothermia, while localized injury is frostbite. Although there is much confusion in the literature regarding the myriad of clinical terms used to describe localized injury, the correct term is frostbite.

HISTORICAL PERSPECTIVE

A myriad of historical events discuss legions of armies exposed to frigid temperatures sustaining enormous numbers of cold-induced casualties. While Hippocrates may have described some of the symptoms and sequelae of frostbite (cold injuries), it is reasonable to assume that they were not prevalent in ancient Greece. In 210 BC, Xenophon reported on the injuries suffered by Spartan soldiers during a retreat across the Carduchion mountains after abandoning Alexander's armies. In 218 BC, Hannibal lost almost 50% of his 46 000 man army to cold injuries in only 15 days when they crossed the Pyrenean Alps. Dr James Thatcher, in 1778, wrote that 10% of General Washington's army had been abandoned and left to perish in the severe winter during his campaign against the British.[1] Contrary to these accounts, it was not until 1805 that the first authentic report was published on the effect of cold injury.[2] The first decisive chronicle of mass casualty occurrence was the report by Baron de Larrey, Surgeon-in-Chief of Napolean's army, during the winter invasion of Russia in 1812–1813.[3] Larrey, in his writings, made the following statement: 'When some external part of the body is caught by cold, instead of submitting it to heat, which provides gangrene, it is necessary to rub the affected part with substances containing very little calorick – for it is well known that the effect of calorick on an organized part that is almost deprived of life is marked by an acceleration of fermentation and putrefaction.'[3] Larrey originated the concept of using friction massage with snow or ice while avoiding heat in the thawing process, encompassing the idea that cold injuries were similar to burn injuries. Consequently, when soldiers with cold injuries rapidly rewarmed their extremities over roaring fires (150–170°F; 65.5–76.6°C) after long expeditions, they only renewed the trek and refroze their extremities the next day. Larrey diagnosed that warming was good; however, he cautioned against the use of excessive heat, and finally (eventually) pinpointed the freeze-thaw-freeze cycle. Napoleon left France with 250 000 men and retreated 6 months later with only 350 effective soldiers. The remaining were casualties of cold or starvation.

Throughout the Crimean War (1854–1856), 300 000 French troops experienced 5000 cases of frostbite with 1000 deaths. During World War I (1914–1918), World War II (1939–1945), and the Korean War (1950–1953), at least a million incidents of frostbite occurred. The Germans had to perform 15 000 amputations for cold injuries in the winter of 1942.[4] High altitude frostbites were first reported and recognized in 1943 from the treatment of World War II pilots.[5] Before the 1950s, cold injury treatment basically followed the protocol, advocated by Larrey. In 1956, experimental original studies performed by Merryman prompted Hamill, a Public Health Service medical officer in Tanana, Alaska, to attempt rapid rewarming (at 100°F; 37.7°C) on a patient with frostbite and hypothermia.[6] This was the genesis and has become the foundation of the procedure currently used in Alaska and advocated by Mills.[6]

TEMPERATURE HOMEOSTASIS IN HUMANS

There are no comprehensive statistical data available on the incidence of frostbite. The Royal College of Physicians in London approximated that about 10% of all elderly British home residents were hypothermic, but no analogous data were obtainable for frostbite.[7] Frostbite is much more predominant during military maneuvers and is classified as a hazard for mountain climbers and Arctic explorers. Even in the nonadventurous civilian population, Mills accumulated 500 cases in Alaska by 1963, Cook County Hospital in Chicago accumulated 843 cases between 1962 and 1972, and Detroit Receiving Hospital in Detroit had treated 154 patients between 1982 and 1985.[8–11]

Physiologically, the human is a tropical being, suited more to giving off heat than absorbing it. When at rest and naked, his neutral surrounding temperature is 28°C; with an environmental drop of only 8°C, his metabolic rate must increase by double in order to avoid a lowering of body temperature. The Arctic fox, on the other hand, can maintain a steady thermal state in an environment whose external temperature is –40°C and by increasing its metabolic rate, can contend with an external temperature of −120°C. Getting dressed in response to declines in temperature is not a reflex, but requires a logical decision. If one's capability to decide or act is marred, there is a risk of cold-induced injury.[12] Intoxication has been involved in many cases of frostbite.[13] Investigators noted that mental instability or alcohol intake directly led to cold injury in 50% of their patients. The consumption of alcohol encourages peripheral vascular dilation and increases heat loss. This could possibly make an exposed part more susceptible to cold injury.

The type and duration of cold contact are the two most important factors in establishing the extent of cold injury.[14] Contact with wood or fabric is clearly not as perilous as direct contact with metal, especially with wet or even moist skin. Cold alone is not nearly as hazardous a freezing constituent as is wind coupled with cold.[15] Air alone is a poor thermal conductor, and this is the basis for the wind-chill index. For example, an ambient temperature of −6.7°C with a 45 mile per hour wind has the same effect as −40°C temperature with a 2 mile per hour breeze.[14] Thus, it is essential to think in terms of heat loss, not cold gain. Frostbite strikes when the body is unable to preserve heat or prevent heat loss.

Because many severe cases of frostbite occur at high altitudes, it has been assumed that, with increased altitude, physiologic changes occur which make individuals more predisposed to frostbite. Present data indicate that a decrease in atmospheric pressure is inconsequential with respect to susceptibility to frostbite. The physiologic function of the reticular endothelial (RE) system has little or no influence on the cold injury.[14] Deep loose snow, on the other hand, was thought to insulate from the cold; but it may actually contribute to frostbite. The temperature beneath deep snow is often much lower than that at the surface. In one expedition as recounted by Washburn, it appears that members of his party found it inordinately difficult to keep their feet warm, despite a clear, sunny, −16°C day with little wind. However, one member of the team unintentionally dropped a thermometer in the snow and observed that it registered −25.6°C. Therefore, feet must be protected appropriately.[14]

Development of frostbite does not only depend simply upon a decrease in temperature and the duration of exposure, but can work in concert with wind chill, humidity, or wetness. Water in the stratum corneum can terminate supercooling by initiating water crystallization not only in the stratum corneum, but also in the underlying tissue. Therefore, damp is conducive to the development of frostbite because it permits crystallization to eliminate supercooling after about half of the exposure time necessary for dry skin. This is corroborated by clinical observation as 'it has been found that hypercooling displays itself in lesser degree in skin that remains unwashed. Washing the skin advocates freezing, while applying to the skin a spirit or anointing it with oil discourages it. The ability to supercool would seem to be associated with the relative dryness of the horny layers of the integument. It is well documented that Arctic explorers do not wash during an expedition.'[16]

The amount and adequacy of protective clothing needed varies with the environmental conditions; clothing may contribute to a lack of conservation of body heat. Snug-fitting clothing may induce constriction which impedes blood circulation and reduces the benefit of heat-retaining air protection. Wet clothing provides transmission for heat from the body into the outer environment because moisture is a thermal conductor far superior to air by a factor of about 25.[13] Clothing which transmits moisture away from the body is more protective if an outer wind-resistant layer abates heat loss. Moreover, this wind-resistant layer should retain the same communication capabilities, otherwise clothing will still get damp. Clothing which reduces the quantity of surface area moisture should reduce cold-injury risk. Mittens are far more protective than gloves, since gloves create a greater surface area and prevent air circulation between the fingers. Eighty percent of overall total body heat loss will occur through the exposed head and neck areas. Furthermore, improperly fitted boots infamously generate frostbite injuries.

Decreased local circulation is a primary contributor to cold-induced injuries. Cigarette smoking causes vasoconstriction, impaired cutaneous blood flow, and tissue necrosis in random skin flaps.[17] Investigators documented smoking-induced arteriolar vasoconstriction and demonstrated reduced blood flow in a nude model which resulted in a similar outcome.[18] Even though red blood cell velocity increased, the resultant effect was a reduction in blood flow in the surface microcirculation during and immediately following smoking. Chronic smokers, however, do not seem to be more susceptible to frostbite. Other drugs known to have vasoactive attributes may also be associated with cold-induced injuries. Furthermore, disease states which change tissue physiology, such as atherosclerosis or arthritis, are likewise implicated.

Clinical observations of a cold-induced injury of an individual who has experienced a previous cold injury is put in a high-risk category amid subsequent cold exposure.[19,20] For obscure reasons, frostbite predisposes an individual, so that consecutive cold exposure, even of a minor degree, induces more rapid tissue damage.[13] Military studies emphasize that long periods of immobility contribute to the extent of cold injury.[13] Motion produces body heat and improves circulation, especially in endangered limbs.

FROSTBITE INJURY

A cold-induced injury has been classified into four pathological phases:[21]

1. *Prefreeze phase:* this is secondary to the chilling process, prior to the crystallization of ice. Changes are caused by transendothelial vasoplasticity and plasma leakage. Tissue temperature varies from 3 to 10°C. Cutaneous sensitivity is predominantly eliminated at 10°C.
2. *Freeze–thaw phase:* this confirmation involves actual ice crystal architecture (composition). Tissue temperature declines to a freezing point as the surrounding environment temperature drops below −15°C to −6°C. Because of the underlying emanation of heat energy, skin must be supercooled to −4°C to freeze. Without circulation, the skin temperature will decline at a rate in surplus of 0.5°C/min. After it is thoroughly frozen, the tissue expeditiously exhibits poikilothermy. The sensitivity of tissue to freezing varies, and it is based on the endothelium, bone marrow, and nerve tissue which appear to be more sensitive than muscle.
3. *Vascular stasis phase:* this causes alterations in blood vessels, which include spasticity and dilatation, and subsequently leads to plasma leakage, stasis coagulation, and shunting.
4. *Late ischemic phase:* the final result of thrombosis and arteriovenous shunting is autonomic dysfunction, gangrene, and ischemia.

There may be an overlap among these phases.[21] The changes which occur during each phase vary with the swiftness of freezing, continuance, and extent of injury. It is appropriately clear to divide these pathologic changes which occur in the frost bite injury into those resulting from immediate cellular injury and those from collateral cellular effects. Changes due to immediate tissue injury encompass:

- extracellular ice formation
- intracellular ice formation
- cell dehydration and shrinkage

- abnormal intracellular electrolyte concentrations
- thermal shock
- denaturation of lipid–protein complexes.[22]

Cells which are exposed to a retarded rate of cooling create ice crystals extracellularly in the cellular interspaces. Swift cooling creates intracellular ice crystals which are more fatal to the cell and less favorable for cell survival. In a cold injury, a slower freezing rate does not create intracellular crystals;[23] however, the extracellular ice formed is not without problems. It drags water beyond the cell membrane, initiating intracellular dehydration. The hypothesis of cellular dehydration was primarily suggested in 1929 by Moran[24] and finally confirmed by Merryman's investigations of 'ice crystal nucleation'.[25] Cellular dehydration creates an alteration or variation of protein structure via an elevated electrolyte concentration, modification of membrane lipids, variation of cellular pH, and imbalance of biochemical hemostasis.[26,27] This phenomenon eventually creates a conspicuous and toxic elevation of electrolytes within a cell, and initiates an incomplete shrinkage and disintegration of the vital cell membrane. This is obviously incompatible with cell survival. The complete content of moisture within a cell is not freezable. A small amount of unfrozen water, 'bound water', makes up to 8–10% of the amount of moisture which is firmly held and is noticeable in the protein complex inside the cell. It is immaterial how rapid or noticeable a cold injury occurs, as this confined moisture will remain liquid. With temperatures below –20°C, practically 90% of available water is frozen.[22]

Sudden chilling has been hypothesized to be incongruent with life; however, the severity of this phenomenon is questionable. Another poorly understood concept is the mechanism by which subzero temperatures induce denaturation of lipid–protein complexes. One theory proposes detachment of lipids and lipid proteins from the cell membrane as a corollary to the solvent action of a toxic electrolyte concentration within a cell.[28,29] There is no real indication supporting an alteration of enzyme activity during freezing; however, DNA synthesis is definitely inhibited.[30] Further, there is indirect evidence that ox liver catalase is inactivated due to denaturation and the alteration of the chemical configuration of lactic acid dehydrogenase after freezing and thawing.[31,32] Indirect cellular damage is dependent on progressive microvascular insults which are more grim than the direct cellular consequence. This is sustained by the observation that skin tissue exposed to a standard freeze/thaw injury, which usually produces necrosis *in vivo*, survived as a full-thickness skin graft when transplanted to an uninjured recipient site.[33] Uninjured full-thickness skin, on the other hand, did not survive when transferred to a recipient area pretreated with the same injury. Consequently, direct skin injury is reversible. The progressive nature of injury is most probably dependent on microvascular changes.

About 60% of skin capillary circulation stops in the temperature range of 3–11°C, and 35–40% of blood flow also is impeded in the arterioles and venules.[34] Capillary patency is primarily restored in thawed tissue, while blood flow decreases 3–5 minutes later. Approximately three simultaneous phenomena happen after thawing:

- transient and initial vasoconstriction of arterioles and venules;
- resumption of capillary circulation and blood flow; and
- barrages of emboli racing through microvessels.[22]

Eventually, this causes progressive tissue loss as observed in the distal lying random flap and the no reflow phenomenon. For both injuries, there is the additional effect of the metabolites and the liberation of the oxygen free radicals which all have been shown to be deleterious and contribute to tissue loss. This may also be the case in frostbite injury.[35]

Significant evidence indicates that the initial alteration of a cold injury is actually an injury to the vascular endothelium.[22] Seventy-two hours post-injury, there is a divestiture of the vascular endothelium with the capillary walls in concert with a significant fibrin deposition. The endothelium may be completely destroyed, and fibrin may permeate the arteriole walls.[22] Ultrastructural aberrations of endothelial cells after the thaw period have been observed by electron microscopy in capillaries of the hamster cheek pouch after exposure to subzero temperatures.[36] The endothelial injury was confirmed by demonstrating fluid extravasation from vessels almost contiguously after thawing.[37] As in other forms of trauma, vascular endothelial cells dilate and project inward into the lumen before they lyse. Venules appear to be more susceptible to a cold injury than other vascular structures; this is probably due to lower flow rates. Arterioles, with a flow rate approximately twice that of venules, are less impaired by freezing and develop stasis later than is the case for venules. Capillaries manifest the least direct effects of cold injury; however, their flow rates are rapidly interrupted due to their location between the arterioles and venules. Generalized stasis and discontinuance of flow are observed at a phase of the injury within 20 minutes after freeze and thaw.

Since Cohnheim had observed tissue transformations in cold injury which were comparable to those seen in other inflammatory states, Robson and Heggers hypothesized that progressive ischemia in frostbite may be due to the eicosanoid mediators responsible for progressive dermal ischemia in a burn wound.[38] They assayed blister fluid from cases of frostbite hands and measured levels of PGE_2, PGF_{2a}, and thromboxane. The vasoconstricting, platelet-aggregating, and leukocyte-sticking eicosanoids (PGF_{2a} and thromboxane A_2) were conspicuously elevated. The investigators suggested that the massive edema, subsequent to the cold injury, was due either to leakage of proteins precipitated by the release of these eicosanoids or to leukocyte adherence in the capillaries and augmented hydrostatic pressure. Recent studies have confirmed the analogy between cold injury and the burn wound.[35]

Experimenting with a minimal cold-injury model in the hairless mouse, severe endothelial injury was observed.[39] In addition, the progression of endothelial injury, vascular dilatation, vascular incompetence, and erythrocyte extravasation was confirmed. This led to the theory that eicosanoid metabolites, which may be generated from severely damaged endothelial cells, are significant in progressive tissue loss. Significantly absent from *in vivo* and microscopic observations were vascular spasm, thrombosis, and fibrin deposition, all of which have formerly been involved as pathophysiologic mechanisms. A rabbit ear model demonstrated enhanced tissue survival following inhibition of the eicosanoid cascade at all levels.[40] The most enhanced tissue salvage resulted when specific thromboxane A_2 inhibitors were employed. This has now been demonstrated to be effective therapy in clinical situations.[9]

Frostbite Symptoms

The severity of frostbite symptoms is usually dependent on the severity of the injury. In the civilian environment, frostbite most often occurs more commonly on the extremities. It can also occur on the nose or ears, and has been described in joggers on the scrotum and penis.[14] Mere insensitivity followed by tingling after rewarming does not comprise bona fide frostbite. Even in its blandest form, true frostbite does injure affected tissues. For most patients, the initial clinical presentation is coldness of the injured extremity, with insensitivity evident on over three-fourths of patients. This eventually makes the involved part feel clumsy or missing and has been accredited to the ischemia following vicious vasoconstriction. When insensitivity is primarily present, it is repeatedly followed by extreme pain during the rewarming procedure.

Palpitating pain begins 2–3 days after rewarming and persists for a variable period, even after the tissue eventually becomes demarcated (22–45 days). About 1 week later, a victim consistently notices a residual tingling feeling, presumably generated by ischemic neuritis. For this reason, this feeling tends to continue longer than other symptoms. The severity of the damage consistently defines the extent of neuropathologic injury. There may be an enormous variation of symptoms, with some patients who never notice pain at the onset of the injury. In patients with no tissue loss, symptoms consistently abate within 1 month, while in patients with tissue loss, incapacity may surpass 6 months. In all cases, symptoms are aggravated by a warm environment. Other sensory deficiencies include involuntary burning and electrical current-like feelings. The burning feeling repeatedly occurs early in presentation and usually ebbs within 2–3 weeks. This feeling is not observed in patients with tissue loss. In patients with no tissue loss, it may recur upon boosting activity, or, in feet, by wearing shoes. The electrical current-like feeling is almost ubiquitous in patients with tissue loss. It consistently begins 2–4 days after injury, persists for about 6 weeks, and is especially unpleasant in the evening hours. All frostbite patients have some degree of sensorial loss for at least 4 years after injury and possibly indefinitely.

The clinical presentation of frostbite may be deceptive.[5,8] Only a few patients are admitted with tissue still frozen. Initially, an extremity appears yellowish-white or mottled blue. It may be insensible and appear frozen solid. Regardless of how deep the injury may be, the extremity may seem frozen. With rapid rewarming, there is almost instantaneous hyperemia, even with the most harsh injury. Sensitivity returns after thawing and continues until the blebs appear. At this point, an effort should be made to assess the severity of the injury. Irrespective of 'degrees' of injury, one usually differentiates between superficial and deep injuries. Even these differences are somewhat factitious, since the primary treatment of frostbite is identical. After the injury is rewarmed, edema occurs within 3 hours and lasts 5 days or longer, depending upon the severity of the case.[5] Vesicles or bullae form 6–24 hours after rapid rewarming.[5,41] During the first 9–15 days, seriously frostbitten skin forms a black, hard, and consistently dry eschar whether vesicles are present or not.[5] Mummification delineates an apparent line of demarcation in 22–45 days.[5]

Favorable prognostic signs encompass sensitivity to pin prick, normal color, warmth, and large clear blebs which occur early and tend to extend to the tips of digits. Detrimental signs embody small dark blebs which occur late and do not extend to the digit tips, the lack of edema, and the presence of cyanosis which will not blanch with pressure.[42] Methods which have been used to approximate the dimensions of injury and forecast the ultimate loss include: intravenous radioisotope scanning, angiography, routine roentgenography, and digital plethysmography. These modalities have also been suggested for calculating the vascular response to vasodilators and distinguishing tissue boundaries for surgical management. No prognostic method is positively accurate in the primary post-thaw period, and a delay of 2–3 weeks is essential in order to surpass the period of transient vascular instability.

Management

Hurley is quoted as saying in 1957: 'Tissue cells can be affected by freezing in three different ways: 1) a certain number of cells are killed; 2) a certain number remain unaffected; and 3) a large number are injured but may recover and survive under the right circumstances.'[43] Evidently, the major therapeutic approach must be focused on the salvage of as many cells in category three as is feasible. Frostbite therapy is aimed individually at the prethaw and post-thaw intervals. If a patient is referred from a nearby facility, no attempt at field rewarming is indicated. Vigorous rubbing is contraindicated as it is considered potentially harmful. During transport, the extremity should not be purposely rewarmed and should be protected from slow partial rewarming by keeping the patient away from extremely warm campfires and car heaters. All constricting and damp clothing must be replaced by dry, loose garments. The extremity should be padded and splinted for protection, but no other therapy is recommended. While there is a parallel between the length of time tissues are frozen and the amount of time necessary to thaw tissue, there is no direct parallel between the length of time tissue is frozen and ensuing tissue damage. Consequently rapid transport of frostbite patients within 2 hours is essential. Otherwise, rapid rewarming must be initiated and the patient must be transported with protective dressings so as to obviate refreezing. Blisters must be left intact. Patients with extended transport periods are at greater risk for recurrent injury. All efforts must be made to avoid further refreezing, because this generates a more severe result than delayed thawing. A patient who must walk through snow should do this ahead of thawing frostbitten feet. While in transit, the extremities must be elevated and tobacco smoking forbidden.[6] Alcohol consumption is also detrimental. Upon arrival in the emergency department, rapid rewarming must be started contiguously. Concomitant traumatic injuries or medical problems must be diagnosed. Systemic hypothermia must be rectified to at least the core temperature, 34°C, prior to frostbite therapy. Fluid resuscitation as a rule is not an issue with frostbite injuries, as only one case of rhabdomyolysis and acute renal failure has been described.[44]

Therapy is focused on the specific pathophysiologic effects of the frostbite injury, by either blocking immediate cellular damage or thwarting progressive microvascular thrombosis and tissue loss. Immediate cellular damage is dealt with by rapid rewarming of all degrees of frostbite with immersion in gently circulating warm water between 40 and 42°C. Adherence to this precise temperature range is essential, since rewarming at lesser temperatures is not beneficial for tissue survival,[9,45] and rewarming at elevated temperatures may exacerbate the injury by inducing a burn wound.[46] Hot tap water (50–60°C) will create profound discomfort and potential tissue damage. Frozen extremities must be rewarmed until the injured skin becomes pliable and erythematous at the most distal parts of the frostbite injury. This normally requires less than 30 minutes. Active motion throughout rewarming is advantageous; however, massage may compound the injury. Intense pain may be experienced while thawing, and unless otherwise contraindicated, parenteral analgesics are administered. Immediate return of skin warmth and sensitivity with the obvious erythematous color is a favorable sign, while the continuation of cold, anesthetic, and pale skin is detrimental. Rapid rewarming alters the direct injury of ice crystal formation in the tissue, but it does not obviate the progressive phase of the injury. McCauley *et al.* have designed a therapeutic protocol based on the pathophysiology of progressive dermal ischemia which has been quite successful in diminishing the prolongation of local and systemic thromboxane by injured tissues.[47,48]

Therapeutic Protocol

1. Patients should be admitted to a specialized treatment unit if possible.

2. Acute frostbite patients needing hospitalization must not be discharged or transferred to another facility unless it is necessary for specialized care. All transfer arrangements must provide protection for the patient from cold exposure.
3. Upon admission, the affected area(s) is immediately rewarmed at 40–42°C consistently for 15–30 minutes or until thawing is complete.
4. Upon completion of rewarming, the involved parts are treated as follows:
   (a) White blisters are debrided and topical treatment with *Aloe vera* (Dermaide aloe) q6H is initiated.
   (b) Hemorrhagic blisters are left intact and treatment with topical *Aloe vera* (Dermaide aloe) q6H is initiated.
   (c) The injured part(s) are elevated with splinting as required.
   (d) Tetanus prophylaxis is executed.
   (e) Analgesics: morphine or meperidine IV or IM is delivered as indicated.
   (f) Ibuprofen 400 mg PO every 12 hours is administered.
   (g) Penicillin G 500 000 units every 6 hours IV for 48–72 hours is administered.
   (h) Hydrotherapy is executed daily for 30–45 minutes at 40°C (104°F). The solution should meet the following protocol:
      (i) big tank capacity – 425 gallons; fill capacity approximately 285 gallons; NaCl, 9.7 kg; Ca hypochlorite solution, 95 ml;
      (ii) medium tank capacity – 270 gallons; fill level capacity, 108 gallons; NaCl, 3.7 kg; Ca hypochlorite solution, 36 ml;
      (iii) small tank estimate – 95 gallons; fill level capacity, 72 gallons; NaCl, 2.5 kg; KCl, 71 g; Ca hypochlorite solution, 24 ml.
5. Kodachrome for documentation is essential upon admission, at 24 hours, and serially every 2–3 days until discharge.
6. Patients are released with explicit instructions for protecting the injured areas; and follow-up occurs weekly until wounds are stabilized. If being discharged with closed wounds, the patient is educated to use wool socks, wear a hat, and use mittens instead of gloves to reduce the loss of heat between the digits. The patient is given instructions concerning the evasion of reinjury. It is explained to the patient that he/she is more prone to refreezing, so he/she must avoid exposure to cold, wear warm clothing and shoes or boots if venturing outside. Specific attention must be made to provide protection to the previously injured area. Similar instructions are given to patients who are discharged with open areas. They are also taught to keep the affected extremity elevated and to take ibuprofen 400 mg PO every 12 hours. *Aloe vera* is applied to the affected areas, or scarlet red is used if the open areas are insignificant.

All frostbite cases, except for minor ones, should be admitted to a hospital. Victims with minor injuries should be admitted only if, after rewarming, warm surroundings cannot be provided for the patient. No patient should ever be released into subfreezing weather. Even with a warm car waiting, the patient should be allowed to leave only if he/she is appropriately clothed (i.e. stocking cap, wool mittens, and wool socks).

Since the majority of frostbite injuries require admission to the hospital, an explanation of the protocol is warranted. The white or clear blisters which are consistent with a superficial injury are debrided so as to prevent further contact of the eicosanoid metabolites with the damaged underlying tissues. Unlike the clear blisters, hemorrhagic blisters mirror structural damage to the subdermal plexus. It is worthwhile to drain the eicosanoid-containing fluid from these blisters, while debridement will permit desiccation of the deep dermis and allow conversion of the injury to full-thickness. Therefore, hemorrhagic blisters are left intact. A specific thromboxane inhibitor is applied to the wound surface to prevent further synthesis of this vasoconstricting mediator. Aspirin was originally given systemically to inhibit the production of the eicosanoids. However, the correct dose of aspirin is not known; consequently, it was replaced by a more specific eicosanoid inhibitor, ibuprofen.[9,48] Ibuprofen not only inhibits the eicosanoid cascade, but also has the additional advantage of fibronolysis. Elevation of the extremity minimizes dependent edema. Edema inactivates the normal streptococcal properties of the skin, and parenteral penicillin is recommended during the edema phase of the injury.[11] Tetanus prophylaxis is also given if suggested by history. Tetanus killed thousands of Napoleon's soldiers in the Russian campaign. There has been a report as recently as April 1985 implicating tetanus in a frostbite injury. Since frostbite primarily involves injuries to the extremities, it is essential that appropriate physical and occupational therapy be started early. Daily hydrotherapy for active and passive range of motion is essential in the preservation of function.[49]

Until 1957[50] hardly anything was recorded about the long-term sequelae of frostbite injuries. Blair and colleagues reviewed 100 veterans from the Korean conflict 4 years post-injury. In order of diminishing frequency, they described excessive sweating, pain, coldness, insensitivity, abnormal skin color, and stiffness of the joints. Additionally they observed frequent asymptomatic defects of the nails, including the ridges and inward bending of the edges. Predominantly, the degree of long-term disability was affiliated with the severity of the original injury. Symptoms were more severe in cold than in warm weather.[51] This is attributed to the fact that the blood vessels do not respond as well to stress.[52] Blood vessels which are previously injured do not contract when exposed to cold as efficiently as do normal vessels, and do not dilate as efficiently when vasoconstriction is inhibited.

It is likely that hyperhidrosis is concomitantly a cause and result of frostbite. Hyperhidrosis connotes the presence of an aberrant sympathetic denervation. Susceptibility to cold and predisposition to recurring cold injury would intimate hyperhidrosis. Blanching and pain upon successive cold exposure may be an annoyance or severe enough to suggest a diagnosis of Raynaud's phenomenon. Virtually without exception, a painful, shiny, cyanotic, and sweaty extremity becomes warm, dry, and functional with sympathetic interruption. Intriguingly enough, Shoning scrutinized the changes in the sweat gland of the Hanford miniature swine post-frostbite injury in order to establish the etiology of hyperhidrosis.[53,54] She observed that the injured sweat gland alterations were of two types: atrophy with necrosis and squamous metaplasia. One might suspect that hyperhidrosis would be absent from any histologic documentation.[53,54] The late divergent changes in skin color, including depigmentation of dark skin and erythrocyanosis appearance in light skin, are consistent as results of ischemia.[51] Correspondingly, the nail abnormality is compatible with ischemia. None of these sequelae usually requires therapy. Late signs of joint stiffness and pain on movement are comparatively common and are really related to the underlying scars and mechanical abnormalities engendered by the variety of amputations. 'Punched out' flaws in subchondral bone of injured extremities have been observed. Localized areas of bone resorption usually appear within 5–10 months post-injury and may involuntarily heal. Vascular constriction is likely to be the determinant for these lesions. This bone involvement in immediate proximity to joint surfaces may offer an explanation for these joint symptoms.

Frostbite effects on untimely closure of epiphyses in the growing hand have recently been reemphasized.[55] The amount of early closure is consistent with the severity of the frostbite and observed in partial-thickness injuries. In the digits, early closure occurs more frequently from a distal to proximal direction. Less often involved has been the thumb. In only 2% of cases does partial epiphyseal closure cause angular deformity. One of the distinctive features of frostbite is the astonishing salvage possible in a seemingly badly injured extremity. Therefore, amputation should only be executed with great conservatism and should be delayed as long as possible. The line of demarcation may not be decided conclusively for weeks or months post-injury. As long as secondary sepsis does not interfere, patience often rewards both the patient and surgeon with maximum length of a functional limb. This is especially true for the upper extremities.

PREVENTION

Ordinarily, frostbite can be averted by experienced leadership, good physical condition, satisfactory food, and use of intelligent equipment. Presumably the two most important basic factors in the prevention of frostbite are the heat-producing ability of the body and the efficiency of the measures to preserve heat once it has been generated. The best primary defense against frostbite is a strong healthy body.

No data exist to support the idea that high altitude enhances sensitivities based on alterations in blood viscosity. Correspondingly, living conditions at high altitudes can additionally jeopardize a victim to a frostbite injury. Cold becomes more fierce as do the force and ferocity of storms. Shelter is less available and less protective. Sleep deprivation, deficient diet, modified digestion, and nervous tension all contribute more to an enhanced degree of fatigue than usually experienced at lower heights. Hypoxia diminishes the ability to reason with a tendency to make one indolent, careless, indecisive, and deficient in normal insight and judgment.[45] The body depends on the same amount of oxygen for various tasks irrespective of the altitude; however, at higher altitudes, the body must utilize more air in order to profit from the same amount of oxygen. Individuals must cautiously adjust their activity; otherwise, they will not only deplete the body, but also cool it. High quantities of heat can be eliminated through the lungs by panting and overexertion, which also contribute to fatigue.[56] Further, since injured local circulation is a major cause of frostbite, anything which induces a mildly antagonistic effect on normal peripheral circulation, such as tobacco or alcohol, should be avoided. Smoking results in altering degrees of redundant vascular spasm, thus diminishing normal peripheral circulation.

REFERENCES

1. Smith D J, Robson M C, Heggers J P. Frostbite and other cold-induced injuries. In: Auerbach P S, Geehr E C, eds. *Management of Wilderness and Environmental Emergencies*. St Louis: CV Mosby, 1989: 101–18.

2. Zingg W. The management of accidental hypothermia. *Can Med Assoc J* 1967; **96:** 214.

3. Larrey D J. *Memoirs of Military Surgery*. Vol 2. Baltimore: Joseph Cushing, 1814.

4. Vaughn P B. Local cold injury-menace to military operations. A review. *Military Med* 1980; **145**(5): 305.

5. Orr K D, Fainer D C. *Cold Injuries in Korea during Winter of 1950–51*. Fort Knox, KY: Army Medical Research Laboratory, 1951.

6. Mills W J. Out in the cold. *Emerg Med*. Jan. 1976; **18:** 134.

7. Fox R H, Woodward P M, Exton Smith A N, *et al.* Body temperature in the elderly: a national study of physiological, social and environmental conditions. *BMJ* 1973; **1:** 200.

8. Boswick J A, Thompson J D, Jonas R A. The epidemiology of cold injuries. *Surg Gynecol Obstet* 1979; **149:** 326.

9. Heggers J P, Robson M C, Manavalen K, *et al.* Experimental and clinical observations on frostbite. *Ann Emerg Med* 1987; **16:** 1056.

10. Kyosola K. Clinical experiences in the management of cold injuries: a study of 110 cases. *J Trauma* 1974; **14**(1): 32.

11. Mills W F Jr. Summary of treatment of the cold-injured patient. *Alaska Med* 1973; **15**(2): 56.

12. Cold Hypersensitivity. *BMJ* 1975; **1:** 643.

13. Knize D M. Cold injury in reconstructive plastic surgery. In: Converse J M, McCarthy J G, Littler J W, eds *General Principles*. 2nd ed. Vol 1. Philadelphia, WB Saunders Co, 1977: 516–30.

14. Washburn B. Frostbite – what it is – how to prevent it – emergency treatment. *N Engl J Med* 1962; **266:** 974.

15. Wilson O, Goldman R F. Role of air temperature and wind in the time necessary for a finger to freeze. *J Appl Phys* 1970; **29**(5): 658.

16. Lewis T. Observations on some normal and injurious effects of cold upon the skin and underlying tissues: III. Frostbite. *BMJ* 1941; **2:** 869.

17. Lawrence W T, Murphy R C, Robson M C, *et al.* The detrimental effect of cigarette smoking on flap survival: an experimental study in the rat. *Br J Plast Surg* 1984; **37:** 216.

18. Reus W F, Robson M C, Zachary L, *et al.* Acute effects of tobacco smoking on blood flow in the cutaneous micro-circulation. *Br J Plast Surg* 1984; **37:** 213.

19. Mills W J, Whaley R. Frostbite: a method of management. In: *Proceedings of the Symposium on Arctic Biology and Medicine: IV. Frostbite*. Fort Wainwright, Alaska: Arctic Aeromedical Laboratory, 1964.

20. Whayne T J, DeBakey M F. Cold injury, ground type. Washington, DC: US Government, 1958.

21. Kulka J P. Vacomotor microcirculatory insufficiency: observations on non-freezing cold injury of the mouse ear. *Angiology* 1961; **12:** 491.

22. Zacarian S A. Cryogenics: the cryolesion and the pathogenesis of cryonecrosis. In: Stone D, Clater H, eds *Cryosurgery for Skin and Cutaneous Disorders*. St Louis: CV Mosby 1985; **7:** 27.

23. Merryman H T. The exceeding of a minimum tolerable cell volume in hypertonic suspension as a cause of freezing injury. In: Walstenholme G, O'Connor M Sr, eds *The Frozen Cell*. London: Churchill, 1970: 51.

24. Moran T. Critical temperature of freezing living muscle. *Proc R Soc B* 1929; **105:** 177.

25. Merryman H T. Mechanisms of freezing in living cells and tissues. *Science* 1956; **124:** 515.

26. Mazur P. Causes of injury in frozen and thawed cells. *Fed Proc* 1965; **24**(Suppl 14–15): 5.

27. Mazur P. Studies in rapidly frozen suspension of yeast cells by differential thermal analysis and conductometry. *Biophys J* 1963; **3:** 323.

28. Lovelock J E. Physical instability in thermal shock in red blood cells. *Nature* 1954; **173:** 659.

29. Lovelock J E. The denaturation of lipid-protein complexes as a cause of damage by freezing. *Proc R Soc Biol* 1957; **147:** 427.

30. Johnson B E, Daniels F Jr Enzyme studies in experimental cryosurgery of the skin. *Cryobiology* 1974; **11:** 22.

31. Marhert C L. Lactate dehydrogenase isozymes: dissociation and recombination of subunits. *Science* 1963; **140:** 1629.

32. Shikama K, Yamazaki I. Denaturation of catalase by freezing and thawing. *Nature* 1961; **190:** 83.

33. Weatherly-White RCA, Sjostrom B, Paton B C. Experimental studies in cold injury. *J Surg Res* 1964; **4:** 17.

34. Rinfret A P *Cryobiology in Cryogenic Technology*. New York: Wiley, 1962.

35. Bulkley G B. The role of oxygen free radicals in human disease processes, *Surgery* 1983; **94:** 407.

36. Rabb J M, Renaud M L, Brandt P A, *et al.* Effect of freezing and thawing on the microcirculation and capillary endothelium of the hamster cheek pouch. *Cryobiology* 1974; **11:** 508.

37. Zacharian S A, Stone D, Clater H. Effects of cryogenic temperatures in the microcirculation in the golden hamster cheek pouch. *Cryobiology* 1970; **7:** 27.

38. Robson M C, Heggers J P. Evaluation of hand frostbite blister fluid as a clue to pathogenesis. *J Hand Surg* 1981; **6:** 43.

39. Bourne M H, Piepcorn M W, Clayton F, *et al.* Analysis of microvascular changes in frostbite injury. *J Surg Res* 1986; **40:** 26.

40. Raine T J, London M D, Goluch L, *et al.* Antiprostaglandins and antithromboxanes for treatment of frostbite. *Surg Forum* 1980; **31:** 557.

41. Miller J W, Danzl D F, Thomas D M. Urban accidental hypothermia: 135 cases. *Ann Emerg Med* 1980; **9**(9): 456.

42. Mills W J Jr. Clinical aspects of frostbite injury. In: *Proceedings of the Symposium on Arctic Medicine and Biology: IV. Frostbite*. Fort Wainwright, Alaska: Arctic Aeromedical Laboratory, 1964.

43. Hurley L A. Angioarchitectural changes associated with rapid rewarming subsequent to freezing injury. *Angiology* 1957; **8:** 19.

44. Rosenthall L, Schechter D S, Sarot A, *et al.* Frostbite with rhabdomyolisis and renal failure: radionuclide study. *Am J Roentgenology* 1981; **137:** 387.

45. Fuhrman F A, Crissman J M. Studies on gangrene following cold injury. VII. Treatment of cold injury by immediate rapid rewarming. *J Clin Invest* 1947; **26:** 476.

46. Mills W J, Whaley R, Fish W. Frostbite: experience with rapid rewarming and ultrasonic therapy. *Alaska Med* 1961; **3:** 28.

47. McCauley R L, Hing D N, Robson M C, *et al.* Frostbite injuries: a rational approach based on the pathophysiology. *J Trauma* 1983; **23:** 143.

48. McCauley R L, Heggers R L, Heggers I P, *et al.* Frostbite: methods to minimize tissue loss. *Postgrad Med* 1990; **88**(8): 67.

49. Edstrom L E, Robson M C, Headley B J. Evaluation of exercise techniques in the burn patient. *Burns* 1977; **4**(2): 113.

50. Mitchell H H, Edman M. *Nutrition and Climatic Stress with Particular Reference to Man*. Springfield, IL: Charles C Thomas, 1951.

51. Blair J R, Schatzki R, Orr N D. Sequelae to cold injury in one hundred patients: follow-up study four years after occurrence of cold injury. *JAMA* 1957; **163:** 1203.

52. Simeone F A. Surgical volumes of the history of the United States Army Medical Department in World War II; cold injury. *Arch Surg* **80:** 296.

53. Schoning P, Hamlet M P. Experimental frostbite in Hanford miniature swine. 1. Epithelial changes. *Br J Exp Pathol* 1989; **70**(1): 41.

54. Schoning P, Hamlet M P. Experimental frostbite in Hanford miniature swine II. Vascular changes. *Br J Exp Pathol* 1989; **70**(1): 51.

55. Weuzl J E, Burke E C, Bianco A J Jr. Epiphysical destruction from frostbite of the hands. *Am J Dis Child* 1967; **114:** 668.

56. Pugh G. Expedition to Cho Oyo. *Georgr J (London)* 1953; **119:** 137.

CHAPTER FORTY

CHEMICAL INJURY

STEPHEN M. MILNER, LINDSEY T. A. RYLAH, THUAN T. NGUYEN, ROBERT J. REDELMEIER, EDGAR J. PIERRE AND DAVID N. HERNDON

INTRODUCTION

A chemical injury may be encountered in all walks of life. Many chemicals are stored in households ranging from those used to clean kitchens and bathrooms, to hair and laundry bleaches. More dangerous exposures may follow occupational use of industrial chemicals. Most injuries will be accidental, but the criminal use of chemicals to assault others is not uncommon. In a 10-year survey from Jamaica, out of a total of 4234 admissions, 13.3% (562) were due to chemical burns of which 236 (42%) were due to interpersonal violence.[1] Amongst military personnel, recent reviews have shown a predominance of injuries due to white phosphorous.[2] Although most physicians are unlikely to encounter casualties of chemical weapons, the proliferation of these agents during the last decade has increased the risk to both military and civilian populations. For this reason an account of current thoughts on management of vesicular agents is included in this text.

It would be impossible to address the many thousands of chemicals which may be encountered. Exposure to elements and their compounds can cause dermal wounds appearing similar to those induced by thermal injury; however, the mechanism of action may be very different and the treatment should, wherever possible, be tailored to the offending substance. Delaying treatment for such injuries until resuscitation has been successfully completed may be harmful, as the chemical may have a prolonged action and produce serious metabolic effects. In this chapter, common agents are classified. The type of injuries, the basic principles of management, and specific recommendations for treatment are examined in a pragmatic fashion. The complications arising from exposure to these chemicals and the supportive measures needed during treatment are also described.

The colour plates for this chapter appear between pp 264 and 265.

PATHOPHYSIOLOGY

The body has very few specific defense and repair mechanisms for thermal and chemical burns. There are similarities between chemical and thermal burns; namely, that both involve protein denaturing and produce wounds which look superficially alike. On the other hand, important differences exist. Thermal injuries are typically produced by very short-term exposure (seconds) to intense heat which is relatively quickly stopped. Chemical injuries are more likely produced by longer (minutes) exposure to chemicals, and this exposure may still be continuing in an emergency room.

Chemically, there are also fundamental differences between the two types of injury. Proteins are oligopolymers of amino acids, ranging in length from 60 to 8000 amino acid units. Protein polymer chains form single helices, fold back on themselves or assume other structures as dictated by the order of the constituent amino acids. There are two structural forms of biological proteins: single helix linear protein chains found in cell membranes, muscles, and other connective tissues; and globular proteins serving as enzymes and in other metabolic roles. These biologically active structures unfortunately are rather fragile since they are not formed by chemical bonds, but rather by weaker forces such as hydrogen bonding and van der Waals' forces. Application of heat or chemicals, especially pH disturbances, can cause the structures to fall apart. In thermal injuries, there is a rapid coagulation of protein due to irreversible cross-linking reactions, whereas with chemical burns the protein destruction is continued by other mechanisms. The commonest mechanism is hydrolysis which is driven by pH disturbances. Thus, there is an additional problem of restoring tissue pH in order to stop cellular damage. These mechanisms may continue so long as traces of the offending agent are present, especially in the deeper layers.

The degree of tissue damage as well as the level of systemic toxicity is determined by the chemical nature of an agent, its concentration, the duration of skin contact, and the mechanism of action.[3] Chemical injury is classified either by the mechanism of action on skin or by the chemical class of the offending agent. A cross-reference of these two classifications along with a broader clinical picture makes it more likely that an appropriate treatment will be instituted.

Mechanisms of Action

With the exception of concentrated or fuming sulfuric acids, thermal injury rarely plays more than a minor role in chemical injury. The main mechanisms of action on living tissue have been placed into six categories.[4] The cells may be damaged by: (1) reduction, (2) oxidation, (3) corrosion, (4) protoplasmic poisons, (5) a chemical which causes desecration or (6) tissues may be damaged by vesicant activity.

Reduction

Protein denaturation is caused by the reduction of the amide linkages following exposure to reducing agents. Heat may also be a product of a chemical reaction, thereby causing a mixed picture. Reducing agents are rather rare and highly reactive chemicals. The reducing agents more likely to be encountered are alkyl mercuric compounds, diborane, lithium aluminum hydride, and other metallic hydrides.

Oxidation

Some agents cause damage by inserting an oxygen, sulfur, or halogen (most often chlorine) atom to otherwise viable body proteins. In general, this destroys a protein's ability to function. Sometimes, the oxidation product can have very untoward effects as it becomes a competitor for active metabolic sites. Common examples are sodium hypochlorite, potassium permanganate, all peroxides, and chromic acid.

Corrosive agents

Some agents corrode the skin and cause massive protein denaturing. As a class, they act in a variety of ways but they tend to produce a soft eschar which may progress to shallow indolent ulceration. Phenols are the commonest corrosive agents encountered; the hydroxides of sodium, potassium, ammonium, and calcium follow as close seconds.

Protoplasmic poisons

Some poisons produce their effects by causing the formation of esters with proteins or by the binding or inhibition of the inorganic ions which are necessary for normal, healthy cellular function. Ester formers are typified by formic and acetic acids, while metabolic competitors or inhibitors include oxalic and hydrofluoric acids.

Desiccants

The damage of desiccants is caused by water being extracted from tissues by hygroscopic agents. The damage is often exacerbated by heat production as these reactions are usually exothermic. Concentrated or fuming sulfuric acid is the best known desiccant.

Vesicants

These are characterized by their ability to produce cutaneous blisters and are potent chemical warfare agents. They include mustards, arsenicals, and halogenated oximes. Mustards are alkylating agents and the damage to DNA renders them toxic to proliferating cells. Recent evidence, however, suggests that alkylation of DNA may not be the critical step so far as skin injury is concerned.[5] Following death of the basal cells, proteases are released from lysosomes, causing the epidermis to separate from the dermis. The result is a blister with the basement membrane on its dermal side. Lewisite, for example, acts by inhibiting several important enzyme systems, the most important of which is the pyruvate dehydrogenase complex.[6]

Chemical Classes

The chemical class of a noxious chemical is based on the chemical reactions which the chemical is prone to initiate. Acidity/basicity, or the ability to influence pH is one of the most important characteristics of an injurious chemical, and one which must be considered in effective wound management. It should also be noted that concentration plays an important role in the reactivity of a chemical. In general, concentrated solutions (>70% wt) are more viscous, more reactive, more hygroscopic, and liberate more heat during lavage or neutralization.

Acids

Acids are proton donors, so they release hydrogen ions and reduce pH from a neutral 7 down to values as low as 0. Hydrogen ions are reactive and will protonate any amine or carboxylic site. This will cause a protein structure to collapse. After time, hydrogen ions will catalyse protein hydrolysis into constituent amino acids. Mineral acids may also have other effects as seen in concentrated sulfuric acid injuries where there is heat generation and desiccation, producing a mixed injury. Phosphoric acid, for instance, can produce a similar mixed injury by also chelating calcium.

Bases

Bases are proton acceptors. The major type to cause injury are mineral alkalis. Bases will strip hydrogen ions from protonated amine groups and carboxylic groups. This will cause protein structure collapse and, in common with acids, bases will catalyse protein hydrolysis. Bases can also cause a mixed injury by forming salts and soaps, causing tissue destruction as seen in the corrosive group (see above). Ammonia, the hydroxides of sodium and potassium, and lime are the most common agents of this type to cause injury.

Organic compounds

A wide range of organic compounds will damage protein by direct chemical reactions and heat production. They may also act as solvents and disrupt the protein structure. Such agents include phenol and petroleum-based compounds.

Inorganic agents

Apart from the mineral acids and alkalis referred to above, highly reactive elements damage skin by direct binding and salt formation as well as heat production. Sodium, phosphorus, lithium, and chlorine are excellent examples. Some salts, especially fluoride, can also cause damage.

General Principles of Management

Emergency Care

A thorough history is mandatory to enable recognition of a responsible agent. Prompt treatment is essential if tissue damage is to be minimized. All clothing serves to entrap a chemical against the skin and should be completely removed. A wound should be thoroughly irrigated with water. Speed is essential. Lavage effectively dilutes a chemical already in contact with the skin, washes unreacted agent from the surface, and helps correct the hygroscopic effects which certain agents have on tissues.[7] Lavage has been shown to reduce hospital stay and reduce the extent of full-thickness injury.[8] That early irrigation increases its effectiveness has been amply confirmed clinically[8] and experimentally with the rat model using subcutaneous pH probes.[9]

Lavage should be done with copious quantities of fluid. Large quantities are necessary since some strong acids and caustics can contaminate large quantities of fluids. For example, 10 ml of 98% sulfuric acid will reduce the pH of 12 liters of water down to 5.0. To increase lavage effectiveness, and to avoid the use of excessive quantities of lavage fluid, the lavage site should be kept drained in order to remove the earlier, more concentrated washings. This can be done by either suction or periodic sponging. When possible, monitoring of the spent lavage solution pH will give a good indication of lavage effectiveness and completion.

There has been considerable discussion about the use of neutralizing solutions. Some of these, such as neutralizing sulfuric acid burns with sodium hydroxide, are the chemical analog of treating thermal burns with liquid nitrogen! Control of the amount of strong neutralizing solutions is the key difficulty. The early use of neutralizing solutions is further contraindicated by the heat generated when concentrated chemicals are neutralized. On the other hand, neutralizing solutions may be very useful when correctly applied. The solutions used should be of the buffered variety, with a pH around 6. This has been shown to be useful if applied after ten minutes of intensive irrigation with water.[9]

Metabolic Support

A victim must be monitored according to the severity of the injury. The major complication of chemical injury may be a gross metabolic upset. This is most likely to occur from pH disturbances following large exposure to strong acids or caustics. Blood gas and electrolyte analysis should be performed at regular intervals during the first 36 hours at least, or until metabolic stability has been assured. Any compromise in the patency of the airway must be treated aggressively by tracheal intubation. If oxygen transport is at risk, oxygen therapy and mechanical ventilation must be instituted. Surgery can take place as soon as a patient is stable. If the condition of the patient continues to deteriorate, a decision must be made as to whether urgent surgery is indicated. Continuous progression or deepening of a wound and progressive metabolic deterioration, including renal and liver failure, would lead to this course of action.

Analgesia must be adequate and relevant. If opiates are needed, large doses may be necessary. Respiratory depression is an unlikely but obvious consequence of high doses of opioids and must be monitored; respiratory support may be unavoidable in a few cases. Support of major systems must be instituted early rather than late as salvage of a failed system may prove impossible.

Any patient having 'copious lavage' is in danger of suffering from induced hypothermia. It is wise to monitor core and peripheral temperatures during this maneouver and maintain room temperature between 31 and 33°C and the lavage water temperature as near to body temperature as possible.

Care of a Burn Wound

Following adequate lavage and debridement, chemical burn wounds are covered with topical chemotherapeutic agents or one of the proprietary skin substitutes and appropriate dressings. Follow-up may be prolonged, as chemical injuries tend to heal more slowly than conventional thermal burns. For deep dermal and full-thickness burns, current practice employs tangential excision or scalpel excision to the level of the investing fascia and split-thickness skin grafting. Careful use of selected buffered neutralizing agents may be of use during these procedures if the presence of residual agent is suspected.

Specific Agents

If an injury has been caused in an industrial setting, it is likely that the causative agent is known. The following list of chemicals (in alphabetical order) is not definitive, but it provides an inventory of the commonest agents to cause chemical 'burns'. Each agent is presented with a specific emergency treatment, if indicated. The medium- and long-term treatment will only be discussed if it is different from normal burn care.

Acetic Acid

This acid is a protoplasmic poison and very similar to the assorted acids (see below). Glacial acetic acid, nearly 100% pure acid, is the usual offender. Vinegar, a 5% solution of acetic acid, is usually benign unless scalding hot.

Alkali (Strong)

Multiple chemical agents are involved in caustic alkali burns. Lime, potassium hydroxide, and sodium hydroxide are the most common agents causing chemical injury. Accidental injury occurs in infants and toddlers. Among chemical burns, alkali injuries occur frequently and are likely to cause severe symptoms. The mechanism by which these alkali injuries are caused is due to three factors:

1. saponification of fat causes fatty tissue to lose its function with increased damage due to heat reaction;
2. extraction of considerable water from cells causes damage because of an alkali's hydroscopic nature; and
3. alkalis dissolve and unite with the proteins of the tissues to form alkaline proteinates, which are soluble and contain OH ions and

these ions cause further chemical reactions which initiate deeper injury of the tissue.[10]

The extent of the damage caused by an alkali substance depends on its concentration, amount, condition and time of contact with the skin, tissue permeability, heat, and sensitivity of the injured region. As these factors become greater, the extent of the damage becomes greater.[11]

As with other chemical burns, alkalis are capable of deep penetration, and can cause severe pain. For treatment, it is necessary to remove the causative substance as quickly as possible by washing with large volumes of water. Washing is presumed to cause dilution and elimination of a chemical substance, attenuation of the chemical reaction, and suppression of any raised tissue metabolism; to have an anti-inflammatory action; to suppress the hygroscopic action; and to return skin pH levels to normal.[11]

The initial treatment for burns caused by strong alkaline solution is copious irrigation with water. Water may carry away any heat by dilution so as to prevent further damage. In lime burns, the dry lime must be brushed away before washing in order to minimize the production of heat. The most readily available material for removing a chemical agent is water, and it is extremely important to remove a chemical agent as rapidly as possible. Attempts to neutralize an alkali agent are not recommended. Therefore, washing with large quantities of water is the preferred treatment. Until the substance is removed, it continues to destroy tissue. In general, injuries which are not promptly washed with copious volumes of water, when admitted later to a hospital, are deep. It is very difficult to determine the depth of tissue damage on admission to a hospital because chemical burns are different from thermal burns. Because the corrosive material blackens the skin, rapidly converting it to a firmly adherent, hard, dry eschar, a true assessment of the depth of an injury can only be made in retrospect, as spontaneous healing, or nonhealing, occurs.[12]

Ocular damage is a common sequel to alkali injury. Damage is related to the pH: the higher the pH, the greater the damage to the eye, with the most significant injury occurring around pH 11–11.5. The corrosive agent trickles down the eyelid and enters the acanthi. Alkalis penetrates quickly and, with little resistance, saponify plasma membranes, denature collagen, and cause vascular thromboses in the conjunctiva, the episclera, and even in the anterior uvea.[13] Very small volumes of alkali material can cause significant damage. The sequelae of corneal lime burns include scarring and opacification of the comea with resultant loss of visual acuity, corneal neovascularization, ulcer formation, and perforation.[13] Other sequelae of untreated or very severe alkali burns include epithelial erosions, secondary glaucoma, progressive cicatrization which occludes the ducts of main and accessory lacrimal glands and causes destruction of conjunctival goblet cells so as to cause dry eyes, cicatricial entropion, and trichiasis.[14]

Such damage may be made worse by repeated attempts to wipe off the chemical agent with the hands or inadequately washing the eyes. The policy is to treat with topical anesthetics followed by copious irrigation, induction of cycloplegia and mydriasis as soon as possible. Antibiotics, such as gentamicin and/or chloramphenicol, are effective topically. Cysteine, a collagenase inhibitor, is applied every 2 hours in order to prevent perforation. Topical steroids are applied four times per day after complete epithelialization has taken place.[15]

Assorted Acids

Tungstic, picric, sulfosalicylic, tannic, trichloracetic, and cresylic acids are all strong protoplasmic poisons. They form hard eschars which may help spare underlying tissues from damage. Tannic acid has been used in the past as a treatment for thermal injury.[16] These acids are absorbable and cause metabolic symptoms and are both renal and hepatic toxins. Most have pungent, suffocating odors and have wide industrial usage. They can be found in solution and in crystalline forms.

Alkyl Mercuric Compounds

Ethyl and methyl mercuric phosphates are primary irritants but are likely to progress to form blisters and erythema. This process will continue while the chemical is in contact with the skin. Blisters will also cause a wound to progress unless they are deroofed and the blister fluid evacuated. Free mercury is released and is found in the blister fluid. After a large or lengthy exposure, this free mercury will be absorbed and may cause systemic effects. An exposed area should be washed, followed by debridement and removal of the blister fluid, and copious lavage of the wound again. Systemic mercurial poisoning is treated with chelating agents and systemic support (see Chromic acid and dimercaprol treatment).

Cantharides

Sometimes called 'Spanish Fly', these agents may be used by certain cultures as an aphrodisiac for both farming animals and humans. These are vesicants which produce papules of 0.5–1.0 cm in diameter with severe histamine release. The edema causes tissue hypoxia which worsens the resultant partial-thickness injury associated with skin contact. Treatment is simply with water lavage.

Cement

Cement is really an alkali, but it differs in enough ways to warrant a separate mention. When mixed with water, sand, and gravel, it becomes more abrasive and is known as concrete. Injuries are not infrequently found in construction workers and do-it-yourself enthusiasts. Cement (calcium oxide) penetrates clothing and reacts with sweat, and an exothermic reaction takes place. The dry powder is very hygroscopic and will cause a desiccation injury if not exposed to moisture. Hydrated calcium oxide becomes calcium hydroxide. An injury progresses as with a strong alkali, and the critical substance responsible for skin damage is the hydroxyl ion.[17] A victim may not know until many hours later that a bum has been sustained as it is often a painless occurrence, under clothing. Treatment consists of removal of contaminated clothing and washing an affected area with soap and water. Surgical excision is likely to be required as these injuries are often deeper than they first appear.

Chromic Acid

A powerful oxidizing agent, chromic acid is used in the cleaning of other metals. The active chemical is chromic trioxide (CrO_3) in a solution of strong sulfuric acid. If a sample is examined, it is a pungent viscid yellow liquid. Contact will cause protein coagulation, blister formation, and ulceration. Ingestion will lead to gastroenteritis which will become severe very rapidly with vertigo, muscle cramps, peripheral vascular collapse, and coma. A nephritis will follow and is associated with glycosuria. The lethal dose is between 5 and 10 g. Primary treatment of contact areas comprises water lavage to dilute the acid. Washing with a dilute solution of sodium hyposulfite, followed by a rinsing with a buffered phosphate solution is the treatment of choice and should be available if this agent is in common use. The buffered solution is made by adding 70 g monobasic potassium phosphate and 180 g dibasic sodium phosphate to 850 ml of water. Systemic manifestations are to be treated with 2, 3-Dimercapto-1-propanol (British antilewisite or dimercaprol) 4 mg/kg by deep intramuscular injection every 4 hours for 2 days, followed by 2–4 mg/kg daily, for about a week along with support for the failing organ systems.

Dichromate Salts

The dichromate salts are highly corrosive and act in a similar manner to proton donators. They produce a soft yellow colored coagulum with deep indolent ulcers. The lethal dose is between 50 and 100 mg/kg body weight depending on the route of entry. These salts remain active for long periods of time after exposure. Additional symptoms of violent gastroenteritis, vascular collapse, muscle cramps, vertigo, and coma may be experienced if ingested. Multiorgan failure may follow. Emergency treatment with water lavage is mandatory. Other more specific treatments include: washing with 2% hyposulfite solution; lavage with a buffer (i.e. 7% potassium dihydrogen phosphate and 18% disodium hydrogen phosphate in water); surgical removal may also be considered.

Dimethyl Sulfoxide (DMSO)

One very powerful solvent may serve as a vehicle to carry other agents. It can solubilize normally insoluble organic agents and greatly aggravate their absorption into tissues and produce deep wounds. By itself, DMSO has only very mild toxicity, but since it is usually used as a solvent, clinicians should ascertain what solute it carries. As this substance is water soluble and not exothermic, the treatment of choice is water lavage along with any specific treatment for the solute.

Formic Acid

Despite the common use of this organic acid for industrial descaling and as a hay preservative,[18] dermal injury is rare. All patients injured by formic acid should be hospitalized, if only for observation, because cutaneous absorption from injured areas can cause metabolic acidosis, intravascular hemolysis, hemoglobinuria, and renal failure as well as pulmonary complications, including ARDS.[19] Vomiting and abdominal pain are usual; and although the cause is unknown, necrotizing pancreatitis has been described as a complication of formic acid ingestion. Elevated serum amylase in formic acid poisoning has not been reported. Acidosis should be corrected with intravenous sodium bicarbonate. Minor hemolysis requires no treatment, but mannitol diuresis is recommended where hemolysis occurs after deep burns. Where extensive absorption of formic acid has occurred, hemodialysis should be considered. The wound has a greenish hue and is followed within 48 hours by gross edema and blister formation. Wounds tend to be deeper than they initially appear and are best treated by surgical excision.

Hydrocarbons

Petrol burns are seen in patients trapped under vehicles following road traffic accidents. The solvent properties of hydrocarbons promote cell membrane injury and dissolution of lipids, resulting in skin necrosis.[2] Symptoms present with erythema and blistering (**Plate 11**). Burns tend to be superficial and heal spontaneously.[20] Grafting is usually not necessary although full-thickness burns do occur. If absorbed systematically, toxicity can cause respiratory depression. If ignited, deep thermal injury is common.

Hydrochloric Acid

One strong acid protonates skin proteins into their chloride salts. While hydrochloric acid is in contact with tissue, a wound will progress and the acid will continue to denature protein. Shallow ulcers form and are overlaid by a coagulum of damaged skin. Hydrochloric acid fumes can result in a pneumonitis type inhalation injury, or airway obstruction, caused by edema formation in the glottic region.

Hydrofluoric Acid

Hydrofluoric acid is a toxic substance used widely in both industrial and domestic settings. It is one of the strongest inorganic acids known. It has been in industrial use since its ability to dissolve silica was recognized in the late seventeenth century. In 1720, the first crude preparation of hydrofluoric acid was discovered by an English glassmaker. In the 1800s, hydrofluoric acid was used for cleaning sand, fluoride ion from castings, and etching glass. In 1974, 375 000 tons of hydrofluoric acid were produced. The dual mechanism of injury makes hydrofluoric acid burns among the most severe and lethal. Hydrofluoric acid produces dehydration and corrosion of tissue due to free hydrogen ions which induce skin necrosis. A fluoride ion complexes certain bivalent cations, primarily calcium and magnesium, to form insoluble salts. Systemic absorption of fluoride anion from hydrofluoric acid leads to complexication of positively charged cations like calcium and magnesium.[21] As cellular calcium is bound and immobilized, cell death occurs. If untreated, inbound fluoride will produce liquefaction necrosis and decalcify bone. The binding of free fluoride anions to free calcium and magnesium forms insoluble salts and may occur at a rate which exceeds the body's ability to mobilize bone calcium and magnesium into serum. Fluoride anion may inhibit the Na-K-ATPase enzyme of the cell membrane, leading to a massive potassium efflux.[22] The resultant ionic shifts, particularly of potassium, are thought to be responsible for the excruciating pain associated with hydrofluoric acid burn. It has been postulated that conjugation with fluoride ions results in a depletion of available calcium. This causes local nerve endings to release cellular potassium and discharge frequently.[23]

The severity of hydrofluoric acid burn is a product of concentration, surface area involved and the duration of exposure. The National Institutes of Health – Division of Industrial Hygiene has classified hydrofluoric acid burns on the basis of hydrofluoric concentration in the offending agent.[24] Concentrations of greater than 50% always cause immediate pain with apparent tissue destruction. Concentrations of 20%–50% result in a burn becoming apparent within several hours of exposure. Dilute concentrations of less than 20% may take up to 24 hours to become apparent. The skin initially appears erythematous; and with long exposure and stronger concentration, skin assumes a gray appearance with a cheesy-yellow substance beneath the skin. Without therapy, injury will progress to full-thickness skin loss with decalcification of underlying bone.

Systemic manifestation

The systemic manifestation of hydrofluoric acid exposure comes primarily from hypocalcemia, serum hypocalcemia (less than 0.62 mmol/l with normal being 2.23–2.57 mmol/l) or hypomagnesemia (less than 0.65 mmol/l with normal being 0.65–1.05 mmol/l).[25] The hypocalcemia seen in hydrofluoric acid exposure is silent. It does not produce the typical signs of hypocalcemia. The serum calcium level and the electrocardiogram are reliable indicators of hypocalcemia.[26] In addition, the hypocalcemia induces cardiac arrhythmia such as refractory ventricular fibrillation which is particularly resistant to treatment.[27] We report a fatal case of severe systemic toxicity in a 50-year-old male with hydrofluoric acid burns. A 50-year-old man was exposed to 20% hydrofluoric acid oil mixture at 300°F (149°C). The patient was admitted to the Blocker Burn Unit with initial evaluation in the tub room, where burn wounds were irrigated with water and calcium gluconate. The patient was alert, but became less responsive, and finally no blood pressure or pulse could be detected. Initial laboratory studies yielded values of serum sodium at 141 mmol/l, potassium at 4.0 mmol/l, calcium 1.6 mg/dl, ionized calcium 0.96 mg/dl, phosphorus 2.2 mg/dl, and magnesium 0.7 mg/dl. This patient sustained a sudden onset of ventricular fibrillation. Closed chest compression was begun, and he responded to cardioversion, epinephrine, and calcium chloride. An epinephrine drip was required at 150 mg/kg/min. The patient remained conscious. Calcium chloride, phosphorus, potassium and magnesium were given in an attempt to normalize serum electrolytes. The patient continued to exhibit sustained multiple episodes of ventricular fibrillation, which necessitated further cardioversion and chest compression. Four hours after admission, total calcium was 3.8 mg/dl and ionized calcium was 2 mg/dl. During the next hour, fibrillation became refractory to DC cardioversion and all attempts to control arrhythmia were unsuccessful. The patient became asystolic, despite correction of electrolyte abnormalities. It has also been stated that the tendency of patients to die of refractory ventricular fibrillation may be due to a direct toxic effect of fluoride ions on the myocardium. Fluoride ions cause a direct activation of myocardial adenylate cyclase which results in an increase in cyclic adenosine monophosphate formation with subsequent myocardial irritability and potentially fatal arrhythmias.

Patients with significant exposure need to be placed on cardiac monitors; have intravenous access established; and have rapid and serial evaluations of calcium, magnesium, and other electrolytes. Physicians should be prepared to administer large doses of IV calcium chloride. Frequent assessment of serum calcium, magnesium, and potassium levels as well as continual cardiac monitoring are necessary for optimal management of electrolyte abnormalities. Electrocardiogram changes such as Q-T prolongation, may provide valuable evidence of hypocalcemia.

The induction of metabolic alkalosis with sodium bicarbonate will enhance renal excretion of fluoride ions. Fluoride can also be removed by hemodialysis or cation exchange. Hemodialysis may be used after excessive fluoride absorption to remove fluoride anion and correct abnormal serum chemistries.[27,28] The volume of distribution (V_d) of fluoride is 0.5 l/kg, plasma protein binding is negligible, and the molecular weight is low. Thus, hemodialysis is effective in removing over 80% of the body stores of this agent within 4 hours. Speed is the key to the treatment of hydrofluoric acid exposure. The initial care is the same as for chemical burns. This includes:

- complete disrobing of a patient;
- immediate copious irrigation of an affected area with tepid water;
- an attempt to identify the offending agent; and
- treatment of systemic toxicity when present:[29]

It is important not to delay initiation of irrigation. Neutralizing the agent is time consuming and is not recommended. Neutralizing agents may produce an exothermic reaction which can cause thermal injury. After initial stabilization is complete, there are a variety of methods to eliminate fluoride ions. A wide variety of treatment methods have been devised to treat hypocalcemia caused by hydrofluoric acid exposure, and most are designed to bind free fluoride ions at the site of injury.

Topical application of calcium gluconate-based gel is now accepted as a rapid, effective, and noninvasive method of initial therapy. In 1932, Wellman and Fredenhagen began using calcium gluconate gel, otherwise known as hydrofluoric burn ointment, as a topical therapy for hydrofluoric acid exposure. It is a mixture of 3.5 g of 2.5% calcium gluconate with 5 oz of a water-soluble lubricant such as K-Y jelly. This is applied and massaged into the skin four to six times a day for 3–4 days. Injection of calcium gluconate into deep tissue layers is also an effective method of binding fluoride anions. Described in 1939, the injections should be carried out using a 27- or 30-gauge needle. The subcutaneous tissues under the involved skin should be injected from sites on the periphery of the lesion. A dose of 0.5 ml/cm^2 of 10% calcium gluconate is used.[30] Although calcium chloride has more milliequivalents per ml of calcium, it is contraindicated for subcutaneous infiltration due to its tissue irritating properties.[31] This method has been shown to result in dramatic relief of pain and immediate improvement of lesion appearance. Pain relief is often immediate from calcium alone. It is controversial whether local anesthetic should be used with calcium injections. It is felt that the return of pain indicates a need for further injection of calcium treatment.

Special considerations

Digital and hand burns deserve special mention as they are frequently seen. Because of the lack of subcutaneous space, relatively little solution can be injected without compromising tissue perfusion. Anderson and Anderson advocated a palmar fasciotomy to the injected fingers in order to avoid potentially dangerous high pressure tissue.[32] Digital burns involving highly concentrated hydrofluoric acid are a difficult problem. Large amounts of neutralizing agent need to be placed in a limited tissue space. Koehnlein and colleagues were the first to describe intra-arterial infusions of calcium gluconate as a treatment for severe hydrofluoric acid burns of the limbs.[33] Recently, Vance and associates found that intra-arterial infusion of calcium gluconate was of value in certain circumstances, such as for burns to the thumb, index and middle fingers. The basic technique used by Vance and colleagues[34] consists of the following:

- percutaneous cannulation of the radial artery with a long catheter;
- insertion of the catheter proximally several centimeters into the radial artery;
- obtaining an arteriogram to confirm blood supply to the injured area;
- infusion of dilute solution of calcium salts with a pump apparatus over 4-hour period (10 ml of a 10% solution of calcium gluconate or calcium chloride in 40–50 ml of 5% dextrose).

If pain returns after four hours of observation, the infusion is repeated until the patient is symptom free. The advantages of intra-arterial therapy is its the ability to deliver large doses of calcium. Disadvantages include the invasive vascular procedure necessary and the need for hospitalization with monitoring of the infusion.[21]

Eye exposure can lead to extensive damage by hydrofluoric acid vapor alone, but liquid hydrofluoric acid causes the most severe damage. McCulley and colleagues report that many of the topical modalities used in the treatment of hydrofluoric acid cause injury to the eye experimentally. Immediate one-time irrigation with water, isotonic saline, or magnesium chloride is found to be effective. Irrigation with calcium chloride causes an increase in corneal ulceration.[35] Rapid copious washing of the eyes should be followed by administering an ice pack. The eye should be irrigated with 1% calcium gluconate every 2–3 hours for 48–72 hours. Recovery usually occurs in 4–5 days. If ocular perforation is suspected, an ophthalmologist should be consulted.

Patients with significant burns of the face or around the mouth must be watched closely for swelling of oral and pharyngeal mucosa. All patients suspected of hydrofluoric acid inhalation should receive 100% oxygen. Administration of 2.5–3.0% calcium gluconate solution through a nebulizer or through an intermittent positive pressure breathing device is recommended.[30] If pulmonary edema develops, a patient should be placed on intermittent positive pressure breathing (IPPB) with positive end-expiratory pressure (PEEP). Pulmonary reaction to hydrofluoric acid continues for up to 3 weeks, and patients must be closely monitored. Radiological studies and pulmonary function tests are of great assistance in evaluating the long-term effects of hydrofluoric acid exposure. Dyspnea during mild and heavy physical activity may occur for as long as 7–9 months. Corticosteroids may need to be administered for as long as 3 months in order to control inflammatory episodes.[29]

First aid treatment as previously described should be initiated immediately after ingestion of hydrofluoric acid. Milk of magnesia (2 oz) may help bind free fluoride ions. Gastric lavage, using lime water or milk, may be undertaken using a gastric tube. A patient should be watched closely for signs of systemic fluoride toxicity and hypocalcemia. Gastroenterologic consultation is advisable.[29] Hydrofluoric acid is a toxic substance, which can cause significant, lethal injury due to its fluoride toxicity. It is important to be aware of the possibility of workers presenting with such burns. Health care professionals must be educated in the latest treatment of hydrofluoric acid burn and, as a preparation measure, must inquire of local companies whether workers are exposed to hydrofluoric acid or other toxic materials. This liquid has a wide industrial use including petroleum refining, glass etching, rust removal and in the semiconductor industry.

Hypochlorite Solutions

Found both in household and industrial preparations, hypochlorite solutions are used as bleaches, disinfectants and deodorizers. They are occasionally used to purify drinking water and in swimming pools. Their use is declining with the growing awareness of the vast damage which they are causing to the environment. They are potent oxidizing agents in a strongly alkaline solution and cause corrosion and protein coagulation in the skin and mucous membranes. The active ion is hypochlorous (OCl^-), but free chlorine (Cl_2) is also present. The concentration of the solution affects the outcome more than the duration of exposure. Commonly available solutions are 4–6% and are only lethal for adults when a large body surface area is exposed. An exposure to 30 ml of a 15% solution must be considered highly dangerous. Skin, eyes, and mucous membranes become irritated in exposed regions. Systemic symptoms include vomiting (which may resemble coffee grounds), dyspnea, hoarseness of voice, edema of the airway, confusion, cardiovascular collapse, cyanosis, and coma. Peritonitis or mediastinitis may complicate the course.

Lewisite

See vesicants.

Mustard

See vesicants.

Muriatic Acid

This is the name given to commercial grade hydrochloric acid which is often used to prepare metals before soldering. Slower acting and producing much less heat than sulfuric acid, muriatic acid is otherwise very similar, and the treatment is the same.

Nitric Acid

This is another strong acid and the mode of action and treatment are the same as for hydrochloric acid. Concentrated nitric acid can also produce organonitrate compounds which are metabolic competitors.

Oxalic Acid

Contact with oxalic acid causes chalky white indolent ulceration. Half a gram per kilogram body weight may be lethal. It binds calcium salts and inhibits many enzyme chains and prevents muscle contractions. It is a strong 'protoplasmic' poison. Calcium salts should be applied to a wound, and the injured area should be lavaged with water. If absorption has occurred, intravenous calcium gluconate or calcium chloride in a 10% solution should be administered. The plasma ionized calcium level should be monitored and signs of muscular dysfunction should be anticipated. Respiratory support and blood gas chemistry manipulation should be instituted early.

Phenol

Phenol is an aromatic hydrocarbon derived from coal tar. It was discovered in 1834 and initially used in crude form for the treatment of sewage. Phenol is a physiologic product of metabolism. Following ingestion or absorption through skin, phenol is bound to albumin irreversibly. In acute phenol exposure, a rapid rise in phenol levels is seen followed by a sudden fall after the exposure ceases. The antiseptic action of phenol on human wounds was first demonstrated by Lemaire in France in 1864[36] and Lister in Scotland in 1867.[37] Phenol was recommended as a spray for antisepsis in the operating room. The germicidal action of phenol was evaluated in 1881 by Koch.[38] The use of phenol in medicine has become very limited, as a number of seriously adverse effects and death have been reported in the literature.

In cases of intoxication, the cytotoxic effects of phenol burns induce cardiovascular symptoms such as ventricular arrythmias.[39] Phenol (carbolic acid) toxicity is most frequently noted following acute ingestion or chronic dermal application. Ingestion of as little as 1 g may cause death. Skin damage may result after prolonged contact. It produces necrosis and is followed by gangrene. The most frequent adverse effects from contact with phenolic disinfectants seem to be dermatitis and depigmentation.[40] Following the use of resorcinol (a phenol derivative, 1,3-dihydroxybenzene), allergic contact dermatitis has been noted. A rusty red pigmentary dermatitis has been reported in industrial workers exposed to resorcinol.[41]

Acute poisoning by phenol absorption through the skin is becoming more frequent, and fatalities have been reported. It is important to handle these accidents promptly. It has been proven that a copious amount of pure water has a remarkable decontamination capability.[41] It can prolong the time it takes for phenol exposure to become lethal by up to three times. Undiluted polyethylene glycol (PEG; molecular weight 300 or 400) is considered the best solvent;[42] however, it has not been found to be more effective than copious water irrigation. Thus, no time should be wasted with the time consuming application of PEG. PEG application should be started soon after the initial water irrigation. The area should be repeatedly sponged with PEG soaks. Decontamination personnel should wear rubber gloves. In animals, Schütz shows that PEG 400 has a superb decontamination capability.[43]

Intravenous administration of sodium bicarbonate has been reported to be effective prophylactically as well as therapeutically. Studies in dogs reveal that there is no possibility of influencing the dissociation of phenol in blood. Infusion of sodium bicarbonate and Tris buffer do not alter phenol levels in tested animals. As the antagonistic effect of alkaline substances is not due to a change of blood pH, another mechanism, still to be discovered, must be responsible for this phenomenon.[44] As phenol burns may appear innocuous it is important to reemphasize the hazardous and life-threatening effects of exposure to this specific substance. Immediate recognition of the severity of phenol burns and correct initial treatment may save the lives of phenol burned patients.

Phosphoric Acid

This mineral acid is in widespread industrial use. Sometimes it is used in very concentrated 93% solutions. Treatment should be as for sulfuric acid (see below) initially, but should switch to phosphorus treatment once lavage is complete. Phosphate ions are strong calcium binders and serum electrolytes should be monitored (see below)

Phosphorus

Phosphorus is an incendiary agent used in a variety of weapons such as hand grenades, mortar bombs, and artillery shells. Thus, their burns are mainly seen in military personnel but may be encountered by manufacturers of fireworks and fertilizers.[45] White phosphorus ignites in the presence of air. On contact with skin it causes a burn which will progress until all the agent is oxidized or starved of oxygen by immersion in water. The combustion products from burning phosphorus are a variety of oxides and polyphosphates, many of which tightly bind calcium ions. The wounds are typically severely painful, necrotic, yellowish in color and have a characteristic smell of garlic (**Plate 12**). Embedded phosphorus must be expected if an explosion has occurred. Clothing may ignite and so must be removed.

Immediate treatment involves removing all of a victim's clothing, thoroughly irrigating the area with saline solution or water, and removing any easily identifiable particles. The burns should then be covered in saline- or water-soaked dressings and kept moist during transportation until the patient reaches a specialist unit. Here, specific therapy can be instituted by irrigation with copper sulfate in a 0.5% solution. This causes the formation of a black film of cupric oxide on the surface above the embedded agent which impedes oxidation and facilitates identification and removal of white phosphorus. Stronger solutions than 1% have resulted in intravascular hemolysis and renal failure.[46] The solution should be freshly prepared, applied as a brief wash, and then removed by water lavage. If available, ultraviolet light can be used to fluoresce the embedded particles for identification. Even small burns will necessitate fluid therapy. Large electrolyte disturbances are possible. Hypocalcemia and hyperphosphatemia, associated with cardiac arrhythmias and sudden death, have been reported.[47] An electrocardiograph must be closely monitored and serum calcium and phosphate levels regularly measured until metabolic stability is guaranteed.

Potassium Permanganate

This is an oxidizing agent which, in dilute solutions, is only mildly irritating to the skin. More concentrated solutions cause a brown discoloration, which will progress to a thick, brown/purple coagulum. The dry crystals are highly corrosive. Systemic effects are rare and usually mild as it is poorly absorbed. If ingested, death may occur due to airway obstruction from edema formation.

Sulfuric Acid

Sulphur trioxide yields sulfuric acid on contact with water. Both are proton donors, powerful desiccants, and have widespread use in industry. Contact will be painful and will result in the release of vast quantities of heat which will add to the insult. The skin is blackened, forming a hard dry eschar under which deep indolent ulceration may form (**Plate 13**). Ingestion is rare but may result in airway obstruction, visceral perforation, cardiovascular and respiratory collapse, and death. Initial treatment is accomplished via copious lavage with water and supportive measures when necessary. The tendency for these burns to involve limited areas and be deep makes them most suitable for early eschar excision and grafting.[48]

Vesicant Chemical Warfare Agents

Vesicant agents include sulfur and nitrogen mustards, lewisite and other arsenicals, and the halogenated oximes. These compounds affect not only skin but also all epithelial tissue with which they come into contact, particularly the eyes and respiratory tract. Early symptoms ascribed to mustard gas include an ocular burning sensation and a feeling of suffocation associated with a burning throat.[49] After 4 hours, erythema is seen; in 12–48 hours, blistering appears, accompanied by severe pruritus which has a predilection for moist areas such as the axillae and perineum (**Plate 14**). The blisters tend to rupture, discharging an amber serous fluid and leaving painful shallow ulcers. Greater exposure produces coagulative necrosis of skin, with either no blistering or 'doughnut blisters' surrounding a central necrotic zone.[50] This will be accompanied by severe conjunctivitis, corneal erosion, and necrotizing bronchitis. A secondary respiratory infection may develop over the next few days which, coupled with associated marrow suppression, can prove fatal. Lewisite (2-chlorovinyl-dichloroarsine) is the best known arsine. It is more powerful than the mustards and symptoms occur sooner. Eye irritation is produced immediately and sneezing, salivation and lacrimation follow rapidly. Nonlethal chronic exposure may lead to arsenical poisoning. Exposure to phosgene oxime, the commonest halogenated oxime, has the immediate effect of stinging, likened to that produced on contact with a stinging nettle.[51] Within a minute, the affected area becomes swollen, with blisters soon forming. An eschar will form after 1 week, but healing is often delayed beyond 2 months. Contamination of the eyes is extremely painful and may result in permanent blindness. Inhalation causes irritation and coughing, hypersecretion, and pulmonary edema.

Treatment for exposure to a vesicant agent

The only prophylaxis against these agents are butyl rubber gloves, boots, and a respirator. The clothing of a victim must either be removed or decontaminated with Fuller's earth powder. Eyes can be irrigated with water but, if available, 1.26% sodium bicarbonate solution or 0.9% saline should be used. Upon reaching a treatment facility, patients must have all their clothing removed if this has not already been done, and all the exposed areas must be cleaned with copious water lavage. Attendants should also be suitably protected, and contaminated clothing must be placed in special bags.

Itching can be treated with sedatives (benzodiazepines or phenothiazines). Antihistamines may be tried. Blisters should be deroofed and dressed with topical antimicrobials; however, silver sulfadiazine is incompatible with dimercaprol (British antilewisite). The mustard blister fluid is harmless.[52] Early excision and grafting in mustard burns has not yet proven to be of any value; however, deep necrotic lesions seen with the other agents are best treated as thermal injury. Dimercaprol, a chelating agent, is a specific antidote for lewisite poisoning. It is available as ointment for skin lesions, as drops for eye applications (5–10% in oil), and in an intramuscular preparation for systemic toxicity. Other chelating agents such as:

- DMSA – mesodimercaptosuccinic acid,
- DMPS – 2,3-dimercapto-1-propanesulfonic acid sodium,
- DMPA – *N*-(2,3-dimercaptopropyl) phthalamidic acid

have a higher therapeutic index, are water soluble, and are effective orally. There is no specific antidote to mustard poisoning although some evidence exists that sodium thiosulfate and cysteine may afford some protection if administered early.[53]

Affected eyes should be irrigated, treated with antibiotics, and inspected at the earliest time by an ophthalmologist. Respiratory injury requires symptomatic treatment according to its severity. Inhalation of high-dose steroids is controversial at present. Severe exposure will lead to agranulocytosis or aplastic anemia.[54] The pancytopenia seen after 7 days with the Iranian casualties did not appear to be helped by transfusion of relevant blood products.[55] Bone marrow transplantation may prove useful, although of little practical value with large numbers of casualties. The effect of bone marrow stimulants such as oxymetholone and lithium carbonate is unknown but may be considered. Fluid replacement must be carried out dynamically with adequate cardiovascular monitoring. The maximum fluid loss occurs during blister formation and not necessarily in the first 24 hours.

Critical Care Aspects

The systemic consequences of a chemical injury must not be underestimated. They must be anticipated and treated early which will increase the chances of survival greatly.

The Airway

The airway can be involved in a chemical injury in many ways. Ingestion will cause contact burns in the upper airway, inhalation of gaseous material may affect the airway from the mouth to the alveoli, and induced histamine release or other immunological events may cause swelling of the airways and/or bronchospasm. The airway can be divided practically into three regions. If the injury is to the face and lips only, with no intraoral exposure, airway problems are unlikely. If there is any injury from the lips down to the larynx, it is wise to protect the airway during resuscitation as edema can progress rapidly and cause airway obstruction. Sloughing of dead epithelium may also be a problem. A patient should be sedated and intubated but may be allowed to breathe spontaneously on humidified, oxygen-enriched air. The patency of the airway should be assessed regularly, and a patient should be extubated only when it is safe to do so. It must be remembered that a tracheal tube is easy to remove when no longer needed but may prove impossible to insert when required in an emergency. Finally, if the lower airway is involved (that is below the vocal cords), intubation, mechanical ventilation, and oxygen therapy are indicated. This will allow the blood gas chemistry to be optimized and adequate oxygen concentrations to be delivered to the vital organs.

The Cardiovascular System

Cardiac output must be maintained at an adequate level in order to deliver oxygen. The absorption of an offending agent may result in direct myocardial depression and a fall in systemic vascular resistance. This will result in inadequate tissue perfusion. Inotropic support should be instituted early before irreversible failure occurs. The drugs of choice are dopamine, dobutamine, and norepinephrine (noradrenaline). Systemic vascular resistance can be manipulated using these drugs, and a combination may prove beneficial. Intense vasoconstriction may occur if high doses are used. This will result in poor skin oxygenation and a wound may progress in either depth or area. Future developments may include the use of nitric oxide inhibitors and other specific cellular messengers and end transmitters.

The Renal System

Dialysis may be used to remove noxious chemicals and their byproducts if performed early. If renal function is impaired, adequate oxygenation and cardiac output must be insured. All drugs given should be of low renal toxicity unless no alternative can be prescribed. Hemofiltration techniques or dialysis should be instigated, as fluid overload will only worsen the renal function and cause edema throughout the body. Early intervention may circumvent later problems.

The Liver

Any absorbed chemicals will pass through the liver. There may be a direct toxic effect, causing necrosis, or the effects may be secondary. A fall in cardiac output will decrease liver blood flow and, likewise, oxygenation, exposing it to the noxious elements for longer and making it more vulnerable to damage. If the renal system cannot deal with the chemicals, then, again, the liver will suffer. Support with charcoal filtration and support for the other systems is all that can be offered.

Conclusion

It is a vital concept to understand that a team approach must be made to the treatment of a chemically injured patient. All information must be channeled through one person who will have the overall picture at his or her disposal and can make the relevant decisions. This arrangement will offer the best chance of survival for patients exposed to chemical agents.

References

1. Personal communication J M Brandey to L T A Rylah, 1993.
2. Mozingo D W, Smith A D, McManus W F, Pruitt B A, Mason A D. Chemical burns. *J Trauma* 1988; **28:** 642–7.
3. Fitzpatrick K T, Moylan J A. Emergency care of chemical burns. *Postgrad Med* 1985; **78:** 189–94.

4. Jelenko C 3d. Chemicals that 'burn'. *J Trauma* 1974; **14**(1): 65–72.

5. Papirmeister B. *Medical Defence against Mustard Gas: Toxic Mechanisms and Pharmacological Implications.* Boca Raton: CRC Press, 1991.

6. Mellor S G, Rice P, Cooper G J. Vesicant burns. *Br J Plast Surg* 1991; **44:** 434–7.

7. Bromberg B F, Song I C, Walden R H. Hydrotherapy of chemical burns. *Plast Reconstr Surg* 1965; **35:** 85–95.

8. Leonard L G, Scheulen J J, Munster A M. Chemical burns: effect of prompt first aid. *J Trauma* 1982; **22:** 420–3.

9. Yano T, Hata Y, Matsuda I, Matsuda H. Effects of washing with a neutralising agent on alkaline skin injuries in an experimental model. *Burns* 1994; **20:** 36–9.

10. Mozingo D, Smith A, McManus W, Pruitt B, Mason A. Chemical Burns. *J Trauma* 1988; **28**(5): 642–7.

11. Leonard L, Scheulen J, Munster A. Chemical burns: effect of prompt first aid. *J Trauma* 1982; **22**(5): 420–3.

12. Lazarus G S, Brown R S, Daniels J R, *et al.* Human granulocyte collagenase. *Science* 1968; **159:** 1483.

13. Pfister R R. Chemical injuries of the eye. *Ophthalmology* 1983; **90:** 1246.

14. Pavan-Langston D (ed.), Burns and trauma. In: *Manual of Ocular Diagnosis and Therapy*. Boston: Little Brown and Co, 1985:

15. Havener W H. *Ocular Pharmacology*, 4th ed. St Louis: C V Mosby, 1978: 573.

16. Cope Z. General treatment of burns. In: *Medical History of 2nd World War: Surgery.* London: HMSO, 1953: 288–312.

17. Pike J, Patterson A, Arons M S. Chemistry of cement burns: pathogenesis and treatment. *J Burn Care Rehabil* 1988; **9:** 258–60.

18. Sigurdsson J, Bjornsson A, Gudmundsson S T. Formic acid burn – local and systemic effects: report of a case. *Burns* 1983; **9:** 358–61.

19. Naik R B, Stephens W P, Wilson D J, *et al.* Ingestion of formic acid-containing agents – report of three fatal cases. *Postgrad Med J* 1980; **56:** 451.

20. Hunter G A. Chemical burns of the skin after contact with petrol. *Br J Plast Surg* 1968; **28:** 337–41.

21. Mistry D, Wainwright D. Hydrofluoric acid burns. *Am Fam Physician* 1992; **45**(4): 1748–54.

22. McIvor M. Delayed fatal hyperkalemia in a patient with acute fluoride intoxication. *Ann Emerg Med* 1987; **16:** 118–20.

23. Klauder J V, Shelanski L, Gavriel K. Industrial uses of compounds of fluoride and oxalic acid. *Arch Ind Health* 1955; **12:** 412–19.

24. Division of Industrial Hygiene, National Institutes of Health. Hydrofluoric acid burns. *Ind Med* 1943; **12:** 634.

25. Baltazaar R, Mower M, Reider R, *et al.* Acute fluoride poisoning leading to fatal hyperkalemia. *Chest* 1980; **78:** 660–2.

26. Mayer T G, Gross P L. Fatal systemic fluorosis due to hydrofluoric acid burns. *Ann Emerg Med* 1985; **14:** 149–53.

27. McIvor M, Cummings C, Mower M, *et al.* Sudden cardiac death from acute fluoride intoxication: the role of potassium. *Ann Emerg Med* 1987; **16:** 777–81.

28. Yolken R, Konecy P, McCarthy P. Acute fluoride poisoning. *Pediatrics* 1976; **58:** 90–1.

29. Flood S. Hydrofluoric acid burns. *Am Fam Physician* 1988; **37**(3): 178–82.

30. Dibbell Dg, Iverson R E, Jones W, Laub Dr, Madison M S. Hydrofluoric acid burns of the hand. *J Bone Joint Surg Am* 1970; **52:** 931–6.

31. Cavarati E M. Acute hydrofluoric acid exposure. *Am J Emerg Med* 1988; **6:** 143–50.

32. Anderson W J, Anderson J R. Hydrofluoric acid burns of the hand: mechanism of injury and treatment. *J Hand Surg* 1988; **13A:** 52–7.

33. Koehnlein H E, Seitz H D, Achinger R. *Abstract of Fifth International Congress of Burn Injuries, Stockholm, Sweden, 1978.*

34. Vance M V, Curry S C, Kunkel D B, Ryan P J, Riggeri S B. Digital hydrofluoric acid burns: treatment with intraarterial calcium infusion. *Ann Emerg Med* 1986; **15:** 890–6.

35. McCulley J P, Whiting D W, Petitt M G, Lauber S E. Hydrofluoric acid burns of the eye. *J Occup Med* 1983; **25:** 447–50.

36. Lemaire J. De L'acide Phenique de son Action sur les Végétaux les Animaux les Fements. 2nd ed. Paris: Germer-Baillière, 1865: 754.

37. Lister J. On a new method of treating compound fracture, abscess etc. *Lancet* 1867; 326, 357, 387, 507.

38. Koch R. Uber Desinfktion. *Kaiserlichen Gesundheistamte Mittheilungen* 1881; **1:** 234.

39. Miller F G. Poisoning by phenol. *Can Med Assoc J* 1942; **46:** 615.

40. Saunders A, Geddes L, Elliott P. Are phenolic disinfectants toxic to staff members? *Aust Nurses J* 1988; **17:** 25.

41. Abbate D, Polito I, Puglisi A, *et al.* Dermatosis from resorcinol in tyre makers. *Br J Ind Med* 1989; **46:** 212.

42. Brown V K H, Box V L, Simpson B J. Decontamination procedures for skin exposed to phenolic substances. *Arch Environ Health* 1975; **30:** 1.

43. Schütz W. Phenoldermatosen (in German): *Berufsdermatosen* 1959; **7:** 266.

44. Bennett I I, James D F, Golden A. Severe Acidosis due to phenol poisoning. Report of two cases. *Ann Intern Med* 1950; **32:** 214.

45. Summerlin W T, Walder A I, Moncrief J A. White phosphorous burns and massive haemolysis. *J Trauma* 1967; **7:** 476–84.

46. Cioffi G C, Rue L W, Buescher T M, Pruitt B A. A brief history and the pathophysiology of burns. In: R. Zaitchuk ed. *Textbook of Military Medicine*. Office of the Surgeon General, Department of the Army, USA, 1989.

47. Bowen T E, Wheelan T J, Nelson T G. Sudden death after phosphorus burns: experimental observations of hypocalcemia, hyperphosphemia, and electrocardiographic abnormalities following production of a standard white phosphorus burn. *Ann Surg* 1971; **174:** 389–95.

48. Sawhney C P, Kaushish R. Acid and alkali burns: considerations in their management. *Burns* 1989; **15:** 132–5.

49. Willems J L. Clinical management of mustard gas casualties. *Ann Med Milit (Belg)* 1989: 3 (suppl): 1–61.

50. Papirmeister B, Feister A J, Robinson S I, Ford R D. The sulfur mustard injury: description of lesions and resulting incapacitation. In: *Medical Defence against Mustard Gas*. Florida: CRC Press Inc, 1990: 13–42.

51. Vesicants. In: *NATO Handbook on the Medical Effects of NBC Defensive Operations*. AMedP-6 Part III – Chemical. Amended final draft. (NATO Unclassified).

52. Sultzberger M B, Katz J H. The absence of skin irritants in the contents of vesicles. *US Navy Med Bull* 1943; **43:** 1258–62.

53. Papirmeister B, Feister A J, Robinson S I, Ford R D. Pretreatments and therapies. In: *Medical Defence against Mustard Gas*. Florida: CRC Press Inc, 1990.

54. Vedder E B. *The Medical Aspects of Chemical Warfare*. Baltimore: Williams and Wilkins Co, 1925.

55. P Rice. Personal communication 1993.

CHAPTER FORTY-ONE

RADIATION INJURIES AND MASS CASUALTIES

STEPHEN M. MILNER, THUAN T. NGUYEN, DAVID N. HERNDON AND LINDSEY T. A. RYLAH

INTRODUCTION

Exposure to ionizing radiation can follow one of three patterns. First, it can be the result of a small scale accident (e.g. in a laboratory and where resources will be available to cope); second, it can be due to a large industrial accident (e.g. the nuclear reactor explosion in Chernobyl, USSR in 1986), where resources may be stretched in coping; and third, exposure may follow the detonation of a nuclear device in a military conflict where resources are totally overwhelmed or unavailable and associated multiple and combined injuries also exist.

This chapter discusses the effects of exposure to ionizing radiation and the acute radiation syndrome. Triage and care protocols are considered according to known and projected prognostic factors. The complications that arise specifically with this injury and the supportive measures that need to be taken are also addressed. Finally, the problem of mass casualties is examined, and protocol recommendations are made. The pathophysiology of chronic exposure to ionizing radiation and malignancy are not discussed.

INCIDENCE

A significant radiation accident is one in which an individual exceeds at least one of the following criteria:[1]

- Whole body dose equal to or exceeding 25 rem (0.25 Sv).
- Skin dose equal to or exceeding 600 rem (6 Sv).
- Absorbed dose equal to or greater than 75 rem (0.75 Sv) to other tissues or organs from an external source.
- Internal contamination equal to or exceeding one half the maximum permissible body burden (MPBB) as defined by the International Commission on Radiological Protection (this number is different for each radionuclide).
- Medical misadministrations, provided they result in a dose or burden equal to or greater than the criteria already listed above.

Radiation accidents should be reported to the Radiation Assistance Center/Training Site (REAC/TS) at Oak Ridge Associated Universities in Oak Ridge, Tennessee 37831–0117 (Tel. (615)576–3130). It is funded by the US Department of Energy (DOE). Each event is recorded in a registry log book and assigned a sequential four-digit registration number. The foreign registry is an incomplete list of generally anecdotal reports of accidents occurring in other countries around the world.

The number of accidents, number of persons involved, as well as the number of fatalities, in the United States and world wide is shown in **Table 41.1**. There have been a total of 103 fatalities recorded by the Registry world wide.[1] The number of radiation accident fatalities world wide by each 5-year period since 1945 are shown graphically in **Figure 41.1**.[1] One-half of the fatalities have occurred in the last decade during which time the rate has been almost five fatalities per year. A majority of these radiation deaths occurred as a result of the Chernobyl accident. The classification of radiation accident by device for the period 1944 until January 1994 is shown in **Table 41.2**.[1] The frequency of accidents by time is shown in **Figure 41.2**. The majority of major radiation accidents are due to radiation devices. This may be an x-ray machine or even

Table 41.1 Major radiation accidents: human experience (1944–December 1993)

Location	No. of accidents	No. of persons involved	Significant exposures	Fatalities
US	232	1305	776	30
Non-US	135	132 012	2005	73
Total	367	133 317	2781	103

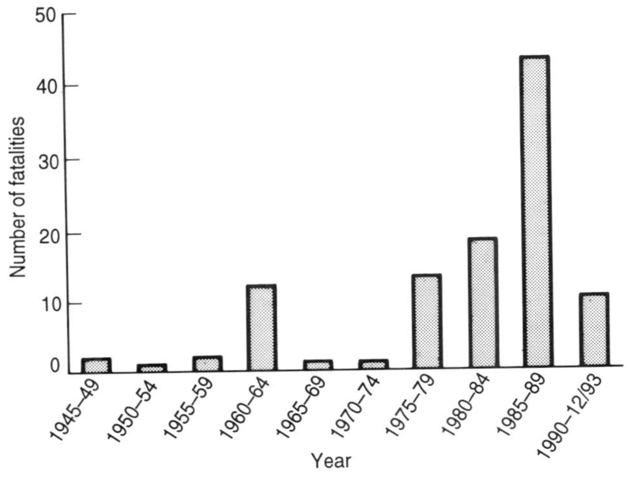

Fig. 41.1 The number of fatal radiation accidents world wide for 5-year periods from 1945 to 1993.

Table 41.2 Major radiation accidents world wide (1944–1994) classed by 'device'

Criticalities		18
Critical assemblies	6	
Reactors	7	
Chemical operation	5	
Radiation devices		272
Sealed sources	184	
x-ray devices	67	
Accelerators	20	
Radar generators	1	
Radioisotopes		77
Transuranics	26	
Tritium	1	
Fission products	10	
Radium spills	2	
Diagnosis and therapy	26	
Other	12	
Total		367

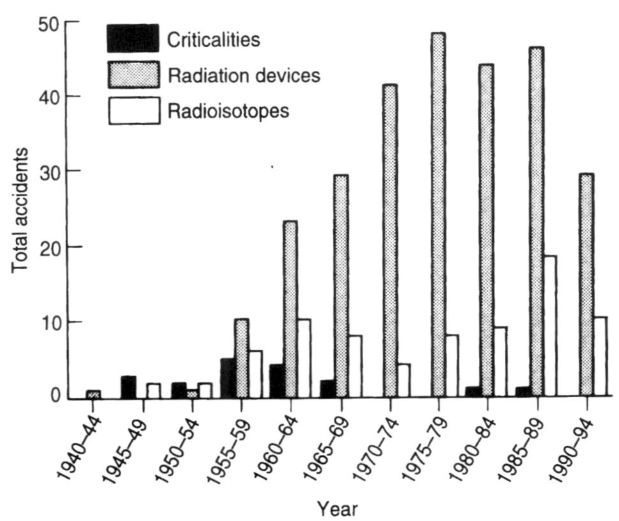

Fig. 41.2 The frequency of radiation accidents between 1940 and 1994 based on classifications of etiologies: those related to nuclear criticality accidents, those resulting from radiation devices, and those involving radioisotopes from unsealed radioactive materials.

an accelerator; however, most devices involved in accidents are encapsulated, highly radioactive sources used for industrial radiography. Next most frequent accidents are radioisotope accidents which involve radioactive materials which are unsealed such as tritium, fission products, radium, and free isotopes used for diagnosis and therapy. Uncommon criticality accidents occur when enough fissionable material, such as enriched uranium, is brought together to produce a neutron flux high enough that the material will undergo a nuclear reaction (become critical).

PATHOPHYSIOLOGY

Several important differences exist between nuclear and conventional high explosive weapons. Significantly from a biological point of view, a nuclear reaction releases enormous amounts of thermal and ionizing radiation.

Thermal Effects

Exposure to radiant heat from a detonation gives rise to flash burns. The clinical picture may range from an erythema of the exposed areas (most commonly face, hands, arms and legs), to a charring of the superficial layers of the skin. Secondary flame burns may be present following the ignition of a victim's clothing or environment. Exact information about the cause of fatalities in a nuclear blast is not available, but from the nuclear attack on Japan during World War II, it has been estimated that 50% of deaths were due to burns and some 20–30% were flash burns.[2]

The physicians at Hiroshima and Nagasaki observed that the 'flame' burn wound seemed to heal at first. However, between 1 and 2 weeks later, a serious relapse occurred. Wound infection set in; there was a disorder in granulation tissue formation; a gray, greasy coating would form on the wounds. Thrombocytopenia resulted in spontaneous bleeding both into the wound and elsewhere. Histologically, the normal collection of leukocytes delineating a necrotic area were found to be absent due to agranulocytosis and gross bacterial invasion was evident;[3] both of these changes obviously affected the prognosis of these otherwise relatively small injuries.

Radiation Effect

Damage to biological tissue by ionizing radiation is mediated by energy transference. This can be the result of exposure to electromagnetic radiation (e.g. x-rays and gamma (δ) rays) or particulate radiation (e.g. beta (β) particles or neutrons). The transference of this energy results in the formation of highly reactive chemical products including free radicals (such as the hydroxyl radical). These can further combine with normal body chemicals to form active moieties (e.g. with water to form hydrogen peroxide) which in turn will combine with cellular components to cause intracellular and molecular damage. The primary targets are cellular and nuclear membranes and DNA.

The morbidity of radiation is dependent on its dose, the dose rate, and the sensitivity of the exposed cell. The most sensitive cells are those which divide rapidly such as bone marrow, skin, and the gastrointestinal tract. The susceptibility of the cells is proportional to their ability to divide, the least sensitive being those of the central nervous system. The unit or dose measurement is the gray (Gy) which is the equivalent of 100 rad. The effect of acute exposure has been quantified as the acute radiation syndrome.[4]

The Acute Radiation Syndrome

The clinical course of acute radiation syndrome (ARS) usually begins within hours of exposure. Prodromal symptoms include nausea, vomiting, diarrhea, fatigue, fever, and headache. A latent period then follows, the duration of which is related to the dose. This is followed by hemopoietic and gastrointestinal complications. The ARS can be subdivided into three overlapping sub-syndromes which are related to the dose exposure.

Hemopoietic syndrome

This syndrome may occur after an exposure of between 1 and 2.5 Gy. The bone marrow is the most sensitive tissue and pancytopenia develops. Opportunistic infections result from the altered immune state of granulocytopenia. The time course of thrombocytopenia is broadly similar to that for granulocytopenia, and spontaneous bleeding results. A progressive anemia will develop. Hemorrhage and infection is the usual cause of death.

Gastrointestinal syndrome

This syndrome requires a larger dose exposure, usually in the range of 8–12 Gy. Severe nausea and vomiting associated with bowel cramps and watery diarrhea occur within hours of irradiation. There is a shorter latent period of 5–7 days, which reflects the turnover time of the gut epithelium (3–5 days). The epithelial damage results in loss of transport capability, bacterial translocation with sepsis, bowel ischemia, and bloody diarrhea. Large fluid imbalances can result in hypovolemia, acute renal failure and anemia from both bleeding and the loss of erythropoiesis. Critical exposure will lead to rapid deterioration with unrelenting bloody diarrhea, fever, refractory hypovolemic shock, and death.

Neurovascular syndrome

An exposure to a dose of 30 Gy or greater can cause a total collapse of the vascular system superimposed on the aforementioned syndromes. This may be due to the massive release of mediator substances, but destruction of endothelium is more probable.[5] This syndrome can progress rapidly with variable neurological symptoms, respiratory distress, cardiovascular collapse, and death.

THE COMBINED INJURY

The combination of a thermal injury with a radiation injury is said to have a synergistic effect on the outcome. Several animal experiments have shown that there is a significant increase in mortality when a standard burn wound model is irradiated. This is over and above that expected from either injury alone.[6,7]

Triage

Triage is the initial classification of casualties into priority groups for treatment and is essential in the management of large numbers of casualties. Those patients unlikely to survive should not be allowed to overwhelm available resources; efforts must be made to insure that adequate treatment reaches those who are most likely to survive. As ionizing radiation is not immediately life threatening, any associated injury should be treated first. The assessment of exposure will be made clinically and later by its biological effect.

If large scale casualties are encountered, triage may need to be draconian. In conventional warfare with limited resources, 50% of soldiers with thermal injuries of up to 70% TBSA will be expected to survive (**Table 41.3**). This survival rate should be bettered in a smaller civilian major accident. Thus burns alone over 70% TBSA should receive expectant treatment and those under 20% can have their treatment delayed. If there has been a significant exposure to radiation as well as a thermal injury, individuals with over 30% TBSA burns are unlikely to survive without the use of major resources.[8]

Table 41.3 Survival rates with major resources available

Burn alone	<70% TBSA	50% survival
Burn alone	>70% TBSA	Probably fatal
Burn plus radiation	<30% TBSA	May survive
Burn plus radiation	>30% TBSA	Probably fatal

TBSA, total body surface area.

TREATMENT

The treatment of any burn requires massive support from a dedicated team. This will be available for small accidents. With larger accidents or a nuclear attack, the number of victims could swamp the services; treatment facilities may be destroyed; normal supply channels could be drastically reduced, if present at all; production, distribution and transportation of supplies may be greatly impaired; and local care workers may also be the victims.

First Aid

The victims must be evacuated from the source of radiation in order to limit exposure. Normal resuscitation procedures must be followed (i.e. airway, breathing, circulation, etc.). Contaminated clothing must be removed, and the skin must undergo decontamination by rinsing with water and soap or detergent if possible. Patients with symptoms of ARS should preferably be sent to specialist centers with facilities which are able to treat bone marrow failure.

Assessment

Assessment of thermal injury has been covered already. Exposure to radiation can be estimated clinically, by noting the onset of symptoms of ARS, supported by biological parameters. If a patient sustains a fall in lympohcyte count of 50% or a count less than 1×10^9/liter in a time period of 48 hours post-exposure, then a moderate dose of radiation has been encountered.[9] This is an unreliable prognostic value when both burn and radiation injury have been sustained. Levels of serum amylase and diamine oxidase (produced by intestinal villi) are useful biological dosimeters. Amylase levels are only reliable when the salivary glands have been exposed and diamine oxidase has not yet been fully assessed in humans. Lymphocyte chromosomal analysis allows very accurate measurement even at low levels of exposure; however, the need for the test to be performed in cell cultures in laboratories over 48-hour incubation would render this test impractical with large numbers of casualties.[10]

Care of the Irradiated Patient

Where possible, a history should be obtained from the patient or others. Factors such as age, concurrent medical problems, smoke inhalation, and multiple trauma will affect the prognosis. With this in mind, a full physical examination is carried out to exclude other injuries. Victims of radiation exposure may not appear to differ clinically from the thermally injured and should receive the same care. Those exposed to lethal doses of radiation will exhibit early signs of radiation sickness and should be triaged accordingly.

All patients should be given adequate analgesia. Opiates or opioids are the drugs of choice. They must be titrated to effect and administered by the intravenous route. Early nausea and vomiting will be distressing and must be treated with available antiemetic drugs. Prochlorperazine has to be given by intramuscular injection but the newer agent, ondansetron, may prove successful as it is used against the similar symptoms encountered in radiotherapy and chemotherapy. It can also be used in children.

After the patient has been cleaned, decontaminated, and debrided, the extent of any thermal burn and its depth can be ascertained more accurately. Patients with thermal burns in excess of 40% TBSA or with associated inhalation or major trauma should be treated expectantly in a mass casualty situation. They should be made comfortable and be given adequate analgesia and/or sedatives if available and thought appropriate. Resuscitation should be the same as that for an uncomplicated thermal injury. Any resuscitation formula can be used, but it must be closely monitored and altered as necessary to maintain an adequate urine output. The fluid requirement will be increased as fluid is sequestered into damaged internal organs, especially the gut. Fluid losses from diarrhea and vomiting may also be excessive and need to be replaced.

Care of the Burn Wound

The patient is bathed gently so as to remove loose nonviable skin, the remnants of burnt clothing, and any other external debris which may be contaminated with radioactive material. The major problems which will be experienced with a radiation burn and/or thermal injuries are those associated with sepsis, fluid imbalance and a nonhealing wound.

Burns are best treated closed because of the high risk of sepsis in immunosuppressed patients whose wounds are susceptible to dehydration, colonization, and portal entry of organisms. Topical chemotherapeutic agents can be used and regularly applied as prescribed. Early tangential excision and split skin grafting provide early wound closure, decreased burn wound colonization, and sepsis and shortened hospital stay.[11,12] Dubos *et al.*[13] performing early excision and grafting of burns in irradiated monkeys, have shown that healing occurred fully by the end of the second week, although histologically there was a slight delay in the healing process. This technique has advantages where the potential to develop septic wounds is great. The authors recommend excision and grafting of deep thermal burns. Information regarding the grafting of radiation burns is not yet available, but the procedure is probably best delayed. The procedure, however, is not without risks. Blood loss in excess of 300 ml/% TBSA excised presents an increased anesthetic hazard.

Treatment of Complications

Hematological

Blood and platelets are administered in order to maintain an adequate hemoglobin concentration and a platelet level of 20×10^9 per liter. If surgery is contemplated, this level should be raised to 75×10^9 per liter. All blood products should be irradiated to avoid graft versus host disease.

Bone marrow transplantation is the treatment of choice following total body irradiation. It should be performed between 3 and 5 days post-exposure as the immunosuppression is at its peak. The use of hemopoietic growth factors such as granulocyte colony stimulating factor (G-CSF) and granulocyte-macrophage colony stimulating factor (GM-CSF) have shown increased survival in animals and primates, but their success is not yet proven in humans.[14]

Infection

The immunosuppression associated with irradiation makes a victim susceptible to exogenous and endogenous pathogens. Exogenous infection can be limited by adequate aseptic technique and nursing the patient in a sterile environment. Selective decontamination of the gastrointestinal tract will lessen the problem of translocation of bacteria from this source to the blood. Monitoring the patient adequately will allow the early diagnosis of sepsis and its treatment before it becomes well established. The antibiotic chosen should reflect the current pattern of susceptibility and nosocomial infections in that particular unit at that time. Combination therapy will be required where there is a profound neutropenia. With the large fluid losses and shifts, gentamicin is not recommended unless there is no other choice. Therapeutic levels will be difficult to obtain without risking toxicity and there are now safer broad spectrum antibiotics (imipenem, ceftazidime and ciprofloxacin). If Gram-positive infection is suspected, vancomycin or the newer and safer teicoplanin should be administered. If there is an inadequate response, an antifungal agent must be added. The use of fresh frozen plasma, gammaglobulin solutions and monoclonal antibodies is at present speculative, but if resources allow and a patient's condition is not stabilizing, these agents should be considered.

Cardiovascular collapse

This complication may occur due to the exposure, sepsis, fluid loss, or hemorrhage. The patient should be given adequate fluid resuscitation, the airway must be protected, and oxygen therapy must be instituted. Sedation and mechanical ventilation will decrease the oxygen debt which will inevitably occur. Inotropic support may become necessary and should be started as early as possible accompanied by relevant cardiovascular monitoring. Agents which manipulate the release of nitric oxide may become available in the near future and may turn out to be the agents of choice in the treatment of septic shock. Invasive cardiovascular monitoring will aid in the treatment of volume replacement, but invasive intravenous lines must be inserted in aseptic conditions, be kept meticulously clean, and be changed regularly. They must be removed when no longer indicated.

Respiratory failure and renal failure

Oxygen therapy and mechanical ventilation should be instigated at the earliest possible time. This subject is more fully discussed elsewhere. Renal failure also requires early attention. Its effects are covered fully in another chapter.

Mass Burn Casualties

Burn-injured patients should ideally be managed individually with treatment tailored to their personal needs; however, with mass casualties, following monumental disasters, whether natural or otherwise, lack of experienced staff, paucity of equipment and insufficient time to perform all relevant tasks, may make this an impossible goal. Nevertheless, every medical facility should be prepared at a moment's notice to cope with such situations. The handling of mass casualties is not confined to hospitals and the success of medical support will depend on adequate planning. It is informative to consider past disasters where mass casualties have involved large numbers of burned patients.[15] These have fared badly over the last 30 years and have included the circus fires in Nitroi, Brazil,[16] in 1961 and at Bangalore[17] in 1981 and the camping ground explosion in 1978 at Los Alfaques[18] where more than 400, 100, and 200 victims died, respectively. European disasters have been smaller but have included the Bradford Football Stand Fire[19] in 1985 and the Ramstein Air Show disaster[20] in 1988.

Clinical management must continue throughout the chain of evacuation and can be divided, for descriptive purposes, into that occurring at the site of injury, at a receiving (trauma or accident and emergency) center, and at a specialist burns unit. At each site the overall management of large scale burn disasters revolves around the three principles of triage, treatment, and transport.

On Site

First Aid Stations

These stations should be placed as close as possible to the disaster area and should be capable of dealing with waves of walking wounded and stretcher cases.

Treatment

At this level, treatment of casualties may be limited to maintenance of airway, management of respiratory problems, commencement of intravenous infusions, protection of the burn wound (e.g. by Clingfilm), and analgesia. Escharotomy should be carried out for full-thickness circumferential burns and antitetanus prophylaxis given.

Triage

Casualties are sorted on the basis of treatment priorities and depend on:

- The general condition of each patient, the extent and depth of the burn injuries, and his/her ambulatory status.
- Availability of facilities and personnel in the adjacent hospitals.

All patients undergoing triage must be adequately labeled. This will enable them to be identified according to their group. Large colored labels that are waterproof should be attached to each victim. The label will denote the triage group, treatment and drugs administered, and time given. Cases can be graded as follows:[21]

A. Ambulant patients with less then 10% burns – wounds are dressed and treatment is continued as an out-patient unless there is a reason for admission (i.e. extremes of age, deep burns requiring surgery, areas requiring special nursing).
B. 10–30% burns – after first aid these patients can be moved to distant hospitals initially, so as not to overload burn centers.
C. Serious burns involving 30–50% TBSA – these patients may be saved by energetic measures and should be transferred immediately to specialist centers for optimum treatment of shock and respiratory problems.
D. More than 50% TBSA burns, especially those with respiratory burns and the elderly, are unlikely to survive. These patients should be transferred to the nearest hospital but admitted to a separate ward.

In any disaster, it is advisable to group similar injured casualties in the same installations. Certain hospitals near the disaster should be designated as 'burn centers' and all cases requiring immediate and intensive care should be sent to these institutions.

Transport

The transportation of burned patients between the site of injury and the receiving hospital is known as primary transport. The initial call will reveal the location, the number of injuries, and the approximate time of the incident. This information will aid in decisions regarding the personnel, vehicles, equipment, and protective clothing that must be sent. On arrival at the scene, vehicles must be parked where they are out of danger and not blocking essential access or exits.

Most burned patients can be safely transported provided that they are properly stabilized and accompanied by competent medical personnel. A patient's physiology should be monitored throughout the journey.[22] Treatment including additional analgesia must be continued en route as necessary. Transfer itself can exacerbate the existing deleterious physiologic changes. The parameters which should be monitored continually during transfer are listed in **Table 41.4**.

Table 41.4 Parameters to be monitored continually during patient transfer

Respiratory rate and pattern
Heart rhythm and rate
Capillary refill time
Blood pressure
Level of consciousness
Blood and fluid loss
Oxygen saturation
Drugs and fluids administered

Accepting Hospital

Triage

Cases greater than 50% TBSA probably will not survive in the mass casualty situation. They should be made comfortable with adequate analgesia and sedation if thought necessary. They should be treated after patients in the more salvageable groups (see above).

Treatment

Mass nuclear casualties have been discussed previously. When supplies and facilities are overloaded, compromises will be necessary. These are:

- Plasma and blood products are reserved for cases with associated trauma. Electrolyte solutions are effective in uncomplicated burns for the first 24 hours.

- Local wound care. Exposure method may be useful in this situation.
- Grafting. Lack of operating space may be a problem. Patients whose wounds can be covered by a single grafting procedure take priority in order to allow for early discharge. Temporary biological cover may be necessary with larger burns until space becomes available.

Away from the site of the disaster, opportunity is taken to carry out the 'secondary survey', a full examination from head to foot. A full history is recorded and an assessment of the extent of the burn and associated injuries is included. A clinical respiratory evaluation, together with arterial blood gases and fiberoptic bronchoscopy (if practical), enables an early decision to be made as to whether a patient requires intubation and ventilation. This decision can be made by analysis of frequent arterial Po_2 measurements on a constant FIO_2 to detect early shunting. A pulse oximeter may provide a more practical substitute for arterial catheterization.

If the casualty is unconscious, attention must be paid to the possibility of associated head and neck injury as well as pneumothorax and carbon monoxide poisoning.[23] The burn wounds are then cleaned with a mild antiseptic solution and debrided. The extent and depth of burns are then estimated, which, together with the weight of the patient, can be used to guide intravenous fluid resuscitation along well established formulas. Success is measured by careful cardiovascular monitoring, aiming to produce a urine output in the range of 0.5 ml/kg/h in adults and 1.0 ml/kg/h in children.

Ideally each patient should have his fluid requirements calculated on an individual basis. When large numbers of casualties are involved, problems can occur in applying the standard formulas.[24] To obviate this problem, the Burn Wheel has been developed[25] to assist nonexperienced personnel in prescribing fluid to adults and children during the first 8 hours.

Transport

Transfer from a receiving hospital to the Burns Unit is known as secondary transport; it is well established that full assessment and resuscitation before moving a patient is invaluable in preventing cardiovascular and respiratory disasters.[26,27] A full examination may reveal other injuries (e.g. a ruptured spleen which could prove fatal if not diagnosed). Biochemical and hematologic parameters are optimized. For example, abnormal potassium predisposes to arrhythmias. Equally, transferring a hypoxic patient increases morbidity and mortality. Airway problems need to be definitively managed before transport. Any suggestion of airway involvement must alert health care providers to the need for intubation. There is no place for intubated patients breathing spontaneously during transfer. Adequate analgesia, sedation, and muscle relaxation should be given so that pain, anxiety, or restlessness do not interfere with the clinical picture. Attention must be paid to the wound, the immobilization of fractures, and the need for escharotomy before transport is commenced. All the necessary drugs and equipment needed during transfer must be available. It is wise to assume that the journey time will be twice that normally encountered so that enough drugs and oxygen are available in case of delays. All documents including drugs and fluids administered must be taken with the patient. A contemporaneous record of events during the journey must be kept.

Tertiary Referral Center

At a burn center, a patient is reassessed. Physiologic stabilization is obtained and those with lesser injuries may be transferred to peripheral hospitals with their treatment plan so as to reduce the strain on the facilities of the burn center. Similarly, cases found to require grafting at a later date can be sent back to the unit so that a two-way traffic is established. It is important that only those needing the tertiary center should remain there. Transportation between tertiary referral centers is very similar to that already mentioned.[28]

Summary

Treatment of radiation injury, whether or not it is combined with a thermal injury, will take up a great deal of resources. With few casualties, adequate treatment should not present a problem. If, however, there are large numbers of casualties such as would occur in a major nuclear accident or military conflict, resources will be limited or simply not available. Triage will limit treatment to those with less than 30% TBSA thermal injury with radiation and no other problems. Others should be made comfortable with analgesia and antiemetics, if available. Intravenous fluids may be limited, and the victims may be advised to take oral fluids consisting of balanced salt solutions and maintain a large urine output. Evacuation of survivors will take days and a natural selection will occur. Full intensive care support will be needed and available only if small numbers are involved. Those that survive and show signs of regeneration of tissues will warrant late surgical intervention. Aplastic anemia, immunosuppression, hemorrhage and sepsis will be major problems for survivors. Planning for mass casualties is important. Well trained personnel, preset protocols, specialized transport, and adequate supplies of documents, drugs, and disposables will insure minimal mortality and the proper use of facilities.

References

1. DOE/REAC/TS Radiation Accident Registries, personal communications and unpublished data.
2. Glasstone S, Dolan P J, eds. Biological effects. In: *The Effects of Nuclear Weapons*. Washington, DC: Dept. of Defense and Dept. of Energy, 1977: 541–628.
3. Oughterson A W, Warren S. *Medical Effects of the Atomic Bomb in Japan*. New York: McGraw-Hill Book Co, 1956.
4. Alt L A, Forcino C D, Walker R I. Nuclear events and their consequences. In: Walker R I, Cerveny T J, eds. *Medical Consequences of Nuclear Warfare*. Alexandria, Virginia: Defense Nuclear Agency, 1989.
5. Kelleher D. Acute effects of ionizing radiation. In: *United States Navy, Royal Navy Workshop on Nuclear Warfare Combat Casualty Care*. 1983: 71–80.
6. Brooks J W, Evans E I, Han W T, *et al*. The influence of external body radiation on mortality from thermal burns. *Ann Surg* 1953; **136**(3): 533–4.
7. Alpen E L, Sheline G E. Combined effects of thermal burns and whole body X irradiation on survival time and mortality. *Ann Surg* 1954; **140:** 113–18.
8. Becker W K, Buescher T M, Cioffi W G, McManus W F, Pruitt B A. Combined radiation and thermal injury after nuclear attack. In: Browne D, Weiss J F, MacVittie T J, Madhavan V P, eds. *Treatment of Radiation Injuries*. New York: Plenum Press 1990.
9. Browne D, Weiss J F, MacVittie T J, Madhavan V P, eds. Consensus summary. *Treatment of Radiation Injuries*. New York: Plenum Press, 1990.
10. Walden T L, Farzaneh M S. Biological assessment of radiation damage. In: Walker R I, Cerveny T J, eds. *Textbook of Military Medicine*. Vol 2. Virginia: TMM Publications, 1989.
11. Burke J F, Bondoc C C, Quinby W C. Primary burn excision and immediate grafting: a method shortening illness. *J Trauma* 1974; **14:** 389–95.
12. Gray D, Pine R, Harnar T, Marvin J, Engrav L, Heimbach D. Early surgical excision versus conventional therapy in patients with 20 to 40 percent burns. *Am J Surg* 1982; **189:** 147–51.
13. Dubos M, Neveux Y, Monpeyssin M, Drouet J. Impact of ionizing radiation on respone to thermal and surgical trauma. In: Walker R I, Gruber D F, MacVittie T J, Conklin J J, eds. *The Pathophysiology of Combined Injury and Trauma*. Baltimore: University Press, 1985.

14. Antin J H. Use of rhGM-CSF in bone marrow failure. In: Browne D, Weiss J F, MacVittie T J, Madhavan V P, eds. *Treatment of Radiation Injuries*. New York: Plenum Press, 1990: 11–18.

15. Barclay T L. Planning for mass burns casualties. Royal Society of Medicine Services. Round Table Series No 3. In: Wood C, ed. *Accident and Emergency Burns: Lessons from the Bradford Disaster 1986*. Oxford: Alden Press, 1986: 81–8.

16. Pitanguy I. Treatment of victims from the great catastrophe of the Gran Circus at Niteroi (Brazil). In: Wallace A B, Wilkinson A W, eds. *Research in Burns*. Edinburgh: E & S Livingstone, 1966: 216–21.

17. Das RAP. Circus fire at Bangalore. *Burns* 1983; **10:** 17–29.

18. Arturson G. The Los Alfaques disaster: a boiling liquid expanding vapour explosion. *Burns* 1981; **7:** 233–51.

19. Sharpe D T, Roberts A H N, Barclay T L, *et al.* Treatment of burns casualties after fire at Bradford City Football Club ground. *BMJ* 1985; **291:** 945–9.

20. Seletz J M. Flugstag-88 (Ramstein air show disaster): an army response to a MASCAL. *Milit Med* 1990; **155:** 153–5.

21. Low Chee Ann W. Mass casualty organization in burn disasters. *Med J Malaysia* 1977; **31:** 349–52.

22. Edbrooke D L, John R E, Murray R J. Transportation. In: Rylah L T A, ed. *Critical Care of the Burned Patient*. Cambridge: Cambridge University Press, 1992.

23. Safar P, Pretto E A, Bircher N G. Resuscitation medicine involving the management of severe trauma. In: Baskett P, Weller R, eds. *Medicine for Disasters*. London: John Wright, 1988: 36–87.

24. Milner S M, Rylah L T A. Burn casualties in war: a simplified resuscitation protocol. *Br J Hosp Med* 1993; **50:** 163–7.

25. Milner S M, Rylah L T A, Bennett J D C. The Burn Wheel: a practical guide to fluid resuscitation. *Burns* 1995; **21:** 288–90.

26. Bion J F, Edlin S A, Ramsey G, McCabe S, Ledingham I McA. Validation of a prognostic score in critically ill patients undergoing transport. *BMJ* 1985; **291:** 432–4.

27. Ehrenworth J, Sorbo S, Hackel A. Transport of critically ill adults. *Crit Care Med* 1986; **14:** 534–7.

28. Ellis A, Rylah L T A. Transfer of the thermally injured patient. *Br J Hosp Med* 1990; **44:** 206–8.

CHAPTER FORTY-TWO

42

Exfoliative and Necrotizing Conditions of the Integument

Maureen Hollyoak, Michael J. Muller and Manuhbai H. Desai

Introduction

Patients with acute, severe exfoliative and necrotizing conditions of the integument develop significant problems with wound infection, sepsis, nutrition, and pain. These are similar to those seen in patients with major burns. Burn centers provide expertise in the treatment and management of critically ill patients with skin loss from all causes, not solely from thermal injury. This chapter describes the pathophysiologic processes of severe exfoliative skin disorders, their diagnosis, and treatment offered by burn units.

Severe Exfoliative Disorders

Erythema multiforme (EM), Stevens–Johnson syndrome (SJS), and toxic epidermal necrolysis syndrome (TENS), have comprised the spectrum of the same disease state and are defined in **Table 42.1**.[1,2] Incidence of hospitalization for toxic epidermal necrolysis/Stevens–Johnson syndrome/erythema multiforme has been reported to be 4.2 per million persons per year.[3] These exfoliative disorders occur in all age groups; however, the incidence is increased in the elderly and in females.[1,4–7] TENS is often fatal (25–80%) early in the course of the disease with sepsis being the

Table 42.1

	Erythema multiforme	Stevens–Johnson syndrome	Toxic epidermal necrolysis
Prodrome	Absent	High fever, malaise	High fever, malaise
Acute phase	4–8 days	4–8 days, sensation of skin burning or tenderness	Sudden onset, 1–2 days sensation of skin burning or tenderness
Skin lesions	Symmetrical, primarily located on the extremities, some target lesions without blisters	Variable distribution, individual vesicles on an erythematous base, Nikolsky's positive	Diffuse generalized epidermal detachment, absence of target lesions, large confluent plagues >10% TBSA, Nikolsky's positive
Mucosal involvement	Absent or limited to one surface, usually oral	Severe, two or more surfaces involved	Severe, two or more surfaces involved
Histo-pathology	Dermoepidermal separation, mononuclear perivascular cell infiltrate, small areas of epidermal detachment associated with target lesions	Dermoepidermal separation, more intense dermal infiltrate, areas of epidermal detachment	Dermoepidermal separation, minimal dermal infiltrate, large areas of epidermal detachment
Recovery	1–4 weeks	1–6 weeks	1–6 weeks
Mortality	0%	0–38%	25–80%

most frequent cause of death. *Pseudomonas* and *Staphylococcus* are the predominant organisms involved. Pulmonary embolism and gastrointestinal hemorrhage are other causes of death.[4,8] The prognosis of TENS/SJS is worse than that of a burn victim with the same extent of skin loss.[8] Mortality is increased significantly in those patients at the extremes of age, percentage of denuded skin, and serum urea nitrogen levels.[8,9] SJS is associated with a mortality rate of 0–38%.[8,10] Erythema multiforme is not generally associated with patient mortality.[10]

Etiology

TENS and SJS have similar etiologic agents. TENS, however, has a much higher percentage associated with antecedent drug therapy. Drugs are implicated in 77–94% of cases of TENS.[11,12] Antibacterials (29%), anticonvulsants (15%), analgesics (5%), and nonsteroidal anti-inflammatory agents are implicated.[1,13–16] Attempts to identify drugs suspected of having caused exfoliative necrolysis by skin test and laboratory tests have seldom been rewarding.[8] Upper respiratory tract infections, pharyngitis, otitis media, or viral illness are frequently reported.[4–6,17–19] *Mycoplasma pneumoniae* and herpes simplex virus have been implicated in the cause of EM and SJS, but not TENS.[5,20] It can be difficult to differentiate some prodomal symptoms as due to viral or other infectious agents, or due to the disease process. Recently, the incidence of HIV infection in patients with toxic epidermal necrolysis has risen.[21,22] Twenty-two percent of cases of toxic epidermal necrolysis are HIV positive compared to the prevalence of HIV in the general population of 1%.[21] Whether this increase is due to their immunocompromised state or the many drugs these patients receive, particularly sulfonamides, is debated. No history of drug ingestion or preceding illness is noted in these patients. Many of these cases may actually suffer from lack of patient recall because of severity of disease or the patient's age. Idiopathic cases accounted for only 4% of TENS.[12]

Morphology/Histopathology

Skin biopsy is essential for diagnosis. Skin manifestations vary from patient to patient and with the age of a lesion (**Figure 42.1**). Skin lesions may evolve to a different stage of development with recurrent attacks of erythema multiforme in a single patient.[23] Advancing edges of the target lesions show scattered necrotic keratinocytes in the epidermis and mild dermal inflammation. In older lesions and central zones of target lesions, the dusky appearance corresponds to areas of extensive keratinocyte necrosis, often the formation of subepidermal bullae and dermoepidermal separation. The surrounding erythematous zone shows papillary dermal edema, vascular dilation with endothelial cell swelling and perivascular mononuclear cell infiltrate.[7] Extravasated erythrocytes may be seen in the surrounding papillary dermis. The reticular dermis is normal.

Epidermal and dermoepidermal suppressor/cytotoxic T lymphocytes in addition to dermal infiltrates of helper T lymphocytes have been demonstrated.[24–26] Hertl has confirmed that these epidermal cells are cytotoxic T cells.[27] Langerhan cells appear to be reduced in the epidermis, although numerous dermal macrophages are observed.[28] A more intense dermal cell infiltrate is present in Stevens–Johnson syndrome, especially in postherpetic cases.[20,24] Dendritic lymphoid cells are observed opposed to damaged dermal macrophages and necrotic keratinocytes. Further, at the point where the cytoplasmic processes contact the keratinocyte, the plasma membrane of the keratinocyte is absent.[28] Aberrant expression of HLA-DR on keratinocytes has been observed, a phenomenon which has been observed in many other inflammatory skin disorders.[25]

Immunofluorescence microscopy has demonstrated IgM and C3 along the dermoepidermal junction and dermal vessels in cases of postherpetic Stevens–Johnson syndrome and erythema multiforme.[20,24] There have been only two reports of basal cell immunoflurescence in toxic epidermal necrolysis.[28,29] The pathogenesis of toxic epidermal necrolysis is not completely understood. Type IV delayed hypersensitivity reaction, keratinocyte cytotoxicity mediated by a lymphocytic substance, type II cytotoxic reaction and nonimmunologic mediated necrolysis are all possible mechanisms along with predisposing factors of infection and genetic susceptibility.[16,30] Positive patch tests in patients with toxic epidermal necrolysis have been used to support the delayed hypersensitivity hypothesis.[26] This view is somewhat at odds with the fact that HIV patients display increased frequency of toxic epidermal necrolysis.[15,16]

Suppression/cytotoxic T-cell infiltrates are observed in the epidermis in toxic epidermal necrolysis[26,28] and graft versus host disease.[31] It is hypothesized that cytotoxic T cells recognize drug metabolites which are complexed with the MHC–I molecule on the surface of keratinocytes, migrate into the epidermis, react with keratinocytes, and cause epidermal necrolysis. The occurrence of sicca syndromes in patients with toxic epidermal necrolysis and graft versus host disease further supports the autoimmune theory.[32] The observation of blebbing of the keratinocyte plasma membrane in toxic epidermal necrolysis is considered a reliable morphologic finding of cytotoxic T-lymphocyte cytolysis.[28] Further, the observation that cyclophosphamide aids toxic epidermal necrolysis patients supports this theory, as cyclophosphamide is known to inhibit cytotoxic T-lymphocyte activity.[28] Type II cytotoxic reactions involve the binding of either IgG or IgM antibodies to a cell-bound antigen. The antigen–antibody complex then activates the complement cascade and results in the cell destruction. This mechanism is not generally supported as nuclear fragmentation, common to keratinocytes of toxic epidermal necrolysis patients, is not a consequence of complement-mediated cytolysis.[28,29,33] Nonimmunological mechanisms include keratinocyte injury by either drug, drug metabolite, or toxic products derived from a drug in the epidermis.[16,21,22]

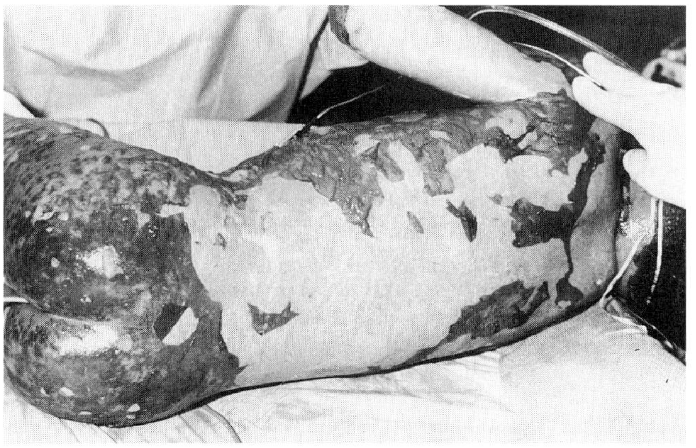

Fig. 42.1 Topical epidermal necrolysis (TEN) is characterized by massive sloughing of the epidermal tissue.

Clinical Features

A prodromal phase of toxic epidermal necrolysis/Stevens–Johnson syndrome is frequently identified and usually consists of a low-grade fever, malaise, and cough; all of these are suggestive of a respiratory tract infection. These symptoms may precede any cutaneous manifestation by 1–21 days.[5] Morbilliform eruptions or discrete erythematous or purpuric macules may evolve into a generalized erythroderma.[30] Later, vesicles and large bullae emerge from areas of erythema. Patients may exhibit diffuse red erythema immediately followed by epidermolysis.[8] Nikolsky's sign: desquamation of epidermis in sheets on light digital pressure, is positive. Generally a lag period of only 1–3 days is observed from initiation of drug until skin eruption.[28]

Two or more areas of mucosa involvement are typical of Stevens–Johnson syndrome or toxic epidermal necrolysis. Mucosal involvement precedes skin lesions by 1–3 days in one-third of cases.[7] Several sites are usually affected, in the following order of frequency: oropharynx, ocular, genitalia, and anus. Most toxic epidermal necrolysis patients have multiple mucosal lesions, and they generally persist longer than cutaneous lesions.[8]

Complications

Toxic epidermal necrolysis is frequently associated with serious complications. The skin does reepithelialize from the dermal elements without scarring; however, abnormal pigmentation is common (**Figure 42.2**). Nail plates are frequently lost and nail regrowth may be abnormal or absent.[7] Mucosal membrane erosions may result in cicatricial lesions causing phimosis in men and vaginal synechiae in women. Oropharyngeal involvement is common and generally results in severe dysphagia.[34] The onset of intestinal symptoms generally occurs concurrently with the cutaneous lesions.[35] Toxic epidermal necrolysis induces esophagitis with frequent subsequent stricture formation.[21] Gastrointestinal erosions resemble ulcerative or pseudomembranous colitis macroscopically, and massive hemorrhage requiring resection has been reported.[4,8,17] Intestinal involvement worsens the prognosis.[8,35] Pulmonary involvement is associated with increased mortality.[34] Involvement may range from diffuse erythema to extensive confluent alterations covered by fibrinous exudate.[30,34] Epiglottal swelling, necessitating intubation, has been reported.[34] Desquamation of alveolar lining cells has been reported and these patients therefore require frequent tracheobronchial toilet.[35] Subclinical interstitial edema is often noticed and 30% of cases progress to frank pulmonary edema.[7] Bronchopneumonia was found to be the most frequent complication, occurring in 50% of patients.[10,17] Pulmonary embolism is an important cause of death in patients with toxic epidermal necrolysis.[8] Hepatitis and hepatocellular necrosis are also described.[7,30]

Hypoalbuminemia, increased erythrocyte sedimentation rate leukocytosis, thrombocytopenia and normochromic and normocytic anemia are common.[10,34] Leukopenia is frequent and a poor prognostic sign.[6–8,17] Transient depletion of T-helper lymphocyte (CD4+) is part of this phenomenon. Ocular sequelae are the most severe long-term complications and occur in half the survivors. Pseudomembranous or membranous conjunctivitis resulting from coalesced fibrin and necrotic debris can lead to opacification, secondary infection, and blindness.[2] Keratoconjunctivitis sicca, Sjögren-like syndrome, ectropion, entropion, trichiasis, and symblepharon can also occur.[32]

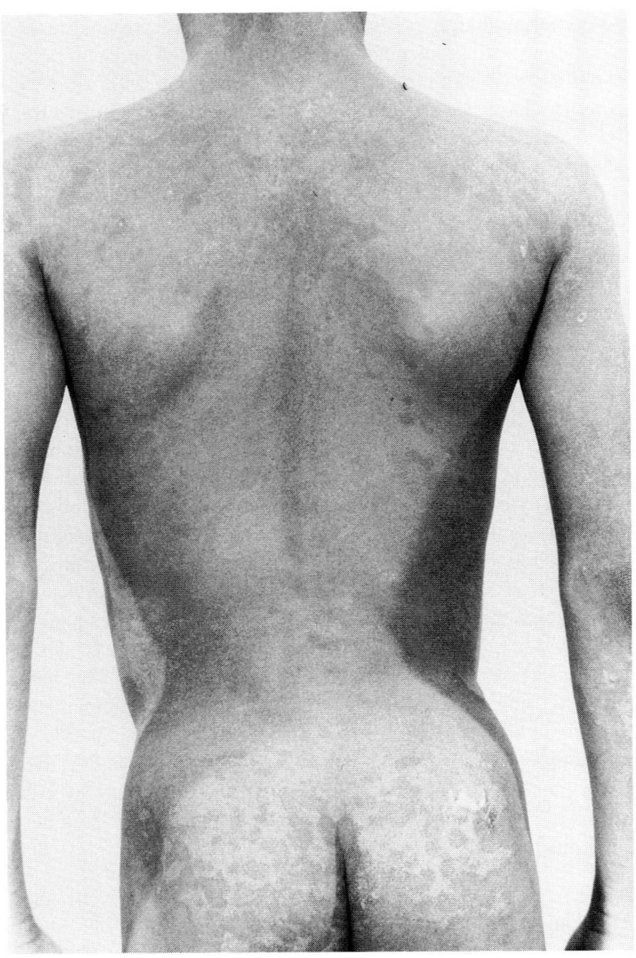

Fig. 42.2 One year post-TEN, wounds are completely closed with minimum of residual scarring.

Management

Toxic epidermal necrolysis is a life-threatening disease and such a patient is best managed in an intensive care burn unit where vigorous fluid resuscitation, nutritional support, wound care, physical therapy, and social services are provided routinely.[4,6,14,17,30]

Surgical Approach

Debridement and application of biological or synthetic dressings are essential.[4,13,14,36] Debridement is best undertaken under general anesthesia as soon as diagnosis is established. Blood loss associated with debridement is minimal, so over-resuscitation must be avoided. Sloughed epidermis should be removed in order to reduce bacterial growth and exposed dermis should be covered. Biological dressings, such as cadaver allograft (homograft) and porcine xenograft, greatly reduce the pain, decrease fluid loss, promote healing, and reduce the risk of sepsis (**Figure 42.3**).[4,13,14,36,37] Porcine xenograft adheres well to the skin and is commercially available in large quantities.[14,36] Homograft is more likely to become vascularized and therefore reduce the number of graft changes.[4,38] All biological or synthetic dressings must be secured. Grafted areas must be immobilized and protected from shear forces. In children, Steinmann pins to suspend extremities are useful.[14] In adults and children, continuous rotation or air fluidized (Clinitron) beds are frequently utilized.

Topical Therapy

As separation occurs at the dermal–epidermal junction, varying depths of viable dermis remain. If this dermis can be protected

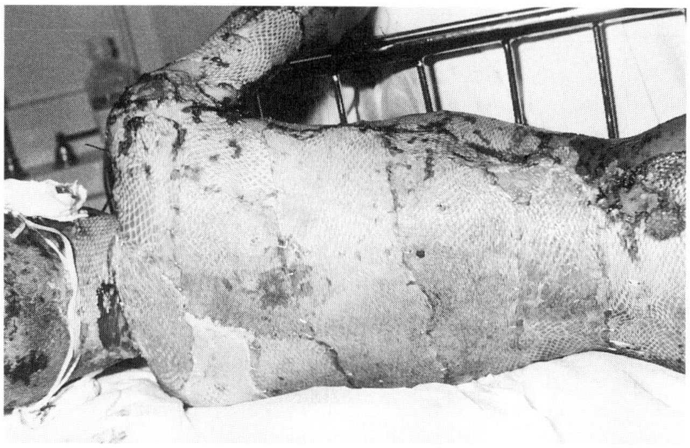

Fig. 42.3 As with many partial-thickness wounds, biological dressings do much to encourage reepithelialization and reduce the pain associated with these wounds.

from toxic detergents, desiccation, mechanical trauma, and wound sepsis, then rapid resurfacing by proliferation of epithelium from the skin appendages will occur.[13] Rapid bacterial proliferation with invasive wound sepsis leads to full necrosis. Hydrotherapy and topical antimicrobials provide debridement and infection control which should be initiated early in the course of the disease.[5,19]

Topical agents used include silver sulfadiazine cream,[23] silver nitrate 0.5% solution,[7,17,19] chlorhexidine gluconate 0.5% solution,[7] and polymyxin-bacitracin ointment.[5] Silver sulfadiazine is widely used but may exacerbate the disease process due to its sulfur content. It has an inhibitory effect on epithelialization and self-limited leukopenia occurs. Silver nitrate 0.5% solution has little chance of contributing to an ongoing allergic reaction, and epithelialization is not inhibited. Frequent dressing changes are required, and serum electrolytes and osmolarity must be carefully monitored. For patients in whom delayed treatment has resulted in contaminated wounds, silver nitrate soaks can reduce contamination and prepare the wound for eventual biological dressing. Chlorhexidine gluconate is rapidly bactericidal and effective against gram-positive and gram-negative organisms, including *Pseudomonas*, and has a low incidence of sensitivity.

Corticosteroid Therapy

Corticosteroid treatment of toxic epidermal necrolysis patients has promoted much controversy. They have been used because of the delayed hypersensitivity reaction or antibody-dependent cytotoxicity theories of pathogenesis.[30,39] The practice of administering high-dose continuous corticosteroid throughout the course of the disease has fallen into disfavor by many authors.[5–7,21,30,31,40–42] The lack of randomized, controlled, prospective trials has made rational assessment of its worth difficult. Many authors feel that steroids enhance the risk of sepsis,[14,17] increase protein catabolism, delay healing,[8] cause severe gastrointestinal bleeding,[8,13,17] prolong hospitalization,[41] and increase mortality.[6,17,43] Lyell himself states that the indication for the use of steroids in the treatment of toxic epidermal necrolysis is vague.[21]

One study found no decrease in the progression of Stevens–Johnson syndrome with steroids, but instead found significant morbidity.[43] In a prospective, although not randomized study, increased survival (66%) was seen in matched patients who did not receive steroids compared to only 33% survival in those who did receive steroids.[17] Pediatric Stevens–Johnson syndrome patients treated with steroids had a longer hospital stay and a complication rate of 74% with steroids compared to 28% in those without steroids.[41] Another study demonstrated 80% mortality associated with steroid therapy which was reduced to 20% when steroids were withheld.[6] Furthermore, toxic epidermal necrolysis has been documented in patients who were receiving corticosteroids for preexisting diseases.[7,13,15] Corticosteroids may have a place in the treatment of toxic epidermal necrolysis during the erythrodermic stage of the disease, before major skin loss has occurred. It cannot be overemphasized that once more than 20% total body surface area has sloughed, steroid therapy is contraindicated.[40]

General Therapy

Suspected drugs should be discontinued immediately. Administration of pain medication is of high priority and antipyretic agents may be required. Consideration should be given to the use of empirically successful broad spectrum antibiotics if neutropenia exists, as these patients are prone to a higher incidence of septic complications. The white blood cell count generally returns to normal levels after 2–5 days. The cause of this immunosuppression is unclear; it may be part of the primary disease or a secondary event.[39] This situation is, however, the only one in which such antibiotic therapy is indicated. 'Prophylactic' antibiotics only promote resistance and *Candida* overgrowth. Oral nystatin prevents intestinal overgrowth of *Candida* and decreases the risk of *Candida* sepsis.[17,39] Frequent monitoring of urinary tract, respiratory tract, skin, and catheters allows early identification of organisms and allows detection of increasing concentrations of organisms early.

Environmental temperature should be raised to 30–32°C. This will allow a reduction in metabolic rate. Heat shield and infrared lamps are beneficial in patients' rooms, tub rooms and operating rooms. Stress ulceration prophylaxis is advisable. Mouth erosion, resulting in severe dysphagia, can be alleviated by the use of viscous lidocaine or cocaine rinses. Oral debris should be removed and the mouth sprayed with antiseptic several times a day.[40] Ocular involvement should be assessed daily by an ophthalmologist. Conjunctival crusting can be minimized by the use of saline every hour. Any adhesions should be broken using a blunt instrument and bland eye drops or ointment applied frequently.[5,13] Documented ocular infections are treated with antibiotics instilled frequently (10–24 times daily). Following recovery, Schirmer's test should be performed.[5,40] Pulmonary involvement requires close supervision with careful toileting, incentive spirometry, mobilization, and coughing so as to prevent infections and complications. Progress should be monitored by daily blood assessment, chest x-ray, and bacteriological culture to help determine if antibiotics are indicated or respiratory support required. Measures to prevent thromboembolism, such as low-dose heparin, should be instituted.

Intravenous fluid replacement is required. Patients do not develop the massive edema evident in burned patients, and fluid resuscitation formulas employed in the management of thermal injuries are therefore excessive.[7,13,14,30,36] Ringer's lactate solution is given at a rate determined by the patient's condition and urine output, remembering to reduce volume once wound coverage is accomplished. Colloid is administered if serum albumin is less than 2.5 g/dl and central line placement avoided wherever possible because of the risk of sepsis. Invasive lines are removed as soon as possible, and oral and nasogastric routes are then utilized.

Nutritional Support

Enteral nutrition should be commenced on admission. Due to the frequent presence of oral mucosal ulcerations, patients may be reluctant to take nutrition orally, and a nasogastric route may then be required. Unlike burned patients who have significantly elevated metabolic rate, these patients appear to have metabolic rates slightly above basal requirements.[13,39] Weight stabilization and a positive nitrogen balance have been achieved in adults with 2500 kcal/day.[13] If gastrointestinal function becomes impaired or sepsis intervenes, requirements may increase. Total parenteral nutrition is to be avoided. Patients with toxic epidermal necrolysis and Stevens–Johnson syndrome demonstrate limitation in mobility, decreased strength, postural and gait deviation, contractures, and impaired coordination. Patients should, therefore, be monitored and treated throughout the course of the disease by a physiotherapist.[44]

Necrotizing Soft Tissue Infections

Staphylococcal scalded skin syndrome, necrotizing fasciitis, and purpura fulminans are examples of a group of conditions which are characterized by extensive soft tissue loss, critical rapid onset, illness, and death. Early, accurate diagnosis is essential to initiate appropriate action, such as extensive surgical excision in the case of necrotizing fasciitis or crepitant soft tissue infections. Burn care centers have much to offer these patients as extensive skin loss is their hallmark.

Staphylococcal Scalded Skin Syndrome

Staphylococcal scalded skin syndrome is the most severe condition which is caused by exfoliative staphylococcal toxins and is characterized by systemic signs and symptoms and generalized involvement of the skin (**Figure 42.4**). It is important to make a diagnosis early and particularly to differentiate it from toxic epidermal necrolysis which has a different management and much greater mortality. Staphylococcal scalded skin syndrome is predominantly a disease of infancy (Ritter's disease) and early childhood with most cases occurring before the age of 5 years.[45] Newborn nurseries are often the sites of outbreaks. Nursery or maternity staff may be the source of epidermolytic toxin producing *Staphylococcus aureus*. Adult staphylococcal scalded skin syndrome syndrome is rare and usually associated with compromised renal function.

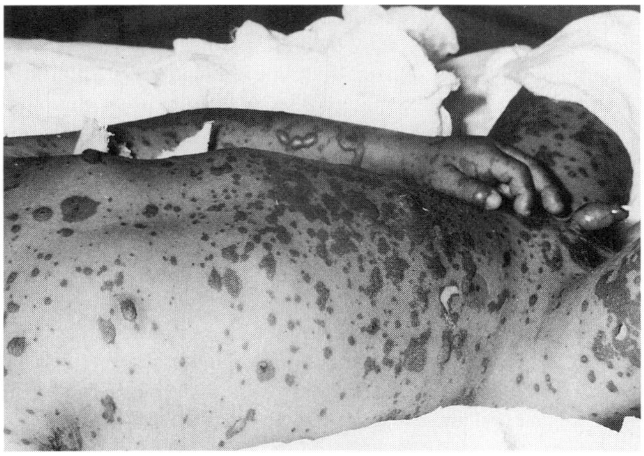

Fig. 42.4 Staphylococcal scalded skin syndrome (SSSS) is characterized by diffuse, erythemic lesions with bullae formation (see left forearm). Epidermis is shed in great sheets with minimal abrasion. The wounds are partial-thickness and heal without surgical intervention.

Mortality is generally only 4%, but can be much higher in adults (40%).[45,46]

Two distinct epidermolytic toxins (A and B), are responsible for the blistering in staphylococcal scalded skin syndrome.[21] Most toxigenic strains of *Staphylococcus aureus* are identified as group 2 phage.[47] The exfoliative toxin is metabolized and excreted by the kidneys and hence those with renal immaturity (children) or renal compromise are predisposed to this disease. The exfoliative toxins produce blistering by disrupting the epidermal granular cell layers through interdesmosomal splittings. The exact mechanism of action of the toxins has not been determined, although it is felt that the toxins directly affect desmosomes, perhaps by proteolysis.[45]

Diagnosis of staphylococcal scalded skin syndrome can be made rapidly with a skin biopsy. The characteristic intraepidermal level of splitting is seen, with the split occurring at the granular layer level (stratum granulosum) with no epidermal necrosis or inflammatory cells in the corium.[45] Immunofluorescent studies of the skin are negative.[47] A Tzanck preparation from a scraping of the base of a freshly denuded area will reveal the affected cell population, i.e. acanthocytic keratinocytes.[47] Bullae, denuded skin and blood are usually sterile, however, and staphylococci can usually be cultured from nares, conjunctiva, or pharynx.[48]

Management

Onset may be marked by fever, malaise, and irritability. Scarlatiniform erythema is often accentuated by flexural and periorificial areas.[45] The skin is generally tender to touch, and sheets of skin may peel away in response to minor trauma (Nikolsky's sign). Blisters appear within 24–48 hours and rupture, leaving a characteristic moist erythematous epidermal base. Severe mucosal involvement is not often seen.

Antibiotics are commenced as soon as the diagnosis has been made. Since the majority of group 2 staphlylococci show resistance to penicillin, semisynthetic penicillinase-resistant penicillin analogs are indicated (e.g. methicillin). Administration of steroids to these patients is contraindicated.[47] Fluid resuscitation is usually required although less volume is required compared to that for a burned patient with a similar involved area. Requirements should be guided by urine output, hemodynamic parameters, and electrolyte and colloid status.

Until barrier function is restored, patients should receive appropriate wound dressings aimed at preventing secondary wound infection. Topical agents are soothing and bacteriostatic. Alternatively, large areas are more effectively managed with the placement of biological or synthetic dressings. They have the advantage of eliminating the need for frequent dressing changes which can be particularly traumatic for young children. Fatalities do occur in very young and adult patients, usually from sepsis or electrolyte imbalance.[47] Complete wound healing within 7 days is usually observed, and scarring and altered pigmentation are not common.

Necrotizing Fasciitis and Bacterial Myonecrosis

Necrotizing fasciitis (NF) is a soft tissue infection which is characterized by widespread necrosis of fascia and subcutaneous tissue which may progress to muscle and skin necrosis. Overall mortality may still be as high as 50%.[46,49] Most cases of necrotizing fasciitis are due to polymicrobial infections including both anaerobic gram-positive cocci and gram-negative bacillus.[49] *Streptococcus, Staphylococcus, Enterococcus*, and *Bacteroides* are commonly found. Bacterial myonecrosis can also result from infection with many bacterial species. Clostridial gas gangrene results in severe systemic toxicity and higher mortality than for necrotizing fasciitis. There is frequently the presence of a prior deep contaminated wound. Streptococcal myositis has a mortality rate of between 80 and 100%.[50] Risk factors for both necrotizing fasciitis and bacterial myonecrositis have been identified as diabetes mellitus, intravenous drug use, age greater than 50 years, hypertension, and malnutrition/obesity. The presence of three or more of these risk factors was found to give a predictive mortality rate of 50%.[51] (See **Figure 42.5**.)

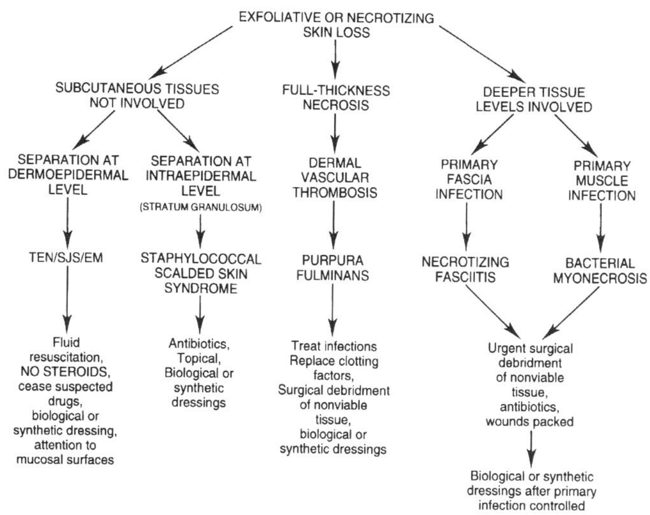

Fig. 42.5 Flowchart of management of exfoliative and necrotizing conditions of the integument.

Diagnosis

Early recognition is extremely important. Initial findings may be localized pain and edema with no discoloration of the skin. Later, induration and erythema may be evident. Paresthesia of overlying skin and eventual dusky discoloration and local blistering may occur. Severe toxemia may develop, usually out of proportion to the local signs. Severe systemic signs are characteristic of myonecrosis. Gas may be evident in subcutaneous tissues on x-ray. CT and MRI imaging may help in the diagnosis and provide information on the nature and extent of the infection.[52] Frozen section biopsies may provide histologic evidence of infection.[53] Microbiological specimen and Gram stains are very important in making a diagnosis and guiding antibiotic treatment later. The distinction between NF, myonecrosis, and other soft tissue infections can often only be made during surgery.

Management

The key to successful management of necrotizing infections is early diagnosis and radical surgical intervention. Adequate fluid resuscitation and nutritional support are also required. Preoperative broad spectrum antibiotics are commenced, although high-dose penicillin is appropriate for clostridial infections. Surgical exploration involves excision of all necrotic tissues. When more than one operation is required to remove infected necrotic tissue, mortality increases from 43% to 71% and highlights the importance of adequate debridement initially.[54] In patients with many risk factors, consideration should be given to amputation of the extremity involved, especially those with myonecrosis. Wounds are packed open with antiseptic soaked dressings and are changed frequently. Kaiser and Cerra have reported unsatisfactory results with either early application of porcine xenografts or burn wound topical antimicrobials.[55] Only when sepsis has been adequately controlled should wounds be closed.

Secondary infections must be prevented by management as for a burn wound. Biological or synthetic dressings offer the advantages of decreased pain, decreased fluid loss, and prevention of secondary infection. Frequently, large areas of skin and soft tissue loss result from this disease and will eventually require extensive surgery to achieve adequate closure. Some authors advocate the use of hyperbaric oxygen and claim that it results in decreased mortality and reduced need for debridement; however, adequate controlled trials are still lacking.[42] Hyperbaric oxygen therapy, if used, should be as an adjunct to radical surgery and antibiotics and should not delay or curtail debridement.

Purpura Fulminans

Purpura fulminans (PF) is a term that describes an acute syndrome of rapidly progressive hemorrhagic necrosis of the skin due to dermal vascular thrombosis associated with vascular collapse and disseminated intravascular coagulation (DIC).[56] It may occur in individuals with:

- dysfunction of the protein C anticoagulant system;
- acute severe infection; or
- idiopathic, with no coagulation dysfunction or infection.

It has been associated with meningococci, Gram-negative bacilli, staphylococci, streptococci, and *Rickettsia* organisms. The skin necrosis begins in a region of dermal discomfort which rapidly progresses to evanescent flush, followed by petechiae. Hemorrhagic bullae progress to frank skin necrosis. The process generally involves the skin and subcutaneous tissues, sparing muscle. Skin involvement is frequently an early manifestation of the disease process; skin biopsy will, therefore, allow an earlier diagnosis.[56] Mortality in the acute phase is 18–40%.[57]

Management is directed at halting progression, preventing secondary infections, and removing nonviable tissue. Heparin and replacement of clotting factors have proven useful to stop intravascular clotting.[57] Volume replacement to correct shock from blood extravasation and sepsis is required. Limb vascular and compartmental pressure should be monitored closely to enable early escharatomy and/or fasciotomy. Skin lesions resulting in blisters only should be treated conservatively with topical treatment (e.g. silver sulfadiazine) so as to prevent secondary infection. Once tissue has become nonviable it should removed as soon as the patient is stabilized. Small areas can be covered with autografts but large areas may require allografts or xenografts. Patients may require limb amputations and many will require revisions for progression of disease.[58]

Conclusion

These inflammatory and infectious conditions of the skin and graft tissues represent a major challenge. The team approach to their care is essential, and wound management is paramount. Burn units are ideally suited to dealing with patients with these conditions and should be considered as the appropriate site of referral for these critically ill patients.

REFERENCES

1. Patterson R, Dykewicz M S, Gonzales A, *et al.* Erythema multiforme and Stevens–Johnson syndrome: descriptive and therapeutic controversy. *Chest* 1990; **98:** 331–6.

2. Wilkins J, Morrison L, White C R. Occulocutaneous manifestations of the Erythema multiforme/Stevens–Johnson syndrome/toxic epidermal necrolysis spectrum. *Dermatol Clin* 1992; **10:** 571–82.

3. Chan H C, Stern R S, Arndt K A, *et al.* The incidence of erythema multiforme, Stevens–Johnson syndrome and toxic epidermal necrolysis. *Arch Dermatol* 1990; **126:** 43–7.

4. Halebian P, Corder V, Herndon D, Shires G T. A burn center experience with toxic epidermal necrolysis. *J Burn Care Rehabil* 1983; **4:** 176–83.

5. Prendiville J S, Hebert A A, Greenwald M J, Esterly N B. Management of Stevens–Johnson syndrome and toxic epidermal necrolysis in children. *J Pediatr* 1987; **115:** 881–7.

6. Kim P S, Goldfarb I W, Gaisford J C, Slater H. Stevens–Johnson syndrome and toxic epidermal necrolysis: a pathophysiologic review with recommendations for a treatment protocol. *J Burn Care Rehabil* 1983; **4:** 91–100.

7. Roujeau J C, Chosidow O, Saiag P, Guillaume J C. Toxic epidermal necrolysis (Lyell syndrome). *J Am Acad Dermatol* 1990; **23:** 1039–58.

8. Revuz J, Penson D, Roujeau J C, *et al.* Toxic epidermal necrolysis: clinical findings and prognostic factors in 87 patients. *Arch Dermatol* 1987; **123:** 1160–6.

9. Scully M C, Frieden I J. Toxic epidermal necrolysis in early infancy. *J Am Acad Dermatol* 1992; **27:** 340–4.

10. Ruiz-Maldonado R. Acute desseminated epidermal necrosis type 1, 2 and 3: study of sixty cases. *J Am Acad Dermatol* 1985; **13:** 623–35.

11. Guillaume J C, Roujeau J C, Revuz J, *et al.* The culprit drugs in 87 cases of toxic epidermal necrolysis (Lyell syndrome). *Arch Dermatol* 1987; **123:** 1166–70.

12. Roujeau J C, Guillaume J C, Fabre J P, *et al.* Toxic epidermal necrolysis (Lyell syndrome): incidence and drug etiology in France, 1981–1985. *Arch Dermatol* 1990; **126:** 37–42.

13. Heimbach D M, Engrav L H, Marvin J A, *et al.* Toxic epidermal necrolysis: a step forward in treatment. *JAMA* 1987; **257:** 2171–5.

14. Marvin J A, Heimbach D M, Engrau L H, Harner T J. Improved treatment of the Stevens-Johnson syndrome. *Arch Surg* 1984; **119:** 601–5.

15. Correia O, Chosidow O, Saiag P, *et al.* Evolving pattern of drug-induced toxic epidermal necrolysis. *Dermatology* 1993; **186:** 32–7.

16. Saiag P, Caumes E, Chosidow O, *et al.* Drug-induced toxic epidermal necrolysis (Lyell syndrome) in patients infected with the human immunodeficiency virus. *J Am Acad Dermatol* 1992; **26:** 567–74.

17. Halebian P H, Madden M R, Finkestein J L, *et al.* Improved burn center survival of patients with toxic epidermal necrolysis managed without corticosteroids. *Ann Surg* 1986; **204:** 503–11.

18. Adzick N S, Kim S H, Bondoc C C, *et al.* Management of toxic epidermal necrolysis in a pediatric burn center. *Am J Dis Child* 1985; **139:** 499–502.

19. Yetin J, Bianchini J R, Owens J A. Etiological factors in Stevens-Johnson syndrome. *South Med J* 1980; **73:** 599–602.

20. Howland W W, Golitz L E, Weston W L, Huff J C. Erythema multiforme: clinical histopathologic, and immunologic study. *J Am Acad Dermatol* 1984; **10:** 438–46.

21. Lyell A. Toxic epidermal necrolysis (the scalded skin syndrome): a reappraisal. *Br J Dermatol* 1979; **100:** 69–86.

22. Goldstein S M, Wintroub B W, Elias P M, Wuepper K D. Toxic epidermal necrolysis: unmuddying the waters. *Arch Dermatol* 1987; **123:** 1153–5.

23. Huff J C, Weston W L, Tonnesen M G. Erythema multiforme: a critical review of characteristics, diagnostic criteria and causes. *J Am Acad Dermatol* 1983; **8:** 763–75.

24. Merot Y, Gravallese E, Guillen F J, Murphy G F. Lymphocyte subsets and Langerhans' cells in toxic epidermal necrolysis. *Arch Dermatol* 1986; **122:** 455–8.

25. Villada G, Roujeau J C, Clerici T, *et al.* Immunopathology of toxic epidermal necrolysis. Keratinocytes, HLA-DR expression, Langerhans cells and mononuclear cells: an immunopathologic study of five cases. *Arch Dermatol* 1992; **128:** 50–3.

26. Miyauchi H. Hosokawa H, Akaeda T, *et al.* T-cell subsets in drug-induced toxic epidermal necrolysis. *Arch Dermatol* 1991; **127:** 851–5.

27. Hertl M, Merk H F, Bohlen H. T-cell subsets in drug-induced toxic epidermal necrolysis. *Arch Dermatol* 1992; **128:** 272.

28. Heng M C, Allen S G. Efficiency of cyclophosphamides in toxic epidermal necrolysis: clinical and pathophysiologic aspects. *J Am Acad Dermatol* 1991; **25:** 778–86.

29. Stein K M, Schlappner O L, Heaton C L, Decherd J W. Demonstration of basal cell immunofluorescence in drug-induced toxic epidermal necrolysis. *Br J Dermatol* 1972; **86:** 246–52.

30. Parson J M. Toxic epidermal necrolysis. *Int J Dermatol* 1992; **31:** 749–68.

31. Paller A S, Nelson A, Steffen L, *et al.* T-lymphocyte subset in the lesional skin of allogenic and autologous bone marrow transplant patients. *Arch Demartol* 1988; **124:** 1795–801.

32. Roujeau J C, Philippoteau C, Koso M, *et al.* Sjögren-like syndrome following toxic epidermal necrolysis. *Lancet* 1985; **1:** 609–11.

33. Hensen E J, Claas F H J, Vermeer B J. Drug-dependent binding of circulating antibodies in drug-induced toxic epidermal necrolysis. *Lancet* 1981; **2:** 151–2.

34. Wahle D, Beste D, Conley S F. Laryngeal involvement in toxic epidermal necrolysis. *Otolaryngol Head Neck Surg* 1992; **6:** 796–9.

35. Chosidow O, Delchier J C, Chaumette M T. Intestinal involvement in drug-induced toxic epidermal necrolysis. *Lancet* 1991; **337:** 928.

36. Taylor J A, Grube B, Heimbach D M, Bergman A B. Toxic epidermal necrolysis: a comprehensive approach. *Clin Pediatr* 1989; **28:** 404–7.

37. Sowder L L. Biobrane wound dressing used in the treatment of toxic epidermal necrolysis: a case report. *J Burn Care Rehabil* 1990; **11:** 237–9.

38. Birchall N, Langdon R, Cuono C, *et al.* Toxic epidermal necrolysis: an approach to management using cryopreserved allograft skin. *J Am Acad Dermatol* 1987; **16:** 368–72.

39. Halebian P H, Shires G T. Burn unit treatment of acute, severe exfoliating disorders. *Ann Rev Med* 1989; **40:** 137–47.

40. Revuz J, Roujeau J C, Guillaume J C, *et al.* Treatment of toxic epidermal necrolysis: Creteil's experience. *Arch Dermatol* 1987; **123:** 1156–8.

41. Ginsburg C M. Stevens–Johnson syndrome in children. *Pediatr Infect Dis* 1982; **1:** 155–8.

42. Riseman J A, Zamboni W A, Curtis A, *et al.* Hyperbaric oxygen therapy for necrotizing fasciitis reduces mortality and the need for debridement. *Surgery* 1990; **108:** 847–50.

43. Rasmussen J E. Cause, prognosis and management of toxic epidermal necrolysis. *Compr Ther* 1990; **16:** 3–6.

44. McDonald K, Johnson B, Prasad J K, Thomson P D. Rehabilitative considerations for patients with severe Stevens-Johnson syndrome and toxic epidermal necrolysis: a case report. *J Burn Care Rehabil* 1989; **10:** 167–71.

45. Resnick S D. Staphylococcal toxin-mediated syndromes in childhood. *Semin Dermatol* 1992; **11:** 11–18.

46. Canoso J J, Barza M. Soft tissue infections. *Rheum Dis Clin North Am* 1993; **15:** 235–9.

47. Elias P M, Fritsch P, Epstein E H. Staphlococcal scalded skin syndrome: clinical features, pathogenesis, and recent microbiological and biochemical developments. *Arch Dermatol* 1977; **113:** 207–19.

48. Itani O, Crump R, Minouni F, *et al.* Ritter's disease (neonatal staphylococcal scalded skin syndrome). *Am J Dis Child* 1992; **146:** 425–6.

49. Patino J F, Castro D. Necrotizing lesions of soft tissue: a review. *World J Surg* 1991; **15:** 235–9.

50. Steven D L. Invasive group A streptococcal infections. *Clin Infect Dis* 1992; **14:** 2–13.

51. Francis K R, Lamaute H R, Davis J M, Pizzi W F. Implications of risk factors in necrotizing fasciitis. *Am J Surg* 1993; **59:** 304–8.

52. Sharif H S, Clark D C, Aabed M Y, *et al.* MR Imaging of thoracic and abdominal wall infections: comparison with other imaging procedures. *Am J Roentgenol* 1990; **154:** 989–95.

53. Stamenkovic I, Lew P D. Early recognition of potentially fatal necrotizing fasciitis: the use of frozen-section biopsy. *N Engl J Med* 1984; **310:** 1689–93.

54. Freischlag J A, Ajalat G, Busuttil R W. Treatment of necrotizing soft tissue infection: the need for a new approach. *Am J Surg* 1985; **149:** 751–7.

55. Kaiser R E, Cerra F B. Progressive necrotizing surgical infections: a unified approach. *J Trauma* 1981; **24:** 349–52.

56. Adcock D M, Hicks M J. Dermatopathology of skin necrosis associated with purpura fulminans. *Semin Thromb Hemost* 1990; **16:** 283–92.

57. Chasan P E, Hansbrough J F, Cooper M L. Management of cutaneous manifestations of extensive purpura fulminans in a burn unit. *J Burn Care Rehabil* 1992; **13:** 410–13.

58. Genoff M C, Hoffer M M, Achauer B, *et al.* Extremity amputation in meningococcemia induced purpura fulminans. *Plast Reconstr Surg* 1992; **89:** 878–81.

Rehabilitation

CHAPTER FORTY-THREE

PREVENTION AND TREATMENT OF DEFORMITY IN BURNED PATIENTS

E. BURKE EVANS, M. IRMA ALVARADO, SHEILA OTT AND KIMBERLEYE MCELROY

PREVENTION AND TREATMENT OF MUSCULOSKELETAL DEFORMITY SECONDARY TO BURNS

With burns, as perhaps with no other order of trauma, there is urgent need for immediate and aggressive initiation of patient specific rehabilitation programs. Distribution and depth of burn so clearly define and predict the patterns of deformity from wound and scar contracture that it is possible on burn day 1 to design a program and to establish short-term and long-term goals. The more extensive the burn, the greater the rehabilitation challenge. A seriously burned extremity in an otherwise modestly burned patient is much easier to restore to function than an extremity similarly burned in a patient with full-thickness burns involving trunk, neck, and head as well as other extremities. Among seriously burned patients, the immediate and primary treatment goals will always be preservation of life and wound coverage. These basic treatment priorities, however, do not preclude the development and implementation of an aggressive rehabilitation program.

In addition to wound and scar contracture factors, other considerations in the genesis of musculoskeletal deformity in burns are: the assumption of positions of comfort by a patient, imposed positions that favor deformity, reluctance or inability of a patient to participate in a rehabilitative program, loss of motor function and gravity. The means for prevention of deformity are: proper positioning with or without splints; exercise to maintain range of joint motion, muscle strength, and muscle tone; and early mobilization. This chapter describes by body region commonly encountered musculoskeletal deformities associated with burns and discusses principles of prevention and treatment.

Spine

Contracture resulting from unilateral or asymmetric burns of the neck, axilla, trunk, and groin will cause lateral curvature of the spine (scoliosis). The level and amplitude of curvature will vary with the site and severity of the contracture. In addition, pelvic obliquity accompanying asymmetric hip or knee flexion contracture will impose a lateral lumbar curve. With none of the scoliotic curves associated with burns is there an intrinsic spinal deformity; permanent spinal deformity will never result if the extrinsic cause, i.e. scar contracture, is eliminated. On the other hand, if the contracture is allowed to persist through several years of growth, the vertebral deformity will become structural and permanent (**Figure 43.1a,b,c**).

As long as a patient is recumbent, lateral curvature can be prevented by maintaining straight alignment of the trunk and neck. Often, however, the curve is insidious in onset and will not be recognized until a patient begins to walk. Trunk list observed early in the ambulation period can be simply a transient accommodation to pain and wound tightness, but a persistent list may herald the development of scoliosis. Once there is an established asymmetric contracture, it is difficult by therapeutic means to stretch it out, so it is probably better to deal surgically with a deforming scar early than to permit scoliosis to persist. Standard pressure garments now in common use are said to prevent scar hypertrophy and to accelerate scar maturity. To the extent that they are effective in scar control, they may act to reduce the occurrence of lateral curve of the spine.

Exaggerated thoracic kyphosis secondary to anterior chest and neck burn is difficult to prevent because the recumbent position cradles the back and encourages protraction of the scapulae. The two-plane contracture extending from chin and neck to thorax and from shoulder to shoulder anteriorly pulls the chin down, flexes the neck and pulls the scapulae forward. Protraction of the scapulae alone may cause a normal thoracic kyphosis to appear to be exaggerated. If the protraction posture is not corrected, however, it tends to become habitual, and the final result features a prominent and rounded thoracic spine (**Figure 43.2a,b**). As this spinal deformity in its genesis is linked to neck and shoulder contractures, the measures for its prevention and correction will be discussed in the section dealing with neck and shoulders.

Exaggeration of spinal lumbar lordosis is rarely related to overlying burn of the back. On the other hand, full-thickness burns of the abdomen are occasionally deep enough to compromise or even eliminate abdominal muscle function. In this circumstance, the pelvis, for lack of support of anterior motors, will roll forward and lumbar lordosis will increase (**Figure 43.3**). Hamstring and gluteus

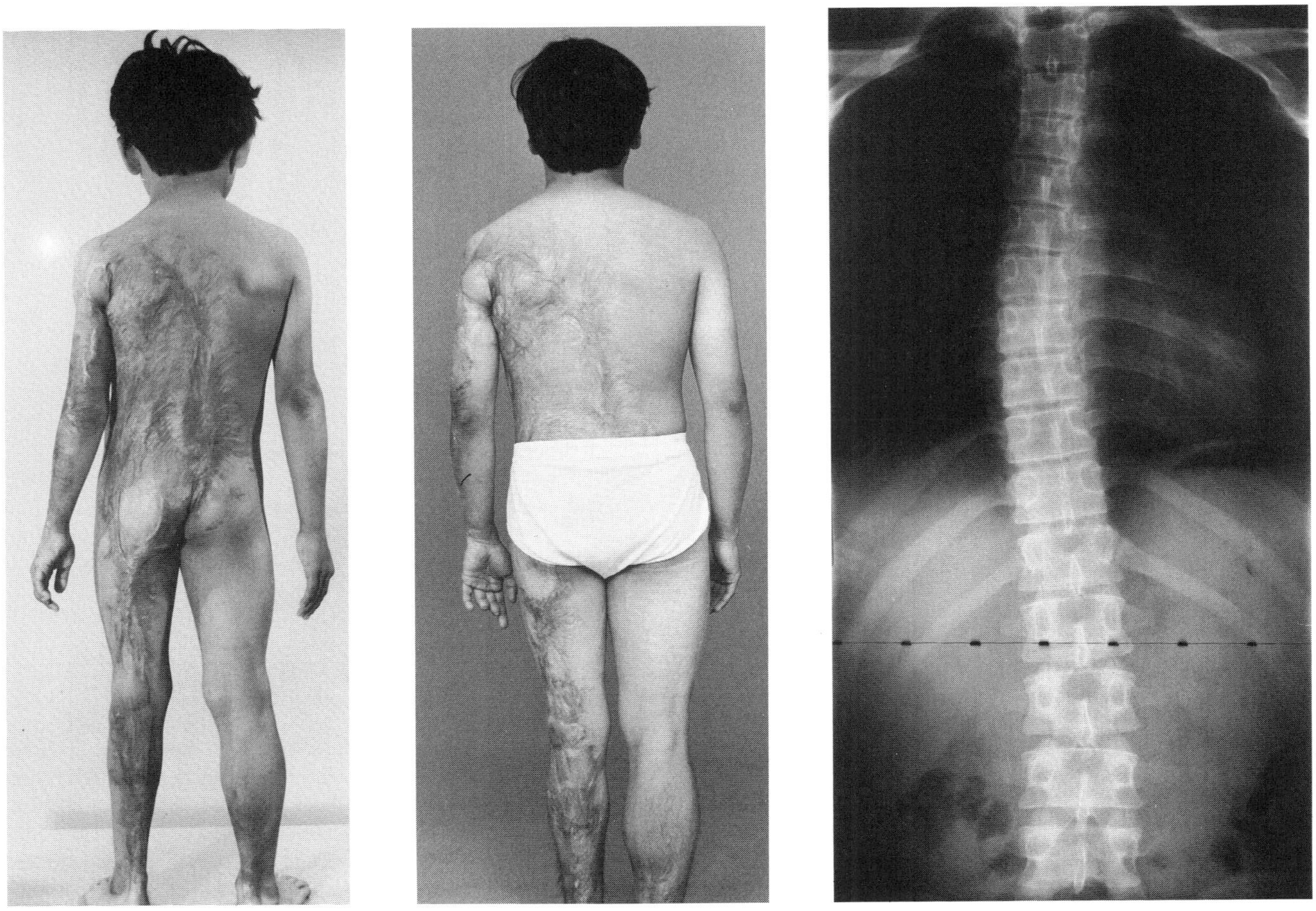

(a) (b) (c)

Fig. 43.1 (a) Six years after 45% TBSA burn involving mainly the left side of the chest and trunk, a 7-year-old male stands with a trunk list to the right which compensates for a scar-imposed unbalanced thoracic spinal curve convex to the right. (b,c) At age 17 spinal alignment has improved. Thoracic asymmetry and shift of the trunk toward the left are due to fixed structural thoracic scoliosis extending from the third thoracic vertebra through the first lumbar vertebra.

maximus muscles, though strong posterior stabilizers of the pelvis, cannot compensate for loss of abdominal muscle power. If all abdominal muscles are lost, viscera will protrude, shifting the center of gravity forward. To compensate and achieve balance, a patient must lean backwards, further increasing the lumbar lordosis. There is no way to prevent this sequence if abdominal muscle function is lost; since surgical correction often is not practical, the only treatment recourse may be sturdy external abdominal support to relieve the burden of protruding viscera.

Neck and Shoulder Girdle and Axilla

In the discussion of thoracic kyphosis, it was noted that burns bridging from chin and neck to thorax and from shoulder to shoulder anteriorly lead to dropping of the chin, flexion of the neck, and protraction of the scapulae. Whether or not the burn extends laterally on the neck, the contracture will elevate and externally rotate the scapulae as well. If there is bridging scar of the axilla that restricts glenohumeral abduction, the scapulae will further elevate and rotate with any active or passive effort to abduct the arm. This clear interrelationship of potential contractures expresses a need for separate management of neck, shoulder, and axillary scarring and for segregation of glenohumeral and scapular motion in exercise programming. If scapulae are habitually protracted and the neck is not completely extensible, balance and level gaze will be gained by spine extension which shifts the thorax posteriorly and hyperextends the lumbar spine.

Positioning for prevention of contracture requires that the head be in the midline position with the neck at neutral or in slight extension. The amount of neck extension must not be so great that traction on the chin causes the mouth to drop open. To encourage scapular retraction, it is sometimes helpful to place a small vertical towel roll posteriorly between the scapulae. Such a roll can be effective only if a patient is on a firm mattress. A transverse transmental pin and 1–2 pounds of traction through a traction bow may be used to keep the chin elevated after surgical release of a neck contracture. The pin will correct mandible retraction at the same time. Long-term traction, however, is not advised as it may erode the bone and may cause protraction of the mandible.

Elevation of the arms should be in the neutral plane or in line with the glenoid at approximately 15–20 degrees of horizontal flexion. In this plane, as much as 80 degrees of elevation may be attained before scapular rotation is imposed. If the arm is elevated in the coronal plane, scapular rotation is more likely to take place

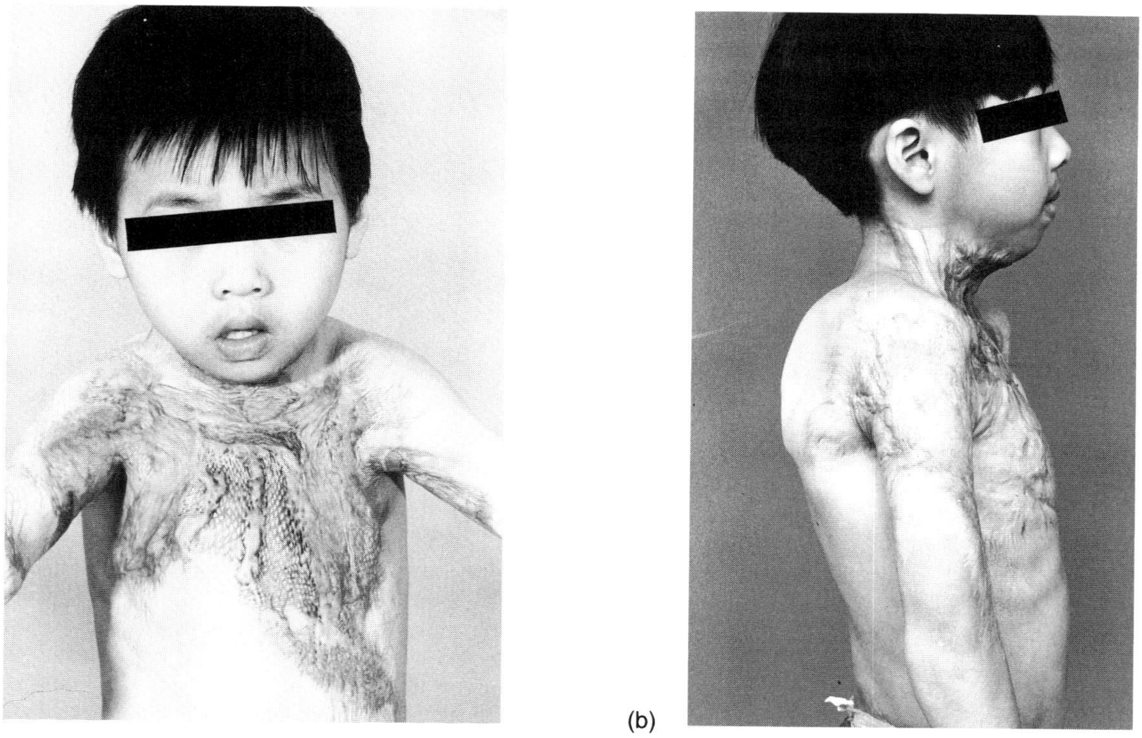

(a) (b)

Fig. 43.2 A 3-year-old boy as he appeared 14 months after a full-thickness anterior burn of neck, chest, and shoulders. Scar contracture has flexed the neck and protracted the scapulae. (b) Three years later, after several release and graft procedures, the shoulders remain protracted, the scapulae are winged, and the thoracic kyphosis is exaggerated.

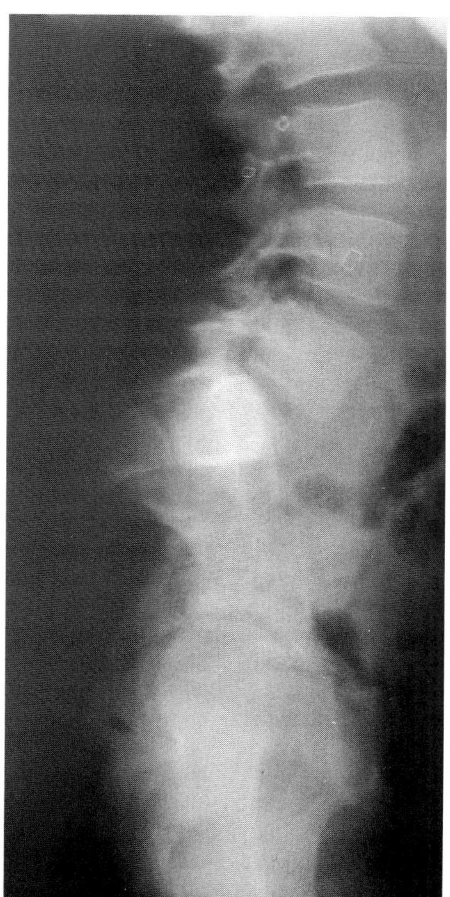

with fewer degrees of abduction. Additionally, abduction in the coronal plane places the glenohumeral joint in relative extension and uncovers the head of the humerus, rendering it more liable to anterior subluxation if the position is chronically held. With primary healing of an axillary burn or with healing following graft, prevention of axillary contracture becomes more difficult. Pressure with axillary pads and figure of eight wrapping and static abduction splints are methods in common use.

Elbow

With severe burns involving the upper extremity, the elbow will be held in flexion. This position favors flexion contracture and threatens posterior exposure of the joint if there is dorsal full-thickness burn. Thus, full extension is the protecting position for the elbow. If the joint remains exposed posteriorly, extension may have to be rigidly maintained for several weeks. If the joint is not exposed, mobilization into increasing flexion range can begin very soon after the burn. The elbow is integral to the so-called delivery system for the hand, and elbow range to full or near-full flexion is more important for overall function than range to full or near-full extension. Flexion is required for grooming, eating and toileting, while extension is needed for reach and stabilization. Radial head rotation for pronation and supination is less often affected by burn than flexion and extension, but forearm rotation is essential for accurate hand placement. Any rehabilitative program must seriously address that function.

Fig. 43.3 In this 17-year-old male, 3 years after a 90% TBSA burn, total loss of abdominal musculature has resulted in pronounced forward pelvic tilt, an almost horizontal sacrum, and an exaggerated lumbar lordosis.

Wrist and Hand

The usual posture of the unsupported burned hand is wrist flexion, metacarpophalangeal extension, interphalangeal flexion and first metacarpal extension and adduction. Metacarpophalangeal extension is imposed to some degree by dorsal swelling of the hand, and the overall posture may be the position of greatest comfort. If the hand rests unsupported on the bed, all features of the deformity may be positionally reinforced with the first metacarpal being pushed farther into extension and adduction. The overall appearance is of an intrinsic minus or claw deformity (**Figure 43.4a,b,c**).

If, in the acute burn phase, the wrist is securely supported in extension, the metacarpophalangeal joints of digits 2 through 5 will tend to fall into flexion because of gravity if the forearm is pronated or the hand elevated and because of the reciprocal tenodesing action between digital flexors and extensors. The first metacarpal will likewise fall forward into flexion. Wrist extension is, thus, basic to control of hand and digit position and to prevention of hand and wrist deformity. Among the digits, the second and fifth most easily drift into metacarpophalangeal extension because each has a proper extensor and has relative functional freedom from the third and fourth digits. The fifth is occasionally pulled into extreme abduction and extension by scar contracture. The thumb may become similarly displaced and, to a lesser degree, the index finger. The severe displacement of these digits gives a grotesque, but characteristic deformity (**Figure 43.5a**).

For adults, adolescents, and older children, preventive static positioning with a custom orthoplast splint can be relatively efficient. There are, however, two common faults in custom splints which are designed to gain metacarpophalangeal flexion and to position the thumb in flexion and abduction. If the transverse fold of the splint is not proximal to the metacarpophalangeal joints of digits 2 through 5, the splint will impede rather than favor metacarpophalangeal flexion. If the thumb component of the splint applies volar rather than medial pressure, the metacarpophalangeal joint will extend and the metacarpal will become correspondingly more adducted. The metacarpophalangeal joint should be maintained in slight flexion and pressure from the splint should be applied just to the medial surface of the digit. Any degree of first metacarpal adduction contracture increases the likelihood that the proximal phalanx will be pushed into hyperextension and eventually subluxation by the splint. Once wrist and digital contractures are established, severity of contracture and maturity of scar determine if the deformities can be best managed by splinting or by skeletal traction or if they will require surgical release followed by splinting or traction (**Figure 43.5b,c**).

Hip

When anterior burns extend from abdomen to thigh, hip flexion is the position of comfort. If the hip is fixed in any degree of flexion, posture will be modified. Bilateral symmetric contractures impose increased lumbar lordosis or knee flexion or both. Asymmetric contracture will cause pelvic obliquity and scoliosis. In adults and older children, thighs are more likely to be held in adduction than in abduction, whereas in preambulatory infants, the secondary component of the contracture may be abduction. Thus, for the hips, the preventive position is full extension and symmetric abduction

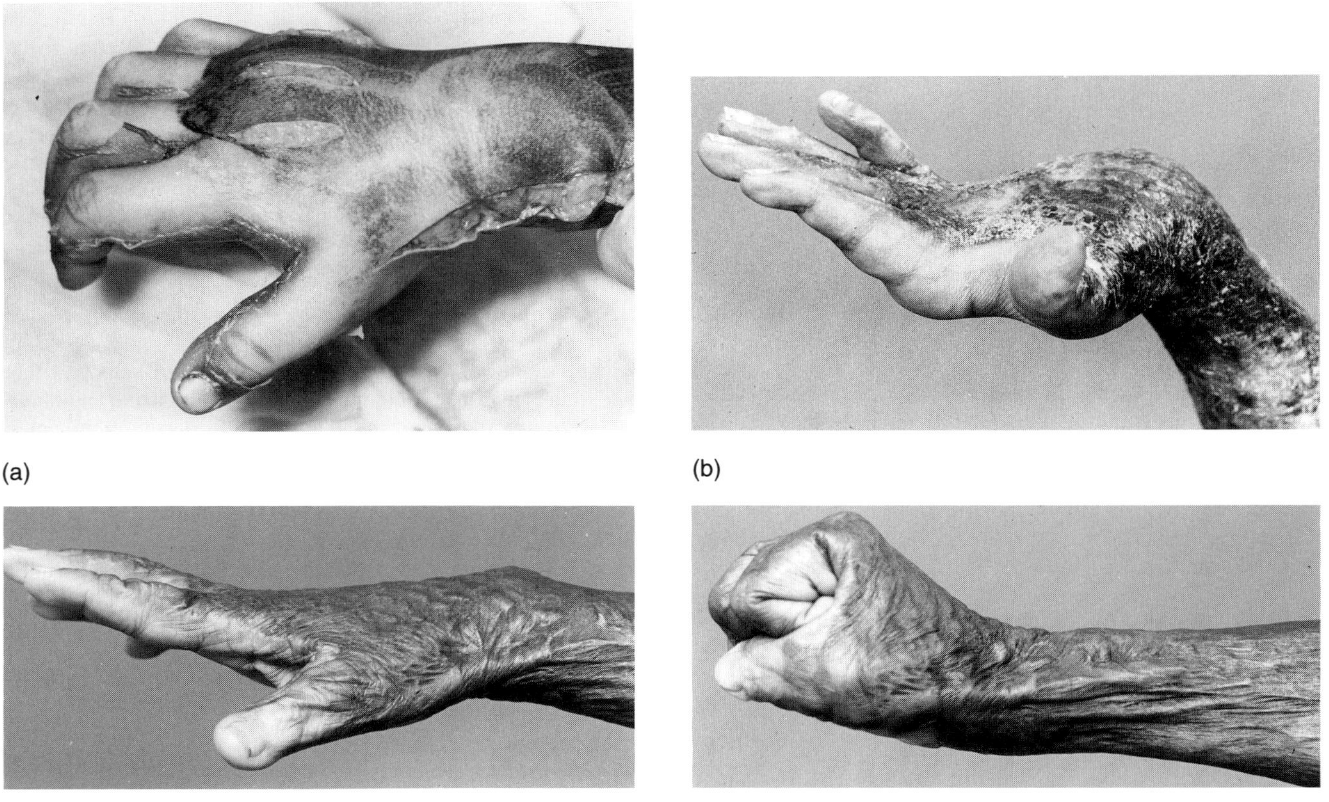

(a) (b) (c)i (c)ii

Fig. 43.4 (a) Edema following a full-thickness burn of the dorsum of the right hand of a 4-year-old boy – imposed metacarpophalangeal extension and digital flexion just 1 day after a 73% TBSA burn. (b) Two months after burn, the hand shows the common progression of the deformity with wrist flexion and fixed hyperextension of all metacarpophalangeal joints. (c)(i,ii) Three years after burn, and following release and grafting procedures, there is functional range of motion and minimal residual deformity.

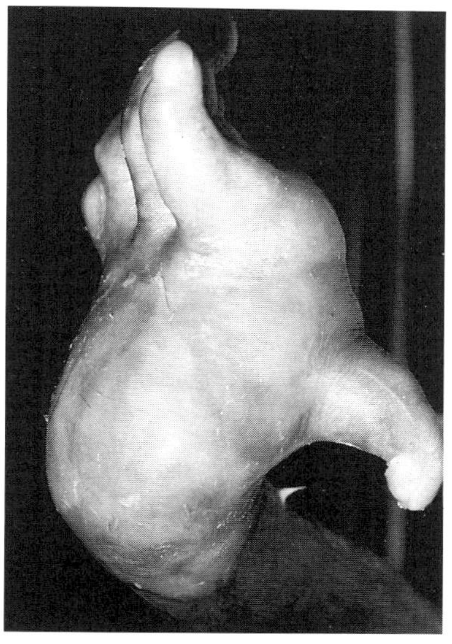

(a)i

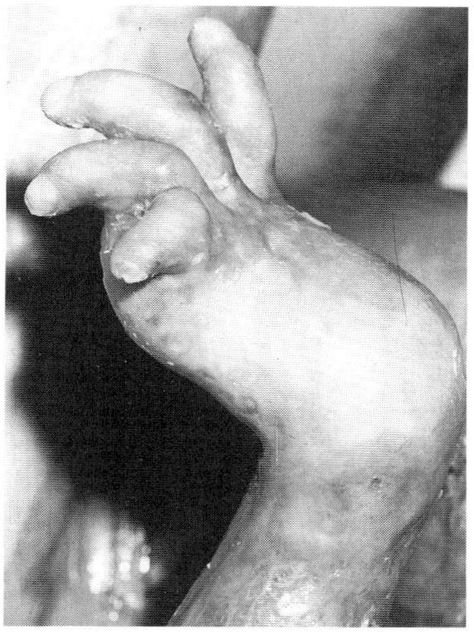

(a)ii

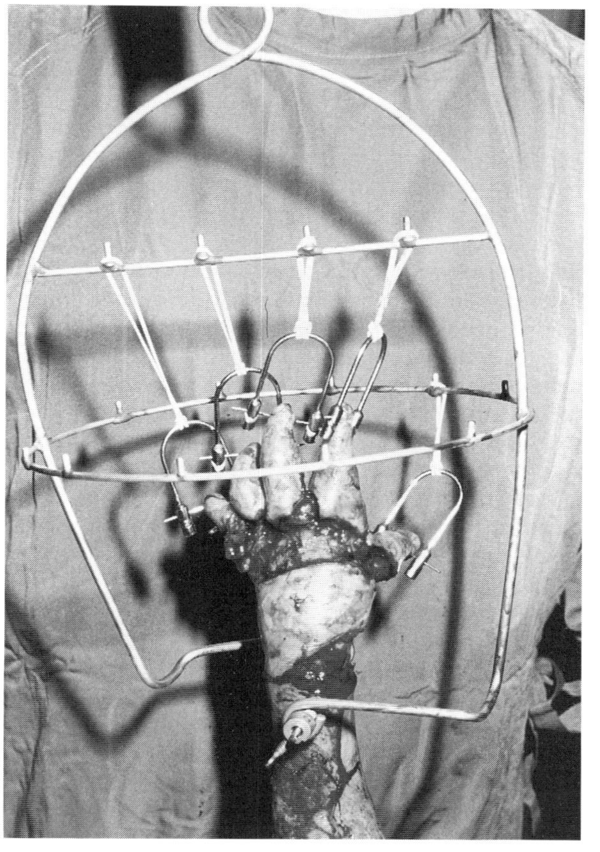

(b)

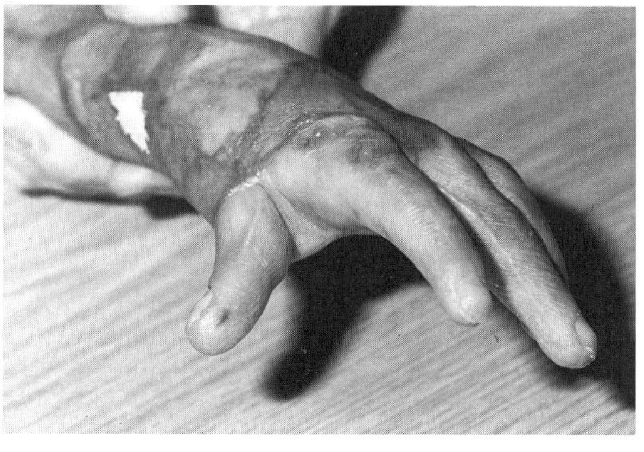

(c)i

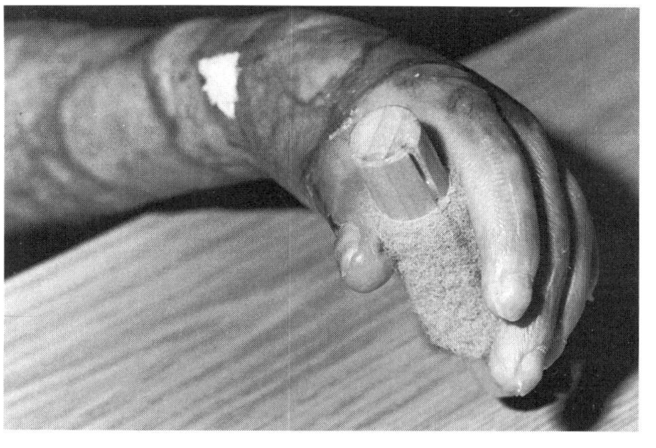

(c)ii

Fig. 43.5(a)(i,ii) Severe wrist flexion and digital extension deformities of the left upper extremity of a 6-year-old boy 7 months after 40% TBSA burn. (b) After surgical release of wrist and digits and split-thickness autogenous skin grafting, the corrected position was maintained with digital pin traction in a halo splint proximally fixed at the wrist. (c)(i) Six months after surgical release, there is active wrist extension to neutral, and digital grasp and release have been restored. The skeletal traction splint was removed 2 weeks after its application when an exercise program was begun. (ii) Position was maintained at rest with an orthoplast splint.

of 15–20 degrees. Full hip extension is difficult to attain and maintain if a patient is on a soft surface or if lower extremities must be elevated for management of leg and thigh wounds. Subtle hip flexion contractures can be easily overlooked when a patient stands, because there may be only a slight increase in lumbar lordosis or forward or lateral shift of the trunk. If established hip flexion contractures are not surgically corrected, posture is likely to be permanently altered with scoliosis or exaggerated lordosis.

Knee

Whether deep burn crossing the knee is mainly anterior or posterior, a patient will more often than not flex the knee. Deep anterior burns may expose the joint, occasionally destroying the patellar tendon. Deep posterior burns result in bridging scar formation. The protective position for the knee is full extension to be maintained by splint or skeletal traction until there is efficient quadriceps function and a patient is ambulatory. Thereafter, night splints must be used until scar contracture is no longer a threat.

Persisting bilateral knee flexion contracture will impose hip flexion. Persisting unilateral contracture may impose pelvic obliquity and scoliosis. As with the hip, posture alteration may be so subtle as to be overlooked. Correction of even a slight contracture should be a surgical priority as should elimination of a soft bridging scar band that does not prevent complete willful knee extension but causes a patient habitually to hold the knee in slight flexion.

Foot and Ankle

Ankle equinus is the most frequently occurring deformity involving the foot. Initially, it is related more to gravity and failure to support the foot at neutral (90 degrees) at the talotibial joint than to the early effect of the burn. Loss of deep and superficial peroneal nerve function will compound the problem by encouraging the foot to drift into inversion as well as equinus because of loss of dorsiflexion and eversion motors. In the end, the total deformity for the unsupported foot may be ankle equinus, hind-foot inversion, and forefoot varus and equinus. Ankle equinus quickly becomes a resistant deformity so that within a few days or even hours the foot can no longer be positioned at 90 degrees of dorsiflexion. Eventually the contractures of scar, muscle, and capsular structures combine to fix the deformity.

Equinus deformity and the attending inversion and forefoot varus can be prevented by accurate and unyielding support of the foot in neutral alignment at 90 degrees or greater of dorsiflexion. If a patient must be nursed prone, the feet must be allowed to fall free from the mattress. Static splinting is often unsuccessful because of a patient's desire and tendency to plantar flex strongly, displacing the splint and leading to ulcers of the heel and toes and at splint edges. A stable foot board may be effective if the feet are kept securely and totally against it. For large burns and particularly for circumferential burns of the lower extremities, skeletal suspension incorporating calcaneal traction will support the foot at neutral if the traction pin is placed in the calcaneus well behind the axis of ankle motion. This balanced traction system demands that the knees be supported in flexion with tibial pins at the level of the tibial tubercle. Calcaneal pins will not prevent forefoot equinus if the traction must be employed for several weeks; in this case, proximal pull through dorsal pins in the first or first and second metatarsals may be required for support of the forefoot. Transmetatarsal pins are useful as well when calcaneal traction is not sufficient to correct equinus.

Minor established equinus deformity will yield with a standing and walking program. At the outset, graduated heel lifts may be used to accommodate the deformity. If a patient must be bed confined, skeletal traction through the calcaneus may be the quickest and most efficient way to correct the deformity. Traction is effective even if scar contracture contributes to the deformity. Serial corrective casts or splints alone are useful mainly for minor contractures. Splints are best used for static recumbent positioning in a standing and walking program. For fixed, unyielding deformity, scar release combined with tendoachillis lengthening with or without posterior capsulotomy is a standard surgical procedure which yields inconsistent results. The correction achieved is often just to neutral or slightly more. The Ilizarov system has been used with generally satisfactory immediate results in severe cases. Once correction is achieved, if there are no dorsiflexion motors and if the range of ankle motion is only a few degrees, ankle fusion may, in the end, yield the best functional result.

The most common intrinsic deformity of the foot is extreme extension of the toes due to dorsal scar contracture. This deformity is insidious in onset and is difficult to prevent as there is no type of nonskeletal splinting which will hold the toes flexed. In its extreme, the deformity includes dorsal metatarsophalangeal subluxation which may involve one or all toes depending on the location of the scar. The metatarsal heads become prominent on the plantar surface and walking may be painful. Correction of the deformity requires dorsal surgical release of the contracture, manual correction of the deformity, and intrinsic or extrinsic pinning of the digit or digits in an overcorrected position. Recurrence of deformity after surgical correction is common.

Dorsal scar contractures extending from leg to foot to toes may pull the foot into marked inversion if the scar is medial or into eversion if the scar is lateral. The fifth and first toes may be separately displaced by the same scar bands. These contractures must always be surgically corrected. Their persistence will lead to bone defor-

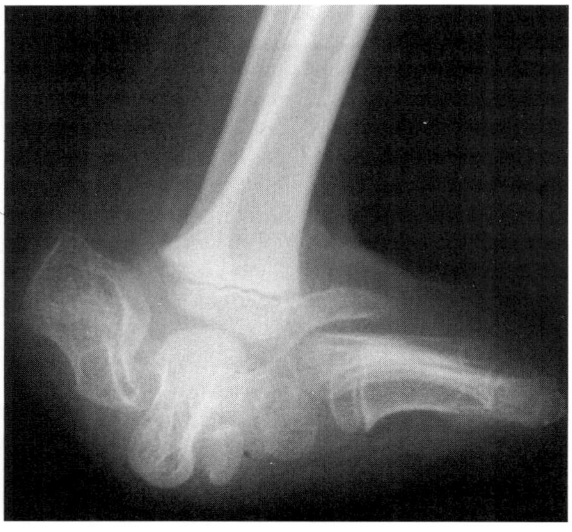

(a)

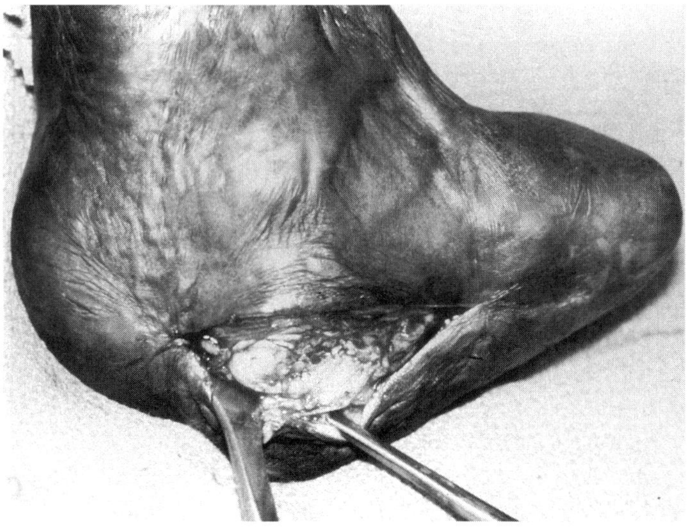

(b)

Fig. 43.6 (a) Extreme rocker-bottom deformity of the left foot of a 7-year-old boy 6 years after a 35% TBSA burn. The deformity is too far advanced for surgical reconstruction. (b) The head of the talus was removed to relieve painful weight-bearing pressure.

mity in a growing child and will permanently adversely affect foot and ankle function. Even slight inversion, whether imposed by scar contracture or motor weakness, will increase pressure on the lateral border of the foot, leading to callous formation and a painful, inefficient gait. Occasionally the base of the fifth metatarsal is so offensive as to require partial surgical ostectomy.

When there is both anterior and posterior scar contracture, the talus will remain aligned with the calcaneus in a relatively plantarflexed position as the midfoot and forefoot are pulled into dorsiflexion. The result is so-called rocker bottom foot with the head of the talus acting prominently as the principal weight-bearing feature (**Figure 43.6a,b**). This deformity, once established, defies correction by usual surgical means because of the shortage of soft tissue and because vessels and nerves cannot be stretched to accommodate to the corrected position. The Ilizarov system may offer a partial solution to the problem.

Pressure Systems in Burn Scar Management

Pressure therapy for scar management is a very old and established component of a recovering burn patient's continuing rehabilitation program. Extensive historical notes on the earliest references to scarring are provided by Linares and colleagues who attribute the first full medical description of scars to Petz in 1790.[1] They also state that the first medical reference to the use of pressure for treatment was written by Johnson in 1678 referring to the work of Ambroise Paré in the sixteenth century.[1] Other historical events noted by Linares *et al.* are: first known accounts of the use of pressure for treatment of children, 1859; use of elastic bandages, 1860; adhesive plaster for pressure, 1881; and use of traction to treat scars, 1902. Linares' review includes descriptions of Nason's work in 1942 in which he noted that ischemia produced by pressure arrests the overproduction of scar tissue, 'where the imprint of the elastic of an undergarment or a belt may be seen – no keloid is present.'[1] Another historical review by Ward[2] reveals that Blair in 1924 reported the positive influence of pressure on healing wounds. Nason's application of the 'constant pressure' principle included developing a type of neck splint made of a piece of dental impression compound or a piece of heavy felt strapped tightly over the scar for 6–8 weeks and possibly longer. Later, various splints were developed utilizing pressure and immobilization.[1]

As pressure therapy for scar management was applied, observations that pressure is not applicable to the face, neck, anterior chest and portions of the back have been reported.[1] These assertions continue and are supported by current literature, reiterating that no pressure is received in concave areas and decreased pressure is recorded in areas of large radii of curvature,[3] such as the axilla.[4] In the 1960s, Dr Paul Silverstein and Dr Duane Larson observed the influence of pressure on healing burns. These observations led to the manufacture of customized pressure garments and the conforming principles of splinting that revolutionized scar management in the 1970s, and continue to date with some modification, to be the standard today.[1,2]

The acute nature of a burned patient's illness can last from weeks into months with a therapeutic regimen which may extend beyond 2 years after the initial trauma.[3] Rehabilitation begins as soon as a patient is resuscitated and continues through the remainder of hospital treatment, discharge, and beyond. When the deep reticular portion of the dermis is disturbed, hypertrophic scarring begins. Collagen fibers develop to bridge the wound, forming an immature active scar which appears as a red, raised, rigid mass which may take years to reach maturity. Hypertrophic scars become apparent 6–8 weeks after wound closure. The clinical significance of the scar varies with the anatomical site.[4] The biochemical characters of hypertrophic scars, mature scars, and normal skin have been extensively investigated by Hayakawa.[5–8] His investigations imply that collagen and connective tissue synthesis is increased for at least 2 years after wound closure. With maturation and pressure therapy, the hypertrophic scars soften and become flatter due to a balance between collagen synthesis activators and the process of collagen degradation.[9]

The use of pressure therapy in the form of custom-made lycra garments is a well established procedure, designed to minimize the overgrowth of the healed area by limiting the supply of oxygen and nutrients and to hasten the maturing of a scar.[4,10] As long as the scar is active, it can be influenced by pressure and positioning; whereas the mature scar can be corrected only by surgical intervention. Deep, partial-thickness burns, requiring skin grafting across joint surfaces, tend to result in hypertrophic scarring involving the flexor surface. These flexion deformities can be avoided through a consistent program of pressure therapy in addition to positioning and exercise until the burn scar reaches maturity. There remains much debate about the amount of interface pressure which is indicated for adequate scar treatment. Recent research indicates that 15–40 mmHg is the therapeutic range necessary for influencing scar maturation, although some authors report good clinical results from as little as 4 mmHg and others advocate pressures up to 55 mmHg.[1]

The therapist's choice of pressure media and scar management programs is determined by the particular patient population served, available resources and the therapist's experience and expertise. In treatment planning and provision, the therapist considers the extent and location of the burn injury, its clinical management, a patient's developmental and comprehension level as well as a patient's or family's ability to don and doff a garment. Not all burns require the use of pressure garments. Patients with burn wounds which heal within 7–14 days do not need pressure therapy. Those patients whose wounds heal within 14–21 days are closely monitored for pressure therapy needs and generally advised to use pressure garments. Early application of pressure garments is necessary, commencing within approximately 2 weeks post-grafting or when spontaneous healing occurrs.[6] A prospective study of patients at risk for hypertrophic scarring indicate that prophylactic compression therapy is beneficial.[11]

Scar suppression can begin immediately through the use of elastic wrap pressure to secure burn dressings and splints. After split-thickness autografts are applied and adhere, elastic wrap pressure continues. Tubular compression sleeves, Tubigrip™, may also be substituted for wraps at this time. Both forms of pressure dressings provide vascular support and control hypertrophic scarring, thus aiding in prevention of burn scar contracture. Tubigrip™ is a continuous tube of material with a single elastic thread spiraling through the weave of the fabric. The therapist should be aware that any alteration, such as cutting holes in the tubular sleeve, changes the continuous compression gradient supplied by the support. The therapist will also note the appearance of the scar over which the tubular compression is applied, observing depressed lines where the elastic thread runs within the sleeve. Tubigrip™, applied over a facepad, is recommended for early control of facial scarring, when a patient may not be able to tolerate other forms of pressure. It is not recommended that Tubigrip™ be applied directly to the face, as the pressure may distort the facial features. Tubular compression sleeves are available in a selection of sizes to fit a variety of anatomical circumferences. Various prefabricated garments such as gloves, vests, and pants are also available. This type of pressure media allows modifications, can be changed frequently, and may be a preferred method of pressure when a patient or family has difficulty learning the elastic wrapping method; it also may be provided at lower cost.[12]

Other options for early application of pressure on forming scars over the hand and digits can be accomplished by using Coban™, a self-adherent wrap. This form of pressure is excellent for controlling edema, decreasing scarring between the web spaces of the hand and foot, and providing pressure to the fingers when the shear force of a glove cannot be tolerated. The therapist can apply Coban™ in a distal to proximal direction (one begins first with the fingers by creating a web space insert, and then over the hand through maximal grip and prehensile joint excursion). Leaving the fingertips exposed allows a patient to use the sense of touch at a critical time in recovery.[13] Precautions taken for excessive circumferential pressure will deform the interosseous structures of the healing hand and further deplete muscle strength. The therapist must be vigilant in wound and skin inspection and must monitor active range of motion and hand strength. This intervention prepares a patient's hand for application of a custom made glove if needed (**Figure 43.7**). Many manufacturers of custom-fit antiburn scar supports also produce interim (noncustom) supports for use prior to the fitting of a custom support for long-term use.[2] Donor areas, from which skin has been harvested for grafting, may scar and are managed in the same manner as the hypertrophic burn scar. If the donor area appears reddened and a patient is scratching, a protective covering, such as elastic wrap or Tubigrip™, can be prescribed in order to prevent scratching which contaminates a wound and causes additional open areas.

A patient undergoing sequential skin grafting procedures in order to achieve wound coverage is a challenge for the therapist due to the various stages of wound healing in different areas of the body. The therapist, during this period, uses multiple forms of pressure media to counteract the scarring process. The use of elastic wraps, adhesive compression dressings, tubular sleeves and interim garments usually precedes an application of custom-made garments. Application of the custom-ordered garments can be delayed due to fragile healing epithelium which can cause chronic blisters and open lesions over joint surfaces. After a patient's body weight stabilizes and wounds are mostly healed, custom-made pressure garments can replace the interim media. A successful pressure program calls for continuous gradient pressure to the active burn scar. Two sets of pressure garments permit laundering of the one set while the other is worn. Pressure garments are removed only for bathing and sometimes during exercise, should they interfere with movements.

Commercially available pressure garments can be ordered to cover all body areas and come with options for providing more or less pressure to body areas as needed. Additional considerations made for design and color may be important in facilitating patient compliance, social acceptance, and patient self-esteem.[14] The therapist should look for a reputable company which provides support for both therapist and patient. Many companies provide measurement materials, forms, and trained staff to come to a burn clinic. The most frequent reason therapists give for choosing a pressure garment company is time expenditure in the process of obtaining a burn scar support. The fit of the custom-made support, the company's willingness to manufacture nonstandard supports, availability of special options, and cost of the supports were all selection criteria cited in a national survey of therapists and pressure support manufacturing companies.[15]

Elastomer inserts are used for unyielding burn scars or in areas which require additional pressure for scar suppression. Common areas requiring increased pressure application are body areas which are concave such as the face, neck, anterior shoulder, small of the back, antecubital or popliteal fossae, sternum, palm of the hand or

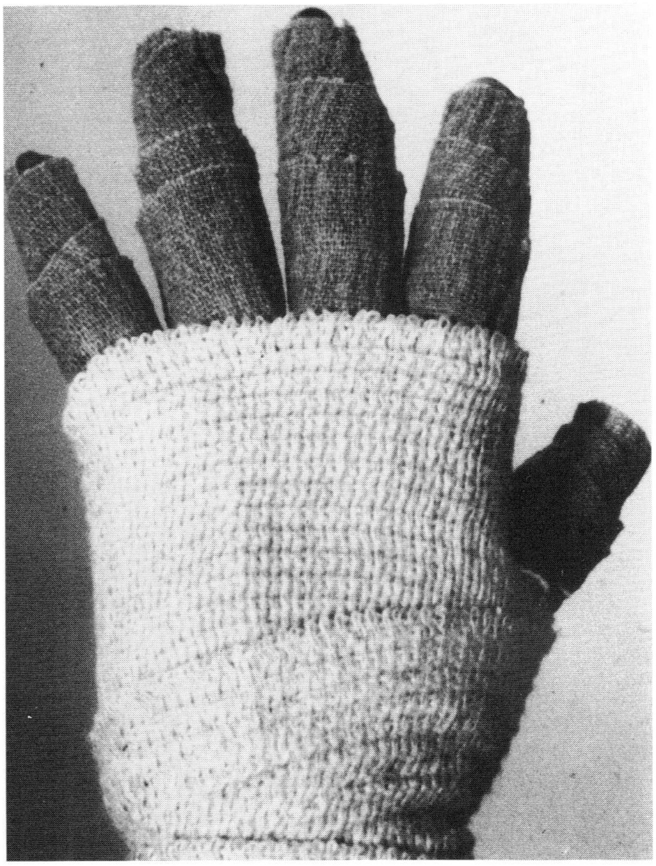

Fig. 43.7 A Coban wrap can be used to decrease edema in hands and arms.

arch of the foot, and digit web spaces. The inserts are worn under pressure dressings, garments and splints. These materials may be graded for progressive pressure in order to accommodate unyielding burn scars.[17] Scar management in areas where it is difficult to fit thermoplastic materials requires the use of a flexible silastic insert or silicone gelsheet. Silicone elastomer products come in a variety of forms including putty, sheets, and Otoform™. Silicone gelsheets can be applied with adhesive tape at the edges and worn under other pressure systems.[18]

Silicone gelsheets act as soothing occlusive barriers and are effective in suppression of burn scars with associated chronic open lesions and/or dry, irritated scars. Following treatment with gelsheets, the scars appear smoother and more supple. Silicone gelsheet is applied to wounds after bathing and is washed to reapply. They are changed on alternate days. Length of wearing time is dependent on scar response, so if they are applied early, wearing time may be as brief as 2–5 months. Form-fitting face masks were developed by Paderewski in 1968 to maintain pressure on facial scars and to hold facial features in position.[1] A silastic face pad (**Figure 43.8**), insert, or clear plastic face mask (**Figure 43.9**) provides consistent conforming pressure to the facial features, particularly for scars around the nose and mouth.[20] The silastic face pad or inserts are worn under a pressure garment.

Burn scar massage is employed when a physician and therapist have determined that the healed burn wound or skin grafted area can tolerate the application of friction. The therapist may perform a paraffin treatment to the scarred area prior to the use of massage. The paraffin helps lubricate and soften the scar while relaxing the joint for range of motion exercise to follow. Scars in the palm of the hand or between the digits may respond to manual massage and the use of a roll-on type of lubricant and pressure application. The therapist must be mindful of a patient's response and skin condition, as early application of friction may cause blistering which results in open lesions.

Specific elements of a patient and family education program should address the necessary hygiene and laundering requirements for all pressure wraps, garments, and devices as well as skin care instruction including the use of lubricants and sunscreens. Any lubricant which does not irritate a patient's skin is acceptable; and those which do not contain perfumes and do contain a sun protection factor (SPF) of at least 15 are recommended.[21] A patient's intolerance to any of the myriad of pressure devices such as thermoplastic materials, silicone, foam, lycra, etc. may also be a cause of skin irritation and chronic breakdown; so patient and therapist may have to explore optional media in order to continue a consistent scar suppression program.[22]

Burn scar suppression methods and a pressure therapy program must be maintained as long as there is evidence that the burn scars have not matured. Patients should be monitored on a regular basis until skin grafts mature, 1 year or more, and there is no evidence of hypertrophic scar activity.[23] Patient compliance is a prime determinant of outcome. Therapists' knowledge of objective research and creative use of available pressure media to discover what will work for a particular patient may be the most important contributing factors to a patient's eventual success.

EXERCISE AND AMBULATION

Exercise

An underlying principle of physical recovery is that the promotion of purposeful activity in patients with dysfunction requires the application of professional hands directed by minds abundant with relevant information.[23] Therapeutic exercise is motion of the body or its parts to relieve symptoms or to improve function.[24] The need for exercise to enhance mobility of the burn patient begins acutely and continues throughout the months of healing. It is painful, and extensive therapy is required during and long after the acute hospital stay. The results are, for the most part, dependent upon a patient's and family's understanding, involvement, and dedication to the treatment.[22] The therapist is challenged to be creative and insightful enough to enlist a patient's cooperation and participation in tedious and painful, purposeful activity over a long period of time.

The goals of exercise in burn treatment are:

- reduction of the effects of edema and immobilization;
- maintenance of functional joint motion and muscle strength;
- reduction of scar.

Scar contracture causes high resistance to passive stretch, and burn scars which cross joints, if left untreated, will prevent motion.

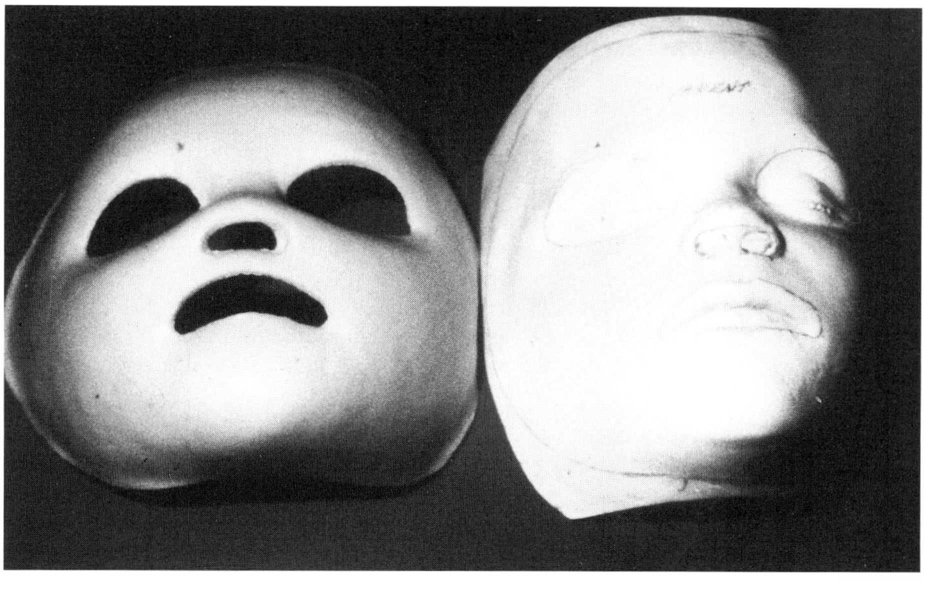

Fig. 43.8 A Moulage elastomer mask provides pressure to the face so as to prevent scarring and contracture and to preserve facial features.

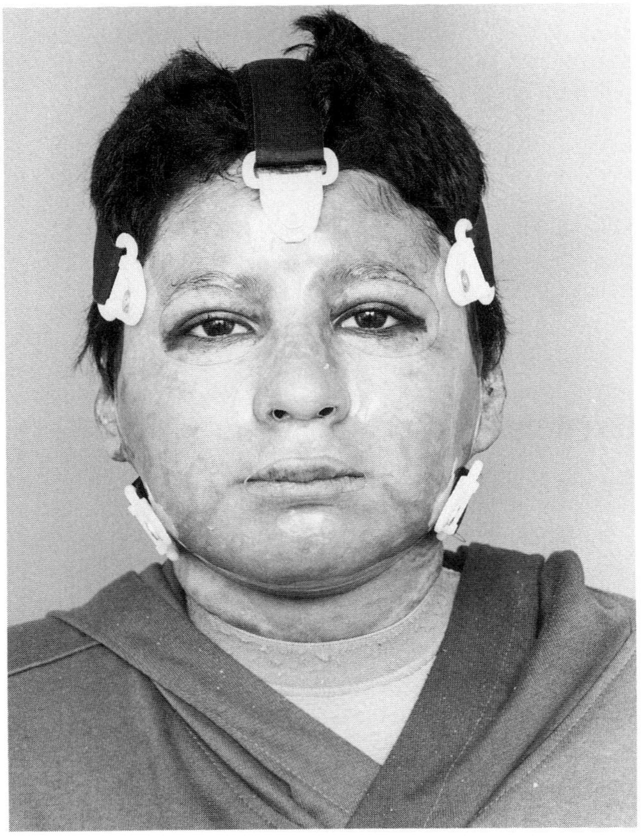

Fig. 43.9 A Uvex clear face mask (where the eyes are left open and uncovered and the mouth is closed) provides pressure to the face so as to prevent scarring and contrature and to preserve facial features.

Muscle and fibrous contracture of the joint structure can cause the deformity to become irreversible. The therapist should educate both a patient and a patient's support group as to how to maintain a patient's functional mobility. For maximum benefit, all instruction should be simple, concise, and pertinent to the individual being treated. Both verbal and written instructions, as well as detailed demonstrations, are necessary. A patient and caregivers should be given time to practice in the presence of a therapist. Early education reduces apprehension and provides a message that therapy is an ongoing evolutionary process.[22]

Exercise sessions depend upon a patient's physical, psychological, and medical status. In the conservative treatment of burn wounds, a vigorous physical therapy program is instituted immediately so as to maintain function.[25] Exercises are generally discontinued for 4–5 days in joints involving autografted areas. Escharotomies, heterografts, and synthetic dressings are not contraindications for exercise.[26] Early mobilization to prevent edema, proper exercise techniques, and accurate documentation of function are more important than the type of wound closure.[25]

Scar contracture and joint mobility limitations are the result of the shortening of immature connective tissue. Therapy aims to prevent deformity and the subsequent limitation of movement. In circumferential burns, both the flexor and extensor surfaces are at risk of contracture. Exercise in conjunction with splinting should promote antagonistic movements around those joints and, thus, the most mobile result.[22] Treatments are tailored to each individual patient and the mobility problems of each with independent living as the ultimate goal from acute admission throughout rehabilitation. To achieve the ultimate goal, objectives include:

- stretching of healing skin;
- maintaining or regaining normal joint range of motion;
- preserving motor skill coordination;
- maintaining or regaining strength and endurance to minimize muscular atrophy; and
- promoting functional independence.[26] There are a variety of exercise techniques which can be incorporated into a therapy session to accomplish these objectives. Exercise techniques can be described in four categories: stretching, strengthening, cardiovascular, and functional activity exercises.

'Stretching' exercises are performed with a slow, prolonged force. Gentle, sustained stretch is more effective than multiple repetitive movements in gaining length of burned tissue. An indication of effective stretching is that the scar tissue will blanche. If the scarring extends across more than one joint, each joint should be stretched singularly, and then the skin stretched as a whole across the involved joints. 'Passive' exercise is a form of stretching exercise which is performed without voluntary muscle contribution. It is a slow, gentle stretch provided by an outside force with the prime result being the stretching of tissue. There is no muscular action, and thus, there are no gains in muscle strength. The use of a continuous passive motion (CPM) device has been documented to be an effective modality for improving joint range of motion.[28] Recent advances have shown CPM treatment to be a viable option because of its benefits to soft tissue remodeling, joint nutrition, wound healing, and venous dynamics.[28,29] All passive exercise should be performed cautiously when there is evidence of bone or tendon exposure.

'Strengthening' exercise improves the muscles' ability to perform work. Strengthening exercises utilize muscular power and will cause an increase in muscle strength. 'Active' exercise is performed independently by a patient. This is the form of exercise most recommended because it stretches healing skin and provides a strengthening component. Frequent exercise performed actively by a patient promotes the greatest increase in movement. 'Active-assistive' exercise utilizes the same principles; however, a patient is 'assisted' by an outside force (therapist or assistive device) to achieve the full range of motion. A patient will develop improvements in strength and range of motion, but not equal to those provided by active exercise. Active-assistive exercise is suggested for those patients who are too weak to perform a full range of motion exercise independently. In 'resistive' exercises, manual or mechanical resistance is applied to a movement. A variety of modalities offer resistance, ranging from traditional weights to innovative combinations of rubber bands. Resistive exercises can begin in an 'assistive' fashion with minimal resistance and assistance provided to complete the range of motion.

'Cardiovascular' exercises are designed to improve a patient's endurance level. These activities are performed for prolonged periods of time with minimum resistance and can be designed to involve activities which are enjoyable for a patient.

'Functional' exercise includes those activities which incorporate all types of the above-mentioned exercises. They are designed to improve the coordination and performance of patients in tasks which are relevant to activities of daily living. For example, eating requires both coordination and strength as well as stretching to take hand to mouth. Performing functional activities is generally rewarding to patients. The goal and purpose are clearly defined and understood. Completion of these tasks requires concentration and appears to distract a patient from the pain of movement. Completion of a functional task also seems to provide a feeling of accomplishment and encouragement to a patient who wants to regain independence.

Some basic physiology principles should be kept in mind when a patient is exercising. The average pulse rate should not exceed 60–75% of the predicted maximum heart rate. In adults, the systolic blood pressure should not exceed 225–230 mmHg. The diastolic blood pressure should be monitored and exercise stopped if the values suddenly and rapidly increase 20 mmHg or more or exceed 130 mmHg. A patient should not become dyspneic or exhibit labored breathing. The nonburned skin of a patient should be closely watched; and it should not become increasingly pale, cool, or moist. An increase in body temperature, malaise, fatigue, and heat prostration should be avoided.[22]

Exercise begins immediately postburn. For a patient being treated conservatively, movement helps maintain strength and range of motion, and aids in circulation and healing. For a patient who has been grafted, isometrics can be performed during the immobilization period. The benefit of isometrics is that a patient does not 'forget' how to contract the muscle, a common phenomenon with periods of prolonged immobilization. Isometric exercise also helps in maintaining muscle strength, though not as profoundly as active strengthening exercise. When skin grafts have become stable, active exercise is begun. Active exercise is initially performed by allowing a patient to limit the intensity by pain. It is followed by passive stretching exercise and strengthening to maintain mobility.

Exercise can be performed with dressing and wraps in place. Care should be taken when dressings are applied so that joint range of motion is not restricted. Dressings which have been correctly applied will minimize discomfort and promote movement, while dressings applied too tightly will limit mobility, increase pain, and may create pressure-induced neuropathies. Exercise can also be performed while a patient is in the tub where the buoyancy of the water and the absence of confining dressings can make exercise less painful. Exercise initially is painful and the very first repetition is often the most difficult. Discomfort is due to stretching skin which has lost its natural lubricating mechanism and has become dry and tight. Movement itself decreases pain. Each subsequent repetition will be easier as the skin stretches, and the muscle pumping action of active movement helps resolve edema, thus significantly reducing pain.

Specific movements can be targeted to prevent burn scar contracture. The position of comfort becomes the position of contracture. Based on knowledge about typical contractures, the following movements are encouraged: neck extension and lateral flexion, shoulder abduction and flexion, elbow extension and supination, metacarpophalangeal flexion, interphalangeal extension, wrist extension, knee extension, ankle dorsiflexion, and metatarsophalangeal flexion (**Table 43.1**). Exercise sessions may be indicated three to four times daily for more involved areas. Patients should be encouraged to exercise between therapy sessions.

Table 43.1 Movements to counteract the position of comfort/contracture

Joint	Movement
Neck	Extension Lateral flexion Rotation
Shoulder	Flexion Abduction
Elbow	Extension Supination
Metacarpal	Flexion
Interphalangeal	Extension
Wrist	Extension
Knee	Extension
Ankle	Dorsiflexion
Metatarsal	Flexion

Ambulation

To walk again following a burn injury is an important goal shared by patients of all ages. The benefits of ambulation are:

- to help maintain range of motion;
- to maintain strength in the lower extremities;
- to prevent thromboemboli;
- to maintain bone density via weight-bearing; and
- to promote independence in functional activities.[22]

Ambulation exercise can also help with preventing decubiti, provide mild cardiovascular conditioning, and increase appetite. Ambulatory patients have fewer problems with lower extremity contractures and endurance.[26]

Opinions differ as to when ambulation can begin. A patient's medical status, including the stability of skin grafts, is usually the prime indicator for commencement of ambulation. As with other exercise, proper positioning facilitates proper gait.[22] A patient who has been allowed to assume a position of comfort will have difficulty extending the hips and knees during ambulation. The ankles may be tight, limiting plantigrade position when in the upright position. If the joints are in the normal alignment, the amount of pain and energy are greatly reduced.

All wounds must have the proper dressings prior to ambulation. Lower extremity burn wounds should be wrapped with elastic bandages in order to facilitate capillary support. Wrapping will decrease edema and therefore decrease pain and promote healing. The extremity should be wrapped distally from the toes proximally to the groin crease. The foot should always be included to avoid excess edema. Those extremities which have had skin grafting generally have less graft loss when there is a second elastic wrap to provide further support. Lower extremity donor sites are less painful when wrapped with elastic bandages. Wrapping which incorporates the 'figure of eight' pattern has been reported to provide better pressure than the spiral wrap,[22] perhaps due to increased vascular support.

The use of a tilt table (**Figure 43.10**) can assist in beginning ambulation for those patients who may have difficulty assuming the upright position. There are a variety of reasons that erect positioning may prove difficult; for example, extended periods of bedrest which influence blood pressure or ankle tightness may inhibit plantigrade position. The tilt table can be used to overcome these obstacles and assist a patient with early ambulation.

Patients tend to perform much better when given an achievable goal such as walking a specific distance or to a certain place. Children do well when provided with a desired incentive such as a toy or game. Frequent rest periods may be necessary secondary to decreased endurance levels or increased pain. Patients should be encouraged to ambulate further distances each day. Care should be taken to avoid prolonged periods of standing so that hypotension does not develop. The lower extremities, even when properly wrapped for support, will show signs of vascular insufficiency

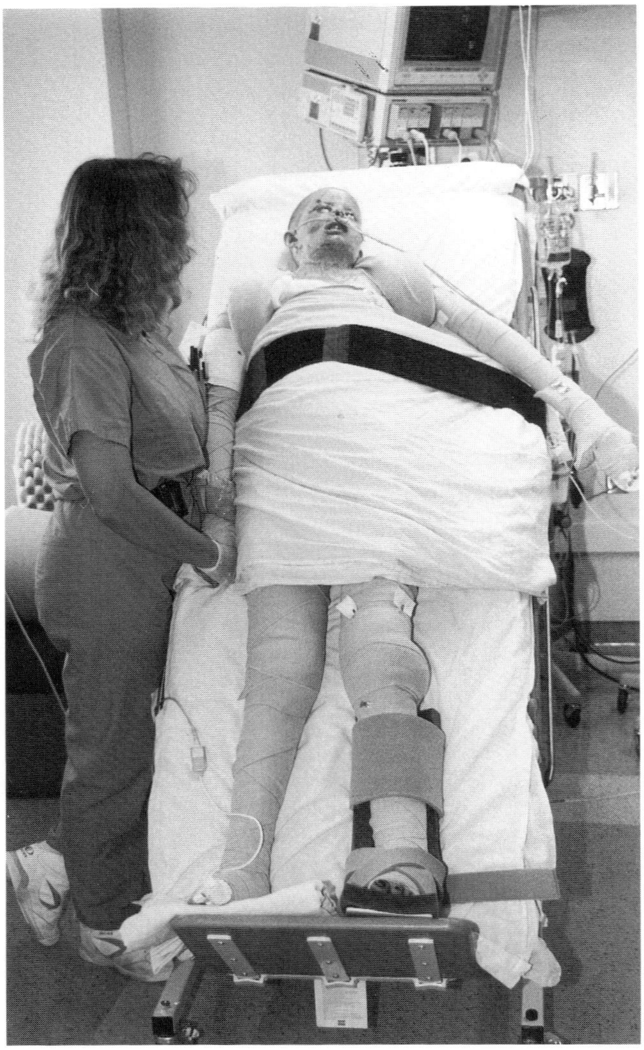

Fig. 43.10 A patient is placed on a tilt table before beginning ambulation in order to accustom the patient to a vertical position.

when dependent for too long a period of time. The use of assistive devices, i.e. crutches or walkers, is discouraged because the legs need the muscle pumping action to prevent edema.[22] Exercise and ambulation are integral parts in the rehabilitation of burn patients. Both allow a patient to resume a life style as active and independent as possible.

References

1. Linares H A, Larson D L, Willis-Galstraun B. Historical notes on the use of pressure in the treatment of hypertrophic scars and keloids. *Burns* 1993; **19**(1): 17–21.

2. Ward R S. Pressure therapy for the control of hypertrophic scar formation after burn injury, a history and review. *J Burn Care Rehabil* 1991; **12**(3): 257–62.

3. Cromes G F, Helm P A. The status of burn rehabilitation services in the United States: results of a national survey. *J Burn Care Rehabil* 1992; **6**(6): 656–62.

4. Reid W H, Evans J H, Naismith R S, *et al.* Hypertrophic scarring and pressure therapy. *Burns* 1987; **13**(suppl): S29.

5. Hayakawa T, Hino M, Fuyamada H, *et al.* Lysyl oxidase activity in human normal skins and postburn scars. *Clin Chim Acta* 1976; **71:** 245–50.

6. Hayakawa T, Hino M, Fuyamada H, *et al.* Prolyl hydroxylase activity in human normal skins and post-burn scars. *Clin Chim Acta* 1977; **75:** 137–42.

7. Hayakawa T, Hashimoto Y, Myokei Y, *et al.* Changes in type of collagen during the development of human post-burn hypertrophic scars. *Clin Chim Acta* 1979; **93:** 119–25.

8. Hayakawa T, Hashimoto Y, Myokei Y, *et al.* The effects of skin grafts on the ratio of collagen types in human post-burn wound tissues. *Connect Tissue Res* 1982; **9:** 249–52.

9. Abston S. Scar reaction after thermal injury and prevention of scars and contractures. In: Boswick J A, ed. *The Art and Science of Burn Care.* Rockville: Aspen Publishers, 1987: 360–1.

10. Linares H A, Larson D L, Baur P S Jr. Influences of mechanical forces on burn scar contracture and hypertrophy. In: Krizek T J, Hoopes J E, eds. *Symposium On Basic Science In Plastic Surgery.* Vol 15, pp101. St Louis: CV Mosby, 1976.

11. McDonald W S, Deitch E A. Hypertrophic skin grafts in burn patients: a prospective analysis of variables. *J Trauma* 1987; **27:** 147–50.

12. Kealey G P, Jenson K L, Laubenthal N, Lewis R W. Compared compliance efficacy and cost of elastic nylon pressure garments with cotton elastic nylon pressure garment Tubigrip. *J Burn Care Rehabil* 1990; **11:** 334–6.

13. Ward R S, Tuckett R P. Sensory thresholds quantitive threshold changes in cutaneous sensation of patients with burns. *J Burn Care Rehabil* 1991; **12:** 569–75.

14. Thompson R, Summers S, Rampey-Dobbs R, Wheeler T. Color pressure garments vs traditional beige pressure garments: perceptions from the public. *J Burn Care Rehabil* 1992; **13:** 590–6.

15. Ward R S. Reasons for the selection of burn-scar-support suppliers by burn centers in the United States: a survey *J Burn Care Rehabil* 1993; **14**(3): 360–7.

16. Gallagher J, Goldfarb W, Slater H, Rososky-Grassi M. Survey of treatment modalities for the prevention and treatment of hypertrophic burn scars. *J Burn Care Rehabil* 1990; **11**(2): 118–20.

17. Van den Kerchove E, Boechx W, Kochreyt A. Silicone patches as a supplement for pressure therapy to control hypertrophic scarring. *J Burn Care Rehabil* 1991; **12**(4): 361–9.

18. McNee J. The use of silicone gel in the control of hypertrophic scarring. *Physiotherapy* 1990; **76:** 194–7.

19. Quinn K J. Silicone gel in scar treatment. *Burns* 1987; **13:** 533–40.

20. Derwin-Baruch L. UVA therapists meet the challenge of scar management. *OT Week* 1993; **April 15:** 15–17.

21. Hurwitz S. The sun and sunscreen protection: recommendations for children. *J Dermatol Surg Oncol* 1988; **14**(6): 657–60.

22. Johnson C L. The role of physical therapy. In: Boswick J A, ed. *The Art and Science of Burn Care.* Rockville: Aspen, 1987: chapter 34, p 304.

23. Wolf S L. Morphological functional considerations for therapeutic exercise. In: Basmajian J V, ed. *Therapeutic Exercise.* 4th ed. Baltimore, MD: Williams & Wilkins, 1984: Chapter 2.

24. Licht S. History. In: Basmajian J V, ed. *Therapeutic Exercise.* 4th ed. Baltimore, MD: Williams & Wilkins, 1984: Chapter 1.

25. Robson M C, Smith D J, VanderZee A J, Roberts L. Making the burned hand functional. *Clin Plast Surg* 1992: **19**(3) pp. 663–71.

26. Fisher S V, Helm P A. Rehabilitation of the patient with burns. In: DeLisa, Gans, Currie, *et al.* eds *Rehabilitation Medicine Principles and Practice.* 2nd ed. Philadelphia: J B Lippincott Company 1993: Chapter 53.

27. Covey M H, Dutcher K, Marvin J A, Heimbach D M. Efficacy of continuous passive motion (CPM) devices with hand burns. *J Burn Care Rehabil* **9**(4): pp. 397–400.

28. Salter R B, Hamilton H W, Wedge J H, *et al.* Clinical application of basic research on continuous passive motion for disorders and injuries of synovial joints: a preliminary report. *J Orthop Res* 1983; **1**(3): pp. 325–42.

29. Lynch J A. Continuous passive motion: a prophylaxis for deep vein thrombosis following total knee replacement. *Orthop Trans* 1984; **8**(3): p.400.

CHAPTER FORTY-FOUR

Treating Deformities Via Positioning and Splinting, Using Skeletal Suspensions and Traction, and with Prosthetics and Orthotics

Sheila Ott, Kimberleye McElroy, M. Irma Alvarado, E. Burke Evans, Jason H. Calhoun, Dan Morgan and Les Hannon

Positioning by Splinting for Functional Outcome

Prevention of deformity is the best cure; however, when prevention fails, other interventions must be pursued. Positioning and splinting offer a variety of prophylactic techniques. External and internal fixators can sometimes reverse deformities caused by scarring in burned patients. When limbs become completely nonfunctional or must be amputated, then resulting deformities or disabilities can be accommodated via prosthetic and orthotic devices. Prevention is the route of choice, but when an impass is encountered, alternative interventions can produce functional results.

Prevention by positioning and splinting is the best answer to many challenging problems faced by patients and therapists treating burns. Desired positions for parts of the body can be summarized in table format (**Table 44.1**). Positioning is implemented upon admission[1] and constant monitoring of a patient's position is imperative. When a patient undergoes a grafting procedure, recommendations for immobilization can range from 4 to 10 days depending on the surgeon's preference. Monitoring of a patient by a therapist during this phase of recovery is extremely important so as to enhance graft take while facilitating functional recovery.

The decision of which thermoplastic splint material to use varies according to preference of therapist or physician. The splint should be cleaned daily, using a mild detergent,[2] in order to prevent infection.[3] When applying a splint, wrapping distal to proximal will assist in controlling edema of extremities. When patients understand the rationale of their positioning program and can actively participate in positioning techniques, splinting devices may be switched to use at night only.[1] Assessment of positioning and splinting during out-patient recovery is important for addressing ever-changing joint positions. Positioning and splinting can be eliminated only after a patient's scars have matured and range of motion is functionally maintained. Serial casting is used in some cases when all other methods of intervention have proven unsuccessful.[6]

As one of the most functional components of the body, the hand receives special attention when burned. With such delicate but complex structures in the hand, various factors need to be considered when deciding on appropriate intervention. Acutely, a therapist will assess burn depth, edema, exposed soft tissue or associated

Table 44.1 Acute intervention

Splinted area	Desired position
Hand	Wrist 15–40 degrees extension, MCPs 70–90 degrees flexion, IPs full extension, thumb abducted and opposed
Elbow	Extension
Axilla/shoulder	90–120 degrees abduction with 20 degrees horizontal adduction
Head and face	Elevate bed at 45 degrees
Neck	Extension/neutral
Foot/ankle	Neutral/dorsiflexion
Knee	Extension
Hip	Abduction/extension
Trunk	Midline

injuries and hand dominance. In treating an edematous hand, it is important to position the hand above the heart in order to control edema, although elevation should not exceed 30 degrees as greater elevation may compromise the vascular supply to the hand.[3] Pillows, troughs, bedside tables or skyhooks can be easily used to elevate the hand.

The burned hand is commonly splinted in the following position: 15–40 degrees of wrist extension, 70–90 degrees of metacarpophalangeal joint (MP) flexion, full extension of the proximal interphalangeal joints (PIPs) and distal interphalangeal joints (DIPs), and the thumb is opposed and abducted radially[4] (**Figure 44.1**). The thumb can also be positioned in a splint using palmer abduction. When a patient presents with a palmer burn, it is suggested that the digits of the hand be positioned in extension so as to prevent 'cupping' of the palm and to preserve the palmer arch.[4] This can be done by splinting either dorsally or volarly. Wrist cockups can be used when the wrist needs support, leaving the fingers free to move. Splint-wearing schedules for a hand will vary depending upon recovery of a patient and procedures which a patient undergoes. Patients who have undergone sheet grafting and/or have circumferential burns with or without grafting procedures may be placed into a 'ukulele' or 'banjo' splint or a 'hay rake' skeletal traction device. 'Webbing' between the digits is best treated with the use of inserts made of silicone elastomer which are worn under pressure gloves,[1] or with the use of foam or custom-made web spacers which attach to a Velcro strap around the wrist. An abduction hand splint can be fabricated to place the fingers into abduction, thereby stretching the web space. C-bar splints are introduced to stretch the web space between the thumb and index fingers.[4] The recovery stage of the burn patient will influence the choice of using various dynamic splints. Knucklebenders and dynamic three-point splints are two of the types of prefabricated finger splints available. Finger gutters can be provided to protect a digit which has exposed tendon or joint.

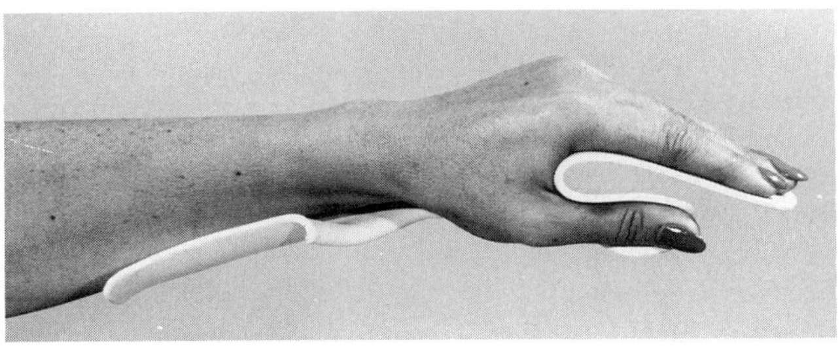

Fig. 44.1 A resting hand splint puts the limb in a position which will promote function and prevent edema.

In positioning the elbow, the desired goal is to place the elbow in extension with the forearm in neutral when fabricating a splint. This position can be achieved through the use of an elbow conformer or a three-point extension splint placed over the flexor surface of the arm. Support to the posterior surface of the elbow is recommended in order to prevent hyperextension. Emphasis on supination is recommended so as to enhance functional outcome. A supination splint can be custom made or purchased commercially to achieve greater supination, if needed.

Maintaining appropriate positioning of the axilla/shoulder can prove troublesome because a patient must undergo many procedures throughout the day which require changing positions. It is important to place a patient's shoulder(s) in 90–120 degrees of abduction[2] with 20 degrees of horizontal adduction in order to prevent undue stress on the brachial plexus.[3] To position the shoulder, the use of foam wedges, troughs (**Figure 44.2**), airplane splints (either conforming or rod supporting), and/or bedside tables can be utilized. A figure of eight wrap (**Figure 44.3**) can be used over axilla pads to assist in the positioning of the shoulders once the grafts have adhered and a patient can be upright and out of bed. The wrap is fashioned by using foam crescents folded in half, which are placed under the axilla. The crescents are wrapped on a patient in a figure of eight pattern (**Figure 44.4**), beginning on the scapula, passing over the shoulders and under to the other side of the body, with the steps repeating until all of the elastic wrap has been used.

Positioning of the head and face acutely requires careful attention in order to reduce edema. The bed should be positioned with the head elevated at 45 degrees. In the later stages of recovery, a patient's face, mouth and nose may begin to contract and scar, depending on the depth of the burn to that area, creating a need for

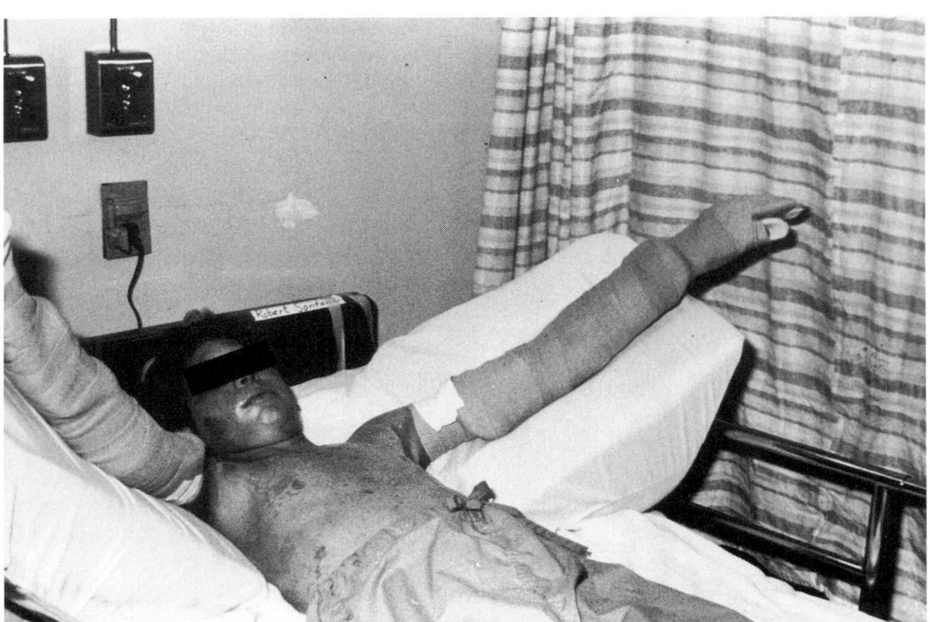

Fig. 44.2 Arm troughs provide shoulder abduction and elevate upper extremities so as to promote function and prevent edema.

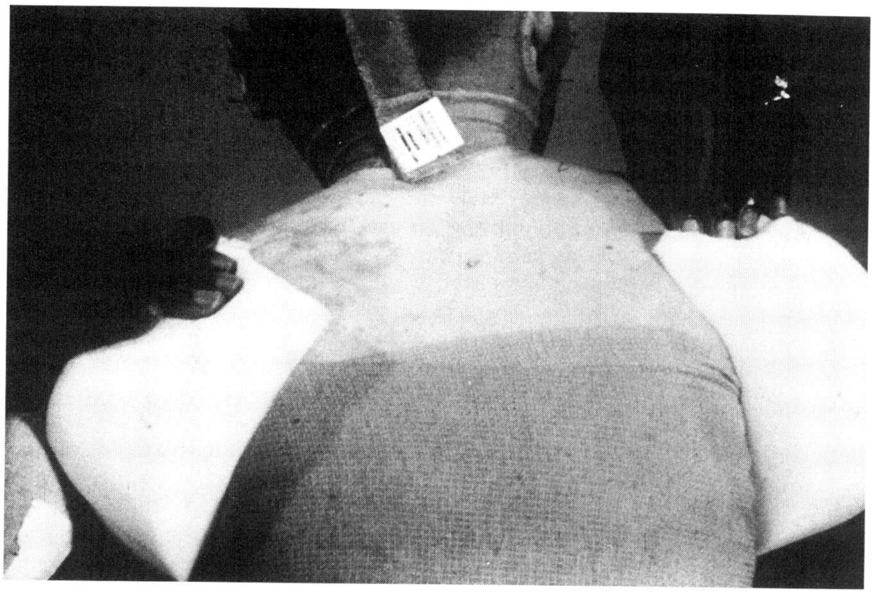

Fig. 44.3 Pads are used in a figure of eight wrap.

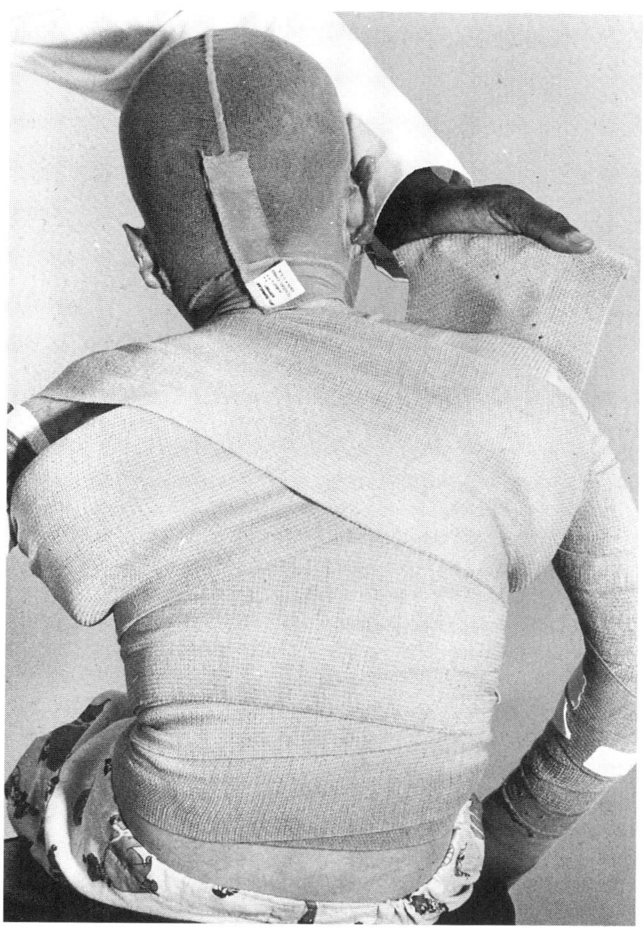

Fig. 44.4 A completed figure of eight wrap provides pressure so as to reduce scarring and provides slight abduction so as to promote later function.

splinting. Face masks are often provided to control scarring and contracture via the use of pressure. The nares can be splinted using nasal obturators. The mouth can be positioned with a mouth-spreader to stretch the commissures, or by using stacked tongue blades between a patient's teeth.

Anterior neck burns require careful monitoring. The focus, when positioning the neck, should be to keep the neck in extension and properly aligned so as to prevent lateral scar banding. The use of pillows is highly discouraged as they can place the neck in flexion and become a source of pressure to the ear. If the ears are burned, pressure increases the likelihood of further damage, i.e. pressure necrosis and chondritis.[5] Ear protectors can be fabricated of high density foam and applied specifically to single out the ear for protection. Proper positioning can be achieved with the use of an anterior neck conformer (**Figure 44.5**) which should be worn at all times. A patient is encouraged to remove the conformer only for periods of up to 1 hour, such as for bath or exercise, in order to attain maximum benefit. Use of a neck conformer for extended periods of time is common, as it is an area of the body which needs assistance to maintain adequate positioning.[1] Hard or soft neck collars can be used depending on the need of a patient. A UVEX neck splint can also be used in this area. Watusi rings can be valuable in providing pressure to the neck, especially when lateral banding occurs. When a patient is in bed, placing the neck in extension off a short mattress is an excellent method for preventing flexion and providing a stretch. Placing a rolled up towel on the posterior surface of the neck when stretching a patient on a mat, or even allowing a patient to hold the head off the mat, is yet another way to provide a good stretch.

Ankle splints are not indicated for all patients with foot burns.[3] Patients who are able to ambulate achieve the ultimate goal of preventing deformity by keeping the ankle in plantigrade position. Patients who are unable to ambulate, however, or patients with exposed tendon or bone, may benefit from some form of positioning. Splinting the ankle in neutral can prevent disabling deformities which might otherwise occur. Prefabricated ankle splints are available for purchase or can be custom made. The focus is to promote dorsiflexion. While a patient is wearing an ankle splint, one must religiously monitor the heel for tissue breakdown. A well-padded footboard is another means available for providing neutral positioning of the ankle while a patient is on bed rest. Prevention of metatarsophalangeal hyperextension is important for the preservation of total function of the foot. This can be achieved through the use of a footplate for night wear and orthopedic shoes for day wear.

As with the elbow, the knee may be splinted with either a conformer or a three-point extension splint. The desired outcome is to prevent knee flexion contracture; thus the splint is fabricated on the

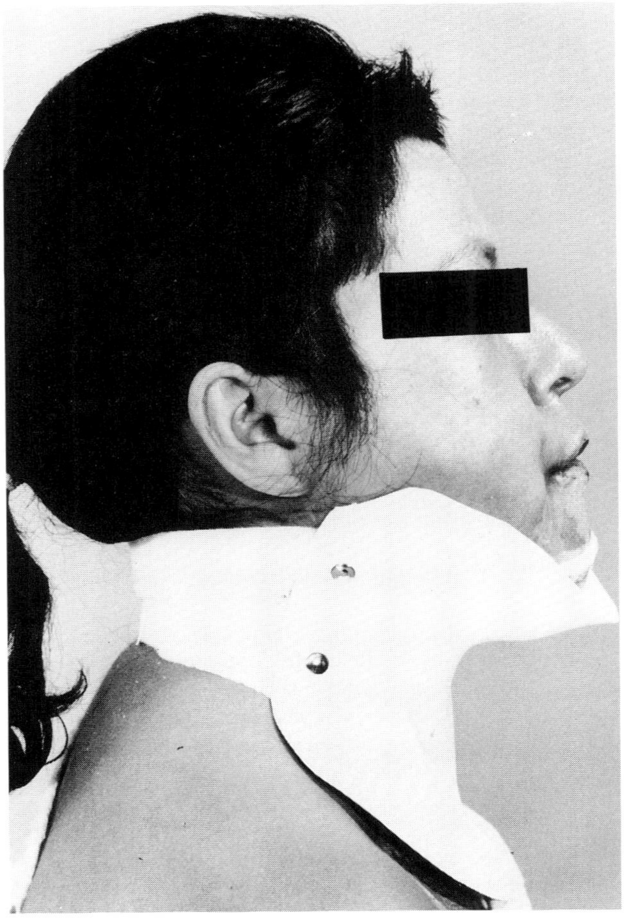

Fig. 44.5 An anterior neck conformer helps prevent scarring and flexion contractures.

posterior aspect of the lower extremity with the knee extended. Elevation of the burned lower extremity is beneficial in decreasing edema, but care should be taken to avoid placement of pillows under the popliteal fossa which would facilitate flexion or under the heel which could cause pressure necrosis. Knee immobilizers are also commonly used when positioning the lower extremity. Care should be taken to protect the common peroneal nerve from undue pressure or excessive stretch. The common peroneal nerve can be placed on a stretch when a patient is in the 'frog leg' position; proper positioning is extremely important to prevent this injury which profoundly complicates rehabilitation.[7]

Splints are rarely required to position the hip or the trunk. Foam wedges to maintain hip abduction or a foam mattress are readily accessible if needed to assist in positioning. A good positioning technique to promote hip extension is to place a patient prone, but care should be taken to support the head, monitoring all other joints in the antideformity positions, and observing for pressure necrosis. Hip spica splints or casts or a Denis Browne bar (commonly seen in the pediatric population) are other sources for positioning the hip. The trunk should be positioned to encourage alignment of the trunk with the hip and shoulders. This is especially important if burns are on the lateral surface of the trunk.

To maximize functional outcome, positioning must begin on hospital day 1 and continue throughout out-patient follow-up. To assure appropriate follow-through, therapists must educate all persons who are involved with a patient's rehabilitation (especially the family and the patient) about the crucial need for positioning and splinting. The therapist's creativity and determination to improve upon current norms have been vital to progress in burn rehabilitation.

Skeletal Suspension and Traction and Stabilization Systems in Burn Management

Skeletal suspension and traction systems have been used to a limited extent in burn management for a number of years. The early reports of Larson[8] and Evans[9–11] described the use of skeletal suspension for positioning and for extremity elevation in open wound management and of skeletal traction for the prevention and correction of contracture. The later reports of Harnar[12] and Youel[13] deal mainly with the management of hand burns with the skeletally anchored digital traction splints bearing the names banjo, halo, and hay rake. Evans[14] has reported using a rigid external fixator for treatment of an exposed unstable knee, and Calhoun[15] has recorded his experience with the use of the llizarov system in the correction of severe burn contracture deformities. Of significant interest are current practices in burn care which are based on the use of transosseous metal pins.

Skeletal Suspension and Traction

The adaption of skeletal suspension and traction systems to burn management grew out of earlier experience with traction to correct elbow and knee contractures of patients with rheumatoid disease and of traction and suspension as definitive means for treating certain extremity fractures. In its earliest application to burn management, skeletal suspension was used for extremity elevation only to facilitate wound care. From this experience evolved better defined traction systems, including those expressly designed for hands and feet.

Upper Extremity

For suspension or traction of an upper extremity, pins may be directed through distal radius or through second and third metacarpals. The radial pin is directed from dorsal to ventral, 1–2 cm proximal to the radioulnar joint, exiting the bone between the median nerve and the radial artery alongside the flexor carpi radialis. The traction bow must extend beyond the hand. Hand support can be supplied with a thermoplastic splint or padded grasp bar attached to the bow. The transmetacarpal pin is introduced anterolaterally in the second metacarpal just proximal to the head and is directed so as to exit the posteromedial surface of the third metacarpal, at the same level. Transfixation of the two functionally fixed units does not inhibit digital or palmar motion. If the hand is burned, suspension of the extremity can be achieved with one of the skeletally anchored traction splints which position wrist and digits through pins in the distal phalanges or hooks attached to the nails (**Figure 44.6b,c**).

Lower Extremity

For lower extremity suspension or traction, pins are introduced through a distal femur, proximal tibia, distal tibia, calcaneus and first and second metatarsals (**Figure 44.6a**). A femoral pin is inserted from lateral to medial, at or just above the condylar flair. The tibial pin is inserted at the level of the tibial tubercle, sufficiently posterior to that structure to traverse securely two cortices. The distal tibial pin is introduced laterally, proximal to the growth

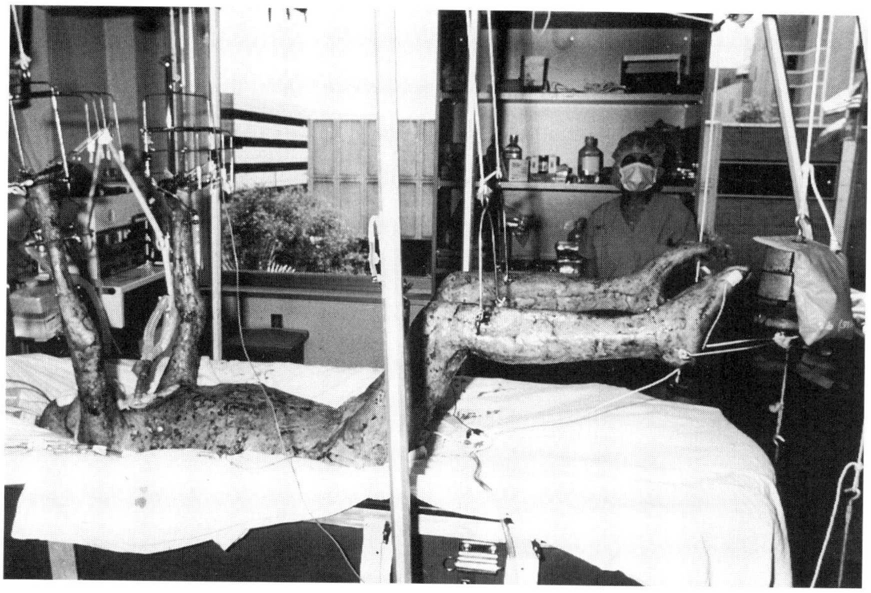

(a)

Fig. 44.6 (a) This 16-year-old male with 94% mainly full-thickness total body surface burn and comatose from anoxic brain injury was placed in skeletal suspension and traction after an initial excision and grafting procedure. Pins were inserted in wrist, hands, tibiae and calcanei. Forefoot equinus was controlled with foam slings (not shown) rather than transmetatarsal pins. Traction was discontinued on the sixty-third postburn day. (b) On postburn day 14 the hand is shown as positioned in hay rake splint with pins through distal radius, second and third metacarpals, and distal phalanges of all digits. The wrist is in approximately 20 degrees of extension, metacarpophalangeal joints in 90 degrees of flexion and digits two through five in interphalangeal extension. The thumb is in metacarpal abduction and flexion and in metacarpophalangeal extension. When grafts were secure, traction was released twice daily for exercise.

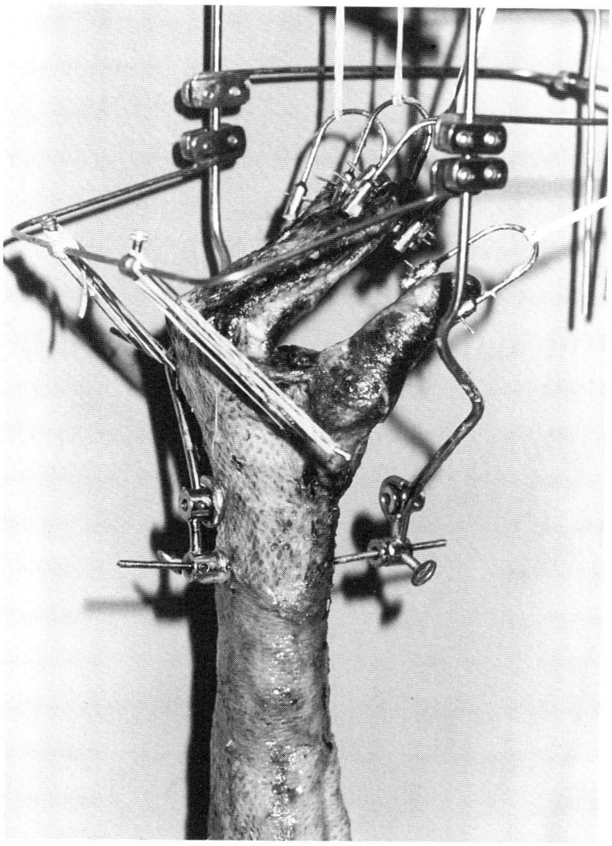

(b)

plate in children and 1–1.5 cm proximal to the talotibial joint in adults. Placement of the calcaneal pin depends upon the reason for insertion. If the pin is only for elevation of the extremity, it is placed transversely in the calcaneus, from lateral to medial, in line with the axis of motion of the talotibial joint, so as to allow free active motion of that joint. If the pin is being used to gain or maintain dorsiflexion of the talotibial joint, it is placed well posterior to the axis of motion (**Figure 44.6a,d**) The transmetatarsal pin is inserted inferomedially into the shaft of the first metatarsal, just proximal to the head. It is directed to exit the dorsolateral surface of the second metatarsal at the same level. This pin is used when calcaneal traction is insufficient to maintain ankle dorsiflexion, when there is threat of development of forefoot equinus, or simply to control rotation of the leg. Skeletally anchored traction splints can be used as for hands to control or position digits.

In the suspension mode for both upper and lower extremities, distal weight is such as to maintain the desired position of the extremity when a patient is asleep or inactive, but is not so great as to prevent active motion or functional exercise. In the traction mode, weight must be sufficient for constant uniform pull in order to correct contracture or to maintain surgically gained position. With lower extremity suspension or traction, a proximal tibial pin is always required to control rotation of the extremity and to prevent hyperextension of the knee. In the management of a patient with extensive burns, lower extremity weights for proximal tibia and calcaneus can be alternately increased or decreased to favor flexion or extension of the knee. In the upper extremity, elbow flexion can be gained just by decreasing distal weight. Occasionally when there is an elbow extension contracture, it is necessary to insert an olecranon pin for traction in order to gain elbow flexion.

Technique

Threaded Steinmann pins are preferred for major bones, with non-threaded pins being used solely for digital traction. Pin size depends on patient size and anticipated weight load. The pin must be strong enough not to bend when traction is applied. When a pin bends with traction, it becomes less efficient and it more quickly erodes the cortical bone. For only one of the usual pin sites is there hazard in insertion: the distal radial pin, whether inserted on volar or dorsal surface, must deal with radial artery and median nerve. With insertion from dorsal to volar, the pin enters the bone just radial to the extensor bundle so as to emerge between the nerve and artery. Just as the pin penetrates the volar cortex, the speed of the drill should be slowed a great deal to avoid ensnaring artery or nerve. With the dorsal approach, the artery, if ensnared, would be lifted from the bone, whereas with the volar approach, it would be

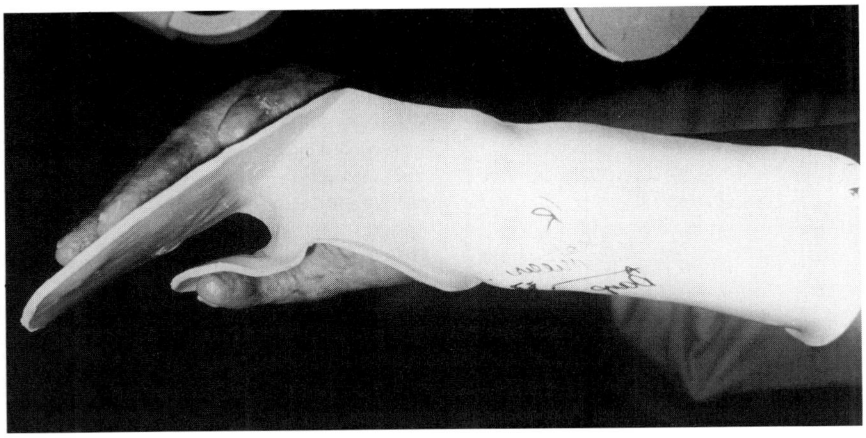

(c)

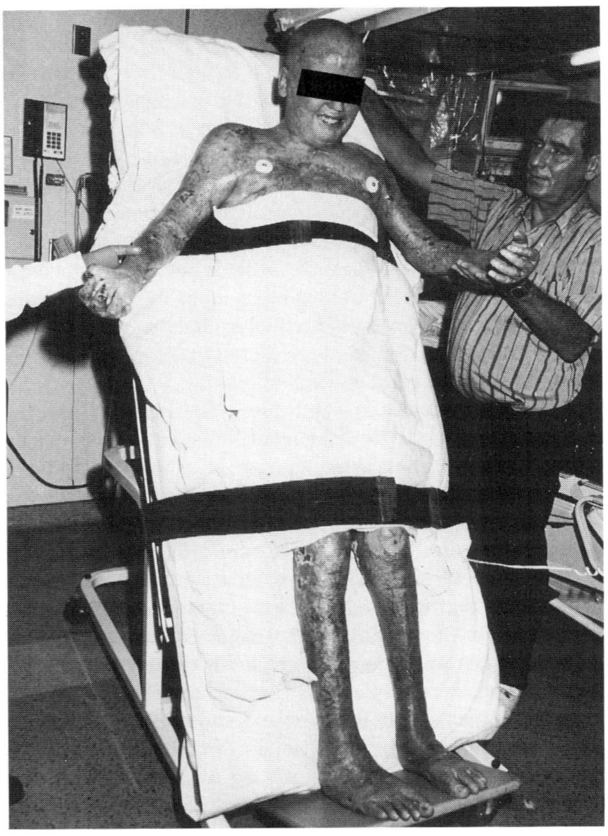

(d)

Fig. 44.6 (c,d) The same 16-year-old male. (c) When traction was removed hand position was maintained with a thermoplast splint. (d) In a standing table, 4 months after burn, feet, ankles, hands and wrists remain in good position. Patient has emerged from a coma.

pulled toward the bone. There is no record of acute injury with pin insertion of either the radial artery or the median nerve.

Complications

Complications recorded by Youel among 1128 extremities in 626 patients treated with skeletal suspension and traction included 30 pin track infections and 14 bone infections.[13] The overall infection rate was 4.0%. This is a low incidence considering the population treated. In fact, it is likely that all pin sites become infected to some extent regardless of the quality of pin site care. If traction for any condition is continued for several weeks, there will be trabecular concentration along the pin tracks. If this denser bone becomes nonviable because of infection along the track, it will separate from the surrounding bone to form a so-called cigarette sequestrum. This kind of bone infection is usually benign and, like simple pin track infection, will resolve after the pin is removed. A diagnosis of osteomyelitis requires positive culture of curetted bone in addition to radiographic changes. The organisms in all infections of pin site origin are those found on the surface wounds. *Staphylococcus* and *Pseudomonas* are the most common. Only one of Youel's 14 cases of osteomyelitis required surgical debridement. All others responded favorably to an average of 2 weeks of antibiotic therapy. Infection related to skeletal pins will always be more common in patients with acute burns than in those whose burn wounds have healed. Youel's study confirms this expected difference. Pin site infection can be kept to a minimum if pins are observed closely for loosening and the pin sites are kept clean and open. Loose pins should be replaced with larger ones at the same site or a new site chosen.

With prolonged transmetacarpal pin traction, a synostosis may develop along the pin track between the second and third metacarpals. This phenomenon is more likely to be observed in patients who develop heterotopic bone at other sites. There is no reason to remove the bridging bone, as the two affected metacarpals make up the fixed part of the hand.

Rigid External Fixators

In acute burn states, rigid external fixators are useful in the management of fractures and for the stabilization of exposed and unstable major joints. The advantage of rigid external fixation for fractures as compared to balanced free skeletal traction is that a patient can be easily moved for wound management. The disadvantage is that the four or more transosseous pins required to align and immobilize the fracture can complicate management of wounds of the affected extremity.

For exposed and/or unstable major joints there is no more secure or accurate way to gain and maintain alignment than with an external fixator (**Figure 44.7a–c**). It is not necessary to use a commercial fixator; as one fabricated of stock metal components or of methyl methacrylate filled plastic tubing and threaded pins will work very well. The advantage of a commercial product is its being readily adjustable. For elbow or knee stabilization, there must be at least four pins traversing eight cortices: two above and two below the joint. For the knees of larger patients, it is better to have six pins through 12 cortices. Commercial unicortical screw systems for fracture stabilization may in burn treatment be as useful for unstable joints as for fractures if need for fixation is relatively short term. There is the concern that in the rapidly demineralizing bone of seriously burned patients, pin purchase in only one cortex might not give continuing stability. In a fixed system, just as with free traction pin, loosening and untidy pin sites are the prime causes of pin site and pin track infection.

In chronic burn states, a rigid pin system is occasionally useful for maintaining skeletal position after contracture release and grafting. The best example of this application is with reestablishment of the first intermetacarpal space after first metacarpal extension–adduction contracture (**Figure 44.8a–c**). Multiple pin fixation is distinctly better than transmetacarpal pinning because it permits fine adjustment and is secure enough for free movement of the metacarpophalangeal and interphalangeal joints of the first and second digits. There are commercial external fixation systems for small bones; however, the most practical system combines commercial threaded pins with methyl methacrylate filled plastic tubing.

Ilizarov External Fixator

The Ilizarov system seems to be ideally suited for correction of chronic skeletal deformities in burns in which there is extreme fixed malposition, tight and unyielding soft tissue contracture, diminishing articular cartilage space, shortened blood vessels and nerves, and loss of skeletal length. Surgical correction is often out of the question because of inadequate soft tissue and because shortened nerves and vessels cannot tolerate an abrupt major stretch. On the other hand, these same structures seem to tolerate well the spaced micro-incremental stretch imposed by the Ilizarov external fixator. In his report, Calhoun lists four major foot and ankle deformities (equinus, cavus, rocker-bottom, and toe dislocation) as indications for use of the Ilizarov system in burn contracture management[7] (**Figure 44.9a–c**). Of the 27 patients treated with the Ilizarov fixator since 1988 at the Shriners Burns Institute, Galveston Unit, only two involved the upper extremity.

An advantage of the Ilizarov system is that the fixation is stable enough to permit a patient to bear weight on an affected lower extremity. In that respect, it is a functional device. On the other

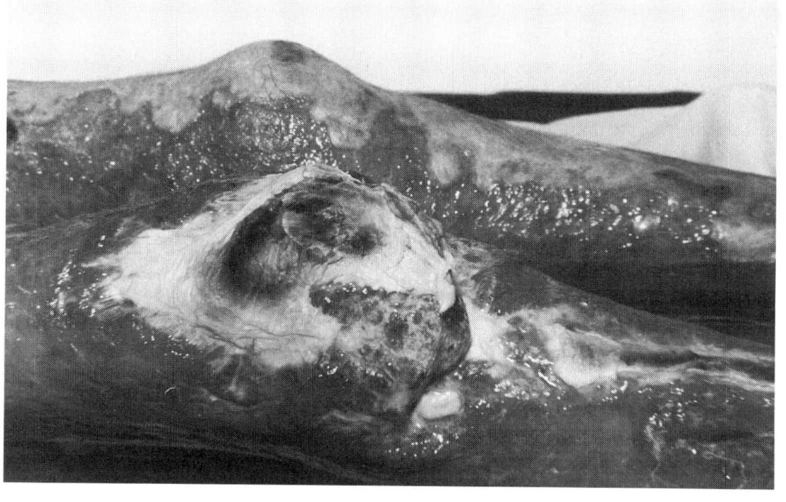

(a)

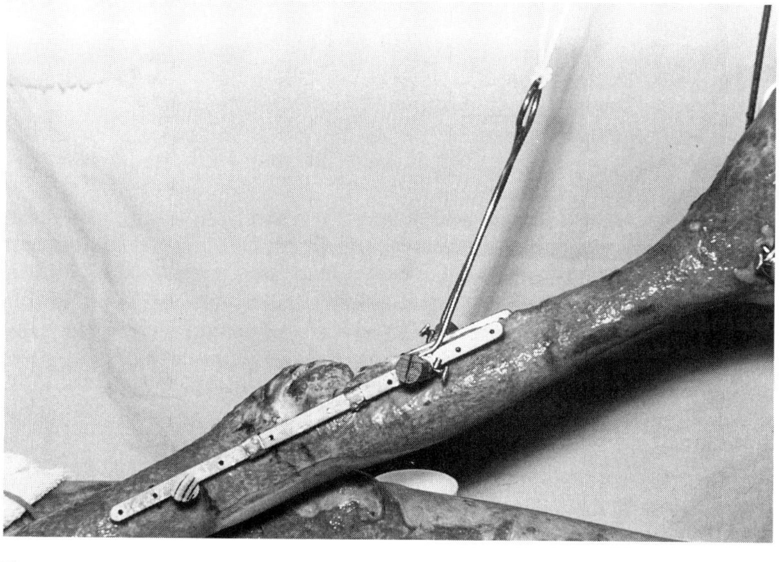

(b)

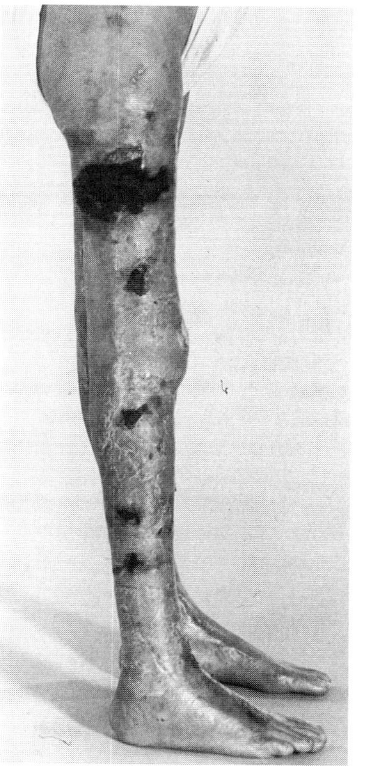

(c)

Fig. 44.7 (a) Widely exposed right knee joint and anterior tibia in an 8-year-old girl, 30 days after a 41% total body surface area burn. (b) For repeated wound debridement and to facilitate eventual wound closure, the knee was stabilized in extension with four pins through medial and lateral external splints fabricated of stock strap aluminum. (c) Four months after burn, the right knee joint and tibia were completely covered with autogenous skin grafts. The knee was completely extensible and could be flexed 30 degrees. The external fixator was removed 2 months after application.

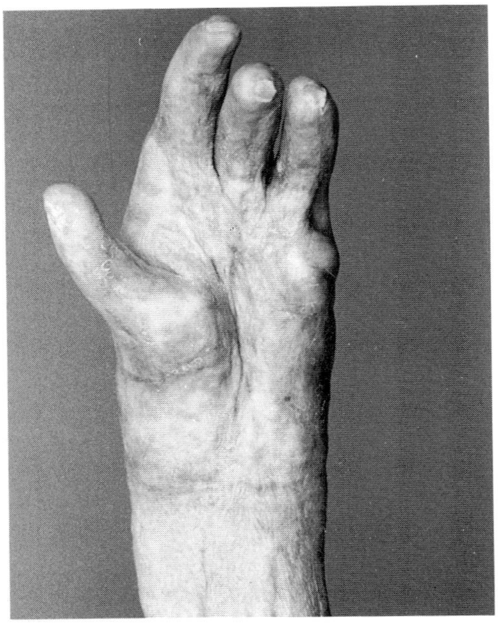

(a)

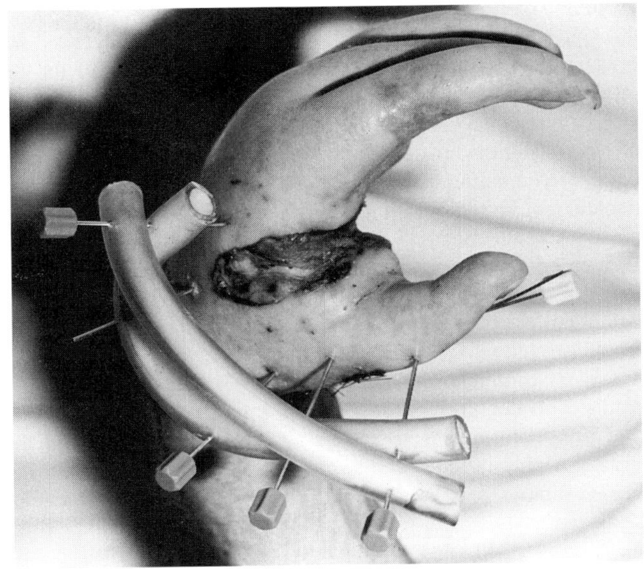

(b)

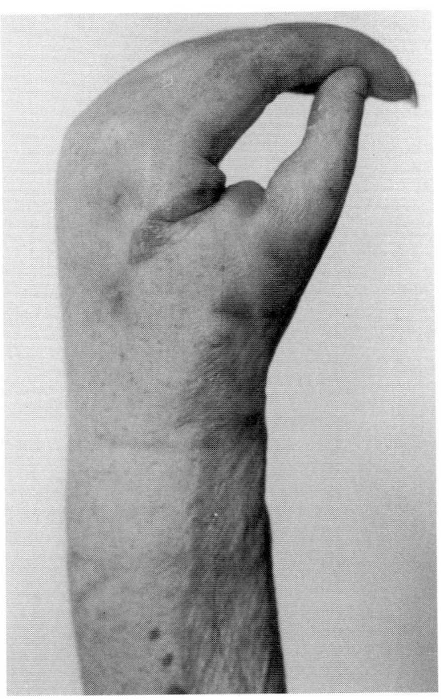

(c)i

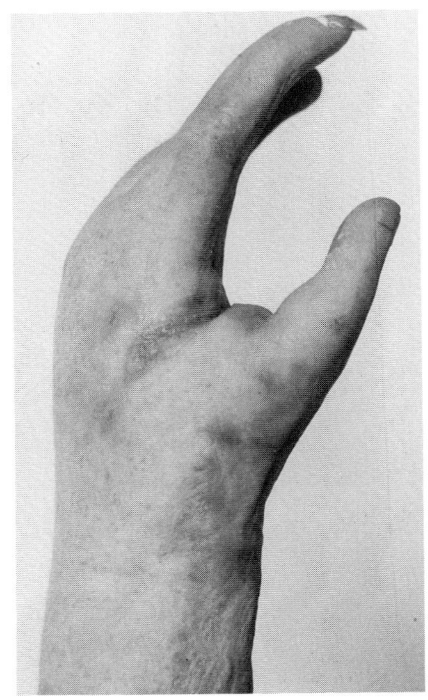

(c)ii

Fig. 44.8 (a) Left hand of a 15-year-old female, 1 year after a 53% TBSA burn. The fifth digit has been amputated at the metacarpophalangeal joint. The first metacarpal has become fixed in flexion and adduction. The first metacarpophalangeal joint is subluxated in extension. (b) The first metacarpal has been freed from the palm and the first metacarpophalangeal and subluxation has been reduced. The thumb ray is held in metacarpal abduction and flexion and in metacarpophalangeal flexion by terminally threaded pins stabilized by two methyl methacrylate filled plastic tubing splints. (c)(i,ii). Two months after corrective surgery, grasp and pinch have been restored. External fixators were removed six weeks after application. Position is maintained with splint and through active and passive exercise.

hand, to gain correction of deformity requires that the device be in place for a long time. Among the 27 patients cited above, the average fixator time was 2.5 months. As with other means of skeletal fixation, infection about the pins is a common complication which is readily controlled with antibiotics or with pin removal. In general, immediate results of correction of burn deformity with the Ilizarov fixator are satisfactory; however, the final attained position cannot be considered to be stable. After removal of the fixator, maintenance of position may require casts, expressly fabricated splints, or braces and aggressive physical therapy. Among children, recurrence of deformity with growth is common. Motor weakness or absence further complicates rehabilitation. In children, the deformity may gradually recur with growth necessitating reapplication of the device. If after correction there is minimum or no

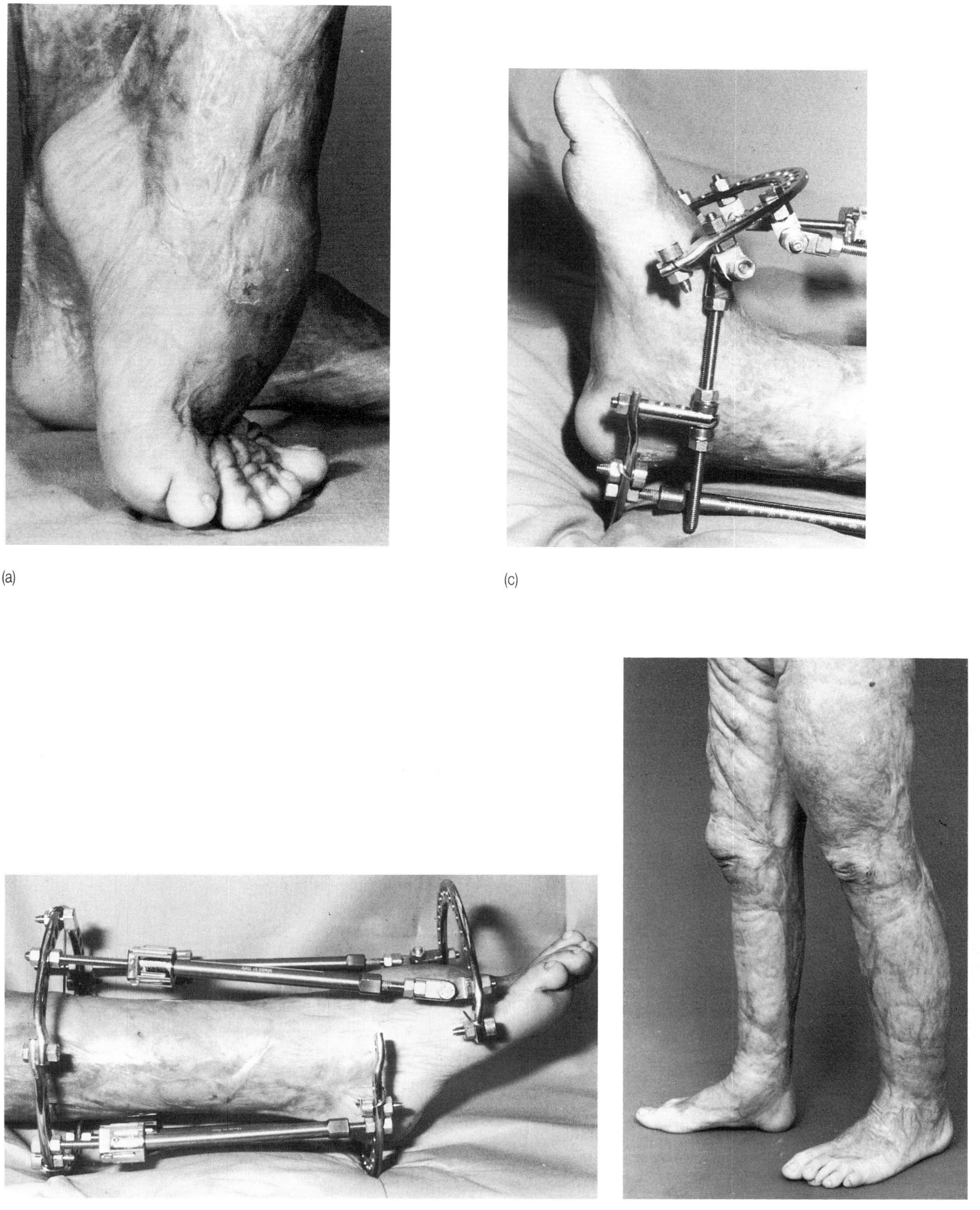

(a) (c) (b) (d)

Fig. 44.9 (a) Extreme equinus deformity of the right foot and ankle of an 11-year-old male, 8 years after a 92% TBSA burn. The deformity was due to scar and triceps surae contracture. (b) To correct an equinus deformity, Ilizarov components were applied so as to gain anterior shortening through a distal transmetatarsal pin and posterior lengthening through a distal calcaneal pin. (c) Correction to 5–10 degrees above neutral was attained in 6 weeks. Walking on the affected extremity was permitted throughout correction period. No soft tissue release was required. The Ilizarov components were removed 13 weeks after application. (d) Four years after removal of the Ilizarov fixator, correction has been maintained and there is active dorsiflexion of 10 degrees from neutral.

motion in a major joint, fusion is the best way to prevent deformity and to gain maximum stable function.

Prosthetic and Orthotic Intervention

The Prosthetist's Role

To date, little has been published regarding prosthetics relating to thermal injury, yet patients with burn injuries can present interesting problems which are simultaneously the same as with other patients and yet unique. Patients who have suffered severe burns have complex, long-term problems and considerable self-care to provide. The challenge to the orthotist and prosthetist is to design a device which is maximally useful to a patient who may have multiple limitations. To be useful, a device must be as easy to use as possible. Simplicity often determines whether the device is successful or discarded by a patient.

Planning for Function

Prosthetic rehabilitation begins with surgery and progresses to splinting, exercise therapy, preparatory, and then definitive prosthetics. Surgeons performing amputations must be familiar with optimal levels for function and growth. Consultation with rehabilitation team members prior to surgery regarding the planned surgical level, weight-bearing areas and alternatives can provide useful information in providing a patient with optimum function while using a prosthesis.

Additional Multiple Involvement

Many burned patients have severe limitations in the function of intact extremities which affect their ability to utilize a prosthesis. Their limitations and strengths are important considerations when planning treatment. For example, functional status has been improved in patients with considerable knee instability secondary to burn trauma by performing below-knee rather than above-knee amputation, stabilizing the knee with prosthetic components, and allowing knee stability to improve over time with the formation of scar tissue. Salvaging part of the forearm where there is an active elbow flexor and no extensor, or even extremely limited range of motion, can provide increased function both with and without a prosthesis compared to a higher amputation level with better skin coverage. Limited function of the contralateral extremity, especially the hand, will affect decisions regarding amputation, amputation level, and reconstructive surgery. Severely burned patients may need to use their remaining functioning extremities differently than patients without total body involvement. Prosthetic rehabilitation should enhance adaptation.

Prosthetic Components

Standard prosthetic texts are useful in providing broad basic information and explanation of the many components available and their use.[16,17] Components for various regions are described below.

Hand

Improved techniques of plastic surgery of the partial hand have greatly reduced the need for partial hand prosthesis other than those for cosmesis. On the other hand, opposition posts can be useful for patients awaiting further surgical improvement.

Below elbow

- Wrist flexion units, especially when there is contralateral upper extremity involvement.
- Distal cushions in below-elbow sockets.
- Padding – which can be attached to a harness ring so as to distribute pressure from straps.
- Rapid adjust buckles for donning and doffing for patients with limited range of motion at the glenohumeral joint.
- Cross-chest straps for patients with protracted scapulae and/or scarring and poor definition in the deltopectoral area.

Above elbow and shoulder level

A flexible thermoplastic inner socket provides reduction in shear stress at trim lines and enhanced adjustability and socket replacement.

Lower extremity

Choice of prosthetic components for the lower extremity is based on a patient's functional ability and physiology pertaining to the maintenance of skin integrity. When these criteria are satisfied, cosmesis is addressed. Severely burned patients may exhibit muscle weakness not usually seen at the same amputation levels in the nonburn patient. These should be noted and compensation such as increasing stability of a prosthetic knee through alignment or components should be provided.

Below knee

Proximal weight-bearing components such as knee joints/thigh lacer or ischial–gluteal weight-bearing brims can be helpful with patients who have problems tolerating full weight bearing on the amputation stump or who have the sagittal plane leverage which a below-knee residual limb can provide but lack the frontal plane stability at the knee. They also assist a patient with diminished thigh strength. For partial feet, several types of prostheses have been utilized. Pressure, especially for dorsal foot burns, should be incorporated into the prosthesis or the shoe so as to inhibit hypertrophic burn scar formation. Where bony overgowth and bone spurs occur, the use of suspension sleeves is recommended. Extra socket depth with replaceable distal cushions is helpful. Knee joints and thigh lacers can be useful for patients whose skin will not tolerate full weight-bearing pressure. The thigh lacer can be longer and extend more proximal for increased pressure distribution.

Above the knee

Neoprene-type suspension belts are well tolerated. Suction, especially suction using 'hypobaric sheaths', can work if no excessively deep scarring is present. Where scarring occurs, the sockets are contoured to the shape presented. Ischial containment with utilization of large surface areas, increased stump to socket stability, and flexible inner sockets are routinely prescribed.

Socket Fitting

Burned patients can be fitted with prostheses relatively early, 7–20 days post-graft, in our experience. Long waiting periods for scar maturation are counterproductive to overall patient rehabilitation.[18,19] With early fitting, some skin problems will be encountered, but in our experience, these have not been of major significance. Occasionally, x-rays may be used to determine the internal bony anatomy of the residual limb relative to the soft tissue shape. The most productive approach, however, has been to apply socket pressures in the standard manner with subtle reductions in modifications to weight-bearing areas which are covered with delicate or unpliable skin. Abrupt changes in contour must be avoided to compensate for decreased skin elasticity.

Soft materials used as socket interface or bridging of the socket wall across sensitive areas can increase friction and skin tension. Low frictional plastic sockets have been satisfactory. Silicone gel or urethane socket inserts, because of extra bulk, weight and replacement expense (especially with still-growing pediatric patients) are not used unless other methods are unsuccessful. Distal cushions made from the usual prosthetic materials such as silicone foam are used. On occasion, patients have removed the distal cushions on their own, and no distal edema problems have been noted.

Initial Prosthetics

Initial and early prosthetic treatment of an upper extremity amputee includes splinting for prevention of contracture. A splint may be extended past the distal end of a residual limb to match the length of the whole limb, thus assisting a patient in retaining the concept of length. This is especially useful for patients whose active participation in a rehabilitation program is delayed. A preparatory prosthesis is provided when early definitive fitting is not prudent, e.g. when reduction of stump volume is anticipated or when fitting over bulky dressings is necessary. For young children, a socket with harness/cable and PVC tube extension has been used.[20] The distal tube is filled with plastic resin, drilled, and tapped to accept a prosthetic device. Friction is provided through a set screw on the side of the distal tube. Wrist flexion units can be added, but they add weight and require maintenance, as well as careful training by an occupational therapist. Unless this component significantly increases a patient's function, it may be more of an irritant than an aid. Standard figure of eight harnessing can be used to attach a prosthesis. To distribute pressure, pads are placed under the harness from C7 to the distal scapular area and extend laterally the width of the back.

Preparatory weight-bearing treatment is provided through an air bag system, utilizing air bags designed for stabilization of a lower extremity. Containers have been fabricated from laminated plastics or polypropylene, using neoprene on the distal end or SACH (solid ankle cushion heal) feet with adapters built into the containers. Treatment is usually begun on a tilt table, progressing to standing and then ambulation in the parallel bars. The system is self-suspending on most below-knee amputees. A belt with attachment straps on the container has been used for above-knee cases.

Definitive Prosthetics

Knowledge about a patient's prosthetic ability, work, and recreational activities will have accrued by the time of definitive fitting. Most patients welcome the opportunity to provide feedback regarding changes in components or changes for function and fit with the definitive prosthesis. Information is provided to a patient regarding available options. Some patients will sacrifice cosmesis for hi-tech, maximum function such as a thermoplastic socket with a frame for a hydraulic knee and energy return foot with no cosmetic covering. Others will part with some function in order to achieve a desired level of cosmesis. The current array of the available prosthetic socket/weight bearing and suspension combinations as well as application and use of the many component combinations is beyond the scope of this chapter. In general, the simplest system which will provide a functional-cosmetic level which can be accepted by the amputee is the best choice.

Prosthetic Examples

The following figures display creative prosthetic use to provide function and ambulation for amputees.

Figure 44.10

The circumstances of a tibial traction pin preclude the use of the air bag and postpone fitting a prosthesis. For such patients, an ischial weight-bearing brim is provided with orthotic side bars which extend past the residual limb to a double adjustable ankle joint attached to a stirrup. The stirrup is drilled, a nut welded over the hole, and a SACH foot attached.

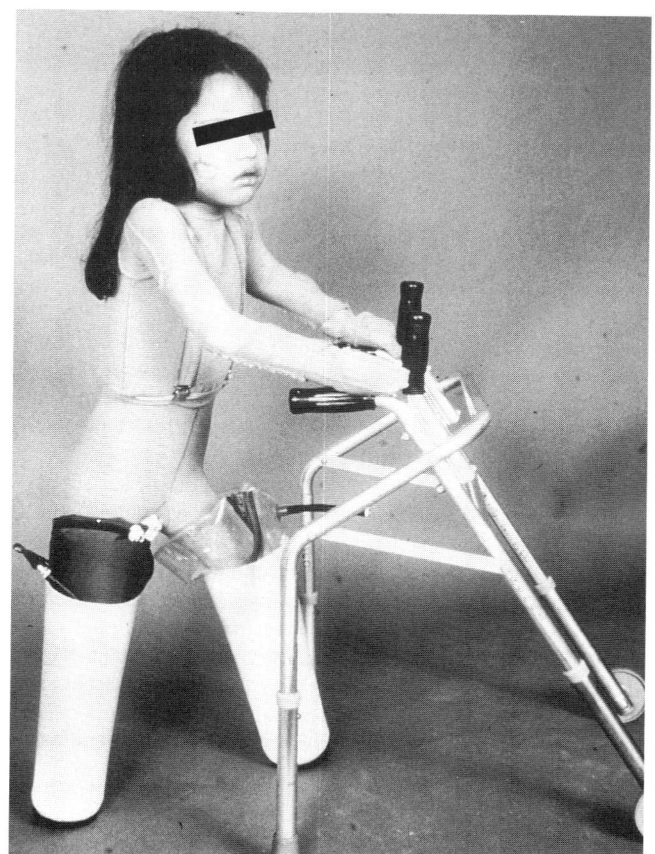

Fig. 44.10 This girl is walking on a set of temporary prostheses which employ air bags surrounding the partially healed stumps. These air bag prostheses allow the patient to begin weight bearing and practice walking before full healing has occurred.

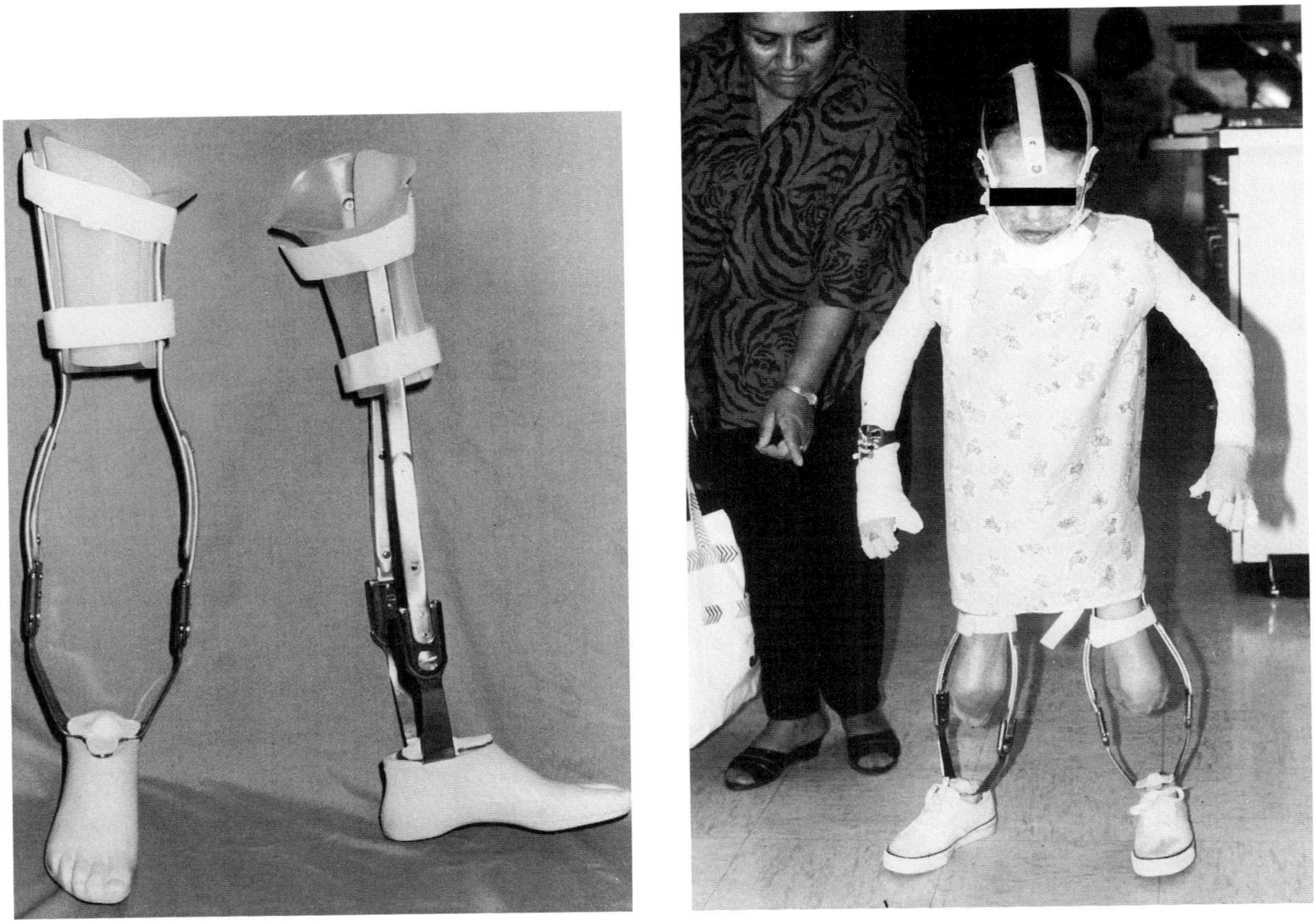

(a) (b)

Fig. 44.11 (a) When the skin at the stump is too fragile to permit weight bearing, a hybridized prosthetic/orthotic device such as this can allow a patient to begin walking (b) by shifting the weight to a proximal site (in this case the ischium) when it cannot be borne distally.

Figure 44.11

For donning, the distal part of the brim is trimmed anteriorly and posteriorly to allow a brace to be rotated and slid proximally. The traction pin is laced to the uprights in a manner which prevents bell-clapping of the distal extremity in the device, but allows slight proximal–distal migration during swing and stance phase.

One patient received an Ilizarov device to lengthen the bones in bilateral above-knee stumps. To assist beginning ambulation for this patient, an aluminum plate fashioned in the shape of the lower ring of the Ilizarov was drilled and tapped to accept a prosthetic pyramid-type endoskeletal adapter. The aluminum plate was bolted to the lower ring, and an endoskeletal system attached in the usual manner. Rocker bottoms of a design often used for initial gait with bilateral above-knee amputees were used. In these rocker bottoms, the posterior part angles upward and extends to prevent a patient from falling backwards. The anterior part is shorter and rounded to allow ease of forward progression.[21] Full weight bearing was achieved with this technique.

Figure 44.12

When a patient is ready to progress from the air bag, a preparatory prosthesis is fitted in the usual manner, using thermoplastic materials. There is often little or no distal pressure tolerance, and skin traction from weight bearing can cause skin breakdown. Therefore, adjustable prosthetic alignment components are mandatory. Because the initial attempts at ambulation are often painful, it is helpful to progress a patient through the air bag system prior to fitting with a preparatory prosthesis so that initial prosthetic ambulation can be a more positive experience.

Posture and positioning of an extremity is often poor, but can progress rapidly. Therefore, adjustable prosthetic alignment components are mandatory. Superficial abrasion will occur, especially in the early phases of full weight bearing. It is not necessary to modify the socket in response to each one. Relief can be provided over bony prominences as long as an abrupt change in contour is not created. If the abrasion is in 'pressure-tolerant' soft tissue, it may heal with continued weight bearing in the prosthesis. All other causes, such as suspension, proper donning, residual limb volume, and prosthetic sock management should be checked and optimized before modifying a socket in these areas.

Figure 44.13

Some patients will continue to use their preparatory prosthesis for extended periods of time while other areas of the body are treated. Prior to definitive fitting, body weight, residual limb volume, wear, and use patterns should be stable in order to optimize the long-term result with the definitive prosthesis. Return clinic visits should

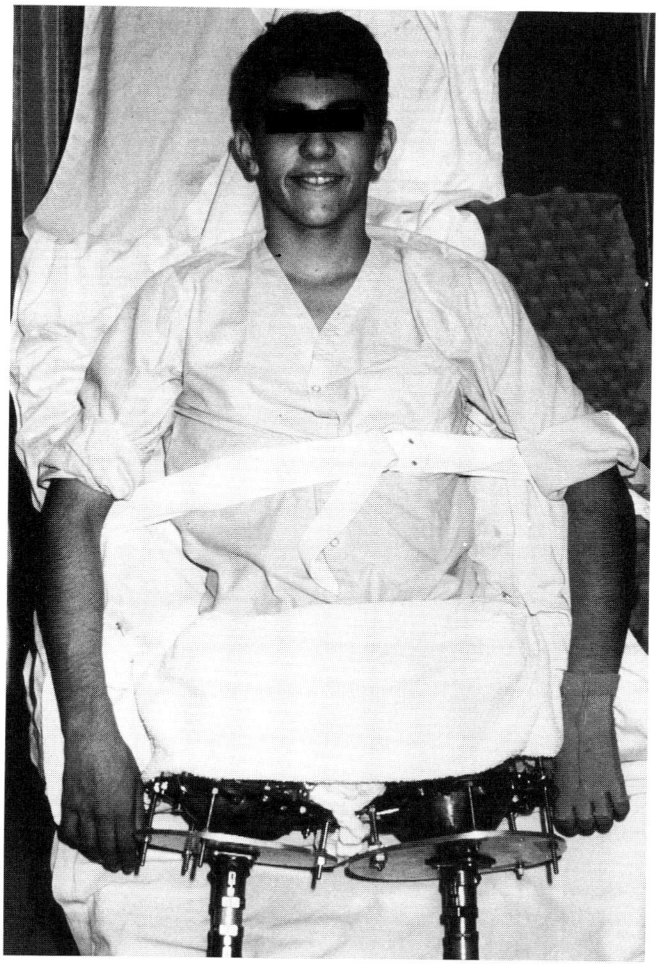

Fig. 44.12 When a bilateral amputation occurs high above the knee, a prosthesis cannot readily be fitted. An orthotic external fixator can be used to lengthen the bones and reduce contractures. In this case the 2–3 inch bones were stretched to about 6 inches while prosthetic pillions were attached to the orthotic fixators in order to allow some weight bearing before the lengthening and healing processes were complete.

include prosthetic evaluation. Children may require length adjustments even prior to definitive fitting. Other patients may leave the hospital with the prosthetic knee locked and may need additional therapy and prosthetic alignment for improved ambulation with swing phase knee flexion.

The Orthotist's Role

The orthotist's role in treating thermally injured persons is much like treating any other person with orthopedic problems. The deformities involving soft tissue and the structural and mechanical nature are addressed by the same forces which are harnessed and applied to other orthotic users. There are some differences in the approach to these patients. These differences are applied to all phases of recovery from acute through post-rehabilitation. The problems associated directly with burns are also discussed in this chapter. A computer search from July 1993, back to 1966, reveals very little information to use as reference material. Most prescription, design, and fabrication criteria can be found in standard orthotic texts used in the United States. Rehabilitation relating to orthotics starts with a recognition of a functional deficit which is treatable with external support or correction. A rehabilitation team will review and evaluate a patient for his/her individual needs. The nature of the deficit is a factor which must be approached by the orthotist using standard orthotic principles with nonstandard techniques. The burned skin itself will not allow direct pressure to the convexity of the deformity without skin breakdown in many cases.

Two common problems are associated with orthotic management of a burned patient:

- Poor skin integrity.
  - (a) Often the skin has been grafted over sites which require pressure to achieve true three-point pressure systems.
  - (b) The skin may have not been burned badly enough to require grafting, yet it has been damaged enough to make it intolerant to even mild pressure.
- Volume fluctuations of the body.
  - (a) In acute burns, edema is a factor which will require good judgment for the right decision on specific orthotic treatment. In acute injuries, the volume of a lower extremity may change several times per day. After fascial excision, problems with edema control may not be resolved for long periods of time; while in the case of tangential excision, edema may be resolved fairly rapidly. The edema situation is very individualized; it may resolve in a short period of time or it may be a long-term problem.

Additional problems which may have an influence on the type of orthosis used include:

- Seams in pressure garments. Pressure garments usually have a closure or a seam. The zipper is the most commonly used closure for pressure garments, as it is the strongest and easiest to use. Unfortunately, the zipper is usually placed anterolaterally on the lower extremity garments. This presents a problem, with the most common equinovarus deformity, if the zipper passes over the lateral malleolus. Seams do not generally present the same type of problems which zippers do. Only rarely have we had to address problems with seams in thermally injured patients.
- Projected duration of orthotic treatment.
- Geographic location or a patient's proximity to other outpatient facilities for follow-up and modifications to an orthosis.
- Language and social barriers. One must be able to communicate to the patient and family concerning how to use the treatment provided. Social mores may result in compliance problems with a patient and family.
- Proximal levels of involvement may also be a factor in deciding what type of orthosis should be used. If ground reaction forces cannot be controlled to provide stability of the knee from below the knee, then bridging the knee joint will be required.

The kinetic chain of the lower extremity is disrupted by significant burn to this area of the body. Skin contractures present a unique problem to the orthotist. All of the other orthopedic problems created by thermal injury are usually compounded initially by poor skin integrity and later by skin contractures. In some cases, a neurological component frustrates a treatment plan. Upper motor neuron problems are much more difficult to resolve in thermally injured patients, as there tends to be a great deal of spasticity. In spastic patients, corrective forces which must be applied will be

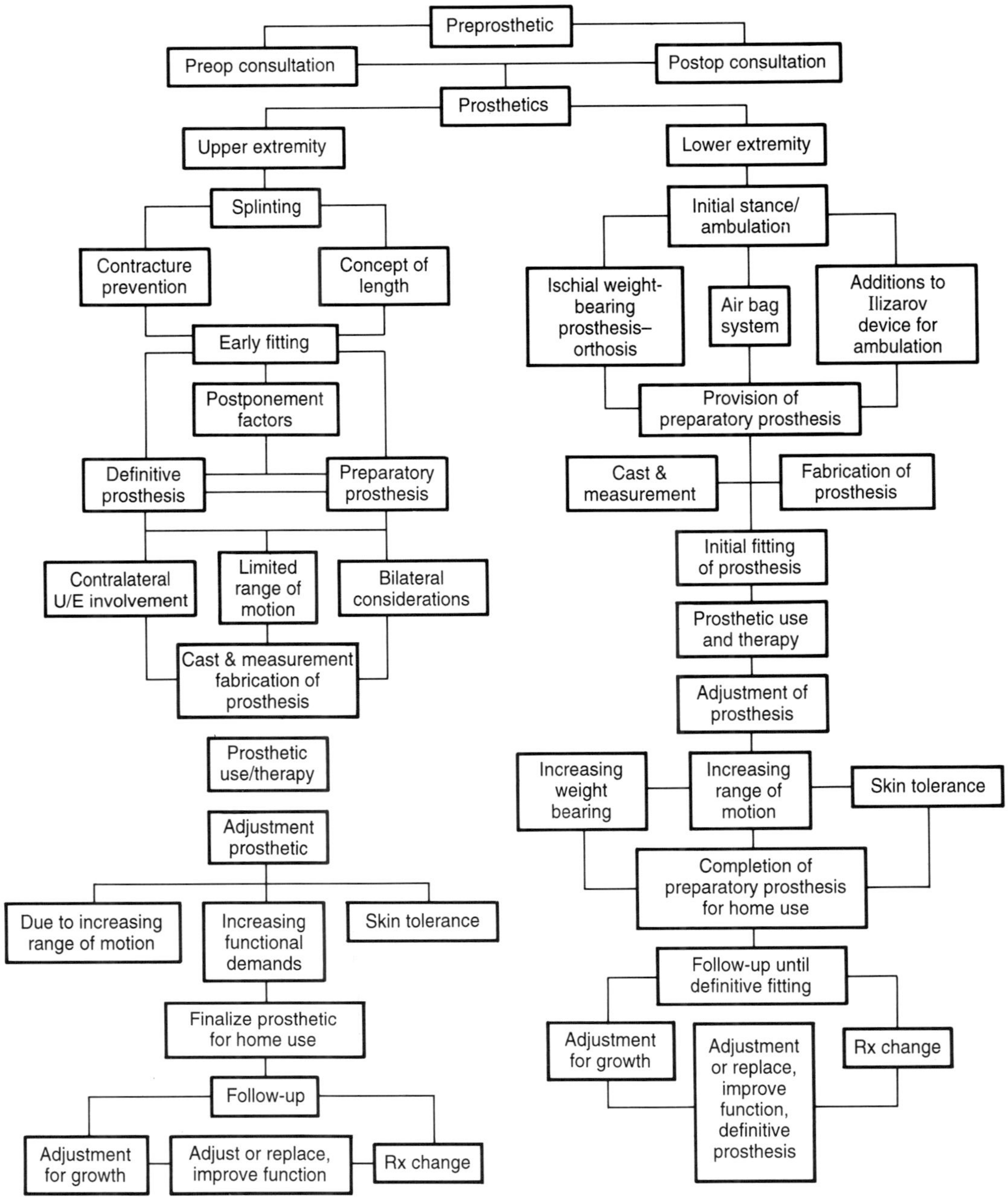

Fig. 44.13 Algorithm showing the process of prosthetic evaluation and fitting.

greater than in cases of lower motor neuron problems without spasticity. Paralytic patients also present added challenges.

Treatment of the Foot

The orthotic treatment of a foot is dependent on the nature of a burn injury. A plantar surface burn may not be treated by an orthotist, while dorsal or circumferential burns may be treated. Acquired absence of toes whether medial, distal, or lateral is often treated by the orthotist. The foot may not be burned at all, but there may be severe burns proximal to the foot which cause deformities and deficit distally and may need an orthosis. Shoes tend to play a great role in the treatment of the foot in thermally injured persons. As long as edema is an issue, a shoe which is accommodative is required. Commercially available surgical shoes and boots are of optimal use, as they are easily modified, provide good support, and will allow for edema and subsequent loss of edema. Commercially available athletic shoes are often employed in the treatment of foot burns.

Many shoe modifications may be used to augment the treatment of a foot. Arch pads and molded foot orthoses are often employed to keep the skin on the plantar surface of the foot stretched out in the case of a circumferential foot burn. The addition of a tongue pad which extends distally over the toes is used to prevent dorsal toe contractures and to distribute pressure evenly over the foot. Shoes often have to be modified in order to fit over external fixators during contracture reduction procedures. When a fixator is being used to reduce an equinus position, a compensatory heel elevation should be added to allow full and even weight bearing on the plantar surface of the foot. This elevation will be removed gradually as the contracture is reduced. The fixator has strategically placed pins which pass through the foot in the frontal plane to make sagittal plane corrections. These pins may be located through the heel and the forefoot. Channels must be cut into the shoe to appropriately clear the pins, and additional closures will have to be added in order to secure the shoe to the foot during ambulation.

Foot Orthoses

Foot orthoses are often used for positioning a foot when a patient is recovered and out of the hospital. The basic types used are plantar supports and the University of California Biomechanical Laboratory Type (UCBL). The UCBL is referred to as a full foot orthosis. The plantar orthosis is usually used in specific cases such as:

- when the plantar surface of the foot needs contact to keep the skin stretched out and to prevent skin contracture;
- when the skin cannot tolerate corrective forces which the full foot orthosis provides;
- when only the sagittal and frontal plane corrections are indicated; and
- when even weight redistribution is required as an accommodation.

This type of orthosis is usually fabricated from one of the closed cell polyethylene foam materials of medium or firm density. As in basic orthotic principles, the flexible plantar orthosis is used because transverse plane corrections are not warranted or cannot be achieved due to skin intolerance or skeletal factors which will not allow correction.

The full foot orthosis is employed for triplanar corrections. The skin must be in good shape and a wearing schedule must be provided to insure success. It is best to use standard casting techniques to correct the *pes plano valgus* or *pes cavo varus* foot. It may be of great benefit to use synthetic casting tape, as it is much stronger and will not delaminate when casting a foot into a corrected position. The negative model may be removed from the foot and trimmed into the shape of the foot orthosis and applied to the inside of a shoe. A patient may walk on this in order to establish whether he/she can tolerate it, and whether the orthosis will produce the desired result prior to fabrication.

Sometimes a modified Denis Browne Bar is attached to shoes while a patient is still preambulatory. If properly used, this device can address all three planes of motion. A T-bar is added to the Denis Browne Bar so as to hold the foot and ankle in dorsiflexion whether a patient is supine or prone, addressing the sagittal plane. The toe-in and toe-out settings can be adjusted to address the transverse plane motion. If leg abduction is required, the specific length of the bar can be established prior to fitting.

Leg Length Discrepancies

Both functional and anatomical leg length discrepancies are seen often in burn victims. Anatomical shortness of a lower extremity may be a result of direct trauma along with a burn; or in the case of children, there may be an interruption to the skeletal growth plate. The anatomical leg length discrepancy may also be a predisposing factor. This type of leg length discrepancy should be treated with a shoe lift only. The functional leg length discrepancy will include soft tissue contractures. Reduction of the contractures will resolve the problems, but shoe elevations which are gradually decreased are part of the treatment. A dorsiflexion contraction, placing the foot into the calcaneus position, is a problem seen with regularity in burn victims. In order to make the foot plantigrade, a patient has to flex the knee and hip, thus shortening the affected side. An anterior elevation may be utilized to resolve this problem conservatively.

Ankle–Foot Orthoses

The ankle/foot complex is a difficult problem for any orthotist in severe cases. Thermal injury compounds this problem. Most cases will involve the equinovarus foot. The talocrural, subtalar and midtarsal joints are the largest and most identifiable joints with which the orthotist should be concerned regarding this problem. The keys to success in treating the equinovarus foot for the orthotist are good preparation by a rehabilitation team, and any adequate preparatory system. A minimum of a three-point pressure system is required. The problem with using a three-point pressure system in burns is poor skin integrity. Most burn scar contractures are very persistent and require long-term, low intensity stretch to be resolved. The area at the lateral malleolus and on the lateral side of the foot generally requires the most pressure. Often this area has been burned and may or may not have been grafted. Applications of pressure garments to this area require that the corrective forces be spread out with the greatest possible pressure-bearing surface.

Both conventional and thermoplastic systems are frequently used when treatment includes the talocrural joint. The conventional double upright ankle–foot orthosis is used primarily because of the difficult management of edema. Again, a surgical boot or shoe is used to accommodate edema. Because the prevalent equinovarus position, a lateral T-strap is added. The dorsiflexion assist ankle joint is employed to gradually reduce the equinus position on a daily basis. The springs are removed from the ankle joint and pins are added in order to maintain contracture reduction or reduce contractures. It is not recommended that excessive toe-in toe-out positions of the shoe on the brace be used to enhance transverse plane corrections. Most of the patients that use this type of orthosis can not tolerate triplanar corrections because of edema and poor skin integrity. These patients are usually acute to post-acute status and may or may not be stable. The thermoplastic ankle–foot orthosis is the treatment of choice when edema is under control and the skin is in good shape. A problem with pressure garment zippers and seams can be resolved. An impression of the lower extremity can be taken with the pressure garment on, and heavy seams and zippers can be marked. An appropriate channel must be made into the orthosis to contain the zipper. This should be done during fabrication. A 2.5 cm × 0.5 cm strip of firm density closed-cell foam should be placed directly on the positive model where the zipper channel is desired. The rest of the lay-up material and the malleolar pads will have to be placed over the channel strip. When the vacu-formed orthosis is removed, the strip will remain on the positive model, thus, creating the channel for the zipper. A patient and family should be instructed in donning a pressure garment and ankle–foot orthosis so that the zipper is placed in the channel every time the orthosis is donned. The zipper is usually placed over the lateral malleolus. Again, with the very common equinovarus deformity, this presents a problem. To maintain contracture reduction, an adequate three-point pressure system must be incorporated into this orthosis. A long anterior trim line which extends from the lateral side half way between the anterior tib tendon and the apex of the lateral malleolus must be utilized in order to prevent skin breakdown. The pressure must be applied over a great area on the lateral side of the foot and ankle. This can be achieved with the zipper channel in place. The configuration of any ankle–foot orthosis should be chosen by using standard orthotic principles. Articulating ankle and ankle–foot orthoses which can be adjusted from at least 10 degrees plantar flexion into slight dorsiflexion are quite helpful to reduce, maintain, and sometimes prevent contracture. Appropriate padding is necessary over bony prominences to prevent skin breakdown. This padding should be added during the fabrication process.

Knee–Ankle–Foot Orthoses

A knee–ankle–foot orthosis (KAFO) is generally indicated when there is extreme knee instability. The sagittal plane knee instability is less common than are frontal and transverse plane instabilities in thermally injured persons. Sagittal plane problems which must be addressed by a KAFO are severe but correctable genuvarum and genuvalgum, and these deformities should be treated as such.

Transverse plane problems should be addressed when taking an impression for a KAFO by using theoretical line of progression. Edema should dictate the decision on whether to use a conventional double upright KAFO or a thermoplastic KAFO. It is suggested by the authors that the use of synthetic casting tape, again, would be a good diagnostic procedure to determine whether a KAFO is required or not. If a proper three-point pressure system and ground reaction forces are harnessed by casting for an AFO, then a KAFO may not be required. If casting a patient in a corrected position from the knee down and if during ambulation it is noticed that the ground reactive forces and corrective position are not adequate, then a patient should be cast up to the height of the standard KAFO. Usually, synthetic casting tape will not delaminate. The impression taken with synthetic casting tape is difficult to remove. Skin condition and body size should dictate the use of this method. The deformities that burn patients tend to have will not always follow the pattern that the kinetic chain dictates. Scar contractures and direct trauma to skeletal and soft tissue structures will account for unusual deformities.

Hip–Knee–Ankle–Foot Orthotics

Transverse plane problems at the hip level are common. Elastic derotational straps are frequently used. The use of these straps is limited to ambulation and is quite effective. The straps should be placed on the posterior section of the waist belt and brought around the leg at the thigh level once, and the level below the knee once, in order to adequately derotate this extremity. These straps, thus, pull the leg into alignment from a turning inward or outward.

Conclusion

The orthotist and prosthetist should have a good working relationship with the rehabilitation team as well as with each other. Often the orthotist is called in on a prosthetic case when a hybridized appliance is needed. This would be indicated in a case such as a below-the-knee amputation which does not have adequate skin integrity to tolerate weight bearing at the residual limb or even somewhat proximal to it. The use of an ischial weight-bearing cuff, with a KAFO or similar orthosis attached to it, may be the best choice, especially in an acute stage. The KAFO ischial weight-bearing prosthosis* will have to include double-action ankle joints and SACH foot with a stirrup adapted to it to make ambulation easier in the sagittal plane.

* 'Prosthosis' is a term coined by the authors of this chapter who have used this particular type of appliance on several occasions.

References

1. Leman C J. Splints and accessories following burn reconstruction. *Clin Plast Surg* 1992; **19**(3): 721–31.
2. Wright M P, Taddonio T E, Prasad J K, Thomson P D. The microbiology and cleaning of thermoplastic splints in burn care. *J Burn Care Rehabil* 1989; **10**(1): 79–83.
3. Covey M H. Occupational therapy. In: Boswick J A, ed. *The Art and Science of Burn Care*. Rockville: Aspen Publishers, Inc 1987: 285–98.
4. Howell J W. Management of the acutely burned hand for the nonspecialized clinician. *Physi Ther* 1989; **69**(12): 1077–90.
5. Harries C A, Pegg, S P. Foam ear protectors for burnt ears. *J Burn Care Rehabil* 1989; **10:** 183–4.
6. Bennett G B. Serial casting: a method of treating burn contractures. *J Burn Care Rehabil* 1989; **10**(6): 543–5.
7. Calhoun J H, Evans E B, Herndon D N. Techniques for the management of burn contractures with the Ilizarov fixator. *Clin Orthop Rel Res* 1993; **280:** 117–24.
8. Larson D L, Evans E B, Abston S, Lewis S R. Skeletal suspension in traction in the treatment of burns. *Ann Surg* 1968; **168**(6): 981–5.
9. Evans E B. Orthopedic measures in the treatment of severe burns. *J Bone Joint Surg [Am]* 1966; **48:** 643–69.
10. Evans E B, Larson D L, Abston S, Willis B. Prevention and correction of deformity after severe burns. *Surg Clin North Am* 1970; **50**(6): 1361–75.
11. Evans E B, Larson D L, Yates S. Preservation and restoration of joint function in patients with severe burns. *JAMA* 1968; **204:** 843–8.
12. Harnar T, Engrav L, Heimbach D, Marvin J. Experience with skeletal immobilization after excision and grafting of the severely burned hands. *J Trauma* 1985; **25:** 299–302.
13. Youel L, Evans E B, Heare T C, Herndon D N, Larson D L, Abston S. Skeletal suspension in the management of severe burns in children. *J Bone Joint Surg [Am]* 1986; **68:** 1375–9.
14. Evans E B. Musculoskeletal changes complicating burns. In: Epps C H Jr, ed. *Complications in Orthopaedic Surgery*. Vol 2. Philadelphia: J B Lippincott Co, 1978: 113–58.
15. Evans E B, Calhoun J H. Musculoskeletal changes complicating burns. In: Epps C H Jr, ed. *Complications in Orthopaedic Surgery*. Vol 2. Philadelphia: J B Lippincott Co, 1994: 1239–78.
16. Bowker J H. In: Michael J W M, ed. *Atlas of Limb Prosthetics: Surgical Prosthetic and Rehabilitation Principles*. St Louis, MO: C V Mosby, 1992.
17. Pritham C H. *Cumulative Volume of Clinical Orthotics and Prosthetics*. Alexandria, VA: The American Academy of Orthotists and Prosthetists 1988: 8(3)–12(3).
18. Malone J M, Fleming L L, Roberson J, *et al.* Immediate, early and late postsurgical management of upper-limb amputation. *Rehabil Res* 1984; **21:** 33–41.
19. Fletchall S, Hickerson, W. Early upper extremity prosthetic fit in patients with burns. *J Burn Care Rehabil* 1991; **12:** 234–6.
20. Fletchall S, Tran T, Ungarao V, Hickerson W. Updating upper extremity temporary prosthetics. Thermoplastics. *J Burn Care Rehabil* 1992; **13:** 584–6.
21. Anderson M H, Bray J J, Hennessy C A. The construction and fitting of lower extremity prostheses. In: Edwards J W, ed. *Orthopedic Appliances Atlas*. Ann Arbor: The American Academy of Orthopaedic Surgeons 1960: 305.

RECONSTRUCTION

CHAPTER FORTY-FIVE

45

Medical Therapy and Surgical Approach to the Burn Scar

Robert L. McCauley and Maureen Hollyoak

Introduction

The survival of patients with major thermal injuries has dramatically increased in recent years. Presently children under 14 years of age have a better than 50% chance of surviving burns greater than 90% of the total body surface area.[1] Unfortunately, the human does not heal through a process of tissue regeneration. Consequently, scarring, as a result of such injuries, is the rule. Such burn scars remain a lasting reminder of the insult for both a patient and the outside world.

In 1968, Janzekovic introduced the concept of early tangential excision and skin grafting and demonstrated superior esthetic and functional results when compared to more conservative methods of excision and grafting at 3 weeks.[2] Today, early excision of a burn wound and coverage with skin grafts is the treatment of choice in acute burn care.[3–5] Indeed, as challenges in burn care begin to highlight issues related to functional rehabilitation and quality of life, management of the burn wound and its impact on scarring becomes a more focused issue.

Scar tissue is the result of a complex sequence of events of repair and a consequence of serious injury. If an injury is of sufficient depth, the formation of a scar proceeds through a maturation process which involves hypertrophy. Linares *et al.* have detailed the histologic patterns of burn scars quite extensively. Needless to say, such hypertrophic burn scars are undesirable regardless of their impact on function. The incidence of hypertrophic burn scars have been sporadically reported to be between 26 and 63%.[6–8] A number of factors have been implicated in their development. Development of hypertrophic burn scars may be a multifactorial process; delayed wound healing, infection, genetic predisposition, and familial tendencies have been previously implicated.[9,10] The impact of such scarring in children has significant implications both esthetically and functionally.[8,11] As with all scars, hypertrophic burn scars are prone to contract and may produce functional limitations as well as visual disfigurements. Prioritization and systematic planning of the reconstructive needs in these patients may alleviate some disfigurements and improve function, but they do not completely eliminate scarring. Longitudinal assessment of the quality of life of patients surviving massive thermal injury suggests that visible scars may have significant impact on the psychological adjustment of an individual.[8,11–13]

Etiology

Clinical assessment of the depth of a burn wound can be difficult, even in the most experienced hands.[14,15] While several reported, noninvasive techniques have improved our clinical assessment of burn wound depth, it is clear that burns which involve the reticular dermis are more prone to hypertrophic scarring. Obviously, wounds which are deeper require a longer healing time. Deitch *et al.* observed a 33% incidence of hypertrophic scarring in wounds which heal between 4 and 21 days and a 78% incidence of hypertrophic scarring in burns which require more than 21 days to heal. Any factor which delays the healing process can predispose one to hypertrophic scarring.[16–22] Infection can prolong the inflammatory phase of wound healing and subsequently prevent wound contraction.[23,24] Many organisms produce toxins which inhibit epithelial migration and digest tissue proteins and polysaccharides present in the dermis.[21] Moniguchi and Fujimoto hypothesize a relationship between hypertrophic scar and cross-links of collagen.[25] They demonstrated increased levels of pyridinoline cross-linkages in hypertrophic scars when compared to mature scars on normal skin. In 1984, Eyre demonstrated that the main cross-linking processes between collagen subunits involved aldehyde residues.[9] Lewis demonstrated that although the incidence of both hypertrophic scarring and a deficiency in aldehyde dehydrogenase-2 are increased in the oriental population, there is no correlation between these two phenomena.[10]

Immunological factors which affect hypertrophic scarring have been scrutinized considerably.[26–28] Controversy exists as to whether immunological differences exist between patients with normal scars and those with hypertrophic burn scars. In 1978, Cohen *et al.* reported increased tissue levels of IgG in keloids.[29] Later, Kischer *et al.* demonstrated increased levels of IgG, IgA, and IgM in hypertrophic scars.[30] The significance of these findings, however, is still unclear. Further investigations into the immunological nature of hypertrophic scars have been characterized by the demonstration of the anomalous expression of HLA-DR antigens on keratinocytes and fibroblasts. Castagnoli *et al.*, using immunoperoxidase staining of skin sections, noted the expression of class II antigens in keratinocytes and fibroblasts from hypertrophic burn scars.[26] Moreover, an abundance of Langerhans cells and IL-2R positive cells infiltrated these lesions, supporting the hypothesis of a cell-mediated immune phenomenon. Castagnoli *et al.* further characterized the role of cytokines in hypertrophic scarring, noting reduced levels of TNFα cells in such lesions. As evidenced by such reports, the role of wound depth, time of healing, infection, genetic predisposition, familial disposition, and immunological factors all have been implicated in hypertrophic scarring. The pathophysiology and mechanisms responsible for this phenomenon, however, have yet to be defined.

Characteristics of Hypertrophic Burn Scars

Hypertrophic burn scars are a consequence of injury to the reticular portion of the dermis.[31] They are characterized by a reddened, elevated, hard mass of skin occurring over and limited to the original wound site. As these scars mature, they become paler, thinner, and softer. In the early stages of formation of the hypertrophic scar, the collagen fibers show no specific overall orientation and a reduced collagen diameter. An abundance of fibroblasts and numerous mast cells are present. Later, a curvilinear pattern of collagen formation develops and there is increased vascularization with irregular patterns. Then, the bundles of collagen increase in thickness and progress from whorl-like arrangements to distinct nodules. The nodule consists of tightly packed collagen with reduced interstitial space. As these nodules increase, the cell population and vascular complex reduce. There is usually a lack of elastic tissue. With maturation, the thick hyaline fibers of the nodules become elongated, and parallel the surface of the skin. As the number of fibroblast cells drop, there is a marked decrease in vascularization and fibrosis increases.[31] Sympathetic innervation of larger vessels apparently only occurs in fully matured hypertrophic scars. This suggests a link between reinnervation and maturation.[32] Immature hypertrophic burn scars demonstrate approximately twice the rate of collagen synthesis compared with normal scars; however, this approaches normal scar levels after 2–3 years.[33] Collagen content, on the other hand, is initially lower in immature hypertrophic burn scars. After 2–3 years, collagen content increases to much higher levels compared with normal scar. Proteoglycans (PG) are ubiquitous components of the extracellular matrix which are thought to be involved in the regeneration of collagen fibril diameter. Dermatan sulphate proteoglycans (DS-PG) have been shown to influence the *in vitro* formation of collagen fibers. Hypertrophic burn (HB) scars contain more PG of varying molecular weights and mucopolysaccharides consistent with a more metabolically active scar compared to nonHB scars.[34–36]

Evaluation of Hypertrophic Burn Scars

Evaluation of hypertrophic burn scars has been a topic of considerable debate. The need for the development of objective parameters to compare various institutional studies in the management of these lesions is essential. Although most clinicians confine visual assessment of these scars to color and thickness. More objective parameters of scar thickness, their mechanical properties, and vascularity are important in the evaluation of various modes of therapy for clinical outcome.[37–41]

Hambleton *et al.* used ultrasound scanning to measure the thickness of hypertrophic scars following burn injury.[37] This study correlated measurements of hypertrophic scars by direct measurement of skin thickness using calipers with that observed by ultrasound measurements using a Dermascan A by Cortex Technology. Their study confirmed that no significant differences existed between the two methods with a good correlation observed between ultrasound and direct measurements of skin thickness ($r = 0.97$). Clark *et al.* felt that the mechanical properties of hypertrophic scars were important for scar assessment and maturation.[38] Using a quasi-static extensometer, these authors measured *in situ* elasticity and strain to correlate their clinical assessment of grading hypertrophic scar.

Since hypertrophic scars sustain an elevated blood flow, laser Doppler analysis has been used in the evalution of these lesions.[40,41] Hoseda *et al.*, using a LD 5000 perfusion monitor with 5 mW helium–neon laser with a wavelength of 632.8 nm, evaluated 16 burned patients with less than a 30% TBSA burn in an attempt to identify which patients would develop early hypertrophic scars.[41] Their data showed that, at 3-week intervals, patients with hypertrophic scarring had increased microcirculatory blood flow when compared to those with nonhypertrophic scars. These authors suggested its use primarily in the evaluation of scar maturation.[39] Leung *et al.* published their results on the use of the laser Doppler for the evaluation, clinical grading, assessment and scar maturity.[39] Although blood flow values were arbitrarily assigned from 0 to 5, with 5 being the maximal flow recorded, vasodilation and vasomotor indices correlated with the clinical grading of scars.

Grading of hypertrophic burn scar remains an unsolved system. Correlation of such scars with functional impairment can further complicate the issue. Such inconsistencies in the grading process have a significant impact on the interpretation of clinical data from various institutions concerning the management of hypertrophic burn scars. Most studies refer to the 'flattening' and 'lightening' of burn hypertrophic scars as the end point. Little attention, however, is given to the pretreatment stratification of hypertrophic burn scars. Earlier studies by Clark *et al.* attempted the clinical grading of scar tissue from O (normal skin) to 5 (hard, thick, purple).[38] Leung *et al.* further defined the clinical grading of such hypertrophic scars based on color, consistency and thickness[39] (**Table 45.1**). Although such stratification is still somewhat subjective, it does serve as a template around which more objective systems may be developed.

Table 45.1 Clinical grading of hypertrophic scars

Grade	Color	Consistency	Thickness
I	Slightly pink	Very soft	Very thin
II	Pink	Soft	Thin
III	Red	Firm	Moderately thick
IV	Purple	Hard	Thick
V	Deep Purple	Very hard, blisters	Very thick

Medical Management of Hypertrophic Burn Scars

Historical Approaches

The difficulties in treatment of burn scars is manifested by a multiplicity of therapeutic methods employed since early times. Compression therapy has been used for centuries to treat hypertrophic scars.[42] The first reference to compression therapy is attributed to Ambroise Paré in the 16th century.[43,44] He advised: 'if the scar is too big, or high, it shall be plained by making convenient ligation and straight bending to the part a plate of lead rubbed over with Quicksilver'. In 1835, Raynor further popularized the use of pressure to improve the appearance of hypertrophic burn scars. In 1896, Verneul described improvements in the management of hypertrophic scars using elastic bandages to provide continuous pressure.[44] These principles of compression with and without splinting in the management of hypertrophic scars subsequently reappeared and were refined throughout the twentieth century by Unna, Guerin, Martin, Pauchet, and others. Acceptance of the concepts of pressure, positioning, and splinting in the management of hypertrophic scars did not, however, gain widespread acceptance until Larson *et al.* published their results from the Shriners Burns Institute in Galveston in the 1970s.[42]

In addition to pressure, multiple lotions and medicines have been utilized. Honey, itself sterile, has been used since ancient times as an adjunctive method to accelerate wound healing. Inhibition of the growth of both gram-negative and gram-positive organisms is attributed to its low pH. It is still used in some underdeveloped countries, where it is claimed to result in faster healing times and reduce hypertrophic scarring.[45]

Linoleic acid, an essential fatty acid, has been topically used to reduce hypertrophic scar formation. Jelenko *et al.* attributed the effect to an improvement in barrier function and water conservation in the wound.[46] It appears that considerable differences exist in the lipid content of epidermis over hypertrophic burn scars, not simply the deficiency of linoleate.[47] In addition, essential fatty acid deficiency did not alter the normal course of cutaneous wound repair in rats, despite all the cutaneous alterations produced by this condition.[48] This agent has, therefore, not obtained universal use. Topical vitamin E preparations are commonly used by the lay public to improve healing and scarring. Despite the documentation of the function of vitamin E as an antioxidant and anti-inflammatory agent, no human study has shown beneficial effects on scar quality. In addition, 20% of patients demonstrate adverse reactions to vitamin E.[49,50]

Current Nonsurgical Approaches

Compression

All methods are generally more effective when prophylactic treatment is commenced before wound hypertrophy occurs.[51,52] Poor compliance is a problem with all methods and apparently defies patient stratification. Pressure can be applied in essentially four methods as follows.

Elasticized bandages ('Ace Wraps'). Properly applied elastic wraps are a good method of applying effective, inexpensive pressure early. They are applied in a figure of eight pattern distal to proximal. A distinct advantage lies in the early application of this dressing even in patients with open wounds. Pressure varies with each application, and the patient's sensation of tightness. Ridges are often evident, indicating uneven pressure distribution. In general, ace wraps serve as an immediate, but temporary, form of compression therapy.

Tubular Compression Bandages (TCB) (Tubigrip, Dermafit). The TCB has several important advantages over other compression modalities.[53] Like elastic wraps, it can be applied immediately over open wounds or dressings. The amount of pressure delivered is uniform and consistent and pressure can be increased 1.9 times by doubling the TCB.[54] In addition, TCBs can be changed and modified as often as needed with no delay in treatment. Finally, it is a relatively inexpensive mode of treatment. In a prospective, although not randomized, trial, Rose and Deitch claimed that TCB was effective in preventing and treating hypertrophic scars.[51] Caucasians had better results than African American patients. Flat body areas had a higher incidence of good results. Failures occurred at sites of mobility, such as groin, head–neck or axilla. In addition, better results were obtained when pressure was applied prophylactically (89% good or satisfactory results), compared to delayed therapy (72% good or satisfactory results).[51]

Ready-Made Garments (Jobst®) and Custom-Fitted Garments. Ready-made garments can be ideal interim garments before custom-fitted garments arrive. They are less expensive, but accurate fit is infrequent and they tend to require many adjustments. Accurate patient measurement is required for a good fitting gradient pressure garment. There is an inevitable delay in a garment's availability, and they tend to be expensive. Weight alterations in adults and growth spurts in children alter a garment's fit. They are required to be worn 23–24 hours a day and are discontinued only when no further response is evident or the hypertrophic scar has matured.[42,55] Irregular contours, such as the side of nose, axilla, sternum, or breast may not only require prolonged compression therapy but, occasionally, a special design to assure uniform compression.

Although the use of pressure to treat hypertrophic scar is almost universal, it is important to note that no study fully validates the mechanisms by which it works nor have adequate controlled clinical trials been conducted. Many theories have been proposed. Larson *et al.* showed that nodules did not develop under pressure treated areas.[42] Kischer and Shetlar demonstrated rents in the endothelial cell cytoplasm and concluded that the degenerating perivascular satellite cells could be a secondary result of hypoxia.[56] Baur *et al.* proposed that pressure reduced blood flow to the scar, reducing α_2-macroglobulin levels. Collagenase-mediated collagen breakdown, normally inhibited by α_2-macroglobulin, could then progress with less interference.[57] Further, pressure is important for reduction and stabilization of mast cells and, hence, for prevention of their products which cause hydration of acid glycosaminoglycans and decrease deposition of mucinous ground substance.[58] It has been shown that the rate of collagen synthesis is lower in pressure-treated hypertrophic scars than in untreated hypertrophic scars. Within 12 months of pressure treatment, the greater the pressure applied, the more rapid was the decrease in synthetic rate. After 12 months, the rate of remodeling was not alterable.[59]

Baur *et al.* maintained that a pressure greater than 24 mmHg was essential in order for capillary pressure to be exceeded.[57] Although this has never been proven scientifically, more recent research indicates that 15–40 mmHg induces more rapid maturation of hypertrophic scars.[59] Considerable debate remains in this area. The Oxford pressure monitor has been used to assess garment–scar interference interface pressures. A wide range of pressure values between different garments and body parts, all less than capillary pressure, are obtained with this device.[60] Cheung *et al.* documented an average garment–scar interface of 5–15 mmHg. High pressures were noted on the chin and shin regions. Wearing the garment continuously for 4 weeks resulted in a 50% drop from the initial pressure reading.[55] Despite the beneficial effects, the adverse effects of sustained high pressure on growing tissues is a concern. Pressure has been, in part, implicated in skeletal growth arrest.[61] The Oxford pressure monitor device uses a pneumatic electrode which causes some distortion of the garment. More advanced devices which allow more effective monitoring of static and active related pressure changes may be indicated in the future. In general, many physicians feel that compression therapy is not indicated in wounds which heal without surgical intervention in less than 10 days. Wounds which require 14–21 days to heal usually will require compression therapy.

Silicone gel sheets

The problem of managing scars in positions with anatomical depressions or high mobility prompted an Australian group to search for a medium other than pressure. In 1982, they reported silicone gel sheets as offering good clinical response.[62] Silicone gel sheets are held in place by tape, bandages or beneath pressure garments. It is generally recommended that the pad be removed briefly twice a day and the scar beneath the pad be cleaned gently. Approximately 10% of patients will develop a rash or superficial erosions which generally respond to a reduction in exposure to the silicone gel sheet (e.g. 12 hours per day).[63] Silicone elastomer can be used for difficult areas with multiple irregular contours. Once the liquid elastomer is mixed with a catalyst it hardens to form a rubbery consistency.[64]

Many units have demonstrated improved scar maturation with silicone gel sheets; however, these investigations were not randomized, controlled studies.[62,64–67] Some studies have used patients as their own controls with mirror adjacent scar sites. Patients with established hypertrophic scars and fresh surgical incisions had silicone sheets applied for 2- or 1-month periods respectively. Hypertrophic scar elasticity improved after 1 and 2 months and clinical improvement lasted for 6 months. Surgical incisions demonstrated less scar volume at 1 and 2 months.[68] Silicone cream containing 20% medical grade silicone oil has recently been used as a dressing for meshed skin grafts with improved cosmetic results.[69] Silicone gel provides a medium for delivering drugs directly to a scar surface. Ofloxacin impregnated gel has been used favorably on split-thickness skin grafts.[66]

The mechanism of action of silicone gel sheets remains undetermined. Investigations into both the physical and chemical effects of this agent have been a subject of recent investigations.[62,69] Quinn eliminated the physical effects of the gel's mode of action by studying differences in pressure, temperature, oxygen tension, hydration, and occlusion.[65,70] The chemical effects of the gel appear to be more important. Earlier studies by Quinn showed that a low molecular weight silicone leaked out of the gel. It is proposed that perhaps either this fluid penetrates the stratum corneum and alters the chemical structure of hypertrophic scars, or, alternatively, the gel, itself, may act as a stratum corneum and, therefore, restore homeostasis to the burn scar, reducing capillary hyperemia and fibrosis. Histologic studies of hypertrophic scars treated with silicone gel sheets show no evidence of inflammation or foreign body reaction.

Steroids

Triamcinolone acetonide is the most frequently used steroid which is administered intralesionally with a fine gauge needle. In 1965, Maguire reported the first successful regression of a keloid from intralesional injections of triamcinolone.[71] Since that time the use of triamcinolone as an alternative method in the management of hypertrophic scars has been widespread.[72–77] Triamcinolone acts by enhancing collagen degradation by increasing the amounts of soluble collagen. Houck *et al.* demonstrated that cortisone may activate or further enhance collagenase activity and thereby decrease the next accumulation of collagen.[72] Side effects of triamcinolone injection included atrophy, depigmentation, and telangiectasia. Grisolia *et al.*, in a study of 44 children with burn hypertrophic scars who were tested with triamcinolone hexacetonide, demonstrated good or acceptable results in 84.1% of the cases.[75] Nicolai *et al.* recommended steroid injections for narrow lesions and pressure treatment for broad lesions. If there was no response after 6 months or the lesion recurred, surgery was recommended.[76] Tang recommended intraoperative and postoperative injections in the management of hyperproliferative scars.[77] Unfortunately, no clinical trials with long-term follow-up can document the efficacy of steroid injections in hypertrophic scars.

Current Surgical Management

The surgical management of hypertrophic burn scars must take into account whether or not functional impairment complicates the problem. In patients with no functional impairment, pressure remains the first line of therapy with or without steroid injections. Once these lesions have matured several surgical options exist to further minimize the visibility of the scar. One must bear in mind that recurrence of hypertrophic burn scars after surgical revision is not uncommon.

Incision and primary closure

Simplicity is often a virtue. Direct closure and primary healing is desirable whenever possible in burn reconstruction. Although intralesion excision and primary closure of hypertrophic scars have been advocated in the past, very few data exist for comparison to extralesional excisions of hypertrophic scars. Engrav *et al.*[70] attempted to compare these two modalities of treatment.[78] They demonstrated that intralesional excision resulted in narrower and more aesthetically acceptable scars. Seventy-seven percent of intralesional excisions resulted in improved scars as compared to only 36% of extralesional excisions. Although this study points in the right direction for the comparison of two modes of treatment, the conclusions reached are based on observation rather than on hard core data. Subsequent investigations by Engrav *et al.* extended into the partial excision of immature, hypertrophic donor sites, skin grafts, and burn scars as a method to improve appearance.[79] Unfortunately, mature scars did not benefit from this method of treatment.

Support for the intralesional excision of burn scars comes from considering the metabolism of the scar. Hypertrophic scars contain more proteoglycan and mucopolysaccharides consistent with a more metabolically active tissue.[34,35] Hypertrophic scars were shown to have higher collagen concentrations compared with normal scars for at least 8 years after wounding.[33] Incised wounds continue to synthesize and deposit collagen rapidly for prolonged periods despite stable collagen content.[80] Scar tissue contains large amounts of collagenase demonstrated in wounds as old as 31 years.[81] Scurvy can result in disruption of healed scars due to inhibition of collagen synthesis and the then excess collagen destruction by collagenase.[82] Wounds which are reopened gain strength more rapidly than primary wounds.[81] Thus, this prolonged metabolic activity of wounds can be utilized by incising old wounds, not excising them, that is utilizing the secondary healing phenomena.

Scar realignment

Redirection of hypertrophic scar will often be all that is required to correct contraction and improve appearance. If excessive scarring is created by its direction across tension lines, correction needs to realign the new scar in the line of minimal resting tension.[83,84] Double triangular transposition skin flaps (Z-plasty) is a technique which utilizes excess skin lateral to the scar in order to gain length in the line of the scar. It is frequently used in the management of burn scar contractures. Multiple Z-plasties, parallel or at varying angles, can be utilized in managing extensive hypertrophic burn scar contractures. Y-V advancement flaps can also be utilized to break up the line of contracture of a scar and utilize excess surrounding skin.

Total excision and resurfacing

When defects exist which can not be directly sutured due to size or position, other techniques may be required. Total excision of a hypertrophic scar followed by skin grafting is an option utilized in hypertrophic scar reconstruction. McCauley *et al.* reported that radical excision, jet lavage, and resurfacing of large areas of infected hypertrophic burn scars with sheet split-thickness skin grafts in children resulted not only in the eradication of the chronic infection but also eliminated further hypertrophic burn scar formation.[85]

Summary

The management of hypertrophic burn scars remains complex. Without functional impairment, medical therapy remains the treatment of choice. Compression therapy has been the mainstay of nonsurgical management of hypertrophic burn scars. Increasing evidence has suggested that the use of silicone gel may be equally effiacious. Future trends in the nonsurgical management of hypertrophic scars have suggested that the effects of interferon-γ on the reduction of collagen production by fibroblast cells may be transferred into the clinical arena as another treatment option; however, such studies are still in a stage of infancy.[86–89] Surgical management of hypertrophic burn scars have indicated that small linear scars may benefit from intralesional excision if such scars are within the lines of minimal tension. Larger areas, which become either secondarily infected or are associated with functional impairment, usually require early excision and resurfacing with either skin flaps or skin grafts.

References

1. Heggers J P, McCauley R L, Herndon D N. Antimicrobial therapy in burns part I. *Surg Rounds* 1992; **15**(7): 613–17.

2. Janzekovic Z. Concepts of early excision and immediate grafting in burns. *J Trauma* 1970; **10:** 1103–8.

3. Bonaldi L A, Frank D H. Pathophysiology of the burn wound. In: Achaver B M, ed. *Management of the Burned Patient.* Los Altos, CA: Appelton and Lange, 1987: 25–38.

4. Herndon D N, Parks D H. Comparison of serial debridement and autografting and early massive excision with cadaveric skin overlay in the treatment of large burns in children. *J Trauma* 1986; **26**(2): 149–52.

5. Herndon D N, Gore D C, Cole M, *et al.* Determinants of mortality in pediatric patients with greater than 70% full thickness total body surface area thermal injury treated by early total excision and grafting. *J Trauma* 1987; **27**(2): 208–12.

6. Deitch E A, Wheelman T M, Rose M P, Clothier J, Cotter J. Hypertrophic burn scars: analysis of variables. *J Trauma* 1983; **23**(10): 895–8.

7. Parks D H, Evans E B, Larson D L. Prevention and correction of deformity after severe burns. *Surg Clin North Am* 1978; **58:** 1279–89.

8. Spurr E D, Shakespeare P G. Incidence of hypertrophic scarring in burn-injured children. *Burns* 1990; **16**(3): 179–81.

9. Eyre D R, Paz M A, Gallop P M. Crosslinking in collagen and elastin. *Ann Rev Biochem* 1984; **53:** 717–48.

10. Lewis W H P, Sun K K Y. Hypertrophic scar: a genetic hypothesis. *Burns* 1990; **16**(3): 176–8.

11. Sawyer M A, Mende K, Zuker R. The burned child – scarred for life: a study of the psychosocial impact of a burn injury at different developmental stages. *Burns* 1983; **9**(3): 205–13.

12. Bjarnason D, Phillips L G, McCoy B, *et al.* Reconstructive goals for children with burns: Are our goals the same? *J Burn Care Rehabil* 1992; **13:** 389–90.

13. Brou J A, Robson M C, McCauley R L, *et al.* Inventory of potential reconstructive needs in the patient with burn. *J Burn Care Rehahil* 1989; **10**(6): 555–60.

14. Fujii T. Local treatment for extensive deep dermal thickness burn and follow up study. *Acta Chir Plast* 1990; **30**(1): 46–56.

15. Robson M C, Barrett R A, Leitch I O W, Hayward P G. Prevention and treatment of postburn scar and contracture. *World J Surg* 1992; **16:** 87–96.

16. Gulbis E, Marion A M, Dumont J E, *et al.* Prostaglandin formation in bacteria. *Prostaglandins* 1979; **18:** 397–400.

17. Dudgeon L S, Goadby H K. The examination of the tissues and some observations on the blood platelets of rabbits at intervals of five minutes and later, after intravenous inoculations of *Staphylococcus aureus* and Indian ink. *J Hyg* 1931; **31:** 247.

18. Selomkin J S, Jenkins M K, Nelson R D, *et al.* Neutrophil dysfunction in sepsis. II. Evidence for the role of complement activation products in cellular deactivation. *Surgery* 1981; **90:** 319–27.

19. Daato M, Lehtonen O P, Niinikosk J. Granulation tissue formation in experimental wounds inoculated with *Staphylococcus aureus. Acta Chir Scand* 1985; **151:** 313–18.

20. Bendy R H, Nuccio P A, Wolfe E, *et al.* Relationship of quantitative wound bacterial counts to healing of decubiti: effect of topical gentamicin. *Antimicrob Agents Chemother* 1964; **4:** 147–55.

21. Lawrence J C. The bacteriology of burns. *J Hosp Infect* 1985; **6**(Suppl B): 3–17.

22. Robson M C, Edstrom L E, Krizek T J, *et al.* The efficacy of systemic antibiotics in the treatment of granulating wounds. *J Surg Res* 1974; **16:** 299–306.

23. Rudolph R. The effect of skin graft preparation on wound contraction. *Surg Gynecol Obstet* 1976; **142:** 49–56.

24. Corps B V N. The effect of graft thickness, donor site and graft bed on graft shrinkage in the hooded rat. *Br J Plast Surg* 1969; **22:** 125–35.

25. Moniguchi T, Fujimoto D. Cross linking of collagen in hypertrophic scar. *J Invest Dermatol* 1979; **72:** 143–9.

26. Castagnoli C, Stella M, Magliacani G, Alasia S T, Richiardi P. Anomalous expression of HLA class II molecules on keratinocyte and fibroblasts in hypertrophic scar consequence to thermal Injury. *Clin Exp Immunol* 1990; **82:** 350–4.

27. Kischer C W, Shetlar M R, Shetlar C L, Chavapil M. Immunoglobulins in hypertrophic scars and keloids. *Plast Reconstr Surg* 1983; **71:** 821–30.

28. Castagnoli C, Stella M, Berthod C, Magliacani G, Richiardi P. TNF production and hypertrophic scarring. *Cell Immunol* 1993; **147:** 51–63.

29. Cohen I K, McCoy B J, Mohanakumar T, Diegelmann R F. Immunoglobulin, complement, and histocompatibility antigen studies in keloid patients. *Plastic and Reconstructive Surgery* 1979; **63:** 689–915.

30. Kischer C N, Shetlar M R, Chrapil M. HS and keloids: a review and new concept concerning their origin. *Scanning Electron Microsc* 1982; **4:** 1669–713.

31. Kischer C W, Thres A C, Chrapil M. Perivascular myofibroblasts and microvascular occlusion in hypertrophic scars and keloids. *Hum Pathol* 1982; **13:** 819–24.

32. Page R E, Robertson G A, Pettigrew N W. Microcirculation in hypertrophic burn scars. *Burns* 1983; **10:** 64–70.

33. Craig R D P, Schofield J D, Jackson D S. Collagen biosynthesis in normal and hypertrophic scars and keloids as a function of the duration of the scar. *Br J Surg* 1975; **62:** 741–4.

34. Scott P A, Winterbottom N, Dodd C M, Edwards E, Pearson C H. A role for disulfide bridges in the protein core in the interaction of proteodermatan-sulfate and collagen. *Biochem Biophys Res Commun* 1986; **138:** 1348–54.

35. Shetlar M R, Dobrkovsky M, Linares H, Villaranti R, Shetlar C L, Larson D L. The hypertrophic scar: glycoprotein and collagen components of burn scars. *Proc Soc Exp Biol Med* 1974; 298–300.

36. Swann D A, Garg H A, Hendry C J, *et al.* Isolation and partial characterization of dermatan sulfate proteoglycan from human post-burn scar tissue. *Collagen Rel Res* 1988; **8:** 295–313.

37. Hambleton J, Shakespeare P A, Pratt B J. The progress of hypertrophic scars monitored by ultrasound measurements of thickness. *Burns* 1992; **18**(4): 301–30.

38. Clark J A, Cheng J C Y, Leung K S, Leung P C. Mechanical characterization of human postburn hypertrophic skin during pressure therapy. *J Biomech* 1987; **20**(4): 397–41.

39. Leung K S, Shea A, Clark J A, Cheung J C Y, Leung P C. Microcirculation in hypertrophic scars after burn injury. *J Burn Care Rehabil* 1989; **10:** 436–44.

40. Ehrlich H P, Kelley S F. Hypertrophic scar: an interruption in the remodeling of repair – a laser doppler blood flow study. *Plast Reconstr Surg* 1992; **90:** 993–88.

41. Hosada A, Holloway G A, Heinbach D M. Laser Doppler flowmetry for the early detection of hypertrophic burn scars. *J Burn Care Rehabil* 1986; **7**(6): 496–9.

42. Larson D L, Abston S, Evans E B, Dobrkovsky M, Linares H A. Techniques for decreasing scar formation and contractures in the burned patient. *J Trauma* 1971; **11**(10): 807–23.

43. Linares H A, Larson D L, Willis-Galstaun B A. Historical notes on the use of pressure in the treatment of hypertrophic scars or keloids. *Burns* 1993; **19**(1): 17–21.

44. Johnson T. In: Clark M, ed. *The Works of that Famous Chirurgeon Ambrose Paré*. London: 1678: 519.

45. Subrahmanyan M. Topical application of honey in treatment of burn. *Br J Surg* 1991; **78:** 497–8.

46. Jelenko C, Wheeler M L, Scott T H. Studies in burns X. Ethyl linoleate: the water holding lipid of the skin. A. The Evidence. *J Trauma* 1972; **12:** 968–72.

47. Shakespeare P G, Strange R E. Linoleic acid in hypertrophic scars. *Burns* 1982; **9:** 7–12.

48. Porras-Reyes B H, Schreiner G F, Lefkowith J B, Mustoe T A. Essential fatty acids are not required for wound healing. *Prostaglandins, Leukot Essent Fatty Acids* 1992; **45:** 293–8.

49. Parsa F D. Vitamin E: facts and fallacies. *Plast Reconstr Surg* 1988; **81**(12): 300–1.

50. Jenkins M, Alexander J W, MacMillian B G, Waymack J P, Kopcha R. Failure of topical steroids and vitamin E to reduce postoperative scar formation following reconstructive surgery. *J Burn Care Rehabil* 1986; **7**(4): 309–12.

51. Rose M P, Deitch E A. The clinical use of a tubular compression bandage, Tubigrip, for burn scar therapy: a critical analysis. *Burns* 1985; **12:** 58–64.

52. Kloti J, Pochon J P. Long-term therapy of second and third degree burns in children using Jobst compression suits. *Scand J Plast Reconstr Surg* 1979; **13:** 163–8.

53. Judge J C, May R, Declement F A. Control of hypertrophic scarring in burn patients using tubular support bandages. *J Burn Care Rehabil* 1984; **5:** 221–4.

54. Robertson J C, Drett J E, Hodgson B, Druett J. Pressure therapy for hypertrophic scarring: preliminary communication. *J R Soc Med* 1980; **73:** 348–54.

55. Cheung J C Y, Evans J H, Leung K S. Pressure therapy in the treatment of post burn hypertrophic scar – a critical look into its usefulness and fallacies by pressure monitoring. *Burns* 1984; **10:** 154–63.

56. Kischer C W, Shetlar M R. Microvasculature in hypertrophic scars and the effects of pressure. *J Trauma* 1979; **19:** 757–62.

57. Baur P S, Larson D L, Stacey T R, Barratt G F, Dobrkovsky M. Ultrastructural analysis of pressure treated human hypertrophic scars. *J Trauma* 1976; **16:** 958–62.

58. Kische C W, Bailey J F. The mast cell in hypertrophic scars. *Rep. B101. Tex Med* 1972; **30:** 327–31.

59. Reid W H, Evans J H, Naismith R S, Tully A E, Sherwin S. Hypertrophic scarring and pressure therapy. *Burns* 1987; **13:** 529–32.

60. Harries C A, Regg S P. Measuring pressure under pressure garments using the oxford pressure monitor. *Burns* 1989; **15**(3): 187–9.

61. Leung K S, Cheng J C Y, Clark J A, Leung P C. Complication of pressure therapy for post burn hypertrophic scars. Biomechanical analysis based on 5 patients. *Burns* 1984; **10:** 434–8.

62. Perkins K, Davey R B, Wallis K A. Silicone gel: a new treatment for burn scars and contractures. *Burns* 1982; **9:** 201–4.

63. Ahn S T, Monafo W W, Mustoe T A. Topical silicone gel for the prevention and treatment of hypertrophic scar. *Arch Surg* 1991; **126:** 499–504.

64. Van Der Kerckhove E, Boeckx W, Kochugt A. Silicone patches as a supplement for pressure therapy to control hypertrophic scarring. *J Burn Care Rehabil* 1991; **12**(4): 361–9.

65. Quinn K J. Silicone gel in scar treatment. *Burns* 1987; **13:** S33–S40.

66. Sawadar T, Yotsuyanagi T, Ara M, Sone K. Experiences using silicone gel tie-over dressings following skin grafting. *Burns* 1990; **16**(5): 353–7.

67. Ohmori S. Effectiveness of silastic sheet coverage in the treatment of scar keloid (hypertrophic scar). *Aesthetic Plast Surg* 1988; **12:** 95–9.

68. Ahn S T, Monafo W W, Mustoe T A. Topical silicone gel: a new treatment for hypertrophic scars. *Surgery* 1989; **106**(4): 781–7.

69. Sawadar Y, Sone K. Benefits of silicone cream occlusive dressing for treatment of meshed skin grafts. *Burns* 1992; **18**(3): 233–6.

70. Quinn K J. The application of silicone gel for treatment of hypertrophic scars and burn wounds and consideration of the 'ideal' burn dressing. Ph.D. Thesis, University of Strathclyde, Glasgow.

71. Maguire H C. Treatment of keloids with triamcinolone acetonide injected intralesionally. *JAMA* 1965; **192:** 325–6.

72. Houck H C, Sharma V K, Carillo A L. Proposed mode of action of corticosteroids of the corrective tissue. *Nature* 1965; **206:** 158–60.

73. Gallen J L, Goldstein I M, Snyderman R. *Inflammation: Basic Principles and Clinical Correlates*. New York: Raven Press, 1988: 21–251.

74. Ketchum L D, Cohen L K, Masteer F W. Hypertrophic scars and keloids: a collective review. *Plast Reconstr Surg* 1974; **53:** 140–54.

75. Grisolia G A, Danti D A, Santoro S, Panozzo A, Bonini A, Panpaloni A. Injection therapy with triamcinolone hexacetonide in the treatment of burn scars in infancy: results of 44 cases. *Burns* 1983; **10:** 131–4.

76. Nicolai J P, Bos M Y, Bronkhorst F B, Smale C E. A protocol for the treatment of hypertrophic scars and keloids. *Aesthetics Plast Surg* 1987, **11:** 29–35.

77. Tang Y W. Intra and postoperative steroid injections for keloids and hypertrophic scars. *Br J Plast Surg* 1992; **45:** 371–3.

78. Engrav L H, Gottlieb J R, Millard S P, Walkinshaw M D, Heinbach D M, Marvin J A. A comparison of intramarginal and extramarginal excision of hypertrophic burn scars. *Plast Reconstr Surg* 1988; **81**(1): 40–4.

79. Engrav L H, Gottlieb J R, Millard S P, Walkinshaw M D, Heinbach D M, Marvin J A. Partial excision of residual burn lesion. *J Burn Care Rehabil* 1987; **8**(5): 398–402.

80. Madden J W, Peacock E E. Studies on the biology of collagen during wound healing III: dynamic metabolism of scar collagen and remodeling of dermal wounds. *Ann Surg* 1971; **174:** 511–20.

81. Madden J W, Arem A J. Wound healing: biologic and clinical features. In: Cohen I K, Diegelmann R F, Lindbled W J, ed. *Wound Healing: Biochemical and Clinical Aspects*. Philadelphia, PA: W B Saunders, 1992.

82. Cohen L K, Kesier H R. Disruption of healed scars in scurvy the result of a disequilibrium in collagen metabolism. *Plast Reconstr Surg* 1976; **57:** 213–15.

83. Daniel R K, Kerrigans C L. Principles and physiology of skin flap surgery. In: McCarthy J G, ed. *Plastic Surgery: General Principles*. Philadelphia: W B Saunders, 1990: 275–328.

84. Hodges P L. Surgical flaps. *Selected Readings in Plastic Surgery*. Dallas: South Western University, 1992; **7:** no. 3.

85. McCauley R L, Rutan R C, Ortiz V B, Herndon D N, Robson M C. Management of infected hypertrophic burn scar in children with total excision and sheet skin graft coverage. *Proc Am Burn Assoc* 1993; **25:** 153.

86. Duncan M R, Berman B. Gamma interferon is the lymphokine and beta interferon the monokine responsible for inhibition of fibroblast collagen production and late but not early fibroblast proliferation. *J Exp Med* 1985; **162:** 516–27.

87. Granstein R D, Murphy G F, Margolis R J, Byrne M H, Amento E P. Gamma interferon inhibits collagen synthesis *in vivo* in the mouse. *J Clin Invest* 1987; **79:** 1254–8.

88. Granstein R D, Deak M R, Jacques S L. The systemic administration of gamma interferon inhibits collagen synthesis and acute inflammation in a murine skin wounding model. *J Invest Dermatol* 1989; **93:** 18–27.

89. Larrabee W F, East C A, Jaffe H S, Stephenson C, Peterson K E. Intralesional interferon gamma treatment for keloids and hypertrophic scars. *Arch Otolaryngol Head Neck Surg* 1990; **116:** 1159–62.

CHAPTER FORTY-SIX

46

LONGITUDINAL EVALUATION OF A BURNED CHILD

ROBERT L. MCCAULEY, MARTIN C. ROBSON, DAVID N. HERNDON, E. BURKE EVANS AND PATRICIA E. BLAKENEY

INTRODUCTION

Patients with large total body surface area burns are surviving acute hospitalization in ever-increasing numbers.[1-3] This rate of survival is further increased if the victim is young and has not sustained inhalation injury or pre-hospitalization shock. The key factors in the survival of these patients have been improvements in resuscitation, control of infection, improved nutritional support, and early excisional therapy. In pediatric burned patients, such an approach has been instrumental in decreasing in-house morbidity and in-house length of stay. As our ability to save patients with ever-increasing total body surface area burns improves, our concept of total rehabilitation of the patient population becomes of tantamount importance.

The care of massively burned children involves several medical disciplines. A multidisciplinary approach to patient needs in a systematic fashion, after survival of the acute injury, provides a mechanism for coordination of long-term care and assessment of rehabilitation and reconstructive needs. The complex reconstructive needs of such patients dictate the development of a mechanism by which reconstruction can proceed in a rational and orderly fashion. At Shriners Burns Institute–Galveston, a form devised by the American Burn Association Rehabilitation Committee was modified and used to design an inventory form to record potential reconstructive needs and to allow systematic planning for future operations. This form is intended to cover all body regions with subdivisions into anatomical units (**Figure 46.1**). The coordination of these efforts by plastic surgeons, general surgeons, orthopedic surgeons, respiratory therapists, physical therapists, and occupational therapists has been proven to be of significant importance in the long-term rehabilitation of these patients. In 1989, Brou *et al.* demonstrated the usefulness of this inventory of potential reconstructive needs in 25 patients with a mean total body surface area burn of 71%. The total number of potential reconstructive needs was 512, of which 235 were in the head/neck region. The average number of problems per patient was 21.[4]

Although it is clear that the identification of specific problems associated with reconstruction and rehabilitation of a burned patient are brought to the forefront using this inventory, such an assessment lacks the critical elements in the global assessment of patient well-being. Burn injury in a child clearly initiates a series of events which may alter not only the normal physical growth and development but may have a significant impact on the psychological development of these patients. Longitudinal evaluation of these parameters assumes that the concept of the 'whole person' is not lost and that our care remains humane.

To date, very few data exist which offer a multidisciplinary approach to the overall care of a burned patient in a longitudinal fashion. Consequently, problems associated with overall growth and development of the soft tissues, muscle, and bone as well as the long-term effects of burn injury on cardiopulmonary development, nutritional, immunological, and psychosocial development are quite limited. Very little is known of the long-term follow-up of growth patterns in children who have sustained major thermal injuries. Only recently have the psychological traumas due to the emotional upheaval associated with major thermal insult been documented in the pediatric population.[5-8] Once the difficult and monumental task of rehabilitation is initiated, progress may be severely limited by abnormalities associated with problems in growth and development of skin, bone, and muscle; recovery from neurovascular insults; integumentary disfigurements; reduced cardiopulmonary reserves; nutritional abnormalities; and/or immunological problems. These problems can further complicate integration back into society. Difficulties in attaining rapid improvement, because of the extent of the burn injury and the associated problems, may push a patient into a period of depression which could further complicate rehabilitation. Consequently, therapy in these patients must include a psychosocial component as well as a clearly conceived and rational program for physical reconstruction and rehabilitation.

OVERALL GROWTH AND DEVELOPMENT

Growth Delay

Normal linear growth and weight gain in pediatric patients are dependent upon a number of factors. The prenatal environment, adequate nutritional intake, and an emotionally nurturing household environment are crucial. Major catastrophic illnesses have been known to produce profound arrests in growth and development in children. Current trends in the management of massively burned children may include multiple operations and prolonged

Scalp	Grade	R	L
1) scalp alopecia			
2) exposed skull, unstable skin			
3) other			
Eyebrows			
4) eyebrow alopecia			
5) other			
Eyelid			
6) upper lid ectropion			
7) lower lid ectropion			
8) entropion districhiasis			
9) epicanthal folds			
10) lacrimal duct injury			
11) other			
Nose and nasolabial fold			
12) tip			
13) ala and columella			
14) bridge			
15) hypertrophic scar			
16) contracture			
17) other			
Mouth			
18) upper lip ectropion			
19) lower lip ectropion			
20) commisure contracture			
21) other			
Chin and Mandible			
22) chin scar			
23) microgenia			
24) mandibular hypoplasia			
25) TMJ ankylosis			
Ear			
26) ear loss			
27) cup deformity			
28) other			
Cheek			
29) contracture			
30) pigmentation change			
31) other			
Neck			
33) contracture			
33) hypertrophic scar			
34) other			

Please refer to the back for instructions

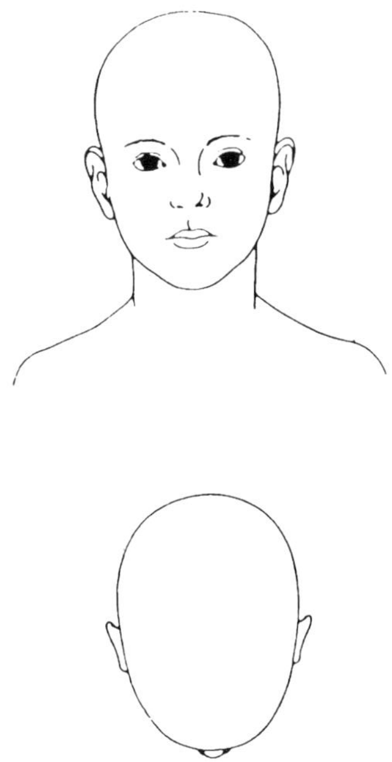

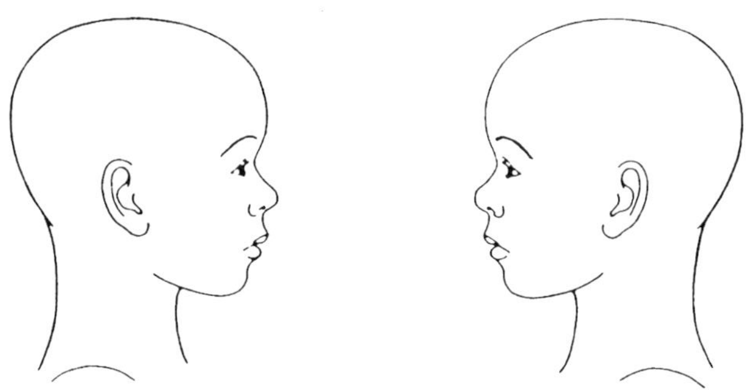

Axilles	Grade	R	L
35) contracture (a)			
36) other			
Elbow contracture			
37) flexion (b)			
38) extension (c)			
39) medial/lateral			
40) other			
Wrist contracture			
41) flexion (d)			
42) extension (e)			
43) radial (f)			
44) ulnar (g)			
45) other			
Hand			
46) digit amputation			
47) boutoniere			
48) swan neck or mallet			
49) IP lateral contracture			
50) MP flexion contracture (h)			
51) MP extension contracture (i)			
52) MP lateral contracture			
53) thumb CMC (j)			
54) thumb MP and IP (k)			
55) hooding of web space			
56) burn syndactyly			
57) palmar contractures			
58) other			

(a-k) Please refer to the back for instructions

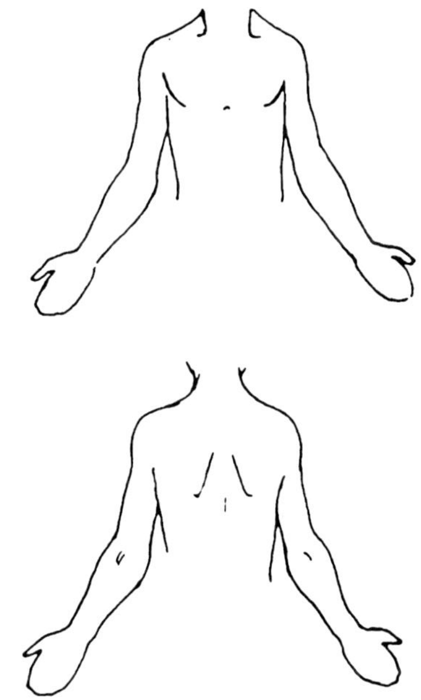

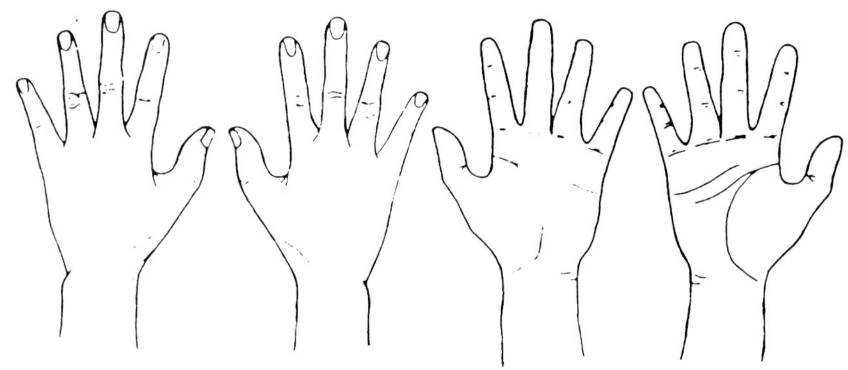

Trunk	Grade	R	L
59) kyphosis			
60) scoliosis			
61) lordosis			
62) breast, nipple, areola			
63) abdominal scar			
64) other			
Perineum			
65) penile scars/deformities			
66) vulvar scars/deformities			
67) perineal contractures			
68) anal stenosis			
69) anal incompetence/prolapse			
70) other			
Hip and Thigh			
71) contractures (l)			
72) amputation/stump			
73) other			
Knee and Leg			
74) contractures (m)			
75) unstable skin			
76) osteomyelitis			
77) amputation/stump			
78) other			
Ankle and Foot			
79) equinus			
80) varus			
81) valgus			
82) cavus			
83) calcaneus			
84) unstable heel pad			
85) toe hyperextension			
86) toe hyperflexion			
87) toe/foot amputation			
88) other			

(l-m) Please refer to the back for instructions

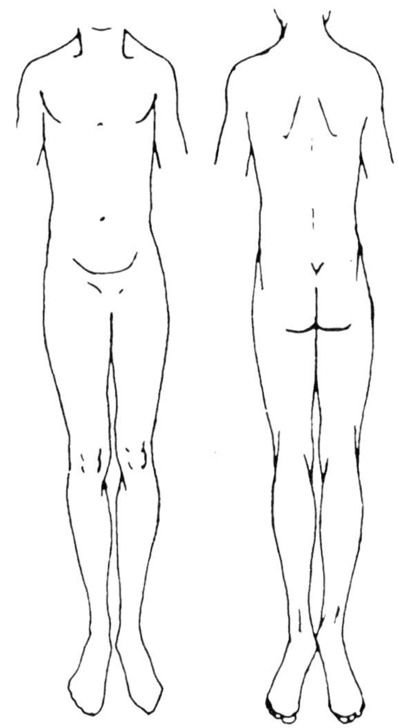

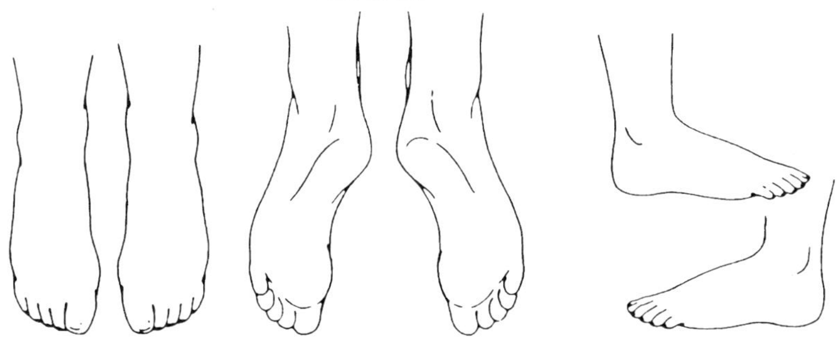

INSTRUCTIONS

I) Identify the patient's abnormality and check the appropriate box (R) for right and (L) for left or both for single or midline structures. Use the empty space in each line to write additional information.

II) Use the diagram to draw the observed abnormality when needed for more detailed information.

III) Signal each abnormality in the diagram by writing the corresponding number.

IV) Grade each observed abnormality as (S) for severe, (Mo) for moderate, and (Mi) for mild.

V) Some items have specific grading criterial such as:

(a) Shoulder abduction (normal ROM 0 to 180 degrees)
Severe: 0 to 60 degrees
Moderate: 0 to 120 degrees
Mild: 0 to 180 degrees

(b) Elbow flexion (normal ROM 0 to 150 degrees)
Severe: 100 to 150 degrees
Moderate: 50 to 100 degrees
Mild: 0 to 50 degrees

(c) Elbow extension (normal ROM 150 to 0 degrees)
Severe: 0 to 50 degrees
Moderate: 0 to 100 degrees
Mild: 0 to 150 degrees

(d) Wrist flexion (normal ROM 0 to 70 degrees)
Severe: 60 degrees or more
Moderate: 60 to 20 degrees
Mild: 20 to -20 degrees

(e) Wrist extension (normal ROM 0 to -60 degrees)
Severe: -60 degrees or more
Moderate: -60 to -40 degrees
Mild: -40 to -20 degrees

(f) Wrist ulnar deviation (normal ROM 0 to 30 degrees)
Severe: 30 degrees or more

(g) Wrist radial deviation (normal ROM 0 to 20 degrees)
Severe: 20 degrees or more

(h) MP flexion (normal ROM 0 to 90 degrees)
Severe: 90 degrees or more
Moderate: 90 to 45 degrees
Mild: 45 to 0 degrees

(i) MP extension (normal ROM 90 to 0 degrees)
Severe: less than 0 degrees

(j) Thumb CMC
Severe: no opposition or pinch possible
Moderate: lateral pinch only
Mild: opposition present

(k) Thumb MP and IP
Severe: no opposition or pinch possible
Moderate: laters. pinch only
Mild: opposition present

(l) Hip
Severe: affects gait and posture
Moderate: affects sporting activities
Mild: no functional impairment

(m) Knee
Severe: affects gait and posture
Moderate: affects sporting activity
Mild: no functional impairment

Fig. 46.1 Inventory form for potential reconstructive needs.

hospitalization. In cases of fascial excision, subcutaneous fat layers in the injured area are also removed. Fat stores are further depleted in providing energy for the process of gluconeogenesis from existing protein stores for dietary supply.

In 1990, Rutan *et al.* demonstrated a dampened growth curve for both height and weight in male and female patients who had sustained major thermal injury.[9] The growth velocities were delayed up to 3 years after burn injury. Even after the return to normal growth velocities, the burned patients lagged behind age- and sex-matched peers. The implication of this growth delay and its impact on the psychological development of children has yet to be elucidated.

Breast Development

It is clear that further longitudinal assessment of soft tissue development is needed. Female patients who sustain significant injuries to the anterior chest wall ultimately wonder about breast development especially if the nipple areola complex has been injured. In 1988, McCauley *et al.* documented the growth and development of 28 burned patients with significant injury to the anterior chest wall involving the nipple areola complex.[10] The mean age at the time of the burn injury was 5.9 years with a mean follow-up of nearly 9 years. At this time, patients were treated with either epluchage or delayed tangential excision. This study provided the first longitudinal assessment of breast development in adolescents with burns. It also documents that, with conservative management of tissue during the acute phase of injury, chances of breast development are optimized. Second, even with loss of the nipple areola complex, the underlying breast bud is rarely injured. Such studies bring to light the impact of acute management on subsequent growth and development of children and clearly demonstrate the need for acute burn surgeons to preserve tissue in critical areas.

Integument

Hypertrophic scar formation and wound contracture are the sequelae of burn wound healing. Compression therapy which was popularized in the late 1960s and early 1970s to minimize scarring and contractures continues to be the mainstay for the non-surgical management of hypertrophic scar formation.[11–13] The lack of clear-cut objective parameters to characterize hypertrophic scars clinically has hampered our ability to be more objective in the use of compression therapy. Documentation of the use of sheet grafts versus 2:1 or 3:1 skin grafts on the subsequent growth and development of children is seriously lacking in the literature. Although it is believed that the use of mesh grafts have an impact on the frequency of wound scar contracture, this has not been objectively documented in the literature. The medical and surgical management of hypertrophic scar formation has been detailed in another chapter of this text.

Truncal Burns

The long-term effects of circumferential truncal burns on growth and development have so far been ignored. Problems associated with postprandial discomfort in patients with extensive abdominal burns with contractures are easily relieved with incisional releases and the addition of skin grafts. Long-term documentation of the effects of circumferential truncal burns on pregnant women have only recently been published.[14] McCauley *et al.* documented the absence of prenatal complications associated with mature circumferential truncal burns. In seven patients with 14 pregnancies, the mean time of follow-up from burn injury to the first pregnancy was more than 12 years.

Skeletal Changes

There is, indeed, a paucity of studies which document growth and development of burned children in the head/neck region. In 1991, McCauley *et al.* documented significant delay in the development of the mandible in children who had been burned in the head/neck region and required compression therapy to assist in the maturation of burn scars or skin grafted areas.[15] Delineation of the contributions of the burn itself versus the compression therapy required to assist maturation could not clearly be determined. Such study does, however, bring to light the subsequent impact of delay in bone growth which is associated with thermal injury.

Skeletal changes associated with burn injury have been reported by a number of authors. Bone atrophy or osteoporosis has been reported by Evans *et al.* in more than 900 children treated at the Shriners Burns Institute in Galveston, Texas in 1966.[16] Bhattachara *et al.* have documented that smaller bones and joints were more prone to damage than larger joints. Joint contractures and joint dislocations were noted in 10% of the patient population.[17] Jackson *et al.* reported growth arrest due to epiphyseal plate injury in burned children.[18] Amputation was required in cases where inadequate blood supply for limb survival or irreparable nerve damage were documented. Klein *et al.* subsequently documented significant decrease in bone density in children who sustained at least 40% body surface area burns.[19] Such documentation occurred years after patients had recovered from the initial insult.

Heterotopic Bone Formation

Heterotopic bone formation has been reported by a number of authors. Indeed, decrease in joint mobility can develop from heterotopic bone later in acute hospitalization or during recovery. Although the etiology of heterotopic bone formation is unknown, it is known that it does not necessarily occur over burned tissue. The incidence of heterotopic bone formation varies between 1% in a retrospective study to 23% in a prospective study.[18,20,21] It is clear that we lack knowledge not only about factors which influence the development of heterotopic bone but also remain ignorant of factors which contribute to the successful surgical management and postoperative care of these patients. Consequently, surgical outcome tends to be less than optimal, and recurrence rates remain high.

Musculoskeletal Development

Joint contractures remain the most frequent muscular skeletal complication in children. Bhattachara noted a 10% incidence in a group of 50% patients.[17] Sixty-four percent of these contractures were in patients younger than 10 years of age. Jones *et al.* noted that patients with tangential excision down to fat had better joint mobility at 1 year post-injury than did those with excisions to fascia.[22] Subsequent verification of the study by other investigators is absent from the surgical literature. It is apparent that in children requiring fascial excision, the development of contour deformities secondary to hypertrophy of the remaining fat cells is not the only problem. Marked differences in muscular development in the upper and lower extremities attest to the previously unrecognized importance of adequate soft tissue coverage for muscular development. The exact mechanisms responsible for arrested muscle growth are poorly defined.

Cardiopulmonary Reserve

Patients who sustain inhalation injury have an increase in morbidity and mortality; however, the patients who survive such a pulmonary insult and proceed to recover from their burns show significant abnormalities in cardiopulmonary reserve.[23–25] Exercise testing has been used in the evaluation of treatment of healthy and ill patients in order to assess ability to tolerate various activities. Although some patients temporarily suffer the effects of disuse atrophy secondary to prolonged periods of immobilization, muscle atrophy becomes of less importance in the detection of cardiopulmonary compromise at a later date. Cisar, in 1986, found that 10 adult burned patients gained normal cardiopulmonary fitness following discharge. In these patients, the mean total body surface area burn was 32.4%.[26] Subsequent studies by Mlcak *et al.* have documented significant cardiopulmonary compromise in exercise tolerance in burned children with more than 40% total body surface area burn.[23] The effects of chronic pulmonary disease on delayed growth and development is well documented in the literature in patients with chronic illnesses. A similar problem, however, for burned patients is not well documented. Desai *et al.* documented greater demands of the respiratory system in burned children with inhalation injury when subjected to treadmill stress testing as compared to their counterparts without inhalation injury.[24] An earlier study by Mlcak *et al.* demonstrated that in 40 children with a mean total body surface area burn of 44%, exercise testing revealed an increased V_D/V_T ratio consistent with uneven ventilation/perfusion relationships 2.5 years after injury.[25] Further ventilatory limitations to exercise were documented when resting spirometry and lung volumes showed a 45% incidence of abnormal lung function in patients more than 2 years after injury. Clearly, cardiopulmonary compromise is an important parameter in the long-term well-being of patients. Yet, only recently has severe cardiopulmonary disease been recognized. Consequently, the relationship of the severity of this problem to associated growth delays in burned children has yet to be scrutinized.

Psychosocial Development

Current literature about the longitudinal sequelae of psychosocial development of patients with burn scars is scarce compared to reports of other aspects of burn care.[5–8] The paucity of objective empirical data from clinical series demonstrates the lack of importance which has been attached to the psychosocial development of burned children. To embrace the whole person concept of burn care, psychosocial development must be an integral part of burn care.

Case studies, anecdotal reports, and the lack of control groups of patients for comparisons make the data regarding psychosocial adjustment difficult to interpret. Some investigators have suggested that facial disfigurements leads to greater problems in psychosocial adjustment when compared to burns in other areas; additionally, female patients appeared to do less well when compared to their male counterparts.[27,28] A later study by Abdullah *et al.* reveals that pediatric burned patients with visible scars may harbor grave self-deprecating feelings while they superficially appear to be adjusting to their injuries quite well. In this study, male patients did not appear as well adjusted as their female counterparts. Confusion in the literature is likely to continue until more objective studies with longitudinal outcome indices are defined.

Immunology

Although virtually no data exist on the longitudinal assessment of immunological function in burn patients, the literature is replete with information attesting to the loss of immune function acutely in patients with major thermal injury. Nineteen patients who were immunized up to 2 years before sustaining major thermal injuries were studied for 2 years after injury. Unpublished data from this group suggested that, indeed, no differences in immune function could be detected in this group as compared with normal control individuals.[29]

Summary

Clearly, the longitudinal effects of burn injury with an emphasis on 'whole person' rehabilitation is in a stage of infancy. As more studies documenting the prolonged effects of burn injury on patient growth and development continue, the physiological and psychosocial alterations associated with burn victims will ultimately foster improved methods of overall patient care. Better care is the goal, so further longitudinal studies are important.

References

1. Burke J F, Bandoc C C, Quinby W C. Primary excision and immediate grafting: a method for shortening illness. *J Trauma* 1979; **14:** 389–95.

2. Herndon D N, Parks D H. Comparison of serial debridement and autografting and early massive excision with cadaveric skin overlay in the treatment of large burns in children. *J Trauma* 1986; **26:** 149–52.

3. Herndon D N, Barrow R E, Rutan R L, Rutan T C, Desai M H, Abston S. A comparison of conservative versus early excisional therapies in severely burned patients. *Ann Surg* 1989; **209:** 547–53.

4. Brou J A, Robson M C, McCauley R L, *et al.* Inventory of potential reconstructive needs in the patient with burns. *J Burn Care Rehabil* 1989; **10:** 550–60.

5. Abdullah A, Blakeney P, Hunt R, *et al.* Visible scars and self esteem in pediatric burn survivors. *J Burn Care Rehabil* 1994; **15:** 164–68.

6. Blakeney P, Herndon D N, Desai M H, Beard S, Wales-Seale P. Long-term psychosocial adjustment following burn injury. *J Burn Care Rehabil* 1988; **9:** 661–5.

7. Herndon D N, LeMaster J, Beard S, *et al.* The quality of life after major thermal injury in children: analysis of 12 survivors with >80% total body–70% third degree burns. *J Trauma* 1986; **8:** 609–19.

8. Wright L, Fulwiler R. Long-range emotional sequelae of burns: effects on children and their mothers. *Pediatr Res* 1974; **8:** 931–4.

9. Rutan R L, Herndon D N. Growth delay in post-burn pediatric patients. *Arch Surg* 1990; **125:** 392–5.

10. McCauley R L, Beraja V, Rutan R L, *et al.* Longitudinal assessment of breast development in adolescent female patients with burns involving the nipple areola complex. *Plast Reconstr Surg* 1989; **83:** 676–80.

11. Larson D L, Abston S, Evans E B, Dobrkosky M, Linares H A. Techniques for decreasing scar formation and contractures in the burned patient. *J Trauma* 1971; **11:** 807–23.

12. Kloti J, Pochon J P. Long-term therapy of second and third degree burns in children using Jobst compression suits. *Scand J Plast Reconstr Surg* 1979; **13:** 163–8.

13. Robertson J C, Drett J E, Hodgson B, Druett J. Pressure therapy for hypertrophic scarring: preliminary communication. *J R Soc Med* 1980; **73:** 348–54.

14. McCauley R L, Stenberg B A, Phillips L G, Blackwell S J, Robson M C. Long-term assessment of the effects of circumferential truncal burns in pediatric patients on subsequent pregnancies. *J Burn Care Rehabil* 1991; **12:** 51–3.

15. McCauley R L, Fairleigh J F, Robson M C, Herndon D N. Effects of facial burns on facial growth in children: preliminary report. *Proc Am Burn Assoc* 1991; **23:** 137.

16. Evans E B. Orthopedic measures in the treatment of severe burns. *J Bone Joint Surg [Am]* 1966; **48:** 643–9.

17. Bhattachara V, Singh J, Sinha F, *et al.* Macroradiographic study of post-burn contracture of limbs. *Burns* 1984; **10:** 379–87.

18. Jackson D M. Destructive burns some orthopedic complications. *Burns* 1981; **7:** 105–22.

19. Klein G L, Herndon D N, Rutan T C, *et al.* Long-term reduction in bone mass and increased fracture risk in children following severe burns. *J Bone Miner Res* 1993; S232.

20. Heslop J. Heterotopic periarticular ossification in burns. *Burns* 1982; **8:** 436–8.

21. Schiele H. Radiographic changes in burns of the upper extremity. *Diagn Radiol* 1972; **104:** 13–17.

22. Jones T, McDonald S, Deitch E. Effect of graft bed on long term functional results of extremity skin grafts. *J Burn Care Rehab* 1988; **9:** 72–4.

23. Mlcak R P, Desai M H, Carp S S, *et al.* Increased physiological dead space/tidal volume ratio during exercise in burned children. *Proc Am Burn Assoc* 1991; **23:** 24.

24. Desai M H, Mlcak R P, Robinson G, *et al.* Does inhalation injury limit exercise endurance in children convalescing from thermal injury? *J Burn Care Rehabil* 1993; **14:** 16–20.

25. Mlcak R P, Desai M H, Robinson E, *et al.* Cardiopulmonary stress testing in children convalescing from thermal injury. *Proc Am Burn Assoc* 1991; **23:** 161.

26. Cisar C, Staley M, Gillespie R. Physical fitness adaptations of the severe burn patient after discharge. *Proc Am Burn Assoc* 1986; **25:** 23.

27. Goldberg R T. Adjustment of children with invisible and visible handicaps: congenital heart disease and facial burns. *J Counsel Psychol* 1979; **21:** 428–32.

28. Blades B, Mellis N, Munster A M. A burn specific health scale. *J Trauma* 1982; **22:** 872–5.

29. Unpublished data.

CHAPTER FORTY-SEVEN

Overview of Burn Reconstruction

Martin C. Robson

Introduction

'Beauty is only skin deep.' The very denial in this statement emphasizes the importance of appearance in society today.[1] Body image is a basic part of personal identity. It incorporates physical characteristics with an individual's attitude toward these characteristics. It emanates from both conscious and subconscious sources.[2] These sources are established by perceived standards of how people look and what is normal. Thus, the final outcome is determined separately by a patient and by society as a whole.[2] In the integumentary system involved in burn injury, even though the processes of wound healing have apparently progressed normally, proliferative scar formation may result. This can occur even though a physician understands normal wound healing and performs all therapeutic maneuvers correctly. Still, too much collagen is laid down with the end result of proliferative scar formation.

Wound Healing

What causes normal wound contraction to result in contracture and hypertrophic scars so frequently seen after burns? It appears that the normal wound healing process begins and seems to continue. It does not shut off, so normal wound contraction becomes contracture and ends with a hypertrophic scar. It is important to remember that contraction is a normal part of the physiology of wound healing; therefore, it is neither possible nor desirous to prevent wound contraction.[3] On the other hand, one may be able to prevent the abnormal continuation of wound contraction which leads to a contracture and deformity. One way to reduce contracture and hypertrophic scar formation is to minimize the time in which normal wound contraction takes place. We can reduce the amount and the intensity of the inflammation. In the burn wound, we can excise and close the wound very early so as to decrease the inflammatory phase.[3] It is desirable to reduce this time because it has been demonstrated that hypertrophic scars are related to the amount of time that a wound is allowed to remain in the inflammatory phase before it moves into the proliferative phase.[4] The inflammatory phase should be reduced not only in wounds healing by secondary or tertiary intention but also in those healing by primary intention. This emphasizes the need for successful skin graft 'take' at the time of initial excision and grafting during the acute care of the burn wound.[3] Another technique for decreasing hypertrophic scar is to minimize or eliminate a deficiency of tissue. In closing burn wounds initially, it is important to make sure that an adequate amount of tissue is placed. Whenever possible, this means using sheet grafts instead of meshed grafts or postage stamp grafts.[3] Despite aggressive and improved acute care, healing of burns too frequently leaves residual deformities. Wound contraction, a normal and necessary part of healing, promotes distortions which produce visual disfigurement and functional limitation. A wound continues to contract until it achieves a comfortable position or an equal opposing force.[5]

Reconstruction

All members of a burn team should participate in the overall reconstruction planning; otherwise, reconstruction degenerates into a series of technical exercises which can achieve only a limited goal.[2,6] Psychological support, splinting, exercises, and pressure garments all affect the surgical result. A patient must also be included in this planning and understand the surgical objectives.[7] Dreams of miracles too often overshadow realistic goals and expectations. Along with other members of a burn team, a physician encourages a patient through the difficult acute period. This can lead to a false optimism on a patient's part because he or she assumes that once this initial period is conquered, everything will return to 'normal'. Even the most honest physician implicitly encourages a patient through this period while privately thinking that the final result will be far from satisfactory. Thus, a patient often will wonder, 'When does the plastic surgery begin?'[8] Preoperative discussion minimizes postsurgical depression by improving patient acceptance. This ultimately helps integrate a patient back into society.

Timing of Reconstruction

If possible, reconstruction is postponed until wounds have matured.[3] Frequently, postponement is not possible if the deformity is progressive or causing a functional deficit. In these cases, reconstruction is initiated early. An example of this might be a severe ectropion of the eyelid. This early reconstruction is usually undertaken to correct significant tissue deficiency. In planning, appreciation of this deficiency is important. In fact, the diagnosis of a true tissue deficiency may be the most important step in reconstruction.[2]

The surgical plan involves recreating the initial tissue loss and then adding appropriate tissue.

Priorities for Reconstruction

Reconstruction proceeds stepwise, with priorities given to certain anatomical areas. The first priority must always remain the prevention of deformity.[2,3] Obviously, this receives great emphasis in acute therapy, but the importance of postoperative splinting or pressure garments must be remembered after each reconstructive procedure.[4] Lack of attention to these details jeopardizes optimal functional and aesthetic results. The next priority is reconstruction of active function.[2,3] The final priority is restoration of passive function.

Although functional reconstruction is afforded the first operative priority, resurfacing procedures of lesser priority may be combined with these functional reconstructions.[2,3] What should be reconstructed becomes clear when one considers a patient as a whole.[9] Confusion occurs when an inexperienced surgeon views a contracture amenable to flap reconstruction as an isolated event unrelated to age, life style, occupation, and physical demands.[3] The complications of a major burn often require multiple procedures and can take several years to reconstruct. A surgeon should document every deformity with possible surgical alternatives and then assign priorities. Brou *et al.* designed a very useful inventory (illustrated in Chapter 46) for potential reconstructive needs to allow a more systematic evaluation guided by body regions, divided into anatomical units.[10] All the somatic abnormalities caused by burns are included, as well as a system for grading severity of the defect. Additionally, a donor tissue surveillance form has been reported to further coordinate a systematic method of management.[11] A priority rating for use of the available tissue ranges from function salvage, through improvement of function, to cosmetic. Restoring function, obviously, is a higher priority than improving cosmetic appearance; however, cosmetic reconstruction will also help a patient improve his/her activities of daily living, improve function, or return to a job.

After the reconstructive needs are prioritized according to anatomical body region and functional severity in order to compile a priority list of reconstructive needs, the list is matched with the available donor tissue sites and a preliminary operative strategy is formulated. Then a patient, parent, surgeon priority survey is consulted to match desires with feasibilities.[7] Once the priorities of reconstruction have been determined, multiple diverse techniques are available. Simplicity is often a virtue.[3]

Closures

Whenever possible, closure of wounds by direct approximation and primary healing is desirable, whether dealing with a primary injury or a reconstructive procedure. Often, however, defects exist which cannot be directly sutured. In such situations, grafts or flaps are required. Traditionally, closure by grafts is considered first; then the possibilities of local flaps and distant flaps are evaluated, choosing the simplest method which will produce the desired result. In burn reconstruction, the Z-plasty, which is in reality two random flaps, often is considered before a skin graft.[3] More recently, with better understanding of the safety of axial and musculocutaneous flaps, these have assumed a more prominent place in the hierarchy of techniques. In addition, reconstruction by the free tissue transfer using microvascular anastomosis has become increasingly common. Skin expansion techniques are also rapidly gaining popularity. It is clear that direct closure, grafts, flaps, free tissue transfer, and tissue expansion comprise the armamentarium of the reconstructive burn surgeon; each must be understood to be properly utilized.

Direct closure

Direct closure in burn reconstruction is the simplest form of scar revision following excision of the scar.[3] Scar formation is the fundamental phenomenon of wound healing in most human tissues, including the dermis. An understanding of normal wound healing and insight into the factors which make a scar less than optimal are both essential to planning scar revisions.[3] All scars proceed through the inflammatory, proliferative, and maturation phases of wound healing, and will therefore require time to reach their final appearance. A normal scar which appears hypertrophic at 6 weeks may be quite satisfactory after 6–12 months. If the mature scar is not satisfactory, application of the basic principles of reconstruction can then be expected to result in an improved scar.

The most common reasons for unacceptable scars are an unfavorable direction of the original wound in regard to the normal lines of skin tension, failure of proper dermal approximation, and a pathologic extension of normal wound contraction which results in a contracture.[3,12] If the excessive scarring was due to an improper direction of the original wound, the wound direction should be realigned so that the new scar will fall in the lines of minimum resting tension.[3] These lines, in general, will run perpendicularly to the fibers of the underlying muscle. Realigning a scar to the minimum resting skin tension lines will often allow it to become almost invisible. When a wound is reapproximated, the dermis is carefully approximated with an inverted suture. This supports the tissues until the tensile strength of the new collagen is sufficient to prevent spreading of the scar. Although a degree of wound contraction is a normal part of wound healing, contracture is preventable. Placing the direction along the lines of minimum resting tension will greatly help.

The Z-plasty technique

The line of contracture can be lengthened either by excising the old scar as an ellipse, thus elongating each side of the wound slightly, or by adding tissue by introducing a Z-plasty, skin graft, or a flap. This is a technique by which two triangular skin flaps are interchanged in position to gain length along a scar or skin fold at the expense of the adjacent tissues.[3] It is used in burn reconstruction so frequently that it almost can be viewed as an extension of the direct closure technique. Understanding the geometry and principles of the Z-plasty allows the reconstructive surgeon to lengthen a contracted scar, obliterate a web contracture, add to an area of deficient tissue and change the direction of the scar, thus giving him an important technique of scar revision.[13] The incisions are designed with three lines of equal length: a central member, and two limbs extending from its ends to resemble the letter Z or its mirror image (**Figure 47.1**). The angles formed by the limbs with the central member can vary depending on the desired final result; angles of 60° can be shown mathematically to give the maximum practical increase in length. When the flaps are mobilized and transposed, the flap bases lie along the line formerly occupied by the central member, resulting in a gain in length. This gain in length is approximately 25% for 30 degree angles, 50% for 45 degree angles and 75% for 60 degree angles.

Skin Grafting

When reconstructive needs are such that excision and direct closure are insufficient, skin grafting is the next most common technique.[3]

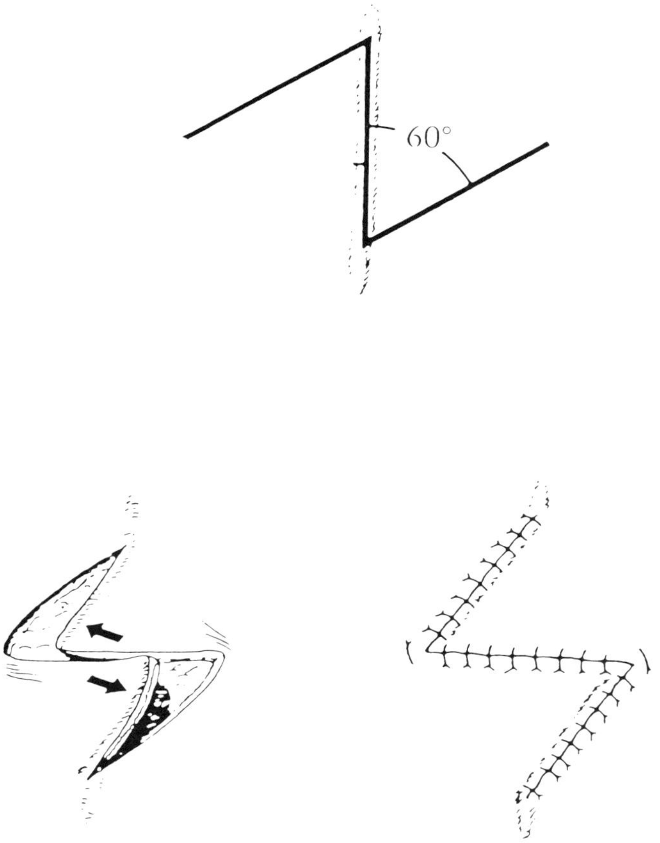

Fig. 47.1 Z-plasty design, transposition, and inset.

When a scar contracture is incised or excised, the wound edges will retract widely and the tissue deficiency will become apparent. A split-thickness or full-thickness skin graft will replace the deficiency and improve the scar. Skin grafts are also useful for scar revision in areas where previous scars or skin grafts are of poor quality or have a poor color match.[3] Following excision, a carefully tailored full-thickness skin graft will improve quality and color match. Skin grafts remain the mainstay of burn reconstruction. These grafts may be of the split-thickness, full-thickness, or composite variety depending on the specific needs of a patient. A split-thickness or partial-thickness skin graft includes epidermis and part of the dermis. A full-thickness skin graft includes epidermis and full thickness of the dermis. A composite graft, although not strictly a skin graft, includes the full thickness of the skin and a portion of the underlying tissue such as subcutaneous tissue, muscle, cartilage, or bone.[12]

Split-thickness skin grafts

These can vary in thickness depending on the amount of dermis included. Thin split-thickness grafts contain little dermis and are cut only to the level of the subpapillary vascular plexus. Medium split-thickness grafts contain most of the dermis, approximately three-quarters thickness. The thickness of the graft is relative, depending on the age and sex of a patient and the region of the body of the donor site.[12] Clinically, the translucency of the graft and the pattern of bleeding from the donor site help determine the thickness. The thicker the graft, the more opaque it becomes. A thinner translucent graft will come from a bed with many closely spaced, fine, bleeding points of the subpapillary plexus.[12] For thicker grafts a deeper layer is cut, leaving a bed with fewer larger vessels from the dermal plexus. Split-thickness skin grafts are best used to cover large denuded surfaces occurring after contracture release or excision of unacceptable burn scar (**Figure 47.2**). They are also used when recurrent wound contraction is of lesser consequence. A great advantage of these grafts is that their donor sites heal themselves from the remaining skin appendages, such as hair follicles and sweat glands.[12] This allows harvesting of the grafts of almost any size needed to close a defect. They can also be harvested from previously healed partial-thickness burn wounds or donor sites.

The thickness of a graft is a matter of preference of the surgeon, but several guidelines are helpful. The thinner the graft, the higher is the chance of survival on the recipient site. Thinner grafts have fewer cells to be nourished prior to establishment of the blood supply. Also, since the undersurface of the graft has a higher density of vessels, vascular ingrowth can proceed more rapidly. Further, the donor site of a thin split-thickness graft will epithelialize more rapidly. Thin grafts have disadvantages which must be considered by the reconstructive surgeon. The thinner the graft, the more the interface of the fibrous tissue between the graft and the recipient site will contract during the maturation phase. Therefore, the wound beneath a thicker split-thickness graft will contract minimally, if at all. Thicker grafts will more closely resemble their donor site in color, texture, and hair distribution.

Full-thickness skin grafts

These tend to resemble normal skin better than split-thickness grafts. They provide more padding, a better color match, a more

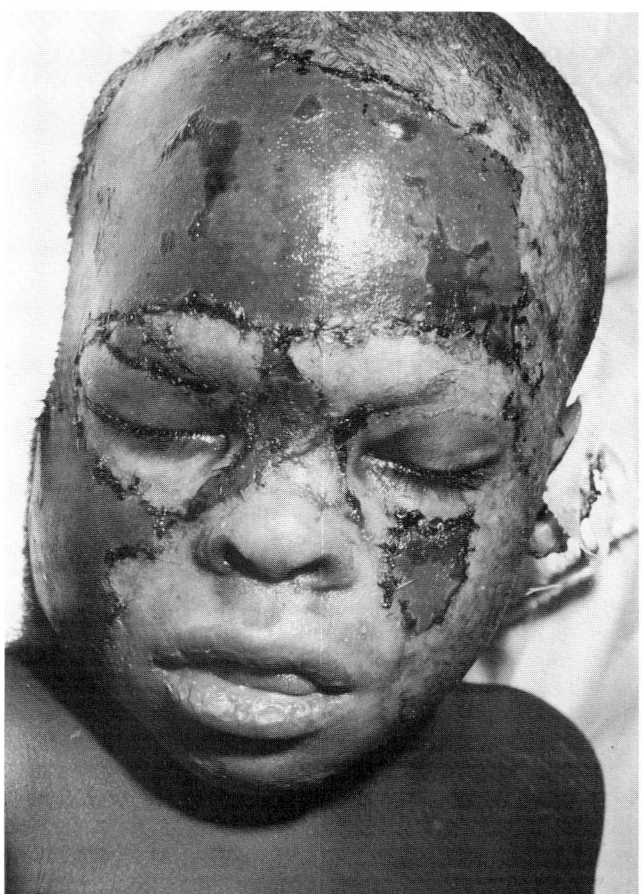

Fig. 47.2 Split-thickness graft to resurface areas of unacceptable scar.

nearly normal hair pattern, and inhibit wound contraction in the recipient site.[12] Because they require near ideal conditions for survival, they must be placed in a vascular recipient site. Their thickness requires more nourishment prior to the establishment of vascular integrity. The major disadvantage of full-thickness grafts is that their donor sites cannot heal spontaneously since no skin appendages are left behind. Therefore, the size of the graft is limited to dimensions which will allow primary closure of the donor site. If this practice is not followed, the donor site from a large full-thickness graft must be closed by a split-thickness graft.[12] Only rarely is this approach used for burn reconstruction, since donor sites are often limited in a burned patient.

Composite graft

Occasionally, a defect requires underlying supportive tissue as well as skin. Most frequently this is reconstructed with a flap, which will be discussed later. If the area is small enough, a skin graft containing underlying tissue (a composite graft) can be used. The risk of non-vascularization of this type of graft severely limits its usefulness. If no portion of the graft is more than 0.5 cm from the wound edge, the survival rate is good.[12] The blood supply to a composite graft comes through its margin instead of its base, which accounts for the strict size limitation. Despite these limitations, the composite graft may be the first choice in reconstruction of areas of the face such as the nasal alae.

Choice of donor site

When skin grafts of any variety are chosen for reconstruction, choosing a donor site requires some thought. The color, texture, vascularity, thickness, and hair-bearing nature of the skin varies from one area of the body to another.[3] The nearer the donor site is to the recipient site, the more closely the skin will match. Skin grafts to the face taken from above the clavicle tend to retain their natural blush state, whereas those from below the clavicle tend to take on a yellowish or brownish hue.[3,12] The donor site of a split-thickness skin graft is like a partial-thickness burn or deep abrasion. It must be protected from trauma and bacteria in order to epithelialize satisfactorily.

Postoperative care

Finally, postoperative care of a skin graft is as important as the grafting operative technique. The graft should be inspected by 48–72 hours after placement, using an aseptic technique. Any fluid found beneath the graft should be aspirated or evacuated by making a small nick in the graft to express it.[12] If fluid is not removed by 96 hours, evidence has been presented that the graft epithelializes on the undersurface, preventing satisfactory vascularization.[14] The graft must be immobilized and protected for at least 5–7 days. Edema should be prevented in the recipient bed for 4–6 months. This becomes of great practical importance in grafts applied to the lower extremity. In this situation, support such as an elastic stocking is required to overcome the hydrostatic pressure until the collagen of the graft is totally incorporated into the extremity.

Reconstruction Using Flaps

Burn deformities and defects are best corrected by excision, primary approximation, or Z-plasty whenever possible. Skin grafting is usually thought of as a second choice. Cases do exist, however, where skin grafting is either not possible or not desirable. The area in need of reconstruction, such as bare bone or tendon, may lack the vascularity necessary to support a skin graft. Tissue to reconstruct these defects must carry its own blood supply. When two surfaces must be reconstructed, an inherent blood supply is obviously necessary.[3] An example of this is the full-thickness loss of an eyelid or lip. There are also situations where a skin graft could theoretically close a defect but would not serve the final purpose as well as vascularized composite tissue.[3] This occurs when deeper tissue is desired for contouring but the defect is too large for a composite graft or when padding is required over a bony prominence. Occasionally a skin graft can correct a deformity or close a defect but is not the most desirable type of reconstruction. If future surgery will be necessary beneath a reconstructed area; if near-normal sensation is required of a reconstructed tissue, or if a hoped-for esthetic result cannot be achieved by a skin graft, then a skin graft is not the best choice. In all of these circumstances, reconstruction can be better effected by a flap.

A skin flap by definition is a segment of skin and subcutaneous tissue which is transferred from its original position on the body to another site while maintaining its own inherent vasculature for nourishment.[12] In some cases of burn reconstruction, deeper tissue such as muscle or bone is carried with the skin flap. All flaps have a ‘pedicle’, which is their vascular base of attachment.

In order to understand skin flaps, a thorough knowledge of their blood supply is necessary. There are two main anatomical patterns of blood supply to the skin. The first of these depends upon vessels from the aorta or its major branches which lie deep to the muscles.[12] Perforating branches through the muscles along fascial planes become the musculocutaneous and fasciocutaneous arteries and terminate by supplying the dermal–subdermal plexus of the skin. This vascular pattern forms the predominant blood supply to the skin. In the other anatomical pattern, vessels from the aorta or its major branches form direct cutaneous arteries which lie superficial to the muscles and parallel to the skin for long distances and supply the dermal–subdermal plexus directly.[12]

Cutaneous or random pattern flap

This is a flap based on a blood supply from musculocutaneous arteries penetrating perpendicularly into its base, supplying the length of the flap through the longitudinal dermal–subdermal plexus[12] (**Figure 47.3**). The surviving length of this flap is limited by the perfusion pressure in the vessels. Since these flaps lack an anatomically recognized arteriovenous system, they have strict length limitations. The length cannot survive beyond the blood supply of the dermal–subdermal anastomotic plexus perfused by the perforating musculocutaneous arteries without special conditioning of the flap.[12]

Cutaneous pattern flaps can be subclassified as local flaps or flaps from a distance. The Z-plasty and its modifications are literally two or more interpolated cutaneous flaps; however, beyond the Z-plasty, they have lost their great utility for burn reconstruction except for the face. Local flaps in the face are still excellent if there is an adjacent unscarred area to serve as donor tissue. Although great amounts of tissue were once moved from far distant sites on the body by the ingenious use of tubed pedicles and delay procedures, those methods have been almost totally supplanted by free flaps and skin expansion.

Axial or arterial pattern flap

This receives its blood supply from a direct cutaneous artery which enters its base and runs longitudinally within the flap.[12] (**Figure**

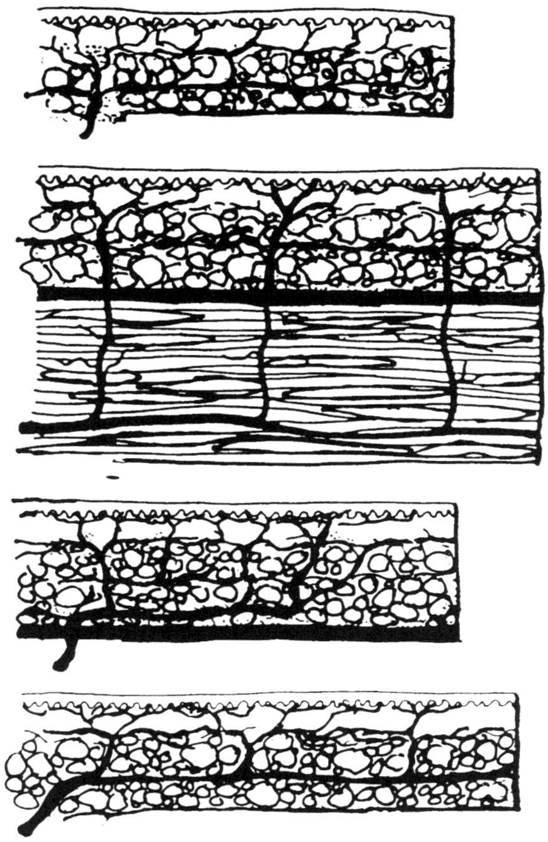

Fig. 47.3 A random flap (top) has a muscular perforator artery, cut from the underlying muscle. If the muscle is included (second from top), the flap is musculocutaneous and brings its own blood supply. The length of an arterial flap (bottom two figures) is dictated by the length of the artery.

47.3). The length of the flap is determined by the length of the direct cutaneous artery supplying it, plus an additional random portion at the termination of the artery supplied by the dermal–subdermal plexus. Since axial or arterial pattern flaps are supplied by a specific longitudinal arteriovenous network, traditional length : base width ratios play no role in the designing of the flap. In fact, no skin is necessary at the base of these flaps, and the artery and vein alone can serve as the base of pedicle.[12] This type of axial flap is called an island flap. Often, the nerve is preserved with the vessels in the pedicle, making it a neurovascular island flap.

Axial flaps can be very useful in reconstructive surgery for burns. The key to their use is an exact knowledge of the anatomy of the direct cutaneous arteries. Since the skin is unimportant in the flap's base, the pivot point becomes the artery itself and the arc of the flap can be 360 degrees within the reach of the artery.[12] This type of flap is particularly useful for reconstruction of facial parts such as the ears and eyebrows, and for the upper extremity. The recent description of the radial forearm flap is a classic example of the island neurovascular island pedicle flap.

Musculocutaneous or myocutaneous flap

This third type of flap has been described more recently. If a muscle is adequately supplied with blood flow through a single dominant vascular pedicle, the muscle with its overlying skin and subcutaneous tissue can be raised as a flap and transferred as a unit on the segmental vascular pedicle[12] (**Figure 47.3**). In this case, a large area of skin can be transferred on multiple muscle perforators which are fed by the pedicle without the limitations imposed on cutaneous or random flaps. Likewise, a fasciocutaneous flap may be raised by including the vascularized fascia in the same way. This type of flap can be quite helpful to reconstruct patients with massive burns where most of the body surface consists of healed skin grafts over fascially excised muscles. Raising the muscle as the blood supply to the previously applied skin graft obviates the lack of cutaneous or axial vessels in the skin.

Free flap

Any of the types of flaps can be transferred by dividing its vascular pedicle and reanastomosing it in a recipient site.[12] When this technique is used, the flap is classified as a free flap. A free flap is not considered a graft since vascularization and nourishment is immediately reestablished through the pedicle. With the advent of microvascular surgical techniques in the late 1950s, it became feasible to anastomose arteries and veins of less than 1 mm diameter.[3,15] Therefore, experimental transfers of skin flaps were performed in the 1960s; by 1973 the first successful free flap was reported in a human.[15]

Microsurgical technique, understanding of flap physiology, and the definition of skin territories have rapidly improved over the past 20 years. This has allowed the almost routine successful free transfer of composite tissue from distant areas.[3] Free flaps have great utility in cases involving a burned patient in which local tissue is not available because it is included in the area of injury. In addition, although most acute wound closures and late reconstructions can be effected by split-thickness skin grafts, there are occasionally cases in need of reconstruction in which the underlying bed following contracture release will not support a graft which would benefit from subcutaneous padding so as to achieve a more esthetic result.[15] Similarly, subcutaneous tissue is desirable if future tendon or bone reconstruction will be necessary beneath the reconstructed integument.[3] With a greater number of surgeons mastering the technique of microsurgery, the methodology is being more frequently applied to severely burned patients. When used judiciously, it should help to solve many of the problems which previously resulted in limb amputation. As free flaps are used more frequently in the acute postburn period, reconstruction will be effected at the time of the initial operation.

Expanded skin

Another type of flap is now available. Expansion of skin can now be performed to yield tissue for reconstruction. Based on the observations that tissue expands in biological conditions of pregnancy and obesity and pathologic conditions such as tissue overlying neoplasms, Neumann used a subcutaneous balloon to artificially expand an area of the skin to reconstruct an ear.[16] After more frequent reports of tissue expansion, animal experiments by Cherry and his associates reviewed the biology of the phenomenon.[17] It appears that gradual stretching of the skin can usually occur with minimal risk of cell necrosis and dermal rupture. Epidermal cells appear to be essentially unaltered, and the thickness of the epidermis remains unchanged. The dermis thins, and there is an increase in the number of fibroblasts and myofibroblasts. There is marked thinning of the subcutaneous tissue and atrophy of muscle both above and below the expander. None of these changes would seem to be detrimental in using expanded skin for reconstruction.[3,15]

In a situation of insufficient unburned skin, any chance of damaging the skin to be used for reconstruction must be viewed from a perspective of proper risk : benefit ratio.[15] Despite this worry, there are areas in which burn scars cannot be adequately reconstructed with conventional means.[3] These include areas of alopecia on the scalp and the male face, where expanded hair-bearing adjacent skin

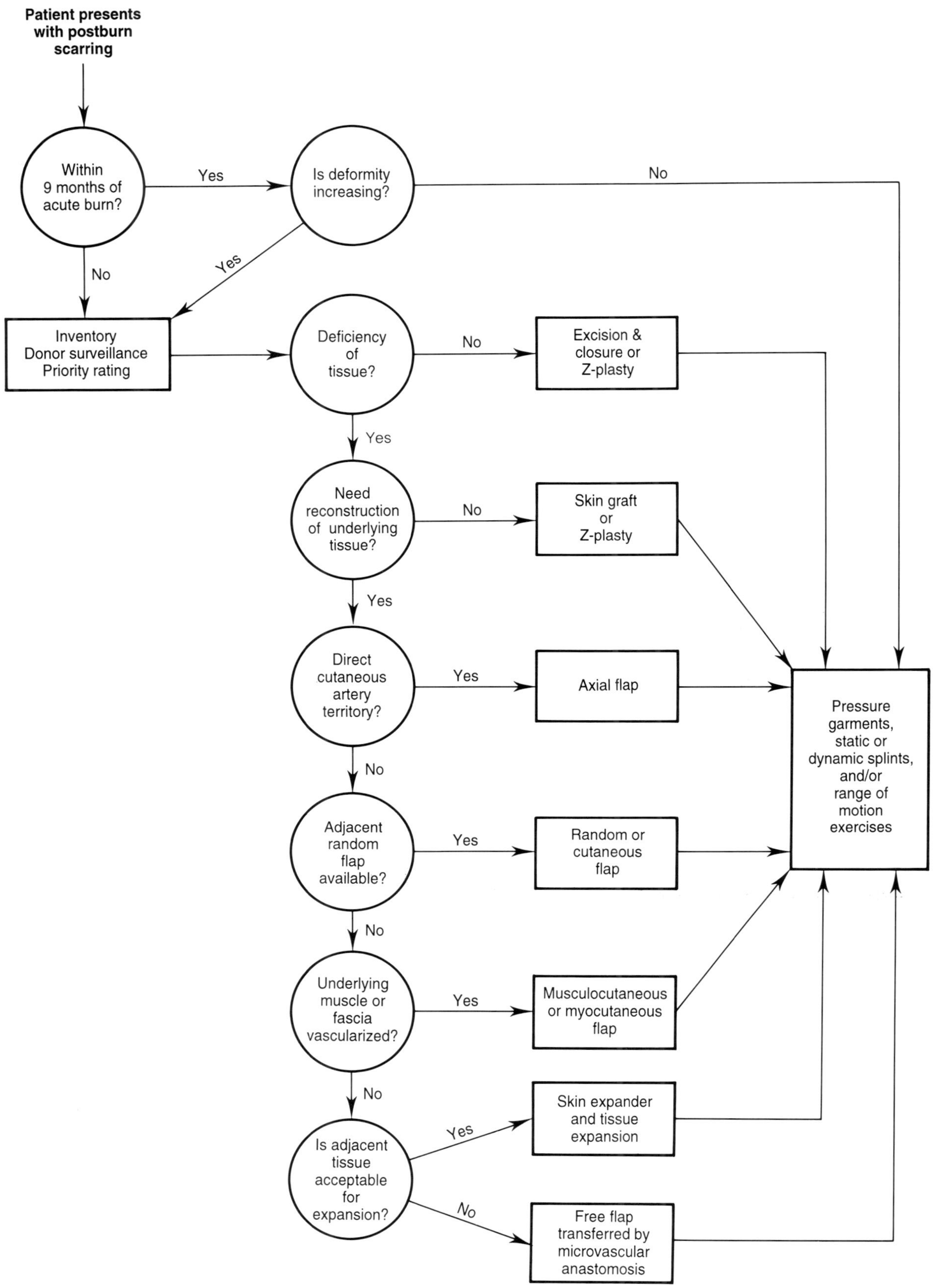

Fig. 47.4 Algorithm outlining series of decisions required on patient presenting with postburn scarring.

would seem ideal. Other burn deformities of the head and neck call for reconstruction with skin of similar color, tone, texture, thickness, and composition.[3] In these cases, results with tissue expansion are frequently far superior to those possible with available alternative techniques.[3,15,18] Once the methods available for burn reconstruction are understood and technically mastered, they can be applied to all parts of the body as needed; however, the principles remain the same: perform a careful evaluation and inventory of deformities, prepare a detailed prioritized plan, and proceed using the principles enumerated here.

Postoperative Principles for Reconstruction

Regardless of what type of operative reconstruction is required on what specific anatomical body part, there are some postoperative principles. Pressure is an effective adjunct in the control of scar maturation. Kischer has shown that in hypertrophic scars treated with pressure, the collagen nodules common in untreated hypertrophic scars disappear and the collagen bundles become oriented parallel to the skin.[19] Pressure garments customized to an individual should be applied as soon as possible after wound healing is completed so as to prevent further shortening of the collagen. Measurements should be taken before healing is complete, as it takes time to receive custom-made garments. The pressure gradient garments may last 1–3 months, depending on activity and weight change; however, they should be replaced before they are completely worn out and lose their effectiveness. Pressure is continued from 6 to 24 months or until it is clinically apparent that the scars have matured and redevelopment of deformity is unlikely. In addition to the pressure garments, the use of flexible elastomer in such concave areas as the axilla, clavicle, neck, hand, and inferior chest has been extremely helpful in producing smooth, nonerythematous healed wounds.[9] The silicone is spread directly on the body part and covered with a compression garment. This technique is also very useful if tried early on fresh scars. Increased skin pliability and range of motion have been noted with its use.

Reconstruction of a burned patient can restore more function as well as result in a subjective and objective sense of greater worth for the patient. It is well known that there may be little correlation between the severity of the physical defect estimated by the physician and the functional limitation perceived by a patient. This is equally true of aesthetic appearance. Because of this, many patients become depressed and ultimately resort to social isolation. Therefore, it is no longer enough to be technically able to perform the reconstructive procedures described or have the judgment to choose the appropriate type and timing of the reconstruction. A surgeon must also be a sympathetic physician who not only reconstructs a patient anatomically and functionally, but also considers the cosmetic or esthetic result and how it will aid the patient in total rehabilitation.[2]

Summary

Postburn reconstruction is complicated by the frequent occurrence of multiple reconstructive needs in a single patient. This chapter presents a simple, comprehensive approach to burn scar reconstruction. The primary aim of the surgeon is to prevent burn scar deformity by rapid wound closure, correction of tissue deficiencies, and assiduous attention to postoperative splinting and compression therapy. The initial step in managing secondary deformities is to identify and prioritize reconstructive needs. Reconstruction is then performed in a stepwise fashion aiming to restore active function first, followed by passive function, and finally addressing esthetic reconstruction. Reconstructive techniques are applied in a hierarchy from simplest to most complex (**Figure 47.4**). Primary excision and closure of scars by reorienting the scar to the lines of relaxed skin tension can significantly improve appearance. The use of Z-plasty, flap repair, and tissue expansion are also reviewed. Skin expansion, in particular, has become the standard management of postburn alopecia and, although associated with a relatively high complication rate, has significantly improved the aesthetic appearance of patients. The reconstruction of a burned patient is often a long process which requires multiple procedures. The approach presented here advocates a stepwise, prioritized approach aiming at both maximum function as well as optimal appearance.

References

1. Bernstein N R. *Emotional Care of the Facially Burned and Disfigured.* Boston: Little, Brown & Co, 1976.

2. Robson M C, Smith D J. Reconstruction of the burned face, neck and scalp. In: Boswick J A, ed. *The Art and Science of Burn Care.* Rockville: Aspen Publishers, Inc, 1987: Chapter 43.

3. Robson M C, Barnett R A, Leitch I O W, Hayward P G. Prevention and treatment of postburn scars and contracture. *World J Surg* 1992; **16:** 87–96.

4. Robson M C. Disturbances of wound healing. *Ann Emerg Med* 1988; **17:** 1274–8.

5. Larson D L, Abston S, Evans E B, *et al.* Techniques for decreasing scar formation and contractures in the burn patient. *J Trauma* 1971; **11:** 807–23.

6. Bernstein N R, Robson M C. *Comprehensive Approaches to the Burned Person.* New Hyde Park, NY: Medical Examination Publishing Co, Inc, 1983.

7. Bjaranson D, Phillips L G, McCoy B, *et al.* Reconstruction goals in burn children: are our goals the same? *J Burn Care Rehabil* 1992; **13:** 389–90.

8. Constable J D. The limitations of esthetic reconstruction. In: Bernstein N R, Robson M C, eds. *Comprehensive Approaches to the Burned Person.* New Hyde Park, NY: Medical Examination Publishing Co, Inc., 1983: Chapter 18.

9. Salisbury R E, Petro J A, Winski F V. Reconstruction of the burn patient. In: Boswick J A, ed. *The Art and Science of Burn Care.* Rockville: Aspen Publishers, Inc, 1987: Chapter 41.

10. Brou J, Robson M C, McCauley R L, *et al.* Inventory of potential reconstructive needs in the burn patient. *Proceedings of the 21st Annual Meeting of the American Burn Association, 1989.* New Orleans, 83, p. 122.

11. Brou J A, Ortega M T, McHugh T P, *et al.* Donor tissue surveillance and priority rating in burn reconstruction. Presented at *Plastic Surgery Educational Foundation Senior Residents Conference, 1990,* New York.

12. Robson M C, Parsons R W. Reconstructive and plastic surgery. In: Cushieri A, Giles G R, Moossa A R, eds. *Essential Surgical Practice.* Bristol, England: John Wright and Sons, Ltd, 1982: Chapter 22.

13. Koss N. The mathematics of flap design. In: Krizek T J, Hoopes J E, eds. *Symposium on Basic Science in Plastic Surgery.* St Louis: C V Mosby, 1976: 274.

14. Littlewood A H M. Seroma: an unrecognized cause of failure of split-thickness skin grafts. *Br J Plast Surg* 1960; **13:** 42–6.

15. Robson M C, Smith D J, Heggers J P. Innovations in burn wound management. In: Habal M B, Morain W D, Lewin M L, Parsons R W, Woods J E, eds. *Advances in Plastic Surgery.* Chicago: Yearbook Medical Publishers, 1987: 149.

16. Neumann C G. The expansion of an area of skin by progressive distention of a subcutaneous balloon. *Plast Reconstr Surg* 1957; **19:** 124–30.

17. Cherry G W, Austad E, Pasyk K, *et al.* Increased survival and vascularity of random pattern skin flaps elevated in controlled, expanded skin. *Plast Reconstr Surg* 1983; **72:** 680–5.

18. Gottlieb L J, Parsons R W, Krizek T J. The use of tissue expansion techniques in burn reconstruction. *J Burn Care Rehabil* 1986; **7:** 234–7.

19. Kischer C S. Collagen and mucopolysaccharides in the hypertrophic scar. *Connect Tissue Res* 1974; **2:** 205–13.

CHAPTER FORTY-EIGHT

Reconstruction of the Head and Neck

W. Glenn Lyle, Robert L. McCauley and Martin C. Robson

Introduction

Burns of the head and neck have always presented a challenge to a burn team. With improved acute care, a higher percentage of more severely injured patients are surviving their burns. Victims of smoke inhalation often have associated severe facial burns. Historically, these patients were nonsurvivors, but with advances in respiratory management, more of these individuals are surviving and subsequently require reconstruction. The goal of acute treatment and reconstruction is no longer mere survival but a meaningful and worthwhile life.[1] As Bernstein states, 'without their faces, human beings would hardly be human at all.'[2] With this in mind, the success of reconstruction of the head and neck ultimately lies in esthetic as well as functional outcome.

Despite advances in acute care, residual deformities after healing of facial burns often result as wound contraction promotes distortions which produce disfigurement and functional limitations. These events add insult to what has already been a devastating injury. The importance of the face in an individual's personal identity is obvious. Body image is a basic part of personal identity; for the face, it is not a static picture but a series of visual interactions incorporating unique physical characteristics and subtle movements which make up human expression. It emanates from both conscious and subconscious sources.[2] A person with facial disfigurement must work out a new identity and recapture his/her self-esteem. New coping mechanisms are developing to maintain one's identity, but our society places such a strong value in appearance that it is extremely difficult to make these readjustments.[3] It is the role of the reconstructive surgeon to assist a patient in renewing his self-esteem by restoring facial form to as normal as possible.

Successful reconstruction of the face and neck is the result of a group effort by all the members of a burn team. Psychological support, exercise therapy, splinting, and pressure garments all affect the surgical outcome. Without such a concerted effort, reconstruction is merely a series of technical exercises which achieve only a limited goal. When planning the procedures, a patient should be included in the decision making; the surgical objective and rationale should be explained. Frequently, unrealistic expectations result from the constant encouragement that burn team members naturally provide to patients in order to help them through the difficult acute period. To avoid post-surgical depression, preoperative discussions should paint a realistic picture of the expected outcome and explain the limitations of reconstruction. Reconstruction ideally should be postponed until wounds are fully mature; frequently this is not possible as deformity may be progressive, leading to a functional deficit. If this is the case, early reconstruction is indicated to correct true deficiency of tissue. The diagnosis of tissue deficiency may be the most important step in surgical planning. The surgical procedure recreates the initial tissue loss and adds appropriate tissue in its place. Priorities are given to certain anatomical areas and should proceed in a stepwise fashion.[1]

The first priority of burn reconstruction is the prevention of deformity, whether it be from the acute injury or after late reconstruction. All reconstruction efforts should utilize postoperative splinting and pressure garments. Failure to do so may jeopardize the optimal functional and aesthetic result. The next priority is reconstruction of active function such as eyelids, oral commissures, and the neck.[1] The final priority is restoration of passive function which includes the nose, perioral area, periorbital areas, cheeks, forehead, and ears. Reconstruction of functionally important areas can be combined with resurfacing of areas of less priority so as to minimize the number of procedures a patient undergoes.[1]

Prevention of Deformity

The need for reconstructing burns of the head and neck is largely determined by the depth of injury and depends on the quality of acute care given to the burn. Prevention of deformity will negate the need for further procedures, and meticulous technique and planning of the initial resurfacing can avoid problems in the future. The majority of facial burns will heal spontaneously, owing to the rich vascularity and abundance of adnexal structures. With this in mind, all but the most obvious full-thickness burns should be observed and treated conservatively for a period of 2–3 weeks prior to consideration of grafting. During this period, attention should be paid to minimizing edema by elevating the head of the bed and preventing infection and subsequent conversion to a full-thickness wound by covering the affected areas with moist topical antimicrobials. In addition, deformities of the nose and mouth can be prevented by careful measures to secure nasogastric tubes and endotracheal tubes without tension and the resultant pressure necrosis which such tension can cause. Ear burns, if they are deep, should be treated with mafenide acetate, as it will penetrate the eschar and provide antimicrobial protection to the cartilage.[4] Precautions should be taken to avoid any pressure on a burned ear. These burns should be treated conservatively to allow spontaneous healing by epithelialization and contraction. Deformities can be addressed at a later date.

While this interval passes, a majority of patients will undergo debridement and grafting to other areas and, with a few notable exceptions, the face does not take priority in the planning of resurfacing. Those patients with isolated facial burns should also be treated conservatively for this same period, and physicians should avoid the temptation to perform early grafting on all but the most obvious full-thickness burns. Deeper burns which have healed spontaneously should be managed with compression garments until they mature, a process which may take 6–24 months (**Figure 48.1**). During this period, patients need encouragement to maintain compliance, and assurances that this period of waiting, although uncomfortable, will often obviate the need for reconstruction or at least improve the outcome of any required procedures.

Resurfacing of burns to the head and neck, whether done in the acute stage or later, should be guided by the esthetic units of the face.[5] Some authors have varied their technique so as to better camouflage the scar junctions,[6] but the overall goal is to restore facial symmetry to reestablishment of esthetic units. These units serve as basic guidelines; however, if a large area can be covered with a large, thick split-thickness graft, this might avoid junction lines and improve overall facial appearance[7] (**Figure 48.2**).

The quality of a graft determines the final appearance of a reconstruction. Thick split-thickness grafts with good color and texture match are ideal, but often donor sites are lacking. The facial skin is the best match, but acceptable donor areas may be unavailable. Upper eyelid skin can be utilized for mild to moderate ectropion releases for the contralateral eyelid. Occasionally, nasolabial fold or preauricular skin may be suitable for perioral grafts. Postauricular skin can be quite useful but retains a pink color in Caucasians. Scalp skin often provides large amounts of skin with excellent color match. Moderate thickness grafts will not transfer hair or alter the donor site's ability to grow hair; however, this donor site may have been cropped several times for other areas, and alopecia can result if care is not taken.[8] The next best color match lies in the skin above the nipple line, including the supraclavicular area, the neck, and the upper back and chest. Owing to the irregularities of contour in these areas, saline expansion and a drum dermatome may be required to harvest split-thickness grafts.[9] The use of other locations for donor sites usually results in an unacceptable color match and a patchwork appearance. If superior donor sites are lacking, the entire reconstruction should be performed utilizing skin of like color or texture, even if it is not from a 'blush' area.[1]

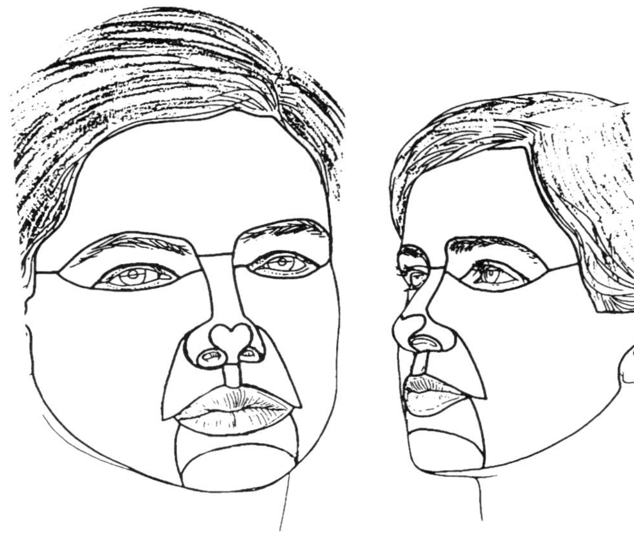

Fig. 48.2 Facial aesthetic units.

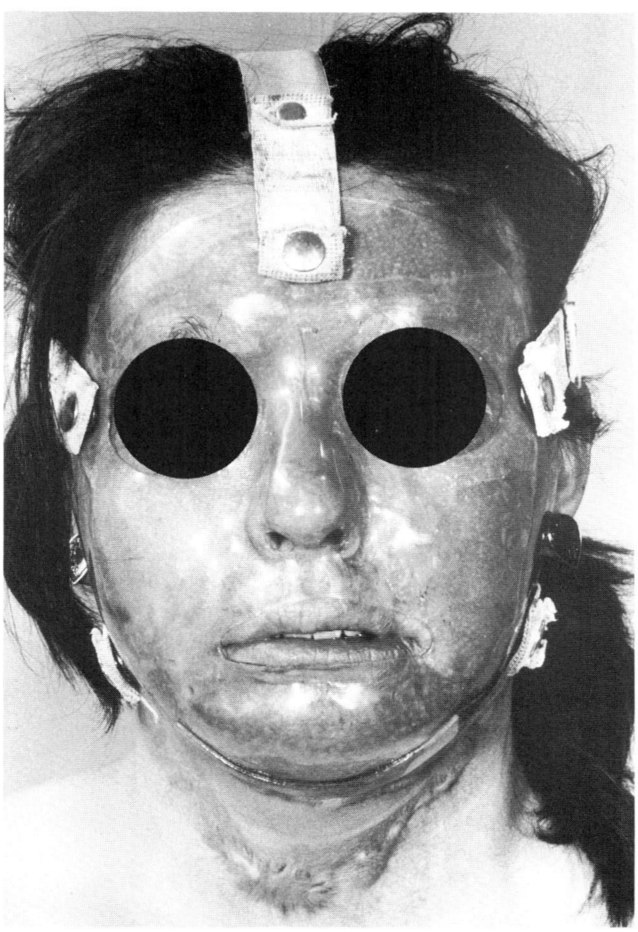

Fig. 48.1 Uvex compression mask to prevent hypertrophic scan.

Local flaps can, on occasion, serve to resurface small burned areas of the face. Feldman has had excellent results utilizing thin skin flaps from the neck or shoulder area.[10] These flaps require numerous delays, however, and are more difficult than traditional grafting. The use of tissue expanders in the head and neck area will provide tissue of excellent texture and color match, and have been used to resurface neck and cheek defects.[11] Disadvantages of this technique include expander infection and exposure, as well as the need for at least two procedures to accomplish the reconstruction.

Reconstruction of Active Function

Eyes

Because the eyes are a focal point of interpersonal communication and in order to provide protection of vision, eyelid reconstruction must take priority in an evaluation of facial burns. Often the eyelids must be reconstructed before the remainder of the burn wound is healed, especially if the cornea cannot be protected by conservative measures such as contact lenses or irrigations. Tarsorrhaphies, utilized frequently in the past, are rarely indicated as they destroy the smooth contour of the eyelid margin.[12]

Ectropion is the most common eyelid defect and should be classified as either intrinsic or extrinsic. Intrinsic ectropion is caused by a defect in the eyelid itself, whereas extrinsic ectropion is caused by contracture of surrounding facial tissues. Upper and lower lid ectropions should be released separately, in most cases, to allow as much tissue as possible to be added. Despite this strategy, scar contracture often intervenes, necessitating further secondary release and grafting. Priority should be given to the lower lids which require stability more than motion. This support can be provided by full-thickness grafts with or without cartilage grafts for additional stability. More extensive cases require flap reconstruction with mucosal grafts for the conjunctiva.[12] The lower lid ectropion release is performed by incising 1–2 mm inferior to the lid margin and extending medially to the medial canthus or nasal area or, if necessary, laterally to the lateral canthal region, and above the transcanthal line. The resultant crescent-shaped defect is bluntly released from the underlying scar, taking care to avoid injury to the orbicularis oculi muscle. This should allow the lid margin and punctum to lie in contact with the globe. The full-thickness graft will mimic a sling and, with healing, will support the lid with minimal chance of recurrence.[1]

The upper eyelids primarily require motion and flexibility which are well provided by split-thickness skin grafts. The upper lid release is performed 7–10 mm superior to the lash line and should extend laterally onto the temporal area above the transcanthal line. Restoring this natural upper eyelid fold will avoid the sad appearance which results if the release is carried too far inferiorly. Tie-over dressings are used to secure the grafts with additional retraction sutures taped to the cheek or forehead for additional immobilization. Retraction sutures are removed in 3 days, and the dressing and sutures are removed from the graft after at least 5 days for split grafts and 7–10 days for full-thickness grafts. Absorbable sutures can be substituted to secure the graft in order to avoid the discomfort of suture removal.[12]

Less commonly encountered eyelid deformities are usually amenable to local flaps. Epicanthal folds can result from the burn itself or the simultaneous release of upper and lower eyelid ectropions. This deformity can usually be released with local flaps such as double opposing Z-plasties.[13] More severe burns can result in further shortening of the palpebral fissure which necessitates a medial canthoplasty. Direct injury or distortion from an associated nasal burn will often cause eversion of the punctum. Careful attention to the punctum must be given when releasing this area. Lacrimal probes should be utilized to avoid injury to the duct and allow release of the punctum to restore continuity with the lacrimal lake. Failure to do so may result in epiphora and corneal exposure.

Mouth

Burns of the mouth and perioral area can interfere with basic function such as eating, drinking, and speaking, while also altering appearance and facial expression. Deformities of the lips, vermilion, and oral commissure must be restored with the goals of restoring oral competence and achieving facial symmetry.[1] Procedures which violate adjacent esthetic units will result in an unfavorable patchwork appearance. To avoid this, commissure integrity should be restored prior to resurfacing the cheek and lips. Correction of the microstomia should take priority to facilitate orotracheal intubation, allow eating and proper speech, and enable dental care to be given.

Like eyelid ectropions, lip ectropions and other perioral deformities can be intrinsic or extrinsic. For example, neck contractures frequently cause lip ectropion and distortion of the commissure which are often corrected or improved by a neck release. Lower lip ectropions which remain after neck release are managed by excising the esthetic unit, leaving a prominence to highlight the chin, and resurfacing with a thick split-thickness graft (**Figure 48.3**). Care must be taken to completely free the vermilion from the underlying tethering scar, and often some excess vermilion must be excised. Adequate neck splinting and pressure garments are essential to avoid recurrence.

Ectropion of the upper lip is best corrected by excising the entire esthetic unit from nasolabial fold to nasolabial fold. The area of the philtrum should have epidermis only removed to allow the philtral columns to remain prominent. Placing two separate skin grafts in this area with their seams secured along the column will often restore a suitable appearance.[1]

Contracture of the columella can be lengthened by the use of

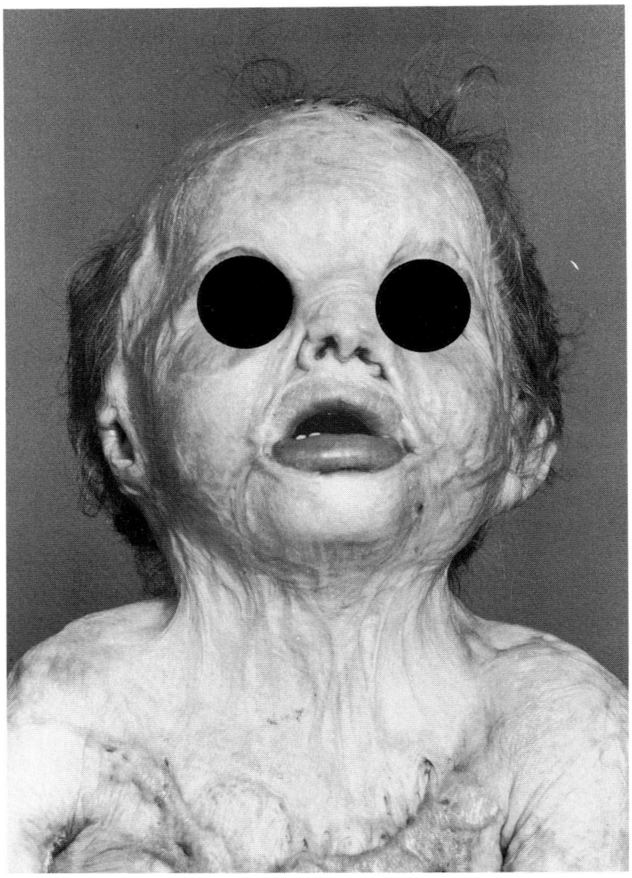

Fig. 48.3 Lower lip ectropion excised and grafted as a single aesthetic unit.

forked flaps.[14] While alar defects should be released, definitive reconstruction should be delayed until nasal reconstruction is performed. Electrical cord injuries result in the most common true commissure burn. The use of dynamic or static splinting early in the acute management of these injuries has reduced the need for late surgical correction.[15] When late surgical intervention is necessary, oral symmetry can be achieved with commisuroplasties such as those described by Gilles and Millard.[16] Thermal burns of the perioral area often result in simple webbing of the commissures which can be corrected with Y-V mucosal advancement flaps.

Neck

Neck reconstruction often takes priority over other areas, depending on the severity of disfigurement. Early neck release may be necessary so as to facilitate intubation for elective procedures and to avoid emergency releases under less controlled conditions. A transverse incision in the operating room under local anesthesia or accom-

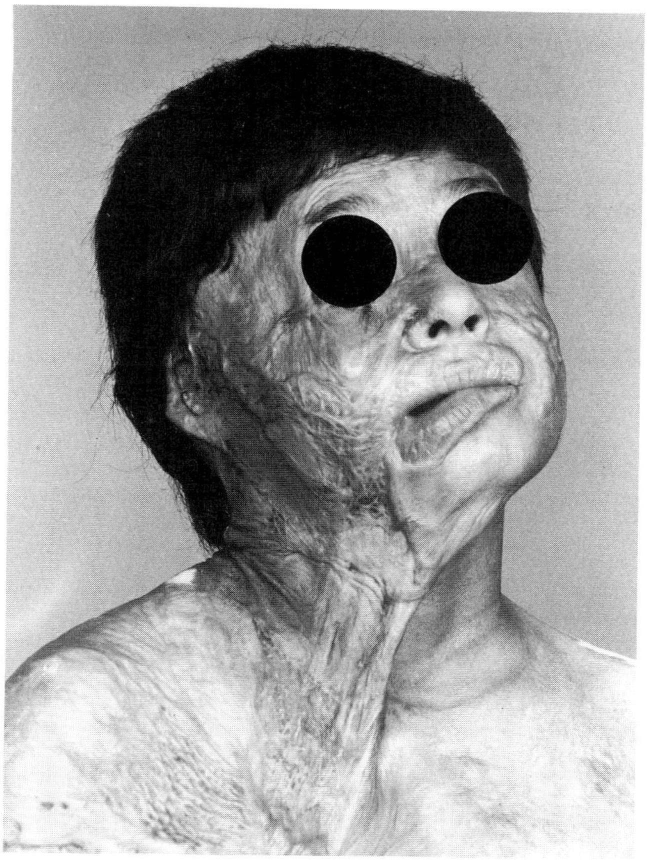

(a)

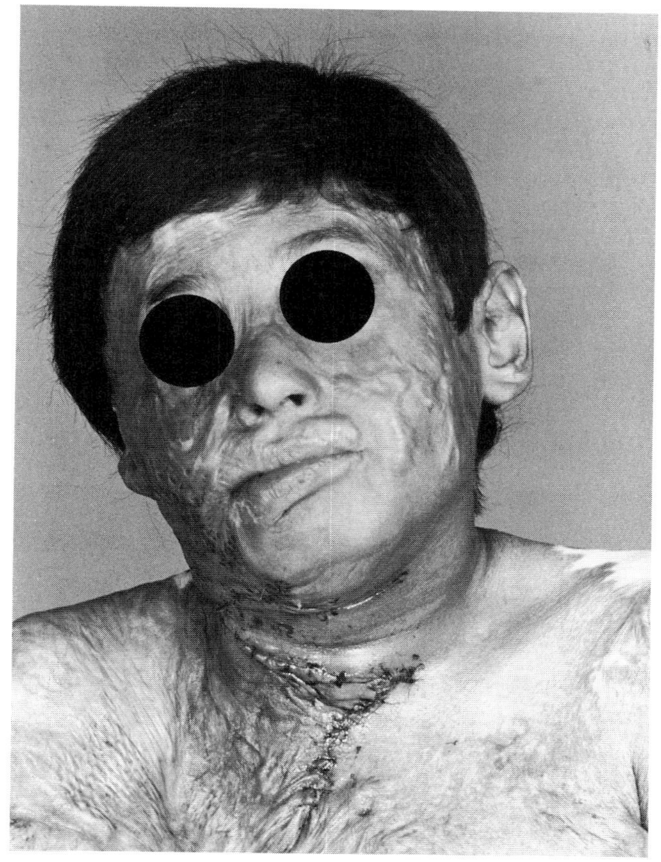

(b)

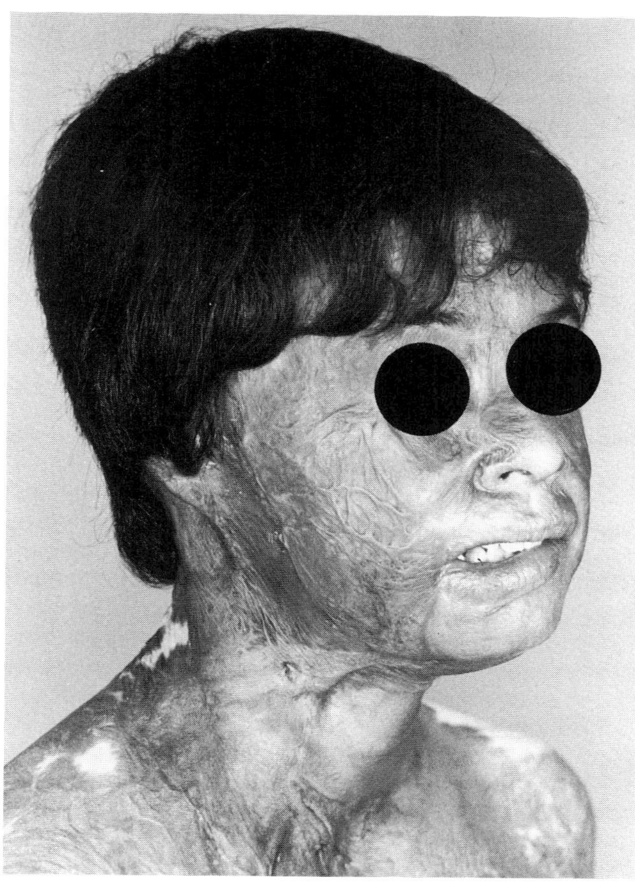

(c)

panied by ketamine anesthesia allows a patient to be intubated prior to definitive scar removal and resurfacing.[17] Neck contractures may affect mandibular growth in younger children and should be released early for this reason. In addition, contractures in this area can affect adjacent areas such as the face and shoulders. Therefore, early release may prevent deformity and facilitate physical therapy.

There are essentially three separate categories of neck contracture:

- those associated with a wide isolated scar;
- a scar contracture involving burned skin with intervening normal skin; and
- a burn scar contracture involving most of the neck skin.[1]

Isolated bands can usually be released with simple single or multiple Z-plasties if they are not too extensive (**Figure 48.4**). These isolated scars are usually vertically oriented, and the transposed flap leaves the scar in the normal resting skin tension lines of the neck and restores the normal chin–neck angle.

More extensive neck contractures, as in the second category, may require total excision of a scar. Because of the laxity of neck skin, a much larger defect than expected will result after release. Smaller defects can be closed with thin skin flaps but, as is most often the case, neck contour must be restored by resurfacing the defect with thick split-thickness grafts. It may even be necessary to extend the release into normal adjacent skin in order to allow unrestricted motion.[1] A tie-over dressing is utilized and the patient is kept at bed rest with the neck extended until the dressing is removed. An orthoplast splint is applied after bolster removal and

Fig. 48.4 (a) Isolated neck contracture released with (b) Z-plasty with (c) good long-term results.

must be continued for at least 4 months (**Figure 48.5**). Soft tissue expansion may eventually prove to be an ideal alternative to grafts in providing normal color and contour; however, at present, associated complications are significant.[11]

Severe neck contracture of the third category is rarely released with incision and grafting. Total excision and grafting is more often required. Release of platysmal scarring is necessary to insure full neck extension. As in the previous category, normal skin may need to be excised to prevent lateral banding. The neck esthetic unit extends to the midlateral line of the neck, a line from the mastoid process down the sternocleidomastoid muscle to midneck, and then posteriorally, paralleling the anterior border of the trapezius until it reaches the clavicle. Again, large split-thickness skin grafts are required to resurface the defect with tie-over dressings and postoperative splints. Any adjacent areas of burned chest or face should be excised and resurfaced at this time as well.[1]

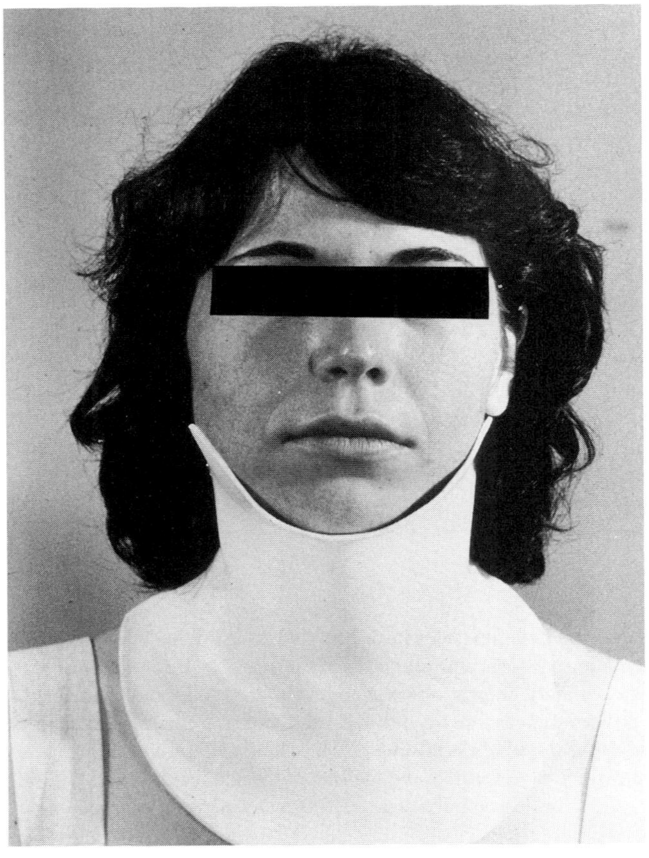

Fig. 48.5 Splint utilized to maintain neck release.

Reconstruction of Passive Function

Nose

After correcting deformities associated with active function of the face, restoration of those structures involved in passive function can be undertaken. The nose should take highest priority in this regard, as it assumes such a prominent focal point on the face. Nasal burn deformities can be quite complex, and the results of reconstruction are often less than satisfactory. Therefore, it is important to make accurate diagnoses of the underlying problems prior to attempting nasal reconstruction. Nasal burns often are allowed to heal spontaneously, resulting in a thin shiny nose with eversion of the nares. Nasal bones are rarely involved, but cartilaginous structures are frequently destroyed or severely distorted. Deformities of the alae and columella are often due to contracture of adjacent burned tissue and may be corrected by appropriate releases of offending scar bands. Residual contour defects still may remain and are very difficult to restore. The first step to nasal reconstruction is resurfacing the dorsum as a unit in concert with release of the nostril borders, which will help lengthen the nose.[1]

Nostril rims can be replaced with composite grafts from the ear helix. The nasal dorsum and rims can also be reconstructed as a single unit using composite grafts of ear cartilage and unburned postauricular skin as a full-thickness graft.[18] Small rim defects may be corrected with release along the superior margins of the lower lateral cartilages and composite grafts of thick skin and fat, which can be harvested from the gluteal crease. If the nasolabial fold is unburned, nasolabial flaps may also correct alar defects.

Often cartilaginous support is missing, requiring a conventional Converse scalping flap.[19] In patients with unburned skin of the forehead, medial forehead flaps augmented by tissue expansion can provide the ideal color and texture match of glabrous skin (**Figure 48.6**). Rarely, distant flaps such as the Tagliocozzi medial arm flap or free tissue transfer may be required for total nasal reconstruction with rib or cranial bone grafts in order to provide additional struts for projection. As the functional areas have been reconstructed, few esthetic units remain. The forehead and cheeks should be resurfaced with large split-thickness grafts as single units. Tie-over bolsters may be utilized or, if several units are being reconstructed

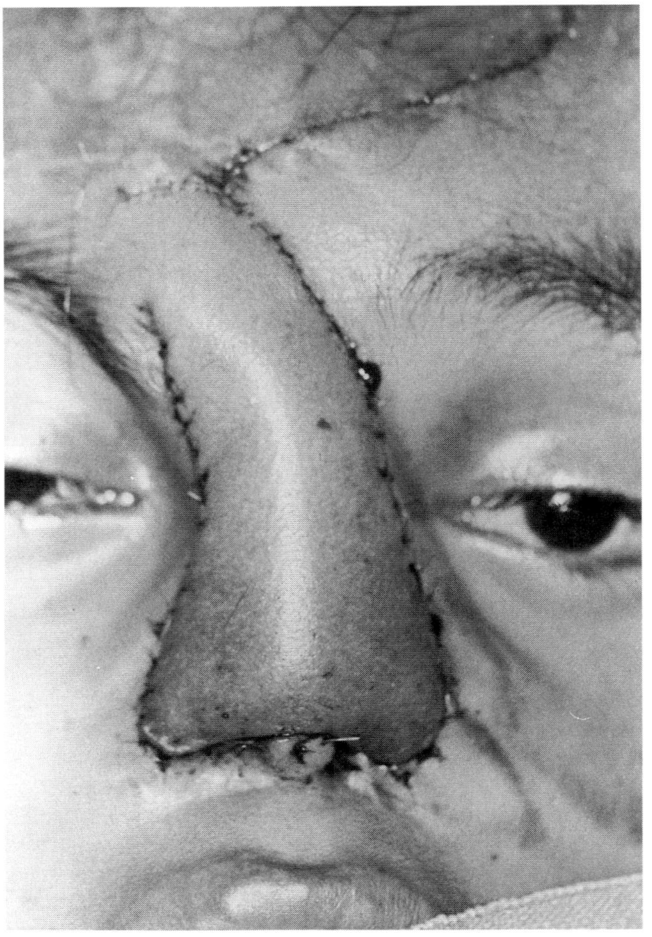

Fig. 48.6 Medical forehead flap to reconstruct nose.

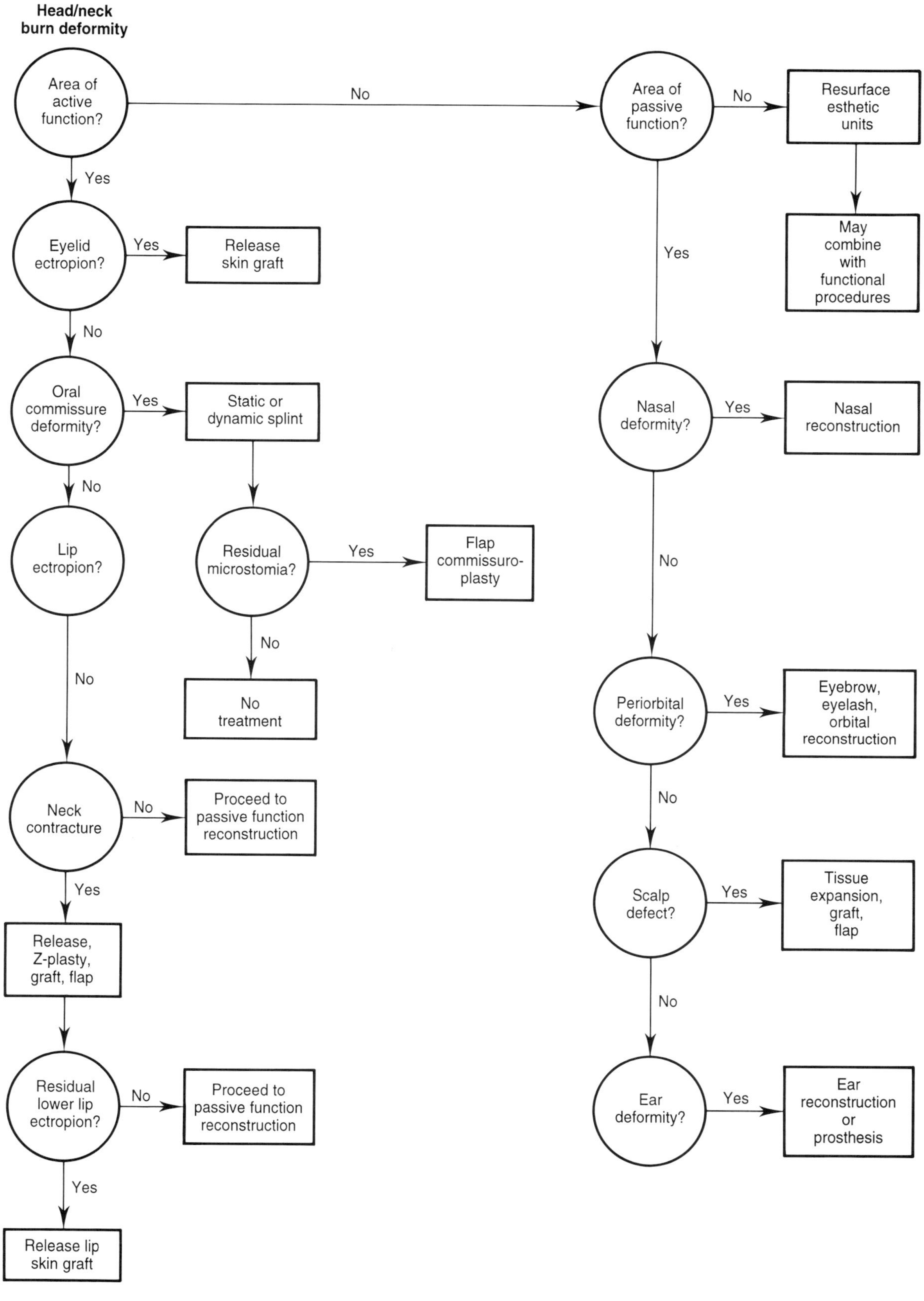

Fig. 48.7 Algorithm or decision tree for reconstruction of the burned head and neck.

simultaneously, preoperatively fashioned facial moulages can provide for immediate postoperative splinting.

Eyebrow alopecia can be satisfactorily camouflaged with makeup in females, but males often desire alternative means. These important visual features can be restored with arterialized island flaps of hair bearing tissue from the scalp based on a branch of the superficial temporal artery. Simpler techniques utilizing composite scalp grafts from the temporal or parietal area can often provide suitable results. Care should be taken to make these narrow (< 5 mm), and close attention should be paid to preserving hair follicles so as to insure hair growth. Otherwise recurrent eyebrow alopecia results. Eyelashes can be replaced by similar methods.[1]

Scalp

Scalp defects can be corrected with local flaps, expansion or free flaps, and will be discussed in the chapter on scalp alopecia.

Ear

Ear defects can often be well hidden by hair styling, and this structure does not serve as prominently in facial appearance as the previously mentioned structures. Often, individuals with ear deformity do not even desire reconstruction, especially after having undergone multiple previous procedures. With this in mind, the ear should be the final priority in head and neck reconstruction. Reconstruction of the ear should be delayed to allow for normal scar maturation. Correction of lesser ear deformities depends upon the quality of postauricular skin. Local flaps and Z-plasties from these areas can be utilized to correct minor defects. Helical rim reconstruction with tubed preauricular, postauricular, or cervical flaps may be required, while smaller defects can be managed with chondrocutaneous advancement flaps such as those described by Anita and Buch.[20] Local flaps with small conchal cartilage grafts may suffice to replace partial ear loss.

Total ear reconstruction remains a challenge and selected individuals, such as older patients who are unable to tolerate more extensive procedures or patients with inadequate donor tissues, may be better served with prosthetic devices. Ear prostheses are often quite unsatisfactory as a result of poor fit, poor adherence, problems with hygiene, or problems with color match. Some of the problems may be overcome with osteointegrated implants and should be considered, particularly in young patients.[1] Total ear reconstruction is best undertaken utilizing the temporalis fascial flap as described by Brent.[21] In many cases, one-stage reconstruction can be accomplished. Carved autologous costal cartilage grafts placed under this flap and covered with skin grafts is the preferred method to provide support. Silastic frameworks, although convenient, risk extrusion and infection. Alternatively, if adjacent tissue is unburned, tissue expansion may provide an ideal coverage for the underlying framework. External auditory canal stenosis may require local flaps for correction, as described by Macomber.[22] Stents are required to prevent restenosis. If the canal is obliterated, reconstruction is not undertaken.

Summary

Facial reconstruction should be undertaken with proper planning, assigning priorities based on function (**Figure 48.7**), and paying meticulous attention to detail in order to achieve the best esthetic result. Ultimately, a more functional face results along with the restoration of a patient's subjective and objective sense of identity. Despite the best efforts by the reconstructive surgeon, the patient's perception of limitations and severity of residual deformities is often quite different from the physician's. Patients may become depressed and eventually resort to social isolation. Therefore, the surgeon must not only be technically proficient at these procedures, but also must be sympathetic and use proper judgment in the timing and extent of reconstruction. Total rehabilitation of a burned patient must take into account the functional as well as the esthetic results. It is with our face, which mirrors our emotions, that we interact with others in our world. As Raymond Mortimer said in his 'Essay on clothes': 'If we really had any modesty it is our faces we should conceal. By comparison our legs are anonymous, our bellies uneventful.'[23]

References

1. Robson M C, Smith D J. Reconstruction of the burned face, neck and scalp. In: Bostwick J A, ed. *The Art and Science of Burn Care.* Rockville: Aspen Publishers, Inc, 1987: 373–83.

2. Bernstein N R. *Emotional Care of the Facially Burned and Disfigured.* Boston: Little, Brown & Co, 1976.

3. Bernstein N R. Trial by fire: the uncharted life course of burned people. In: Bernstein N R, Robson M C, eds. *Comprehensive Approaches to the Burned Person.* New Hyde Park, New York: Medical Examination Publishing Co, Inc, 1983: 49–77.

4. Kucan J O, Robson M C. Care of the burned ear. In: Wachtel T, ed. *Burns of the Head and Neck.* Philadelphia: W B Saunders Co, 1983.

5. Converse J M, McCarthy J G, Dobrkovsky M, *et al.* Facial burns. In: Converse J M, ed. Philadelphia: W B Saunders Co, 1977: 1595–642.

6. Frank D H. Reconstruction of head and neck burn injury. In: Wachtel T, Dean D H, eds. *Burns of the Head and Neck.* Philadelphia: W B Saunders Co, 1984: 158.

7. Kobus K. Late repair of facial burns. *Ann Plast Surg* 1980; **5:** 191–204.

8. Brou J, Vu T, McCauley R L, *et al.* The scalp as a donor site revisited. *J Trauma* 1990; **30:** 579–81.

9. Warpeha R L. Resurfacing the burned face. *Clin Plast'Surg* 1981; 258–9.

10. Feldman J. Reconstruction of the burned face in children. In: Serafin D, Georgaide N, eds. *Pediatric Plastic Surgery.* St Louis: C V Mosby Co, 1984: 552–632.

11. Marks M W, Argenta L C, Thornton J W. Burn management: the role of tissue expansion. *Clin Plast Surg* 1987; 543–8.

12. Smith D J, Robson M C. Eyelid burns. In: Spoor T C, Nesi F A, eds. *Management of Ocular, Orbital and Adnexal Trauma.* New York: Raven Press, 1988: 427–35.

13. Converse J M, Smith B. Repair of severe burn ectropion of the eyelids. *Plast Reconstr Surg* 1959, **23:** 21–6.

14. Millard D R Jr. Columella lengthening by a forked flap. *Plast Reconstr Surg* 1958; **22:** 454–7.

15. Silverglade D, Zacher J B, Ruberg R L. Improved splinting of oral commissure burns: results in 21 consecutive patients. *Ann Plast Surg* 1982; **9:** 316–20.

16. Gilles H D, Millard D R Jr. *Principles and Art of Plastic Surgery.* Boston: Little, Brown & Co, 1957.

17. Wilson R D, Knapp C, Traber D L, *et al.* Safe management of the child with a contracted neck: a new method. *South Med J* 1970; **63:** 1420–5.

18. Baker D. Massive chondrocutaneous grafts for nasal reconstruction. Presented at The American Association of Plastic Surgeons, Chicago, 1984.

19. Converse J M. Reconstruction of the nose by the scalping flap technique. *Surg Clin North Am* 1959; **39:** 335–65.

20. Antia N H, Buch M S. Chondrocutaneous advancement flap for the marginal defect of the ear. *Plast Reconstr Surg* 1967; **39:** 472–7.

21. Brent B, Byrd H S. Secondary ear reconstruction with cartilage grafts covered by axial, random, and free flaps of temporoprietal fascia. *Plast Reconstr Surg* 1983; **72:** 141–52.

22. Macomber W B, Wang M K H, Leuder H W. Reconstruction of the traumatically stenosed external auditory canal. *Plast Reconstr Surg* 1958; **22:** 168–73.

23. Mortimer R. Essay on clothes. In: Brophy J, ed. *The Human Face Reconsidered.* London: Harrap, 1962.

CHAPTER FORTY-NINE

Correction of Burn Alopecia

Robert L. McCauley

Introduction

Burns to the head and neck represent some of the more challenging problems in acute wound care, subsequent rehabilitation, and reconstruction. The defects are not easily hidden. Initial reports documented a 25% incidence of burn injuries involving the head and neck region.[1] In 1989, Brou *et al.* noted that defects in the head and neck region constituted 235 of 517 (45%) problems in 25 pediatric patients with a 71% mean TBSA burn.[2] In a more recent study of 194 pediatric burned patients, alopecia was noted in 32% of the patient population.[3] Although this study documented a 61% incidence of burn alopecia in patients with burned scalps who ultimately required use of the scalp as a donor site, it was difficult to determine if the alopecia occurred because of the burn itself or because of the harvesting to scalp skin grafts. Regardless of the etiology, alopecia in burned patients continues to pose a significant problem for the reconstructive surgeon.

Approaches to Correction of Alopecia

Reconstruction of scalp defects with the use of excision and primary closure has proven to be applicable in regions with small defects.[4,5] Indeed, several excisions have been reported to be successful in the correction of burn alopecia, less than 15% of the hair-bearing scalp. In 1977, Huang *et al.* reported that the use of primary excision and/or rotation flaps was useful in the correction of defects covering 15–20% of the hair-bearing scalp.[1] These methods remain useful in the correction of small scalp defects; however, larger defects require more involved surgical techniques.

In 1968, Ortichochea introduced the four-flap technique for reconstruction of scalp defects.[6] This was subsequently modified to the three flap scalp reconstruction in 1971.[7] Although it is difficult to gauge the extent of alopecia covered using these techniques, these methods have been quite useful in the correction of moderate size alopecia defects. The primary disadvantage associated with the use of these techniques relates to the use of blood transfusions, the extensive scarring which results from mobilization of the multiple scalp flaps, and their inability to close very large defects.[8] Also taking advantage of the profuse vascular supply of the scalp, Juri *et al.* used a variety of monopedicled scalp flaps to cover segmental areas of alopecia, especially in the frontal region.[9–11] The use of this pedicled flap was limited in that size of the alopecia segment to be corrected was small. The clinical application of tissue expansion to the closure of large scalp defects without excessive scarring revolutionized our approach to this problem.

Tissue Expansion

Skin expansion is based on the dynamic fashion in which living tissue responds to a constant mechanical stress load. The growth of the gravid uterus and our ability to gain or lose massive amounts of weight, demonstrates the ability of the skin to develop independently. Tissue expansion represents a medical application of the normal physiologic process for the correction of significant traumatic defects using adjacent, identical tissue.

As part of the exotic esthetics of various cultures, tissue expansion has achieved significant social implications in a variety of societies throughout the world. The enlarged lips of the Acadian women were primarily developed to accentuate their own sense of beauty. The elongated necks that were subsequently produced in the Padugung women of Burma also attest to the exotic aesthetics associated with tissue expansion.[12]

Clinical uses of soft tissue expansion did not gain significance until 1905 when bone lengthening by distraction resulted in expansion of soft tissue.[13] These experiments were initially conducted by Codivilla with subsequent follow-up by Putti in 1921.[14] The first reported clinical case of pure soft tissue expansion occurred in the reconstruction of a traumatic ear defect by expansion of post-auricular skin using a subcutaneous balloon.[15] In 1975, Radavan and Austed, working independently, developed the concept of soft tissue expansion using a silicone implant.[16–18] Although Radavan became the first surgeon to gain extensive experience in the use of silicone expanders, Austed first reported the laboratory and clinical experience with tissue expanders prior to subsequent clinical use.

Biology of Tissue Expansion

Histologic Studies of Skin

Experimental data on the biology of tissue expanders have resulted from animal experimentation.[18–20] Subsequent human studies were noted to be similar to the animal data.[21] Initial studies by Paysk *et al.* showed that, although cellular retraction was normal, the epidermis appeared thicker and was associated with the loss of rete ridges. Histologic examination of the dermis revealed a thinner dermis. Also noted was an increase in dermal collagen content with breakage of elastic fibers; however, no significant changes in skin appendages were seen. Electron microscopy also documented the absence of significant physiologic changes of skin associated with soft tissue expansion.

Vascular Supply of Expanded Skin

Several investigators have observed a significant increase in vascularity associated with soft tissue expansion both histologically and clinically. Cheng *et al.* noted an increase in the surviving length of expanded skin flaps when compared to delayed skin flaps.[22] Sasaki *et al.*, using labeled microspheres, confirmed these earlier studies while also documenting an increase in blood flow associated with expanded skin flaps.[23] The ability of soft tissue to expand is based on several physiological properties. The skin has a constant ability to adapt, although this depends primarily on the amount and distribution of structural proteins and tissue fluids. Collagen fibers become parallel with the stretching of the tissue. Although elastin fibers are important for recoil after stretching, collagen fibers lengthen permanently.

Clinical Application in Burn Alopecia

The role of tissue expansion in the correction of pediatric burn alopecia has slowly become recognized as the gold standard with which other reconstructive methods must be compared. With the increased survival of children suffering massive total body surface area burns, reconstruction of significant defects have become quite a challenge.

In 1978, Huang *et al.* classified the extent of burn alopecia as it related to the correction of this problem. At this time, the authors used primary excision and rotation flaps as a means to either eliminate or camouflage burn alopecia. These investigators felt that alopecia greater than 15% of the hair-bearing scalp was not amenable to correction with serial primary excision. A major thrust in the clinical application of tissue expansion for the correction of burn alopecia developed with the 1984 report of Manders *et al.*[24] This group of investigators demonstrated the efficacy and safety of soft tissue expansion in the correction of scalp defects in pediatric patients.[24] Later reports confirmed the feasibility of tissue expansion in the correction of burn alopecia despite moderately high complication rates.[24–27] Subsequently, McCauley *et al.* further classified burn alopecia based on not only the pattern of the alopecia but also the extent of the alopecia.[28] This classification was designed as a means by which reconstructive efforts could be designed so as to correct specific problems of burn alopecia (**Table 49.1**). In this report, patients with types IA and IB burn alopecia

Table 49.1 Classification of burn alopecia

Type I	Single alopecia segment
	A Less than 25% of the hair-bearing scalp
	B 25–50% of the hair-bearing scalp
	C 50–75% of the hair-bearing scalp
	D 75% of the hair-bearing scalp
Type II	Multiple alopecia segments amenable to tissue expansion placement
Type III	Patchy burn alopecia not amenable to tissue expansion
Type IV	Total alopecia

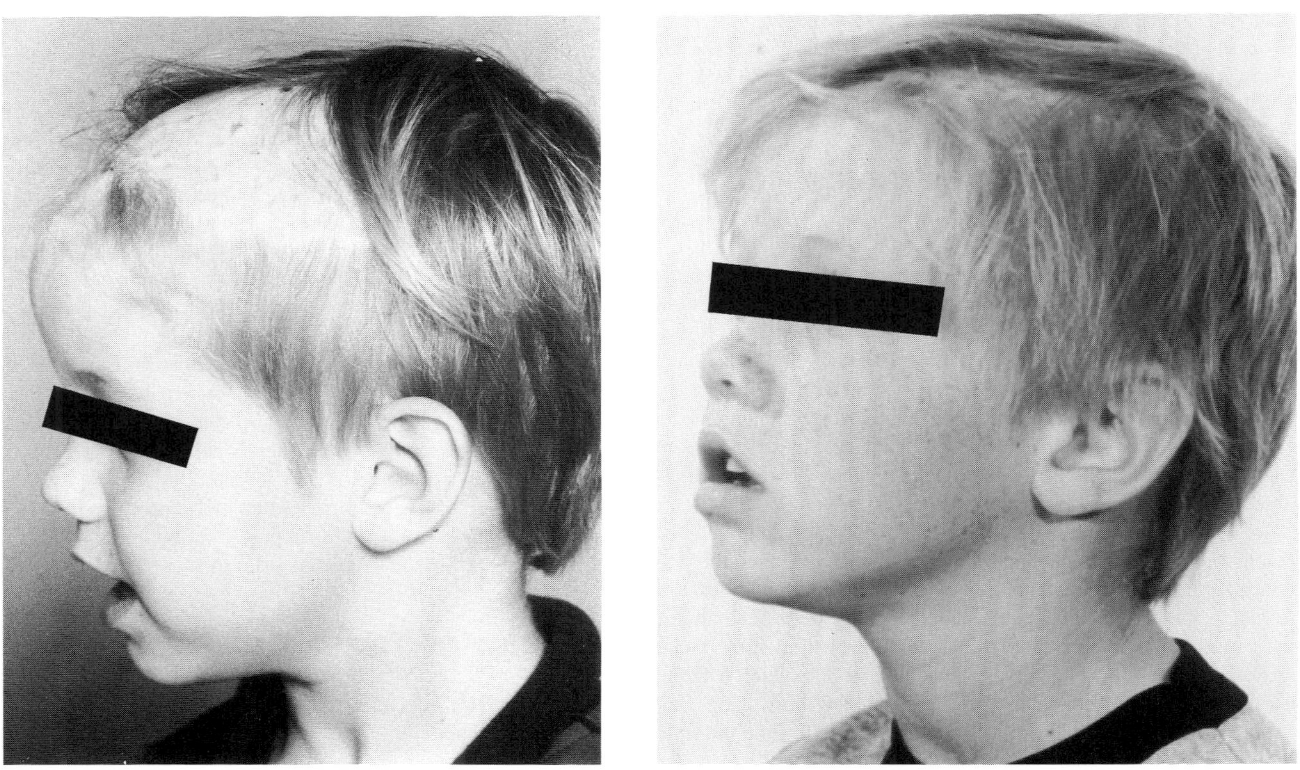

(a) (b)

Fig. 49.1 (a) Preoperative view of 6 year-old white male with type 1A burn alopecia. (b) Postoperative view after correction of alopecia with a single expansion.

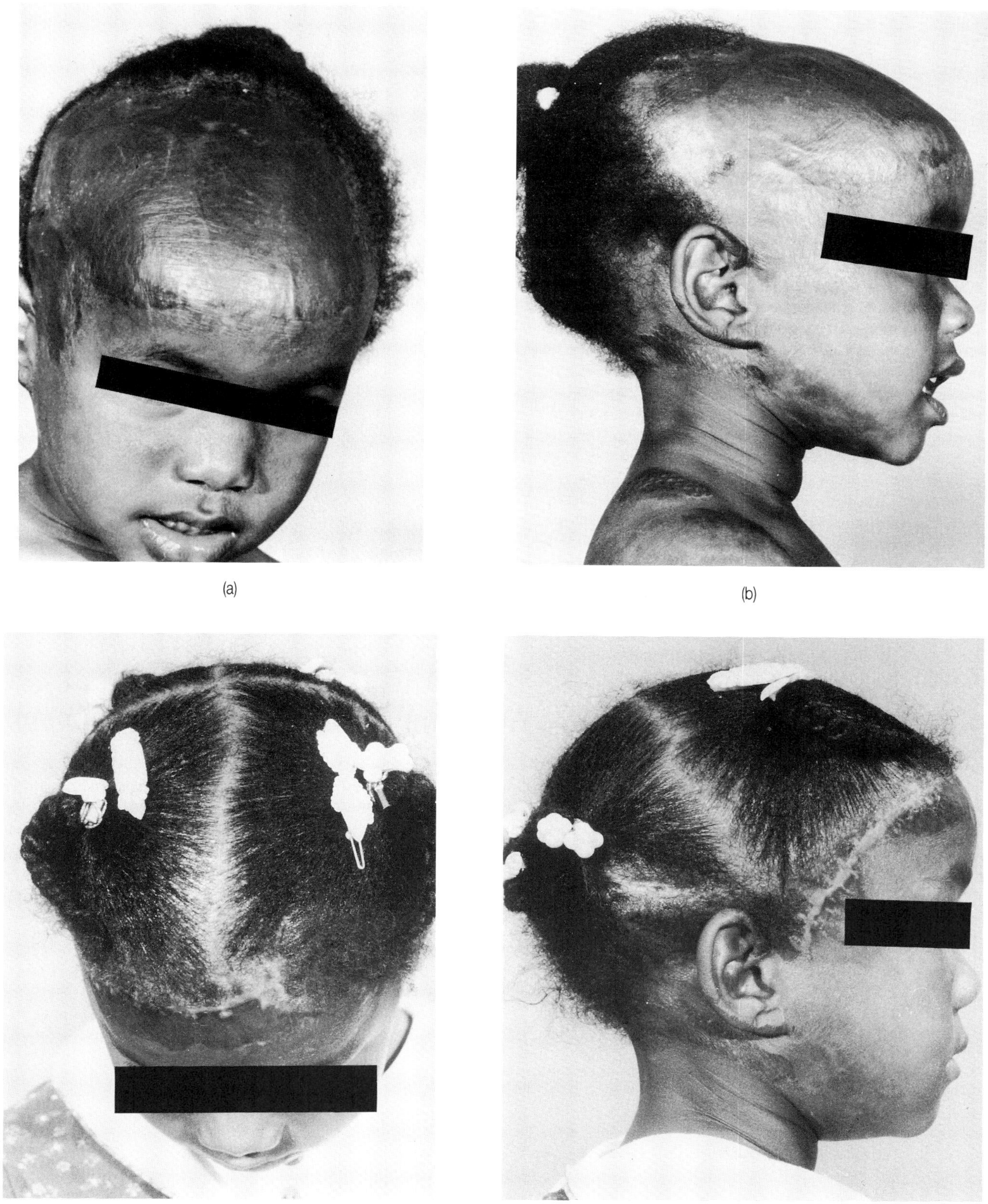

(a) (b) (c) (d)

Fig. 49.2 (a,b) Preoperative views of a 6-year-old black female patient with type IC burn alopecia. (c,d) Postoperative views after correction using sequential expansion.

were corrected via a single expansion, although over inflation of the scalp expander may be required (**Figure 49.1**). Patients with type IC and ID burn alopecia required sequential expansion in order to obtain complete coverage (**Figure 49.2**). Patients that presented with type II burn alopecia were corrected with a single expanded scalp flap; however, patients with type IIB, C or D required multiple expanders if the adjacent alopecia segment could accommodate an expander. Alternatively, if the hair-bearing segments could not accommodate an expander, this tissue was incorporated around the larger expanded flap. Once the wound matured, the anterior portion of the uniform hair-bearing scalp was lifted and advanced as a single flap. Obviously patients with type III and type IV burn alopecia were not candidates for tissue expansion.

Complications

Complications associated with tissue expanders can be subdivided into those which are major and those which are minor. Major complications have been reported to be as low as 3% and as high as 40%.[24–26,28,29] It appears that the incidence of complications associated with tissue expanders continues to remain around 15–20%. The major complications are usually defined as those which require removal of the expander. Such complications may be secondary to infection, exposure of the expander from traumatic extrusion, wound dehiscence, or erosion of an envelope fold or reservoir through the skin.[27] Implant failure, which requires removal of the implant, also is considered a major complication as would be ischemia of the expanded scalp flap, resulting in necrosis. Manders *et al.* reported a major complication rate of 24%.[8] Several investigators have reported similar complications ranging from 17 to 24%.[25,28] Minor complications have been documented with these patients and have been defined as poor compliance, intolerance of the injection to fill the expanders, and alterations in the early preoperative plans secondary to incomplete coverage following expansion. Rates of such minor complications have been reported to be between 17 and 40% with a mean still in the range of 20%.[8,25]

Conclusion

It is clear that tissue expansion has become a permanent member in the armamentarium of the reconstructive surgeon for the correction of soft tissue defects. This role in the correction of burn alopecia has been one with tremendous impact. Numerous reports detailing the success of tissue expansion in the reconstruction of scalp defects are available. With so many burn injuries occurring to the head and neck, reconstructive surgeries, such as those designed to correct alopecia, are becoming more common and are experiencing new improvements in technique.

References

1. Huang T T, Larson D L, Lewis S R. Burn alopecia. *Plast Reconstr Surg* 1977; **60:** 762.

2. Brou J A, Robson M C, McCauley R L, *et al.* Inventory of potential reconstructive needs in the burn patient. *J Burn Care* 1989; **10:** 555.

3. Brou J A, Vu T, McCauley R L, *et al.* The scalp as a donor site: revisited. *J Trauma* 1990; **30:** 579.

4. Paletta Fu. Surgical management of the burned scalp. *Clin Plast Surg* 1982; **9:** 167.

5. Vallis C P. Surgical management of cicatricial alopecia of the scalp. *Clin Plast Surg* 1982; **9:** 179.

6. Ortichochea M. Four flap scalp reconstruction technique. *Br J Plast Surg* 1967; **20:** 159–71.

7. Ortichochea M. New three flap scalp reconstruction technique. *Br J Plast Surg* 1971; **24:** 184–8.

8. Manders E K, Schendon M J, Fussey J A, *et al.* Soft tissue expansion: concepts and complications. *Plast Reconstr Surg* 1984; **74:** 493–504.

9. Juri J. Use of parieto-occipital flaps in the surgical treatment of baldness. *Plast Reconstr Surg* 1975; **55:** 456.

10. Juri J, Juri C, Arufe H N. Use of rotation scalp flaps for the treatment of occipital baldness. *Br J Plast Surg* 1978; **61:** 23.

11. Juri J, Juri C. Aesthetic aspects of reconstructive scalp surgery. *Clin Plast Surg* 1981; **8:** 243–54.

12. Saszki G. Tissue expansion. In: Jurkiewicz M J, Krizek T J, Mathes S, Ariyan S, Saszki G, eds. *Plastic Surgery: Principles and Practice* St Louis: C V Mosby, 1990; Chapter 50, p. 1608.

13. Codiville A. On the means of lengthening the muscle and tissues in the lower limbs which are shorted and high deformity. *Am J Orthop Surg* 1905; **2:** 353.

14. Putti, V. Operative lengthening of the femur. *JAMA* 1921; **77:** 937.

15. Neumann C G. The expansion of an area of skin by progressive distention of a subcutaneous balloon. *Plast Reconst Surg* 1957; **19:** 124.

16. Austed E D, Thomas S V, Pasyk K. Tissue expansion: dividend or loan? *Plast Reconstr Surg* 1986; **78:** 63.

17. Radavan C. Tissue expansion in soft tissue reconstruction. *Plast Reconstr Surg* 1984; **74:** 491.

18. Austed E D, Pasyk K A, McClatchey K D, Cherry G W. Histomorphometric evaluation of guinea pig skin and soft tissue after controlled tissue expansion *Plast Reconst Surg* 1982; **70:** 704–10.

19. Pasyk K A, Austed E D, McClatchey K D, Cherry G W. Electron microscopic evaluation of guinea pig skin and soft tissues expanded with a self-inflating silicone implant. *Plast Reconst Surg* 1982; **70:** 37.

20. Pasyk K A, Argenta L C, Hasseh C. Quantitative analysis of the thickness of human skin and subcutaneous tissue following controlled expansion with a silicone implant. *Plast Reconstr Surg* 1988; **81:** 516.

21. Pasyk K A, Argenta L C, Austed E D. Histopathology of human expanded tissue. *Clin Plast Surg* 1987; **14:** 435–45.

22. Cherry G W, Austed G D, Pasyk K A, McClatchey K D, Romich R J. Increased survival and vascularity of random pattern skin flaps elevated in controlled, expanded skin. *Plast Reconstr Surg* 1983; **72:** 680–5.

23. Sasaki G H, Pang C Y. Pathophysiology of skin flaps raised on expanded skin. *Plast Reconstr Surg* 1984; **79:** 59–65.

24. Manders E K, Graham W P, Schendon M T, Davis T S. Skin expansion to eliminate large scalp defects. *Ann Plast Surg* 1984; **12:** 305–12.

25. Neale H W, High R M, Billmon D A, *et al.* Complications of controlled tissue expansion in the pediatric burn patient. *Plast Recontr Surg* 1988; **82:** 840–5.

26. Buhrer D P, Huang T T, Yee H D. Treatment of burn alopecia with tissue expanding in children. *Plast Reconstr Surg* 1988; **82:** 840–5.

27. Ortega M T, McCauley R L, Robson M C. Salvage of an avulsed expanded scalp flap to correct burn alopescia. *South Med J* 1988; **23:** 220–3.

28. McCauley R L, Oliphant J R, Robson M C. Tissue expansion in the correction of burn alopecia: classification and methods of correction. *Ann Plast Surg* 1990; **25:** 103–15.

29. Sasaki G H. Intraoperative sustained limited expansion (ISLE) as an intermediate reconstructive technique. *Clin Plast Surg* 1987; **14:** 563–71.

CHAPTER FIFTY

50

Reconstruction of the Trunk and Genitalia

Robert L. McCauley

Introduction

Recent studies, used to develop an inventory of reconstructive needs in burned children, have documented that burns of the torso and lower extremities eventually result in a significant number of problems. Brou *et al.* in an evaluation of 25 patients with a mean body surface area burn of 71%, documented 70 problems associated with the trunk and perineum.[1] In 1993, Burns *et al.* analysed the reconstructive management of patients with greater than 80% total body surface area burns. In the 28 patients analysed, there were 564 needs identified.[2] This correlated well with previous studies documenting approximately 20 reconstructive needs per patient when the total body surface area burn was at least 70%. The trunk was noted to be the most frequently identified area of injury in the torso/lower extremity region. Indeed, this region was only second to the hand as the most frequently injured anatomical unit. Further examination of truncal injuries clearly identified the breast as the most frequently identified area of reconstruction needs. Subsequent analyses of the donor tissue surveillance form revealed that the necessary donor sites for reconstruction were often not available or were of poor quality when at all feasible. Consequently, it became quite clear that a stepwise plan of action for reconstruction could not be followed. Indeed, patient and family desires must be combined with a projected realistic outcome in order to determine the most judicious and efficacious use of available donor sites.

Historical Issues

Evaluation of the management of burns to the truncal region requires longitudinal analysis of parameters of growth and development in order to assess the efficacy of variations in acute burn wound management. Over recent years, an increase in the survival of burned patients has been associated with better resuscitation, improved antimicrobial therapy, and early excisional therapy. Such data are well documented in the burn literature and remain the standard of care today.[3–7] Longitudinal assessment of earlier methods of burn care, which included delayed excision and epluchage, exhibited an increase in hospital morbidity and mortality of burned patients. The conservative management of tissue over the torso proved to be quite beneficial in female patients who survived this type of management. In 1989, McCauley *et al.* documented the conservative management of burn tissue over the anterior chest wall, involving the nipple–areola complex, which resulted in normal breast development even with nipple loss.[8] This retrospective study, which analysed burn therapy nearly 20 years earlier, revealed that, indeed, conservative management of the nipple–areola complex in these patients was uniformly beneficial. On the other hand, 71% of these patients required incisional releases of the anterior chest wall to assist in breast development. The importance of this study lies in the observation that, even with loss of the nipple–areola complex, the breast bud itself is rarely injured. Although burn management prior to 1970 was quite conservative, the longitudinal effects of blunt eschar separation resulted in maximum tissue preservation which evolved into flexible, mature burn scars.

Even with today's advanced surgical techniques, reconstruction of the breast mound, itself, rarely matches the shape and contour of a normally developed breast. Often it is difficult to evaluate the development of young females who have lost their nipple–areola complex as they proceed to develop in their adolescent years. Many of these patients require frequent follow-up in order to document the early stages of breast development and to plan surgical correction should entrapment of the developing breast in burn scar become a problem. During this period of time, pressure garments are often worn in order to assist the maturity of burn scars to accommodate the subsequent developing breast. Many of these patients will require an incisional release to allow the developing breast to remain free. Subsequent maturation of skin grafts not only results in blending in with injured tissue but also allows the tissue over the breast to immediately become more relaxed.

In patients who require global fascial excision of the anterior chest wall, breast development will not occur. In such patients, maturity of the tissue over the anterior chest wall is of paramount importance if reconstructive methods are to be successful at a later date. Many of these patients will require tissue expansion and subsequent placement of some muscular prosthesis to give the appearance of developing breasts.

The unilateral chest wall burn presents a significant problem. In children, the uninjured side will proceed with uninhibited breast development whereas the burned side may require surgical procedures in order to assist a developing breast. The development of breast asymmetry and contour deformities are quite common. The burned breast tends to be fuller and does not have the natural ptosis associated with a matured female breast. Mastopexy of the uninjured breast is often performed in order to relieve the grade II or greater ptosis, to realign the nipple–areolar complex, and to give the uninjured breast a fuller appearance.

Multiple breast releases, conducted to assist development, may result in multiple contour deformities. The lack of fullness and accentuated asymmetry of the infraclavicular may require reconstruction using pedicled fasciocutaneous flaps or a latissimus dorsi musculocutaneous flap. Even if the level of the nipple–areola complexes is similar, medial or lateral displacement of the nipple may be of significant concern to the patient. If breast contracture is a problem, medial or lateral incisional releases and coverage with skin grafts will allow better nipple positioning. On the other hand, if breast contracture is not a problem, isolated repositioning of the nipple–areola complex is indicated.

Reconstruction of the nipple–areola complex is a significant problem and represents the second stage of breast reconstruction. Although many techniques are available, most have been fraught with loss of nipple projection within 6 months. Evaluation of various techniques in the burned breast are still lacking. Recent studies by McCauley *et al.* have documented the safety of using the 'skate' flap as described by Littler. Longitudinal assessment of this procedure has shown that nipple projection is maintained although contraction does occur.[9]

Perineal Burn Management

The acute management of perineal burns is well documented at the Shriners Burns Institute–Galveston, and protocols for the management of out-patients are well publicized.[10,11] Rutan *et al.*, in a 20-year review of more than 5500 pediatric patients hospitalized at the Shriners Burns Institute in Galveston, showed only 1% of these patients sustained burns to the perineum or genitalia. Boys tend to outnumber girls 3:1 with a majority of these patients having greater than or equal to a 40% total body surface area burn. Other investigations have documented the efficacy of conservative management of genital and perineal burns.[12,13] These wounds are treated with topical antimicrobial agents in an open manner. Sharp debridement, particularly over the penis, is discouraged. Urinary catheters are frequently used during the resuscitative periods for the first 48–96 hours, when concomitant injury to the urethra has been ruled out. When required, urinary diversion has been accomplished through suprapubic catheterization. Long-term urethra catheterization has been associated with ureterostenosis which contributes to urinary tract infections.

Burn scar contractures of the perineum and genitalia are the most frequent long-term sequelae of burn injuries. Perineal webbing can present significant problems with limitation in hip range of motion as well as hooding of the external genitalia. More extensive burns involving the buttock region can also result in perianal stenosis or hooding which may impede fecal evacuation. Alghanem *et al.*, in a retrospective review, documented the 5% incidence of rectal prolapse which was related to malnutrition, diarrhea and constipation.[10] Manual reduction and correction of the instigating factors led to correction of this problem in all patients. Reconstruction of the perineal burn scar bands can usually be accomplished with multiple Z-plasties in order to correct banding genitalia hooding. Patients who present with perianal stenosis may have entrapped unburned tissue in this region.[12] Reconstruction can be accomplished with an incisional release of burn tissue from the perineum body to the coccyx through the stenotic orifice and the eversion of the unburned tissue from the anus. Lateral excision of burn scar tissue will allow recreation of the gluteal folds and access to a normal uninjured anus.

Reconstruction of the male external genitalia represents one of the most challenging problems for reconstructive surgeons. Problems may be minor, as in those which can be corrected using Z-plasties or skin grafts to restore function. Major problems in patients are secondary to partial or total loss of the penis. Fortunately, problems associated with full-thickness injuries to the penis in burn patients are relatively few. Consequently, except in electrical injuries, conservative management of burned tissue in this region is the rule.[13–15] The subsequent contractures over the penis are small; however, reconstruction of the penis may be required in the acute phase if a patient complains of significant pain during erection. Here, the immature scar is treated by an incisional release and, if possible, full-thickness skin graft to alleviate this problem. Complete loss of the penis is a devastating problem and challenges every reconstructive surgeon. Documentation of urinary excretory function is essential in evaluating such patients for further reconstruction. The use of rectus abdominus myocutaneous flap for penal reconstruction is well published.[14,15] However, significant problems have been associated with the development of urethral stenosis. In addition, erotic sensation appears to be limited, although with the subsequent placement of a penal implant, intromission is accomplished. A more recently developed technique using the radial artery forearm flap with coaptation of sensory branches of the cutaneous nerves from the forearm to the pudendal nerve has been associated with much improved erotic sensation.[15,16] Stenosis of the urethra continues to be a problem. The use of full-thickness strips of bladder to line the neourethra may improve or eliminate problems associated with urethra stenosis.

Summary

Problems associated with reconstruction of burns to the truncal region continue to represent a challenge. Entrapment of breast tissue in burn scars in female patients can be eliminated with skin grafts. Contour problems which are associated with developing breasts may be corrected with the use of skin grafts and/or fasciocutaneous flaps. Improved symmetry of the breast is of significant importance for patients who have unilateral burns of the breast. Reconstructive techniques, including mastopexy and reduction mammaplasty, may be required in order to obtain symmetry. In patients requiring fascial excision of full-thickness burns over the anterior chest wall, tissue expansion and subsequent placement of submuscular saline implants have been quite successful for breast reconstruction.

Management of wounds to the perineum and genitalia during the acute phase should be conservative. Perineal burn scar bands remain the most frequent complication associated with burns in these areas. Contractures are corrected with the use of multiple Z-plasties. Total effacement of the gluteal folds and perianal stenosis can be addressed with lateral excision of the burned tissue and eversion of the normal tissue. Penile reconstruction continues to remain a significant challenge. Staged pedicle flap reconstruction has been replaced with the use of musculocutaneous flaps and free tissue transfer with subsequent placement of penile implants. Indeed, as we continue to scrutinize the severity and frequency of problems associated with burns in the truncal regions of pediatric patients, the complexity and numbers of reconstructive procedures necessary for complete rehabilitation will undoubtedly continue to grow.

References

1. Brou J A, Robson M C, McCauley R L, *et al.* Inventory of potential reconstructive needs in the patient with burns. *J Burn Care Rehabil* 1989; **10:** 555–60.

2. Burns B F, McCauley R L, Murphy F L, Robson M C. Reconstructive management of patients with greater than 80% TBSA burns. *Burns* 1993; **19:** 429–33.

3. Burke J F, Bandoc C C, Quinby W C. Primary excision and immediate grafting. A method for shortening illness. *J Trauma* 1974; **14:** 389–95.

4. Herndon D N, Parks D H. Comparison of serial debridment and autografting and early massive excision with cadaveric skin overlay in the treatment of large burns in children. *J Trauma* 1986; **26:** 149–52.

5. Herndon D N, Gore D C, Cole M, *et al.* Determinants of mortality in pediatric patients with greater than 70% full thickness total body surface area thermal injury treated by early total excision and grafting. *J Trauma* 1987; **27:** 208–12.

6. Herndon D N, Barrow R C, Rutan R L, Rutan T C, Desai M H, Abston S. A comparison of conservative versus early excisional therapies in severely burned patients. *Ann Surg* 1989; **209:** 547–53.

7. Desai M H, Herndon D N, Broemeling L, Barrow R E, Nichols R J, Rutan R L. Early burn wound excision significantly reduces blood loss. *Ann Surg* 1990; **211:** 753–62.

8. McCauley R L, Beraja V, Rutan R L, Huang T T, Abston S, Rutan T C, Robson M C. Longitudinal assessment of breast development in adolescent female patients with burns involving the nipple-areolar complex. *Plast Reconstr Surg* 1989; **83:** 676–80.

9. McCauley R L, Robson M C. Reconstruction of the nipple areola complex in the burned breast using the 'skate' flap. *Proc Am Burn Assoc* 1994; **26:** 14.

10. Alghanem A A, McCauley R L, Robson M C, Rutan R L, Herndon D N. Management of pediatric perineal and genital burns: twenty year review. *J Burn Care Rehabil* 1990; **11:** 308–11.

11. Rutan R L. Management of perineal and genital burns. *JET Nurs* 1993; **20:** 169–76.

12. Alghanem A A, McCauley R L, Robson M C. Gluteal pouching: a complication of perineal burn scar contracture. A case report. *J Burn Care Rehabil* 1990; **11:** 137–9.

13. Culp D. Genital injuries: etiology and management. *Urol Clin* 1977; **4:** 143–6.

14. Edelman C G, Sweet M E, Messing E M, Helgerson R B. Treatment of severe electrical burns of the genitalia and perineum by early excision and grafting. *Burns* 1991; **17:** 506–9.

15. Garner W L, Smith D J. Reconstruction of burns of the trunk and breasts. *Clin Plast Surg* 1992; **19:** 683–91.

16. Kao X S, Kao C L, Yang Z N, Shi H R. One stage reconstruction of the penis with free skin flap: report of three cases. *J Reconstr Microsurg* 1984; **1:** 149–53.

CHAPTER FIFTY-ONE

51

Reconstruction of the Burned Hand

Louis L. Strock, Robert L. McCauley, David J. Smith, Jr and Martin C. Robson

Introduction

> Regardless of all the reparative principles that we have at our disposal, the one and only chance at restoring a hand to functional normalcy may or may not be lost in the initial treatment of the injury.
>
> *W. B. Macomber*[1]

The American Burn Association categorizes hand burns as major injuries, despite the less than 3% total body surface area which each hand represents. The functional importance of the hand cannot be overemphasized, as severe hand burns may leave an individual unable to work or even care for himself. Thus, the management of hand burns must focus on restoration of function with stable soft tissue coverage. This function should include fine pinch and power grip, but is ultimately determined by the individual patient's needs. Although this chapter focuses on hand burns, successful functional outcome is also dependent upon the mobility of the remainder of the extremity. Full motion and positioning of the hand is impossible if significant contracture limits motion of the elbow or axilla.

The potential and ultimate success of reconstruction following hand burns depends upon the initial treatment following injury. Thus, the acute management of the burned hand is central to a discussion of reconstruction. Treatment goals are determined by a variety of factors which include patient age, dominance of the injured hand, and occupation and work habits. The approach to burned hand deformity begins with a detailed functional assessment. Careful evaluation of each structure of the hand and the deformities present will guide the development of a plan for management. The success of reconstruction will depend on the correct assessment of the deformity and treatment goals which meet a patient's needs.

The overriding goal in reconstruction of a burned hand is to maximize and restore function. The best means to make a burned hand functional is to prevent the need for reconstruction and rehabilitation from the outset.[2] Thus, the initial diagnosis and treatment of an acutely burned hand assumes a more important role than attempts to reconstruct a crippled or deformed hand which did not receive the proper early priority. To properly treat a burned hand and avoid deformity, a basic understanding of the anatomy and physiology of the hand and the pathobiology of the effects of thermal injury on its specialized anatomy is required.[3]

Anatomy

The soft tissues and skin of the hand have several unique characteristics. Dorsal skin is thin and flexible, and lies on a thin layer of subcutaneous tissue. While little protection for the underlying extensor apparatus is provided, it does maximize tendon gliding function. Wrinkles over the interphalangeal joints deepen with finger extension and stretch with finger flexion. Longitudinal wrinkling over the metacarpophalangeal joints permits similar movement of the transverse arch of the hand. These adaptive characteristics allow for full flexion and extension without extensive skin redundancy or tightness. The dorsal sweep of the web spaces begins at the level of the metacarpal heads, with an abundance of skin allowing for motion of individual fingers.[4]

Dorsal skin has numerous hair follicles, sebaceous glands, and pigment cells. The hair is most prominent on the ulnar aspect, and is also distributed over the proximal and middle phalanges. Large peripheral veins lie directly beneath the dorsal skin and are important modulators of heat exchange. By contrast, the palmar skin is hairless and has a thick dermis and no pigment cells. There is a keratinized layer above the epidermis which is thickest over the finger pulp and grasping areas, while the dermis and keratin are thinner over the flexion creases of the hand. The topography of multiple whorls, arches, and ridges maximizes grip function by insuring that the ridges are always at right angles to the object being grasped. Stability of grip is provided by numerous fibrous septae which connect the dermis of the palmar skin to the underlying palmar fascia from the volar wrist crease to the proximal finger creases. Cleland's and Grayson's ligaments provide stability distally. Cleland's ligament is a firm fascial structure which connects the skin with the flexor fibro-osseous tunnel, and lies dorsal to the neurovascular bundle. Grayson's ligament stabilizes the palmar skin, but is not as well defined and lies volar to the neurovascular bundle.[4,5]

The extensor mechanism is at risk because of its thin overlying skin, especially at the level of the proximal interphalangeal joint. At this level, the extensor tendon has formed a trifurcation consisting of the central slip and two lateral bands. While the central slip inserts into the base of the middle phalanx, the lateral bands continue distally to the base of the distal phalanx. The transverse retinacular ligament maintains this spatial relationship at the proximal interphalangeal level, which allows for simultaneous extension of the middle phalanx by the central slip and the distal phalanx by the lateral bands. Burn injury may directly destroy the underlying tendon, resulting in a boutonnière deformity, or disrupt the balance between the extrinsic and intrinsic systems.[4]

The fingernail and nailbed are vulnerable to thermal injury. The nailbed is comprised of a soft tissue matrix, immediately beneath the nail, which produces nail migration and regeneration. The nail consists of three layers, each formed by a separate area of the nail fold. Distal growth results from restriction of the nail fold. As each matrix cell flattens to occupy a larger area than when it was in the germinal state, pressure is exerted to direct growth distally. Complete nail growth requires between 70 and 160 days, and occurs at a rate of 0.1 mm/day.[4]

PHYSIOLOGY

The functional capabilities of the hand depend upon its unique architectural construction. The centerpiece of this architecture is Littler's 'fixed unit of the hand'.[6] It consists of the distal carpal row which maintains a fixed transverse arch, and the central second and third metacarpals which form a fixed longitudinal arch projecting from the carpus[6] (**Figure 51.1**). Support is provided for the three mobile units of the hand:

- the thumb and its metacarpal with their wide range of motion at the carpometacarpal joint;
- the index finger with its relative independence of motion; and
- the long, ring, and small fingers with the fourth and fifth metacarpals, which stabilize objects for manipulation by the thumb and index finger and with other hand units for power grasp.[4]

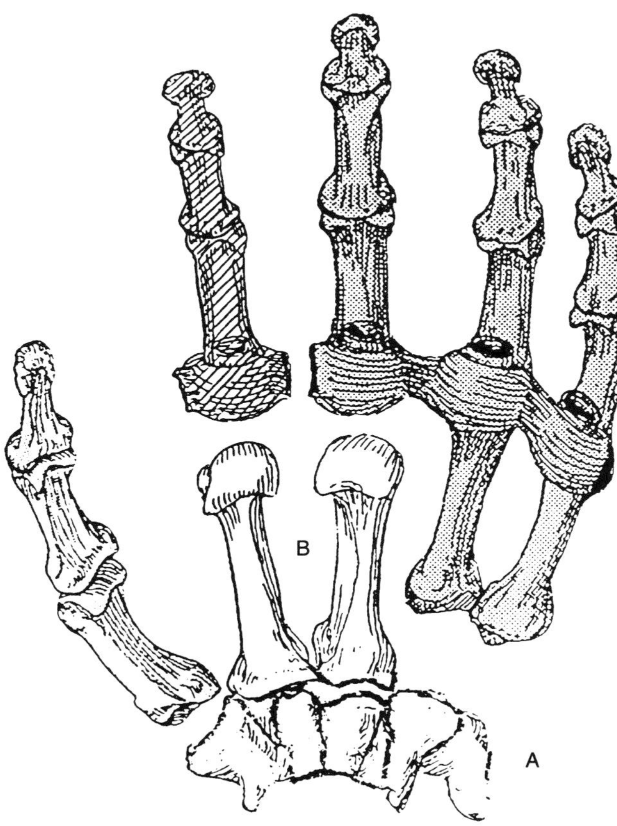

Fig. 51.1 Arches of the hand: A, transverse arch; B, longitudinal arch

While thermal injury may affect the transverse arches of the hand, alterations in flexion and extension are more common. For isolated digital flexion to occur, there is an interplay between the direct effects of the flexor digitorum superficialis, flexor digitorum profundus, lumbrical and interosseus muscles, and the indirect effects of the wrist and finger extensors. Flexion of the metacarpophalangeal, proximal, or distal interphalangeal joints depends upon flexor–extensor interplay for stabilization of the fixation of the remaining joints. Thermal injury may have a profound impact on the function of the hand by disruption of the usual interrelationships between the muscles, tendons, joints, and skin which allow for the hand's varied capabilities.[4]

The hand is central to our ability to evaluate the environment and protect ourselves from injury. Nearly everything we learn about objects which we cannot gain from other senses is gained by hand testing. The main digits for exploration are the thumb along with the index and long fingers, supplied by the median nerve. The median nerve provides the major sensory input to the large area of cerebral cortex which is dedicated to the hand. Additional stimuli testing is provided by the sense of muscular effort, or proprioception. The hand is able to evaluate objects by the combination of the highly refined superficial testing capacity and the complex proprioceptive mechanism.[4]

PATHOBIOLOGY

The pathobiology of a burned hand requires an understanding of the direct effects of heat on tissue, and the unique problems presented by the anatomy of the hand. The pathobiology can be divided into four phases:

- pathologic effects of the heat itself;
- pathologic effects secondary to edema;
- pathologic effects secondary to decreased circulation;
- pathologic effects secondary to bacterial colonization of the wound.[3,4]

The isolated hand burn shows how the comparison of time and temperature reported by Moritz and Henrique can result in injury and cell death with temperatures as low as 43°C (109°F).[7] Extremity burns inspired Artursson to suggest that prostaglandin derivatives have a central role in the progressive deterioration of the zone of stasis.[8] Heggers and Robson demonstrated the presence of PGE_2 and TXB_2 in the blister fluid from burned hands.[9] These studies helped to delineate some of the delayed effects of heat on cells.

Anatomy unique to the hand allows for other direct heat effects not seen elsewhere in the body.[4] Tendons and joints are situated closely beneath the skin over the dorsum of the fingers, making these structures more susceptible to the effects of heat. The nail and nailbed are directly exposed to the heat source. The cylindrical form of the fingers, with their ligaments, such as Cleland's and Grayson's, and the vertical septae of the pulp, limit swelling and volume change in the finger following injury.[4] Edema causes pathologic effects by creating pressure and decreased circulation. Intracellular edema results from disruption of the sodium pump with resultant entry of sodium and water into the cell. Edema also results from the shift from normal homeostasis between PGE_2 and $PGF_{2\alpha}$ toward PGE_2 in the zone of stasis.[9] In all burn injuries over 30% total body surface area, total capillary permeability occurs and can be aggravated by over-resuscitation. Dependence of the extremity can also add to the edema following injury. While the edema usually improves by 72 hours post-injury, persistence results in tissue fibrosis and limitation of range of motion.[10]

There are two areas of the hand which are extremely susceptible to secondary infection.[4] The thin skin overlying the dorsum of the proximal interphalangeal joints makes the tendons likely to be injured or result in an open joint. Decreased blood supply with this injury may also increase the susceptibility to infection with secondary joint injury. The nailbed is the other area which is particularly susceptible to injury. Despite its high vascularity, the nailbed is readily exposed to thermal injury and secondary trauma and infection.

Management of an Acute Hand Burn

Pruitt has reported that over 85% of patients admitted to hospitals following thermal injury have burns of the hands.[11] While a detailed discussion of the management of the acutely burned hand is beyond the scope of this chapter, six treatment principles can be outlined for management which, if followed, will help to prevent deformity and maintain function:

- do no harm;
- maintain circulation;
- prevent infection;
- obtain wound closure;
- preserve or regain motion;
- obtain functional rehabilitation.

These treatment principles, though presented separately, overlap conceptually and temporally.[3,4]

Principle 1: Do No Harm

The admonition 'primum, non nocere' (first, do no harm) is never more appropriate than when dealing with management of a burned hand.[4] Management must focus on preservation of the zone of stasis, which is comprised of cells which are initially injured but are still viable. Do nothing which will lead to further microvascular deterioration in this zone. Avoid maceration, which removes the remaining natural barriers to infection of intact skin. Removal of blister fluid is appropriate, as it contains inflammatory mediators thought to be detrimental to the microcirculation in the zone of stasis.[3,4] This can be done by either debridement of the blister or by aspiration of the fluid. Pharmacologic manipulation of the zone of stasis may be possible through blockade of detrimental mediators. Zawacki showed that desiccation can further injure the zone of stasis and result in a deeper injury.[12] If the blister is broken, one should debride and prevent desiccation.

Principle 2: Maintain Circulation

The circulation can be maintained by preventing microvascular deterioration and by preventing excess edema. Cooling a burned hand, as a first aid measure within the first 30 minutes of a burn injury, has been shown to prevent leukocyte sticking and increase wound perfusion. Cooling of the wound is thought to maintain normal homeostasis between PGE_2 and $PGF_{2\alpha}$, and prevent the formation of thromboxane.[13] Elevation of the burned extremity during transfer and resuscitation is needed to minimize edema formation.

Despite cooling and elevation, eschars proximal to a burned hand may jeopardize distal circulation. Salisbury and Levine show that the intrinsic musculature cannot withstand ischemia.[14] Close monitoring is necessary with early operative decompression instituted for release of circulatory embarrassment. The surgeon should carefully plan surgical escharotomy incisions so as to release areas of compromise early, restore adequate flow, and yet not injure underlying structures. While a decision to perform operative decompression with a patient under anesthesia in an operating room may be made with some reluctance, the procedure attempted in a burn center or emergency department may be inadequate. Blood loss can be surprisingly great and can further increase risk to nerves or vessels underlying the escharotomies.

In an attempt to avoid problems associated with surgical escharotomies in the hand, Krizek reported a noninvasive method of eschar decompression.[15] This medical decompression uses the enzymatic debriding agent, Travase, which causes a proteolytic dissolution of the constricting eschar. A thin layer of Travase is applied in a wet dressing for one hour, and the circulation is reassessed. If total release has not occurred, the procedure is repeated. The authors choose this technique in place of surgical escharotomy and find it most effective for acute burns of the upper extremity. If the burn injury is several hours old or is secondary to an electrical burn, surgical escharotomy may become a therapeutic necessity.

Principle 3: Prevent Infection

Infection in a burned hand can be secondary to several causes. Clostridial infection arising from burns of the hands is rare, but does occur. This infection is totally preventable, as long as tetanus immunoprophylaxis is part of the management plan. The guidelines for tetanus immunoprophylaxis as published by The Committee on Trauma of the American College of Surgeons should be followed.[16]

The normal defense system of the body against the β-hemolytic streptococci is neutralized during the edema phase of the burn wound. Administration of a specific antistreptococcal agent (penicillin or erythromycin), during the edema phase, can prevent sequelae such as streptococcal cellulitis or erysipelas of a burned hand. Heggers and Robson demonstrated the presence of penicillin in the blister fluid of patients who had received the drug, and Hing showed that penicillin penetrates from the systemic circulation into the burn eschar.[9,17]

The normal equilibrium of the bacterial flora of the skin is disrupted by thermal injury. Bacteria which normally reside in sweat glands and hair follicles migrate through burned skin and multiply. Transient organisms which are normally prevented from achieving bacterial lodgement by the intact cutaneous barrier, become capable of proliferation and invasion. As these organisms multiply, they further compromise the blood supply by perivascular compression. An avascular burn wound sepsis results when these bacteria multiply to more than 10^5 organisms per gram of tissue.[18] The resultant infection is not responsive to systemic antimicrobials and is best prevented by topical antimicrobial creams. The selection of a cream for a specific wound can be guided by use of the agar well technique on a homogenate of a burn wound tissue biopsy.[19] Antibacterial liquids can be used as alternatives to creams. Silver nitrate in a 0.5% concentration has been used on burned hands, but requires a bulky dressing which decreases motion. Mafenide acetate has been used as a 5% solution, and is reported to be as effective in the control of bacterial growth, prevention of desiccation, and allowing for motion.[20]

Principle 4: Obtain Wound Closure

The goal in the management of an acutely burned hand is to obtain a wound closed with autogenous tissue which is pliable and durable enough to allow for full function. There are five basic options for wound closure, depending upon the depth of the injury, which include:

- early spontaneous reepithelialization within 14 days;
- early excision of nonviable tissue and grafting;
- delayed spontaneous healing requiring more than 14 days;
- late tertiary closure of the spontaneously healing burn; and
- delayed excision of the burn wound with grafting.[21]

Wound closure for a superficial partial-thickness burn occurs by epithelialization, within 2 weeks if the diagnosis is correct. Treatment is aimed at not impeding epithelialization. Rovee and coworkers have shown that epithelialization proceeds most rapidly in a moist milieu.[22] Thus, biological dressings, water-based creams, and possibly thin-film dressings seem to be justified, as each is aimed at preventing dryness and desiccation. The use of a bilaminate, synthetic dressing (Biobrane®) has been shown to be effective in these wounds.[23] Because burn wound sepsis is not likely to occur in these superficial burns, topical antibacterials are probably not justified after the edema phase, unless used in the form of water-soluble creams to prevent wound desiccation.[4]

Full-thickness burns of the hand generally do not do well regardless of treatment. If only the hands are burned, the author's preference is for early full-thickness excision with preservation of spared dorsal veins and sheet grafting. If accompanied by deep burns over other areas of the body, the hands must be grafted in order of priority. The priority of burned hands is quite high, usually following the head and neck.

The majority of hand burns requiring hospitalization are deep dermal burns. The treatment of these burns has been controversial, initially parallel to that of full-thickness burns. The wound is excised and grafted before infection develops. Alternative treatment followed the advent of topical antimicrobials in the mid-1960s. This allows bacterial control and spontaneous healing, and suggests that most hand burns are deep dermal burns and not full-thickness. This has led to several approaches to deep partial-thickness hand burns.

Surgeons who believed that early wound closure was the key to good hand function advocated early excision and grafting as the preferred treatment for deep dermal burns. Tangential or intradermal debridement techniques, thus, replaced full-thickness excision (**Figure 51.2**). This resulted in shorter periods of hospitalization, cost-saving, better function, and fewer complications. Other surgeons believed that, since dermal elements were present in the majority of hand burns, conservatism was justified. This approach was advocated by Labanter *et al.* and was based on the use of topical antimicrobials and a vigorous physical therapy program to maintain function.[24] The two radically different approaches warranted prospective randomized series to attempt to establish superiority of one of the approaches. Three such trials have been reported and showed the treatments to be of equal efficacy.[25–27]

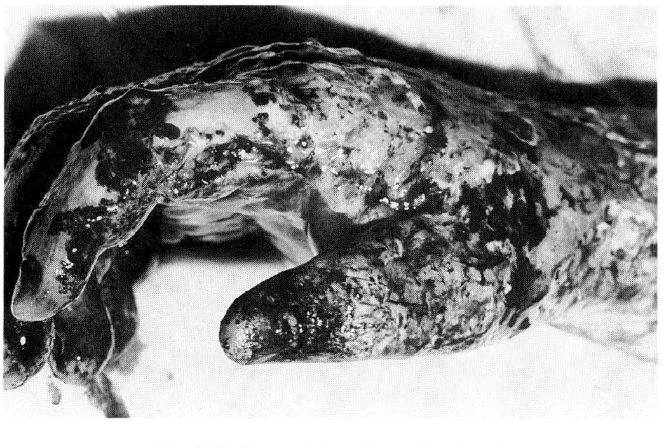

Fig. 51.2 Tangential excision of the hand.

Krizek suggested 'delayed primary excision' as an alternative approach for patients with mixed depth burns which had not healed in 2 weeks.[28] This was based on his observations of spontaneously healed burn wounds, that the new epithelium was fragile and easily abraded because of a lack of rete ridges. As these wounds lacked sweat glands, streptococcal erysipelas was common with its associated pruritis. Since this time, splinting, positioning, and exercising are aggressively applied soon after surgery. Additionally, Robson reported that the use of pressure garments with prolonged anti-streptococcal protection can prevent many of the problems associated with spontaneously healed burns.[29]

The choice of the type of graft applied to the burned hand deserves careful attention. Sheet grafts are indicated, when possible, as ultimate function depends upon timely wound closure and a decrease in the associated inflammatory phase.[4] Nonexpanded 1.5:1 mesh graft is an alternative to sheet grafting.

Unlike dorsal hand burns, palmar burns are rarely excised and usually heal spontaneously.[4] No plane of dissection exists in the palm. Splinting is crucial, with emphasis on maintenance of palmar width.

Principle 5: Preserve or Regain Motion

Proper positioning of the burned hand in the early post-injury period is a major priority. The burned hand initially presents in an intrinsic minus position, with the metacarpophalangeal joints extended or hyperextended, the proximal and distal interphalangeal joints flexed, and the thumb adducted. This is the position of comfort and ultimately results in contracture if not corrected.[4] This position makes physical therapy difficult and is nearly impossible to correct secondarily.

A supervised program of splinting and exercise is started in the early postburn period. If early excision is not chosen, splinting is continued until the edema of the hand resolves. With dorsal burns, night splinting is continued to maintain the position achieved during daily exercise. Static splinting is discontinued when flexion to the midpalmar crease is obtained. Exposed tendons are treated with splinting in order to maintain a lax position and with dressing changes in order to prevent tendon desiccation until permanent coverage is obtained.

The ability of a patient to tolerate an exercise program can be difficult to assess. Careful attention to vital signs is important, as poor tolerance may be indicated by dyspnea, diaphoresis, immediate increase in systolic blood pressure of 20 mmHg, and tachycardia.[30,31] These responses can be due to other factors, ranging from poor nutritional status, hypermetabolism, and electrolyte imbalance, to anxiety, infection, age, and environmental status.[4] While initial progress may be slow, gentle passive and active range of motion exercises are encouraged two to four times daily. Active motion against resistance can be used to increase muscle activity, increase pumping activity, and help to decrease edema. While static splinting maintains position, dynamic splints provide a force against scar contracture. Thus, dynamic splinting may be of use following the edema phase.

Rehabilitation goals during the acute phase include:

- stretching of healing skin;
- maintenance of full range of motion in the joints;
- preservation of motor skill coordination;

- promotion of functional independence; and
- maintenance or return of strength and endurance to minimize muscle atrophy.[4]

These goals are accomplished by range of motion exercises, participation in activities of daily living, and ambulation. Range of motion should be routinely documented and be correlated specifically with the degree of healing.[32] The exercise or splinting program is changed if a patient is noted to plateau or regress.

Principle 6: Obtain Functional Rehabilitation

The final goal is functional rehabilitation. This requires that a patient have adequate and durable skin coverage.[4] If spontaneous healing has occurred, the quality, fragility, and pliability of the closure must be evaluated relative to the patient's specific needs. Webbing, dorsal hooding, and burn syndactyly of the web spaces are best prevented. These complications are avoided by careful grafting techniques, maintenance of proper position post-injury, and proper spacing between the digits.

Compression garments are useful in helping to prevent edema, decrease secondary infection, and protect hands during the collagen maturation phase. Compression gloves appear to be most useful for about 4–6 months after spontaneous healing or grafting with any burn deeper than superficial partial-thickness.[4] Anti-streptococcal medications and lubricants for the skin are useful to obtain the best functional results.[28]

Ultimately, functional recovery is best measured by the ability of a treated hand to perform necessary tasks. This is best evaluated by the use of detailed industrial or domestic task evaluation scales. If a patient cannot perform specific tasks, a determination should be made as to whether the deficit is temporary or permanent. Temporary deficits can be remedied with work-hardening programs, whereas patients with permanent deficits may require vocational retraining.[4]

Clinical Assessment of the Burned Hand Deformity

Few problems in surgery may seem as overwhelming as the evaluation of a patient with a neglected healed burned hand (**Figure 51.3**). While the six principles discussed will usually help a patient presenting with an acute hand burn to maintain function, not all patients receive such attention to hand function during the early post-injury period. A nonfunctional hand with insufficient and inadequate skin coverage, with fixed contractures in the intrinsic minus position, and with decreased sensation, may appear impossible to reconstruct and rehabilitate.[3,4] A stepwise approach, with evaluation of each structure, followed by a list of abnormalities, will begin to unravel the problem.[4] Photographs in many planes and motions and specific measurements of joint mobility aid in the assessment, in addition to radiographs, bone scans, vascular studies, and electromyograms as indicated. One must evaluate the ability of a hand to perform its necessary tasks. Specific and detailed domestic and industrial tasks must be determined for a patient, and the lack of ability to perform these tasks must be recorded.[4]

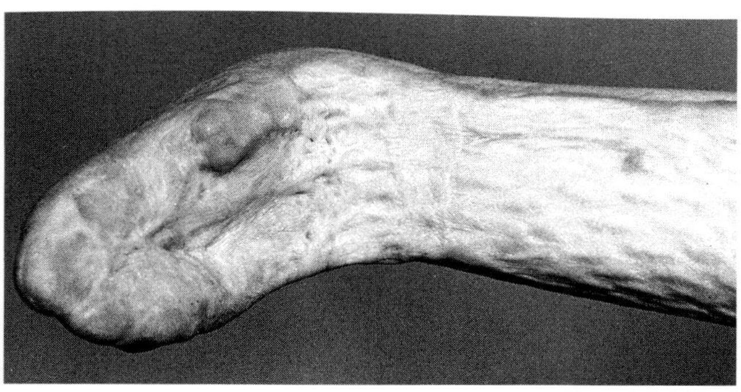

Fig. 51.3 Healed, neglected, mitten hand.

A plan for management must begin with repeated, detailed discussions with a patient.[4] Expectations must be realistic and require the input of family and often a patient's employer. The priorities of a patient and surgeon must coincide. The focus must center on the correction or improvement of each of the injured structures if optimal function is to be achieved. The ability of a surgeon to correct a particular deformity must also be considered in the formulation of a treatment plan.

Reconstruction of Late Problems

Once the deformities and functional deficits have been enumerated and related to specific anatomical structures, reconstruction can begin.[3] The surface covering is always the first priority and must be carefully evaluated to insure that the skin is present in sufficient amount and quality to withstand the demands of everyday life. Frequently, initial wound coverage may have been accomplished using expanded mesh grafts which ultimately fail to provide the desirable long-term properties of skin. These grafts are frequently associated with itching, breakdown, hypertrophy, and contracture.[4]

Dorsal burn scar contractures require the addition of stable tissue coverage. The surgical approach begins with removal of the entire scar, release of residual contractures, and elimination of all unstable scars. Occasionally flap coverage is necessary, if the paratenon is removed or if tendon, joint, or nerve reconstruction is needed. While flaps can be too bulky, use of the lateral arm free flap or the radial artery forearm flap may give more esthetic results. Initial resurfacing with sheet grafts is preferred until such reconstruction is planned. The grafts are best applied transversely with the hand splinted with the wrist in neutral, metacarpophalangeal joints at 90 degrees, and the interphalangeal joints at 0 degrees.[4] Motion is started when the grafts are stable, usually at 5–7 days. The combination of night splinting, daytime active therapy, and compressive garments are important for obtaining optimal results.

One type of contracture is that on the dorsum of the web spaces which results in burn syndactyly. Direct attention to the spacing between digits during the acute injury treatment phase can prevent web space contracture. Since maintenance of the hand in the 'safe' position, with the metacarpophalangeal joints flexed, places the digits in marked adduction, exercises must be prescribed which maintain abduction and spreading in addition to flexion and extension.[3,4] Spacers may also be incorporated into dressings. Burn syndactyly can be corrected using a variety of methods.[33] Larson suggested that pressure garments can remodel immature contracture and overcome the need for surgery.[34] For mature contractures, surgery seeks to accomplish one of three goals:

- break line and add length to a straight-line contracture;
- recreate the web space commissure by use of local flaps; and
- add skin from outside the local area for severely scarred web spaces.[4]

While many authors have suggested that tissue deficiency is the major problem, Krizek *et al.* reported that most cases of burn syndactyly could be successfully treated with local flaps.[33] Extreme webbing with extension to the proximal interphalangeal joint did, however, often require the addition of tissue for successful treatment. The simplest approach to lengthen a straight-line contracture is a Z-plasty. Z-plasties placed side-to-side, in tandem, and employing various angles, such as four-flap and five-flap Z-plasties, are used when the webbing covers a longer distance (**Figure 51.4**). On occasion, skin grafts are added in combination with local flaps, with the local flap preferentially placed on the dominant side and the skin graft on the nondominant side of the digit. This problem is most frequently seen in the thumb–index web space.[4,33]

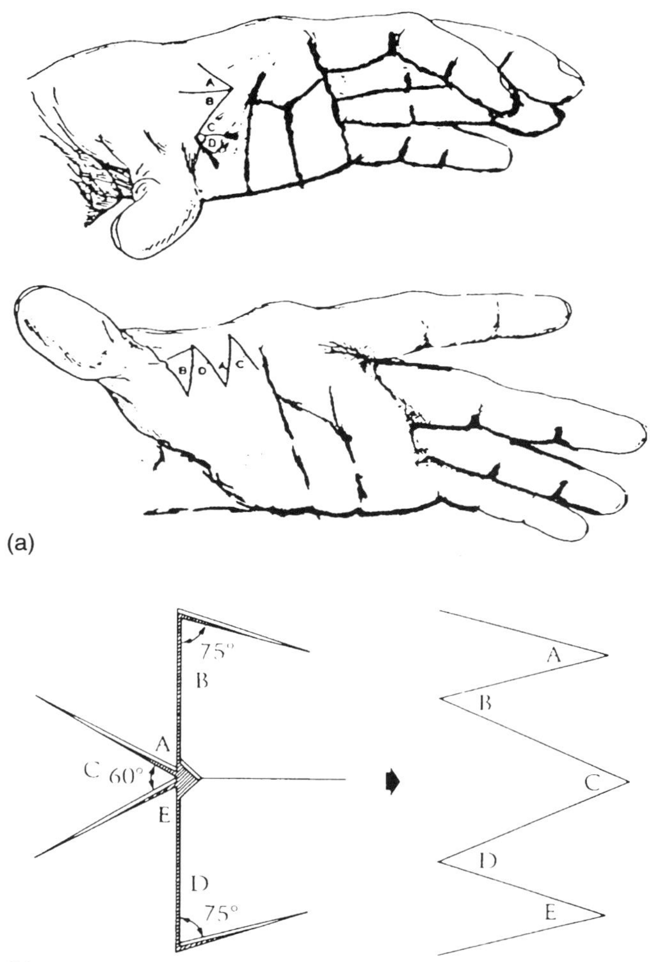

Fig. 51.4 Four-flap (a) and five-flap (b) Z-plasties.

Nailbed complications can be extremely bothersome. Whether the result of the heat injury itself or secondary problems due to ischemia or infection, nailbed problems are frequent. Deformities can include hook nails, grooving, nonadherence, and notching; they result from the heat differential which causes various levels of injury.[35] Usually, the surrounding skin is shiny and flattened, with obliteration of the normal eponychial fold. Bacterial or fungal infection may contribute to partial or complete loss of the nail. The early emphasis is on a conservative, nonsurgical approach. Dermatologic consultation may be helpful in the treatment of infectious complications. In the postburn patient, surgery should not be considered for at least 6 months, as nail growth is often delayed.[4] Split-thickness skin grafts, split nailbed grafts, reverse dermal grafts, and obliteration are all surgical alternatives.

Long-term deformities can result from injury to deeper structures at the time of a burn injury. When blood vessels are involved, long-term problems result from ischemia. Volkmann's ischemic contracture following thermal injury is now rare, largely because of increased monitoring and awareness. Because of the extreme devastation which follows Volkmann's contracture, reconstruction using free muscle transfer may be needed. Particularly difficult to diagnose is ischemic intrinsic contracture. An autopsy study from the US Army Institute of Surgical Research reported the presence of intrinsic muscle necrosis in two-thirds of the completely burned upper extremities in which escharotomies had been performed.[14] These findings emphasize that conventional escharotomy does not protect the deep structures of a hand from ischemia. Intrinsic fasciotomies should be considered in the acute period if the fingers remain in the intrinsic minus position with the metacarpophalangeal joints in hyperextension and the interphalangeal joints in flexion.[3,4] Decompression of the intrinsic muscles is accomplished by incision of the investing fascia through a small dorsal incision placed in the first web space and then between the metacarpals.

In late post-traumatic ischemic contractures involving only the proximal interphalangeal joints, persistent decreased flexion of that joint occurs.[4] While this limitation is often suspected to be caused by residual capsular tightness or post-traumatic synovitis, the presence of intrinsic tightness can be confirmed on physical examination. With the metacarpophalangeal joints extended proximal interphalangeal flexion is restricted when tightness exists. Conversely, with metacarpophalangeal joints flexed, flexion of the proximal interphalangeal joint is improved. Restriction due to capsular adhesions is not altered by a change in metacarpophalangeal position. When the metacarpophalangeal joint is unaffected, therapy is directed toward the improvement of proximal interphalangeal flexion. This can be achieved by surgical release of the oblique fibers of the lateral bands.[4] A more severe deformity which involves both the metacarpophalangeal and proximal interphalangeal joints requires extensive release of the dorsal aponeurosis. If muscle function exists, an interosseous slide may be appropriate. If the muscles are scarred and fibrotic, as is often the case if enzymatic or surgical decompression of the intrinsic compartments was not adequate, release of the interosseous contracture by transection of the tendons proximal to the metacarpophalangeal joints is indicated.[4] Release of para-articular structures which restrict motion is also indicated.

Henderson *et al.* were the first to emphasize the occurrence of peripheral neuropathies in burned patients.[36] Most often, patient complaints included numbness and tingling and an inability to perform motor tasks which involved the median or ulnar nerves or both. They reported a 15% incidence of polyneuropathies in 249 nondiabetic and nonalcoholic burned patients. The neuropathies were most often associated with burn surface area of greater than 20% in adult patients. Helm and coworkers confirmed these results by demonstrating electromyographic and clinical changes of nerve compression syndromes in both burned and unburned extremities.[37] They observed nerve compression in 30% of patients and confirmed that patients with a burn area greater than 20% were more likely to develop a neuropathy.

Frank and Robson have also shown a high incidence of postburn bilateral nerve entrapment syndromes at the wrist.[38] The high incidence of bilaterality suggested that the thermal injury and its treatment may promote or increase the likelihood of nerve compression. This led to the authors' suggestion that the 'safe' position be modified, with the hand splinted during the acute phase with the interphalangeal joints in extension, the metacarpophalangeal (MP) joints in 80–90 degrees of flexion, and the wrist only slightly extended from the neutral position. Splinting during all phases of recovery should avoid wrist hyperextension. Liberal use of nerve conduction studies can help to clarify weakness and sensory changes due to the burn injury itself from those caused by nerve entrapment.

Tendon complications are much more common with extensor than flexor tendons and include disruption and adhesion. Attempts at tenolysis and release of adhesions are rarely successful as scar encases the tendon over the entire distance of the burn and the overlying skin quality is poor.[4] Thus, good quality skin cover must be provided prior to functional tendon reconstruction. Loss of the extensor hood creates the typical boutonnière deformity. Treatment of this deformity in a burned hand requires a different approach. Progressive splinting is rarely helpful because the dorsal skin will not tolerate the pressure without ulceration. Arthrodesis with minimal bone shortening is often the best alternative. With adequate dorsal skin, Elliot's reconstruction, consisting of repair of the central slip and plication of the lateral bands, provides an excellent surgical alternative.[39] Joint problems frequently accompany this deformity, most often metacarpophalangeal tightness. Successful rehabilitation occurs when reconstruction is combined into a single procedure. While McShane has reported success with joint replacement in highly motivated patients,[40] the best functional results often follow carefully chosen fusion combined with procedures for adjacent joint mobility.

Para-articular ossification occurs in 2–3% of severely burned patients, with osseous bridging of the joint occurring in no more than 1%.[41] The incidence ranges from 11% to 13% for burns of the extremities only.[42] This occurs most often at the elbow, with the anterior aspect most commonly involved in children and the posterior aspect more common in adults.[4] Para-articular calcification occurs more frequently when the surface area surrounding the elbow has been burned, but may also occur when the area burned is distant from the elbow. In adults, bridging occurs from the olecranon to the medial supracondylar ridge of the humerus, with range of motion compromised by the sixth week following injury. Bone changes become radiographically evident during the eighth week post-injury. Management depends upon recognition of three facts:

- all para-articular calcification and ossification may increase in dimension as long as granulating wounds remain;
- when the burn has healed and heterotopic bone has not bridged the joint, it will gradually disappear in children or become markedly smaller in adults; and
- as ectopic bone which bridges a joint spares the articulation, adequately removed bone which is removed after the bone has healed will not reform sufficiently to compromise motion.[41]

Thus, once a burned patient has recovered and his wounds are healed, the potential for this form of bone formation is lost.

Partial or complete amputation of the thumb and fingers can accompany severe burn injury to hands. This can result in the most severe of functional deficits, with loss of the ability to grasp or pinch objects. This presents a tremendous reconstructive challenge. When the thumb and fingers are amputated at or just beyond the metacarpophalangeal level, and the thumb metacarpal is preserved, pollicization of the index metacarpal ray may be performed.[43–45] May *et al.* emphasize the value of advancement pollicization in providing improved length and arc of movement and resultant functional advantage.[45] They also emphasize the importance of flap resurfacing of the radial side of the hand prior to advancement pollicization in order to improve the flexibility of the first web space following reconstruction.[45] Metacarpal stacking procedures may also be used to lengthen amputated digits and allow a patient to regain the functional ability to grasp objects (**Figure 51.5**). Microvascular transfer of toe to hand is an alternative approach, particularly when the index finger is functionally intact.

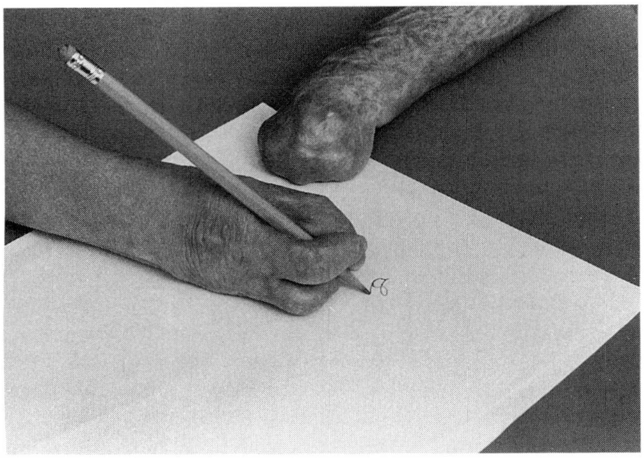

Fig. 51.5 Metacarpal stacking done to give length.

Rehabilitation Following Reconstruction

As with the initial assessment in the acute phase post-injury, successful functional rehabilitation depends upon many factors. There must be repeated and detailed discussions between a patient and a reconstructive team; these discussions should include family members, teachers, and vocational counselors, as indicated. This will help to insure that expectations are realistic and that the priorities of the patient and the reconstructive team coincide. Counseling which can be vital to recovery from an acute injury, is also vital to long-term functional recovery.

Summary

The functional importance of a hand cannot be overemphasized, as adequate hand function can determine whether a person is able to work and care for himself. The principles for successful management of a patient with burns of the hands are outlined in detail, with emphasis on preservation and restoration of function. The potential and ultimate success of reconstruction following hand burns depends largely upon the initial treatment following injury. With this in mind, a detailed discussion for management of acute hand burns is presented.

The approach to a burned hand with deformity is presented, with emphasis on an initial detailed functional assessment of the specific structures involved with the injury. This initial evaluation serves as a guide for the development of a specific plan for management. The ultimate function of the patient with burns to the hands depends upon the magnitude and treatment of the initial injury, the careful evaluation and management of late deformities present, and the willingness of the patient and burn team to work together in establishment of realistic goals and treatment priorities appropriate for the patient's needs (**Figure 51.6**).

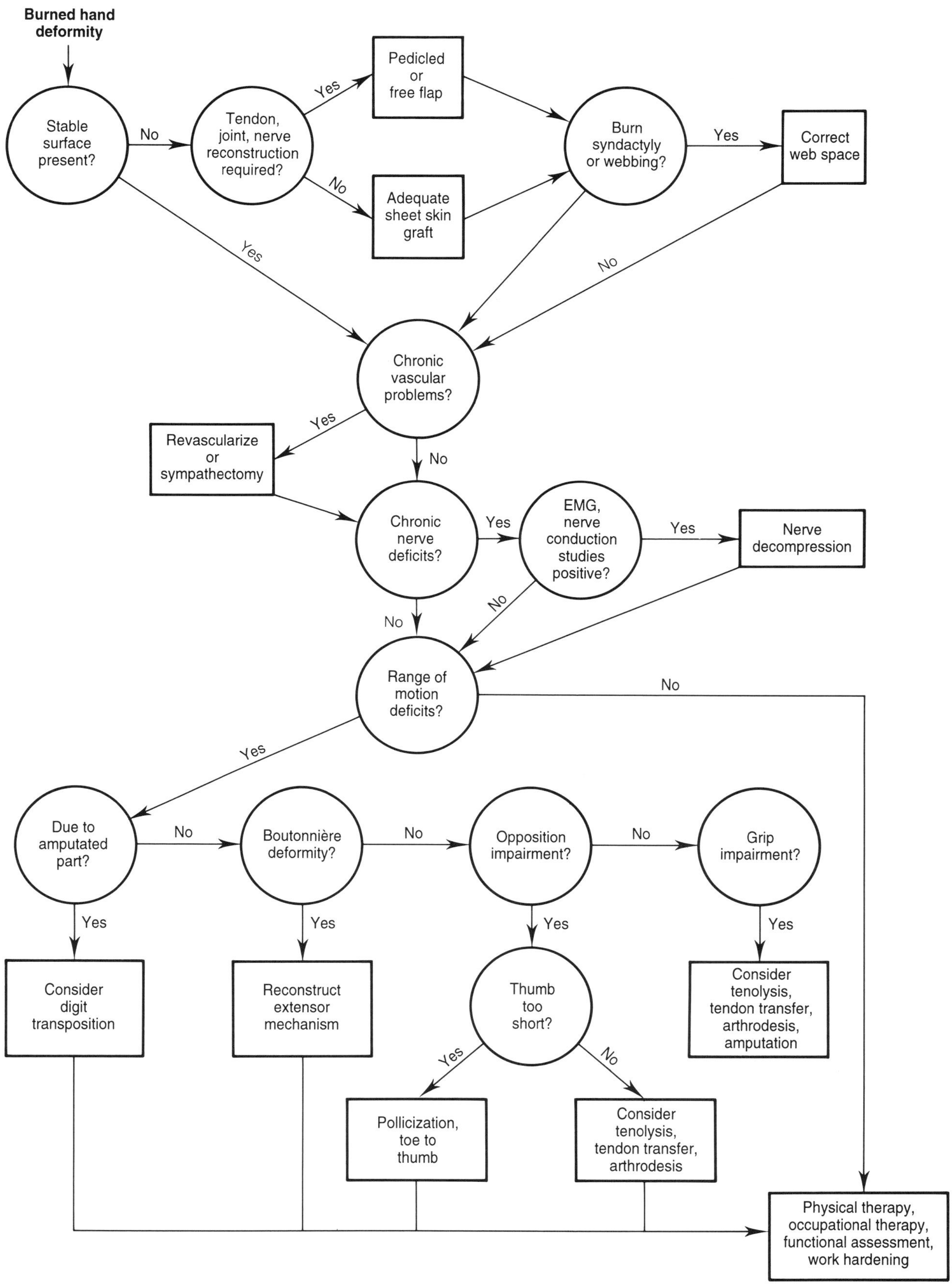

Fig. 51.6 Algorithm for reconstruction of the burned hand deformity.

REFERENCES

1. Macomber W B. Relationship of superficial and deep reconstructive surgery of the hand. *Plast Reconstr Surg* 1950; **5:** 139.

2. Robson M C. Reconstruction and rehabilitation from admission. In: Bernstein N R, Robson M C, eds. *Comprehensive Approaches to the Burned Person*. New Hyde Park, NY: Medical Exam Publishing, 1983; 35–48.

3. Robson M C, Smith D J, VanderZee A J. Making the burned hand functional. *Clin Plast Surg* 1992; **19**(3): 663–71.

4. Robson M C, Smith D J. Burned hand. In: Jurkiewicz M J, Krizek T J, Mathes S J, Ariyan S, eds. *Plastic Surgery: Principles and Practice*. St Louis: C V Mosby, 1990: 781–802.

5. Kaplan E B. Anatomy and kinesiology of the hand. In: Flynn J E, ed. *Hand Surgery*. Baltimore: Williams & Wilkins Co, 1982: 14–24.

6. Littler J W. Principles of reconstructive surgery of the hand. In: Converse J M, ed. *Reconstructive Plastic Surgery*. Philadelphia: W B Saunders, 1977: 3103–53.

7. Moritz A R, Henrique F C. Studies of thermal injury: the relative importance of time and surface temperature in the causation of cutaneous burns. *Am J Pathol* Sept 1947; **23:** 695–720.

8. Artursson G. Arachidonic acid metabolism and prostaglandin activity following burn injury. In: Ninemann J L, ed. *Traumatic Injury: Infection and Other Immunologic Sequelae*. Baltimore: University Park Press, 1983; 57–78.

9. Heggers J P, Robson M C. Prostaglandins and thromboxanes. In: Ninemann J L, ed. *Traumatic Injury: Infection and Other Immunologic Sequelae*. Baltimore: University Park Press, 1983; 79–102.

10. Peacock E E, Madden J W, Trier W C. Some studies on the treatment of burned hands. *Ann Surg* 1970; **171:** 903–14.

11. Pruitt B A. Epidmiology and general considerations. In: Salisbury R D, ed. *Burns of the Upper Extremity* Philadelphia: W B Saunders, 1976: 1–15.

12. Zawacki B E. Reversal of capillary stasis and prevention of necrosis in burns. *Ann Surg* 1974; **180:** 98–102.

13. Raine T J. Cooling the burn wound to maintain microcirculation. *J Trauma* 1981; **21:** 394–7.

14. Salisbury R E, Levine N S. The early management of upper extremity thermal injury. In: Salisbury R D, ed. *Burns of the Upper Extremity*. Philadelphia: W B Saunders, 1976: 36–46.

15. Krizek T J. Emergency nonsurgical escharotomy in the burned extremity. *Orthop Rev* 1975; **4:** 53–5.

16. Committee on Trauma, American College of Surgeons. Tetanus immunization schedule. In: *Advanced Trauma Life Support Manual*. Chicago: American College of Surgeons, 1985.

17. Hing D N. Tissue penetration of parenteral antibiotics in the burn wound. *Surg Forum* 1982; **33:** 604.

18. Robson M C. Burn sepsis. *Crit Care Clin North Am* 1988; **4:** 281–298.

19. Nathan P. A laboratory method for selection of topical antimicrobial agents to treat infected burns. *Burns* 1978; **4:** 177–187.

20. Kucan J D, Hurt A V, Parsons S. 5% mafenide acetate solution in the treatment of thermal injuries. Paper presented at the sixteenth annual meeting of the American Burn Association, San Francisco. April 12, 1984.

21. Krizek T J, Flagg S V, Wolfort F G. Delayed primary excision and skin grafting of the burned hand. *Plast Reconstr Surg* 1973; **51:** 524–529.

22. Rovee D T, Kurowsky C A, Labun J. Local wound environment and epidermal healing. *Arch Dermatol* 1972; **106:** 330–4.

23. McHugh T P, Robson M C, Heggers J P, Phillips L G, Smith D J, McCollum M C. Therapeutic efficacy of Biobrane® in partial thickness and full thickness thermal injury. *Surgery* 1986; **100:** 661–4.

24. Labanter H, Kaplan I, Shaih C. Burns of the dorsum of the hand: conservative treatment with physiotherapy versus tangential excision and grafting. *Br J Plast Surg* 1976; **29:** 352–4.

25. Edstrom L E, Robson M C, Management of deep partial-thickness dorsal hand burns: study of operative vs. non-operative therapy. *Orthop Rev* April 1979; **8:** 27–33.

26. Goodwin C W, McManus W F, Pruitt B A, *et al.* Prospective study of burn wound excision of the hands. *J Trauma* 1983; **23:** 510–17.

27. Salisbury R E, Wright P. Evaluation of early excision of dorsal burns of the hand. *Plast Reconstr Surg* 1982; **69:** 670–5.

28. Krizek T J. Delayed primary excision and skin grafting of the burned hand. *Plast Reconstr Surg* 1973; **51:** 524–9.

29. Robson M C. Care of the healed wound: a prospective randomized study. Paper presented at the Twelfth Annual American Burn Association Meeting 1980, San Antonio.

30. Kozerefsky P M. Exercise and ambulation in the burn patient. In: DiGregorio V R, *Rehabilitation of the Burn Patient*. New York: Churchill Livingstone, 1984; 55–74.

31. Wilmore D W. Nutrition and metabolism following thermal injury. *Clin Plast Surg* 1974; **1:** 603–19.

32. Edstrom L E, Robson M C, Headley B J. Evaluation of exercise techniques in the burn patient. *Burns* 1977; **4:** 113–117.

33. Krizek T J, Robson M C, Flagg S V. Management of burn syndactyly. *J Trauma* 1974; **14:** 587–93.

34. Larson D L. Technique for decreasing scar formation and contractures in the burn patient. *J Trauma* 1971; **11:** 807–23.

35. Zook E G. The perionychium: anatomy, physiology, and care of injuries. *Clin Plast Surg* 1981; **8(1):** 21–31.

36. Henderson B, Koepke G H, Feller I. Peripheral polyneuropathy among patients with burns. *Arch Phys Med Rehabil* April 1971; **52(4):** 149–51.

37. Helm P A, Johnson E R, Carlton A M. Peripheral neurologic problems in the acute burn patient. *Burns* 1977; **3:** 123–5.

38. Frank D H, Robson M C. Unusual occurrence of chronic nerve compression syndromes at the wrists of thermally injured patients. *Orthop Rev* 1979; **8:** 180–3.

39. Elliot R A, Boutonniere deformity. In: Cramer L M, Chase R A, eds. *Symposium on the Hand*. St Louis: C V Mosby, 1971.

40. McShane R. Prosthetic joint replacement and extensor mechanism reconstruction in the burned hand. Presented at the 47th Annual Meeting of the Am Soc Plast Reconstr Surg. Hollywood, FL, 1978.

41. Evans E B, Larson D L, Yates S. Preservation and restoration of joint function in patients with severe burns. *JAMA* 1968; **204:** 91.

42. Edlich R F, Horowitz J H, Rheubanks, Nichter L S, Morgan R F. Heterotopic calcification and ossification in burn patients. *J Burn Care Rehabil* 1985; **6:** 363–8.

43. Littler J W. Neurovascualar pedicle method of digital transposition for reconstruction of the thumb. *Plast Reconstr Surg* 1953; **12:** 303–19.

44. Ward J W, Pensler J M, Parry S W. Pollicization for thumb reconstruction in severe pediatric hand burns. *Plast Reconstr Surg* 1985; **76:** 927–32.

45. May J W, Donelan M B, Toth B A, Wall J. Thumb reconstruction in the burned hand by advancement pollicization of the second ray remnant. *J Hand Surg* 1984; **9A**(4): 484–9.

CHAPTER FIFTY-TWO

Reconstruction of the Foot

W. Glenn Lyle, Linda G. Phillips and Martin C. Robson

Introduction

Burns of the feet can be a source of significant morbidity whether they occur in isolation or associated with other thermal injuries. These injuries are categorized by the American Burn Association as major burns, but today, isolated burns of the feet are still treated on an out-patient basis by many physicians. These burns should be treated by in-hospital care in order to avoid complications such as cellulitis, hypertrophic scarring, and prolonged hospitalization.[1] When presenting as part of a larger burn, foot burns are usually given lower priority by many burn teams and often are covered with widely meshed skin, which may hasten contracture. In addition, the increased hydrostatic pressure associated with dependency will lead to disruption of vascular connections between grafted skin and its donor site. This, in combination with the edema formation which results from lymphatic destruction, leads to graft loss which further worsens future burn scar contractures.[2] Scarring and contractures of the foot cause disabling sequelae which in turn can cause gait disturbances, problems with shoe fit, growth abnormalities, and chronic ulceration.[3] Clearly, prevention of contracture is of the utmost importance in avoiding more extensive reconstruction in the future. Established contractures require reconstruction in order to prevent permanent skeletal and functional deformities.

Anatomy and Physiology

The anatomy of the foot is similar to the hand in many ways. The skin of the dorsum of the foot is loosely connected to the underlying fascia and is rich in lymphatics, veins, and sensory nerves. Deep destruction of this tissue can result in significant edema formation. The superficial location of the extension tendons in this area often results in exposure of bare tendons if excision is too aggressive. Without their vascularized paratenon, these structures will not accept a graft. Tendon excursion may be severely limited by grafting directly on paratenon. The contractile nature of a scar in this area will frequently lead to severe contractures. Movements around the metatarsophalangeal joints are concentrated on dorsiflexion more than plantar flexion, and a resultant dorsiflexion contracture is common.[4] The plantar skin, on the other hand, is firmly held to the underlying plantar fascia by fibrous septa which divide the underlying fat into compartments, preventing movement and providing a shock absorbing effect. The skin of the sole of the foot has a thickened statum corneum which forms callosities. Burns to the plantar surface rarely lead to full-thickness injury and rarely require resurfacing, except in young children. When full-thickness injuries violate this tough skin barrier, a skin graft is necessary. Since the underlying subcutaneous fat is relatively avascular and susceptible to necrosis, graft take on this surface is less than ideal.

Another important feature of the foot is that it possesses both a longitudinal and a transverse arch. The medial longitudinal arch centers on the head of the talus and includes the calcaneal tuberosity, the navicular, three cuneiforms, and the first three metatarsals. Stability is provided by the plantar aponeurosis, which leads to medial instability if it loses its attachment to the base of the proximal phalanx of the great toe. The transverse arch runs medial to lateral and consists of the cuboid, three cuneiforms, and the bases of the metatarsals.[5] Contractures, which are caused by deficiency of tissue of the foot, often need to be released in both planes in order to reestablish the normal weight-bearing relationships of the foot.

The importance of the foot in daily activities of living should be emphasized. The foot strikes solid ground approximately 1800 times a mile while walking, and remains dependent throughout most of an average person's day. Body weight is distributed equally between the ball of the foot and the heel during resting stance, but this balanced distribution is maintained by muscular contraction. Loss of this muscular control will shift the weight disproportionately towards the metatarsal heads. At resting stance, one-half of the body weight borne by the foot is distributed to the metatarsals and one-third of this weight (one-sixth total body weight) is distributed to the great toe. As weight is added to the resting frame, a higher percentage is borne by the first metatarsal.[6] Similarly, with gait changes from walking to running, loads are distributed disproportionately, creating more stress on localized areas of the sole.

Gait, whether walking or running, refers to the cycle of coordinated movements which results in forward progression.[7] The gait cycle is made up of a swing phase and a stance phase. The swing phase takes up approximately 40% of the cycle in walking and begins when the toes push off the floor, and ends when the heel strikes the floor. The stance phase begins with heel strike and ends with push off, and comprises 60% of the cycle. During running, the proportion of time spent in the swing phase increases and the time spent with both feet on the ground (double support phase) is zero. Throughout this gait cycle, a complex interaction between the muscular forces which act on the joints of the foot and sensory feedback from the plantar surface of the foot occurs, which allows for adjustment to varied terrain, establishes balance, and maintains fluid ambulation. The presence of fixed contractures certainly upsets this interaction and the normal distribution of weight which results; it can lead to gait disturbances, joint problems, and skin breakdown.

Prevention – Acute Care

The need for late reconstruction depends in large part on the severity of injury and the quality of acute care given to a foot burn. Prevention of deformity obviates the need for contracture release and can be achieved by adequate tissue coverage and proper splinting. Acute burn injuries should be treated with escharotomies for circumferential burns, and if necessary, strict leg elevation, topical antimicrobials, and splinting. Although controversy exists about the use of systemic antimicrobials, obligate edema associated with burns of the foot and resultant lymphatic destruction warrants prophylactic treatment with an antistreptococcal agent during the acute phase in order to prevent cellulitis.[1] Priority should be given to burns of the foot as early coverage will allow earlier ambulation and rehabilitation. The extremities require prolonged elevation and immobility and this is best done early so as to avoid impeding the progress of recovery.[2]

The primary excision should be performed carefully in order to avoid exposure of underlying tendons and the unnecessary destruction of viable veins and lymphatics of the foot. The expansion ratio of the meshed split-thickness skin graft utilized in the initial grafting procedure also determines the degree of contracture formation. Alison *et al.* showed that skin meshed at a ratio of 1:4 caused more scar formation and an accelerated rate of contracture than that meshed at 1:2.[8] While sheet grafting or meshing at a 1:2 ratio is optimal, donor site availability may be limited and use of such an expansion ratio might not be feasible in a larger burn.

Postoperatively, all grafted feet should be stabilized with splints and the legs should remain elevated until graft take is insured and the wound has achieved enough tensile strength to be stable (usually for 1–2 weeks). The use of skeletal suspension, advocated in the past for severe foot burns,[9] is no longer felt to be necessary for most cases. This is in large part due to the aggressive early excision and grafting techniques, utilized today, which allow a foot to be definitively covered and splinted earlier. There are instances, however, when very deep burns and those with exposed joints and tendons might be best served with skeletal suspension in order to maintain proper positioning and allow local wound care while a patient awaits definitive reconstruction.

Ambulation after reconstruction is progressive and supervised by physical therapists until a patient is fully independent. All lower extremity burns should have circumferential graded pressure support, initially with elastic bandages and eventually with custom-fitted pressure garments. Patients are discharged with orthopedic shoes or high-topped tennis shoes with silicone inserts and/or foot plates (**Figure 52.1**). Splints should be worn while at rest and at night, and should be maintained for 3–4 months in order to prevent Achilles shortening and dorsal contracture.[8]

Established Deformities

Established deformities occur in previously grafted feet as well as in deeper burns which are allowed to heal spontaneously. Pressure garments and splinting should be the first line of therapy,[2] but frequently reconstruction is necessary. The most common deformity consists of gross hyperextension and subluxation of the toes. This deformity is often accompanied by syndactyly of the toes and the rocker bottom foot which results from a dorsal burn scar (**Figure 52.2**). Motion of the toes and the metatarsophalangeal joint is often severely decreased, especially the ability to flex the toes; however, functional disability may be remarkably slight. Frequently, problems with shoe fit and recurrent skin ulceration necessitate intervention.[8]

Mild to moderate linear burn scar contractures of the foot can sometimes be corrected with single or multiple Z-plasties to lengthen the scar.[4] More extensive tissue deficiency is usually the case and requires release and skin grafting. Deficiency of tissue in the transverse or longitudinal plane will determine the need for release of the appropriate arch and often both need release. A transverse release across the dorsum of the foot is performed beginning medial to the first metatarsal joint and carried laterally to the fifth metatarsophalangeal joint. Extension into normal skin is necessary in order to achieve a complete release. Excision of hypertrophic scar may be performed but often is not necessary, as the scar, now released from tension, will remodel and flatten. This maneuver accomplishes release of the longitudinal arch.[8] Utilizing this method, Waymack, Fidler, and Warden reported a 15% recurrence rate of contracture which occurred just over 4 years after the original release in burned children.[10] The recurrence rate was not influenced by graft type (sheet graft or 1:2 meshed graft). They emphasized the importance of diligent postoperative splinting so as to reduce recurrence. While release of the longitudinal arch may suffice to regain function, often the transverse arch must be released by adding a longitudinally directed release parallel to the plane of the metatarsals (**Figures 52.3 and 52.4**). Additional incisions into the web spaces may be necessary in order to complete the release and may be extended to correct syndactyly.[8]

Care must be taken when performing contracture releases so as

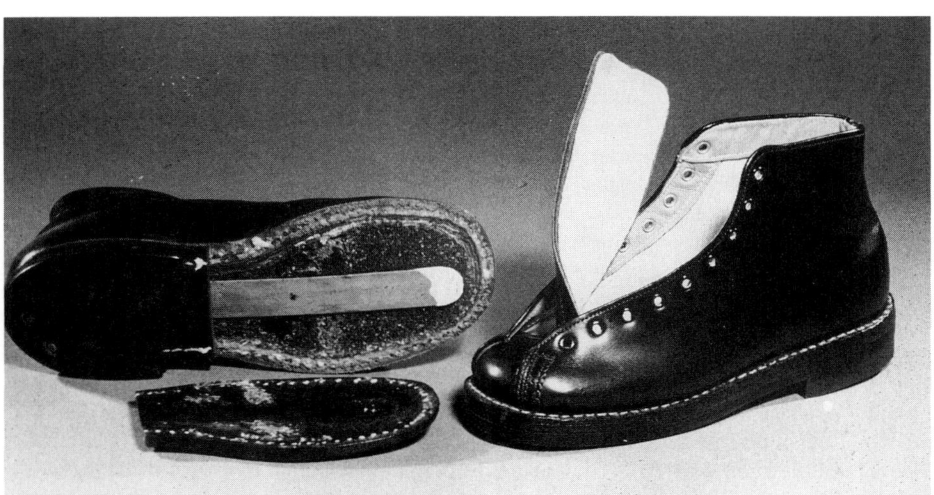

Fig. 52.1 Orthopedic shoes, with reinforcements, can prevent pedal burn scar contracture.

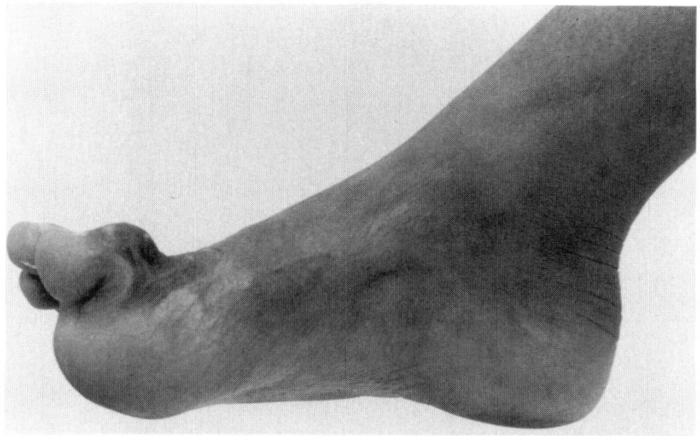

(a)

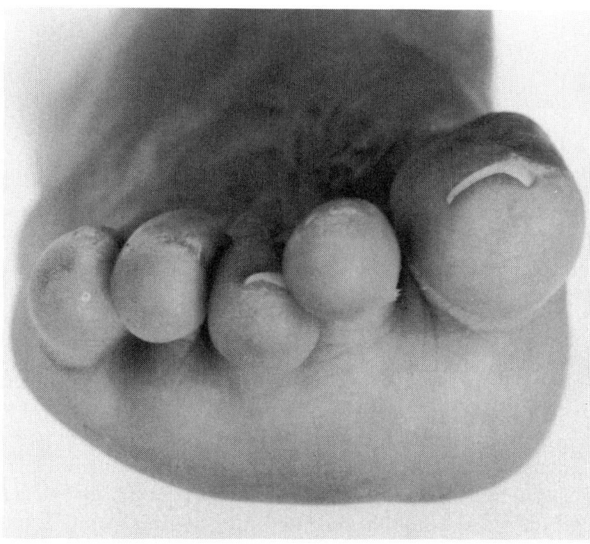

(b)

Fig. 52.2 Dorsal scar contracture causes foreshortening of foot and rocker bottom deformity.

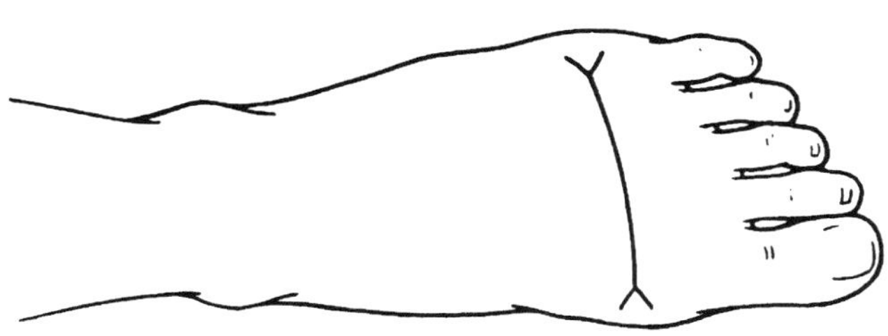

Fig. 52.3 Transverse burn scar release gives length and allows the foot to lie flat in the longitudinal axis.

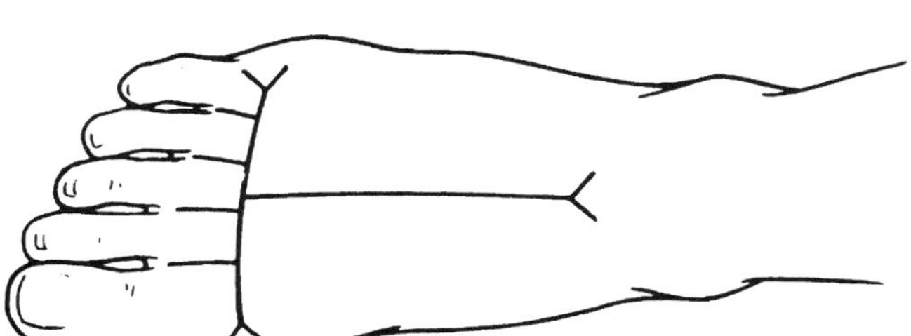

Fig. 52.4 The addition of a longitudinal release restores width to the foot and the normal arch. The addition of interdigital releases corrects burn syndactyly.

to insure soft tissue covering over the tendons. Meticulous hemostasis should be obtained with larger vessels being ligated with fine sutures in order to prevent future lymph leak and graft loss. Wound closure is achieved with moderately thick split-thickness skin grafts so as to decrease scarring and recontracture. Tie-over protects the Achilles tendon and heel. Splints should be fashioned and placed on the operating table prior to extubation in order to insure proper positioning in the plantar flexed position and to prevent shearing. Severe contractures may require joint capsule releases and/or Kirschner wires in order to maintain positioning. Tendon contractures may dictate a need for a two-stage release, with skin grafting followed by aggressive physical therapy for stretching, followed by repeat grafting. Postoperative care is similar to that given after an acute burn with bed rest along with elevation and proper splinting until graft take is insured. Progressive ambulation can be initiated with non-weight bearing at first, followed by graded full weight bearing. Pressure garments should be fitted prior to discharge and worn continuously until wounds mature. Utilizing this approach, releases performed at Shriners Burns Institute in Galveston were associated with a reduction in recurrence. This was felt to be a result of adding the transverse arch release.[8] Burn syndactyly affects the toes in these injuries as well, and can be managed with release and skin grafting, or by a variety of methods outlined for the hand[11] such as Y-V advancement, Z-plasties, and V-M-plasties. Simple release and grafting of foot burn scar contractures will suffice to manage the majority of contractures. More severe contractures which affect underlying bone, ligaments and tendons require more extensive procedures, which may utilize osteotomies, bone resections, and soft tissue flaps. To avoid this, the Ilizarov fixator has been used to correct chronic burn deformities.[12]

The equinus deformity of the foot can be caused by postburn contracture, anterior muscle loss, improper postburn splinting, and tibial growth into scar. Often this deformity is amenable to release of the Achilles tendon by tenolysis, tendon lengthening, or tenotomy. Unstable burned skin in this region may make for unsatisfactory postoperative healing, or insufficient tissue may necessitate complex soft tissue flaps. The Ilizarov fixator can overcome these problems (**Figure 52.5**). It can be affixed in the operating room under general, regional, or local anesthesia (in adults). The frame consists of two tibial–fibular rings, a calcaneal ring, and a metatarsal ring and all are secured to the bone with 1.5 mm pins. Correction is achieved by pushing the calcaneus distally and the metatarsals proximally at a rate of 1–2 mm/day, limited by patient comfort. Periodic x-rays confirm proper progress. Correction usually occurs in 4–6 weeks, and removal of the frame should be followed by a short leg cast for 6 weeks.

More complex equinus deformities require combined procedures with tendon lengthening, arthrodesis, and Ilizarov fixator application. Cavus deformities result from burns of the plantar surface of the foot. Treatment with fascial release or midfoot osteotomies may suffice, but they can also be accomplished with an Ilizarov half-ring frame to distract the calcaneus and metatarsals. The rocker bottom deformity, caused by dorsal burn scar contracture, which can be corrected with soft tissue releases, has also been problematic. More severe fixed contractures, previously treated with osteotomies or fusions, are now being treated with the Ilizarov fixator to recreate the arch. Toe dislocations, causing moderate to severe deformities, were treated with bone resections and amputations in the past, but they can now be treated with the Ilizarov technique by allowing gradual distraction and lengthening of the burn scar. The Ilizarov fixator can be associated with complications which can be avoided with proper pin care, meticulous attention to pin placement, and close patient follow-up so as to detect soft tissue problems. The risk of complications caused by infection, long a concern when external fixation devices are used in burn patients, is surprisingly low.[12]

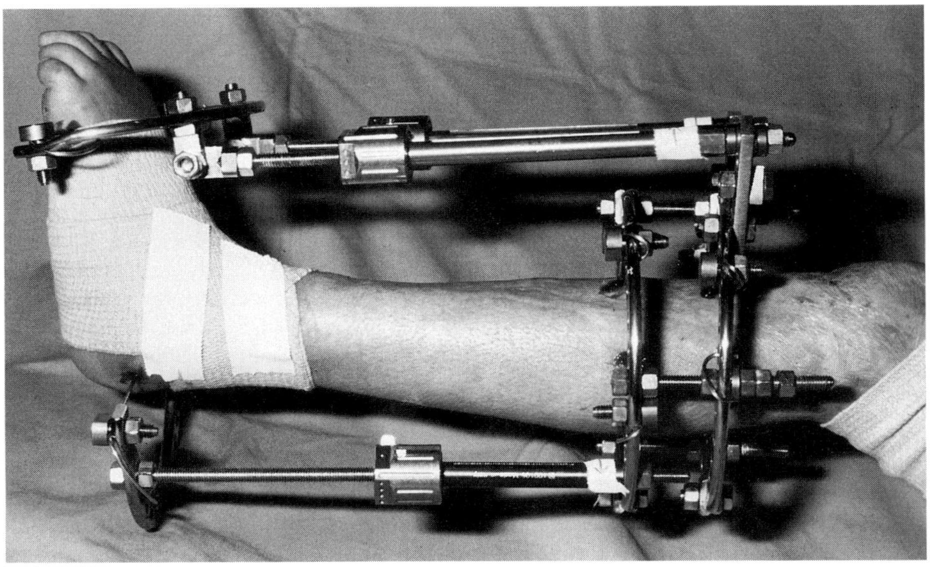

Fig. 52.5 The Ilizarov technique to reverse burn scar contracture.

Deep soft tissue defects can occur anywhere on a burned foot and often accompany electrical injury. Exposed tendons, ligaments, and joint structures are not served by skin grafts and require soft tissue reconstruction. Local flaps are rarely useful as the surrounding tissue is usually burned. Leung has had success with dorsalis pedis pedicled island flaps for ankle defects when the dorsum is unburned.[4] Defects of the heel may be treated successfully with deepithelialized turnover fasciocutaneous flaps as suggested by Ramakrishnan.[13] Cross-leg musculocutaneous flaps may be appropriate for soft tissue defects of a foot, but they require prolonged immobilization and are contraindicated in the elderly.[3]

Without local tissue to reconstruct deep wounds of a foot, the exposed bone, tendon, and cartilage will undergo desiccation, may become infected, and will often require amputation. If allowed to granulate, these wounds will eventually contract, epithelialize, and close; this occurs at the expense of severe joint deformity and soft tissue contracture. In these cases, free tissue transfer can serve to provide excellent soft tissue coverage and preserve function of the foot. The use of free flaps for deep burns of the lower extremity has been described by Harii.[14] Early free flap coverage of fourth degree burns was advocated by Grotting and Walkinshaw, who used latissimus dorsi and transverse scapular free flaps[15] (**Figure 52.6**). For patients who are stable enough to tolerate prolonged operating times, have adequate donor tissue, and have adequate proximal arterial and venous recipient vessels, free tissue transfer may provide the optimal means of reconstruction.

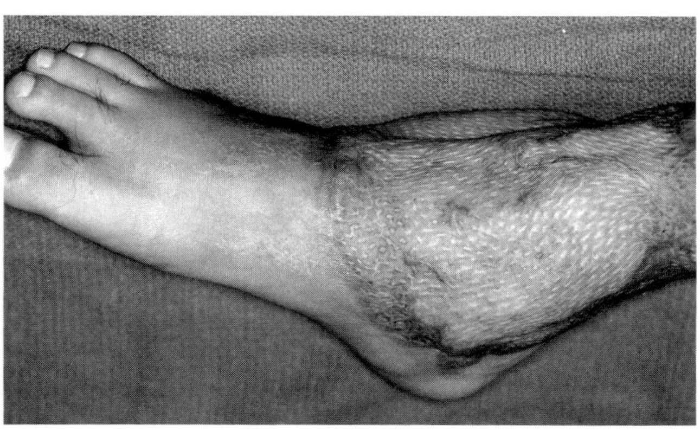

Fig. 52.6 Free flap used to cover exposed ankle joint.

Despite the best of acute care, utilizing timely escharotomies and excisional therapy, the magnitude of the original burn may be so great that the tissues of the feet become nonviable and require amputation. Similarly, supervening infection may threaten the life of the individual, necessitating amputation of the infected limb.[16] These eventualities, even when unavoidable, bring a sense of defeat to both the patient and surgeon alike. Preservation of the maximal length of the burned lower extremity should be the goal of the burn team as long as it does not threaten the life of the victim. With advances in burn care such as topical antimicrobials, early excision and grafting, and temporary allografts, limb salvage can be achieved in all viable lower extremities. Formal amputations should be reserved for only the most obvious nonviable tissues.

Toe burns frequently result in complete mummification of the digits. These should be treated with mafenide acetate in order to prevent progressive infection and be allowed to demarcate in order to preserve viable forefoot tissue. When all toes are severely injured and distal forefoot skin is deeply burned, open transmetatarsal amputation may be warranted. In acute burns, the resultant wound should be left open and undergo delayed closure. Amputations of one or more toes may only have a minor affect on ambulation, affecting pushoff primarily; but amputation of the great toe is associated with a greater loss of function owing to its greater contribution to weight bearing.

Transtarsal amputations at the Chopart level are associated with imbalance of remaining muscles of the foot, an equinus deformity, and unstable weight bearing. Younger patients may tolerate this amputation well with or without a prosthesis. Syme's amputations may be successful, particularly in young patients, but should be performed only if more distal amputation levels cannot be performed.[17] The resultant amputated limb should be pain free, well padded, have full-thickness skin and normal sensation in order to function within a prosthesis. With foot amputations, often all that is required is a shoe insole molded to replace the missing areas of phalanges and metatarsals. This helps maintain the remaining portion of foot in its normal position within the shoe. Syme's amputation can function successfully with a modified solid-ankle–cushion-heel (SACH) prosthesis.[18] All patients requiring amputations should be evaluated by a competent prosthetist for proper prosthetic fit. Frequent follow-up, particularly in a growing child, is mandatory in order to accommodate changes in the affected limb.

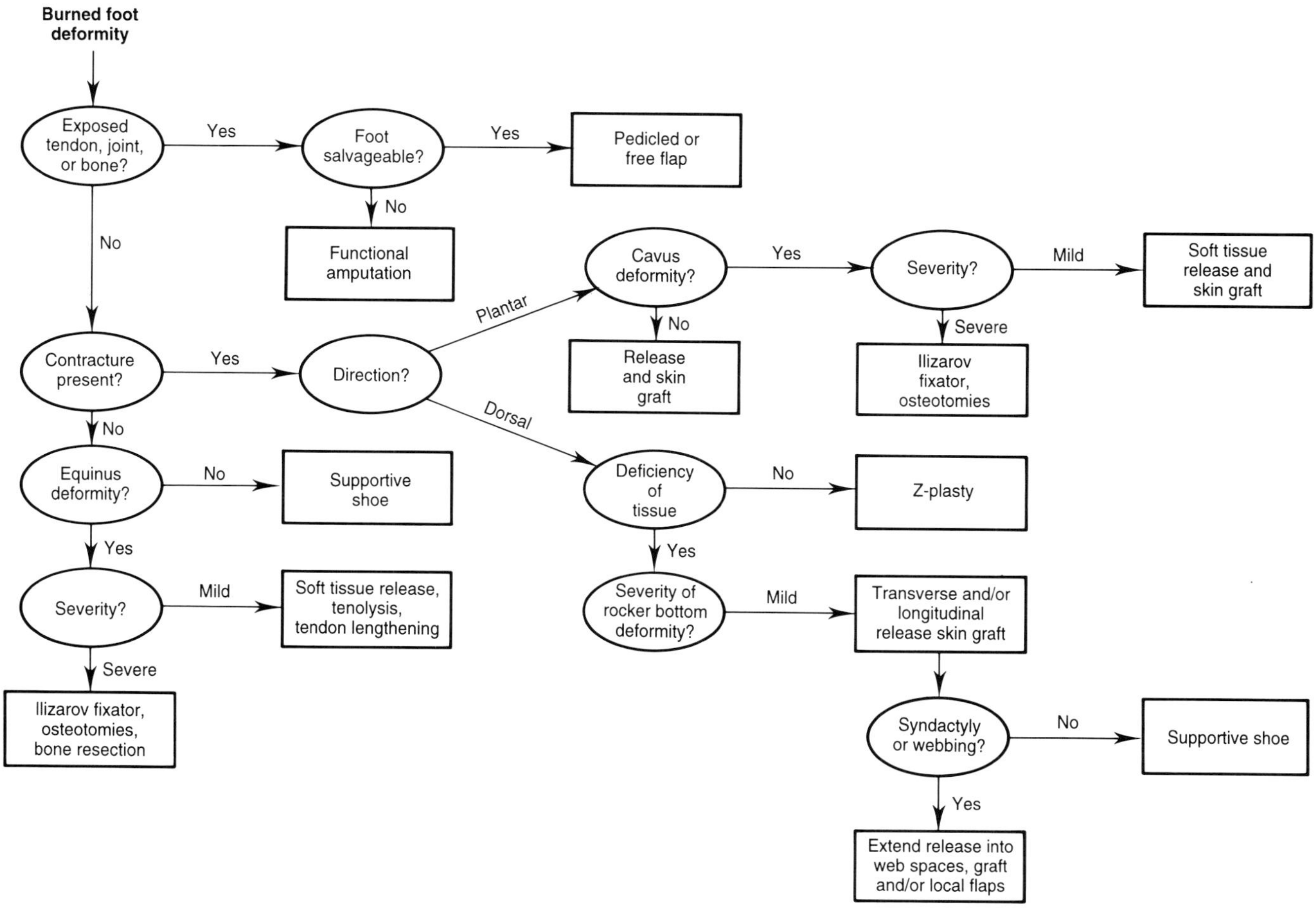

Fig. 52.7 Algorithm for reconstruction of the burned foot.

Summary

Foot burns should be given relatively high priority both in the acute situation and during the reconstructive phase (**Figure 52.7**). Long-term morbidity such as gait disturbances, problems with shoe fit, and recurrent skin breakdown will result without proper initial care or release of established contractures. Orthopedic measures are often necessary in order to overcome severe deformities. All surgical efforts should be supported with proper splinting and pressure garments in the postoperative period. Established contractures usually involve the dorsum of the foot and can often be corrected with transverse and/or longitudinal releases to reestablish the arches. More severe contractures frequently require orthopedic measures, including tendon lengthening, osteotomies, or the Ilizarov fixator. Exposed tendon or joints require local flaps or free tissue transfer. Amputations are performed as a last resort when infection threatens or other reconstructive efforts have failed.

References

1. Zachary L S, Heggers J P, Smith D J Jr, Robson M C, Maniker A, Sachs R J. Burns of the feet. *J Burn Care Rehabil* 1987; **8:** 192–4.

2. Witt P D, Achauer B M. Lower extremity. In: Achauer B M ed. *Burn Reconstruction.* New York: Thieme Medical Publishers Inc, 1991: 134–47.

3. Heimberger R A, Marten E, Larson D L, Abston S, Lewis S R. Burned feet in children: acute and reconstructive care. *Am J Surg* 1973; **125:** 575–9.

4. Leung P C, Cheng J C Y. Burn contractures of the foot. *Foot and Ankle.* 1986; **6:** 289–294.

5. Mann R A. Biomechanical approach to the treatment of foot problems. *Foot Ankle* 1982; **2:** 205–11.

6. Hollinshead W H, Jenkins D B. *Functional Anatomy of the Limbs and Back.* Philadelphia: WB Saunders Co, 1981.

7. Lamont J G. Functional anatomy of the lower limb. *Clin Plast Surg* 1986; **13:** 571–80.

8. Alison W E, Moore M L, Reilly D A, Phillips L G, McCauley R L, Robson M C. Reconstruction of foot burn contractures in children. *J Burn Care Rehabil* 1993; **14:** 34–8.

9. Youel L, Evans E B, Henro T C, Herndon D N, Larson D L, Abston S. Skeletal suspension in the management of severe burns in children. *J Burn Care Rehabil* 1986; **68A:** 1375–9.

10. Waymack J C, Fidler J, Warden G D. Surgical correction of burn scar contractures of the foot in children. *Burns* 1988; **14:** 156–60.

11. Krizek T J, Robson M C, Flagg S V. Management of burn syndactyly. *J Trauma* 1974; **14:** 587–93.

12. Calhoun J H, Evans E B, Herndon D N. Techniques for management of burn contractures with the Ilizarov fixator. *Clin Ortho Rel Res* 1992; **280:** 117–24.

13. Ramakrishnan K M, Jayaraman V, Ramachandran K, Mathivanan T. Deepithelialized turnover flaps in burns. *Plast Reconstr Surg* 1988; **82:** 262–6.

14. Harii K, Ohmori K, Ohmori S. Utilization of free composite tissue transfer by microvascular anastomosis for repair of burned deformities. *Burns* 1975; **1:** 237–44.

15. Grotting J, Walkinshaw M. The early use of free flaps in burns. *Ann Plast Surg* 1985; **15:** 127–31.

16. Winkley J H, Gaspard D J, Smith L L. Amputation as a life-saving measure in the burn patient. *J Trauma* 1965; **5:** 782–91.

17. Clippinger F W. Amputations and limb substitutions. In: Sabiston D C, ed. *Textbook of Surgery.* Philadelphia: WB Saunders Co, 1986: 1488–92.

18. Meier R H. Amputations and prosthetic fitting. In: Fisher S V, Helm P P, eds. *Comprehensive Rehabilitation of Burns.* Baltimore: Williams and Wilkins, 1984: 267–310.

PSYCHOLOGICAL AND SOCIAL ISSUES

CHAPTER FIFTY-THREE

FUNCTIONAL SEQUELAE AND DISABILITY ASSESSMENT

GLENN D. WARDEN

INTRODUCTION

Advances in acute burn care during the past 25 years, in terms of decreased mortality and decreased length of hospital stay, have been truly outstanding and amazing. In 1971, survival statistics at the Institute of Surgical Research in San Antonio demonstrated an LD_{50} (lethal dose resulting in a 50% survival rate) with approximately 40% TBSA (total body surface area) burn. Thus, 50% of the patients with burns of only 40% died. Now, the LD_{50} approaches 80% TBSA, and if no inhalation injury is involved, patients with burn injuries greater than 80–90% of their total body surface area routinely survive. In almost every burn unit in the United States, the length of stay has decreased from nearly 3 days per percent burn to less than 1 day per percent burn. The success can be stated simply: patients with larger, more severe burns are surviving; however, are these patients returning to society to become productive citizens? What is the real outcome of massively burned patients? Do pediatric burned patients become functional adults? How do they function socially later in life? What is the long-term effect on the patients' families and society? Are survival and decreased length of stay really the measure of productivity for our specialty? The real product or measurement of customer service is a patient who can successfully return to society and, even more importantly, be a useful, productive individual who can successfully interact socially within a community. Yes, patients with larger and more severe burns are surviving, but this has created new problems for patients' quality of life. Although the problems are magnified in massively burned patients, they exist even in smaller burns. These problems are best demonstrated in a pediatric burn patient with a 95% total body surface area burn (**Figure 53.1**). Cultured keratinocytes were utilized to achieve wound coverage. The child survived; however, when we examined the patient's current and future reconstructive needs, they totaled 33 potential reconstructive procedures. Thus, the reconstructive problems are monumental in a child with very few donor sites.[3] With regard to survival, the results of this patient are impressive; however, we must ask the question: 'Has the medical expertise in terms of survival progressed past the ability to reconstruct and rehabilitate patients?' Unfortunately, the answer is clearly 'yes'. Are we returning our patients to a society which is not ready financially, psychologically, or socially, to accept them? Again, unfortunately, the answer is clearly 'yes'.

The American Burn Association has made rehabilitation a major emphasis. There is now a standing committee on rehabilitation and it has grown in importance under the direction of Roger E. Salisbury, MD, the twenty-fourth president. Dr Salisbury emphasized the problem of rehabilitation in his 1992 presidential address.[4] He reminded us that rehabilitation of a burned patient is a large, glaring area where quality work remains to be done. It is important and imperative that burn centers evaluate the functional outcome of a thermally injured patient. This is important, not only for disability assessment, but also for evaluation of our medical management. Outcome studies in the 1990s will not only empha-

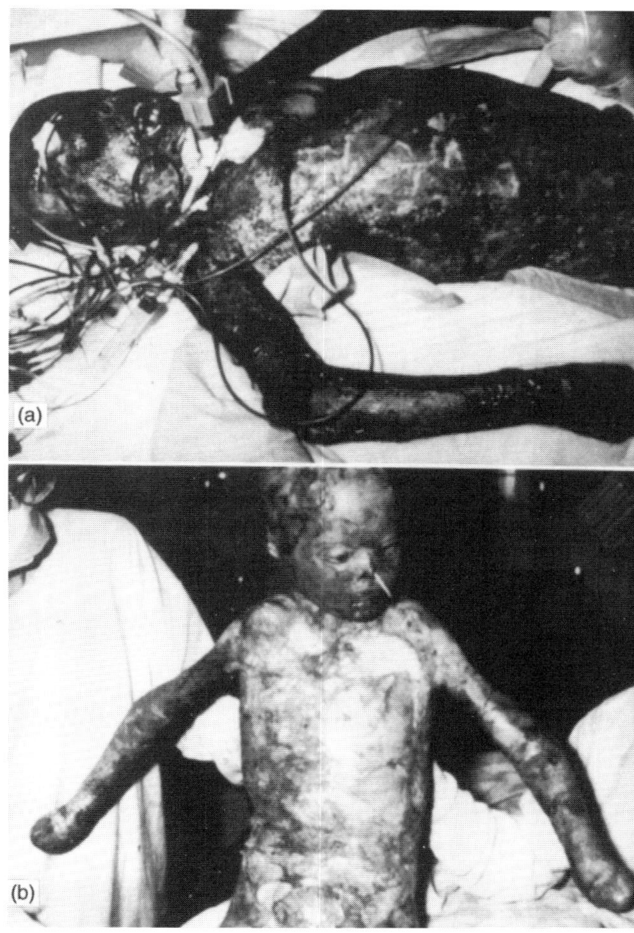

Fig. 53.1 Pediatric burn patient with 95% total body surface area burn (a) at the time of admission and (b) at discharge. Reproduced from ref. 3 with permission.

size survival and hospital stay, but also patient satisfaction and ability to return to work. The purpose of this chapter is to review the functional sequelae and disability assessment following thermal injury.

Basic Considerations – Impairment – Disability – Handicap

The various terms such as 'impairment', 'disability', and 'handicap', appear in laws, regulations, and policies of diverse origin without proper coordination of the ways in which they are used. 'Impairment' means alteration of the individual's health status which is assessed by medical means.

'Disability', which is assessed by nonmedical means, means an alteration in an individual's capacity to meet personal, social, or occupational demands or to meet statutory or regulatory requirements. Simply stated, impairment is what is wrong with the health of an individual, disability is a gap between what the individual can do and what the individual needs or wants to do. An individual who is impaired is not necessarily disabled. Impairment gives rise to disability only when the medical condition limits the individual's capacity to meet the demands which pertain to nonmedical fields and activities. On the other hand, if an individual is able to meet a particular set of demands, the individual is not disabled with respect to those demands, even though a medical evaluation may reveal impairment.

The concept of 'handicap' is independent of both impairment and disability, although it is sometimes used interchangeably with either of those terms. Under the provision of federal laws, an individual who is defined as handicapped has an impairment which substantially limits one or more life activities including work, has a record of such impairment, or is regarded as having such an impairment. As a matter of practicality, however, a handicap may be operationally understood as being manifest in association with a barrier obstacle to functional activity. An individual of limited functional capacity is handicapped if there are barriers to accomplishment of tasks or life activities which can be overcome only by compensating in some ways for the effect of an impairment. If an individual is not able to accomplish a task or activity despite accommodation, or if there is no accommodation which will enable the accomplishment, then in addition to being handicapped, the individual is also disabled. On the other hand, an impaired individual who is able to accomplish a task or activity without accommodation is, with respect to that task or activity, neither handicapped nor disabled. The concept of 'employability' deserves special attention, for, in an occupational setting, if an individual within the boundaries of a medical condition has the capacity, with and without accommodation, to meet a job's demands and conditions of employment as designed by the employer, the individual is employable and consequently not disabled. On the other hand, an individual who does not have the capacity or who is unwilling to travel to and from work, to be at work, and to perform assigned tasks and duties, is not employable.

Their first critical task in carrying out a medical determination related to employability is to learn about a job, specifically the expectations of the incumbent, with respect to performance, physical activity, reliability, availability, productivity, expected duration of useful service life, and any other criteria associated with qualifications and suitability. Sufficient detailed information from a job analysis will provide a basis upon which a physician determines exactly what kinds of medical information are needed and to what degree of detail to assess an individual's health with respect to demand criteria.

Impairment Assessment

Before discussing the medical aspects of evaluating thermally injured individuals, it must be pointed out that no Social Security and Worker's Compensation disability program medical listing exists for burns. Instead, burns must be evaluated under the appropriate body system. Often, more than one system is involved, in other words, musculoskeletal, respiratory, skin, and all must be considered in the final decision. Claims must be aimed primarily at resolving the question of onset, whether the impairment can be expected to last 12 months or end in death. The medical evidence needed to document the existence and severity of a medically determinable impairment due to burns must include a history of the impairment, which describes the origin and course of the condition, dates of confinement, nature of treatment, and the claimant's response; current objective findings such as results of examinations, laboratory tests such as blood pressure, electrocardiogram, x-rays, blood tests, range of motion, medical factual data upon which diagnoses are based; and a description of the objective findings of the claimant's limitations and remaining capacities. In other words, how far can he or she walk, which activities cause shortness of breath or chest pain, what extent of motion is there in affected parts of the body. Regional specialized burn centers treat many serious burns annually. These centers are excellent sources of medical evidence as they maintain complete detailed records regarding the nature of an injury, treatment, complications, and prognosis. Advances in burn care have improved the survival rate in major burns. Efforts to rehabilitate these survivors and improve their quality of life represent a significant challenge for those involved in their care. The rehabilitation of these survivors is unique and multifaceted, and rarely limited to one system. Many individuals will experience some type of long-term physical impairment or mental limitation, and the rehabilitation process may take years to complete. It must be emphasized that impairments resulting from a burn are not restricted to the skin. Complications may affect any body system; thus, the examiner who is assessing individuals for disability must be attentive to the systemic sequelae of burn injury. The evaluation of a burn victim has some unique features. The necessity to consider such subjective factors as heat and cold intolerance, sensitivity to sunlight, pain, chemical sensitivity, and changes in sweating pattern, as well as the more objective considerations of decreased coordination, sensation, strength, and contracture, lends itself to a unique evaluation.

Disfigurement from scarring, a frequent sequela of burns, may not affect performance and thereby, in and of itself, causes no impairment. Scarring represents a special type of disfigurement. Again, no percentage of impairment is assigned for the existence of a scar *per se*; however, scars affect sweat glands, hair growth, and nail growth, and cause pigment changes or contractures and may affect loss of performance and cause impairment. Sensory deficit, pain or discomfort from scars needs to be evaluated, as well as the loss of motion of a scar area. An impairment due to disfigurement from scarring may also create behavioral or psychological impairments which subsequently may be rated. The need for intermittent or continuous treatment of the skin with topical agents and pressure garments can impair a person's function and needs to be considered. There is a surprising lack of published literature which relates to the impairment evaluation of a burned patient. The following are concepts which must be kept in mind when evaluating a postburn patient for impairment and resulting deformities.

Skin

Scars and cutaneous abnormalities which result from the healing of burned tissue may represent a special type of disfigurement. Scars should be described by giving their dimensions in centimeters, and by describing their shape, color, anatomical location, and evidence of ulceration; their depression or elevation, which relates to whether they are soft and pliable or hard and indurated, thin or thick, and smooth or rough; and their attachment, if any, to underlying bone, joints, muscle and other tissues. Good color photography with multiple views of a defect enhances the description of scars.

The tendency of a scar to disfigure should be considered in evaluating whether impairment is permanent or whether the scar can be changed, made less visible, or concealed. Function may be restored without improving appearance and appearance may be improved without altering anatomical or physiologic function. If a scar involves loss of sweat gland function, hair growth, nail growth, or pigment formation, the effect of such loss on performance of an activity of daily living should be evaluated. Furthermore, any loss of function due to sensory pain, any sensory defect, pain or discomfort in a scar should be evaluated.

Burn scar contracture is probably the most frequently seen cause of impairment in a postburn individual. Every burn, regardless of the depth of injury, heals with some element of contracture. Contractile forces continue long after a wound is healed and can result in severe skin shortage. Inadequate skin prohibits movement to a joint's normal arc of motion and will influence not only the joint underlying the contracture, but also those adjacent to the scar. In the early stages of development, burn scar contractures may often be corrected through the use of splints and pressure garments designed to force developing scar tissue into more normal configurations. In spite of the benefits derived from these modalities, they may also function as a type of impairment, both physically and cosmetically. Understanding the splints which individuals must wear and their limitations are important factors in the assessment of disability. Often, surgical means must be employed in order to restore function. When a surgical release of a contracture is performed, the resultant defect can be of considerable size and will require closure by means of a skin graft or flap of tissue. Burn scar contracture frequently requires a series of staged surgical procedures before optimal function and cosmesis are achieved. Recovery from surgical intervention must be followed by an extensive rehabilitation program. If an individual does not participate in a rehabilitation program, contractures will reoccur.

The definition of functional impairment should not be limited to an individual's ability or inability to perform joint range of motion. An extremity can exhibit full active range of motion and still be considered impaired due to poor skin quality. Although much can be done to restore function, the skin is never restored to normal. Scar tissue is less tolerant of the everyday stress imposed on it than normal skin. Scar epithelium is thin, fragile, and prone to chronic ulceration. Regardless of the location, these chronic open areas will not heal and will eventually require skin grafting. This type of lesion can occur at any time, even years after the initial hospitalization. Skin grafts have the same abnormalities as burn scars in that they all involve contracture formation, have loss of sweat gland function, hair growth and altered pigment formation. Although frequently cosmetically more acceptable, skin grafts are still not normal skin. Physical limitations such as cold and heat intolerance, difficulty with sun exposure, altered sensation, or painful scars may prohibit an individual from performing his or her past work or other work.

Musculoskeletal

Functional limitation secondary to burn injury usually results from an anatomical alteration about a major joint. The degree to which the function of a joint is affected is greatly influenced by the amount of soft tissue loss and the degree of pain associated with movement. Full-thickness burns, those involving all layers of skin, may also result in secondary damage to muscle, bone, tendon, and ligaments. In the acute phase of treatment of such injuries, a joint may be exposed, making it vulnerable and susceptible to a chronic infection (known as osteomyelitis), instability, and arthritic changes. Ectopic calcification, the abnormal deposition of calcium around the joints, is usually seen in the elbow, but it can occur in any joint. Symptoms include pain with a significant decrease in motion. These changes in joint structure can be verified by x-ray and will require surgery at a later date for correction. Extensive soft tissue destruction involving the loss of muscle mass as seen in electrical injuries, will require numerous staged procedures in order to restore function. An individual may never be restored to full function and may be excluded from performing certain types of work which exist in the national economy.

Restriction of normal movement by contracture is not limited to the extremities. When a scar occurs over the trunk or anterior chest, severe and chronic postural changes can result which may cause a secondary spinal deformity or altered respiratory functions. Amputations are another leading contributor to postburn impairment. Unlike amputations which are performed for other medical conditions such as peripheral vascular disease, amputations following an extensive thermal injury will often require several staged surgical procedures in order to produce a stump which is capable of accommodating a prosthesis. It is also important to realize that amputations are not confined to the extremities alone but may also involve skin appendages such as the ears and nose. Complicated staged procedures using local or distant full-thickness skin or muscle–skin flaps are required in order to restore function and cosmesis in these areas. An understanding of how long it will take for an individual's function to be restored is an important factor in deciding about the issue of disability.

Special senses and speech

Impairment to the senses of hearing or vision can occur as a result of a thermal insult, secondary to life-sustaining treatments or as a complication of a healing burn. The loss of central or peripheral vision may begin at the time of contact with a burning agent and can cause the destruction of the eyelids and damage to the cornea. A series of surgical procedures must be performed in order to create a functional eyelid. Contracture of the eyelids, more commonly the lower, may develop quickly, resulting in incomplete closure of the eyelid; and potential damage to the cornea can result in conjunctivitis or corneal ulceration. In spite of adequate surgical correction, it is common for such injured individuals to have repetitive episodes of recontracture for up to 2 years post-healing, due to the ongoing scar contracture process. Perioral burns which result in lip eversion and microstomia, or contracture of the mouth, may eventually impair mastication and result in drooling as well as inhibiting an individual from producing speech which can be heard or understood. Hearing impairment due to the acute burn is rare, but there may be a loss of the external ear, or a deafness secondary to the treatment of life-threatening infections with antibiotics.

Respiratory system

Burns which occur in an enclosed space, such as a building structure, often result in some form of inhalation injury to the respiratory system. Impairment may be limited to a temporary need for ventilatory support or extend to permanent respiratory disease. Chronic and recurrent respiratory infections and pulmonary insufficiency may limit an individual's ability to perform his or her past work or other work in the national economy, especially when toxic chemicals or dust are present in the workplace. Patients with severe inhalation injuries may require a tracheostomy long after the burn has healed. Closure of the stoma is often delayed for the purpose of intubation and anesthesia in future reconstructive surgeries. Pulmonary function tests are essential in determining respiratory impairment.

Cardiovascular system

A cardiovascular evaluation should include a good history and electrocardiogram. Patients complaining of chest discomfort thought to be of cardiac origin should have a more extensive workup. There is some evidence of increased incidence of cardiovascular disease in the long-term follow-up of survivors of large thermal injuries.

Neurological system

Neurological impairment caused by a burn may be obvious at the time of admission to a burn center or become clinically apparent up to 2 years following the injury. Patients who are considered at risk include those who have sustained an electrical injury, are predisposed to stroke, or who exhibit signs of peripheral neuropathies secondary to thermal damage. Such patients should be closely monitored for signs of progressive neurological deficit. Electromyography studies will chart the development of degenerative peripheral nerve or spinal cord dysfunction. Dysfunction may be demonstrated in the form of paresis, paralysis, tremor, involuntary movement, or ataxia. Individuals who have suffered an electrical injury may develop a condition characterized by progressive degeneration of fine and gross motor coordination. Resultant complications can range from inability to perform work-related tasks safely to an inability to perform the routine activities of daily living. It is a disease process which takes place over a significant period of time and may worsen after an individual has returned to work. In addition to the motor deficits caused by electrical injury, those individuals in whom a current passed above the level of the clavicle have a high incidence of cataract formation within the first 3 years post-injury.

Hemic and lymphatic

Full-thickness or deeper burns, particularly of the lower extremities, will also cause damage to the lymphatic system. Such injured individuals often demonstrate a lack of normal lymphatic drainage, resulting in chronic edema and the development of stasis ulcers. There can be little or no improvement expected post-healing. External support in the form of elastic garments is necessary to help replace the normal activity of the lymphatic system in reabsorption of fluid. These individuals frequently have difficulty in standing for long periods of time or working in a hot and humid environment.

Digestive system

The digestive system is not usually a problem except in those individuals who have had superior mesenteric artery syndrome, cholecystitis, or peptic ulcer disease during the acute admission. The post-discharge clinical course of these individuals is never predictable; if affected individuals become symptomatic, they should be followed up by a specialist.

Genitourinary system

The genitourinary system may be a problem if deep perineal or buttocks burns occurred. Aside from the obvious psychological problems, partial loss of the penis or scarring of the external genitalia may result in difficulty voiding. A badly scarred perineum or buttocks may make sitting in one position for prolonged periods painful and difficult.

Psychological

The advances of surgical techniques involving early excision and grafting as well as the increased ability to prevent infection allow many patients who would otherwise perish to face life shattered by psychological problems as a result of disfigurement. The onset of a thermal injury is a sudden and frightening experience not only to a patient, but also to his family members. Because of the unexpected nature of onset, all phases of the patient's life style are abruptly changed. Often, the full emotional impact is not felt until the time a patient is discharged from the protected environment of a hospital. At this time, the reality of the emotional, physical, and financial burden of a thermal injury are apparent and must be faced. The extent to which a person can psychologically deal with his injuries varies, as do individual personalities. Each case is unique and must be evaluated as such. Studies on the psychological adjustment of survivors of burns generally reflect a biased adjustment to moderate injuries. Few quantifiable data are available concerning the psychological well-being of long-term survivors of severe injuries. Although most authors conclude that victims of burns make satisfactory adjustments, others report symptoms of the psychopathologic sort which contradict this optimism.[6] Public acceptance is an important problem facing a burned patient. Goffman, in 1963[3], stated that the way that burn disfigured patients have dealt with the world has generally been shown to be affected by society showing negative responses to visible scars. The burn disfigured person has his or her own attitude toward body image with which to deal as well as the attitudes of the people and the culture around him or her. TV and radio have altered not only family standards, but standards of self-perception as well. The young and the beautiful are emphasized. Everyone must be a 'ten', as illustrated by Bo Derek. Patients with burns, like paraplegic or quadriplegic persons, have injuries which can be seen and understood by the public; however, there is also marked ambivalence about a patient with burns as emphasized by the movie industry which has frequently characterized the evil person as being deformed. The Phantom of the Opera is a burn victim; Vincent Price in the House of Wax has burns of his hands; and the popularity of A Nightmare on Elm Street, now in its fifth sequel, depicts Freddie Krueger as evil, deformed, and scarred. The burned patient must deal not only with his burn injury, but also with society's built-in impressions which are fostered early in life through cartoons, advertising, television, and movies. This is especially important in the pediatric burned patient for whom returning to school can be difficult, to say the least. Recent studies from the Shriners Burns Institute–Galveston emphasize that, in pediatric patients with large thermal injuries, the children appear to be adjusting well;[6] however, in-depth evaluation demonstrates grave self-deprecating feelings.[7] These feelings may not surface with the use of present medical evaluation and further refining and modification, in addition to our current techniques, are needed to bring out the latent fears and detrimental feelings in these patients.

Impairment Evaluation

The physical examination of a burn victim is much the same as the disability evaluation for any patient. With the information gathered from the history and physical examination, and using the tables in the American Medical Association's *Guide to the Evaluation of Permanent Impairment*,[1] the physician can arrive at an impairment rating. In addition to the usual range of motion form, a questionnaire regarding the special problems related to burns is useful (**Table 53.1**). The American Medical Association's *Guide to the Evaluation of Permanent Impairment* is difficult, complex, and time consuming. It is helpful to have members of a rehabilitation department, namely physical therapy and/or occupational therapy, be familiar with this evaluation. A combined approach with either an occupational therapist or a physical therapist to evaluate actual objective determination such as range of motion, and a burn surgeon performing the subjective rating for the skin or psychological status, is useful. The objective measurements due to restriction of active motion and amputations are well outlined in the *Guide to the Evaluation of Permanent Impairment*. The techniques of measurement are simple, practical, and scientifically sound. For the examination of upper and lower extremities, a large and small portable goniometer are used. The upper extremity, lower extremity, the spine, and the pelvis are considered a unit of the whole person; and tables are available in the manual to determine impairment ratings of the whole person. The subjective rating for skin or psychological determination is not as precise. The criteria for evaluating permanent impairment of the skin is divided into four classes:

- *Class I impairment of the whole person is 0–5%.* A patient belongs in class I when (a) signs or symptoms of skin disorder are present, and (b) with treatment, there is no limitation or minimal limitation in the performance of the activity of daily living, although exposure to certain physical and chemical agents might increase limitation temporarily.
- *Class II impairment of the whole person is 10–20%.* A patient belongs in class II when (a) signs and symptoms of skin disorder are present, and (b) intermittent skin treatment is required, and (c) there is limitation in the performance of some of the activities of daily living.
- *Class III impairment of the whole person is 25–50%.* A patient belongs in class III when (a) signs and symptoms of skin disorder are present, and (b) continuous treatment is required, and (c) there is limitation in performance of many of the activities of daily living.
- *Class IV impairment of the whole person is 55–80%.* A patient belongs in class IV when (a) signs and symptoms of skin disorder are present, and (b) continuous treatment is required which may include periodic confinement to the home or other domicile, and (c) there is limitation of performance of many of the activities of daily living.

This impairment evaluation is somewhat subjective; however, individual patients can be placed into various categories. The final impairment rating is a combination of the actual objective determinations and the subjective rating for skin and psychological impairment.

Table 53.1 Patient questionnaire related to burn sequelae

Decreased sensation	Yes—	No—	Areas involved ————	
Heat intolerance	Yes—	No—	Areas involved ————	
Cold intolerance	Yes—	No—	Areas involved ————	
Sensitivity to sunlight	Yes—	No—	Areas involved ————	
Sensitivity to chemicals	Yes—	No—	Areas involved ————	
Area of increased perspiration————				
Area of decreased perspiration ————				
Restricted chest motion	Yes—	No—		
Restricted abdominal motion	Yes—	No—		
Loss of hair	Yes—	No—		
Loss of nails or malformed nails	Yes—	No—		
Dysesthesias	Yes—	No—	Where ————	
Hypopigmentation	Yes—	No—	Where ————	
Hyperpigmentation	Yes—	No—	Where ————	
Drug use	Yes—	No—		
Increased alcohol use	Yes—	No—	Amount————	
Donor site scarring	None—	Minor—	Moderate—	Severe—
Approximate body surface area of donor ————%				
Gastric pain	Yes—	No—		
Joint pain	Yes—	No—	Where ————	
Tearing, photophobia	Yes—	No—		
Decreased vision	Yes—	No—		
Shortness of breath	Yes—	No—		
Lack of endurance	Yes—	No—		
Hoarseness or other vocal cord problem	Yes—	No—	Describe ————	

Functional Outcome

Outcome from thermal injury depends upon many factors other than severity of illness; this may include social status, family support, and patient motivation. A determination of impairment combined with disability is an excellent modality to determine outcome. Presently, we perform formal impairment ratings only when asked by insurance companies, social security, worker's compensation, or the legal system. With emphasis on continuous quality improvement and insurance companies evaluating care by outcome determinations, it is important for burn surgeons to document their outcome. Impairment ratings are time consuming; however, they are an excellent way to evaluate outcomes of care. A systematic approach to evaluating outcomes in this manner should be initiated.

Summary

Disability determination is a difficult and by no means objective procedure. It is not within the scope of this chapter to present all the possible complications and resulting impairments secondary to burn injury.[2,5,8] There are certain concepts which must be kept in mind when evaluating a postburn patient for impairment and resulting deformity. Most burn injuries which are significant enough to require admission to a specialized burn care facility will likely result in some type of temporary or permanent disability. Concepts unique to burn patients include:

- the most common complications arise from burn scar contracture and cosmetic deformity, and will require staged surgical procedures for correction;
- rehabilitation may take several years to return a patient to an acceptable level of functioning;
- postburn cosmetic deformity needs to be confined to areas which are socially visible;
- resulting disabilities are not proportional to the extent of cutaneous injury; and
- certain complications, such as neurological degeneration, may not arise until a few years following an injury and are fairly unpredictable.

Many burned patients will have limitations which, individually, fall short of the criteria needed for evaluating disability. It is important to evaluate the comprehensive result of all limiting factors in order to accurately assess the level of disability.

References

1. American Medical Association Committee on Rating of Mental and Physical Impairment. *Guide to the Evaluation of Permanent Impairment.* Chicago: American Medical Association, 1988.

2. Fisher S V. Disability determination. In: Fisher S V, Helm R A, eds. *Comprehensive Rehabilitation of Burns.* Baltimore: Williams and Wilkins, 1984: 401–11.

3. Warden G D. Burn patients: coming of age, the 1993 Presidential Address of the American Burn Association. *J Burn Care Rehabil* 1993; **14:** 581–8.

4. Salisbury R E. Burn rehabilitation: our unanswered challenge, the 1992 Presidential Address to the American Burn Association. *J Burn Care Rehabil* 1992; **13:** 495–505.

5. Salisbury R E, Carr-Collinis J, eds. *Disability Evaluation of the Thermally Injured Patient.* New York: Rehabilitation Committee, American Burn Association, 1988.

6. Herndon D N, Le Master J, Beard S, *et al.* The quality of life after major thermal injury: an analysis of 12 survivors with ≥ 80% total body, 70% third degree burns. *J Trauma* 1986; **26:** 609–19.

7. Abdullah A, Blakeney P, Hunt R, *et al.* Visible scars and self-esteem in pediatric patients with burns. *J Burn Care Rehabil* 1993; **15:** 164–8.

8. Stolov W C, Clower M R. *Handbook of Severe Disability.* Washington, DC: Government Printing Office, 1981.

CHAPTER FIFTY-FOUR

54

Pain Response and Pain Control

Janet A. Marvin, Michael J. Muller, Patricia E. Blakeney and Walter J. Meyer III

Introduction

The first reaction one has to the words 'burn injury' is pain. Whether the injury is a simple sunburn or an extensive second or third degree burn covering a large portion of the body, the mere thought of this type of injury causes one to cringe and think of pain. Yet the management of pain in a patient with a burn injury often is given little thought by burn care professionals. Attempts to manage pain in a patient with a burn injury is frustrating because of the changing physiologic and psychological reactions to the injury. Beecher[1] observed that soldiers burned in battle could perform heroic feats without apparent pain; yet as soon as they were in a safe place their pain was significant. As noted by Choinière, the pain expressed by a burned patient is very variable[2] (see **Figure 54.1**). This great variation from day to day and hour to hour makes it difficult to titrate the medications used in pain management to meet a patient's needs. Thus, a health care professional becomes confused and frustrated in trying to give enough medication to relieve a patient's pain without giving too much and causing potentially significant untoward reactions. Also, fears of causing addiction continue to be voiced by caregivers and even family members and patients in our current 'drug prone society'. Therefore, it is easy to understand the frustration of caregivers and patients related to the management of a burned patient's pain.

Pathology of a Burn Injury as it Relates to Pain

All burn injuries are painful. First degree or very superficial partial-thickness burns may damage only the outer layers of the skin, the epidermis; but they do produce mild pain and discomfort, especially when something such as clothing rubs against the burned area. Moderate to deep partial-thickness or second degree burns result in variable amounts of pain depending on the amount of destruction to the dermis. Superficial dermal burns are the most painful initially. Even the slightest change in air currents moving past the exposed superficial dermis causes a patient to experience excruciating pain. Without the protective covering of the epidermis, nerve endings are sensitized and exposed to stimulation. In addition, as the inflammatory response progresses, with the increase in swelling and the release of vasoactive substances, pain is increased.[3,4]

Areas of deeper partial-thickness burns may display a confusing pattern of pain over the first few days. These areas may show little or no response to sharp stimuli such as a pin prick; yet a patient may complain of deep achy pain related to the inflammatory response. These wounds are more similar to full-thickness burns in their pain response. In a full-thickness burn, the dermis, with its rich network of nerve endings, is completely destroyed. This leads to an initial response of a completely anesthetic wound when a sharp stimulus is present. Yet, patients often complain of a dull or pressure type of pain in these areas. Once the devitalized tissue, i.e. eschar, sloughs and is replaced by granulation tissue, a patient again experiences the sensation of sharp pain to noxious stimuli.

Pain-generating Mechanisms During an Initial Injury

Although no one would question the fact that burn injuries are painful, the dearth of information on the mechanism of pain perception and reports of burn victims accomplishing extraordinary feats after injury[1] leaves many unanswered questions. Meyer and Campbell[3] attempted to study the mechanism of pain after thermal injury. These studies were accomplished in monkeys and humans exposed to a series of thermal stimuli before and after a 53°C 30-second burn to the glabrous skin of the hand. In monkeys, the response of C and A nociceptive afferents were studied and compared to subjective responses by humans. The burn resulted in increased sensitivity of the A fibers, decreased sensitivity of the C

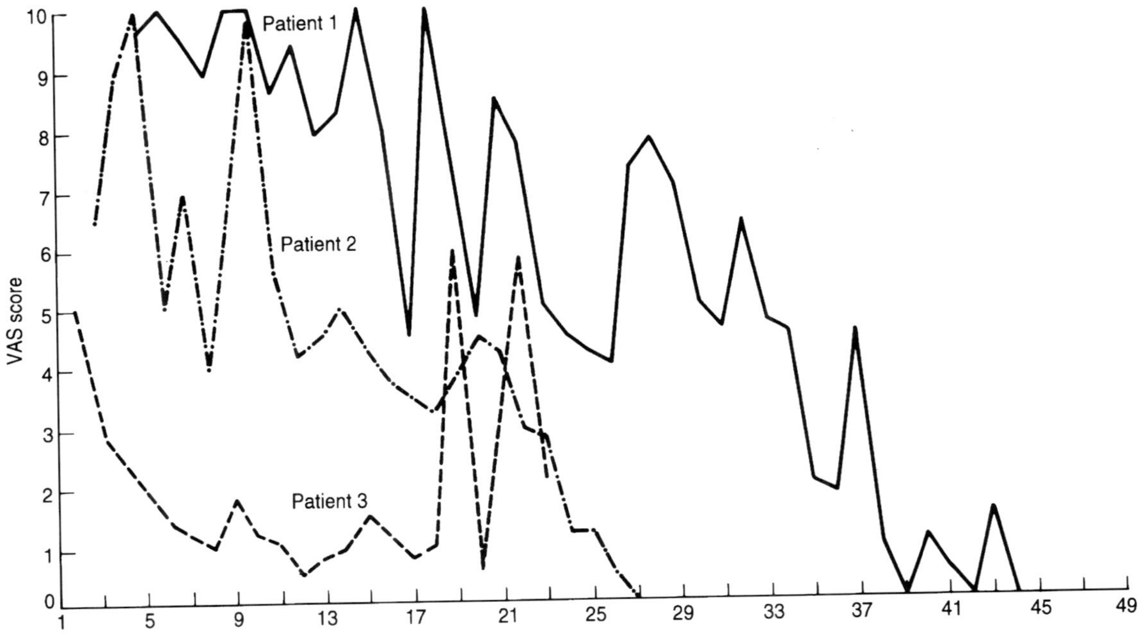

Fig. 54.1 VAS scores for different patients show how variable expressions of pain can be from day to day and from one patient to the next. Reproduced with permission from Choinière et al.[2]

fibers, and increased pain sensitivity (hyperalgesia) in human subjects. This study would suggest that A fibers rather than C fibers are chiefly responsible for the hyperalgesia related to burn injury. To test this hypothesis, Meyer and Campbell[3] used a sphygmomanometer cuff inflated to 250 mmHg 20 minutes after the burn injury. Motor functions and sensitivity to light touch disappeared after 40 minutes. Hyperalgesia at the site was likewise demonstrated, yet pain evoked by the test stimuli applied 5 cm from the injury to uninjured skin was not decreased. It would appear from these experiments that C-nociceptive afferents code for pain intensity of thermal pain near the threshold (43–48°C) of the glabrous skin of the uninjured hand, and that A fibers code for pain above the threshold during a prolonged, intense heat stimulus and for hyperalgesia which resulted minutes after the injury. Preliminary work by the same investigators in other areas of the body did not produce similar results, which could be related to the difference in intensity of A and C fibers in the skin of different areas of the body. Later studies by Campbell *et al.*[4] and Coderre and Melzack[5] confirm that burn injuries not only make an injured area and surrounding tissue more painful but also cause hyperalgesia.

Pain-generating Mechanisms Following an Initial Injury

Even less is known about pain-generating mechanisms after an initial injury than during. As a wound remains unhealed for days or weeks and as various surgical and nonsurgical therapies are applied to a wound during the healing phase, a patient's pain complaints vary considerably. In an attempt to describe the pain experience by burned patients after an initial injury, Charlton and associates[6] used a series of pain measurement tools and standardized psychological tests to measure anxiety and depression. Visual analog pain rating for overall pain in a group of burned patients were skewed towards the low end of the scale, with a median of 1.75 on a 10-point scale in the study by Charlton *et al.* Patients in Charlton *et al.*'s study also completed the McGill Pain Questionnaire. As a group, these patients were comparable to a group of post-herpetic neuralgia patients on the Present Pain Intensity Scale and the Number of Words Chosen Scale, but resembled a group of arthritic patients on the pain rating index.

Choinière *et al.*[2] utilized the visual analog scale (VAS) on a daily basis and asked patients to rate their worst pain for each day. Patients' scores varied widely from patient to patient. Overall pain scores varied widely from day to day in individual patients but gradually declined towards the end of hospitalization. In an effort to elucidate the predictor of pain in these patients, Choinière *et al.* compared pain scores with patient's age, socioeconomic status, and educational level and found no significant correlations. Likewise no significant correlation was found between the pain scores and burn size which was similar to the results in studies by Klein and Charlton[7] and Perry *et al.*[8] Choinière and associates suggest that perhaps these results are related to two issues:

- assessment of the size of the burn wound is usually made only once at the time of injury, thus the measure does not necessarily reflect the current clinical condition of the patients at the time of pain measurement; and
- calculation of the burn does not usually include the superficial first degree burns, which are known to be painful.

Further analysis of their data to include the first degree areas in total extent of burn and limiting the pain measurements to those obtained during the first week postburn showed a positive correlation of pain with burn size ($p < 0.02$). In addition they found that pain scores at rest were significantly correlated with extent of first degree burns ($p < 0.04$) and pain at time of treatments was significantly correlated with extent of second degree burns ($p < 0.02$). No correlation was found with the extent of third degree burns. Atchison *et al.*[9] measured pain scores in children and found a significant correlation between pain scores during the procedure and both the extent of total burn injury and the extent of third degree burn. Issues of concern with the Atchison *et al.* study were that the pain scores spanned the time post-injury from 2 to 117 days in burns from 4% to 93% TBSA, that pain management was constant for the individual child across the entire period of treatment, and that pain medications were not adjusted to a child's weight. These factors raise major concerns about the validity of the data.

Another source of confusion concerning the amount of pain expressed by burn patients is the role played by psychological problems such as anxiety and depression. Charlton *et al.*[6] used the State/Trait Anxiety Inventory to measure anxiety and reported that the study sample of adult burned patients was not particularly anxious. Other studies have suggested that burned patients have increased levels of anxiety, especially related to treatment and outcome and that these levels may increase over time.[10–12] Anticipation of pain related to treatments which occur daily or more often can increase a patient's perception of pain. Anticipatory anxiety related to treatments leads to increased pain, and the increased pain leads to further increases in anxiety. This reaction may explain some findings which suggest that pain increases over time in burned patients.[13–15] Using the Zung Depression Scale to measure depression, Charlton *et al.*[6] found that most patients experienced only mild to moderate depression with few showing moderate to severe depression. Similar results were found by Choinière *et al.*[2] who noted that pain at rest was significantly and positively related to the levels of anxiety or depression, i.e. with elevated anxiety or depression, pain scores at rest increased. Interestingly, all patients hospitalized more than 3 weeks showed an increase in the depression scores. Although these studies demonstrate the great variability in pain expression in burned patients, they do not identify pain-generating mechanisms, either physiologically or psychologically, in a burn-injured patient. Further work in these areas is needed to better understand the great variability of burn pain.

Pain as the Function of the Healing Process

As a deep dermal or full-thickness burn wound heals, either by primary intention from excision and grafting or by secondary intention through granulation tissue and scar formation, the injured neural tissue is reorganized.[16] Reflex neural function returns to a skin grafted burn approximately 5–6 weeks after the burn has been covered by autografted skin.[17] Active vasodilatation, vasoconstriction, and pain sensation all return at this time. These functions also return to the burn wound which heals through scar formation but may take up to 6 months for complete neural reorganization.

Although rare, causalgia, dysesthesia, and phantom pain syndrome can sometimes develop in healing skin. The incidence of these chronic pain syndromes seems to be related to the healing process. Burns which have been excised and grafted on a clean and uniform vascular bed rarely develop one of these chronic pain syndromes. Wounds which heal by granulation and scar formation seem to be more apt to develop a chronic pain problem. Skin biopsies of granulation tissue have clearly shown neuronal tissue entrapment.[17] This pain often subsides over time as the scar tissue matures.

Types of Pain in Burned Patients During the Acute Phase of Treatment

As already noted, the pain expressed by a burned patient is extremely variable. In many studies, burned patients have been asked to rate overall pain, pain at rest, overall procedural pain, and worst pain during the procedure. Such perplexing instructions may account for some of the variability in pain reports. For example, if asked to rate one's overall pain for the day, one would expect this rating to include resting pain, pain during normal activity, and pain during painful procedures. A more reasonable approach may be to ask a patient to rate pain as procedural and nonprocedural pain, giving each type of pain an operational definition. Procedural pain would be pain related to wound care and active or passive stretching of the patient's scar tissue, two activities which seem to cause the worst pain for burned patients. Nonprocedural pain would be the discomfort experienced at rest and while performing activities of daily living. This nomenclature of procedural and nonprocedural pain allows for planning therapies for pain relief, based on the intensity of pain experienced throughout the day. As therapies for pain management are discussed later in this chapter, the importance of differentiating procedural and nonprocedural pain will become increasingly clear.

Measurement of Pain in Burned Patients

Pain Measurement Techniques for an Adult Burned Patient

A variety of pain measurement techniques have been used with adult burned patients. The more common measures include adjective scales (**Table 54.1**), numeric scales (i.e. rating pain on a scale of 0–5, 0–10 or 0–100), and visual analog scales (**Figure 54.2**). Each of these scales measures the sensory component of a patient's pain. Adjective scales and numeric scales are quick and easy to administer because they do not require a visual representation of the scale. The visual analog scale requires a visual representation of the scale to be presented to a patient. Patients must mark or point to the place on the scale which represents their level of pain. This presents a problem for a burned patient whose hands are burned, so some investigators have used a technique of sliding a line or color strip along the scale with instructions to a patient to direct the movement of the slide, stopping at the point representative of the patient's pain. The visual analog scale has been used in a number of studies with a variety of patient samples and has been shown to be a valid method of measuring the sensory component of a patient's pain. The demonstrated validity of the scale allows for comparisons of visual analog pain assessments between studies with different patient samples.

Motivational–affective and cognitive–evaluative components of pain are most frequently measured using the McGill Pain Questionnaire (MPQ).[18] The MPQ consists of 20 sets of adjectives which describe all three components of pain: sensory, affective, and evaluative. Qualitative profiles and quantitative scores for each

Table 54.1 Adjective scales in English and Spanish

0	No pain	0	Nada de dolor
1	Slight pain	1	Dolor leve (ligero)
2	Moderate pain	2	Dolor moderado
3	Severe pain	3	Dolor severo (grave, fuerte)

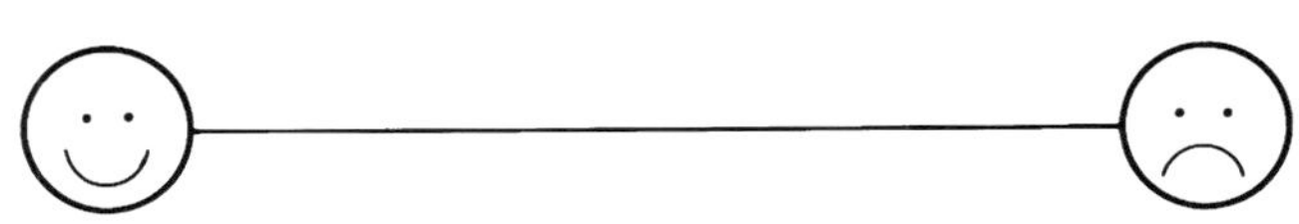

Fig. 54.2 Visual analog scale (VAS) for children to rate their levels of pain from the Varni Thompson Pediatric Pain Questionnaire.[47]

dimension as well as a total pain score can be derived from the selected adjectives. The MPQ has been translated into several languages and has been shown to be a reliable and valid measurement tool. The major problem with the tool is that it takes 10–20 minutes to administer and may not be as useful for frequent, repeated measurements. Many studies have employed this measurement on a daily basis to measure either overall or resting pain.

A major concern in the clinical setting is to use a consistent tool to measure pain and to use it before and 1–2 hours after the administration of a medication for pain relief. For procedural pain management, the same tool should be used to measure pain at the beginning of a procedure (post-premedication), during it, and post-procedure in order to measure the effectiveness of pain management regimens for procedural pain.

Pain Measurement Techniques for Pediatric Patients

The measurement of children's pain is much more complex than it is for adults, especially for preverbal children. For many years it was thought that infants did not feel pain because of incomplete myelinization of the sensory nerves. Anand and colleagues published data in 1987[19] and 1988[20] to suggest that infants do experience pain as evidenced by a variety of physiologic and metabolic responses. Anand and Hickey[21] hypothesize that although Aδ fibers are not completely myelinated and may not be efficient in transmission of pain, unmyelinated C fibers take over the transmission of noxious stimuli. This research has demonstrated the need for pain assessment and management in infants and preverbal children as well as older children.

The assessment of pain in children has included physiologic measurements, behavioral assessment, and patient reports of pain. The physiologic indicators which have been evaluated are heart rate,[17] respiratory rate,[22] blood pressure,[22] endocrine changes,[22,23] and changes in Po_2.[24] None of these shows promise as an indicator for measuring pain in sick children, since all are affected by a variety of stressors in addition to pain.

A number of behavior scales have been devised to measure pain by providing standardized instructions and guidelines for observing behaviors thought to be specific to pain. A number of investigators[25–30] have looked at infants' cries as measurable behaviors which can be observed in order to evaluate pain. Although these studies demonstrate that length of cry, pitch, intensity, and other characteristics of crying may be used to evaluate pain in infants, the analyses of cry are very time consuming and require elaborate audio equipment. Izard *et al.*,[31] Craig *et al.*,[32] and Granau and Craig[29] have attempted to code facial expressions as measures of pain in infants. Their system characterizes nine facial actions involved in the expression of pain, but its use requires videotaping and detailed analyses of an infant's facial movements. Although this method offers excellent research applications, it, like the detailed analyses of crying, is not appropriate for the clinical setting. On the other hand, the studies do provide clinicians with information about various facial actions, as categorized by Granau and Craig, which may be helpful in the clinical identification of pain in infants. Other investigators have devised multidimensional scales which include length of cry, facial expressions, and behavioral states in order to measure pain in infants.[33–35] These scales are easier to use and allow an observer to assess pain as either present or absent without further quantification.

Examples of observational scales which allow for quantification and may be used with toddlers and preverbal children are the CHEOPS (Children's Hospital of Eastern Ontario Pain Scale)[36] and The Observer Scale.[37] The CHEOPS is a scale of six behaviors, each scored on a numeric range; it yields a total numeric score for pain. This scale has been shown to be valid and to have good inter-rater reliability. The Observer Scale is another standardized instrument which categorizes overall pain behaviors or comfort behaviors on a scale of 1–5. The five categories are:

1. laughing, euphoric;
2. happy, contented, playful;
3. calm or asleep;
4. mild–moderate pain: crying, grimacing, restlessness, but can be distracted with toy, food, parent; and
5. severe pain: crying, screaming, inconsolable.

At this time, this scale has not been validated.

Research suggests that simple self-report scales can be used with preschool children. Examples of such scales include the Oucher Scale (photographs of children with various facial expressions).[38–40] Drawing of faces[41,42] have also been used with preschool age children[43] and young school age children (6–8 years).[44] Preschool children have also used the Poker Chip Tool,[45] color scales,[46,47] and a thermometer[48] to report the degree of pain or hurt. These simple tools allow a preschooler to report pain and are easy to use. One caution with the face scales is that a practitioner must help a child differentiate between physical pain and sadness unrelated to pain. Since there is no evidence that any one of these is more valid than another, it is recommended to pick one and use it consistently with a preschooler. When self-report scales are used in conjunction with observational scales, a practitioner gets a better picture of a child's response to pain and pain therapies.

A school-aged child's cognitive development allows more abstract thinking. They can use simple numeric scales 0–5 in the early school years (ages 6–8)[49] and more complex scales 0–10 or 0–100 in the later years (age 9–12), as well as visual analog scales anchored with happy and sad faces,[47] and simple adjective scales.[47,50] In addition to self-reports of pain, observational scales such as the CHEOPS,[36] or the Procedure Behavior Check List[51] can be used with a school-aged child. Again, the important issue is to use consistently one selected scale since no one has been shown to be more valid than others.

Adolescents can think abstractly and can quantify and qualify phenomena and so can use the same scales as adults. One concern with adolescents is that, when they are ill, they tend to regress and thus may require the use of a simpler scale during such times.[52] In summary, there are many measurement tools for pain assessment across the life span which can be useful to the researcher and the clinician. **Table 54.2** presents a list of clinically useful tools according to patient age.

Pharmacologic Management of Pain

Pharmacologic management of burn pain is the mainstay of therapy. Review articles[53–60] recommend a variety of therapeutic modalities for background and procedural pain during the stages of burn treatment. The three stages are:

- the emergency or resuscitative phase (0–72 hours after injury);
- the acute phase (72 hours to 3 or 5 weeks, until the wounds are closed); and
- the rehabilitative phase (from the time of wound closure to scar maturity).

For pain management therapy, the emergency or resuscitative phase applies only to patients with burns greater that 10% total body surface area (TBSA). **Table 54.3** provides a matrix summary

Table 54.2 Recommended clinical pain measurement tools for burned patients

Infants and toddlers	
	CHEOPS[36]
	The Observer Pain Scale[37]
Preschooler	
	Faces drawing[43,44] or Oucher[38–40]
	Pediatric Pain Questionnaire[47]
	CHEOPS[36]
School age child	
	Visual analog
	Numeric scale
	Pediatric Pain Questionnaire[47]
	Procedure Behavior Checklist[51]
Adolescents and adults	
	Visual analog
	Numeric scales
	Adjective scales
	McGill Pain Questionnaire[18]

of therapies which are recommended for procedural and background pain over the three phases of burn care. Also included in this table are the anxiolytic agents which are suggested for use by several authors. A variety of routes or methods of administration are also suggested. The routes or methods recommended not only include the usual intravenous bolus (IVB), intravenous continuous infusion (IVCI), patient-controlled analgesia (PCA), and orally administered agents on a nonpain contingent (NPC) basis.

Emergency Phase

During the emergency phase, the preferred route for most medications is the intravenous route because of potential problems with absorption from the muscles and stomach related to decreased perfusion. Of the agents recommended for the relief of procedural pain, morphine is the most widely used. For procedures, IVB and IVCI are the most common methods used. For extremely painful procedures in both the emergency and acute phase, fentanyl has a major advantage in that it is shorter acting and avoids oversedation following a procedure as might occur with repeated doses of morphine. As with any narcotic, tolerance to fentanyl may develop quickly. Osgood[57] reported the administration of as much as 8000 μg of fentanyl for a burn dressing change after 15 days, following a protocol which begins with 1–6 μg/kg during the procedure.

For background pain, although IV bolus administration has been the norm, PCA and IVCI are being used with greater frequency. Both of these methods allow for greater flexibility in dose titration and should avoid over- and undermedication. Since even the more severely burned patients are usually alert and coherent, the PCA method is the ideal method for titration. PCA can be used with or without a background IVCI. For a burned patient with extensive hand burns, the control cord can be fitted with a padded pedal-type apparatus which can be positioned so that the patient can press it with a foot, elbow, etc.

In addition to the agonist drug, the agonist–antagonist group (Nubain, for example) would appear to offer pain relief with decreased threat of respiratory depressant effects. Osgood[57] suggests that if these drugs are to be used, they should be used initially, since to use these after a patient has been on an agonist for a period of time could precipitate symptoms of withdrawal. In addition to the opiates, analgesic doses of anesthetic agents such as ketamine and nitrous oxide may be used for procedural pain. These two agents, along with anxiolytic agents to be used as adjuncts to pain management, will be discussed later in this chapter.

Acute Phase

During the acute phase, the choice of pharmacological agents used to manage procedural pain encompasses a number of orally administered agents. Of these agents, hydromorphone (Dilaudid) is an

Table 54.3 Pharmacologic therapies for burn pain relief

Emergent Phase	Acute Phase	Rehabilitative Phase
	Procedural	
Morphine (IVB, IVCI)	Morphine (IVB, IVCI, PCA)	For severe pain:
Meperidine (IVB)	Roxanol (oral morphine)	Hydromorphone (PO) (Dilaudid)
Fentanyl (IVB, IVCI)	Meperidine (IVB, IM)	
Hydromorphone (IVB, PO) (Dilaudid)	Fentanyl (IVB, IM)	For mild to moderate pain:
Nalbuphine (IVB) (Nubain)	Hydromorphone (PO) (Dilaudid)	Oxycodone (PO) (Percocet)
Ketamine (IV) (Ketalar)	Nalbuphine (IVB) (Nabain)	Nonsteroidal anti-inflammatory drugs (NSAIDs) with or without narcotics
Nitrous oxide (IH)	Ketamine (IV, IM) (Ketalar)	
Anxiolytics	Oxycodone (PO) (Percocet)	
Diazepam (IV) (Valium)	Anxiolytics	
Lorazepam (IV) (Ativan)	Diazepam (PO) (Valium)	
Midazolam (IV, IVCI) (Versed)	Lorazepam (PO) (Ativan)	
	Alprazolam (PO) (Xanax)	
	Background	
Morphine (IVCI, PCA)	Morphine (IVCI, PCA)	Usually not necessary
Meperidine (PCA)	Meperidine (IVCI, PCA)	Acetaminophen
Methadone (PO, NPC)	Methadone (PO, NPC)	NSAIDs
	Sustained release morphine (PO, NPC) (MS Contin)	
	Acetaminophen (PO, NPC)	
	NSAIDs (PO, NPC)	
	Choline magnesium trisalicylate	

excellent oral agent for the relief of moderate to severe pain when given in equianalgesic doses to morphine. Of concern with this drug is that the period of peak effect varies widely from 45 to 90 minutes; for this reason, the combination of lorazepam given 1 hour before a procedure and hydromorphone given 45–60 minutes before a procedure results in excellent pain control for the majority of adult patients. As with other opiates, tolerance may develop rapidly, so the dose of hydromorphone may need to be adjusted frequently.

To control background pain during the acute phase, the use of PCA of NPC (nonpain-contingent) medication regimens are far superior to the PRN (as requested) method. PRN regimens often result in undermedication by one nurse and overmedication by the next nurse. A patient may become angry and confused about what to expect regarding pain control and may feel realistically helpless in an environment where others decide whether relief is necessary. Allowing a patient to medicate himself as needed usually results in better pain control as well as better staff and patient relationships. An alternative to PCA, which seems to work equally well for background pain is the use of NPC medication regimens. Such regimens may use methadone in a pain cocktail, slow release morphine (MS Contin®), or other oral agents given on a fixed dosing schedule, the frequency of which will depend on the pharmacologic agent.

Rehabilitative Phase

During the rehabilitative phase, most patients complain more of an aching type of pain, similar to arthritic pain. In this case, mild narcotics, acetaminophen, or nonsteroidal anti-inflammatory drugs (NSAIDs) may be used for either procedural (exercise) or background pain. If a procedure will cause severe pain, hydromorphone may be used.

Age of Patient and Pain Management

Since the pharmacologic management of burn pain not only spans the phases of burn care, but also must be tailored to meet the needs of all age groups, it is important to comment on pain management in both the very young and the elderly. There is a tendency to give less medication to young children because 'they don't complain of pain'. It is unlikely that a burn is any less painful in 3-month old than in a 30-year-old; thus, the same therapeutic modalities adjusted for age and size are appropriate for burned children. At the other extreme of age is an elderly patient. Again, the tendency is to give less medication, either because these patients do not complain as much or because they are 'more sensitive' to pain medications. A realistic and important concern with the elderly is oversedation. Studies in nonburned elderly people have shown that with increased age, the efficiency of the clearance mechanism for certain drugs is decreased and repeated doses may lead to drug accumulation. This would suggest that, when managing pain in an elderly burned patient, it is not that the dose *per se* should be decreased, but that the interval between dosing should be lengthened so as to prevent accumulation and oversedation.

Empirical Data Regarding Pharmacologic Management of Pain

The preceding discussion has focused on the reviews and reports of 'how we do it' or the 'bias' of health care professionals in treating burn pain. The following is a review of recent studies of various pharmacologic modalities in burn pain management.

Opioids

Novoa[61] reported, in 1980, that burned patients could tolerate, for procedural pain, higher doses than the usual 10–15 mg IV dose of morphine. She reviewed a 2-year experience in which adults were given from 20 to 35 mg (occasionally as much as 50 mg) of morphine intravenously in incremental doses during debridement. Although the total number of patients treated was not given, she reported only two incidents over the 2 years in which naloxone hydrochloride was needed to correct respiratory depression.

Perry and Inturrisi[62] reported that the pharmacokinetics of morphine in burned patients were not significantly altered in comparison to normals. They found that the $t_{1/2\alpha}$ (apparent distribution half-life in minutes) was 4.3 ± 3.4 (SD) in burned patients vs. $t_{1/2\alpha}$ 1.7 ± 1.2 in normals and that the $t_{1/2\beta}$ (apparent elimination half-life in minutes) was 98.8 ± 20.8 (SD) in burned patients vs. 176.8 ± 70.3 in normal. Likewise, the apparent volume of central compartment, clearance, hepatic extraction, and plasma binding were similar for burned patients and normals. Osgood[57] found in a group of acutely burned children that the distribution and elimination half-life of morphine markedly shortened [$t_{1/2\alpha}$ = 1.2 ± 0.39 (SEM) for burned children vs. 2.2 ± 0.49 minutes in normals; $t_{1/2\beta}$ = 36.9 ± 6.40 for burned children vs. 126 ± 38.18 minutes in normals ($p < 0.05$)] and that the rate of clearance was increased for acutely burned children.

Bloedow *et al.*[63] reported on the pharmacokinetics of meperidine in eleven acute burns (1 week post-injury) and in five convalescent patients (about 6 weeks postburn). The meperidine steady state distribution volume (l/kg) during both the acute and convalescent phases was about half the distribution volume reported in the literature for meperidine in healthy subjects. The meperidine clearance in burned patients (acute, 420 ml/min and convalescent, 600 ml/min) was slower than would be anticipated in the presence of known marked increases in hepatic blood flow in burned patients.

Sandidge[64] reported on the use of methadone in a pain cocktail used on a nonpain contingent basis for the relief of background pain. Using a prospective, double-blind crossover study, 10 male burned patients (age 18–63) with burn sizes ranging from 5% to 20% TBSA were given a pain cocktail. The base contained 650 mg of acetaminophen and 50 mg of hydroxyzine per dose. Either 0.3 mg/kg of methadone/day in four divided doses or no methadone was added in a randomized crossover design. All subjects were allowed to have additional analgesics as requested. There was a significant decrease in pain during the week with methadone as compared to the week without on the following measures: McGill Pain Questionnaire ($p < 0.05$), sensory subscale ($p = 0.02$), affective subscale ($p = 0.02$), evaluative subscale ($p = 0.012$), pain rating index and number of words chosen ($p = 0.039$), visual analog scale (VAS) score of 'pain now' ($p = 0.042$), and 'most pain in past 24 hours' ($p = 0.008$). The one pain score which was not significantly different was 'least pain' in past 24 hours on the VAS scale. When all medications (methadone plus PRN narcotics) were converted to morphine equivalents, there was no difference in the total amount of analgesics taken ($p = 0.278$). Thus, although patients made up for the analgesics in morphine equivalents during the week that methadone was not administered, the quantity and quality of pain was significantly alleviated when methadone was administered.

Concilus *et al.*[65] reported the use of an intravenous methadone infusion to control nonprocedural pain in 17 critically ill burned patients. An initial loading dose of 0.1–0.2 mg/kg/hr was given over 2 hours and then a maintenance infusion of 0.01–0.02 mg/kg/hr was used. Median VAS scores were 70% lower than baseline at 2 hours and 80% lower than baseline at 24 hours. Cardiovascular parameters remained stable. There was a significant drop in respiratory rate from a mean on 19.6 ± 9.8 to 15.5 ± 9.7 at

2 hours but no significant change in $P\text{CO}_2$ (10 of the 17 patients were ventilated). One patient required naloxone because of a drop in respiratory rate from 32 to 16 and a rise in $P\text{CO}_2$ from 39 to 55 mmHg. Another patient with severe respiratory injury required intubation and ventilation, but it is not clear whether her respiratory problems were contributable to methadone or the progression of her inhalation injury, since she had problems with oxygenation as well. Only one patient required additional morphine in the first 24 hours. Additional analgesia was given for procedural pain after 24 hours.

Lee *et al.*[66] reported on the effectiveness of nalbuphine hydrochloride when compared to morphine sulfate in the relief of procedural pain in burned patients. The prospective double-blind, single-dose study compared nalbuphine hydrochloride 0.4 mg/kg to morphine 0.2 mg/kg given intravenously (pre-procedure) and a maintenance dose (during procedure) of up to 0.2 mg/kg of nalbuphine or 0.1 mg/kg of morphine which was administered incrementally during the procedure at the patient's request. The sample consisted of 50 men (25 received nalbuphine and 25 received morphine). There was no difference in the two groups in relation to age, weight, height, size of burn, or American Surgical Association (ASA) classification of the severity of illnesses. There was also no difference in the mean initial dose, number of patient-required maintenance doses, or mean maintenance dose when the 2:1 nalbuphine to morphine equivalency was taken into account. Likewise, there were no differences in adjective or VAS pain scores with either treatment. There was no respiratory depression in either group. The authors concluded that nalbuphine hydrochloride could be used in doses of 2:1 equivalency to morphine in the alleviation of procedural pain.

Sandidge *et al.*[67] compared the use of PCA using morphine or standard therapy which included a methadone pain cocktail with additional analgesia as requested. Seventeen patients age 18–65 years were randomized to receive either PCA or standard treatment. The two groups were compared for age; size of burn; length of stay; pain as measured daily on VAS for 'least pain', 'most pain', and 'pain now'; a McGill Pain Questionnaire every 3 days; and a daily VAS score for nausea. Additionally, all analgesia was converted to morphine equivalents and compared. No significant differences were found between groups on any measured parameter. Thus, PCA was found to be equal in pain relief to a standard regimen when morphine equivalents were comparable.

Wolman *et al.*[68] presented very different results in a study of PCA in 52 adult burned patients. In 10 of 10 patients who were not given an initial bolus of morphine, there was failure to induce or maintain adequate pain relief. In the 42 remaining patients who received an initial bolus of morphine and a minimum of 12 hours of continuous infusion of morphine prior to starting PCA, 30 of the 42 patients asked to exit the study within 24 hours because of inadequate pain relief.

Kinsella *et al.*[69] in 1988, reported on the use of morphine via patient-controlled analgesia in 18 nonseriously burned patients postoperatively and five acutely burned patients. In the postoperative group, PCA was used for 12–24 hours with 'good' results. In the five acutely burned patients, morphine at a mean dose of 3.1 mg/h for a mean duration of 28.3 hours (range 9.5–72 hours) was also reported to give 'good' results.

From the ten studies cited here on the use of opioids, one would have difficulty making decisions about the best drug, the best dosage range, or the best route or method (i.e. PCA, PRM, or continuous infusion) of administration of these drugs in burned patients. As noted in the many review articles, morphine or other opioids are considered mainstays of pain relief in burned patients but many reviewers report less than adequate pain relief for burned patients with the use of opioids. Personal experience has shown that even a PCA regimen must be individualized and frequently adjusted. Important caveats for the use of PCA should include:

- an initial bolus of 5–10 mg of morphine or equivalent dose of other drugs;
- increasing the patient-controlled dose as needed to achieve pain relief (recognizing that tolerance develops at varying rates in individual patients);
- planning for a change in dosing regimens at night to include:
  - (a) giving a bolus dose at bedtime;
  - (b) doubling the patient controlled dose and lengthening the time interval between doses so that when a patient awakens in pain, he or she does not have to lie awake to push a button several times in order to get adequate medication; and
  - (c) if the increased intermittent dosing is not adequate, being lenient with bolus doses or to start a patient on a continuous morphine drip at night.

Fentanyl and its Derivatives

Kyff and Prasad,[70] in a retrospective study, reported on the use on fentanyl (4–8 μg/kg) and midazolam (0.08 mg/kg) in 256 burned patients prior to dressing changes. Both drugs were mixed together in 20 ml of intravenous solution in a micro drip chamber and administered over 5–10 minutes. Patients and staff reported 'superior' pain relief. Therapists reported an improved level of consciousness post-dressing change when patients were expected to participate in therapy. There were no reports of respiratory depression and narcotic reversal was not necessary. Fentanyl and some of its newer derivatives (alfentanil, sufentanil, lofentanil), because of their increased potency, may prove to be very useful for burned patients. To date, in nonburned patients the pharmacokinetic data show great variability, especially with the parent compound fentanyl.[71] Thus, further pharmacokinetic studies, in nonburned as well as burned patients, need to be completed in order to better understand the efficacy and safety of this class of drugs in burned patients.

Nonsteroidal Anti-inflammatory Drugs (NSAIDs)

Two reports[72,73] were found concerning the use of NSAIDs in burned patients. Neither of these studies reported on the use of NSAIDs for pain management, but one study by Wallace[72] reported a significant reduction in body temperature (0.67°C ($p < 0.01$)) and a decrease in metabolic rate (11.4%; $p < 0.01$) with the administration of ibuprofen, suggesting that this drug may attenuate the metabolic response to thermal injury by blunting the temperature elevation associated with burn injuries. A study of the pharmacokinetics of ibuprofen when given enterally to burned patients reports the half-life to vary from 1.4 to 5.1 hours, depending on whether the drug was given by enteral tube with tube feeding ($t_{1/2}$ = 1.4 hours) or orally with a regular diet ($t_{1/2}$ = 5.1 hours).[73] Although ibuprofen was not given for pain control in either study, the results might lead one to ask, concerning the first study, was the decrease in metabolic rate solely related to a decrease in body temperature or was some of the effect a result of better pain control? The second study is also important if one is going to use ibuprofen as part of a pain management regimen. The results would suggest that different dosing schedules might be necessary if a patient is receiving tube feedings or a regular diet. Nonsteroidals, such as ibuprofen, have, in addition to analgesic effects, anti-inflammatory activity which, in some instances, may be advantageous due to the ability to inhibit prostaglandin biosynthesis. This activity is, however, directly associated with some of its side effects which include gastrointestinal bleeding, hypertension, and congestive heart failure.

Because of the significant side-effect profile of nonsteroidal and anti-inflammatory drugs such as ibuprofen, acetaminophen has been considered for the management of chronic pain. In 1991, Bradley *et al.* reported that acetaminophen at a dose of 10–15 mg per kg of body weight given every 4 h (up to a maximum of 4000 mg/day) was equal in efficacy to Ibuprofen at a dose of 10 mg/kg of body weight given every 4 h (up to a maximum of 2400 mg/day). In addition, acetaminophen caused no more side effects and slightly fewer gastrointestinal side effects. Acetaminophen was well tolerated, although there is some long-term concern about renal problems and liver problems with this medication when used in high doses such that blood levels reach 50 μg/ml.

Shriners Burns Institute in Galveston recently completed an analysis of 198 consecutive acutely burned pediatric patients who were treated with a pain management protocol, which utilized acetaminophen scheduled at 10 mg/kg every 4 hours as background management with morphine added for breakthrough pain and procedures such as tubbing. Background pain for 44% of the children was managed with acetaminophen alone, whereas the pain of 48% was managed with morphine. Best response to acetaminophen was in the younger age groups where 68% of the children under 3 years have their pain well managed by acetaminophen. The size of the burn also had a significant influence on the effectiveness of acetaminophen. The smaller the burn, the more likely the positive response. Further, 49% of those with burns of less than 10% responded to acetaminophen alone, whereas only 10% of those with burns greater than 60% could be managed with acetaminophen alone. Studies did not include an analysis of the depth of the burns. It usually included a mixture of severe second degrees as well as third degrees. Acetaminophen can be easily monitored in the blood, and in the authors' experience, 10–15 mg/kg every 4 hours does not cause blood levels to exceed 10 μg/ml; thus it should be safe over a long period of time. It may be given in conjunction with morphine as well as NSAIDs with probably no significant additional side effects. Acetaminophen is rapidly absorbed from the stomach and small bowel and achieves peak analgesic efficacy more rapidly than even aspirin. It is available in elixir and oral drops. One should be aware that, because acetaminophen is packaged in conjunction with hydrocodone in the form of Vicodin, one should be careful to not give acetaminophen in addition to Vicodin.

Antianxiety Drugs

Although studies by Charlton[74] and Choinière[2] would suggest that burned patients are not particularly anxious, antianxiety agents are often used alone or in combination with opioids and other agents for pain relief.[75–77] Martyn *et al.*[78] studied diazepam in burned patients. After a single dose, there was a rapid decline in concentration due to the high lipid solubility and rapid tissue uptake, leading to a shorter hypnotic effect of the drug. Interestingly, the elimination half-life was significantly prolonged for burned patients (72 hours vs. 36 hours for normals). Thus, with repeated administration, the tissue could become saturated and then the termination of the effect would depend more on biotransformation by hepatic enzymes. Hepatic enzyme activity has been shown to be quite depressed in burned patients.[79,80] This may explain the prolonged sedation seen in burned patients with repeated doses of diazepam.

Martyn *et al.*[81] have also studied the pharmacokinetics of lorazepam in burned patients. The study involved burned patients compared to controls matched for age and weight. The burned patients were studied at a mean of 22 ± 4.6 (SE) days post-injury. The data showed that with burn injury there is an increased volume of distribution 2.66 ± 0.55 vs. 1.39 ± 0.1 l/kg ($p < 0.02$); an increased clearance, 4.28 ± 1.20 vs. 1.16 ± 0.1 ml/min/kg ($p < 0.01$); and a significantly reduced half-life, 9.6 ± 1.3 vs. 13.9 ± 0.9 hours ($p < 0.025$).

Stanford[82] reported a case of a previously healthy 30-year-old with a 27% TBSA burn, who exhibited delirium after a 2 mg intravenous dose of lorazepam. For approximately 7 hours after the infusion, the patient exhibited delusional beliefs, confusion, psychomotor agitation, and rapid unintelligible speech. Symptoms did not recur after discontinuation of treatment. Despite this unusual report by Stanford, it would appear from Martyn's work that lorazepam would be superior to diazepam in treating anxiety in burned patients. Martyn suggests that, in addition to the fact that the clearance of lorazepam is faster than diazepam in burned patients, two other features of lorazepam make it a more acceptable drug for burned patients. First, it is metabolized by conjugation (a cytochrome P-450 independent pathway) to a pharmacologically inactive glucuronide metabolite and, second, the unbound volume of distribution is much less that diazepam with clinically effective blood concentrations persisting for many hours and resulting in longer lasting sedation. In addition, unlike diazepam, lorazepam is not affected by the concomitant administration of cimetidine.

Although the pharmacokinetics of midazolam have not been reported in burned patients, it has characteristics in nonburned patients which would seem to make it an attractive anxiolytic agent for burned patients. Midazolam has a more rapid onset than either diazepam or lorazepam; thus, it allows for more rapid titration for effect in an individual patient. The elimination half-life of 2.5 hours is considerably shorter than that of lorazepam (13 hours) or diazepam (36 hours) and should result in a shorter recovery time after a procedure.[83] It is better tolerated by the veins when given intravenously. The anesthetic effect of midazolam is greater than diazepam.[84,85] Elderly patients have a more consistent response to a given dose.[86] Of the three benzodiazepines reviewed, either lorazepam or midazolam would seem to be more appropriate for repeated use in burned patients.

Anesthetic Agents Used in Analgesic Doses for Procedural Pain

Nitrous oxide

Baskett[87,88] reported the use of nitrous oxide in addition to a neuroleptanalgesic (a combination of dehydrobenzperidol and phenoperidine) during burn dressing changes in children. The addition of 50% nitrous oxide was noted to decrease the respiratory depression associated with neuroleptanalgesia alone and provided a safe, short-acting analgesia. In these studies, patients were fasted for 6 hours before the procedure but resumed normal oral intake within 2 hours.

Filkin *et al.*[89] reported results from both a retrospective study and a prospective study on the use of 50% nitrous oxide and 50% oxygen for debridement pain. In the retrospective study, the charts of 52 male patients were reviewed for the number of treatments, the effectiveness of pain relief, and the frequency of side effects. The average burn size was 19% TBSA (range 2–85%), and the mean age was 28 years (range 16–64). The number of treatments varied from one to 52 per patient, with a mean of 12 treatments per patient. Of the 52 patients, only one patient reported no pain relief and requested to discontinue the use of the nitrous oxide. Side effects noted were dizziness, giddiness, increased verbalizations, euphoria, dream-like state, nausea, and nonspecific tremors. Only in two patients were the side effects considered to be significant enough to withdraw the treatment; these occurred in one patient with nausea and in one patient who developed nonspecific tremors. In the prospective study, all patients were given a standard dose of morphine (0.2 mg/kg) pre-procedure. Patients were then randomized to receive either a 50% nitrous oxide 50% oxygen mixture or compressed air for a given study treatment. Patient and patient care staff were blinded as to the treatment condition. Pain scores were taken at 10, 20, and 30 minutes using a four-point adjective scale and at 3 hours post-procedure using a VAS scale. All patients were allowed to use the nitrous oxide mixture in addition to morphine for debridement when they were not being studied. The study was aborted when 80% of the planned 30 patients requested to withdraw from the study because they did not feel that they were getting consistent pain relief on study days, preferring to use nitrous oxide for all treatment.

The conclusions from both of these studies, as well as a retrospective study reported by Marvin[90] in which charts from 130 patients (65 who received nitrous oxide and 65 patients matched for % TBSA burn who did not), were reviewed and found excellent patient acceptance and few side effects. In the study by Marvin, the frequency of specific side effects related to peripheral neuropathy, changes in liver function, and anemia were noted: no patient in either group showed changes in liver function tests while receiving the nitrous oxide mixture. Anemia as a direct side effect of nitrous oxide could not be studied in this patient sample because of the frequent surgical procedures requiring blood transfusions in both groups. The only significant finding was that four patients in the group treated with nitrous oxide had a discharge finding of a neurological disorder which included one carpal tunnel injury, an exposed Achilles tendon, a brachial plexus injury, and 'decreased function related to disuse'. The carpal tunnel injury and the exposed Achilles tendon were directly related to the initial injury. The brachial plexus injury, noted within 24 hours of an operative procedure, was thought to be due to positioning and was resolving at the time of discharge. The fourth patient had been a very uncooperative patient who had decreased hand function attributed to lack of exercise to maintain function. None of these neurological disorders was similar to the polyneuropathies previously reported in relation to chronic nitrous oxide exposure.[91–93]

Hayden *et al.*[94] reported one case of progressive myeloneuropathy in burns related to the use of nitrous oxide. In this case, a 23-year-old male with a 46% TBSA burn, including the legs, trunk, buttocks, and patchy areas on both arms, used a mixture to 50% nitrous oxide and 50% oxygen PRN (as necessary) for a period of 3 months. During this 3 months, he used 40 000 liters of Entonox®. During treatment, the patient developed bilateral foot drop and weakness of grip in both hands. He also complained of electrical shock sensations radiating from the lumbar spine to both feet with sudden neck flexion. He went on to develop diarrhea (four to five bowel movements/day) and was unable to walk without assistance. Post-discharge, he complained of impotency. At 6 months post-discharge, he had experienced gradual return of all function except power and sensation in his lower extremities. The PRN use reported here varies from the once or twice daily use reported by Basket,[87,88] Filkin,[89] and Marvin;[90] it would seem from the report that the patient consumed vastly larger doses. This may well explain the neurological problems seen in this case which were similar to those described with chronic abuse of nitrous oxide.[91–93]

Ketamine

Slogoff *et al.*[95] reported their clinical experience with the use of subanesthetic doses of ketamine for 150 debridement and dressing change procedures in 40 burned patients. Fourteen patients had only one exposure and the remainder had 2–13 exposures. The initial dose was 1.6 mg/kg of ketamine given intravenously. The results showed that patients with one or two exposures had coherent conversation or no vocalization 60% of the time; screaming or vocalization unrelated to stimulation, 34%; and vocalizations in response to stimulation, 5%. In the group that received more than two exposures, coherent vocalizations dropped to 40%, while screaming or vocalization unrelated to stimulation increased to 49% and vocalizations related to stimulation increased to 11%. Involuntary movement was rare in either group: 7% in ≤ 2 exposures and 8% in < 2 exposures. One patient developed upper airway obstruction, which responded to manipulation of the mandible, and one patient experienced unpleasant emergence reactions after each of four procedures but did not refuse further treatment with ketamine. Significant findings in this study were:

- all patients who had more than two procedures required higher doses ($p < 0.001$);
- the duration of analgesia per dose, min/mg/kg was less with subsequent doses ($p < 0.001$; and
- the time to complete orientation was less with subsequent doses ($p < 0.01$).

With the increase in dosage after the second exposure, the actual time of analgesia remained constant at about 15 minutes. All patients had complete amnesia for all procedures.

Martinez *et al.*[96] described a dream state of burned patients treated with ketamine for dressing changes. A randomly selected sample of 15 patients (ten males, five females; age range from 20 to 85 years) were asked to describe their dreams while under the influence of ketamine. All subjects were prepared by either a nurse or a physician in an unstructured interview to discuss the procedure and 'the likelihood that positive thoughts would result in pleasant experiences'. Twelve of 15 subjects stated that they experienced dreams while under the effects of ketamine. Eight of the 12 described their dreams as pleasant. Subjects were also asked to rate their ketamine experience according to a list of descriptions: seven chose 'frightening', eleven chose 'floating', two chose 'beautiful', eight chose 'helpless', two chose 'powerful', and eleven chose 'confusing'.

Two protocols for the use of ketamine in burned patients were published in the *Journal of Burn Care and Rehabilitation* (March/April, 1987). One protocol, from San Francisco General Hospital, allowed a nurse to administer ketamine 2–3 mg/kg body weight intramuscularly for dressing changes under the order and immediate supervision of a physician.[97] The second protocol presented was from the Shriners Hospital for Crippled Children Burns Institute, Galveston, Texas.[98] This protocol actually described the use of ketamine as an anesthetic, not an analgesic agent. The doses used were 1–2 mg/kg body weight, intravenously, or 8–10 mg/kg body weight given intramuscularly. The procedures required administration by an anesthesiologist. A review by Martyn[99] of the use of ketamine in burned patients as an analgesic agent was also presented with the above-mentioned protocols. One salient point from the review is that, in low doses (1–3 mg/kg body weight rectally), ketamine can produce short periods of analgesia (5–30 minutes) for dressing changes. Second, with repeated use, tolerance can develop, so increased doses are required over time. Third, despite the maintenance of laryngeal and pharyngeal reflexes, patients should have nothing by mouth for 4–6 hours prior to administration. The side effects of ketamine include the production of copious upper airway secretions (necessitating the use of drying agents: atropine or glycopyrrolate), hypertension, pulmonary and systemic arterial hypertension, tachycardia, and postoperative emergency reactions. Ketamine is contraindicated in patients with systemic or pulmonary arterial hypertension, myocardial infarction, ventricular failure, history of cerebral injuries, or psychiatric disorders.

More recently, Dimick *et al.*[100] reported on the use of anesthesia-assisted procedures in burned patients. They reported on 109 procedures in 46 patients for staple removal from grafts (34 procedures); massive dressing changes or vigorous debridement (74 procedures); or facial moulage (one procedure). Anesthesia time ranged from 40 to 180 minutes. A variety of different combinations of inhalation and intravenous agents were administered. Ventilation was assisted at the discretion of the anesthesiologist in attendance. Ninety-eight procedures (90%) were uneventful. In the other 11 patients, two patients lost their intravenous access and had to be recannulated; seven patients had systolic blood pressure and/or pulse rate vary more than 20% from baseline and required treatment; two patients required unplanned intubations, but both were extubated at the end of the procedure. Within 2 hours after the procedure, 72% of patients were able to cooperate fully; and within 4 hours, all were able to cooperate fully. They concluded that anesthesia-assisted procedures in a burn intensive care unit could be performed safely with appropriate professional care and monitoring.

Neuropathic or Phantom Pain

Some severely burned children have partial loss of digits or limbs associated with their burns. This adds a different dimension to the management of their pain since these children often have feelings of the existence of these digits or limbs for many years after their loss. This type of pain usually does not respond to traditional pain management with nonsteroidal acetaminophen or opiates. This neuropathic type of pain often does respond to the use of tricyclics or anticonvulsants. Doses of imipramine or amitriptyline of 1 mg/kg body weight often is effective. If the pain does not respond to this, then Tegretol might be utilized in doses which are therapeutic for seizures. Over time, these types of pain become more tolerable and slowly dissipate.

Nonpharmacologic Therapies in Burned Patients

A variety of nonpharmacologic techniques to aid in pain reduction have been used with burned patients. For the most part, the studies that have been reported have involved small numbers of patients, have failed to describe whether the nonpharmacologic technique was employed alone or as an adjunct to pharmacologic modalities, and would appear to be operator dependent. For this discussion, the nonpharmacologic techniques will be divided into hypnosis and other nonpharmacologic techniques which will include behavior modification, stress reduction, distraction, TENS (transcutaneous electrical nerve stimulation), and acupuncture.

Hypnosis in Burn Pain Management

Studies of hypnosis for control of burn pain prior to 1970 included six articles[101–106] that reported 23 cases (one to eight cases per report), resulting in a positive result in 62.5–100% of reports. The age of the subjects ranged from 7 to 45 years. In one report, hypnosis was used as the sole anesthetic for five major surgical procedures in the single case reported.[104]

Since 1970, four studies have been reported with larger numbers of subjects. LaBaw[107] reported using hypnosis as an adjunct to pain control in children 6–16 years of age). Although generally positive results were reported, there were no specific data about the method of judging the results. Shafer[108] reported the use of hypnosis for both anesthesia and analgesia in a group of 20 burned patients with positive results in 70% (14 of 20) of the patients. He noted that most patients who were not good candidates for hypnosis were children and adolescents who were too anxious to be approached. Wakeman and Kaplan[109] reported a controlled study of hypnosis in which two groups of hypnotized burned patients, patients with 0–30% burns ($n = 24$) and patients with 31–60% burns ($n = 18$), were matched with control groups of patients who received 'attention only'. Pain was measured by standard observable criteria, i.e. patients were allowed to decide for themselves how much medication they required. The ages of the subjects were 7–70 years. The results of this study demonstrated that subjects in the hypnotized groups used less medication than the control groups, and that children and adolescents responded better to hypnosis than did adults. Everett *et al.*,[110] with 32 subjects, compared hypnosis plus placebo anxiolytics, lorazepam plus placebo hypnosis, hypnosis plus lorazepam, and placebo hypnosis plus placebo anxiolytics as adjuncts to opioids for pain control during dressing changes. Analysis of pain scores on the visual analog scale (VAS) indicated that there was no significant decrease in pain over consecutive days ($p = 0.08$), and that there was no treatment effect for groups or for any group by repeated measures ANOVA. VAS scores for anxiety showed similar results for effects between groups and within group by repeated measures interaction. Patient anxiety ratings did decrease significantly across groups from baseline to post-treatment ($p < 0.01$. The authors suggested that, although there was no difference between treatment groups in this study, studies including more patients might show an effect. They also suggested that early aggressive pain management with adequate amounts of opioids, individualized to patients, may be adequate for procedural pain management.

Other articles have been published concerning the use of hypnosis in small numbers of burned patients. Margolis and DeClement[111] reported two cases with positive results. Wallace[112] reported on the use of hypnosis in an English burns unit, thoroughly describing the technique and reporting data from a single case which resulted in good control of background pain and partial control of procedural pain. Van der Does *et al.*[113] described the use of hypnosis in a Dutch burns unit where they had used hypnosis in eight patients, but reported data analyses on only four cases. The results demonstrated a reduction in the levels of pain in three of the four patients by 50–64%. In one patient, the pain level increased by 52%. The mean decrease in the four patients was 30% for both overall and worst pain. A 30% reduction in anxiety levels and a modest reduction of medication use were also reported. Patterson *et al.*[114] reported five subjects who underwent hypnosis and compared them to eight historical controls which were matched for initial pain rating scores. They found that the hypnotized group showed reduction in their pain rating scores relative to their own baselines and to the pain curves of historical controls.

Patterson[115] in a review article queried both the efficacy of hypnosis in burn pain control and the cost-effectiveness of this modality. Although his review, as well as our own experience, suggests that hypnosis can be an effective adjunct to pharmacologic control, the question of cost-effectiveness is a concern. Studies, with the exception of Crasilneck,[102] do not address cost; however, the minimum amount of time required of the hypnotist is 30–60 minutes initially if the subject is a good hypnotic candidate, and several visits from a hypnotist may be required. In addition, the procedure is personnel dependent. For hypnotic inductions, audio tapes may be used by good and trained subjects, but a nurse or therapist working with patients should also be trained to aid patients in achieving and maintaining the hypnotic trance. The conflicting reports about the ability of children and adolescents to be hypnotized reflects the differing skills of hypnotists more than differences in children. As long as a skillful hypnotist is available and willing to provide the necessary coverage for a burn care facility, the technique can be utilized with great success; however, it falls quickly into disrepute when a hypnotist leaves or fails to provide continuous coverage.

Nonbehavioral Approaches: TENS

Klimball *et al.*[116] reported that TENS was as effective as a standard dose of morphine based on patient weight (dose not reported) in controlling the pain resulting from the application of Travase®, an enzymatic debriding agent, to a burn wound. Of the 24 patients in the study, 16 were randomly assigned to a treatment group. Using VAS data, there were no differences in pain ratings measured at baseline, every 15 minutes for the first hour, and hourly for 4 hours. This was the only published article found on the use of TENS in burned patients. Via personal communication, the authors are aware that TENS has been used 'successfully' in burn pain management. TENS has been used with moderate success with several patients who sustained electrical burns and continued to complain of phantom limb pain or severe headache in the rehabilitative phase.

Behavioral Approaches

A variety of behavioral approaches have been used to manage burn pain in both adults and children. Stoddard[117] presented several case histories and concluded the following components of an overall treatment plan to diminish pain:

- psychological preparation for procedures;
- parent surrogate and/or consistent caretaking relationships;
- reinforcing denial where appropriate;
- tolerance of regression;
- encouraging adaptive fantasy;
- pharmacologic relief for pain and anxiety; and
- hypnosis, distraction, biofeedback, acupuncture, etc., as adjunctive treatments. Beales[118] also suggests that keeping debridement tools, dressings and wounds out of sight, as well as limiting staff discussion which could give a child clues about painful events, would be helpful.

A classic article by Fagerhaugh[119] focused on teaching patients to endure pain. In this report, burned patients were taught by staff and other patients that complete pain relief through medication was impossible and one must learn to endure pain. Likewise, patients were taught that they must control their expression of pain for the benefit of other patients and the staff. The author further suggests that group work of this nature should be encouraged because it helps patients understand the phases of burn care and burn pain and the methods of distraction that others have found helpful. Patients felt that group support helped to reduce pain by reducing their anxiety. Kueffner[120] likewise concluded that the presence of same-age peers was supportive to a burned child.

Others have tried specific intervention behavioral therapy. Most of these studies are based on small samples and lack rigorous methodology. Examples of studies which involved more that one case study include those of Wernick *et al.*,[121] Cromes *et al.*,[122] Elliott and Olsen,[123] Knudson-Cooper,[124] Kelly *et al.*,[125] and Kavanaugh.[126] Wernick *et al.*[121] used a stress inoculation technique with eight severely burned adults and compared them with a no-treatment group. Stress inoculation consisted of several sessions in which a patient was presented with a rational goal for treatment and with relaxation and distraction techniques which could be used to cope with pain. The control group was not offered any of the techniques for coping with pain. Treated patients showed improvement in measures of unauthorized pain medication requests, physical and emotional self-ratings, 'tanking' ratings, compliance with hospital routine, and state and trait anxiety, while the no-treatment subjects showed little improvement. The author suggested caution in the interpretation of these data, due to the small sample size, the lack of information on reliability and validity of some measures, the subjective nature of the measures, and the lack of blinding of patients and staff to the treatment conditions.

Cromes *et al.*[122] used relaxation training to reduce anxiety and pain in burned patients. They found that when a group of patients ($n = 20$) who were taught relaxation prior to each debridement procedure was compared with a control group ($n = 20$), relaxation training resulted in self-reports of decreased anxiety and pain as well as significant decreases in pulse and blood pressure.

Elliott and Olsen[123] used a reversal design in eight burned children (ages 5–12) with a therapist-coach present and using attention–distraction procedures. Results were compared to times when the therapist-coach was not present. They found a 25–52% reduction in pain behaviors when the therapist-coach was present.

Knudson-Cooper[124] investigated both relaxation therapy and biofeedback training in a group of burned children (ages 7–16). Three groups of nine each, matched for age, sex, and extent of burn, received either biofeedback training, relaxation training, or no intervention. The results indicated that both relaxation and biofeedback reduced observable symptoms of anxiety and self-reports of anxiety and pain in comparison to the control group.

Kelly *et al.*[125] used visual distraction (cartoons) and feedback about behavior during burn treatment (star chart) in two children ages 4 and 6 years. They reported a reduction of 40% in the frequency of pain behaviors occurring during treatment. When the therapies were withdrawn, the frequency of the behaviors increased.

Kavanaugh,[124] in contrast to those who advocate distraction, used a focused-control approach which allowed a child to participate, make decisions about and predict when painful events would occur. In a study of nine children (five controls with standard ward care and four subjects with maximum predictability therapy), Kavanaugh found statistically significant differences with the control group scoring higher in the areas of depression, anxiety, hostility, and stress. This study also suffers from lack of objective data and from small sample size, but presents an interesting and different approach.

More recently Miller *et al.*[127] explored the use of videos as an adjunct to morphine for pain control in a randomized study of 17 adult patients. The videos were composed of scenic beauty accompanied by music. Pain scores were significantly lower in the group that viewed the videos when scores were subjected to multiple linear regression techniques which were adjusted for age, percent partial-thickness burn, and choice of topical antibacterial agent.

These studies and the review article by Tarnowski[128] suggest that a variety of behavioral techniques can be of benefit in the reduction of anxiety and pain in burned patients. Future investigations are needed in order to demonstrate the relative efficacy of behavioral components of treatment and to identify which approaches are most effective with different personality patterns and different ages. Although the costs of behavioral approaches in terms of personnel time may seem high, many of the principles of behavioral techniques can be easily taught to the personnel who will be with the patients anyway. If, as most investigators have reported, the benefits of behavioral management techniques include and extend beyond pain relief, the efficacy of such techniques as adjunctive therapies may be quite satisfactory.

SUMMARY

The state of the art in burn pain management would seem to be based more on personal bias and tradition than on a systematic, scientific approach. As noted above, we have few studies of the pharmacokinetics of opioids and antianxiety drugs in burned patients. Martyn,[55] in a review of pharmacologic studies in burned patients, describes a variety of pathophysiologic changes accompanying burn injury which can alter drug deposition. These changes include cardiovascular changes, alteration in renal and hepatic function, and fluctuations in plasma protein concentration which may render pharmacokinetic studies of nonburned patients not applicable to burned patients. In addition, the number of pharmacokinetic studies of pain-relieving drugs of any kind in young children is virtually nil. Since approximately 35% of all burn injuries occur in children under 16 years, with a great majority of these occurring in children under 2 years, we have almost no information on which to base the use of pain-relieving drugs in burned children. It is no wonder that Perry and Heidrick[129] found great disparity in what burn care staff would order or administer to a young child or an adult with burns of similar size and area of distribution on the body. There is a need for more pharmacokinetic studies in both adults and children with burn injuries.

Similar to the lack of conclusive date about the use of the various opioids or anxiolytic agents, is the lack of scientific data to recommend any of the nonpharmacologic techniques. The most studied single nonpharmacologic modality has been hypnosis, and these studies present conflicting data. Some suggest that children are poor candidates, while others suggest that children are the best candidates for hypnosis. Some studies have used hypnosis as the only technique, while others have reported on it as an adjunct to pharmacologic methods. Thus, the role of this modality is still in question.

How, then, can we provide the 'best' pain management for a burned patient? Probably the first answer to the question is flexibility. Patients show great individual variation in their responses to the variety of agents and modalities presented. A successful approach with a burned patient requires that health care personnel understand the pain associated with the different depths of wounds, the phase of the healing process, and the components of the pain response. For the burned patient during the initial 3–7 days, the more superficial areas give rise to moderate or severe pain, while the full-thickness areas contribute less to the overall pain response.[2] Although moderate to severe pain is usually related to procedures or physical therapy, background pain (or pain at rest) is usually described as mild, or very mild, but may be exacerbated by emotional concerns and anxiety. By the second week postburn, the moderately deep partial-thickness burn with its multitude of skin buds accounts for the majority of the moderate to severe pain. In many burn centers, deep dermal and full-thickness burns are excised and grafted between the third and tenth days postburn. Although this may eliminate the severe pain associated with wound debridement during the second and third week, donor sites are often as painful as the areas of more superficial burns were initially. Dressing changes 3–5 days post-grafting also may be accompanied by the removal of sutures or staples which is usually described by patients as an excruciatingly painful procedure. By the third or fourth week, if the wounds are not mostly healed, anxiety and depression may cause a patient to perceive increased levels of pain. The work of Choinière[1] would suggest that a burned patient's pain varies widely day by day; thus, a fixed regimen of pain management may overmedicate a patient one day and undermedicate the next.

To avoid over- and undermedication in adults, regimens which allow patients to control their own therapy seem most appropriate. For procedural pain, patient control regimens may include self-administered nitrous oxide, PCA, hypnosis, a variety of behavioral approaches, or a combination of these approaches. For background pain, the best control seems to be the use of slow release opioids or methadone pain cocktails or other medications given on a nonpain contingent basis (i.e. every 4–6 hours) with the flexibility to supplement this with PRN or 'as desired' medication. Another approach would be to use PCA with or without a continuous low-dose infusion of narcotics. A variety of nonpharmacologic therapies may also help relieve background pain. The most important aspect to remember with all of these regimens, as mentioned before, is flexibility. The other obvious aspect is to remember that a patient is not only the best person to assess his pain, but he is also the best to evaluate the success of the therapies provided.

Pain management for children with burns is confusing and difficult. The regimens presented in **Table 54.4**[130] may assist one to manage a burned child's pain. It is important to remember that the regimens presented are only guidelines and must be individualized according to patient response. Certain groups of children are excluded from this protocol because they require a very individualized approach. The exclusions are:

- patients with burns greater than 60% TBSA;

Table 54.4 Shriners Burns Institute (Galveston Unit) pain control protocol for children

Pre-tub
- First choice
  - PO midazolam 0.3 mg/kg and PO acetaminophen 10 mg/kg
- If inadequate
  - add PO morphine solution 0.3 mg/kg (if > 15 kg)
- If NPO
  - IV midazolam 0.03 mg/kg and IV morphine 0.03 mg/kg (if > 15 kg)

Pre-therapy
- On request of therapist
  - PO morphine sulphate solution 0.1–0.3 mg/kg or IV morphine 0.01–0.03 mg/kg

Postoperative
- Option A
  - IV morphine infusion via PCA pump (if > 5 years), total dose 10–20 μg/kg/h
  - > 5 years continuous infusion
  - > 8 years continuous infusion and/or self-administered bolus
- Option B
  - Attendant administered bolus slow IV push morphine 0.02–0.05 mg/dose q 2 h (hold if level of responsiveness is decreased)

Background pain
- Oral acetaminophen 10 mg/kg q 6 h if inadequate add oral morphine solution 0.1–0.3 mg/kg q 4 h or MS Contin 0.5 mg/kg PO q 8–12 h

Anxiolytic
- For all non-critical patients – routinely lorazepam PO 0.03 mg/kg q 6 h

Itch
- Dipenhydramine PO 1.5 mg/kg q 6 h or hydrozyzine PO 0.5–1.0 mg/kg q 6 h

NOTE: Taper benzodiazepines and narcotics over 3 days.

- children less than 12 months of age with weight less than 12 kg;
- children with respiratory difficulty for any reason;
- septic patients; and
- children of any age who are below the tenth percentile in weight for age.

Likewise, all patients are started on a bowel regimen at the time that opioids are initiated.

In conclusion, the management of burn pain is both challenging to the health care provider and extremely important to burned patients. Recent studies suggest both physiologic and psychological reasons to successfully manage pain. Kavanagh *et al.*[131] have demonstrated that pain in a burned patient adds significantly to the physiologic demands caused by stress. Schreiber and Galai-Gat[132] as well as Ptacek *et al.*[133] have shown that successful pain management can significantly reduce the occurrence of psychological disorders such as post-traumatic stress syndrome.

REFERENCES

1. Beecher H K. Relationships of significance of wound to pain experience. *JAMA* 1958; **161:** 1609–12.

2. Choinière M, Melzack R, Rondeau J, Girard N, Paquin M J. The pain of burns: characteristics and correlates. *J Trauma* 1989; **29:** 1531–9.

3. Meyer R P, Campbell J N. Myelinated nocueptive afferents account for hyperalgesia that follows a burn to the hand. *Science* 1981; **213:** 1527–9.

4. Campbell J N, Meyer R A, Roya S N. Hyperalgesia: new insights. *Pain* 1984; **Suppl 2:** Abstr 3.

5. Coderre T, Melzack R. Increase pain sensitivity following heat injury involves a central mechanism. *Behav Brain Res* 1985; **15:** 259–62.

6. Charlton J E, Klein R, Gagliardi G. Factors affecting pain in burned patients: a preliminary report. *Postgrad Med* 1983; **59:** 604–7.

7. Klein R M, Charlton J E. Behavioral observation and analysis of pain behavior in critically burned patients. *Pain* 1980; **9:** 27–40.

8. Perry S, Heidrich G, Ramos E. Assessment of pain by burn patients. *J Burn Care Rehabil* 1981; **2:** 322–6.

9. Atchison N E, Osgood P F, Carr D B, Szyfelbein S K. Pain during burn dressing change in children: relationship to burn area, depth and analgesia regimens. *Pain* 1991; **47:** 41–5.

10. Andreasen N J C, Noyes R, Hartford C E, Bordland G, Proctor S. Management of the emotional reactions in seriously burned adults. *N Engl J Med* 1972; **286:** 65–9.

11. West D A, Schuck J M. Emotional problems of the severely burned patient. *Surg Clin North Am* 1978; **58:** 1189–204.

12. Goodstein R K. Burns: an overview of the clinical consequences afflicting patient, staff and family. *Compr Psychiatry* 1985; **26:** 43–57.

13. Savedra M. Coping with pain: strategies of severely burned children. *The Canadian Nurse* 1977; **73:** 28–9.

14. Beales J G. Factors influencing the expectation of pain among patients in a children's burn unit. *Burns* 1983; **9:** 187–92.

15. Mannon J M. *Caring for the Burned: Life and Death in a Hospital Burn Center*. Springfield, IL: C C Thomas, 1985.

16. Ponten B. Grafted skin: observations on innervation and other qualities. *Acta Clin Scan (Suppl)* 1960; **257:** 1–5.

17. Freund P R, Brengelmann, G L, Rowell L B, *et al.* Vasomotor control in healed grafted skin in humans. *J Appl Physiol* 1981; **51:** 168–71.

18. Melzack R. The McGill Pain Questionnaire: major properties and scoring methods. *Pain* 1975; **1:** 277–99.

19. Anand K J S, Sippel W G, Aynsley-Green A. Randomized trial of fentanyl anesthesia in preterm neonates undergoing surgery: effects on the stress response. *Lancet* 1987; **1:** 243–8.

20. Anand K J S, Aynsley-Green A. Does the newborn infant require potent anesthesia during surgery? Answers from a randomized trial of halothane anesthesia. In: Dunbar R, Gebhart G, Bond M, eds. *Pain Research and Clinical Management*. Vol 3 Amsterdam: Elsevier, 1988: 329–35.

21. Anand K J S, Hickey P R. Pain and its effects in the human neonate and fetus. *N Engl J Med* 1987; **317:** 1321–9.

22. Attia J, Amiel-Tison C, Mayer N-N, *et al.* Measurement of postoperative pain and narcotics administration in infants using a new clinical scoring system. *Anesthesiology* 1987; **67:** A532.

23. Szyfelbein S K, Osgood P F, Carr D B. The assessment of pain and plasma B-endorphin immunoactivity in burned children. *Pain* 1985; **22:** 173–82.

24. Williamson P S, Williamson M L. Physiologic stress reduction by a local anesthetic during newborn circumcision. *Pediatrics* 1983; **71:** 36–40.

25. Fuller B. F M signals in infant vocalizations. *Cry* 1985; **6:** 5–10.

26. Fuller B, Horii Y. Differences in fundamental frequency, jitter and shimmer among four types of infant vocalizations. *J Commun Dis* 1986; **18:** 111–18.

27. Fuller B, Horii Y. Spectral energy distribution in four types of infant vocalizations. *J Commun Dis* 1988; **20:** 111–21.

28. Franck L S. A new method to quantitatively describe pain behavior in infants. *Nurse Res* 1986; **35:** 28–31.

29. Granau R V E, Craig K D. Pain expression in neonates: facial action and cry. *Pain* 1987; **28:** 395–410.

30. Johnston C, O'Shaughnessy D. Acoustical attributes of infant pain cries: discriminating features. In: Daubner R, Gebhart G, Bond M, eds. *Pain Research and Clinical Management*. Vol 3, Amsterdam: Elsevier, 1988: 341–7.

31. Izard C E, Heubner R R, Risser D, *et al.* The young infant's ability to produce discrete emotional expressions. *Dev. Psychol* 1980; **19:** 132–40.

32. Craig K D, McMahon R J, Morison J D, Zaskow C. Developmental changes in infant pain expression during immunization injections. *Soc Sci Med* 1984; **19:** 1331–7.

33. Johnston C C, Strada M E. Acute pain response in infants: a multidimensional description. *Pain* 1986; **24:** 373–82.

34. Katz E R, Kellerman J, Siegel S E. Behavioral distress in children with cancer undergoing medical procedures: developmental considerations. *J Consult Clin Psychol* 1980; **48:** 356–65.

35. Mills N, Preston A. Acute pain behaviors in infants/toddlers. In: Funk S, Tornquist E, Champagne M, *et al.*, eds. *Key Aspects of Comfort: Management of Pain, Fatigue and Nausea*, pp. 52–9. New York: Springer, 1989.

36. McGrath P J, Johnson G, Goodman J T, Schillinger J, Dunn J, Chapman J A. CHEOPS: a behavioral scale for rating postoperative pain in children. In: Fields H L, Dubner R, Cerrera F, eds. *Advances in Pain Research and Therapy*. New York: Raven Press, 1985: 395–402.

37. Krane E J, Jacobson L E, Lynn A M, Parrot C, Tyler D C. Caudal morphine for post operative analgesia in children in comparison with caudal bupivacaine and intravenous morphine. *Anesth Anal* 1987; **66:** 647–53.

38. Beyer J, Aradine C. Content validity of an instrument to measure young children's perceptions of the intensity of their pain. *J Pediatr Nurs* 1986; **1:** 386–95.

39. Beyer J, Aradine C. Patterns of pediatric pain intensity: a methodological investigation of self report scale. *Clin J Pain* 1987; **3:** 130–41.

40. Beyer J, Aradine C. The convergent and discriminant validity of a self-report measure of pain intensity for children. *Children's Health Care* 1988; **16:** 274–82.

41. McGrath P A, de Veber L, Hearn M. Multidimensional pain assessment in children. In: Fields H, Dubner R, Cerrero F, eds. *Advances in Pain Research and Therapy*. New York: Raven Press, 1985: 387–93.

42. Tyler D C, Tu A, Douthit J, Chapman C R. Toward validation of pain measurement tools for children: a pilot study. *Pain* 1993; **52:** 301–9.

43. Maunuksela E L, Olkkola K T, Korpela R. Measurement of pain in children with self reporting and behavioral assessment. *Clin Pharmacol Ther* 1987; **42:** 137–41.

44. Bieri D, Reeve R A, Champion G D, Addicoat L, Zeigler J B. The faces pain scale for the self-assessment of the severity of pain experienced by children: development, initial validation, and preliminary investigation for ratio scale properties. *Pain* 1980; **41:** 139–50.

45. Hester N O. The pre-operational child's reaction to immunization. *Nurse Res* 1979; **28:** 250–4.

46. Eland J. Minimizing pain associated with prekindergartener intramuscular injections. *Issues Compr Pediatr Nurs* 1981; **5:** 361–72.

47. Varni J W, Thompson K L, Hanson V. The Varni/Thompson Pediatric Pain Questionnaire. In Chronic musculoskeletal pain in juvenile arthritis. *Pain* 1987; **28:** 23–38.

48. Szyfelbein S K, Osgood P F, Murphy J L, Atchison N E. Comparison of fentanyl plasma levels and pain scores in burn children. Abstract 107. Presented at the 17th Annual Meeting of the American Burn Association, March 27–30, 1985, Orlando, Florida.

49. McGrath P J, Unruh A M. *Pain in Children and Adolescents.* Amsterdam: Elsevier, 1987: 351.

50. Sevedra M, Gibbons P, Tesler M, *et al.* How do children describe pain? A tentative assessment. *Pain* 1982; **14:** 95–104.

51. LeBaron S, Zettzer L. Assessment of acute pain and anxiety in children and adolescents by self-report, observer reports, and behavior checklist. *J Consult Clin Psychol* 1984; **52:** 729–38.

52. Beyer J, Wells N. The assessment of pain in children. *Pediatr Clin North Am* 1987; **36:** 837–54.

53. Marvin J A, Heimbach D M. Pain Management. In: Fisher S V, Helm P A, eds. *Comprehensive Rehabilitation of Burns.* Baltimore: Williams and Wilkins, 1984: 311–28.

54. Marvin J A. Pain management. *Top Acute Care Trauma Rehabil* 1987; **1**(4): 15–24.

55. Martyn J A S. Clinical pharmacology and drug therapy in the burn patient. *Anesthesiology* 1986; **65**(1): 67–75.

56. Mackersie R C, Karaglanes T G. Pain management following trauma and burns. *Anesthesiol Clin North Am* 1989; **7**(1): 211–19.

57. Osgood P F, Szyfelbein S K. Management of burn pain in children. *Pediatr Clin North Am* 1989; **36**(4): 1001–13.

58. Ahrenholz D H, Solem L D. Management of pain after thermal injury. *Adv Clin Rehabil* 1987; **1:** 215–29.

59. Judkin K D. Pain control in burns. *Clin Anaesth* 1987; **1**(3): 635–48.

60. Ross D M, Ross S A. *Childhood Pain: Current Issues, Research and Management.* Baltimore: Urban & Schwarzenberg, 1988; 259–73.

61. Novoa J. Large dose morphine for pain control. Presented at the 12th Annual Meeting of the American Burn Association, San Antonio, Texas, March 27–29, 1980.

62. Perry S W, Inturrisi L E. Analgesia and morphine deposition in burn patients. *J Burn Care Rehabil* 1983; **4:** 276–9.

63. Bloedow D C, Goodfellow L A, Marvin J, Heimbach D. Meperidine disposition in burn patients. *Res Commun Chem Pathol Pharmacol* 1986; **54:** 87–9.

64. Sandidge C H, Marvin J A. Methadone therapy in treating non-procedural pain in burn patients. Presented at the 18th Annual Meeting of the American Burn Association, Chicago, Illinois, April 9–12, 1986.

65. Concilus R, Denson D D, Knarr D, Warden G, Raj P P. Continuous intravenous infusion of methadone for control of burn pain. *J Burn Care Rehabil* 1989; **10**(5): 406–9.

66. Lee J J, Marvin J A, Heimbach D M. Effectiveness of nalbuphine for relief of burn debridement pain. *J Burn Care Rehabil* 1989; **10**(3): 241–6.

67. Sandidge C H, Marvin J A, Heimbach D M. Patient controlled analgesia (PCA) in treating pain in burn patients. Presented at the 19th Annual Meeting of the American Burn Association, Washington, DC, April 29–May 2, 1987.

68. Wolman R L, Lasecki M H, Alexander L A, Luterman A. Clinical trial of patient controlled analgesia in burn patients. Presented at the 19th Annual Meeting of the American Burn Association, Washington, DC, April 29–May 2, 1987.

69. Kinsella J, Galvin R, Reid W H. Patient-controlled analgesia for burn patients: a preliminary report. *Burns Incl Therm Inj* 1988; **14**(6): 500–3.

70. Kyff J V, Prasad J K. Use of intravenous fentanyl and midazolam for dressing changes in burned patients. Presented at the 21st Annual Meeting of the American Burn Association, New Orleans, Louisiana, March 29–April 1, 1989.

71. Mather L E, Phillips G D. Opioids and adjuvants: principles of use. *Clin Crit Care Med* 1986; **8:** 77–103.

72. Wallace B H, Caldwell F T, Cone J B. Ibuprofen lowers body temperature and metabolic rate of humans with burn injury. *J Trauma* 1992; **32:** 154–7.

73. Cone J B, Wallace B H, Olsen K M, Caldwell F T, Gurley B J, Bond P J. The pharmacokinetics of ibuprofen after burn injury. *J Burn Care Rehabil* 1993; **14:** 666–9.

74. Charlton J E, Klein R, Gagliardi G. Factors affecting pain in burned patients: a preliminary report. *Postgrad Med* 1983; **59:** 604–7.

75. Diamond A W. Analgesia for burn dressings. *J R Soc Med* 1982; **75** (Suppl 1): 33.

76. Sotovnikova T, Leikep K, Adamkova M. Problems of anesthesia and analgesia in burns. *Acta Chir Plast* 1977; **19:** 228.

77. Wilson G R, Tomlinson P. Pain relief in burns – how we do it. *Burns* 1988; **14**(4): 331–2.

78. Martyn J A J, Greenblatt D S, Quinby W C. Diazepam kinetics following burns. *Anesth Analg* 1983; **62:** 293–7.

79. Yisheng C, Ngua L, Jingquan S, Yuangpin L. Histopathological and ultrastructural changes in liver tissue from burned patients. *Burns* 1985; **11:** 408–18.

80. Arturson G. Pathophysiological aspects of burn syndrome with special reference to liver injury and alterations of capillary permeability. *Acta Chir Scand Suppl* 1961; **274:** 5–121.

81. Martyn J A J, Greenblatt D J. Lorazepam conjugation unimpaired in burn patients. (Abstract) *Anesthesiology* 1985; **63:** A113.

82. Stanford G K. Postburn delirium associated with use of intravenous lorazepam. *J Burn Care Rehabil* 1988; **9**(2): 160–1.

83. Greenblatt D J, Locniskar A, Ochs H R, Lauren P M. Automated gas chromatography for studies of midazolam pharmacokinetics. *Anesthesiology* 1981; **55:** 176–9.

84. McClure J H, Brown D T, Wildsmith J A W. Comparison of the IV administration of midazolam and diazepam as sedation during spinal anaesthesia. *Br J Anaesth* 1983; **55:** 1089–93.

85. Driessen J J, Booij L H, Vree T B, Crul J F. Midazolam as a sedative on regional anesthesia. *Arzneim Forsch/Drug Res* 1981; **31:** 2245–7.

86. Brophy T, Dundee J W, Heazelwood V, Kawar P, Varghese A, Ward M. Midazolam, a water-soluble benzodiazepine, for gastroscopy. *Anaesth Intensive Care* 1982; **10:** 334–47.

87. Baskett P J F, Hyland J, Deane M, *et al.* Analgesia for patient dressing in children. *Br J Anaesth* 1969; **41:** 684–8.

88. Baskett P J F. Analgesia for the dressing of burns in children: a method using neuroleptanalgesia and Entonox. *Postgrad Med J* 1972; **48:** 138–42.

89. Filkin S A, Cosgrav P, Marvin J A, *et al.* Self-administered anesthesia: a method of pain control. *J Burn Care Rehabil* 1981; **2:** 33–4.

90. Marvin J A, Engrav L H, Heimbach D M. Self-administered nitrous oxide analgesia for debridement: a five year experience. Presented at the 16th Annual Meeting of the American Burn Association, San Francisco, California, April 11–14, 1984.

91. Layzer R H. Myeloneuropathy after prolonged exposure to nitrous oxide. *Lancet* 1978; **2:** 1227–30.

92. Layzer R B, Fishman R A, Schafer J A. Neuropathy following abuse of nitrous oxide. *Neurology* 1978; **28:** 504–6.

93. Paulson G W. Recreational misuse of nitrous oxide. *J Am Dent Assoc* 1979; **98:** 410–11.

94. Hayden P J, Hartemink R J, Nicholson G A. Myeloneuropathy due to nitrous oxide. *Burns* 1983; **9**(4): 267–70.

95. Slogoff S, Allen G W, Wessels J V, Cheney D H. Clinical experience with subanesthetic ketamine. *Anesth Analg Curr Res* 1974; **53**(3): 354–8.

96. Martinez S, Achauer B, Dobkin de Rios M. Ketamine use in a burn center: hallucinogen or debridement facilitator. *J Psychoactive Drugs* 1985; **17**(1): 45–9.

97. Handrop M, Spinella J. Ketamine: featured protocol. *J Burn Care Rehabil* 1987; **8**(2): 148–9.

98. Parker J. Ketamine: review of featured protocol. *J Burn Care Rehabil* 1987; **8**(2): 149.

99. Martyn J A J. Ketamine pharmacology and therapeutics. *J Burn Care Rehabil* 1987; **8**(2): 146–48.

100. Dimick P, Helvig E, Heimbach D, Marvin J A, Coda B, Edward W T. Anesthesia assisted procedures in a burn intensive care unit procedure room: benefits and complications. *J Burn Care Rehabil* 1993; **14:** 446–9.

101. Bernstein N R. Observations on the use of hypnosis with burned children on a pediatric ward. *Int J Clin Exp Hypn* 1965; **13:** 1–10.

102. Crasilneck H B, Stirman J A, Wilson B J. Use of hypnosis in the management of patients with burns. *JAMA* 1955; **158:** 103–6.

103. Dahinterová J. Some experiences with the use of hypnosis in the treatment of burns. *Int J Clin Exp Hypn* 1967; **15:** 49–55.

104. Finer B L, Nylen B O. Cardiac arrest in the treatment of burns and report on hypnosis as a substitute for anesthesia. *Plast Reconstr Surg* 1961; **27:** 49–55.

105. Hartley R B. Hypnosis for alleviation of pain in treatment of burns: a case report. *Arch Phys Med* 1968; **49:** 39–41.

106. Pellicone A J. Hypnosis as an adjunct to the treatment of burns. *Am J Clin Hypn* 1960; **2:** 153–6.

107. LaBaw W L. Adjunctive trance therapy with severely burned children. *Int J Child Psychother* 1973; **3**(2): 80–92.

108. Shafer D W. Hypnosis on a burn unit. *Int J Clin Exp Hypn* 1975; **23:** 1–4.

109. Wakeman R J, Kaplan J Z. An experimental study of hypnosis in painful burns. *Am J Clin Hypn* 1978; **21:** 3–12.

110. Everett J J, Patterson D R, Burns L, Montgomery B, Heimbach D. Adjunctive interventions for burn pain control: comparison of hypnosis and Ativan: The 1993 Clinical Research Award. *J Burn Care Rehabil* 1993; **14:** 676–83.

111. Margolis C G, DeClement F A. Hypnosis in the treatment of burns. *Burns, Incl Therm Inj* 1980; **6:** 253–4.

112. Wallace L M. Hypnosis and pain control on an English burns unit. *Int Care Nurs* 1987; **3:** 50–5.

113. Van der Does A J, Van Dyek R, Spijker R E. Hypnosis and pain in patients with severe burns: a pilot study. *Burns Incl Therm Inj* 1988; **14**(5): 399–404.

114. Patterson D R, Questad K A, de Lateur B J. Hypnotherapy as an adjunct to narcotic analgesia for the treatment of pain for burn debridement. *Am J Clin Hypn* 1989; **31**(3): 156–63.

115. Patterson D R, Questad K A, Boltwood M D. Hypnotherapy as a treatment for pain in patients with burns: research and clinical considerations. *J Burn Care Rehabil* 1987; **8**(3): 263–8.

116. Klimball K L, Drews J E, Walker S, Dimick A R. Use of TENS for pain reduction in burn patients receiving Travase. *J Burn Care Rehabil* 1987; **8**(1): 28–31.

117. Stoddard F J. Coping with pain – a developmental approach to treatment of burned children. *Am J Psychiatry* 1982; **139**(6): 736–40.

118. Beales J G. Factors influencing the expectation of pain among patients in a children's burn unit. *Burns* 1983; **9**(3): 187–92.

119. Fagerhaugh S Y. Pain expression and control on a burn unit. *Nurs Outlook* 1974; **22**(10): 645–51.

120. Kueffner M. Passages through hospitalization for severely burned, isolated school children. *Community Nurs Res* 1976; **7:** 181–97.

121. Wernick R L, Jaremka M E, Taylor P W. Pain management in severely burned adults: a test of stress inoculation. *J Behav Med* 1981; **4**(1): 103–9.

122. Cromes G F, McDonald M, Robinson C. The effects of relaxation training on anxiety and pain during burn wound debridement. Presented at the 12th Annual Meeting of the American Burn Association, San Antonio, Texas, March 27–29, 1980.

123. Elliott C H, Olson R A. The management of children's distress in response to pain medical treatment for burn injuries. *Behav Res Ther* 1983; **21:** 676–83.

124. Knudson-Cooper M S. Relaxation and biofeedback training in the treatment of severely burned children. *J Burn Care Rehabil* 1981; **2**(2): 102–10.

125. Kelly M L, Jarvie G J, Middlebrook J L, McNeer M F, Drabman R S. Decreasing burned children's pain behavior: impacting the trauma of hydrotherapy. *J Appl Behav Anal* 1984; **17:** 147–8.

126. Kavanaugh C. Psychological intervention with the severely burned child: report of an experimental comparison of two approaches and their effects on psychological sequelae. *J Am Acad Child Psychiatry* 1983; **22:** 145–65.

127. Miller A C, Hickman L C, Lemasters G K. A distraction technique for control of burn pain. *J Burn Care Rehabil* 1992; **13:** 576–80.

128. Tarnowski K J, Rasnake L K, Drabman R S. Behavioral assessment and treatment of pediatric burn injuries: a review. *Behav Ther* 1987; **18**(4): 417–41.

129. Perry S, Heidrick G. Management of pain during debridement: a survey of US burn units. *Pain* 1982; **13:** 267–80.

130. Muller M J, Meyer W, Blakeney P E, Marvin J A. A protocol for pain management. Personal communication.

131. Kavanaugh C K, Lasoft E, Eide Y, *et al.* Learned helplessness and the pediatric burn patient: dressing change behavior and serum cortisol and beta endorphins. *Adv Pediatr* 1991; **38:** 335–63.

132. Schneiber S, Galai-Gat T. Uncontrolled pain following physical injury as the core trauma in post traumatic stress disorder. *Pain* 1993; **54:** 107–10.

133. Ptacek J T, Patterson D R, Montgomery B, Ordonez N A, Heimbach D M. The relationship between pain during hospitalization and disability at one month post burn. Abstract 46. Presented at the 26th Annual Meeting of the American Burn Association, Orlando, Florida, April 20–29, 1994.

CHAPTER FIFTY-FIVE

Psychiatric Disorders Associated with Burn Injury

Walter J. Meyer III and Patricia E. Blakeney

Introduction

The knowledge and skills of a psychiatrist are often needed in the pharmacologic management of psychiatric symptoms which commonly occur in conjunction with burn injuries.[1] Psychiatric expertise is also an asset to a burn team in addressing multitudes of psychological issues concomitant to burn injuries. Although a psychiatrist is usually sought as a consultant, a psychiatrist is most helpful to patients and to burn teams as an integrated member of the medical staff.

Preexisting psychiatric disorders are relatively common in the histories of burned patients, and frequently appear to have contributed significantly to the etiology of the injury itself.[2-6] Substance abuse, organic brain dysfunction, hyperactivity, attention deficit disorder, conduct disorders, and personality disorders have been reported as frequently occurring premorbid conditions. A small, but important, number of patients are admitted with serious burn injuries resulting from purposeful self-immolation.[7-9] As described by Stoddard and Cahners[9] and by Raskind,[10] such patients present emotional, as well as physical, challenges to a treatment team. A suspected suicide attempt will almost invariably elicit requests for psychiatric involvement in management and treatment of a patient. Less dramatic indicators of premorbid psychiatric disorders are also identifiable early in a patient's admission and signal the need for psychiatric consultation.

In this chapter we will focus on the psychiatric treatment of common mental disturbances which can be expected to occur as part of a symptom complex which is experienced by any patient who is suffering a serious burn injury. Although preexisting psychopathology alters the expression of a patient's distress and complicates medical management of the patient, the common symptoms described in this chapter are not necessarily indicative of premorbid pathology – yet they can be very distressing to patient, family, and staff if not well managed by both behavioral and pharmacologic therapies. The most commonly occurring psychiatric symptoms discussed in this chapter are delirium, organic psychoses, burn encephalopathy, post-traumatic symptoms, sleep disturbances, pain, and depression, which occur during the critical care phase of burn treatment. Psychiatric problems are often noted as part of the long-term process of recovery from burn injury, i.e. phobias and other anxiety disorders, fully developed post-traumatic disorder, major depression, and dysthymia.

Common Psychiatric Symptoms, Critical Care Phase

Delirium, Organic Psychoses, and Burn Encephalopathy

Organic factors and premorbid conditions contribute to symptoms during the initial part of treatment. Disorientation, confusion, sleep disturbance, transient psychosis, and delirium are commonly observed among adolescent and adult patients.[3,11-14] Causes of these symptoms are usually unclear and multifactorial. Hypertension, hypoglycemia, electrolyte imbalance, sepsis, and/or a variety of organic problems can contribute to delirium. The unusual physical surroundings of an intensive care unit heighten the probability of psychoses. The altered state of consciousness may be transitory, wax and wane over several days, or, with large burns, persist for weeks. The picture may be confused further by a suspected occurrence of anoxia. Delirium has been found to occur more often in males who have a history of substance abuse and with burn injuries over 30% TBSA.[12] A past history of substance abuse is often suspected as contributing to delirium, particularly with adolescent and adult patients. Inhalant abuse or intoxication at the time of a fire are factors to be considered.

In an altered state of consciousness, patients may misinterpret their surroundings, resulting in potentially frightening illusions of reality. A patient may shout about the fire or the accident, describe symbols of death, monsters, or the devil. A patient may misidentify the people in the room, seeing instead absent friends or dead people, or may identify a treatment team as prison guards. The content of the illusions or hallucinations may be so bizarre and morbid as to suggest a schizophrenia, a brief reactive psychosis, or a psychotic depression (e.g. dead bodies, dead people, or angels). Sometimes patients are so frightened by these visions that they try to escape or become combative. Such psychotic symptoms are understandably frightening to a family and disconcerting to even experienced staff.

In our experience, symptoms of delirium and transient psychosis occur rarely among children under the age of 10 years;[14] however, burn encephalopathy, as characterized by lethargy, withdrawal, or coma, is a condition observed in children as well as adults.[15,16] EEGs in such cases typically reveal diffuse, nonspecific slow waves.[15,17]

Causative factors probably are the same as those for delirium.[18] Although Andreasen *et al.*[19] report long-term neurological impairment following burn delirium in adults, other studies (and our own experience) do not find residual neurological effects following delirium or encephalopathy.[11–16] These symptoms, though apparently short-lived, are upsetting to a patient's family and treatment team when they do occur. Proper treatment must first address organic causes of delirium and/or encephalopathy. Vital signs must be stabilized and blood chemistries and glucose normalized. Also, oxygenation should be checked and sepsis investigated and treated. Pain must be addressed. Then psychotropic medications may be administered.

The use of antipsychotic phenothiazines in an acute burn unit is a common approach to address delirium and/or combative, uncooperative behavior such as pulling off dressings, attempting to get out of bed, or striking out at caretakers.[20–23] Pharmacologic control is preferable to physical restraints which tend to exacerbate a patient's distress and worsen the symptoms.[1] Haloperidol (Haldol) is the phenothiazine of choice, as it does not have significant cholinergic side effects. The initial dose is 1 or 2 mg of haloperidol, but doses as high as 5 or 10 mg may be administered. Since phenothiazines do not cause respiratory depression, they may be repeated hourly until symptoms begin to come under control. Usually, phenothiazines are administered in two or three doses per day.

Chlorpromazine (Thorazine) and thioridazine (Mellaril) may be used in place of haloperidol in the dosage range of 25–100 mg per dose. Chlorpromazine and thioridazine have strong sedative effects and interfere with learning, but are less likely than haloperidol to produce associated dystonia, pseudo-Parkinsonism, and akathisia. If more than 2 mg of haloperidol per day are used, attention must be given to simultaneous administration of 1 or 2 mg/day of benztropine (Cogentin) or 2–5 mg/day of trihexyphenidyl (Artane) in divided doses. Benztropine or trihexyphenidyl are used to avoid dystonia, pseudo-Parkinsonism, and akathisia.[21] Occasionally, dystonia takes the form of an oculogyric crisis which resembles an acute neurological catastrophe[24] and can be a true medical emergency if respiration is impaired. These reactions are usually alleviated by 50 milligrams IV diphenhydramine (Benadryl).

There are two severe side effects for which the patient on phenothiazine must be monitored: neuroleptic malignant syndrome and tardive dyskinesia.[21] Neuroleptic malignant syndrome is an acute emergency characterized by hypothermia, severe extrapyramidal effects, and autonomic dysfunction. This can be a life-threatening crisis and must be treated aggressively with supportive therapy, as well as dantrolene and bromocriptine. The long-term side effect of greatest concern for patients who receive phenothiazine is tardive dyskinesia. This reaction can be permanent and is characterized by abnormal, involuntary, irregular choreiform and athetoid movements. Usually, a patient is unaware of the writhing and twisting movements that most often involve the tongue, but can also involve the limbs and the trunk as well. The reaction typically occurs only in individuals who have received phenothiazines for extended periods of time, i.e. longer than 6 months. The risk of occurrence is 2–4% per year over the first 7 years in which phenothiazines are taken. Although it is a very unusual complication in individuals who receive phenothiazines for short periods of time, it has been reported.

Due to the problems which have been associated with phenothiazines, benzodiazepines have been used to a greater extent in recent years for the combative, delirious patient.[21,25,26] The two most commonly used benzodiazepines are diazepam (Valium) and lorazepam (Ativan). Lorazepam (0.03 mg/kg) orally or intravenously, can usually be given every 4–8 hours; for a very combative patient it can be given hourly. A third benzodiazepine which is frequently used is midazolam (Versed) at 0.05 mg/kg IV, typically used in conjunction with morphine for procedures such as tubbing and staple removal. When using the benzodiazepine class of medications, a clinician must balance the desired effects of relaxation with oversedation. Visual and auditory hallucinations may occur if the dose of benzodiazepine is too high. In those cases, it should be reduced or replaced by another type of medication. In cases of excessive anxiety in the presence of adequate pain control, Iorazepam can be added to a patient's treatment. Nighttime doses usually enhance sleep. Diazepam in doses of 2–10 mg per dose, depending on the size of an individual, may be used in place of lorazepam if simultaneous muscle relaxation is desired.[27] Diazepam has an extremely long half-life, 40 hours, and therefore should be used sparingly (see Chapter 54). To avoid excessive sedation by benzodiazepines, a patient should not be awakened for the next dose.

Post-trauma Symptoms

If anxiety is associated with other symptoms of post-traumatic stress, such as hypervigilance or poor sleep, an antidepressant tricyclic such as imipramine should be considered.[14] Beginning doses of imipramine are 25 mg/day unless a person weighs less than 25 kg. The beginning dose is 12.5 mg for those under 25 kg. The dose can be increased rapidly over the next few days to a dose of 1 mg/kg. Further increases should be monitored by blood levels and EKG changes. A dose can be divided and given twice a day, but such division is usually unnecessary. The preferable time of administration is in the evening to aid with sleep. Major side effects of the tricyclics such as imipramine are anticholinergic effects (dry mouth and dry nasal passages, constipation, urinary hesitance, and occasional esophageal reflux).[21] Autonomic complications such as orthostatic hypotension, palpitations, and hypertension have been reported in adolescents with this medication.[20] Cardiac arrhythmias, associated with a prolonged PR interval, can be life-threatening.[28–30] Sudden death has been reported for teenagers and children receiving desipramine and other tricyclics.[31] Amitriptyline or doxepin may be used in place of imipramine. The dosages are similar; however, both these medications cause more sedation than imipramine.[21]

Sleep Disturbances

Patients with significant sleep problems are common in an acute burn unit. When sleep disturbance with nightmares is associated with post-traumatic anxiety, as described above, imipramine is the drug of choice. For an individual patient who is receiving imipramine and still not experiencing adequate sleep, doxepin (a more sedating antidepressant) in similar or slightly higher doses, may be given instead. Sleep problems may be associated with stimulation from the caretaking staff who awaken a patient while checking vital signs and well-being throughout the night. Sometimes lights and televisions are left on throughout the day and night in a patient's room. These environmental factors can be destructive to a patient's sleep–wake cycle. As soon as physiologic conditions allow, a patient should be given as much undisturbed sleep time at night as possible, so as to allow natural sleep cycles to reestablish, and to maintain a normal circadian rhythm. If a patient continues to have significant sleep problems, sleep can be induced with diphenhydramine. Diphenhydramine doses of 1.5 mg/kg are often used throughout the day for itching and may be used alone for sleep at night or as an adjunct to other sleep medications. Usually, doses of 25 or 50 mg in the evening are adequate.

Often, post-traumatic symptoms other than sleep disturbances are not evident. In such cases, chloral hydrate may also be used in doses of 1.5 mg/kg, up to a maximum of 1 g per single dose.[26] Doses of 250 mg are usually adequate for a child; however, we prefer to use benzodiazepine, imipramine, and/or diphenhydramine for sedation and sleep with pediatric patients because deaths have been reported in children taking chloral hydrate for sedation.[26] Also, in our experience, chloral hydrate does not alleviate nightmares as does imipramine.

Depression

For depression, tricyclics have been the medications of first choice and are given as described above by following symptoms and monitoring blood levels. Recently, fluoxetine (Prozac), 20–40 mg, is being used for impulsive, angry patients with depressive symptoms.[28,30] Fluoxetine has the added advantage of being a safer drug for out-patient treatment since an overdose is unlikely to cause significant cardiac problems as have been attributed to the tricyclics.[28] Side effects of fluoxetine include gastrointestinal upset, increased agitation, headaches, and sweating. It has, however, fewer instances of anticholinergic side effects such as constipation. Patients should be monitored for hypomania or mania induced by antidepressant medications. When this occurs, the antidepressant dose should be lowered and lithium therapy should be considered.

Pain

Symptoms of depression and agitation are often related to excessive pain and subside with adequate pain management (see Chapter 54). A patient's experience of pain is related to the extent and depth of injury and influenced by individual responses to analgesia, pain threshold, emotional state, cognitive functioning, cultural beliefs, interpersonal interactions, and expectations.[18,32–34] Chemical analgesics and anesthetics are as important in managing pain with burns as they are with other medical/surgical conditions. Care must be taken to consider the appropriate doses of medication and the most efficacious schedule of administration. Modifications should be continued until good control is achieved.[35,36] Around-the-clock or continuous administration of analgesics achieves better pain control than PRN administration.[37,38] This avoids the period of less than therapeutic levels of the drug with increased discomfort prior to the request for medication and ameliorates a patient's anxiety about whether the medication will be allowed. Postoperatively, patient-controlled analgesia (PCA) pumps are very effective in achieving around-the-clock pain control with minimal undesired side effects for adults and for children.[39,40]

In-Hospital Recuperation

After the initial postburn period, a patient progresses through a series of operative procedures interspersed with days of physical therapy in order to maintain physical activity and range of motion. Immediate operative sites (those grafted and those which donate) are painful. In addition, exercises are painful. A patient's world is one of pain or concern about possible pain in the near future. The major goal of therapy from the psychiatrist's point of view is to control the pain and maximize a patient's participation in the exercises and other aspects of care.

In addition to the pharmacological treatment described above, designing a psychological milieu which supports comfort and security is a primary task.[14] A specific daily treatment schedule is crucial to achieving these goals. The schedule provides specific times for pain medication to insure coverage at times of expected pain (e.g. tubbing and physical therapy), but avoids sedation during family, social, and educational activities. Time should be provided in the schedule for fun and diversionary activities. A pediatric patient must have time scheduled for school and play. Patients must be allowed to have expected 'safe' periods without procedures. Whenever possible, the patient, even a young child, should be included in planning the schedule. The schedule should be posted and followed as closely as possible. In order to motivate a patient to participate at a maximum level in rehabilitation, a reward system can be incorporated, with rewards consisting of special treats as designated by a patient, such as extra videos or going out of the hospital.

As a latency age child, adolescent, or adult recovers, he/she often wants to talk about the accident. A patient begins a long process of 'understanding' what has happened. Part of this process is learning to look at a 'new' self, literally and metaphorically. As part of the treatment plan, a regularly scheduled meeting with a psychotherapist is established. This special time for 'talking' therapy may vary in content from play therapy with a child or light banter with an adult to serious confrontation with the most difficult emotionally charged issues. The reliability of this safe time in which a patient can complain about everybody and everything, express anger, express fear and sadness, can be very therapeutic. It is important for a patient to have someone other than family who is accepting, safe, and neutral with whom to talk.

A patient's experience in adapting to burn injury can be thought of as a grieving process. A patient has experienced a loss of self. Using a familiar paradigm, we can describe a patient as moving through several stages of adjustment to loss: shock, denial, anger, depression, and finally acceptance.[41] This formulation is useful in working with a patient about his/her injury. In our experience, shock and denial predominate during the initial hospitalization; anger and depression often last for years as a patient continues in treatment, faces reconstructive surgeries, and confronts a series of social experiences.

Psychiatric Problems Beyond Acute Hospitalization

A number of approaches have been used to determine the incidence of psychiatric difficulties among survivors of major burns, and these approaches report with surprising consistency that large numbers of survivors do not suffer long-term major psychiatric disorders. Our own work has focused on children and adolescents who are at least 1 year postburn and are either out-patients or have returned for further reconstructive surgery. The novice usually expresses a belief that all burned persons need to see a psychiatrist due to the nature of the injury. One method we have used has been to survey patients with questionnaires pointed at specific psychiatric symptom complexes. For instance, Koon *et al.*[42] surveyed adolescents with the Piers–Harris Children's Self-concept Scale and found that male pediatric burn survivors had significantly higher scores than the normative population. Females described themselves as less popular, although otherwise equal to the norm. Self-esteem did not appear to be related to other burn-related variables (i.e. age at burn or size of burn). With a similar goal of looking for specific symptoms, we hypothesized significant depression and utilized several standardized instruments, including the Suicide Probability Scale (SPS),[43] to assess depressive symptoms. This study revealed no increase above norm in depression or suicidality, but did not reveal significant anger among adolescent burn survivors.

We use a variety of instruments to detect general psychiatric needs among the children that we follow. The Achenbach series of standardized behavioral checklists are useful screening tools.[44–46] They offer validity, reliability, and convenience of administration in a setting such as ours where we must assess many clinical variables in a brief period of time. The Child Behavior Checklist (CBCL)[44] is a 113-item rating of each child's current behavior problems and competencies as perceived by a parent. Complementary to the CBCL are the Teacher Report Form (TRF)[45] and the Youth Self Report (YSR),[46] which provide assessments of the same behaviors by different observers. Our data from these instruments indicate that about 20–25% of the children and adolescents who survive major thermal injury may develop a variety of significant behavioral problems as indicated, but good adjustment is achieved by the majority of individuals.[47,48] Parents usually report more problems than do the children themselves or the teachers.[47,49] In one study, 60 children with burns (35 boys, 25 girls) were surveyed with the Achenbach instruments at least 1 year after burn injury. The parental perception on the CBCL revealed a statistically significant ($p < 0.05$) increase in problems and decrease in competency for most age groups and both sexes when compared with the normal reference population. In contrast, the Teacher Report Form and the Youth Self Report revealed very few differences from the reference population. Burn size did not account for any of the differences. Item analysis of individual questions revealed excessive endorsement by parents of specific items on all scales compared to their respective reference populations.[50] These results could be explained by increased problems of the children following severe burns. Another standardized instrument, the Parental Stress Index (PSI),[51] revealed that parents who reported their children as troubled were themselves more stressed than the normal reference population, not only by their children's behaviors but in areas unrelated to their children.[52] In addition, on a measure of mood state, the Eight-state Questionnaire (8SQ),[53] mothers who reported troubled children more often felt depressed and guilty than did mothers of well-adjusted children.[52] This study emphasizes the need for psychological attention to parents of burned children, as well as to the children themselves.

Using a standardized psychiatric interview for children, Stoddard *et al.* reported a very high incidence of psychiatric disorders among 30 pediatric burn survivors.[54,55] In order to make a fair comparison with other populations, these authors compared the burn survivors with a group of survivors of flood trauma and a community sample. Burned children had significantly more phobic disorders, over anxious disorders, enuresis, encopresis, major depression, post-traumatic stress disorder (PTSD), and substance/ethanol abuse than the comparison groups.[55] Sleep disorders and psychotic disorders were also slightly more common among the burned children. Even though most burn survivors eventually make good adjustments, they can be expected, at some time during the adjustment process, to suffer psychiatric sequelae which might be attenuated by psychiatric treatment.

Phobias and Other Anxiety Disorders

Many patients continue beyond acute hospitalization to have periods during which they appear extremely anxious and express fear. These periods often recur in association with return to a hospital for reconstructive surgeries. Some are so anxious that they are constantly soliciting their families or others for comfort. Generalized anxiety disorder or overanxious disorder of childhood is characterized by the following:

- excessive worry occurring more days than not for at least 6 months about a number of events;
- difficulty in controlling the anxiety;
- the anxiety causes clinically significant distress or impairment in social, occupation, or other important areas of functioning;
- anxiety and worry associated with three or more (only one for children) of the following symptoms (with some symptoms present for more days than not for the past 6 months): restlessness, feeling on edge, easily fatigued, difficulty concentrating or mind going blank, irritability, muscle tension, sleep disturbances.

In a burned patient, difficulty controlling anxiety which is so distressful that it interferes with important functioning, restlessness, and difficulty in concentrating are diagnostic of anxiety disorders since some other symptoms can be related to burn injuries specifically, e.g. being easily fatigued.

Not infrequently, anxiety spills over to other situations and/or becomes focused on specific objects; thus, phobias develop which are characterized by excessive persistent fear in response to specific stimuli. Although adults may express anxiety through 'panic' symptoms such as sweating, palpitations, trembling, or nausea, children may express anxiety by crying, tantrums, freezing, or clinging. A differential diagnosis of these anxiety disorders distinct from post-traumatic stress disorder is difficult and requires a careful interview. Burned patients suffering from post-traumatic stress often see the fire or aspects of their accidents whenever they close their eyes; they dream about their traumas. An overanxious patient is afraid of what might happen; the post-traumatic stress disorder patient fears what has happened. Most burned patients, certainly those who qualify for the diagnosis of generalized or overanxious disorder, benefit from lorazepam therapy in addition to supportive psychotherapy.

Post-traumatic Stress Disorder and Nightmares

Post-traumatic stress disorder (PTSD) is the most common psychiatric disorder seen in survivors of major burns. This disorder is characterized in the *Diagnostic and Statistical Manual of Mental Disorders* (DSM-IV) by the following criteria:

- The person has experienced, witnessed, or was confronted with an event which involved actual or threatened death or serious injury to self or others, and the person's response involved intense fear, helplessness, or horror.
- The traumatic event is persistently re-experienced. Recurrent and intrusive thoughts of the event occur. Burned patients often complain of seeing the fire whenever they close their eyes or when they try to go to sleep. Young children may relive the event over and over again in repetitive play. Nightmares about the event are common; in young children frightening dreams occur without recognizable content. Feeling as if the event were recurring (e.g. flashback) is reported often. Intense reactivity, psychological and/or physiologic, occurs at exposure to internal or external cues which trigger associations with the traumatic incident, e.g. seeing a fire on television.
- There is continued avoidance of stimuli associated with the trauma or numbing of general responsiveness. Persons suffering from PTSD develop flat affect, memory problems, and withdrawal from others. Children's behavior may be regressed; children may lose recently acquired developmental skills such as toilet training or language skills.

- Persistent symptoms of increased arousal, which were not present before the trauma, may develop. These symptoms include sleep disturbance, irritability/anger, difficulty concentrating, hypervigilance, exaggerated startle response, and panic attacks. Patients have periods of feeling afraid and not knowing why.

Nightmares and altered sleep patterns are usually the symptoms first noted. Many of the other symptoms are described when a more complete history is taken. Patients should be given ample opportunity to explore their feelings and fears about the traumatic event. This process may persist for months. In addition, tricyclic medications are helpful in reducing the nightmares and improving the sleep pattern. Our preference among these medications has been imipramine. The initial dose is usually 25 mg at bed time. This may be increased in 25 mg increments until a dose of 1 mg/kg is reached. If the symptoms are still uncontrolled, the dose may be increased stepwise to 3 mg/kg, but only with frequent checking of the plasma level with each increment of dosage increase. Usually a patient's sleep pattern improves quickly. Imipramine therapy must often be continued up to a year longer. When therapy is to be discontinued, the medication should be reduced, for suddenly stopping the medicine will cause a recurrence of sleep disturbance.

Major Depression and Depressive Disorders

Although depression is a reaction most observers would expect of burned patients, it is a rare long-term sequela of burn injury. According to Stoddard,[54] fewer than 50% of the children he surveyed had ever suffered major depression; dysthymia, another depressive disorder, occurred in only 10%. Outcome studies of adult burn survivors show a similar prevalence of major depression.[11,19,56–59]

To diagnose major depression, a patient must have five or more of the following DSM-IV symptoms *for a period of at least 2 weeks, and they must represent a change from previous functioning*:

- depressed mood most of the day (may be an irritable mood in children and adolescents);
- markedly diminished interest or pleasure in most activities;
- significant change in appetite, resulting in either weight loss or gain (for children, failure to make expected weight gains);
- insomnia or hypersomnia;
- feelings of worthlessness or excessive/inappropriate guilt nearly every day;
- fatigue or loss of energy nearly every day;
- diminished concentration or enhanced indecisiveness nearly every day;
- psychomotor agitation or retardation observable by others;
- recurrent thoughts of death, suicidal ideation, suicide attempt or plan.

This is an extremely difficult diagnosis to make during the acute burn period since many of the criteria are linked to physical symptoms. Even beyond the acute phase, the diagnosis is often complicated by grief following the loss of a loved one during a fire, and by sadness at one's altered body. The critical symptoms in a burned patient are depressed mood and anhedonia. Many times a patient's expressed interest in play or plans for the future rule out the diagnosis.

Major depression, with or without grief reaction, should be treated by a team approach. A patient should be involved in scheduled daily activities. Psychotherapy should begin to identify and address appropriate issues. Medication with tricyclics, as described for post-traumatic stress, is often helpful. After checking serum levels, the dose should be increased until it reaches therapeutic levels. This process involves frequent checking of serum levels as the dose is raised. A steady state is usually not reached until a given dose is maintained for 3–5 days. Again, the sleep pattern improves first. Therapy must often be continued for 6 months or longer. When discontinuing therapy, the medication should be slowly reduced rather than stopped suddenly so as to prevent dysphoria and sleep problems.

A smaller percentage of burned patients will develop a milder but more protracted type of depression called dysthymia. This condition must be present *for at least 2 years in adults, or 1 year in children and adolescents in order to be diagnosed.* It is characterized by the following:

depressed or irritable mood;

appetite changes

sleep difficulties;

fatigue;

low self-esteem;

poor concentration or difficulty making decisions; and

feelings of hopelessness.

The same combination of medication and psychotherapy is recommended for dysthymic patients as for major depression.

Summary

Psychiatric symptoms occur commonly as part of the complex systemic response to burn injuries. Psychological and pharmacologic treatment are important in the successful recovery of a burned person, and perhaps mitigate against long-term psychiatric sequelae of post-injury. It is important to note that psychological adaptation is a lengthy process occurring over months or years. During the post-burn years, it is imperative that the burn team assess the mental and affective states of patients while assessing their physical recovery. Although most burned patients eventually make satisfactory adjustments, many continue for a long time to struggle with self-image, anger, and sadness. These disturbances often seem to be expressed through symptoms which are not easily observed by other than intimate friends and family of a patient.[60] Sleep disturbance, fear or withdrawal from previous activities are not behavioral disturbances which necessarily insure that a patient will attract psychiatric attention and treatment. They are, however, unhappy responses which can be ameliorated by treatment. It then becomes a responsibility of the expert in burn care and recovery to be aware of frequently occurring disturbed responses, to ask the right questions in order to assess a patient's status, and to assist a patient in receiving psychological and psychiatric assistance.

References

1. Mendelsohn I E. Liaison psychiatry and the burn center. *Psychosomatics* 1983; **24**(3): 235–43.

2. Ochitill H. Psychiatric consultation to the burn unit: the psychiatrist's perspective. *Psychosomatics* 1984; **25**(9): 689, 697–701.

3. Andreasen N J C, Nayes P, Hartford C. Factors influencing adjustment of burn patients during hospitalization. *Psychosom Med* 1972; **34**(6): 517–25.

4. Noyes R, Frye S, Slymen D, Canter A. Stressful life events and burn injuries. *J Trauma* 1979; **19**(3): 141–4.

5. Darko D, Wachtel T, Ward H, Frank H. Analysis of 585 burn patients hospitalized over a six-year period. Part III: Psychosocial data. *Burns* 1986; **12:** 395–401.

6. Vogtsberger K, Taylor E. Psychosocial factors in burn injury. *Texas Med* 1984; **80:** 43–6.

7. Nielson J A, Kolman P B R, Wachtel T L. Suicide and parasuicide by burning. *J Burn Care Rehabil* 1984; **5**(4): 335–8.

8. Davidson T, Brown L. Self-inflicted burns: a five-year retrospective study. *Burns* 1985; **11:** 157–60.

9. Stoddard F J, Cahners S S. Suicide attempted by self-immolation during adolescence; II Psychiatric treatment and outcome. *J Adolesc Psychiat* 1985; **12:** 266–80.

10. Raskind S M. Suicide by burning: emotional needs of the suicidal adolescent on the burn unit. *Issues Compr Pediatr Nurs* 1986; **9:** 369–82.

11. Steiner H, Clark W. Psychiatric complications of burned adults: a classification. *J Trauma* 1977; **17:** 134–43.

12. Perry S, Blank K. Relationships of psychological processes during delirium to outcome. *Am J Psychiatry* 1984; **141:** 843–7.

13. Patterson D, Everett J, Bombardier C, Questad K, Lee V, Marvin J. Psychological effects of severe burn injuries. *Psychol Bull* 1993; **113**(2): 362–78.

14. Blakeney P, Meyer W J III. Psychological aspects of burn care. *Trauma Q* 1994; **II**(2): 166–79.

15. Haynes B, Bright R. Burn coma: a syndrome associated with severe burn wound infection. *J Trauma* 1967; **7:** 464–75.

16. Antoon A, Volpe J, Crawford J. Burn encephalopathy in children. *Pediatrics* 1972: **50:** 609–16.

17. Hughes J, Cayaffa J, Boswick J. Seizures following burns to the skin: III. Electroencephalographic recordings. *Dis Nerv Syst* 1975; **36:** 443–7.

18. Stoddard F. Psychiatric management of the burned patient. In: Martyn J A J, ed. *Acute Care of the Burn Patient.* Orlando, F L: Grune and Stratton, 1990: 256–72.

19. Andreasen N J C, Norris A, Hartford C. Incidence of long-term psychiatric complications in severely burned adults. *Ann Surg* 1971; **174**(5): 785–93.

20. Teicher M H, Glod C A. Neuroleptic drugs: indications and guidelines for their rational use in children and adolescents. *J Child Adolesc Psychopharmacol* 1990; **1:** 33–56.

21. Schatzberg A F, Cole J O. *Manual of Clinical Psychopharmacology.* 2nd ed. Washington, DC: American Psychiatric Press, 1991.

22. Kiely W F. Psychiatric syndromes in critically ill patients. *JAMA* 1976; **235:** 2759–61.

23. Moore D P. Rapid treatment of delirium in critically ill patients. *Am J Psychiatry* 1977; **134:** 1431–2.

24. Huang V, Figge H, Demling R. Haloperidol in burn patients. *J Burn Care Rehabil* 1987; **8:** 269–73.

25. Coffey B J. Anxiolytics for children and adolescents. Traditional and new drugs. *J Child Adolesc Psychopharmacol* 1990; **1:** 57–83.

26. USP DI Volume I: *Drug Information for the Health Care Professional.* Rockville, MD. United States Pharmacopeial Convention, Inc, 1994.

27. Martyn J A J, Greenblatt D J, Quinby W C. Diazepam kinetics in patients with severe burns. *Anesth Analg* 1983; **62:** 293–7.

28. Glassman A H. The newer antidepressant drugs and their cardiovascular effects. *Psychopharmacol Bull* 1984; **20:** 272–9.

29. Glassman A H, Bigger J T Jr. Cardiovascular effects of therapeutic doses of tricyclic antidepressants. *Arch Gen Psychiatry* 1981; **38:** 815–20.

30. Ryan N D. Heterocyclic antidepressants in children and adolescents. *J Child Adolesc Psychopharmacol* 1990; **1:** 21–31.

31. Popper C W, Elliott G R. Sudden death and tricyclic antidepressants: clinical considerations for children. *J Child Adolesc Psychopharmacol* 1990; **1:** 125–32.

32. Szyfelbein S, Osgood P, Carr D. The assessment of pain and plasma B-endorphin immunoactivity in burned children. *Pain* 1985; **22:** 173–82.

33. Beales J. Factors influencing the expectation of pain among patients in a children's burns unit. *Burns* 1983; **9**(3): 187–92.

34. Charlton J, Gragliardi G, Klein R, Heimbach D. Factors affecting pain in burned patients – a preliminary report. *Postgrad Med J* 1983; **59:** 604–7.

35. Perry S. Undermedication for pain on a burn unit. *Gen Hosp Psychiatry* 1984; **6:** 308–16.

36. Watkins P, Cook E, May R, Ehleben C. Psychological stages in adaptation following burn injury: a method for facilitating psychological recovery of burn victims. *J Burn Care Rehabil* 1988; **9**(4): 376–84.

37. Yaster M, Deshpande J, Maxwell L. The pharmacologic management of pain in children. *Therapy* 1989; **15**(10): 14–26.

38. Colditz P. Management of pain in the newborn infant. *J Pediatr Child Health* 1991; **27:** 11–15.

39. Webb C, Stergios D, Rodgers B. Patient-controlled analgesia as post-operative pain treatment for children. *J Pediat Nurs* 1989; **4**(3): 162–71.

40. Gaukroger P, Chapman M, Davey R. Pain control in pediatric burn – the use of patient-controlled analgesia. *Burns*, 1991; **17**(5): 396–9.

41. Knudson-Cooper M. Emotional care of the hospitalized burned child. *J Burn Care Rehabil* 1982; **3:** 109–16.

42. Koon K, Blakeney P, Broemeling L, Moore P, Robson M, Herndon D. Self-esteem in pediatric burn patients. *Proc Am Burn Assoc* 1992; **24:** 112.

43. Cull J G, Gill W S. *Suicide Probability Scale Manual.* Los Angeles: Western Psychological Services, 1982.

44. Achenbach T M. *Manual for Child Behavior Checklist 4/18 and 1991 Profile.* Burlington, VT: University of Vermont Department of Psychiatry, 1991

45. Achenbach T M. *Manual for the Teachers Report Forms and 1991 Profile.* Burlington, VT: University of Vermont Department of Psychiatry, 1991.

46. Achenbach T M. *Manual for the Youth Self-Report and 1991 Profile.* Burlington, VT: University of Vermont Department of Psychiatry, 1991.

47. Blakeney P, Meyer W, Moore P, *et al.* Social competence and behavioral problems of pediatric survivors of burns. *J Burn Care Rehabil* 1993: **14:** 65–72.

48. LeDoux J, Blakeney P, Meyer W, Herndon D. Relationships between parental emotional states, family environment and the behavioral adjustment of pediatric burn survivors. *Proc Am Burn Assoc* 1994: **26:** 134.

49. Blakeney P, Meyer W, Moore P, *et al.* Psychosocial sequelae of pediatric burns involving 80% or greater total body surface area. *J Burn Care Rehabil* 1993; **14:** 684–9.

50. Meyer W J, Blakeney P, Moore P, *et al.* Inconsistencies in psychosocial assessment of children post major burn. *J Burn Car Rehabil* 1995: in press.

51. Abidin R R. *Parental Stress Index Manual.* Charlottesville, VA: Pediatric Pathology Press, 1983.

52. Meyer W J, Blakeney P, Moore P, Murphy L, Robson M, Herndon D. Parental well-being and behavioral adjustment of pediatric burn survivors. *Burn Care Rehabil* 1994; **15:** 62–8.

53. Curran J P, Cattell R B. *Manual for the Eight-State Questionnaire (8SQ).* Champaign, IL: Institute for Personality and Ability Testing, 1976.

54. Stoddard F J, Norman D K, Murphy M. A diagnosis outcome study of children and adolescents with severe burns. *J Trauma*, 1989; **29:** 471–7.

55. Stoddard F J, Norman D K, Murphy M, Beardslee W R. Psychiatric outcome of burned children and adolescents. *J Am Acad Child Adolesc Psychiatry* 1989; **28:** 589–95.

56. Ward H, Moss R, Darko D, *et al.* Prevalence of post-burn depression following burn injury. *J Burn Care Rehabil* 1987; **8**(4): 294–8.

57. Malt U. Long-term psychosocial follow-up studies of burned adults: review of the literature. *Burns* 1980; **6:** 190–7.

58. Malt U. A long-term psychosocial follow-up study of burned adults. *Acta Psychiatr Scand Suppl* 1989; **80(355):** 94–102.

59. Faber A, Klasen H, Sauer E, Vuister F. Psychological and social problems in burn patients after discharge: a follow-up study. *Scand J Plast Reconstr Surg* 1987; **21**(3): 307–9.

60. Meyer W J, LeDoux J, Blakeney P, Herndon D. Diminished adaptive behaviors among pediatric burn survivors. *Proc Am Burn Assoc* 1994; **26:** 133.

CHAPTER FIFTY-SIX

56

Abuse by Burning

Patricia E. Blakeney and David N. Herndon

Introduction

As a subject of scientific investigation, violence, including that occurring within the family, has received much attention from professionals in sociology, mental health, medicine, and law.[1] Yet most health professionals, themselves devoted to healing and comforting others, are reluctant to believe that human beings will cause serious injury to others, especially to those who are significant members of their own family circles and most especially to those who are helpless, such as young children or elderly parents. The evidence is overwhelming that people do behave brutally, and they do cause injury even to close family members. Sometimes the maltreatment involves burning. The problem of deliberate injury to children by burning has been identified and discussed in the professional literature for about 20 years.[2] Similar aggressive acts toward adults began to be recognized as a concern more recently,[25] and abuse of adults by burning has rarely been documented in empirical studies.

Three articles have been found which report abuse to adults by burning.[2–4] It seems highly probable that burning as a form of violence against adults occurs with much greater frequency than reflected in the literature, but has long been unrecognized. Unless adult patients are asked about abuse, they are unlikely to volunteer the information.[3] As burn care professionals become increasingly sensitive to the problem of abuse to adults, the reported incidence will probably increase dramatically and replicate the pattern observed with child abuse, i.e. the more we ask, the more we will discover.[5]

The authors share the guilt of failing to be attuned to abuse in adults in the same way in which we alert to that possibility with children. Therefore, our clinical experience with known adult abuse by burning is limited to a few flagrant cases. Our experience with child abuse is extensive. Since the literature, as well as our own experience, is heavily weighted with information about child abuse, this chapter also represents that bias. The reader may be, at times, led to believe that the pediatric population is the only target for maltreatment. That is not an intention but rather a reflection of our current knowledge; and we caution the reader, as we remind ourselves, to avoid that misconception. In this chapter, we have integrated our experience with available information to identify risk factors in the total population and to suggest therapeutic approaches to treating the burn wounds, as well as the complex social, interpersonal, and familial issues which both produce injury and complicate the recovery and rehabilitation of a patient (**Figure 56.1**).

Child Abuse Indicators

Reports of child abuse by burning indicate that such injuries account for as many as 20% of burn unit pediatric admissions.[6–14] Most of these injuries occur to children of ages 3 years and under and are scald or contact burns.[7–9,11] Most of these abused children live in poverty-level households headed by a young, single parent who has two or more children.[7,8,11,15] Abused burned children are reported to require longer hospitalization and to have higher rates of morbidity and mortality than nonabused children.[16–18]

Suspicion of child abuse may be prompted by observations of parental behavior. Parents who are not abusive typically report the details of the child's injury spontaneously and express concern about the treatment and prognosis. They exhibit a sense of guilt, ask questions about discharge date and follow-up care, visit the child frequently, and bring gifts. In contrast, abusive parents usually do not volunteer information, but are evasive or contradictory; they seem critical of the child and angry with the patient for being hurt. They do not seem to feel guilty or show remorse. They show no concern about the injury, treatment, or prognosis. They seldom visit or play with the child, do not ask about discharge date or follow-up care, and appear to be preoccupied with themselves and unconcerned about the child.[19]

The following are a list of indicators of child abuse often identified by empirical studies. Any one of these indicators should elicit suspicion. The presence of two or more indicators has been found to identify 60% of abusive situations.[13]

- Child is brought for treatment by an unrelated adult.[9,13]
- An unexplained delay of 12 or more hours in seeking treatment.[8,13,18]
- Inappropriate parental affect: parent(s) appear inattentive to child; lack empathy; may appear to be under the influence of alcohol or drugs.[9,15]
- Attribution of guilt for injury to the patient's sibling or to the patient.[15,20]
- An injury which is inconsistent with the description of the injury.[7,8]

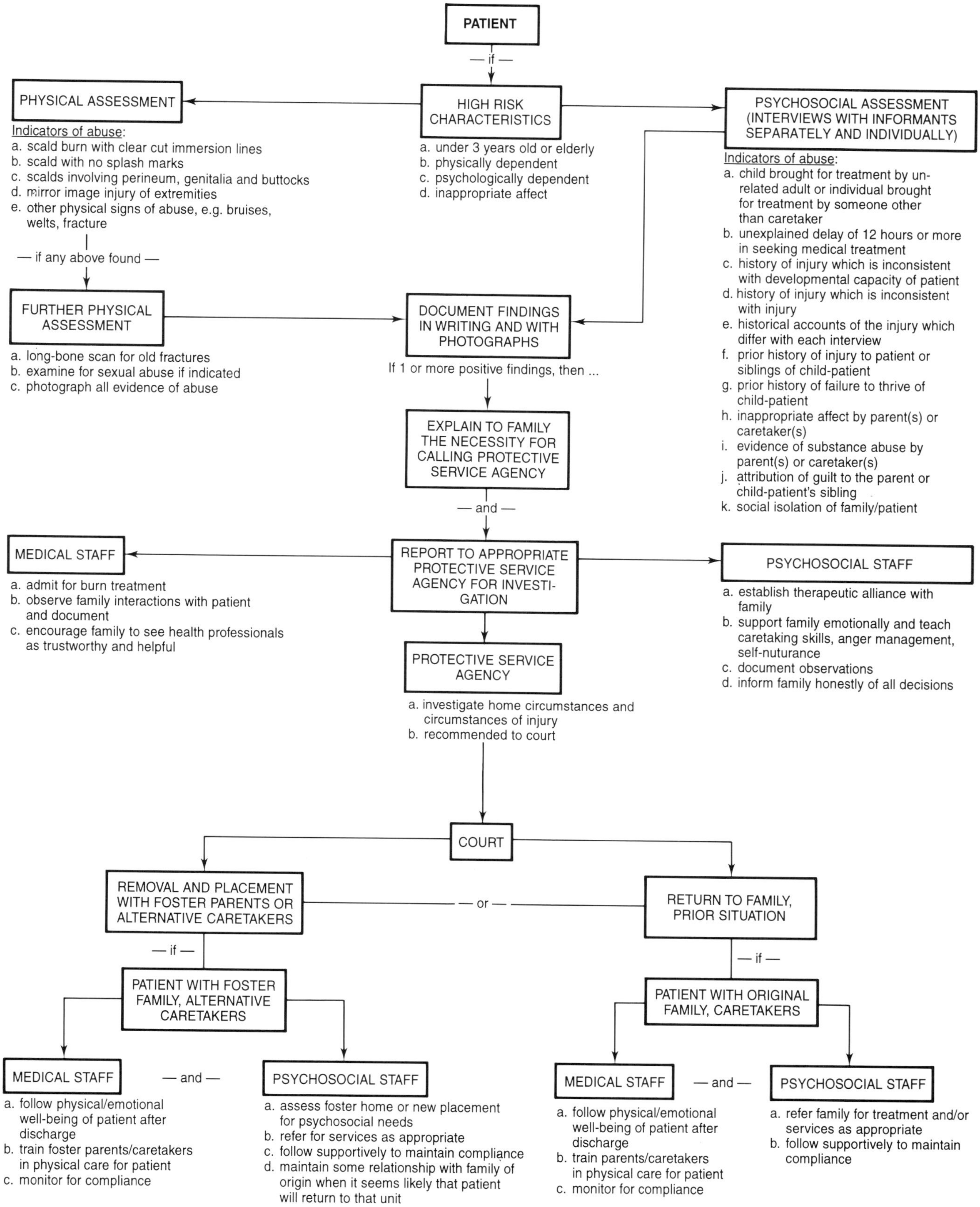

Fig. 56.1 Flow of activities toward treating victims of abuse.

- History of injury which is inconsistent with the developmental capacity of the patient.[7–9,21]
- Prior history of accidental or nonaccidental injury to the patient or to siblings.[15]
- Prior history of failure to thrive.[9,14]
- Historical accounts of the injury which differ with each interview.[8,20]
- Injury localized to genitalia, perineum, and buttocks (because of frequency with which injury occurs related to toilet training).[7–9]
- 'Mirror image' injury of extremities.[7,9]
- Inappropriate affect of child; child appears withdrawn with flattened affect.[9,22]
- Evidence of unrelated injuries, e.g. scars, bruises, welts, fractures.[7,9]

Adult Abuse and Indicators

Abuse by burning of adults is, as noted earlier, much more rarely reported, probably because the index of suspicion for abuse of an adult is low and therefore more rarely investigated. Adult victims are also noted to be reluctant to report the circumstances of their injuries because of their fear of retaliation or because of shame and embarrassment.[23] Two studies describe burn injuries of adults due to violent assault.[3,4] Associated risk factors in these reports were substance abuse and domestic violence. Although Purdue and Hunt[4] report that there was no identifiable burn pattern, Krob *et al.*,[3] describe a pattern of scald injury to the anterior trunk and upper extremity. Males and females seem equally at risk for burning by assault.

Bowden *et al.*[2] describe a population of older adults made vulnerable by physical or mental impairment who were burned by abuse or neglect. All but three of their 26 subjects were burned while living in health care facilities or institutions. Although this single article identifies abuse of the elderly by burning as a problem, it is likely that such abuse occurs with greater frequency than presently documented, and that it occurs within family settings as well as the institutional settings which dominate this Michigan sample. Elder abuse has been identified as a public concern in the United States only in the last 15 years. Relatively little, however, has been written about the subject in spite of the estimated 2.5 million persons who suffer annually.[24] When such abuse does occur within a family, it is often perpetrated by an adult child or spouse of the victim. The abusers are often intoxicated and have a history of being abused as children.[25] Some abusers of the elderly are individuals with no prior history of pathology, but who have become exhausted by the demands of their lives, e.g. caring for an aged parent as well as a spouse and children of their own.[5,23] Passive neglect may also result in injury to an elderly or vulnerable person, particularly if that person is disoriented or is reluctant to ask for attention and physical care.[24]

Risk factors of abuse for adults seem to be similar to those for children and are as follows:

- Physical dependence.[2,5,23]
- Psychological dependence.[23,24]
- Accessibility as a target for abuse as occurs with institutional living or living with a 'caretaker'.[2,24]
- Caretaker(s) with a history of substance abuse, and/or other psychopathology.[5,23,25]
- Social isolation.[24]
- An injury which is not consistent with the story described.[2]
- Conflicting reports of the injury.[2]
- Scalds with clear-cut immersion lines and no splash marks.[2]
- Scalds which involve the anterior or posterior half of an extremity and/or the buttocks and genitals, or exhibit a flexion pattern.[2]
- Other physical signs of abuse/neglect.[2]
- History of related incidents.[25]

Working therapeutically with a family suspected of abusing or mistreating a patient requires skill and diplomacy, not only because of a strong tendency on the part of health care professionals to be angry with anyone who would allow or inflict such maltreatment, but also because suspected perpetrators often appear hostile toward the professional staff. Yet establishing a therapeutic alliance with these families is extremely important, for, no matter how serious the injury, the patient will probably return to that same family, if not at the time of discharge from the hospital, then at a future time.

One careful study[26] aimed at identifying factors which determine which children will be removed from parental custody, shows that the nature of the abuse and a social worker's perception of the severity of maltreatment, as well as child, family, and environmental factors, were poor predictors of those decisions. Referrals to protective agencies from police and the courts are more likely to result in foster home placement of children than referrals from medical or school officials. The single most important determinant is the identity and/or location of the investigating agency. Although not mentioned in that study, our experience indicates that the availability of foster homes is a prime determinant. Agencies in large urban areas are much more likely to recommend foster home placement than agencies in rural areas even though burn injuries by abuse can always be considered as potentially lethal, regardless of where they occur. Even if a child is removed from parental custody, placement will often be made with another family member, such as a grandparent or aunt. Such placement might seem illogical since the families of abusive patients are also probably abusive and since all family members are likely to share similar values and sympathies.[19] Nonetheless, a key provision of the United States Federal law regarding child abuse requires that 'reasonable efforts' be made to prevent removal of neglected and abused children from their homes, and to reunite families when children are removed.[27] The intent of the law is to insure that families are provided with necessary services to enable them to become healthy and nurturing environments; however, 'reasonable efforts' is not defined. Thus, in conjunction with the large caseloads of most caseworkers in protective service agencies and the limited number of available foster homes, abiding by the law frequently results in children continuing to live with the same adults who hurt them. Adults who have been abused within a family often prefer to return to that family setting, especially if they believe that the alternative will be an institution.[23]

In order to protect a patient from further harm and to achieve good recovery and rehabilitation, the professionals who interact with a family suspected of violent abuse must establish therapeutic rapport. As with all patients and families, the therapeutic relationship is initiated at admission and developed through the process of assessment and treatment. To facilitate a positive relationship, psychotherapists must be sensitive to the fear, pain, and sadness which are often the sources of a perpetrators' abusive behavior.[7]

Dynamics of Abuse

It is helpful when dealing with persons suspected of abuse to understand that abuse usually occurs as a multigenerational characteristic which is symptomatic of relationships impoverished of nurturance. Central to understanding abuse is understanding that abusers typically are individuals who were themselves denied adequate parenting and who experienced severe emotional deprivation. The infantile needs of the abuser were unmet; the adult abuser has not learned that it is possible to assert oneself appropriately and to meet one's own needs autonomously. Rather, the abuser looks to external sources in order to meet his needs to be cared for and comforted.

In some situations there are two 'abusers', i.e. the actual perpetrator and the overtly passive observer who does not stop the abuse. Both persons are elements of a psychosocial system that supports abuse, and usually both are from similar backgrounds with similar needs.[28] Although violence may seem anything but passive, it often grows from a nonthinking, passive life position. Violent behaviors can be thought of as expressions of desperation from immature individuals who feel lost and helpless, are incompetent to care for themselves, and are in a constant quest for some external source of comfort. Their own experiences of parental neglect or abuse have taught them to mistrust others so that, as adults, they are typically socially isolated. This further decreases opportunities for comfort or for developing self-efficacy. Feeling helpless and inadequate, and predicting rejection in every interpersonal contact, such people also experience more difficulty in seeking and securing employment; thus they frequently incur a further stress of financial instability.

In an environment devoid of emotional support, abusers passively wait for comfort from a spouse, a lover, or a child. When those 'others' fail to gratify the abusers' needs or when a change in the situation imposes additional stress, these needful persons react in a child-like, nonthinking way to resolve frustration. Physical aggression and violence are often the end results of intense frustration.[19] A child, an elderly person, or a physically dependent adult is commonly an immediate precipitator of stress as well as an easily available target for physical aggression.[19,23,25]

A perceived helplessness and desperate needfulness explains some of the behaviors commonly attributed to abusers. They often fail to seek appropriate and timely medical treatment for an injured child, not only because they fear punishment but because of their learned helplessness and passivity. They discount the seriousness of an injury, as well as their ability to take care of the injury. 'I didn't think it was that bad' is an explanation often given for a delay in seeking treatment. By diminishing the significance, they relieve themselves of responsibility to act. When an abuser does take a child for help, it is frequently first to a relative or neighbor rather than to a physician because the abuser does not believe in her/his own ability to decide whether to seek medical treatment. Abusers are observed to interact inappropriately with their children because they are preoccupied with having their own needs met. A child who is hurt and demanding is unlikely to reward an abuser with feelings of comfort which an abuser seeks, and so the abuser withdraws from the child. If a child is quiet and compliant, an abuser may be observed to ignore the child and sit passively, watching television for long periods until some external force acts as a stimulus to motivate the adult into action.

Justice and Justice[29] describe six erroneous belief systems which most commonly contribute to a family system in which child abuse occurs:

1. If my child cries, misbehaves, or does not do what I want, he or she does not love me and I am a bad parent.
2. My child should know what I want and should want to do it.
3. My child should take care of me like I took care of my parents.
4. My spouse/lover should know what I want and meet all of my needs.
5. If I have to ask, it does not count.
6. I cannot trust anyone.

Although Justice and Justice were writing about families who abuse children, if, as most authorities believe, violence is a multigeneration intrafamily pattern, then it is likely that the belief system attributed to child abusers can be extrapolated to abusers of adults as well. The issues of dependency, lack of trust, felt inadequacy, frustration, and emotional pain recur in situations describing abuse spanning age groups.[23,25,30]

Assessment

Understanding that abuse does occur and that it is an expression of rage stemming from pain and sadness can enable a health care professional to begin the process of assessment as a critical observer and empathetic interviewer. The interviewer must not respond personally to apparent hostility from an informant(s) but must recognize hostility as a defense against fear. Each informant should be interviewed separately, not only to check for conflicting stories, but also because there are likely to be tensions between the informants which inhibit the interviewer's ability to establish a relationship with each individual. The informants should also be interviewed together to provide the opportunity to observe tensions, conflicts, and alliances within a family group.

Interviewing a Pediatric Patient with a Suspicious Injury

Interviews with a child-patient are especially important in cases of suspicious injury. Even children as young as 29 months often relate information with remarkable accuracy.[31] An interview with a child alone should be conducted by a professional who has established rapport with the child. The professional can first ask the child to recall specific past experiences, which are thought to have no relationship to the current suspected abuse, such as a birthday party or Christmas celebration. The descriptions of these events provide some indication of the child's ability to recall and to describe memories either verbally or in drawings. Questions about the specific events leading to injury should initially be very general, e.g. 'how did you get hurt?' and the child should be encouraged to tell the story freely. Specific questions for clarification should be asked only after the child has told the story. If the child seems unwilling to talk about what happened, the interviewer can suggest that the child raise a hand or wiggle a finger to signal that he or she knows something but does not yet want to talk about it. Interviews with a young child are best conducted in several short sessions, giving the child an opportunity to feel safe in the hospital and with the interviewer.[32]

Interviews with an Elderly or Handicapped Adult Patient

When interviewing children or other vulnerable patients, special care must be taken to help them feel safe and comfortable with an interviewer and a hospital setting. The vulnerable adult may be frightened of retribution by his/her caretaker(s) or afraid of being placed in an institutional setting. Abused adults also may be embarrassed and ashamed of their victimization. If the perpetrator is an adult child, the victim may attempt to protect the perpetrator from detection and punishment. The interviewer must assess the circumstances of the injury and establish a relationship in which the patient can trust the hospital staff to act in the best interests of all concerned, i.e. the patient and the perpetrator(s).

Reporting Suspected Abuse/Neglect

State legislatures in the United States first enacted reporting laws in 1963; by 1967, every state had laws mandating professionals who work with children to report suspected abuse or neglect to designated authorities. A Federal law, the Child Abuse Prevention and Treatment Act, was passed in 1974. The laws require professionals to report suspected abuse or neglect of a child when there is evidence that 'would lead a competent professional to believe abuse or neglect is reasonably likely'.[27]

There are no federal programs to specifically address reporting of suspected abuse in adults. Each state has its own set of definitions, reporting laws, and penalties.[23] Professionals who suspect abuse or malignant neglect of an adult should be guided by the same principles as in reporting suspicious injury to a child, comforted by the knowledge that it is the role of the health care professional to report suspicious injury in the interests of helping a patient stay safe and healthy. It is not the health professional's job to prove culpability.

The ultimate decision about whether abuse has actually occurred is left to investigating officials; however, the professionals reporting the incident must document the observed data to provide the investigating officials and/or the courts with the information necessary to intervene appropriately. Professionals should document, for example, observations which render a caretaker's professed ignorance of the cause of an injury questionable or show that an explanation of cause is implausible given the nature of the injury. Observations of inappropriate affect or lack of interest in a child's treatment must be documented. Although any single observation may seem unimportant, a pattern of behaviors described by multiple observations may be very significant in obtaining protection for a victim and help for a perpetrator.[27]

Therapeutic Interventions with Abusive Families

Ironically, professionals of a burn team who identify and report suspected abuse also have an exceptional opportunity to intervene in the dynamic process which has led to the violence. During the days or weeks of a patient's hospitalization, a family is placed in a situation of coerced interaction with the burn team. At this time, the family is also in a state of crisis, i.e. their customary defenses have failed to protect them from external scrutiny. In a state of crisis, when their usual belief systems and defensive behaviors are failing, people are more likely to be amenable to new learning and change than during times of equilibrium.[33] Thus, if members of a burn team can interact with an abusive family in ways which invalidate, or at least cast serious doubt upon, the family beliefs, there is a good possibility that the family system will begin to change. As change is initiated, continued positive support for change can lead to further change.

In order to take advantage of a therapeutic opportunity, the members of a burn care team must relate to abusers with honesty and compassion. This does not mean that the team should approve of the behaviors of the perpetrator(s) nor advocate for the perpetrator(s) to be given another opportunity to harm a victim. The team can, however, work with perpetrators in a manner which encourages them to trust professional help. The team's behavior can demonstrate that not all people are self-serving and that it is possible to relate to others in ways which are more likely to lead to gratification of their needs for nurturance and comfort. To work effectively with these families, it is essential to control the expression of anger on the part of the health care team. The clinician who rages against abusers only reinforces an abuser's view of the world as a hostile, uncaring place against which one must battle for survival. To mitigate one's natural anger toward abusers, it is helpful to remember the sad histories of abusers as victims and to respond to them as the suffering, hurt children they once were. Beneath the hostile, suspicious facade of an adult abuser is a frightened and lonely child who feels hopelessly unworthy of kindness. The clinician who is consistently honest, firm, and compassionate can develop a therapeutic alliance with a perpetrator even while explaining that reports are being made to appropriate investigating agencies. It can be explained that this report is not only mandated by law, but also is a way to obtain helpful services for the family. The clinician then must assist the family during the process of investigation. It is important that the clinician continue to honestly inform the family of decisions which are made as a result of the investigation. Even while explaining that parental rights are terminated or that criminal charges are being filed, a skillful clinician can maintain a therapeutic relationship with the perpetrator(s). By helping the perpetrator(s) perceive the situation as one in which there is hope and opportunity to receive help, the clinician can continue a therapeutic relationship which greatly enhances the likelihood that the abusive family will accept further assistance to continue the process of change.

A burn team can work with community agencies to obtain help for abusive families. Many communities have programs which provide foster grandparents or parent aides, i.e. lay therapists who teach parenting skills and nurture the parent(s).[19,29] There also may be local self-help groups or telephone crisis intervention services for abusive families; concrete services such as financial assistance or transportation are available for most families in need in the United States. If a burn team has succeeded in developing and maintaining the trust of an abusive family, they are in an advantageous position to encourage families whose prior experiences with social service agencies may have left them hostile and suspicious. Even when parental rights are terminated or a patient is removed from the home, the burn team's continued therapeutic support of the abuser(s) is advisable since the victim will likely return to that family eventually. In any event, perpetrators of violence against others are a risk to society, and health professionals have an obligation to use their knowledge and skills so as to diminish that risk.

References

1. Hansen J C, Barnhill L R. *Clinical Approaches to Family Violence*. Rockville, Maryland: Aspen, 1982: 157 pp.
2. Bowden M, Grant S, Vogel B, Prasad J. The elderly, disabled and handicapped adult burned through abuse and neglect. *Burns* 1988; **14**(6): 447–50.
3. Krob M, Johnson A, Jordan M. Burned and battered adults. *J Burn Care Rehabil* 1986; **7**(6): 529–31.
4. Purdue G, Hunt J. Adult assault as a mechanism of burn injury. *Arch Surg* 1990; **125**(2): 268–9.
5. Pedrick-Cornell C, Gelles R J. Elder abuse: the status of current knowledge. *Fam Rel* 1982; **31:** 457–65.
6. Herndon D, Rutan R, Rutan T. Management of the pediatric patient with burns. *J Burn Care Rehabil* 1993; **14**(1): 3–8.
7. Weimer C, Goldfarb I, Slater H. Multidisciplinary approach to working with burn victims of child abuse. *J Burn Care Rehabil* 1988; **9**(1): 79–82.

8. Showers J, Garrison K. Burn abuse. A four-year study. *J Trauma* 1988; **28**(11): 1581–3.

9. Hight D, Bakalar H, Lloyd J. Inflicted burns in children. *JAMA* 1979; **242**(6): 517–20.

10. Hobbs C. When are burns not accidental? *Arch Dis Child* 1986; **61:** 357–61.

11. Kumar P. Child abuse by thermal injury – a retrospective survey. *Burns* 1984; **10:** 344–8.

12. Rossignal A, Locke J, Burke J. Pediatric burn injuries in New England, USA. *Burns* 1990; **16**(1): 41–8.

13. Hammond J, Perez-Stable A, Ward C. Predictive value of historical and physical characteristics for the diagnosis of child abuse. *South Med J* 1991; **84**(2): 166–8.

14. Rosenberg N, Marino D. Frequency of suspected abuse/neglect in burn patients. *Pediatr Emerg Care* 1989; **5**(4): 219–21.

15. Bakalar H, Moore J, Lloyd J. Psychosocial dynamics of pediatric burn abuse. *Health Soc Work* 1981: 27–31.

16. Watkins A, Gagan R, Cupoli J. Child abuse by burning. *J Fla Med Assoc* 1985; **72**(7), 497–502.

17. Campbell J, LaClave L. Clinical depression in pediatric burn patients. *Burns* 1987; **13**(3): 213–17.

18. Purdue G, Hunt J, Prescott P. Child abuse by burning – an index of suspicion. *J Trauma* 1988; **28**(2): 221–4.

19. Justice B, Justice R. *The Abusing Family*. New York: Human Services Press, 1976.

20. Harmel R, Vane D, King D. Burn care in children: special considerations. *Clin Plast Surg* 1986; **13**(1): 95–105.

21. Carrigan L, Heimbach D, Marvin J. Risk management in children with burn injuries. *Journal Burn Care Rehabil* 1988; **9**(1): 75–8.

22. Hammond J, Nebel-Gould A, Brooks J. Frequency of suspected abuse/neglect in burn patients. *Pediatr Emerg Care* 1989; **5**(4): 219–21.

23. Fulmer T. Elder mistreatment: progress in community detection and intervention. *Fam Community Health* 1991; **14**(2): 26–24.

24. Sukosky D G. Elder abuse: a preliminary profile of abusers and the abused. *Fam Violence Sexual Assault Bull* 1992; **8**(4): 23–6.

25. Rathbone-McCuan E. Elderly victims of family violence and neglect. *Soc Casework* 1980; **61:** 296–304.

26. Runyan D K. The emotional impact of societal intervention into child abuse. In: Goodman G S, Bottoms B L, eds. *Child Victims, Child Witness: Understanding and Improving Testimony*. New York: Guilford Press, 1993: 263–77.

27. Myers J E B. *Legal Issues in Child Abuse and Neglect*. Newbury Park, CA: Sage, 1992: 102.

28. Kempe C H. Pediatric implications of the battered baby syndrome. *Arch Dis Child* 1971; **46:** 28–37.

29. Justice R, Justice B. Crisis intervention with abusing families: short-term cognitive coercive group therapy usine goal attainment scaling. In: Roberts A R, ed. *Crisis Intervention Handbook*. Belmont, CA: Wadsworth, Inc., 1990: 153–72.

30. Goldberg H. The dynamics of rage between the sexes in a bonded relationships. In: Hansen J C, Barnhill L R, eds. *Clinical Approaches to Family Violence*. Rockville, Maryland: Aspen, 1982: 61–7.

31. Fivush R. Developmental perspectives on autobiographical recall. In: Goodman G S, Bottoms B L, eds. *Child Victims, Child Witness: Understanding and Improving Testimony*. New York: Guilford Press, 1993: 1–24.

32. Yuille J C, Hunter R, Joffe R, Zaparniuk J. Interviewing children in sexual abuse cases. In Goodman G S, Bottoms B L, eds. *Child Victims, Child Witness: Understanding and Improving Testimony*. New York: Guilford Press, 1993: 95–115.

33. Roberts A R. An overview of crisis theory and crisis intervention. In: Roberts A R, ed. *Crisis Intervention Handbook*. Belmont, CA: Wadsworth, Inc, 1990: 3–16.

CHAPTER FIFTY-SEVEN

Psychosocial Recovery of Burned Patients and Reintegration into Society

Patricia E. Blakeney and Walter J. Meyer III

Introduction

Burn treatment extends beyond patient survival to include the recovery of optimal function of the whole person. The increased likelihood of physical survival of a burn victim heightens concern for potential psychological morbidity for the burn survivor.[1–5] Burn care providers enact, even in emergency circumstances, treatment plans based on an assumption of future life for a patient. Decisions about treatment are influenced by concerns for preserving functional mobility, cosmetic appearance, and psychological well-being of a survivor. Psychological and social issues are integral parts of burn treatment from the time of injury through recovery and rehabilitation of a patient.

Burn survivors experience a series of traumatic assaults to the body and mind which present extraordinary challenges to the human capacity for psychological resilience.[1,3,6,7] Contrary to what might be expected, empirical data regarding the long-term sequelae of burn injury indicate that many burn survivors do achieve a quality of life which is satisfying to them and that most are judged by external criteria to be well-adjusted individuals. Thirty percent of any given sample of adult burn survivors consistently demonstrate moderate to severe psychological and/or social difficulties.[5,7–11] Outcome studies of pediatric burn survivors also indicate that many burned children, even those with the most extensive and disfiguring injuries, adjust well, although the incidence of psychopathology may be somewhat higher than for adults.[7,12–20] Empirical studies, as well as clinical observations and patient self-reports, suggest that burn care of the whole person can be managed to facilitate a survivor's positive psychological adaptation to the challenges of traumatic injury, painful treatment, and permanent disfigurement.[7]

Psychological Treatment Concurrent with Physical Treatment

Clinicians with expertise in human behavior should be involved in the treatment program for all burned patients throughout the process.[3,7,21–24] In this chapter, these experts are called psychotherapists. Every person, however, who interacts with a patient impacts the psychological world of the patient. Any caregiver, including the patient's family, may be the instrument of psychotherapeutic intervention.[7] The role of the expert psychotherapist is to consult with caregivers about psychological and social issues and to suggest therapeutic interventions that any or all can act upon.[24–26] The psychotherapist on a burn team provides direct treatment to patients as appropriate to their changing concerns. As the needs of the patient evolve, the intensity of direct psychotherapeutic intervention varies according to those changing needs.

The family of a patient will always greatly influence a patient's recovery and must be considered as part of a patient's treatment plan. For the psychotherapist on the burn team, the family unit is the 'patient'.[7,26–29] Each individual within a family, including the burn survivor, is an essential element of this unit which must adapt to change. The psychosocial issues and therapeutic tasks for the patient and family are much the same across the spectrum of ages from young children through the elderly, regardless of size and severity of injury.[7,8,12,26,30–34]

Treatment plans and programs must be based on an assumption of life beyond the hospital; however death also occurs on the burn unit, and psychosocial treatment planning includes plans for assisting patients in living to the cessation of life.[7] As part of such a plan, the patient's family must be aided in preparing for and enduring bereavement.[35]

In this event, supporting and enhancing whatever coping strengths the family manifests is the primary task for psychotherapy. Most families initially deny the possibility of death, appearing not to hear an unwanted prognosis. Staff can allow the family to maintain hope while subtly preparing them with honest statements which pose death as an outcome which is possible to accept.[7] Comforting the bereft and helping them to care for themselves, physically and spiritually, are essential elements of a plan that facilitates the family's ability to minister to their patient. Keeping the family informed about changes in the patient's condition and actively supporting, sometimes instructing, them in continuing their relationships with the dying patient help the patient and family through this difficult event. A death occurring in the context of family acceptance is also more easily accepted by staff.

The Pattern of Psychological Recovery

Psychological healing occurs across time commensurate with physical healing in a pattern which is predictable and consistent.[6,7,26–30] Awareness of this pattern allows caregivers to anticipate the emergence of psychosocial issues and to prepare a patient for coping with those issues. Predicting problematic issues for patients enables them to view their concerns in a context of normal reactions rather than symptoms of psychological impairment.[3,7] For convenience in describing this pattern, we have arbitrarily designated five phases of recovery, i.e. admission, critical care, in-hospital recuperation, reintegration, and rehabilitation.

Admission Crisis

At admission, burned patients universally suffer pain and anxiety. Most are experiencing terror, confusion, and psychological shock. Events causing a serious burn injury are frightening, and the patient often believes that death is imminent. The hospital environment can also be confusing and frightening. While the physiologic emergency is confronted, the psychological crisis must also be addressed.[7] At admission, the primary psychological tasks are to establish therapeutic rapport, diminish anxiety, and assess the psychosocial strengths and needs of the patient. The first two tasks are addressed immediately by orienting a patient, by assisting the patient to focus on immediate priorities, and by assuring the patient that the burn team are knowledgeable experts who will provide excellent care. The patient's heightened anxiety can be expected to interfere with their comprehension, so it is usually necessary to repeat statements of reassurance. To prevent the patient from becoming emotionally overwhelmed, it may be necessary to suppress trauma-related content.[36]

Psychotherapeutic rapport is developed as a patient associates the voice or touch of a therapist with increased comfort. Techniques of hypnotherapy or relaxation with focused imagery can be very helpful in quickly assisting a patient to feel more comfortable. Patients during this crisis can be expected to be cognitively and emotionally regressed, and it may be important to respond to them at that regressed level. Touching patients in a soothing rhythm is often the most effective way to maintain a regressed patient's focus and communicate reassurance.[7] Members of the patient's family are also traumatized and may experience difficulty in eating and sleeping for the first several days. They, too, experience difficulty in concentrating and may require frequent repetition of information. They feel a loss of control, a generalized sense of incompetence, and helpless in providing comfort for the patient.

The psychotherapeutic tasks to be accomplished immediately with a family are similar to those for a patient, i.e. to establish a therapeutic relationship and to diminish anxiety. By assisting them in orientation to the hospital and by providing relevant information about the normal responses to trauma, both tasks are broached. Explaining, for example, that most people in this situation have difficulties for a few days in eating, sleeping, and concentrating, communicates empathy and validates that their distress is acceptable and temporary.[3,7] The family members are important components of the therapeutic efforts for the patient, and it is important to say that to them explicitly, beginning to return to them a sense of purpose and control. Even on the day of admission, the staff begins teaching the family by outlining some immediate concerns. Learning about the injury and its treatment helps to restore a family's sense of competence and provides opportunities for them to experience the reality of their roles in helping the patient.

Psychosocial assessment is also begun immediately. Prior physical and psychological health, coping skills, and family/social support are the factors which best predict the responses and recovery of a patient.[7,15,16,37–39] Size or severity of burn, age at injury, and gender of the survivor are important variables in treatment, but have little documented influence on the eventual outcome for a survivor.[12,13,37,40,41] Prior stressful events and coping strategies, risk factors, as well as psychosocial and economic strengths are included in a good history of a patient's premorbid life style. A patient's history, a patient's position in the family, and the family's strengths and weaknesses are critical pieces of information in guiding plans for treatment.

Because a patient will be dependent to some extent on family or other caretakers during recovery, it is essential to identify risk factors in a family group of caretakers.[7] Historical risk factors which may predispose individuals to burn injury and which portend poor prognoses are physical illness, substance abuse, psychiatric illness, behavioral problems, poverty, inadequate social support, and heightened family disruption.[1,42–47] The causes of many burns are, indirectly at least, attributed to these factors which will also complicate recovery and rehabilitation if they are not addressed. In addition to these risk factors, every family has its unique difficulties. The trauma of serious injury exacerbates preexisting problems. Early identification of psychosocial strengths and vulnerabilities, including those which contributed to the circumstances of the burn injury, allows the team to develop treatment and discharge plans which maximize the probability of optimal recovery for a patient.[7] The importance of assessing the circumstances of injury is emphasized in instances of abuse or malignant neglect. In addition, during early assessment interviews with a family, the staff initiates a therapeutic alliance with those who are most likely to be involved in assisting a patient's recovery.

Critical Care Phase

From hospital admission until the majority of open wounds are covered, the emphasis in treatment of a burned patient is necessarily on intensive medical and surgical care to resolve physiologic crises. This period is psychologically critical as well.

A patient experiences great anxiety during much of this time. Fear of death blends into fear of pain and fear of treatment procedures.[27] A multitude of organic factors stemming from both the injury and its treatment as well as premorbid conditions can all contribute to psychological symptoms of disorientation, confusion, sleep disturbance, transient psychosis and delirium which are commonly observed among adolescent and adult patients.[36,48,49] Psychological interventions can diminish anxiety and confusion. Repeated statements of orientation to time, place, and person are mandatory. Objects which are familiar and comforting to a patient can be placed in the patient's view or so that the patient can touch them. The patient's environment should be as soothing as possible. A schedule which approximates a regular wake/sleep cycle helps a patient begin to feel normal.[7,49] Visits from family and friends can provide familiarity and reassurance to a patient.

Staff who interact with patients during this phase must be willing to listen to patients' anxieties and reassure them that the nightmares and vivid memories are normal aspects of recovery.[3] Staff can help patients focus on the present time in which they are safe in the hospital and are healing. When a patient is withdrawn or in a coma, staff must remember that the patient may be hearing although not responding and must take care to talk to the patient. They must also be discreet in what is said within a patient's hearing range. Patients are often listening to determine what will happen to them and, in their altered mental states, they may attribute unexpected meanings to what they hear. Although the staff should persist in attempting to orient a patient, they should not argue about the patient's description of reality. Arguments with a patient who is having vivid illusions, delusions, or hallucinations are usually counterproductive. Psychological interventions are aimed at diminishing anxiety and increasing comfort rather than correcting a patient's perceptions of reality.[7]

Often, the content of the patient's visions can be used to facilitate reassurance and relaxation.

For example, a man in this phase who believed he was on a boat was combative and remained agitated in spite of psychopharmacological attempts to calm him. The psychologist assisted during procedures by talking to the patient about being on the boat in the same manner used to induce hypnotic trance. As the patient engaged in the description of the boat, the psychologist described calming elements of their imaginary surroundings such as the rhythm of the waves, the cool breeze, the warm sun. The patient for these temporary periods could become calm and could follow the psychologist's instructions to allow procedures. Although the patient was, for several days, disoriented and intermittently agitated, the staff were able to provide the care he needed during this critical phase.

Family members during critical-care usually become at ease with the routines of the hospital. They may, however, continue to experience some symptoms of post-traumatic stress, such as intrusive thoughts or avoidance behaviors.[50,51] They remain anxious about a patient's condition and eager for information about the patient's present and future status.[52,53] In addition, as they accept what has happened, they begin to think of other concerns which elicit anxiety. They may find themselves thrust by the burn injury into new roles with new responsibilities. Often, especially if the hospital is at some distance from their home, they are without their customary support systems.

It is helpful to provide a family with information about what they may expect to observe with their burned patient in the immediate future and to guide the family as they respond to the patient. Families need instruction about how they can be helpful.[53,54] They may be reluctant to touch the burned person for fear of causing pain and are usually relieved when encouraged to do so. They may feel uncomfortable in talking aloud to a nonresponsive patient; the staff can suggest that their voices and words are extremely important to the patient even though the patient does not respond. The staff must find ways to allow family members to nurture their patient and provide instructions so that the family can begin to become comfortable in caring for the patient's needs. Staff members of critical-care units are very busy and may, at moments, want to send the family away so that tasks can be completed more efficiently. These first instructions to the family are of critical importance to the future of the patient who needs the expressions of care by loved ones. Taking the time to 'treat' the family is a very important part of treating the patient.

In addition, this 'treatment' facilitates the family's resumption of feelings of competence and control, desensitizes them to the sights and odors of the burned person, and encourages the family to join with the burn team in the healing and rehabilitation of the patient.

A team must also emotionally support the family's defenses. Often family members appear to deny or to cling to delusions about the critical nature of a patient's status or the extent of a patient's injuries. It is important to give a family honest information while allowing them to protect themselves from overwhelming despair.[38] A family must find reason to hope, and the staff can assist them by suggesting realistic and optimistic outcomes. For example, we display in our offices many photographs of burn survivors engaged in a variety of activities such as swimming, going to a prom, wedding pictures, pictures of survivors with their children. The snapshots convey a hopeful message even if nothing is said explicity about them. However, family members of acute patients usually can be observed looking at the photos, and at that point it is easy to discuss which of those survivors had injuries comparable to the current patient. The message to be conveyed is that there is hope for a good outcome and that successful recovery requires arduous and painful work.

Psychotherapeutic work with the family must also identify and plan for management of those family issues which may impede a patient's recovery and rehabilitation. Some of the common issues are financial support, family alliances, historical family events, and beliefs which influence current perceptions and behaviors.[7] Management plans must support, to the extent possible, the physical and emotional well-being of all the members of the family during a period of time in which the burned patient's needs place unusual and urgent demands on the family system.[55]

Psychological factors play a significant role in pain management (see Chapter 54). The scheduling of pain assessments and the choice of assessment tools utilized have psychological relevance. Regular, routine assessments of pain imply to a patient and a patient's family that the medical staff consider discomfort a valid issue which will be treated. This not only validates a patient's concerns but sets an expectancy of relief when pain is a problem. The use of standardized scales provides the message that to experience a range of pain and comfort responses is normal and allows the patient to participate to some degree in mastering discomfort.[7] When the staff assess comfort as routinely as vital signs and indicate that they believe the patients, patients are less likely to feel that they must complain loudly in order to convince the staff that their need for pain relief is legitimate. They also are less likely to feel hopeless and helpless and become depressed.

A supportive milieu which diminishes anxiety also enhances a patient's ability to gain increased comfort with both background and procedural pain. The presence of a supportive person is effective in decreasing pain.[56] Encouraging patient participation in self-care has been demonstrated to be effective in assisting a patient to become more comfortable.[3,57] Particularly, patients who are hypervigilant and reluctant to trust seem to gain mastery over pain when they remove their own dressings or debride their own wounds. Behavioral interventions which enhance a patient's mastery or control in general seem to decrease pain and anxiety. For example, adults and children who are developmentally capable of understanding the relationship of treatment to healing better tolerate procedures when told the reason for each procedure.[58] The choice of words used in explanations of procedures can ameliorate anxiety and reduce the expectancy of pain; for example, one can say 'some people feel a poke; others feel a prick or a tingle – you tell me what you feel' rather than saying 'This is going to hurt now.'[7] Touch can be used as a distraction and to induce relaxation; continuous, rhythmic repetitive stroking of a noninjured and nonthreatening body part accompanied by comforting sounds assists relaxation of adults as well as children, including infants.[7,59] Music therapy can be an excellent adjunct to analgesia.[7] Verbal praise and other tangible reinforcers facilitate learning to cope with painful stimuli by relaxing.[60] Modeling for and instructing a family in soothing a patient is important.[7] While outside the hospital, family members may know well how to calm a patient, they may need instruction and/or encouragement from the staff to be comforting within the hospital. Once involved, family members can be valuable assets in providing the 'placebo' to relieve a patient's distress.

Other nonpharmacologic interventions also can facilitate comfort. Distraction, deep breathing, progressive relaxation, and biofeedback have all been reported to be effective in decreasing pain and distress associated with burn treatment.[60–63] Hypnosis induces a relaxed and focused state of awareness which can be extremely helpful in facilitating comfort for adults and pediatric patients.[63–66] The use of hypnosis as an adjunctive analgesic appears to decrease a patient's use of medication.[66,67] Hypnosis may offer other benefits to a burned patient as well. Some studies suggest that hypnotic suggestions given early postburn modify the physiologic response to the injury and hasten healing.[68–71] Hypnosis also can be used to increase appetite, to decrease regressive behavior, and to enhance a patient's sense of well-being, self-confidence, and body image.[64–66] An inflexible protocol for hypnosis, however, will be no more effective than an inflexible regimen of medications. With each patient, hypnotic inductions and suggestions must be modified so as to facilitate a patient's use of imagery. Some patients will respond well to suggestions of imagining a 'favorite place'; others can more easily imagine switches to 'turn off' sensation in selected body parts. Children aged 3 and over respond well to story telling with suggestions for comfort and mastery interwoven into the story.[72,73]

Providing good pain control enhances a burn care staff's effectiveness in promoting psychological recovery of a patient by allowing the staff to interact in more pleasant ways with happier patients. Comfortable patients who perceive themselves to have some power are less prone to regressive behavior. They are perceived by the staff as more likable which, in turn, reinforces the positive self-regard of the patients.

In-Hospital Recuperation Phase

Paradoxically, as burned patients become physically stronger, open wounds almost healed and grafting near completion, their continued treatment presents additional, and perhaps more difficult, challenges to the burn team. Treatment at this stage cannot simply be imposed upon a relatively helpless patient; now the team must succeed in motivating the patient to participate in treatments and to assume responsibility for recovery. The patient who desires optimal recovery must comply with the medical team's orders and instructions, many of which require significant physical discomfort.

In this phase, patients are just beginning to comprehend the extent of their injuries and to realize that their bodies, changed forever, are no longer congruent with their premorbid self-images. Their anxieties now are increasingly about the future and less about the past and present. Pain continues to be a concern; new experiences of pain must be addressed as patients become increasingly active in rehabilitative exercises. Patients are confronted with the new physical limitations imposed by their injuries; they experience their bodies now as incompetent and disfigured.[7] Patients involved in this struggle shift rapidly in affective behaviors reflecting rapid shifts in cognition. Much of the time, patients experience themselves as the 'preburn self', i.e. the 'real self'. When the body will not move as it did in the past or when the scarred skin is viewed, a patient remembers and grieves.[21] Patients slowly become aware of their changed appearances as they notice that others perceive and respond to them in ways that invalidate their former images. Their concepts about their social roles may no longer fit with society's beliefs. Their pre-morbid identities no longer exist intact and new identities must incorporate remnants of the old, as well as the changed, physical body, thus further stripping them of their identities. In this confusing state, the patient may be expected to act out anger and fear.

In addition to physical limitations, the role of 'hospital patient' imposes a loss of control and autonomy on the survivor. After a period of realistic dependence on others, a patient may be frightened and ambivalent about resuming self-care.[7,38] The demanding schedule necessary for treatment during this period heightens a patient's feelings of inadequacy. A patient becomes easily fatigued yet must continue in a schedule of tasks determined primarily by the burn team, thus providing additional evidence of the patient's loss of autonomy and ability.

Emotional lability and cognitive and behavioral regression are typically observed in patients of all ages during this trying time.[7,74] Perhaps the most difficult behavior for patient, family, and staff is the patient's expression of anger. They, of course, have many reasons to be angry, and they need to express that anger in order to define and direct it adaptively;[7,27] however, there are significant limitations upon the availability of situations in which they can express anger. Patients have almost no privacy, nor can they relieve tension through physical activities such as running. Typically, family members and patient care staff, having devoted much time and energy to the patient, may perceive the patient's angry behavior as a personal and unjust attack by an ungrateful patient. Certainly, the patient will direct rageful temper tantrums toward those who are the safest targets, usually a spouse or parent first and then a nurse or therapist. Angry attacks are best understood as necessary ventilation by the patient rather than sincere evaluations of the family or staff.

Expressions of rage are not only upsetting to family and staff; they also frighten patients who themselves perceive this loss of control as evidence of potential destruction of self or others on whom they are dependent. Following an outburst, a patient typically feels guilty and fears withdrawal of love and support by those who were earlier subjugated to the angry behavior. These fears are added to the patient's fears of being rejected because of the changed appearance. Turning anger now toward self, the patient may feel overwhelmed, hopeless, depressed, and even suicidal. If the hospitalization continues over several weeks, patients experience repetitive frustrations, and tend to feel hopeless and depressed more often.[7,27]

The family during this time must learn how to assist a patient in grieving and accepting the new situation. The family must also assess their changed situations. They must plan and implement adjustments in the family and home environment that will be necessary for the continuation of the patient's recovery and rehabilitation after discharge. Maintaining the integrity of the family unit while making needed adjustments is of high priority and is a challenge. Much of the psychotherapeutic work during this phase is accomplished with the patient and the family together. Staff can model for the family behaviors which demonstrate respect and courtesy for each family member including the patient. A psychotherapeutic challenge of this phase is to accept and validate the patient's emotional demonstrations as normal behaviors in the recovery process while also setting limits on the ways in which the emotional upheaval will be expressed. Early in this phase, as the patient begins to ask about the future, the psychotherapist can describe the predictable pattern of emotional vicissitudes indicating that, should such occur, they are normal; they can be endured and managed. The staff must demonstrate positive regard and acceptance of the patient while also helping the patient to exercise control over destructive behaviors. At times, they must impose external limits to protect the patient.

Another psychotherapeutic task with both patient and family is to titrate their denial with graded presentations of reality.[37] The staff can anticipate and assist a patient in asking questions about future disfigurement and functional abilities, including sexual activity. Without evading questions, a psychotherapist gives honest but hopeful appraisals which emphasize ability and minimize deformity and disability. For example, as a patient voices an unrealistic belief that time and/or plastic surgery will return the former appearance, one can state that burned skin will never look like unburned skin and that there will always be some scarring, but that the appearance will change with time. Allowing patients to hope, even for unrealistic outcomes, protects them from despair and enables them to continue to believe that there are reasons to endure the pain of rehabilitation.[25] Patients and families should be given the information that rehabilitation may require several years to achieve optimal satisfaction but that the painful efforts usually obtain good results.[7]

The therapeutic message to be delivered is that survivors can find ways of achieving whatever goals they set for themselves; the process is lengthy and difficult, and survivors will often feel overwhelmed and hopeless. Expressing sadness and anger is to be expected and accepted; however, such feelings can never be allowed to stop a patient from participating in the necessary regimen to achieve full recovery. Being burned does not relieve a survivor of the responsibility of competence.[7]

Many survivors have endured the process and discovered that they can enjoy their lives even though their early expectations were not, and could not have been, realized.[4] Introducing such a recovered survivor to the recuperative burned patient can be a very helpful intervention at this point.[27] The more experienced survivor can be heard as a trustworthy authority in a way the unburned professional cannot. Visual images of burn survivors telling their stores and presenting themselves in daily life activities on film or video can aid in accomplishing this purpose.[75–77] Groups of patients and/or families of burned patients at varying stages of recovery and rehabilitation have been helpful in providing information, emotional validation, and support as well as reinforcing the concept that it is possible to survive burns and live acceptably happy lives.[7,52,78]

Reintegration Phase

Although plans for a patient's discharge to out-patient status are developed from the time of admission, very specific plans must be made in the last 10–14 days of hospitalization.[7] A major objective at this time is to facilitate a patient's reentry and reintegration into life at home. Returning home signifies social interactions with the larger community of extended family, friends, and strangers. Patients as well as family must prepare for those encounters. Goodstein[38] appropriately labels this the 'social emergency' phase of treatment.

Families and patients alike are ambivalent about leaving the safe environment of the hospital. Patients, including very young children, fear social rejection or ridicule because of their changed appearance.[7,79–81] Family members will probably feel, and may express, a desire to protect their patient from rejection or ridicule. Family members may also express concerns about their abilities to continue the time-consuming physical care of the patient while resuming their usual responsibilities. Patients may doubt their abilities to resume former activities. As discharge approaches, anxieties intensify, and patients can be expected to evidence some regressive behaviors which, in turn, can reinforce the family's doubts.

Psychotherapeutic activities of this phase involve education of patient and family about the difficulties that can be anticipated at discharge. The therapist may assist in problem-solving to develop a repertoire of alternative behaviors to address those problems. Rather than accepting their assurance that problems will not arise, the psychotherapist can characterize such concerns as normal and 'usual', and proceed with a verbal rehearsal of problem solving ... 'just in case' without appearing pejorative. Issues such as recurrence of symptoms of post-traumatic stress, including sleep disturbance and irritability, or fear of resuming sexual activities, should be discussed during the days prior to discharge. This preparatory rehearsal enhances the probability that the patient/family will be less reluctant to ask for help if problems do occur; if problems do not occur, the staff has the opportunity to congratulate the patient/family on their strengths or skills in coping.[7]

Toward the end of in-patient treatment, patients are expected to resume increased autonomy; caretakers are supported in withdrawing assistance to the degree possible. It is helpful at this point to develop with patients/families a daily schedule to guide them in accomplishing necessary tasks. The burn team relinquishes performance of daily care so that the patient/family can assume care to the extent that they will be required to conduct it at home. The patient and family can benefit from the opportunity to rehearse out-patient care while still able to consult with a burn team for direction and support. Rehearsals are opportunities for all involved to experience difficulties in a safe environment and to plan corrective actions.[7]

Important among these rehearsals are those of interpersonal interactions outside the hospital. Burn survivors have reported their most difficult experience at discharge to be observing the reactions of others.[21,81] Patients benefit from the opportunity to experience such reactions before discharge from the hospital. They may leave the hospital for brief outings and return to the hospital for reassurance, encouragement, and praise.[82,83] Patient/family groups can be extremely helpful in the process of anticipating difficulties at discharge and rehearsing solutions while also providing emotional support.[7]

In addition to preparing a patient and family for discharge, the burn team may also prepare the 'community' to which a patient will return. The 'community' may include extended family, neighbors, church groups, social clubs, a patient's workplace or, in the case of a school-age pediatric patient, the school. Instructing those unfamiliar with burns in what to say or do to ease a survivor's reentry may facilitate reintegration.[81–86]

A few well organized reentry programs for pediatric burned patients have been described in the literature.[81,84–86] Although there is no evidence that adult burn survivors are in less need of assistance with reintegrating into their social worlds, published information about organized reentry programs for adults is scarce.[82,87,88] Reentry programs for adults and children involve the same fundamental elements and address the same issues.[81] They educate the community in a developmentally sensitive fashion. They address both the intellectual and emotional aspects of burn injury, provide generic information about burn injuries and burn treatment, and emphasize a survivor's abilities as well as clarify the ways in which a survivor may need assistance. Homemade videotapes can be sent to target groups ahead of a patient, thus allowing a community the opportunity to see and hear the burn survivor, to anticipate difficulties, and to plan coping responses.[81,88] Educational information presented in pamphlets or letters can be directed to those who will play key roles in facilitating a patient's transition from hospital to home community.[89,90] If possible, one or more members of a burn team may visit the home community and speak to targeted groups, answering questions which people may be reluctant to ask of the patient or family. Although there are no empirical data to demonstrate that reentry programs do, in fact, facilitate reintegration, anecdotal reports and clinical experience suggest that survivors have benefited from such efforts.[7,81,91]

Rehabilitation Phase, Post-discharge

Discharge from in-patient treatment does not signify that a patient is well. A burn survivor's wounds are covered with sensitive and fragile skin which is vulnerable to breakdown and requires special care.[7] Dressing changes, exercises, and application of special splints and pressure garments continue. Patients must confront anew their losses and may experience a delayed grief reaction. Upon leaving the protective hospital environment, symptoms of post-traumatic stress which had remitted in the hospital may recur. A survivor must continue in the arduous process of tedious, uncomfortable physical treatments while struggling to comprehend and incorporate the multitude of changes into an image of 'self' which the survivor can accept and value. The process of psychological adaptation may require several months to several years. Empirical data indicate that while the first year or so postburn is fraught with discomfort and distress, much of the difficulty is transient.[4,11] Most burn survivors do eventually adapt well and resume lives of productive activity with satisfactory social interactions.[7,15,37]

The long-term impact on the families of burn survivors has not been well studied, but clinical experience and scanty empirical data indicate the sequelae to be significant. Family members may continue to experience symptoms of post-traumatic stress after a patient has returned home.[50,51] A series of studies at our institution found that parents of recovering pediatric burned patients reported significant depressive symptoms at 2 years post-injury and that they attributed their distress to their burned children.[92–94] Although parental distress appears to improve with time for most, parents of the most troubled burned children continued across time to be troubled themselves.[94] Parents express concerns for their unburned children whom they felt were slighted of attention and time while the burned sibling required the extensive devotion of both. They also note personal financial difficulties attendant to the injury and treatment of the burned child even though their children received medical treatment at a hospital which provides care free of charge to the patient's family.[93]

Burn survivors and families may need psychotherapeutic attention for months or years as they adapt to new roles. Regular monitoring of psychosocial problems is important to early intervention.[7,11]

The psychotherapist must also help the patient to define a new self-image. In the early months or years, a patient is encouraged to overcompensate and enjoy the positive identification of 'hero'. The survivor is commended for rehabilitation gains and social accomplishments. Each victory is celebrated. As a patient's physical and psychological adaptation stabilize, the psychotherapist must assist the patient in resisting the temptation to remain satisfied with the identity of 'heroic survivor'.[7] This role invites a survivor to achieve expectations which are unrealistic and to deny unhappiness or anger or pain. The task of the psychotherapist is to make explicit the expectation that each burn survivor is a human individual who can be strong and competent, optimistic and autonomous, and also can have moments of sadness, despair, or rage. Guiding the patient to accept vulnerabilities and flaws without detracting from the overall positive evaluation of 'self', the psychotherapist insists that the person who has been the 'heroic burn survivor' can become a competent, interesting individual who also once survived a serious burn injury.

The symptoms of disturbance among burn survivors are likely to be such that only intimate friends and family members will observe them, e.g. nightmares or enuresis.[95] Persons with expertise in burn adaptation must ask about such common symptoms and inform the survivors that psychological and psychiatric assistance can alleviate some distress.

REFERENCES

1. Andreasen N J C, Noyes P, Hartford C. Factors influencing adjustment of burned patients during hospitalization. *Psychosom Med* 1972, **34**(6): 517–25.

2. Chang F, Herzog B. Burn morbidity: a follow-up study of physical and psychological disability. *Ann Surg* 1976; **183**(1): 34–7.

3. Vanderplate C. An adaptive coping model of intervention with the severely burn-injured. *Intl J Psychiatr Med* 1984; **14**(4): 331–41.

4. Patterson D, Everett J, Bombardier C, Questad K, Lee V, Marvin J. Psychological effects of severe burn injuries. *Psychol Bull* 1993; **113**(2): 362–78.

5. Ward H, Moss R, Darko D, *et al.* Prevalence of post-burn depression following burn injury. *J Burn Care Rehabil* 1987; **8**(4): 294–8.

6. Mendelsohn I. Liaison psychiatry and the burn center. *Psychosomatics* 1983; **24**(3): 235–43.

7. Blakeney P, Meyer W J. Psychological aspects of burn care. *Trauma Quarterly* 1994; **11**(2): 166–79.

8. Malt U. Long-term psychosocial follow-up of burned adults: review of the literature. *Burns* 1980; **6:** 190–7.

9. Andreasen N J C, Norris A, Hartford C. Incidence of long-term psychiatric complications in severely burned adults. *Ann Surg* 1971; **174**(5): 785–93.

10. Malt U. A long-term psychosocial follow-up study of burned adults. *Acta Psychiatr Scand Suppl.* 1989; **80**(355): 94–102.

11. Faber A, Klasen H, Sauer E, Vuister F. Psychological and social problems in burn patients after discharge: a follow-up study. *Scand J Plast Reconstr Surg* 1987; **21**(3): 307–9.

12. Stoddard F, Norman D, Murphy M. A diagnosis outcome study of children and adolescents with severe burns. *J Trauma* 1989; **29:** 471–77.

13. Stoddard F, Norman D, Murphy M, Beardslee W. Psychiatric outcome of burned children and adolescents. *J Am Acad Child Adolesc Psychiatry* 1989; **28:** 589–95.

14. Tarnowski K, Rasnake L, Linscheid T, Mulick J. Behavioral adjustment of pediatric burn victims. *J Pediatr Psychol* 1989; **14:** 607–15.

15. Blakeney P, Herndon D, Desai M, Beard S, Wales-Sears P. Long-term psychological adjustment following burn injury. *J Burn Care Rehabil* 1988; **9**(6): 661–65.

16. Blakeney P, Portman S, Rutan R. Familial values as factors influencing long-term psychosocial adjustment of children after severe burn injury. *J Burn Care Rehabil* 1990; **11**(6): 472–5.

17. Moore P, Blakeney P, Broemeling L, Portman S, Herndon D, Robson M. Psychologic adjustment after childhood burn injuries as predicted by personality traits. *J Burn Care Rehabil* 1993; **14:** 80–2.

18. Love B, Byrne C, Roberts J, Browne G, Brown B. Adult psychological adjustment following childhood injury: the effect of disfigurement. *J Burn Care Rehabil* 1987; **8:** 280–5.

19. DeWet B, Cywes S, Davies M R Q, Van der Riet L. Some aspects of post-treatment adjustment in severely burned children. *Burns* 1979; **5:** 979–80.

20. Byrne C, Love B, Browne G, Brown B, Roberts J, Steiner D. The social competence of children following burn injury: a study of resilience. *J Burn Care Rehabil* 1986; **7:** 247–52.

21. Knudson-Cooper M. Adjustment to visible stigma: the case of the severely burned. *Soc Sci Med* 1981; **15:** 31–44.

22. Kjaer G. Psychiatric aspects of thermal burns. *Northwest Med* 1969; **68:** 537–541.

23. Morris J, McFadd A. The mental health team on a burn unit. A multidisciplinary approach. *J Trauma* 1978; **18**(9): 658–63.

24. Ochitill H. Psychiatric consultation to the burn unit. The psychiatrist's perspective. *Psychosomatics* 1984; **25**(9): 689, 697–701.

25. Tucker P. The burn victim – a review of psychosocial issues. *Aust N Z J Psychiatry* 1986; **20:** 413–20.

26. Knudson-Cooper M. Emotional care of the hospitalized burned child. *J Burn Care Rehabil* 1982; **3:** 109–16.

27. Watkins P, Cook E, Mary R, Ehleben C. Psychological stages in adaptation following burn injury: a method for facilitating psychological recovery of burn victims. *J Burn Care Rehabil* 1988; **9**(4): 376–84.

28. Tucker P. Psychosocial problems among adult burn victims. *Burns* 1987; **13**(1): 7–14.

29. Shenkman B, Stechmiller J. Patient and family perception of projected functioning after discharge from a burn unit. *Heart Lung* 1987; **16**(5): 490–6.

30. Luther S, Price J. Burns and their psychological effects on children. *J School Health* 1981; **51:** 419–22.

31. Wallace L. Abandoned to a 'social death?' *Nurs Times* 1988; **84**(10): 34–7.

32. Davidson T, Bowden M, Feller I. Social support and post-burn adjustment. *Arch Phys Med Rehabil* 1981; **62:** 274–7.

33. Blumenfield M, Reddish P. Identification of psychologic impairment in patients with mild-moderate thermal injury: small burn, big problem. *Gen Hosp Psychiatry* 1987; **9:** 142–6.

34. Andreasen N J C, Norris A. Long-term adjustment and adaptation mechanisms in severely burned adults. *J Nerv Ment Dis* 1972; **154**(5): 352–62.

35. Stoddard F. Psychiatric management of the burned patient. In: Martyn J A J, ed. *Acute Care of the Burn Patient*. Orlando, FL: Grune and Stratton, 1990: 256–72.

36. Blank K, Perry S. Relationship of psychological process during delirium to outcome. *Am J Psychiatry* 1984; **141:** 843–7.

37. Bowden L, Feller I, Tholen D, Davidson T, James M. Self-esteem of severely burned patients. *Arch Phys Med Rehabil* 1980; **61:** 449–52.

38. Goodstein R. Burns: an overview of clinical consequences affecting patient, staff, and family. *Compr Psychiatry* 1985; **26**(1): 43–57.

39. Roberts J, Browne G, Streiner D, Byrne C, Brown B, Love B. Analyses of coping responses and adjustment: stability of conclusions. *Nurs Res* 1987; **36**(2): 94–7.

40. Byrne C, Love B, Browne G, Brown B, Roberts J, Streiner D. The social competence of children following burn injury: a study of resilence. *J Burn Care Rehabil* 1986; **7:** 247–52.

41. Blakeney P, Meyer W, Moore P, Broemeling L, Hunt R, Robson M, Herndon D. Social competence and behavioral problems of pediatric survivors of burns. *J Burn Care Rehabil* 1993; **14:** 65–72.

42. Darko D, Wachtel T, Ward H, Frank H. Analysis of 585 burn patients hospitalized over a 6-year period. Part III: Psychosocial data. *Burns* 1986; **12:** 395–401.

43. Davidson T, Brown L. Self-inflicted burns: a 5-year retrospective study. *Burns* 1985; **11:** 157–60.

44. Knudson-Cooper M, Leuchtag A. The stress of a family move as a precipating factor in children's burn accidents. *J Hum Stress* 1982; **June:** 32–8.

45. Noyes R, Frye S, Slyment D, Canter A. Stressful life events and burn injuries. *J Trauma* 1979; **19**(3): 141–4.

46. Vogtsberger K, Taylor E. Psychosocial factors in burn injury. *Tex Med* 1984; **80:** 43–6.

47. Wilson G, Buckland R, Sully L. Childhood illness an an etiological factor in burns. *Burns* 1988; **14**(3): 237–8.

48. Haynes B, Bright R. Burn coma: a syndrome associated with severe burn wound infection. *J Trauma* 1967; **7:** 464–75.

49. Steiner H, Clark W. Psychiatric complications of burned adults: a classification. *J Trauma* 1977; **17:** 134–43.

50. Cella D, Perry S, Kulchycky, Goodwin C. Stress and coping in relatives of burn patients: a longitudinal study. *Hosp Community Psychiatry* 1988; **39**(2): 159–66.

51. Cella D, Perry S, Poaz M, Amand R, Goodwin C. Depression and stress responses in parents of burned children. *J Pediatr Psychol* 1988; **13**(1): 87–99.

52. Rivlin E, Forshaw A, Polowyj G, Woodruff B. A multidisciplinary group approach to counselling the parents of burned children. *Burns* 1986; **12**(7): 479–83.

53. Terry D. The needs of parents of hospitalized children. *Children's Health Care* 1987; **16**(1): 18–20.

54. Kasper J, Nyamathi A. Parents of children in the pediatric intensive care unit: what are their needs? *Heart Lung* 1988; **17:** 574–81.

55. Reddish P, Blumenfield M. A typology of spousal response to the crisis of severe burn. *J Burn Care Rehabil* 1986; **7**(4): 328–30.

56. Kelley M, Jarvie G, Middlebrook J, Mceer M, Drabman R. Decreasing burned children's pain behavior: impacting the trauma of hydrotherapy. *J App Behav Anal* 1984; **17**(2): 147–58.

57. Kavanagh C. Psychological intervention with the severely burned child: report of an experimental comparison of two approaches and their effects on psychological sequelae. *J Am Acad Child Psychiatry* 1983; **22**(2): 145–56.

58. Beales J. Factors influencing the expectation of pain among patients in a children's burns unit. *Burns* 1983; **9**(3): 187–92.

59. Baker C, Wong D. Q.U.E.S.T.: a process of pain assessment in children. *Orthop Nurs* 1987; **6**(1): 11–21.

60. Elliot C, Olson R. The management of children's distress in response to painful medical treatment for burn injuries. *Behav Res Ther* 1983; **21**(6): 675–83.

61. Perry S. Undermedication for pain on a burn unit. *Gen Hosp Psychiatry* 1984; **6:** 308–16.

62. Knudson-Cooper M. Relaxation and biofeedback training in the treatment of severely burned children. *J Burn Care Rehabil* 1981; 103–10.

63. Zeltzer L, LeBaron I. Hypnosis and nonhypnotic techniques for reduction of pain and anxiety during painful procedures in children and adolescents with cancer. *Behav Pediatr* 1982; **101**(6): 1032–5.

64. Crasilneck H, Stirman J, Wilson B, McVranie E, Fogelman M. Use of hypnosis in the management of patients with burns. *JAMA* 1955; **158:** 103–6.

65. Schafer D. Hypnosis on a burn unit. *Int J Clin Exp Hypn* 1975; **23**(1): 1–14.

66. Wakeman R, Kapan J. An experimental study of hypnosis in painful burns. *Am J Clin Hypn* 1978; **21**(1): 3–12.

67. Van der Does AJW, Van Dyck R, Spijker R. Hypnosis and pain in patients with severe burns: a pilot study. *Burns* 1988; **14**(5): 399–404.

68. Ewin D. Emergency room hypnosis for the burned patient. *Am Clin Hyp* 1986; **29**(1): 8–12.

69. Hammond D, Keye W, Grant C. Hypnotic analgesia with burns: a initial study. *Am J Clin Hypn* 1983; **26**(1): 56–9.

70. Margolis C. Domarque B, Ehliben C, Shrier L. Hypnosis is the early treatment of burns: a pilot study. *Am J Clin Hypn* 1983; **26**(1): 9–15.

71. May S, DeClement F. Effects of early hypnosis on the cardiovascular and renal physiology of burn patients. *Burns* 1983; **9**(4): 257–66.

72. Olness K. Imagery (self-hypnosis) as adjunct therapy on childhood cancer. *Am J Pediatr Hematol Oncol* 1981; **3**(3): 313–20.

73. Kuttner L. Favorite stories: a hypnotic pain-reduction technique for children in acute pain. *Am J Clin Hypn* 1985; **28:** 289–95.

74. Stoddard F. Body image development in the burned child. *J Am Acad Child Psychiatry* 1982; **21**(5): 502–7.

75. Blakeney P, Washam K, Cahners S, Driscoll E. *Brandon*. Tampa, FL: Shriners Hospitals for Crippled Children, videotape, 1993.

76. Blakeney P, Washam K, Cahners S, Driscoll E. *Megan*. Tampa, FL: Shriners Hospitals for Crippled Children, videotape, 1993.

77. Doctor M E, Burne B, Jarecke D. *Through the Eyes of a Child: Burn Recovery*. Denver, CO: Children's Hospital, videotape, 1993.

78. Cahners S. Group meetings benefit families of burned children. *Scand J Plast Reconstr Surg* 1979; **13:** 169–71.

79. Langlois J H, Downs A C. Peer relations as a function of physical attractiveness: the eye of the beholder or behavioral reality? *Child Dev* 1979; **50:** 409–18.

80. Barden R C. The effects of crania-facial deformity, chronic illness, and physical handicaps on patient and familial adjustment: research and clinical perspectives. In: Lahey B B, Kazdin A E, eds. *Advances in Clinical Child Psychology*. Vol 13. New York: Plenum, 1990: 343–75.

81. Blakeney P. School reintegration. In: Tarnowski K J (ed.) *Behavioral Aspects of Pediatric Burns*. New York, Plenum, 1994: 217–41.

82. Dobner D, Mitani M. Community reentry program. *J Burn Care Rehabil* 1988; **9**(4): 420–1.

83. Stein J. Comments from Maricopa Medical Center, Phoenix. *J Burn Care Rehabil* 1988; **9**(4): 418–19.

84. Cahners S. A strong hospital – school liaison: a necessity for good rehabilitation planning for disfigured children. *Scand J Plast Reconstr Surg* 1979; **13:** 167–68.

85. Doctor, M E. Returning to school after a severe burn. In Boswick J A Jr, ed. *The Art and Science of Burn Care*. Rockville, MD, Aspen Press, 1987: 323–8.

86. Walls Rosenstein D L. A school reentry program for burned children. Part I: development and implementation of a school reentry program. *J Burn Care Rehabil* 1987; **8:** 319–22.

87. Blumerfield M, Schoeps M. Reintegrating the healed burned adult into society: psychological problems and solutions. *Clin Plast Surg* 1992; **19**(3): 599–605.

88. Angermeier J. A desensitization process to facilitate first visits between burn scarred parents and young children. *J Burn Care Rehabil* 1991: **12**(4): 344–5.

89. Shriners Burns Institute. *Back to School Guidelines for Parents*. Cincinnati, OH: Shriners Hospitals for Crippled Children, 1993a.

90. Shriners Burns Institute. *Back to School Guidelines for Parents*. Cincinnati, OH: Shriners Hospitals for Crippled Children, 1993b.

91. Blakeney P, Moore P, Meyer W, *et al.* Efficacy of school reentry programs. *J Burn Care Rehabil* in press.

92. Blakeney P, Moore P, Broemeling L, Hunt R, Herndon D, Robson M. Parental stress as a cause and effect of pediatric burn injury. *J Burn Care Rehabil* 1993; **14**(1): 73–9.

93. Blakeney P, Meyer W, Moore P, Murphy L, Broemeling L, Robson M, Herndon D. Psychosocial sequelae of pediatric burns involving 80% or greater total body surface area. *J Burn Care Rehabil* 1993; **14:** 684–89.

94. Meyer W, Blakeney P, Moore P, Murphy L, Robson M, Herndon D. Parental well-being and behavioral adjustment of pediatric burn survivors. *J Burn Care Rehabil* 1994; **15:** 62–68.

95. Meyer W, Blakeney P, LeDoux J, Herndon D. Diminished adaptive behaviors among pediatric burn survivors. *J Burn Care Rehabil* in press.

CHAPTER FIFTY-EIGHT

58

CASE MANAGEMENT AND THE NURSE CASE MANAGER IN A BURN CENTER

BEVERLY J. MCCOY, ANN CHAVARRIA, VICTORIA GILINSKY, THERESA PICKETT AND JANET A. MARVIN

INTRODUCTION

A nursing case management system is one way to provide planned, coordinated care to meet the needs of a high-risk patient population in a way which minimizes fragmentation and maximizes individualized care. Care coordination and resource management are the two characteristics which set case management apart from other health care delivery systems. Care coordination activities such as scheduling tests, arranging for consultation, and planning for discharge are typical nursing activities which are a part of case management.[1]

Resource management integrates the nurses' clinical and management skills with family and community resources to insure that out-patient care and rehabilitation are available and accessible. The key to success in this area is to identify accurately the needs of a high-risk patient and to link those needs with the most appropriate resources. This requires direct, effective communication skills and the ability to plan, collaborate, and negotiate with a patient, a patient's family, health care team members, and agencies within a community. Sometimes the process includes educating nurses and other health care team members in the hospital and the community about the role of a nurse case manager. Teaching others how to identify a patient or family whose needs are not being met adequately and how to work as a team to individualize a plan to meet those needs is critical to the success of the case manager role.[2]

CASE MANAGEMENT EXPLAINED BY EXAMPLE

Case management was initiated in the Shriners Burns Institute (SBI), Galveston, as a way to organize nursing care and to coordinate the care of the 'burn team'. Typical tasks for the case manager to accomplish with patients and families include initial interventions, assessments of needs and resources, arrangement of referrals, and follow-up (**Table 58.1**). The case managers at SBI, Galveston each carry a case load of 20–30 active patients which includes both in-patients and out-patients. The responsibilities of case managers vary depending on the needs of patients (**Table 58.2**). The responsibilities of the case managers are broad and often require creative solutions to a multitude of problems. No rigid formula can prescribe a proper method for case management in practice. The following case studies illustrate the variety of issues with which case managers deal.

Table 58.1 Nurse case manager: interventions with families and children with burn injuries

Provide crisis interventions for a family coping with loss
Identify family needs and direct them to an appropriate hospital resource person
Collaborate with nursing staff in planning patient care
Assess and identify patient and/or family needs which are not being met and discuss them with a treatment team
Encourage and empower families to learn about wound care and pressure therapy prior to discharge
Assess family resources needed for discharge planning
Anticipate and address questions and/or difficulties commonly encountered when returning home
Collaborate with the treatment team in discharge planning and coordinating needed referrals
Arrange nursing referrals post-discharge. Provide referral agencies with information and education about burn care (which may involve a visit to a child's home and community in order to identify resources and teach specifics about burn care to the community's health care professional)
Monitor patient and family adjustments after discharge with follow-up telephone calls to family and referral sources

Case Study 1

A 4-year-old white male, who will be called WP, sustained a 38% TBSA flame burn from a mobile home fire of unknown origin. WP shared that home with his mother and two younger siblings. A 3-year-old brother, PJ, was also burned in the fire. The mother attempted unsuccessfully to rescue the children, and a neighbor subsequently was able to retrieve them from the fire. The boys were transported to SBI, Galveston accompanied by their mother; within 1 week, the maternal grandfather and the father, who was not living in the home at the time of the fire, arrived at the hospital. While PJ was only moderately injured, WP sustained second and third degree burns circumferentially to both arms, face, and ears as well as an inhalation injury. He underwent several surgeries for excision, debridement, and grafting until the wounds were covered.

Table 58.2 Specific indicators for case management care at Shriners Burns Institute, Galveston Unit

Acute patients
- All patients with over 80% TBSA burn injuries
- Patients with over 50% TBSA burn injuries with limb loss and/or primary language other than English
- All patients being followed by CPS
- All patients needing a nursing referral for home visits post-discharge
- All patients whose family dynamics have the potential to interfere with patient treatment and the accomplishment of desired outcome
- Patients whose family calls back to the hospital more than two times within the first week after discharge

Reconstructive surgery patients
- All patients undergoing surgery for specific procedures which require specialized care at home and are high risk, such as those with:
  - tissue expander
  - Ilizarov placement
  - pin placement
- All patients needing nursing referrals post-discharge
- All patients with a history of having difficulty with follow-up care, i.e. pressure, exercise therapy, wound care and/or failure to return for follow-up appointments as planned
- Post-discharge – if phone calls are received from the family more than two times within one week

Rehabilitation patients
- Patients with > 50% TBSA burn injuries with complicating factors, e.g. hearing loss, amputations, impaired family dynamics, primary language not English, etc.
- All patients being followed by more than one medical service, i.e. ophthalmology, ENT, orthopedics, plastic surgery, and general surgery

During the first week of hospitalization, the Registered Nurse Case Manager (RNCM) became involved with WP when staff nurses reported that his mother and father were arguing loudly while visiting in his room and were verbally attacking staff members who attempted to intervene. Taking into consideration the family's stress resulting from the accident and marital strife, the case manager arranged a patient care conference to review WP's plan of care and to bring some structure to the chaotic communication pattern. Present at the conference were mother, father, grandfather and representatives of all the clinical services providing care to both children. The goals were to:

- review the care plan and the expected family participation;
- formulate a care schedule to be posted in WP's room with specific times for family participation;
- discuss Department of Human Services (home state) involvement;
- elicit questions and concerns from the family, and provide support to both patient and family members;
- initiate discharge planning by assessing resources and family plans.

To streamline communication, the RNCM and the psychologist were the designated resource people and the family was asked to direct questions and concerns to one of them. This plan was successful in providing the structure needed to decrease anxiety and facilitate more effective communication.

WP responded by becoming more verbal and talking about the accident, his fears, what he liked and disliked, and generally finding his way into the hearts of staff members. The music therapist was instrumental in encouraging and maintaining verbalization with daily visits which included song writing and singing. Within a short time, WP's father returned home. When 3-year-old PJ was ready for discharge, the plan was for his mother to return home with PJ. In the meantime the custody issue was being considered by the home state Department of Human Services (DHS) and followed closely by the psychologist and case manager. Still, it was unclear who was going to provide care and a home for WP. His mother returned home, and his grandfather stayed to support and care for WP. As discharge became imminent, the plan developed for the grandfather to take WP to one of the in-hospital apartments for a few days to become accustomed to caring for WP. This became an impossible plan as the grandfather's health began to deteriorate resulting in his departure for hospitalization in his home state.

It was difficult to find a consistent caregiver to take responsibility for this child. His mother was at home caring for PJ; she was not able to return to the hospital for home care instructions needed to care for WP. His father was no longer in the home, and it was clear that his grandfather was too ill to assist. With numerous patient care conferences to review and revise discharge plans and continued communication with DHS, the home care referrals for nursing and physical therapy were made. WP was ready to leave the hospital. Telephone contacts with the Department of Human Services social worker, the home health nurse, and the family resulted in a plan for the RNCM to accompany WP home. This provided opportunities to meet with the caregivers, to explain needed wound care, pressure therapy, and exercises, so that WP's mother could receive demonstrations of proper home care.

The RNCM integrated clinical nursing skills, personal involvement, and resource coordination in an advocacy role for the child and the family. These interventions are reinforced by maintaining telephone contact and by providing care during out-patient clinic appointments. This kind of relationship with a patient provides continuity of care and at the same time allows the RNCM to recognize and reinforce a patient's and family's positive personal coping skills at each developmental stage.

Case Study 2

VJ was a 15-year-old, Hispanic male from northern California, who sustained 95% TBSA burn in June, 1993 from an appliance fire. After receivnig local emergency treatment, he was transported to SBI accompanied by his mother. VJ sustained third degree burns of his face, neck, anterior and posterior trunk, bilateral upper and lower extremities, and an inhalation injury. During the acute phase of hospitalization, VJ underwent repeated surgeries for excision, debridement and grafting; amputations of fingers and toes were necessary on bilateral feet and hands.

At the time of the injury, VJ had been living with his mother, stepfather, and two younger sisters for only a short time. Previously, VJ lived with his father, an itinerant worker, who left VJ alone to provide for himself for weeks at a time. As a result, VJ developed an air of 'tough' independence which the burn injury interrupted; he was completely dependent in a strange place, and he was in constant pain. VJ was angry and lashed out frequently at his mother and staff both verbally and physically. It was important to support VJ's desire for control and independence, but frustrating and discouraging to bear the brunt of his anger. Patient care conferences with the multidisciplinary staff, including a psychiatrist and clinical psychologist, were scheduled frequently by the case manager. Participation in these conferences gave staff members an opportunity to ventilate feelings, support each other, plan strategies to handle the most difficult parts of his treatment, and review treatment goals and progress. VJ's verbal abuse at times was so intense and personal that nurses left his room in tears. A plan which worked well during that most difficult time of his treatment was 'volunteer duty'. Nurses who were able to set limits and handle the insults more objectively volunteered to care for VJ as the rest of the staff supported them and tried to learn more about the difficulty VJ was having accepting help. An important part of the plan was to insure that a nurse who was familiar with the rough Hispanic environment from which VJ had come would care for him as often as possible, for these nursing staff members bonded more easily with VJ.

When Mrs J and VJ became fatigued, they more frequently spoke Spanish, their primary language. It was therefore advantageous to have a bilingual case manager to assist them with communication at the more stressful and difficult times so that they could speak in the language which was more comfortable and familiar. This also helped with the assessment of other treatment issues. For example, VJ experienced severe pain, high anxiety levels, and difficulty in falling asleep. It was part of the case manager's role to elicit information from VJ about his perceptions of all that was happening to him. This was consistently documented and communicated to the team managing the medication needed to decrease the pain, anxiety, and periods of insomnia.

Developing a daily schedule with VJ's participation facilitated consistency with needed treatments, provided VJ with a sense of control, and contributed to the trust which was at last developing between VJ and the team which was caring for him. VJ began to cooperate and to take some responsibility for his daily care and treatments; and the nursing staff was able to resume regular assignment methods. As the time for discharge approached, VJ and his mother became more proficient with the daily care of his wounds. Necessary referrals were made. VJ was discharged to an in-patient rehabilitation hospital near his home in November, 1993, where he and his family received extensive psychiatric evaluation and psychotherapy as part of the overall rehabilitation program.

A review of the 5 months of VJ's hospitalization reveals that not only had VJ progressed, but his case manager had benefited as well, developing skills in problem identification, problem solving, and negotiating. These skills would be used again with VJ and with other patients in the future. VJ was readmitted 2 months later due to chronic open wounds, behavioral problems, and symptoms of depression. The team immediately mobilized treatment strategies which had worked in the past and instant trust was established. VJ indicated that this time he was part of the team from the beginning. One of his first questions was 'how much do I have to eat in order to receive a soda water reward'? The treatment team's reward was to see VJ involved in his recovery and accepting assistance on his long journey to wellness. Case management with VJ continues to be a challenge as team members strive to address his changing needs, support his tenacity, and work through agencies in his home community.

Case Study 3

A 4-year-old white female, called LM, sustained a 77% TBSA burn injury on December 4, 1991. The injury occurred when her brother knocked over a lantern filled with kerosene and a candle nearby ignited the fluid and caused a flash fire. She was rescued by her parents who also sustained minor injuries in the fire.

During LM's acute phase of hospitalization, she underwent multiple surgeries for excision, debridement, and grafting in order to achieve wound coverage. Child Life Therapy assisted LM in coping with hospital treatments, providing emotional support and an avenue of expression through play therapy. Family Services provided counseling and emotional support to the parents in order to help them cope with the results of the accident and with the treatments needed for LM to get well.

Early in the acute phase, nursing staff identified family stressors which were leading to parental withdrawal from the patient. With counseling by Family Services, the parents were encouraged to become involved in LM's care early in the acute phase. Both parents participated in care, but because another sibling was at the hospital with them, one parent had to do wound care while the other watched the sibling. Even with this plan of separation, both parents exhibited much animosity toward each other, blaming each other for the accident. They both demonstrated poor parenting skills and emotional outbursts, and they received minimal support from their extended family. A Child Protective Services (CPS) report regarding the family environment identified stressors:

- Intense marital conflict.
- Inability to demonstrate concern or empathy toward the child and the psychosocial issues related to making an adjustment to the burn injury.
- Poor parenting skills.

The following recommendations were made:

- Monitor the familiy's ability and willingness to provide wound care and compliance with pressure treatments.
- Provide family counseling and parenting classes.
- Assess and evaluate the child's adjustment at home.

At discharge, a home nursing referral and rehabilitation therapy referral was made so that LM would be seen every day. Weekly visits to the SBI clinic were planned because of the parents' inability to comply with discharge instructions, repeated missed clinic appointments, deterioration of the patient's physical progress, and continued family stressors. The patient had to be readmitted to the hospital for corrective surgery to release contractures. The case manager on the reconstructive surgery unit began to follow this patient closely while she was hospitalized for corrective surgeries and continued to follow her after discharge.

During the initial interview with the mother, the case manager noticed that the mother was constantly yelling at her 2-year-old son; LM was fretful and wanted her Jobst garment off; her mother appeared unsure about what she should do. The mother revealed that LM never had immunizations, and when the case manager inquired why she had not received her immunizations she stated, 'LM had been through enough' and she 'didn't want anyone giving her a shot'. The case manager's goals were to develop trust with LM's mother, the primary caretaker, and to establish a relationship with her so she would share her concerns and ask questions. The hope was that by increasing her knowledge of, and hopefully her compliance with, instructions, the care team could promote healing of wounds and minimize burn scar contractures. Additionally, the nurse case manager was also to monitor compliance with scheduled clinic visits, to communicate with the nurse at the home health agency involved in her care, and to answer questions about wound care as needed.

The case manager called Mrs M weekly and sometimes twice a week but many times she would not answer the phone. Her mother informed the case manager that Mrs M sometimes takes the phone off the hook. When she did return calls, she talked as if everything was okay. She requested additional supplies, which were sent, she also stated that she was not fond of the nurse who came out to check on LM, although she was not specific about her complaint.

According to the home health nurse, initially Mrs M complied with wound care and with pressure and exercise therapy instructions, but family stressors continued to increase. Many times the nurse would go to the home to find no one there or Mrs M would refuse to open the door. It became impossible for the nurse and the therapist to follow the patient and perform necessary care. CPS was notified of the deteriorating home situation, and the patient was placed under the care of the Office of Community Services. A representative from that office monitored the situation, and the home health agency continued to assist with her care. LM was eventually placed in the custody of the state, and her mother voluntarily relinquished custody rights for all of her children. Realizing that she needed help, she went to a drug treatment center. The father left home and stated that he was getting a divorce. The two siblings were placed in foster care. LM was placed in a licensed facility which cared for children with medical needs and began to improve considerably. She was eventually placed with a loving foster mother who has been nurturing and meeting her needs, both physically and emotionally. The courts are in the process of terminating the parental rights of the mother and father. On return to clinic appointments, LM is more verbal and outgoing. She makes eye contact when talking, is in second grade, and is doing well.

Conclusion

These three cases demonstrate the variety of activities in which a nurse case manager may participate. The involvement during the initial admission is important, especially for families with complex needs. Close monitoring after discharge with frequent telephone calls and early identification of problems during the rehabilitation phase can often lead to early intervention during home care and provide support to a child-patient, a family, and community agencies. Case management is one method for coordinating all the activities and services needed for a patient with major burn injuries and complex family situations. Nurses are ideal case managers because they have a broad knowledge of the medical, emotional, and social care needs of patients and families.

References

1. Strong A G. Case management and the CNS. *Clin Nurse Specialist*, 1992; **6**(2): 64.

2. Nugent K E. The clinical nurse specialist as case manager in a collaborative practice model: bridging the gap between quality and cost of care. *Clin Nurse Specialist* 1992; **6**(2): 106–11.

CHAPTER FIFTY-NINE

59

PREVENTION OF BURN INJURIES

STUART P. PEGG

INTRODUCTION

Most burns are preventable;[1] however, prevention is difficult to achieve. The main avenues are by legislation and education. Public awareness must be increased by any method possible, from posters to television. Epidemiologic studies should be done to determine predominant causes of burns and 'at-risk' populations. Specific plans for prevention can be developed based on this data.

Few members of a burn team would disagree with the sentiment that most burns can be prevented. There may be exceptions; lightning burns may be a striking example, but even in these instances sensible precautions taken during thunderstorms can do much to lessen the chance of injury. All members of a burn team experience the frustration of admitting a new burn victim and observing that the injury could have been prevented but for a lack of awareness, a lack of judgment, or failure to follow safety guidelines. When a single type of injury occurs repeatedly, the question of prevention is obvious. Why have these injuries not been prevented? The questions often seem more poignant with childhood injuries. Why are children scalded? We know that in 83% of cases, parents were responsible for supervising a child when an accident occurred.[2] Where is the failure in that supervision? A burn team left to care for such a patient knows that there is no substitute for prevention. But prevention is very difficult to achieve. The problems of prevention are to determine an effective strategy, to financially support a prevention campaign, and to evaluate the effectiveness of the campaign. The treatment of burn injuries has improved dramatically, but the basic fact remains that optimal results would be achieved if burn injuries were prevented.

EPIDEMIOLOGY

Establishing an effective prevention program begins with epidemiologic studies of burn injuries. Many surveys have been conducted, some much more sophisticated than others, ranging from burn unit surveys to national data collections. All indicate that the problems to be tackled are huge. In the USA each year, approximately 7500 people die, and 310 000 are seriously injured in fires; it is estimated that about twice that many injuries occur and are not reported.[3] Burn injuries are not so well reported in many other countries. Only by detailed studies from general hospitals, burn units, and national statistics can the size of the overall problem be grasped. Persons involved in planning prevention strategies must assess for themselves the problems to be targeted in their own locale. The predominant causes of injury will vary considerably according to geography, culture groups, and socioeconomic groups.[4] For example, burn injuries from open heating fires may be common in colder countries in winter but are rarely seen in tropical areas. The opposite may be true in relation to barbecue injuries.[5] Identifying the causes of injury is a critical first step to developing prevention strategies.

'AT-RISK' GROUPS

Universally, the very young[6] and the very old are at risk; they are more likely to be burned and less likely to survive (**Table 59.1**). Lower socioeconomic groups appear to be more at risk than those with greater resources.[4,7–9] People with limited financial resources

Table 59.1 At-risk groups

Very young
Very old
Lower socioeconomic groups[4,7–9]
Mentally handicapped[10,11]
Physically handicapped
Illness[5,10]
Alcohol[5]
If poor access to medical treatment

more often use appliances which are not working safely and use makeshift methods of heating and cooking. They also may have more limited access to medical treatment. The mentally and physically handicapped pose a problem not only in the home environment but also in hospitals and nursing homes.[10,11] Other illnesses, such as diabetes and epilepsy, contribute significantly.[5,10] Alcohol abuse accounts for 6.3% of injuries, according to one survey.[5]

Prevention Strategies

Development of prevention strategies begins with knowledge of the target population for a campaign. Although overall public education may be one goal of every prevention program, it is usually more effective to concentrate on one facet of a problem. For example, concentrating resources on educating patients with seizure disorders about the risks of burn injury can be a very effective prevention even though the target population is limited. Efforts to overcome public apathy require strategies to sensitize the public to their own vulnerability. International, professional societies and professional publications, as well as posters, can provide avenues to stimulate efforts at national and local levels.

Legislation

On a national or state government level, much can be achieved by legislation, particularly in the industrial arena in relation to standards of equipment, safety inspections, and safety regulations.[4,12] The low incidence of industrial burns relative to the potential for such injuries is an example of the efficacy of such regulations. Similarly, regulations and standards covering the construction of motor vehicles have done much to decrease injuries. Storage of flammable liquids has been regulated to prevent recurrence of the boiling liquid expanding volume explosion (BLEVE) as happened in the Las Alfaque disaster.[13] The transportation of flammable liquids between states and cities can also be controlled by legislated standards. Compulsory installation of smoke detectors and core circuit breakers, along with standards for electrical wiring of houses can increase the safety of home and work environments. Unfortunately in lower socioeconomic groups and in less educated areas there may be bypassing of electrical work which may not be accomplished by professionals, and this makes these areas vulnerable. A provision concerning guards against electrical fires which are deemed adequate by legislated standards has prevented full-thickness burns to the palm of the hand which used to occur commonly, especially among children.

Flammable clothing is a problem which has been successfully approached by legislation in many areas.[14,15] Standards for children's night wear has done much to reduce thermal injuries. The flammability of carpets and draperies can also be attacked by legislating standards. Hot tap water scalds are still very common causes of death.[16–18] Adequate legislation could greatly reduce these injuries.[19] The use of fireworks in some countries is a frequent cause of burn injuries which can be eliminated by the banning or legislated control of fireworks. In Brisbane, the simple step of banning outdoor rubbish fires eliminated from that city burns to children's feet which were caused by walking through hot coals.

While legislation can play a major role in prevention, it is too important an area to leave only to government officials. All members of a burn team, individually and collectively through professional associations, must participate and enlist aid from diverse sources wherever possible, such as service clubs and the media, as well as by living their own lives in a fashion which will set a good example.

Education

Education may be approached by diverse methods (**Table 59.2**). Although most campaigns start with printed materials (e.g. brochures and posters), the persons targeted as most at risk are often the least likely population to read them; thus they may be ineffective in actually preventing injuries.[20] Television and the news media reach large audiences and can greatly increase public awareness. Although purchased time on television is very expensive, there are avenues to obtain publicity free of charge as part of a current affairs bulletin or news segment. The methods used and the messages must vary considerably dependent upon the cultures of the targeted audiences. The education of children can indirectly influence parents and may offer the additional and gradual effect of reducing burns over the long term as those children grow into responsible adults.[21] It should be noted that while education may increase knowledge, it does not necessarily lead to behavioral and/or life style changes.[22] It has been recommended that successful educational programs commence with young children in the early years of elementary school.[23,24] An exemplary 'KIDSAFE' house can be attached to a hospital to demonstrate safety precautions to preschool and school-age children as well as parents-to-be who may tour through the house (**Figure 59.1**).

Table 59.2 Education methods

Brochures
Posters
Television
News media
Target children
'KIDSAFE' house
Puppet shows
Videos

Puppet shows[25] for children can be produced as part of the school curriculum and to educate children and adults in first aid and burn treatment, as well as in fire/burn prevention and survival. Video recordings of such productions can be made widely available and are not as labor intensive as 'live' productions.[18] In addition to obvious target audiences of school children, baby sitters, home care patients, and child care workers could benefit from such videos.[26,27] Whenever programs are developed, whether by live demonstration, puppet shows, or video recordings, there should ideally be a trained person present to answer questions in age-appropriate language.

Specific Areas

Electrical Burn Injuries

Approximately 9% of burn injury hospital admissions are due to electrical injuries. When one considers the potential damage that can be caused by electricity and society's massive reliance on electricity, then this incidence is relatively low. Such injuries have been prevented by a combination of legislation and education. In highly developed countries strict regulations require that electrical installation be made only by qualified electricians and that electrical appliances be manufactured according to strict standards. Core circuit breakers are installed in houses so that a sudden leakage of electricity will switch the power off; this limits the risk of electro-

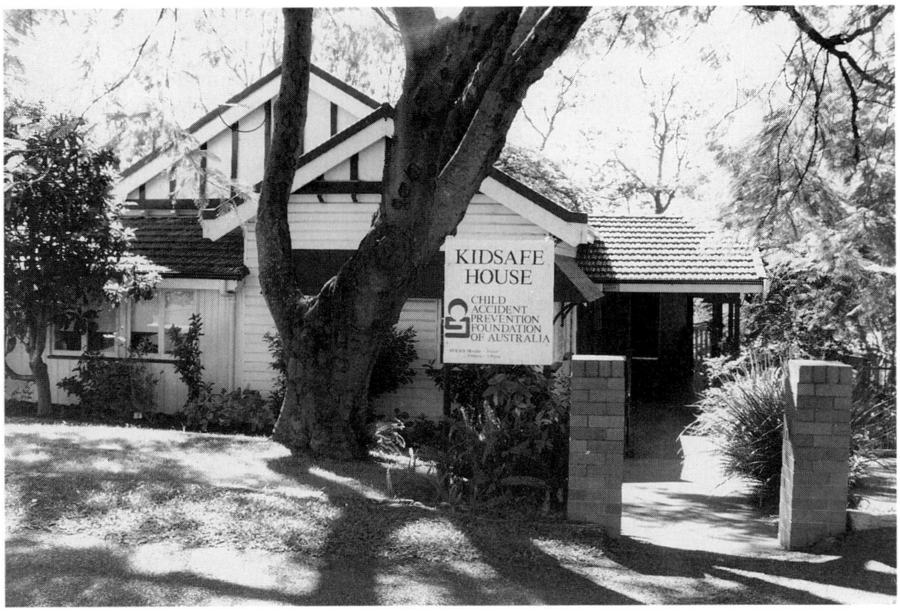

Fig. 59.1 'KIDSAFE house' run by The Child Accident and Prevention Foundation of Australia. Tours of school children and parents are conducted through this house showing various safety measures that can be implemented.

cution and burning. The education of parents and children regarding the hazards of electricity with frequent reminders on television and in the newspapers and magazines have been helpful. The positive effects of such a coordinated approach are evidenced by the uncommon occurrence of injuries to children as opposed to the greater incidence in countries with fewer controls.[28] Electrical burns to the mouth in a pediatric population are reported in the USA but are very rare in Australia where a coordinated program of parental education has been implemented (**Figure 59.2**).

High tension electrical-arc-induced thermal burns, relatively common in industry and in relation to railway overhead cables, are often severe and fatal.[29] In Australia, they occur frequently among teenage boys climbing onto the roofs of railway carriages; with the electrical lines sagging between supports, arcing causes electrical burns, superimposed flame burns, and additional injuries from the fall. Programs to sensitize adolescents to the dangers of their activities and improvements in railway security could help prevent such injuries.

Motor Vehicles

A combination of legislation and regulations have been directed toward manufacturers as well as users of motor vehicles, but motor vehicles are still implicated in many incidents involving severe burns.[30] Strict laws regarding alcohol consumption while operating a motor vehicle have helped reduce the incidence of burns, and laws requiring the use of seat belts have led to decreased deaths following auto crashes. The misuse of gasoline to prime carburetors continues,[31] as do scald injuries from vehicle radiators,[32] although these could be prevented by appropriate vehicle design and public education. Children who are left alone in cars and then play with matches or cigarette lighters invariably sustain severe inhalation injuries.

Motor Cycles

In motor cycle accidents, burns from gasoline are usually severe as the victim is typically very close to the gasoline tank.[33] However, the most common burn injuries related to motorcycles are due to contact burns as skin touches very hot metal. Better vehicular design and use of protective clothing for driver(s) and passenger(s) would limit contact burns and help prevent friction burns. Visors on crash helmets assist in preventing facial burns. Motor cycle clubs and magazines have promoted awareness of burn prevention so successfully that the frequency of these injuries is decreasing. Crashes in motor racing events show well the efficacy of protective clothing (**Table 59.3**).

Table 59.3 Causes of burns from motor cycles and preventive measures

Causes	
	Gasoline[33]
	Hot metal
	Friction
Prevention	
	Education
	Protective clothing
	Vehicle design

Gasoline

The misuses of gasoline cause 7% of burns in children[17] and 23% in adults[5] in Australia. Statistics from other countries reflect similar situations.[34] Gasoline is improperly stored in sheds and garages. Gasoline is also inappropriately used to start barbecues and rubbish fires with disastrous results to the user and bystanders. Gasoline is also the most common flammable agent used in attempted suicides by burning.[35] Such misuse is almost impossible to control by legislation, although legislation has been effective in regulating containers for fuel. Prevention through education programs have not proved successful.[34]

Forest Fires

In hot dry summers, a bushfire is dreaded in Australia in areas prone to such devastation. Similarly, forest fires in the USA have caused much concern. Education in preventing forest fires is paramount, including such programs as 'Smokey' the Bear.[14] Not only should the public be educated to prevent inadvertently starting fires, but household owners need education to protect their buildings. Simple

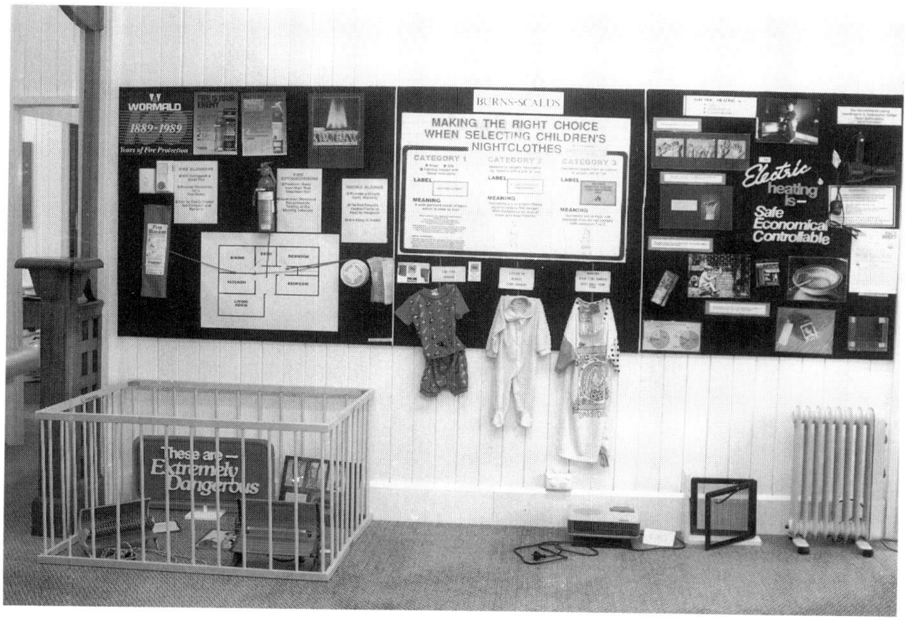
WORMALD
1889–1989
BURNS–SCALDS
MAKING THE RIGHT CHOICE WHEN SELECTING CHILDREN'S NIGHTCLOTHES
Electric heating is— Safe Economical Controllable
These are — Extremely Dangerous

Fig. 59.2 Poster displays showing danger areas and preventative features in relation to electrical burns.

procedures such as removing flammable wastes (e.g. leaves from roofs), maintaining proper guttering, and the use of shutters over windows can do much to prevent houses from burning. Wood shingles instead of nonflammable roof material can create a fire hazard.[3] Increasing public awareness by public education and legislative controls could diminish greatly the risks (**Table 59.4**).

Table 59.4 Aspects of prevention related to forest fires

Education
Smokey the Bear
Prevent fires
Protect buildings
Remove waste
Clear roof
Nonflammable roof[3]
Public awareness

Scalds

Approximately 60% of admissions to children's burn units are due to scalds; 60% are males, and 65% are under 2 years of age.[2] The largest number occurs in the evening when the meal is being prepared or eaten; 82% occur in the patient's own home with 64% occurring in the kitchen.[2] Hot cups of tea and coffee were frequent offenders, and the dangers of a dangling kettle flex (electric cord) are well documented.[36] Fortunately, the majority of these accidents affect small surface areas. A disturbing feature is that 83% occur while a parent is in attendance.[2] In the bathroom, risks of scald injuries are ever-present, and often the scald is much larger and more severe. Most prevention measures in the bathroom have been aimed at preventing access to the hot water tap.[18] Continuous and adequate supervision of the young child in the bath is imperative. The temperature of the water should be tested before a child is placed in the water. The child should not regard the bath as a play area and should not be left unattended by an adult. If the phone rings, the child should be taken out of the bath, wrapped in a towel and taken to the phone.[18]

Most hot water systems are set at temperatures which are too hot because of worries regarding inadequate supplies of hot water. Similarly, solar water systems need mixing valves to limit the temperature, and these valves are readily available[37,38] but not widely used. The effect of legislation to lower the temperature of the water in public buildings to 49°C (120°F) has been shown to be very effective in reducing scalding,[19] but a combination of legislation and education is needed. Parents and doctors must be alerted to the dangers of inhalation of steam with or without chemicals, as when used for treatment of respiratory congestion.[39]

Cooking

Accidents while cooking account for approximately 9% of burn injury admissions,[5] with estimates ranging from 5 to 11%.[40] These occur in both home and commercial cooking areas and often involve cooking in inappropriate vessels.[40] Often fires related to cooking cause houses to burn and persons to sustain severe injuries. Hot grease without flame can also cause severe injuries. Vessels with thermostats should be used for cooking involving oils. Educational material could be supplied with the sale of cooking utensils in order to reduce the risk of thermal injury. The elderly[41,42] are frequently involved with cooking accidents when their clothing ignites while they reach across a stove. Other contributing environmental factors could be identified through investigations and used in designing programs to educate the elderly.

Clothing

In many countries, regulations regarding fabric flammability and the use of fire retardants in clothing have been enacted.[13,14] This concern has extended to the treatment of mattresses, carpets, and furniture. While there have been problems with fire retardants,[14] there has been much success in this area.[13] Changes in the design of children's night wear along with provisions for adequate guards to electrical and open fires have reduced the risks of burns. The benefits of protective clothing have been especially well illustrated in motor racing and motorcycling.

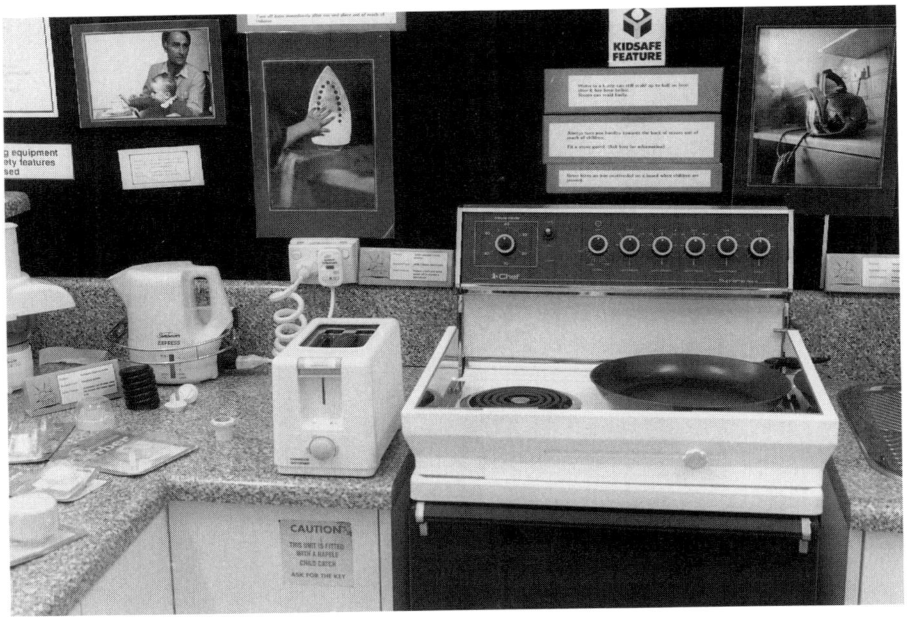

Fig. 59.3 Display showing guard around electric stove, curly cords to the jug with a guard around the jug, handle of fry pan to the back of the stove and other safety features.

Sunburn

In tropical areas, particularly those with large sandy beaches, sunburn is a problem. The body surface areas involved may be large, and the injury may be very painful and quite severe, especially in children. Much of the prevention campaign regarding sunburns has been assumed by anticancer groups with the emphasis on long-term damage and skin cancers. The nightly weather report on television gives the day's ultraviolet ratings. The effects have been positive; sunbathers increasingly avoid the most damaging portions of the day, wearing protective hats, and using good blockout agents (**Table 59.5**).

Table 59.5 Preventive measures for sunburn

Education
Anticancer groups
UV reports on TV
Protective clothes
Hats
Blockout agents

Maritime

Fires do occur at sea where furnace explosions can be lethal; however, maritime laws which regulate safety factors for most large vessels minimize burn injuries at sea. Most burns involving boats occur in pleasure crafts[43] which are subject to less rigorous enforcement of regulations.[43] Carelessness, alcohol intoxication of the crew, and the collection of fumes in the cabin are frequent risk factors in pleasure crafts. Education regarding vessel maintenance and risk factors as well as the provision of firefighting equipment would help to lessen the incidence of injuries. Working through yacht clubs and marinas should render prevention an achievable goal.

Hospitals

Burn injuries in hospitals are not common, but the same injuries that occur in a home can occur in hospital. In addition, there are special high-risk areas in hospitals. For example, an operating theater involves such risks as the use of laser, cautery, chemicals, anaesthetic agents, and heating pads. In nursing homes, many agents can present dangers when combined with the problems of the physically and mentally infirm: hot foods and beverages, carelessness in smoking tobacco, electrical blankets and hot water bottles are potential dangers in patients with physical and mental impairments. The high cost of litigation is an added incentive for prevention campaigns in these institutions (**Table 59.6**).

Table 59.6 Danger areas in hospitals

Operating rooms
Laser
Cautery
Chemicals
Anesthetic agents
Heating pads
Wards – ill patients
Hot foods
Hot beverages
Smoking
Electric blankets
Hot water bottles

Industry

Molten metal burns, electrical injuries, and a multitude of chemical injuries occur in industrial settings.[12] Fire can be a major hazard in factories, and management must establish secure escape routes.[44] Staff should be trained in fire prevention and made aware of the risks from molten metal and chemicals. First aid officers must know which chemicals are in use and the appropriate first aid treatment for each.[45]

Cigarettes

Despite the hazards involved, smoking cigarettes remains a part of the social milieu. The introduction of self-extinguishing cigarettes could help reduce the incidence of house and forest fires.[3,14] Allied to cigarettes are the dangers of matches and cigarette lighters, which are factors in many house and caravan (mobile home) fires resulting in burn injuries and death.[46] Cigarette lighters must not be regarded as toys and must be kept out of the reach of young children. Smoking in bed, especially combined with the use of alcohol and/or sleeping tablets, results in a high mortality and morbidity rate. A smoke detector in the ceiling above the bed could reduce injuries in these cases. Vast education campaigns have helped to reduce the smoking of cigarettes, but a serious problem still remains.

Home Heaters

Gas heaters pose problems as do hot water systems with gas pilot lights and flammable liquids stored nearby.[3] Wood burning stoves for heating may be unsafely installed or have inadequate guards.[3] Faulty fireplace flues can cause house fires. Contact burns, particularly to the hands of children, easily occur from many kinds of heaters, especially kitchen stoves and hot plates. Proper installation and education designed to increase public awareness are needed in the home environment.

Warfare

Burn injuries peculiar to warfare are those associated with explosions of missiles and rockets as well as certain chemicals. Troops must be well trained to prevent injuries to themselves. The use of protective clothing for this purpose is well documented.[47]

Assessment of Results

A prevention campaign can be an expensive operation in terms of time, effort, and financial resources, and it may take years for the results to become apparent.[21] While burn prevention is a long-term strategy, an assessment of the success of a program is essential. This can be done via properly designed and executed prospective clinical trails.[48] Formulae are available to assess the incidence of burn injuries and burn mortality in a given population size. Obviously this may be easier in a large metropolitan population than in a smaller rural population. Such analyses offer a prevention team an opportunity to demonstrate the importance of appropriate statistical analysis. Additionally, an assessment can be done in a less complicated way by pre- and post-testing of the program.[24] For example, a program for school children can be assessed by examination. With an elderly group, a less formal type of evaluation can be used.[49] Assessment gives useful feedback regarding the efficacy of a program, including the effectiveness of legislation in preventing a particular type of burn injury.[13] Ultimately, burn prevention begins at home,[50] and the efficacy of the example set by caregivers can be assessed by the final outcome.

Summary

Etiologies of burn injuries vary from locality to locality depending on customs, socioeconomic conditions, the predominant industries, the level of education of the population, housing standards, and many other factors. To coordinate prevention strategies, epidemiology in areas of concern need to be studied. Campaigns and techniques from other countries can do much to give a headstart to the task of developing strategies to increase public awareness and reduce the incidence of burn injuries. The simple fact remains, however, that while most burn injuries can be prevented, it will take a lot of educating to raise awareness so that complete prevention can be achieved. In the meantime, any opportunity should be grasped to spread the safety message, be it a slot on television or graphic posters in a less literate society. The prevention strategy must be tailored to the local needs. Prevention is better than cure.

References

1. O'Ya H, Ohmori S. Most burns are preventable. *Burns* 1978; **5:** 8–11.
2. Phillips W, Mahairis E, Hunt D, Pegg S. The epidemiology of childhood scalds in Brisbane. *Burns* 1986; **12:** 343–50.
3. Silverstein P, Lack B O. Epidemiology and prevention. In: Boswick J A, ed. *The Art and Service of Burn Care*. Rockville: Aspen, 1987; Chapter 2: 11–17.
4. de Kock M. The Cape Town burn profile. *Burns* 1978; **5:** 210–11.
5. Pegg S P, Gregory J J, Hogan P G, Mottarelly I W, Walker L F. Epidemiological pattern of adult burn injuries. *Burns* 1979; **5:** 326–34.
6. Mason S A, Hillier V F. Decreased awareness of surroundings in childhood thermal injuries. *Burns* 1992; **18**(6): 513–14.
7. Pegg S P, McDonald G P, Tracey-Patti C E, Mayze T D. Epidemiology of burns attending a Casualty Department in Brisbane. *Burns* 1983; **9:** 416–21.
8. Lochaitis A, Iliopoulou E, Komninakis E, *et al.* Burns as a result of domestic accidents and their prevention. *Burns* 1992; **18**(5): 416–18.
9. Slater S J, Slater H, Goldfarb I W. Burned children – a socio-economic profile for focused prevention programs. *J Burn Care Rehabil* 1987; **8**(6): 566–7.
10. Siu S, Lehman M L, Longden L A, Pegg S P. Burn injuries associated with epilepsy. *Proc Div Surg R Brisbane Hosp* 1987; **3:** 41–6.
11. Backstein R, Peters W, Neligan P. Burns in the disabled. *Burns* 1993; **19**(3): 192–7.
12. Pegg S P, Miller P M, Sticklen E J, Storie W J. Epidemiology of industrial burns in Brisbane. *Burns* 1986; **12**(7): 484–90.
13. Arturson G. The Los Alfaques disaster – a boiling liquid expanding vapor explosion. *Burns* 1981; **7:** 233.
14. Langley J, McLoughlin E. Difficulties and bonuses of evaluation: evaluating New Zealand's Children's Night Clothes Act 1977. *Burns* 1988; **14**(6): 435–9.
15. Silverstein P. Burn prevention: recollections. *J Burn Care Rehabil* 1993; **14:** 281–3.
16. Walker A R. Fatal tapwater scald burns in the USA 1979–86. *Burns* 1990; **16:** 49–52.
17. Pegg S P, Gregory J J, Hogan P G M, Mottarelly I W, Walker L F. Burns in childhood – an epidemiological surgery. *Aust NZ J Surg* 1978; **4:** 365–73.
18. Maley M F. Scald burns associated with tap water. *J Burn Care Rehabil* 1989; **10**(2): 172–3.
19. Erdmann T C, Feldman K W, Rivara F P, Heimbach D M, Wall H A. Tap water burn prevention. *Pediatrics* 1991; **88**(3): 572–7.
20. Hammond J, Varas R. Coordinated strategies in burn prevention programs: a case study. *J Burn Care Rehabil* 1990; **11**(4): 376–8.
21. Keswani M H. The prevention of burn injury. *Burns* 1986; **12**(8): 533–9.
22. Linares A Z, Linares H A. Burn prevention: the need for a comprehensive approach. *Burns* 1990; **16**(4): 281–5.
23. Varas R, Carcone R, Hammond J S. A one-hour burn prevention program for grade school children: its approach and success. *J Burn Care Rehabil* 1981; **9**(1): 69–71.
24. Eckelt K, Fannon M, Blades B, Munster A M. A successful burn prevention program in elementary schools. *J Burn Care Rehabil* 1985; **6**(6): 509–10.
25. Morrison M I S, Herath K, Chase C. Puppets for prevention: 'playing safe is playing smart'. *J Burn Care Rehabil* 1988; **9**(6): 650–1.

26. Schmeer S, Stern N, Monafo W W. An outreach burn prevention program for home care patients. *J Burn Care Rehabil* 1988; **9**(6): 645–7.

27. Meyer M. 'Baby-walker' frames: a preventable factor in infant burns. *Burns* 1988; **14**(2): 145–6.

28. Heberal M, Oner Z, Bayraktar U, Bilgin N. Epidemiology of adults' and childrens' burns in a Turkish burn center. *Burns* 1987; **13**(2): 136–40.

29. Koller J. High tension electrical-arc-induced thermal burns caused by railway overhead cables. *Burns* 1991; **17**(5): 411–14.

30. Pegg S P, Mayze T D. Burn injuries associated with road trauma. *Aust NZ J Surg* 1980; **50**(60): 593–6.

31. Abidin M R, Williams M F, Munster A M. Carburetor burns: preventable injuries associated with high morbidity and frequent litigation. *J Burn Care Rehabil* 1990; **11**(5): 451–3.

32. Benmier P, Rosenberg L, Sagi A, Bur Yakar Y. Radiator scald burns: a preventable hazard. *Burns* 1990; **16**(2): 135–6.

33. Pegg S P, Mayze T D. Burn injuries associated with motorcycles. Burns 1983; **9:** 288–91.

34. Williams J B, Ahrenholy D H, Solem L D, Warren W. Gasoline burns: the preventable cause of burn injuries. *J Burn Care Rehabil* 1990; **11**(5): 446–50.

35. Persley G V, Pegg S P. Burn injuries related to suicide. *Med J Aust* 1981; **1:** 134.

36. Burd D A, Burd E. The electric kettle flex – a cause for concern. *Burns* 1985; **12**(2): 136–8.

37. Murray J P. A study of the prevention of hot tapwater burns. *Burns* 1988; **14**(3): 185–95.

38. Stephen F R, Murray J P. Prevention of hot tap water burns – A comparative study of three types of automatic mixing valve. *Burns* 1993; **19**(1): 56–62.

39. Pegg S P, Campbell D C. Children's burns due to cresol. *Burns* 1985; **11:** 294–6.

40. Pegg S P, Seawright A A. Burns due to cooking oils – an increasing hazard. *Burns* 1983; **9:** 362–9.

41. Turner D G, Leman C J, Jordon M H. Cooking-related burn injuries in the elderly. Preventing the 'granny gown' burn. *J Burn Care Rehabil* 1989; **10**(4): 356–7.

42. Lewandowski R, Pegg S P, Fortier K, Skimmings A. Burn injuries in the elderly. *Burns* 1993; **19**(6): 513–15.

43. Shergill G, Scerri G V, Regan P J, Roberts A H N. Burn injuries in boating accidents. *Burns* 1993; **19**(3): 229–31.

44. Benmeir P, Sagi A, Rosenberg L. An example of burn prevention: the 'Urim' factory fire. *Burns* 1989; **15**(3): 252–3.

45. Pegg S P, Siu S, Gillett G. Intra-arterial infusions in the treatment of hydrofluoric acid burns. *Burns* 1985; **11:** 440–3.

46. Maley M P. Children under age five and butane cigarette lighters. *J Burn Care Rehabil* 1988; **9**(4): 423–4.

47. Shafir R, Nili E, Kedem R. Burn injury and prevention in the Lebanon war 1982. *Israel J Med Sci* 1984; **20**(4): 311–13.

48. Peck M D, Maley M. Population requirements for statistical analysis of efficacy of burn prevention programs. *J Burn Care Rehabil* 1981; **12**(3): 282–4.

49. Victor J, Lawrence P, Munster A, Horn D. A statewide targeted burn prevention program. *J Burn Care Rehabil* 1988; **9**(4): 425–9.

50. Varas R, Hammond J S. Burn prevention begins at home – your home. *J Burn Car Rehabil* 1989; **10**(1): 88.

CHAPTER SIXTY

ETHICALLY VALID DECISION MAKING

BRUCE ZAWACKI

INTRODUCTION

Moral decision making in medicine is like breathing: we all do it all the time. Only when it becomes difficult are we even conscious of it.[1] If, in a given case, the cause of breathing difficulty is not obvious, then a formal and sophisticated analysis of the complex physiologic events involved in normal and abnormal breathing may be required in order to clarify and solve, or at least manage, the problem. Similarly, if the decision about what is morally right or wrong to do in a given medical case proves difficult, a formal, critical, and at times in-depth analysis of arguments, assumptions, and decision-making processes will often be necessary. Such a disciplined analysis of morality and moral decision making is what we mean by ethics. Applied to medical problems, it is termed medical ethics.

Ethics proves at times to be difficult, controversial, and changing. But so too are the pathophysiological mechanisms thought to be involved in, for example, the adult respiratory distress syndrome (ARDS). No apologies are necessary, therefore, for the intricacies of some of the diagrams which follow. Despite their apparent complexity, I believe physicians (and patients) will find them 'user-friendly' because the concepts and processes which they depict are familiar; as much as possible the approach in this chapter will be to criticize and clarify with ethical sensitivity the physician–patient interactions which have already become habitual for most of us. In effect, this chapter hopes to examine the familiar in order to help readers appreciate, perhaps for the first time, the ethical dimensions of what they have been doing all along, and to help locate points of difficulty when they are encountered.

Finally, not textbook authors, but *doctor and patient together* are *ultimately* responsible for dealing with a particular problem of dyspnea or of ethical decision making at the bedside. Ethics, at its best, is about personal struggle and achievement, not passive acceptance of 'expert' opinions. This chapter seeks, therefore, to coach both caregivers and carereceivers toward active, synergistic collaboration as well as recognition that the burden of ethical decision making, while always personal, need not always be lonely.

This chapter was adapted from an article entitled *Principios eticos en las unidades de cuidados intensivos* originally published in Spanish in *Tradado de Quemaduras*, First Edition, A Bendlin, 1991, published by Interamerican New Editoral, Cedro 512, Mexico, D.F. 06450.

How?

In a pluralistic democratic society, universally accepted or imposed norms of right and wrong are rare. In such a society, how a decision is made – the process – is extremely important, and very often decisive. In what follows, I have attempted to utilize and improve upon previously published models of 'an ethical work-up'[2–6] and to be as visual as possible in order to help decision makers keep the many steps and perspectives which are involved in their task constantly in view.[7]

As diagrammed in **Figure 60.1**, ethical decision making in a burn center or intensive care unit (ICU) typically involves a four-part transaction.

The Physician's Role (Figure 60.1, part a)

A physician's initial role is to provide to a patient or patient-surrogate the information necessary for valid assent to or refusal of treatment. This involves three steps:[8]

1. The first step is *diagnostic* and answers the question 'What can be wrong?' It is scientific, weighing the probabilities and costs of errors, and after consideration of possibilities produces the most probable diagnosis.
2. The second step is *therapeutic* and answers the question 'What can be done?' It too is scientific (or at least 'professional' and weighs all plausible treatments, their prognoses, pros and cons, finally narrowing them down to 'indicated treatments' with their prognoses and their pros and cons. ('Pros and cons' will be used herein to signify risks versus benefits, prohibitions versus obligations, etc.) Although a physician has a moral obligation to carry out this step competently, this step is *not* a formally moral step in that it does not yet provide a recommendation for which a physician bears responsibility. After all, 'indicated treatments' are those prescribed by textbook authors for textbook cases. They are based on purely pathophysiologic considerations independent of the unique details about, and values of, a particular caregiver and a particular patient.
3. The third step is formally *moral* in that it answers the question 'What should be done?' The presence of the word 'should' explicitly indicates that moral language is being used. Based on

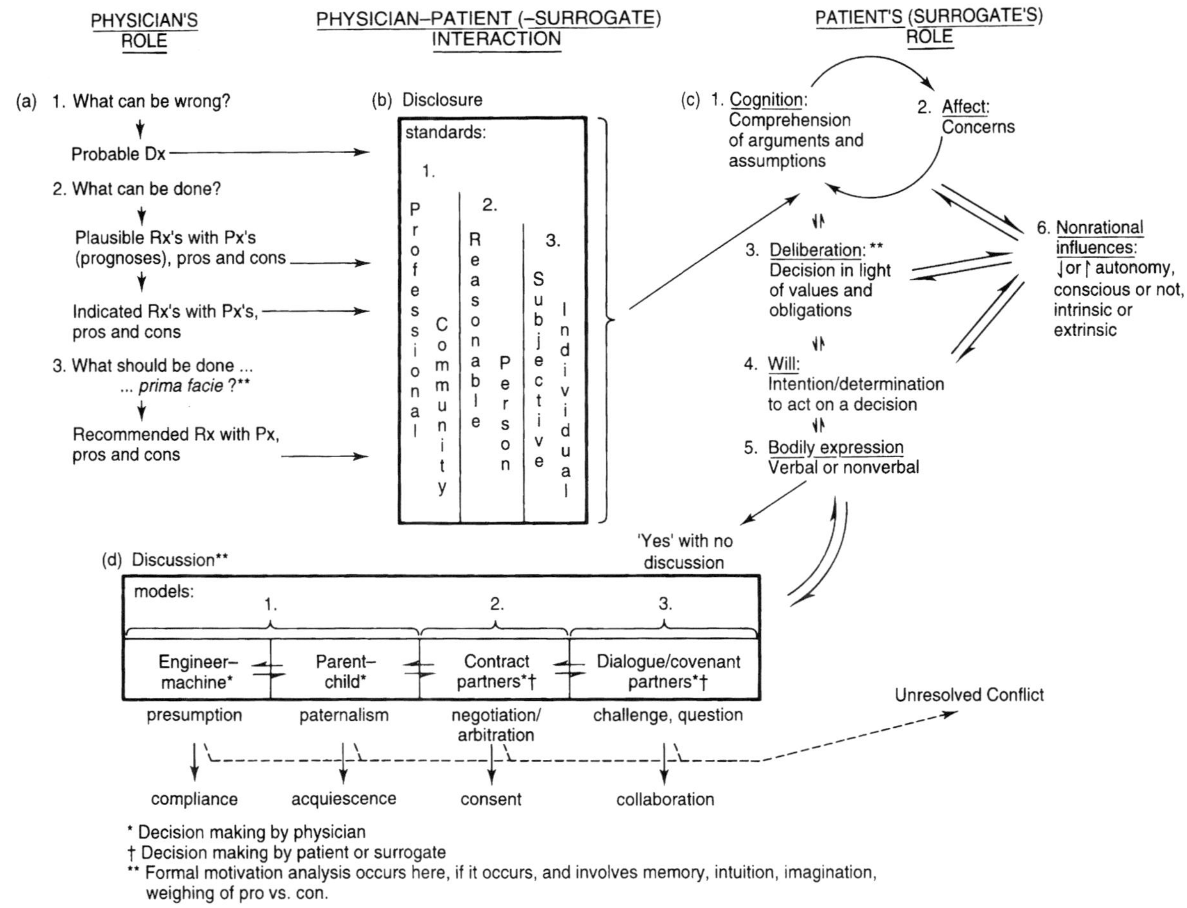

Fig. 60.1 Flow diagram of the process of decision making in the burn center illustrating (a) the three-step initial role of the physician, (b) the initial physician–patient (-surrogate) interaction of disclosure, (c) the role of the patient or his surrogate, and (d) the four common models of physician–patient discussion. As described in the text, the numbered discussion models are logical continuations of the numbered disclosure standards.

an initial evaluation of a patient and his condition (for simplicity masculine pronouns will be used when referring to physicians, patients and/or surrogates) in as much detail as a physician is able to discover about the patient's unique characteristics and values; this step results in a recommended treatment with a prognosis, together with an evaluation of the pros and cons involved. It is prima facie or initial because it is subject to reconsideration and reevaluation after further discussion with the patient or patient-surrogate.

In fashioning a recommendation, a physician deliberates on the information he has developed, weighing the options in the light of his own value system and of what he knows about a patient's system of values and obligations. He then makes a value judgment about what should be recommended, develops an intention to express it, and barring interference, does so. Of course like any other human being, a physician is subject to many unconscious and/or nonrational influences in making decisions. This complex process is at the heart of ethical decision making for *both physician and patient* and will be further detailed below under 'The patient's or surrogate's role'.

The Initial Physician–Patient Interaction: Disclosure (Figure 60.1, part b)

As indicated in **Figure 60.1**, part (a) produces precisely those details of information which are needed by a patient or his surrogate as raw material in considering whether he should assent to a recommended treatment. If there are significant gaps in this information, to that extent the validity of the patient's or surrogate's decision is in jeopardy. Note (**Figure 60.1**, part b) that three standards of disclosure have been developed in the USA, each filtering out less information from the patient than the one before. The *professional community standard* (b)-1 requires revelation of only that which is customarily disclosed by an appropriately trained and experienced physician in a given location. The *reasonable person standard* (b)-2 requires disclosure of what a hypothetical 'reasonable patient' would want to know. The *subjective individual standard* (b)-3 filters out the least amount of information by requiring the physician to provide all that this particular patient, here and now, needs to know in order to decide.[9]

The Patient's or Surrogate's Role

This is to develop valid, autonomous assent to or refusal of a physician's initial recommendation. As illustrated in **Figure 60.1**, part c, the steps involved in decision making by a patient or patient-surrogate are recognizable, on reflection, as what all human beings do everyday in making decisions.[10] First a patient or surrogate tries to comprehend the situation as disclosed to him (c)-1. Almost inevitably (but not always immediately), this evokes some affect or concern (c)-2 which may, in turn, influence cognition. For example, serving not as a responsible physician but as a surrogate for my wife, fears about the incompleteness of my own life without her might encourage me to focus only on hope and make me unwilling or unable even to consider foregoing life support should she be burned and precedent for survival be absent. On the other hand, in part because I believe that absolutely unwavering commitment to an enormously painful and arduous task is necessary in order not to lose courage or miss any opportunity for success, any suggestions that I, as physician, give less than maximal care to a child with a 98% total body surface area (TBSA) full-thickness burn so as to insure every chance of survival, strikes fear and anger into my heart and is likely to trigger, in me, a perception of the individual making the suggestion as disloyal, cowardly, or unreliable. In both cases, initially at least, affect would color cognition significantly and change my *appreciation*[11] of the situation; this can occur in physicians, patients and/or surrogates. After comprehending and appreciating the information disclosed, a patient or surrogate ideally deliberates (c)-3, weighing options in the light of prior values, arriving at what is believed to be an appropriate value judgment of a given option. He then decides whether or not he intends to act on that judgment (c)-4 and finally does or does not express that intention in word and/or deed (c)-5.

Logically these steps run in serial order: cognition/affect–deliberation–intention–behavior. At any point in the process, however, nonrational influences (c)-6 may enhance or diminish a patient's or surrogate's autonomy. For example, 'sleeping on a problem overnight' or receiving encouragement, etc. may increase autonomy; while pain, fear, etc. may decrease autonomy. Whether intrinsic (e.g. hypoxemia or electrolyte abnormality) or extrinsic (e.g. fear of punishment and/or harassment by others), these influences are described as nonrational, not because they cannot be understood, but because they affect decision making biologically, biochemically, socially, etc. rather than be appealing to rationality. Moreover, as indicated by the reversing arrows in **Figure 60.1**, part (c), any step taken may trigger reconsideration and revision of one or more prior steps. For example, arriving at and articulating a decision to discontinue life support may seem acceptable to a patient until a physician announces he will now pull the plug. At that point fear may cause an alert patient to reevaluate his situation (e.g. 'Life on a ventilator isn't *that* bad!'), and he may repeat steps (c)-1 through (c)-5 but this time arrive at a decision to remain on life support measures.

To the extent that the above-mentioned process is carried out effectively, consent to or refusal of a physician's initial recommendation will be more or less valid, that is *informed* (comprehending and appreciating pertinent information), *free* (substantially free of distorting nonrational/emotional influences), *deliberate* (decided after weighing facts and pros and cons in the light of one's value systems), *voluntary* (reflecting a patient's own intentions and determinations, and *expressed* (communicated by verbal or nonverbal means). Clinical determination of the 'decision-making capacity' or 'substantial autonomy'[12] of a patient assesses just these parameters. This is typically done by verifying a patient's comprehension by asking if he can rephrase the information provided to him in his own words, and by asking him to explain why he has made the decision he has. Investigation into the role of nonrational influences may be necessary to assure an autonomous decision, and of course pain should be controlled as much as possible. When in cases of dispute, a court is asked to adjudicate the decision-making capacity of a patient or patient-surrogate, typically a formal hearing occurs and a technical-legal determination of 'competence' or 'incompetence' is sought. Formal adjudication is rarely required in making treatment decisions, however, and the nontechnical term 'decision-making capacity' is more correct in everyday clinical use.

Discussion Between Physician and Patient or Surrogate (Figure 60.1. part d)

If a patient agrees with the recommendation of a physician, no further discussion is necessary. If, on the other hand, further discussion is necessary because of some doubts or questions on the part of the patient or his surrogate, several modes of interaction are possible.[13] In the engineer–machine interaction, a physician makes all the decisions and acts without discussion, forcing compliance from a patient or surrogate. In the parent–child interaction, a patient or his surrogate may be allowed to speak but, like a child, will not be taken seriously, and a physician as a paternalistic figure will demand the acquiescence of the patient. Here also the physician is virtually the only decision maker, the patient or surrogate being overcome typically by the rank and social influence of the physician. On the other hand, physician and patient or surrogate may disagree and be able to negotiate a mutually acceptable compromise or contract resulting in consent by the patient or surrogate (**Figure 60.1**, part (d)-2). Under ideal circumstances, however, not a physical or social overpowering, nor an armistice of wills, but a meeting of minds and reason is achievable through dialogue which allows a mutually committed physician and patient or surrogate to reason together and develop collaborative agreement (**Figure 60.1**, part (d)-3). In part (d)-2 and (d)-3, both physician and patient or surrogate are involved in decision making. Although it is true that, all else being equal, consent and collaboration (the right side of the scale in **Figure 60.1**, part d) are more respectful of the dignity and growth of decision makers than are compliance and acquiescence (the left side of the scale), it must not be supposed that they are always so. Lack of time, suicidal intent, or incapacity to decide on the part of a patient may force use of an engineer–machine or parent–child model at least temporarily. Later, however, with stabilization and/or identification of a surrogate, contract or dialogue may be possible, especially during the rehabilitative phases of care. Thus, as indicated by the reversing arrows between the models (**Figure 60.1**, part d), it is often necessary to move from one model to another at different times with the same or different patients. Chances of synergy in a 'win–win relationship' are enhanced, however, and influence is more rational than nonrational with progress toward the right of the scale. If, despite all efforts, a conflict remains unresolved, in the United States a hospital ethicist, ethics committee,[6] or court may be consulted.

To illustrate how the decision-making process, which is diagrammed in **Figure 60.1**, may work in dealing with a patient with large burns, the case of an 80-year-old with a 90% full-thickness burns may present little problem with completing step (a)-1: his injury is typically easy to diagnose. In considering step (a)-2, among the *plausible* treatments are:

- (i) active involuntary euthanasia without disclosure by administration of, for example, intravenous potassium and barbiturate (this is a *plausible* option for some people even though illegal in all countries, including Holland);
- (ii) no therapy of burn shock, allowing a patient to die with comfort measures only but without necessarily discussing options with the patient or family;
- (iii) treating burn shock to facilitate collaborative discussion about subsequent management with the patient if he becomes competent or with his surrogate if he does not; or
- (iv) fluid therapy of burn shock and massive excision with application of cultured autokeratinocytes whether the patient approves or not.

A review of textbooks on this matter would reveal option (iv) to be the 'indicated' treatment, i.e. 'pointed to' by consideration only of the pathophysiology involved in the case: an engineer–machine relationship. Options (i) and (ii), though *very* different morally are similar to option (iv) in disregarding the value of input from the patient or patient-surrogate and similarly achieve compliance or at best an acquiescent parent–child relationship. Of the options discussed (there are several others), only (iii) attempts to provide the patient or surrogate with an autonomous role by engagement in collaborative ethical dialogue.

If physicians *habitually* treat their patients as engineers do their machines or as parents do their children, they may *habitually* disenfranchise their patients by denying them necessary information. If, whenever possible, an effort is made to enhance patient decision-making capacity by treating shock, removing pain, etc., then giving a patient the requisite disclosure and allowing a valid contribution by the patient is possible, even if only by designating a surrogate. If for some reason a patient's capacity to make a valid decision is diminished and cannot be enhanced, rarely a previously executed 'living will' or a 'durable power of attorney for health-care decisions',[14] which designates a surrogate, may assist in discovering what a patient's wishes might be. If a close friend or family member is available who has some idea what a patient's wishes may have been in the past, then with appropriate precautions that individual or individuals may be helpful in deducing or otherwise discerning the patient's wishes, even without a formal designation of a surrogate. When no such information is available, in most jurisdictions in the United States a decision is appropriately made by seeking what appears to be in the 'patient's best interests'. This term refers to the patient's welfare as well as the physician and other caregivers are able to guess it based on what a reasonable person could be expected to want under these circumstances. In some localities, however, recommendations have been made that such cases go either to an ethics committee or to the courts for review.[15]

While not often considered, the decision-making capacity of a physician is not always perfect. Often distorting nonrational or unreflected-upon affective influences may be minimized or avoided by taking the time to develop a cordial and trust-building relationship with a patient or surrogate before pressing either for consent to a recommendation. Talking with other team members in order to come to a consensus,[16] using a social worker to sort out one's feelings about a case, or simply 'sleeping on a problem overnight' are also helpful.

WHY?

Why do physicians and patients decide one way rather than another in making life and death decisions in the ICU? What impulses, constraints, motivations, etc. influence the decision at which they arrive? Some motivations we invent; more are experienced passively; still more (probably) are unconscious. But as stated by no less an authority than Plato, the unexamined life is not worth living. The mature life of moral responsibility requires that we bring to consciousness all the significant motivations of our important personal decisions so that we can deliberately choose among them.

Of course, insights about why we choose to act this way or that can come at any time even without conscious effort. As part of a formal medical decision-making effort, however, motivation analysis, that is intentional examination and critique of our choices among available options, world views, values, goals, etc., occurs most logically during deliberation and discussion (indicated in **Figure 60.1** by a double asterisk **) and is a task to be faced by the patient or his surrogate as well as by the physician.

Many relationships influence and motivate decisions about life and death in a burn center (**Figure 60.2**). Typically, and day-to-day, we physicians are motivated by world views and values which are limited to the central regions of the diagram: we wear moral blinders which give us 'telescopic vision' to focus technically on a patient as a bearer of diseased organs or organ systems for which we can provide diagnosis, therapy, and prevention. When physicians stereotypically use this limited perception, then short of brain death in a patient, they may habitually direct unlimited effort at cure and control of disease in every case regardless of the decision-making capacity or wishes of the patient or his surrogate. This is especially understandable in difficult cases because, unless caregivers focus intently on cure, success is less likely. In response to this, patients' rights advocates move a step more peripherally in this scheme (**Figure 60.2**) in order to trump the engineer–machine domination of physicians over their patients. They assert that a patient's role as a member of the subcultural reference group called consumers gives him certain rights. Deciding to continue or discontinue maximal therapy for any illness, without even attempting to achieve informed consent, they see as a violation of patients' rights.

As physicians, our response to this consumer-oriented position is also quite typical. If conflict cannot be resolved using the narrow engineer–machine perspective, then we too move one step more peripheral in the scheme to use the power of a different set of subculture groups. We may mobilize nurses, chaplains, and

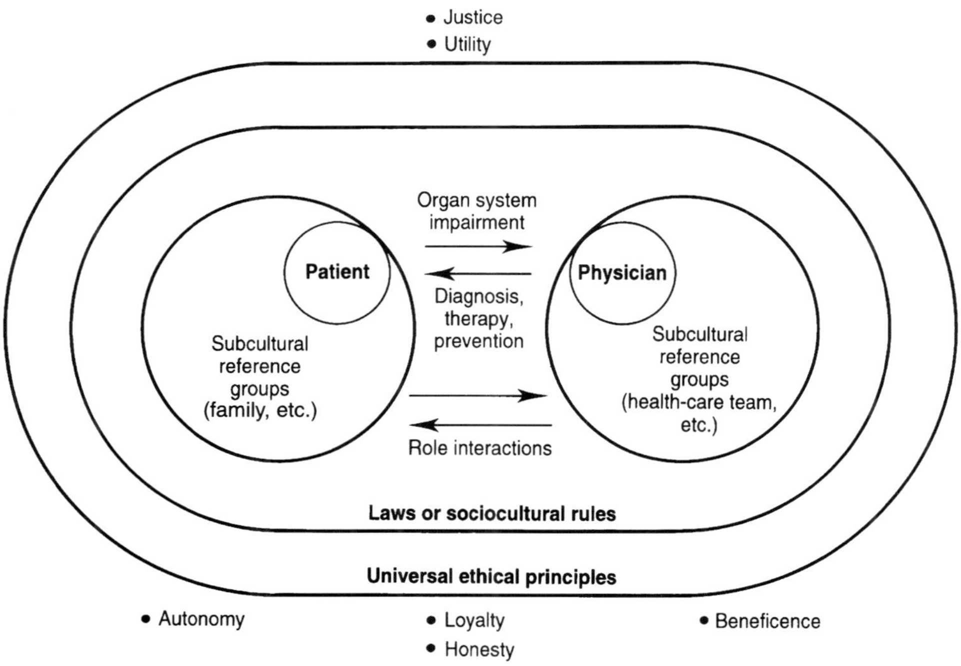

Fig. 60.2 The physician–patient relationship in the burn center seen as part of a system in which not only technical factors, but also roles, laws and ethical principles motivate behavior. Modified from Bloom[17] with permission from the Russell Sage Foundation.

psychiatrists to convince a patient. For support we may turn to colleagues, to hospital administration, to decision-making ethics committees and risk management teams, even to a national medical-specialty consensus statement, all in order to buttress our position and to motivate a patient to agree with us. In response, patients or surrogates may react in kind by seeking a patient ombudsman, consulting an ethics committee, or getting friends to support them. If agreement or compromise is not reached, escalation peripherally to the level of law may occur: the hospital lawyer may be consulted, the family lawyer may give the physician a call, and eventually a lawsuit may even be filed.

Influences which motivate physicians and patients in their decisionmaking can be visualized as a series of complex and constantly changing force fields and conflicting impulses. Ethical principles (the most peripheral ring of forces depicted in **Figure 60.2**) have been articulated in an effort to resolve such conflict at the broadest and most universal level.[18] But clearly, for example, the beneficent desire of a physician to cure an illness may still conflict with the autonomy of a patient or with what is owed in justice to other patients. Ethical and theological theories or schemes have been elaborated throughout all of human history in an effort to reconcile conflicting ethical principles. These models tend to be abstract, rational, general and universal in their language, and are located, even more peripheral than ethical principles, at a point very distant from 'everyday life'. The very multiplicity of such theories demonstrates the lack of consensus and inability of any one of them to resolve the above-mentioned conflicts for prolonged periods of time. Serious students of these problems have no alternative but to live within this vortex of ambiguity and to struggle for reasons and models which seem to make sense. The endpoint chosen, the position temporarily accepted, is usually some sort of compromise or balance, a 'reflective equilibrium'[19] which appears to maximize the welfare and dignity values of those involved and appears least offensive to moral sensibility, is most consistent, least contradictory, etc. Of course, new facts, new visions, etc. may force a conscientious reentry into the firestorm of opposing motivations and rationalizations. The search for clarifying models and analogies is among the most creative activities in ethics and involves what is called the 'moral imagination'. This activity is not limited to grand overarching ethical theories. For example, in considering patients without precedent for survival in a situation of resource scarcity, the physician may be construed as analogous to a defense lawyer doing all that is possible (seeking loopholes if that is what a patient wants) to get maximum treatment for the patient while insuring that all parties respect valid law. This places a physician in the role of patient advocate in opposition to those who would limit treatment in a given case. It also enhances a patient's trust. It is not an unpatriotic position violating the requirements of distributive justice any more than that of the defense lawyer who, in a murder trial, holds an analogous position defending his client against the interests of the state or country in matters of retributive justice.[20]

Analogies, examples, theories, models, etc. like the above are explicitly rational ethical motivators for decision making. They do not use physical fear, social power, or anxiety about legal sanctions in order to obtain agreement but depend upon the rational attraction of a cognitive construction. This is the realm of formal ethical endeavor and creative ethical scholarship, several examples of which will be found below.

WHAT?

In life and death decision making in a burn center, certain characteristics of or labels applied to actions are often cited as sufficient to distinguish right from wrong. What are some of these characteristics, and which, if any, by themselves, are adequate moral criteria?

'Indicated' Versus 'Futile' or 'Hopeless' Treatment

Considering burned patients 'without precedent for survival', a 1979 National Institutes of Health Consensus Exercise[21] concluded that physicians have:

- the duty always to give 'resuscitation' (i.e. fluid therapy for burn shock) if only to avoid stifling therapeutic progress; and
- the authority to do so without obtaining informed consent because 'physical and/or emotional shock ... make it impossible for a victim to contribute to the early decision making process'.

In 1980,[22] and more recently,[23] other authors echoed roughly similar conclusions about various classifications of burned patients. In opposition, a series of papers stated that physicians:

- have the duty not to treat burn shock in patients without precedent for survival, because it is 'futile' to do so; and
- have (with certain exceptions) the authority to proceed in this way.[24–26]

Advocates of patient autonomy and informed consent have claimed both these positions to be paternalistic, i.e. 'benevolent but also treating the patient (or surrogate) as a child who cannot be permitted to determine his or her own welfare or the means to it.'[27] These advocates of informed consent sought to restore decision-making capacity to such burned patients as soon as possible after admission, or, if that could not be accomplished, to let the 'socially designated next-of-kin or other relatives speak for the patient'.[28,29] Since these publications, opponents on all sides of this issue have remained apparently adamant about and immovable from their original positions despite several, virtually annual, public airings of their differences at national meetings.

In an interesting parallel, between 1987 and 1991, a series of papers were published about nonburned patients by individual physicians[30] or specialty groups[31–33] asserting that if a specific intervention (particularly CPR) is in 'general medical opinion ...'[31] or by 'Consensus ... probably on the national level,'[30] considered 'futile', then 'The issue of patient autonomy is irrelevant'[30] and the intervention 'need not be performed or even discussed with the patient and/or his surrogate[31] *even if previously requested by the patient*'.[33] Again, in opposition to this 'paternalist' position, advocates of patient autonomy affirmed the necessity of patient inclusion in such decision-making discussions.[34,35] Despite very insightful efforts at clarification and reconciliation,[36] recent publications give evidence that opponents have become entrenched in their positions despite (or perhaps because of) escalating verbal warfare between them.[37,38]

These debates cannot be resolved here, but (as indicated in **Figure 60.1**, parts (d)-1 and (d)-2) it can be suggested that opponents in both these debates (including the author) have rather stereotypically engaged in an 'engineer–machine' or 'paternalistic' versus a 'consent-based' model of discussion with each other. We have modeled for physicians and patients/surrogates how not to listen to each other, and how to seek to overpower verbally rather than collaborate. I believe it is now time for spokespersons on both sides of both debates to model

- listening, working, collaborating dialogue rather than verbal warfare;

- vulnerable, 'subjective individual' self-disclosure of the assumptions and nonrationalities which we bring to the debate; and
- commitment to win–win rather than win–lose relationships (**Figure 60.1**, part (d)-3).[39] The lessons learned would be worth more than any further searches for 'knock-down' arguments in a verbal warfare which has so far been a Pyrrhic stalemate for all concerned.

Withholding Versus Withdrawing Life Support

When something disturbing occurs, somehow omission bothers us less than commission; we feel more comfortable as observer than participant. Consequently, when life support is foregone, withholding treatment seems less repellent than withdrawing. As Dan Brock points out,[40] a gravely ill unconscious patient with a terminal illness and a 'living will' refusing intubation should not be intubated. But consider what should happen if, without this knowledge the patient is intubated, and the patient's family and physician subsequently announce the terminal illness and present the 'living will' refusing intubation. In this instance, withdrawing treatment is as justified as withholding because of the same considerations: the prognosis and wishes of the patient. Mere accidents of timing should be irrelevant. Because of considerations such as these, there is a widely held consensus among ethicists that a justification adequate to withhold should be adequate to withdraw. A policy always excluding subsequent withdrawal might unjustifiably discourage vigorous initial attempts at full treatment of the seriously ill when information is incomplete.[41]

Ordinary Versus Extraordinary Means

A widely held presumption of patients and courts is that in considering life support measures, ordinary means are necessary and extraordinary means are optional. The problem lies with understanding what different people mean by the word 'extraordinary'. Does it mean unusual, complex, artificial, invasive, costly, burdensome, heroic, etc.?[41] In fact, it appears in practice that the words ordinary and extraordinary express not criteria for distinguishing right from wrong but label a decision made on other grounds. If a treatment is considered to be too burdensome for the benefits offered or is not required by a given ethical system, it is then labeled 'extraordinary' and vice versa for the label 'ordinary'. Because the distinction between extraordinary and ordinary is not fundamental and often confusing, such labels are best avoided unless very clearly defined.

Active Voluntary Euthanasia and Assisted Suicide

So much has been written on this subject that it cannot be reasonably summarized here.[42–46] However, a few comments can be made. First of all, at this writing, in most jurisdictions of the USA, a physician aiding active voluntary or involuntary euthanasia risks a verdict of acting illegally and/or being guilty of murder or manslaughter.[47] It is not certain that such illegal actions will always be prosecuted or punished, especially in certain countries like Holland.

The argument for rational euthanasia as an enhancement of autonomy appears doubtful at best. It is often recommended as a way for dying patients to become masters of their souls and captains of their fate, much as a sea captain is master of a ship. But clearly it does not promote the autonomy of a sea captain in stormy weather to pull down the sails of his ship and 'unplug' its sea cocks below the water line, much less for the captain's to use his own cannon to blow a hole in the hull. Such actions in fact would demolish whatever vestiges of control the captain might still have over his ship. On the contrary, the autonomy of storm-tossed sea captains and terminally ill patients is best promoted by '*removing* obstacles', not by inflicting another which is, by design, insurmountable and fatal.

On the other hand, proponents of active voluntary euthanasia (proposed as an example of 'justified' homicide caused by the physician) and physician-assisted suicide, at times offer persuasive arguments. If one can, in self-defense, kill another's body (for example, as a last resort against involuntary constraint and torture), why is it not allowable, as a last resort, to kill one's own body which because of a severe burn constrains and tortures one? If a patient may justifiably ask a physician as a last resort to amputate a terribly damaged and unbearably painful crushed limb because he does not believe it worth the pain for the predicted level of function and comfort, why is euthanasia or physician-assisted suicide unjustified when the patient believes that a 99% body surface area third degree burn is not worth the pain or predicted level of function and comfort? If physician-caused euthanasia is ruled out because of the unequal power and current impersonality of the relationship between doctor and patient, then physician-assisted suicide eliminates those dangers.[46] Appeals of this kind may be countered by a citation of the dangers to the doctor (e.g. euthanasia may weaken patient trust in doctors, decrease a doctor's drive to exert himself in very difficult circumstances, or devalue the nontechnological, etc.)[44] or to society; but this verbal battle has been waged for years without signs of definitive resolution.

Another approach to the issue of euthanasia is to hear what patients may actually, but implicitly, be requesting when in desperation they ask for death in this way. Such patients '... "merely" need pain control, emotional support, spiritual counseling, respect, enduring relationships, reliable housing, and other attributes of tolerable living ...' during and after hospitalizaiton.[48] As the goals of total burn care outlined in this book are approached, I believe calls for euthanasia and/or physician-assisted suicide will diminish proportionately, and both sides of the debate on this subject seek that outcome.

Foregoing Treatment Versus Foregoing Hygiene

There is a widely held consensus that surrogates of patients may justifiably decide to forego therapy such as dialysis, artificial ventilation, CRP, etc. when patients are in the persistent vegetative state of irreversibly terminally ill with death imminent.[49,50] Can hygienic measures such as food and fluid be justifiably foregone? Is there not a qualitative difference between treatment and nutrition? Foregoing nutrition leads inevitably to death and at what else than death can, for example, discontinuation of gastrostomy feeding be aimed?

Frequently it is stated than gastrostomy feedings are just another technological means by which life is sustained. Since it requires skill, experience, technical knowledge, surgical expertise, etc. to install and maintain, it is therefore a form of medical treatment. But it is no less logical to define treatment and hygiene by their ends. Treatments heal or cure; hygiene maintains health. The ancient Greeks saw the difference when they discerned separate gods for each function: Aescalpius for medicine and Hygeia for hygiene.[41] Although we may grant that certain activities may be physiologically similar, are they morally the same? After all, eating chickens and eating people may both be *physiologically* eating meat, but they are not necessarily equivalent *morally*.

Against this position is the argument that tube feeding may be miserable for a demented patient since it may require tying him down and may violate his previously expressed wishes 'not to be kept alive on tubes'. Patients in the persistent vegetative state may have expressed their wish previously not to be so fed in order to free their families from crushing financial burdens. That there may be an element of heroism in such a decision cannot be denied. With strict safeguards and restrictions, US courts have, on a number of occasions, allowed caregiver compliance with a patient's refusal of fluids and nutrition. Whether they have thereby added grease to an already slippery slope, time alone will tell.

When and Where?

Factual completeness, conceptual clarity, patience, calmness, impartiality, empathy, modesty, autonomy and simplicity are widely accepted as the distinguishing marks of effective and mature moral deliberation.[51,52] The optimum time and most appropriate location for decision making are those which most foster these characteristics. Of course there are times when snap judgments must be made, but to achieve the goals cited, time, dialogue, study and discussion with friends often clarify decision making greatly. If a difficult decision about a course of therapy can be anticipated, it is helpful to delay discussion until after arterial pH and PO_2 as well as pain are controlled but before signs of sepsis set in.[29]

If a patient is asked early to designate a surrogate, and the surrogate agrees to perform that duty, the patient's surrogate should, if possible, be present when the physician and patient discuss diagnosis, prognosis, and the patient's wishes about CPR, dialysis, etc. if appropriate.[29] Currently we discuss such matters whenever a mortality rate of greater than 50% is anticipated. Except for mass disaster situations, however, virtually never should such decisions be made by a patient or family or any single member of the caregiving team prior to full and formal evaluation by the heath care team. If problems develop, counseling with friends, family, pastors, social workers, ethics committee, counseling teams, etc. remains enormously helpful in bringing calmness, trust, honesty, and increased self-knowledge to the discussion.

Who?

'Who decides?' This question is the single most frequent formulation of the major issues involved in life and death decisions in a burn center. It implies that the problem is one of power or authority. Nothing could be more damaging to the prospects of success. More important and productive than the issue of 'Who has the right or power to decide?' is an identity issue: 'Who are you and who is your patient?'

Although rarely recognized as doing so, moral sentiments (i.e. impulses to treat persons not as means only and with justice, beneficence, etc.) arise fundamentally and perhaps exclusively from a personal, one-on-one, vulnerable experience of ourselves and/or others as somehow compelling and intrinsically valuable.[53] Like religious sentiments and experiences, they almost irresistibly demand expression, in morality as poetry, songs, drama, ethics, law, and socialization; in religion as theology, hymns, ritual, scriptures, parables, etc. It is no accident that theology and ethics are among the oldest and most enduring of Western intellectual disciplines: they express our deepest sentiments.

Moral sentiment cannot be taught. Total recall and ability to rehearse all the world's ethical theories and categories cannot produce virtue. The question 'Why should I be moral?' cannot be answered logically. The answer is to experience your patients, care for them not just as a doctor does a patient, but as 'I' Bruce or Juan experience 'Thou', Paul or Maria (see **Figure 60.3**), and the question will be answered experientially. Then the impulse to be just, respectful, beneficent, etc. will arise spontaneously and not as an act of one's reason or will. Of course, we need to remain some distance from our patients, to see them as examples of biological and ethical categories. But that will never be sufficient to produce moral sentiments which arise perhaps exclusively from 'I–Thou' relationships. As Martin Buber put it, '... without *It* (the appreciation of categories rather than individuals) man cannot live. But he who lives with *It* alone (that is without "I–Thou" relationship) is not a man.'[54] A contemporary of Buber's, among the most respected of US physicians, put it another way:

> The treatment of a disease may be entirely impersonal, the treatment of a patient must be completely personal ... for the secret to the care of the patient is in caring for the patient.[55]

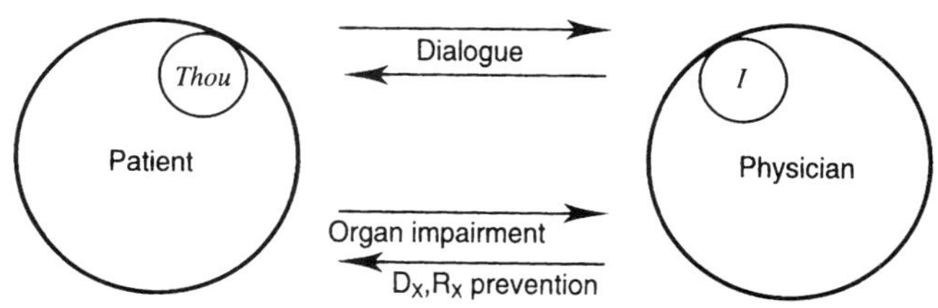

Fig. 60.3 The physician–patient relationship in the burn center suggesting that the terms 'physician' and 'patient' actually designate roles. Only between a particular 'I' and a particular 'Thou' is dialogue possible and a source of moral sentiment.

There are two obvious ways to seek an Archimedian point, i.e. to seek firm ground and a clear view amid the roles, laws and storms of individual and group interest (portrayed in **Figures 60.2** and **60.3**). One way, illustrated by the outermost ring of **Figure 60.2**, is achieved by being very general and abstract as in the development of ethical principles and theories. The other way, illustrated by the innermost rings of **Figure 60.3**, is accomplished by being totally particular and individual, in seeking 'I–Thou' relationships with our patients. It turns out that both are necessary on our moral journey: ethics provides the compass of theory and principles, and the moral sentiment of 'I–Thou' relationships provides the motor or impulse to act on them. In the end, being a 'hard-headed' expert about medicine and/or ethical theories and categories is not enough; we must also have a 'soft heart' for the persons whom the profession of burn care brings into our lives.[56]

References

1. Maguire D C. *The Moral Choice*. Garden City, New York: Doubleday, 1978: 113.

2. Thomasma D. Training in medical ethics: an ethical workup. *Forum Med* 1978; **1:** 33–6.

3. Pellegrino E D, Thomasma D C. *A Philosophical Basis of Medical Practice*. New York: Oxford University Press, 1981: pp 119–52.

4. Jonsen A R, Siegler M, Winslade W J. *Clinical Ethics*. 3rd ed. New York: McGraw-Hill, 1992: 197 pp.

5. Ross J W, Bayley C, Michel V, Pugh D. *Handbook for Hospital Ethics Committees*. Chicago: American Hospital Publishing, Inc, 1986: 25–7.

6. Ross J W, Glaser J W, Rasinski-Gregory D, Gibson J M, Bayley C. *Health Care Ethics Committees: The Next Generation*. Chicago: American Hospital Publishing, Inc, 1993: 17–28.

7. Bresnahan J F. Letter to editor: Moral complexity. *Health Prog* 1989; **70**(4): 9–14.

8. Modified from Pellegrino E D, Thomasma D C. *A Philosophical Basis of Medical Practice*. New York: Oxford University Press, 1981.

9. McCullough L B Informed consent and refusal. In: Civetta J M, Taylor R W, Kirby R R, eds. *Critical Care*. 2nd ed. Philadelphia: JB Lippincott, 1992: 71–6.

10. Gillon R. *Philosophical Medical Ethics*. Chichester: John Wiley & Sons, 1985: 60–6, 119–25.

11. Applebaum P S, Grisso T. Assessing patients' capacities to consent to treatment. *N Engl J Med* 1988; **319:** 1635–8.

12. Faden R R, Beauchamp T L. *A History and Theory of Informed Consent*. New York: Oxford University Press, 1986: 240.

13. Modified from Veatch R M. Models for ethical medicine in a revolutionary age. *Hastings Ctr Rep* 1972; **2**(3): 5–7.

14. California Consortium on Patient Self-Determination. *The PSDA Patient Self-Determination Act Handbook*. Hospital edition. Los Angeles: Pacific Center for Health Policy and Ethics, University of Southern California, Law Center, 1991: 7–17.

15. Los Angeles County Medical Association, Los Angeles County Bar Association, Joint Committee on Biomedical Ethics. Forgoing life-sustaining treatment for adult patients: patients without decision-making capacity who lack surrogates. *LACMA Physician* 1993; **July:** 23–4.

16. Fratianne R B, Brandt C, Yurko L, Coffee T. When is enough enough? Ethical dilemmas on the burn unit. *J Burn Care Rehabil* 1992; **13:** 600–4.

17. Bloom S W. *The Doctor and His Patient: A Sociological Interpretation*. New York: Russell-Sage Foundation, 1963: 63.

18. Beauchamp T L, Childress J F. *Principles of Biomedical Ethics*. New York: Oxford University Press, 1979: 314 pp.

19. Rawls J. *A Theory of Justice*. Cambridge, Massachusetts: The Belknap Press of Harvard University Press, 1971: 20.

20. Zawacki B E. ICU physician's ethical role in distributing scarce resources. *Crit Care Med* 1985; **13:** 57–60.

21. Goldberg M I, Black E A. Technical summary: NIH Consensus Development Conference on Supportive Therapy in Burn Care. *J Trauma* 1979; **19** (Suppl): 855–7.

22. McCrady V, Kahn A. Life and death for burn patients. *J Trauma* 1980; **20:** 356–7.

23. Herndon D N, Rutan R L, Desai M H, Blakeney P, Waymack J P. What size burn should be resuscitated? *Proc Burn Assoc* 1993; **25:** 106.

24. Wachtel T L, Frank H A. Comfort care: an alternative treatment programme for seriously burned patients. *Burns* 1987; **13:** 1–5.

25. Frank H A, Wachtel T L. Life and death in a burn center. *J Burn Care Rehabil* 1984; **5:** 339–42.

26. Hammond J, Ward C G. Decision not to treat: 'Do not resuscitate' order for the burn patient in the acute setting. *Crit Care Med* 1989; **17:** 136–8.

27. Childress J F. *Priorities in Biomedical Ethics*. Philadelphia: The Westminster Press, 1981: 21.

28. Imbus S H, Zawacki B E. Autonomy for burned patients when survival is unprecedented. *N Engl J Med* 1977; **297:** 308–11.

29. Imbus S H, Zawacki B E. Encouraging dialogue and autonomy in the burn intensive care unit. *Crit Care Clin* 1986; **2:** 53–60.

30. Blackhall L J. Must we always use CPR? *N Engl J Med* 1987; **317:** 1281–5.

31. Bone R C, Rackow E C, Weg J G, *et al*. Ethical and moral guidelines for the initiation, continuation and withdrawal of intensive care. *Chest* 1990; **97:** 949–58.

32. Task Force on Ethics of the Society of Critical Care Medicine. Consensus report on the ethics of foregoing life-sustaining treatments in the critically ill. *Crit Care Med* 1990; **18:** 1435–9.

33. Council on Ethical and Judicial Affairs. American Medical Association guidelines for the appropriate use of do-not-resuscitate orders. *JAMA* 1991; **265:** 1868–71.

34. Scofield G R. Is consent useful when resuscitation isn't? *Hastings Ctr Rep* 1991; **21:** 28–36.

35. Lo B. Unanswered questions about DNR orders. *JAMA* 1991; **265:** 1874–5.

36. Tomlinson T, Brody H. Futility and the ethics of resuscitation. *JAMA* 1990; **264:** 1276–80.

37. Schneiderman L J. Medical futility: the duty not to treat. *Camb Q Healthcare Ethics* 1993; **2:** 151–9.

38. Truog R D. Beyond futility. *J Clin Ethics* 1992; **3:** 143–45.

39. Covey S R. *The Seven Habits of Highly Effective People*. New York: Simon and Schuster, 1989: 358 pp.

40. Brock D. Death and dying. In: Veatch R M, ed. *Medical Ethics*. Boston: Jones and Bartlett, 1989: 329–56.

41. Lynn J, Childress J F. Must patients always be given food and water? In: Lynn J, ed. *By No Extraordinary Means*. Bloomington, Indiana: University Press, 1986: 47–60.

42. Wolf S M. Holding the line on euthanasia. *Hastings Ctr Rep* 1989; **Jan/Feb Spec Suppl:** 13–15.

43. Callahan D. Can we return death to disease? *Hastings Ctr Rep* 1989; **Jan/Feb Spec Suppl:** 4–6.

44. Crigger B. Dying well? A colloquy on euthanasia and assisted suicide. *Hastings Ctr Rep* 1992; **Mar–Apr:** 6–55.

45. Capron A M, Michel V, Gomez C F, Kass L R, Callahan D. Euthanasia, California Proposition 161. *Commonweal* 1992; **Sep Suppl Spec:** 1–16.

46. Quill T E, Cassel C K, Meier D E. Care of the hopelessly ill, proposed clinical criteria for physician-assisted suicide. *N Engl J Med* 1992; **327:** 1379–83.

47. Newman S A. Euthanasia: orchestrating 'the last syllable of … time.' *Univ Pittsburgh Law Rev* 1991; **53:** 153–91.

48. Lynn J. Letter to editor: Euthanasia. *N Engl J Med* 1989; **321**(2): 9.

49. President's Commission for the Study of Ethical Problems in Medicine and Biomedical and Behavioral Research. *Deciding to Forego Life-sustaining Treatment*. Washington, DC: US Government Printing Office, 1983: 2–9.

50. The Hastings Center. *Guidelines on the Termination of Life-sustaining Treatment and the Care of the Dying*. Briarcliff Manor, New York: The Hastings Center, 1987: 29.

51. Frankena W K. *Ethics*. 2nd ed. Englewood Cliffs, New Jersey: Prentice-Hall, 1973: 113–14.

52. Brandt R B. *Ethical Theory: The Problem of Normative and Critical Ethics*. Englewood Cliffs, New Jersey: Prentice-Hall, 1959: Chapter 10.

53. Maguire D C. *The Moral Choice*. Garden City, New York: Doubleday, 1978: 72–3.

54. Buber M. *I and Thou*. 2nd ed. New York: Macmillan, 1958: 34.

55. Peabody F W. *The Care of the Patient*. Cambridge, Massachusetts: Harvard University Press, 1931: 12–48.

56. Kreeft P. *The Snakebite Letters*. San Francisco: Ignatious Press, 1991: 96.

INDEX